Foundations *for* Population Health *in* Community/Public Health Nursing

FIFTH EDITION

Marcia Stanhope, PhD, RN, FAAN

Education and Practice Consultant and
Professor Emeritus
College of Nursing
University of Kentucky
Lexington, Kentucky

Jeanette Lancaster, RN, PhD, FAAN

Sadie Heath Cabiness Professor and Dean Emeritus
School of Nursing
University of Virginia
Charlottesville, Virginia
Associate, Tuft & Associates, Inc.

ELSEVIER

ELSEVIER

3251 Riverport Lane
St. Louis, Missouri 63043

Notice

Practitioners and researchers must always rely on their own experience and knowledge in evaluating and
using any information, methods, compounds or experiments described herein. Because of rapid advances in
the medical sciences, in particular, independent verification of diagnoses and drug dosages should be made.
To the fullest extent of the law, no responsibility is assumed by Elsevier, authors, editors or contributors for
any injury and/or damage to persons or property as a matter of products liability, negligence or otherwise,
or from any use or operation of any methods, products, instructions, or ideas contained in the material
herein.

Senior Content Strategist: Jamie Blum
Content Development Manager: Lisa P. Newton
Senior Content Development Specialist: Tina Kaemmerer
Publishing Services Manager: Julie Eddy
Senior Project Manager: Richard Barber
Designer: Ashley Miner

Printed in Canada

Last digit is the print number: 9 8 7 6 5 4 3 2 1

MARCIA STANHOPE, PhD, RN, FAAN

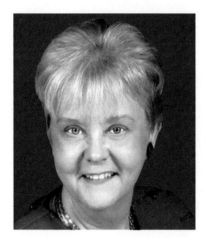

Marcia Stanhope is currently an education and practice consultant for nursing education programs nationally, an Associate with Tuft & Associates, Inc., an executive search firm in Chicago, Illinois; and Professor Emeritus from the University of Kentucky, College of Nursing, Lexington, Kentucky. In recent years, she received the Provost Public Scholar award for contributions to the communities of Kentucky. She was appointed to the Good Samaritan Endowed Chair in Community Health Nursing and held the position for 12 years. She has practiced community and home health nursing, has served as an administrator and consultant in home health, and has been involved in the development of a number of nurse-managed centers as well as the doctorate of nursing practice program nationally. She has taught community health, public health, epidemiology, primary care nursing, policy, and administration courses. Dr. Stanhope was the former Associate Dean and formerly directed the Division of Community Health Nursing and Administration at the University of Kentucky. She has been responsible for both undergraduate and graduate courses in population-centered, community-oriented nursing. She has also taught at the University of Virginia and the University of Alabama, Birmingham. Her presentations and publications have been in the areas of home health, community health and community-focused nursing practice, nurse-managed centers, primary care nursing, and the doctorate of nursing practice. Dr. Stanhope holds a diploma in nursing from the Good Samaritan Hospital, Lexington, Kentucky, and a bachelor of science in nursing from the University of Kentucky. She has a master's degree in public health nursing from Emory University in Atlanta and a doctorate of science in nursing from the University of Alabama, Birmingham. Dr. Stanhope has been the co-author of four other Elsevier publications: *Handbook of Community-Based and Home Health Nursing Practice, Public and Community Health Nurse's Consultant, Case Studies in Community Health Nursing Practice: A Problem-Based Learning Approach,* and *Public Health Nursing-Population-Centered Health Care in the Community.*

JEANETTE LANCASTER, RN, PhD, FAAN

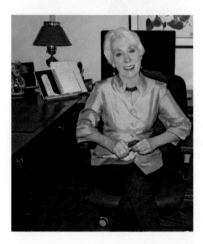

Jeanette Lancaster often serves as a visiting professor in both Taiwan and Hong Kong. She is an associate with Tuft & Associates, Inc. She served for 19 years as the Sadie Heath Cabaniss Professor of Nursing and Dean at the University of Virginia School of Nursing in Charlottesville, Virginia. When Dr. Lancaster stepped down as dean at the University of Virginia, a professorship, grant program for faculty, office suite, and the street in front of the school were named in her honor. From 2008 to 2009 she served as a visiting professor in the School of Nursing at the University of Hong Kong. In spring 2013 and fall 2014, she served as a professor with Semester at Sea and taught cross-cultural health promotion and nutrition as the students, faculty, staff, and life-long learners sailed around the world for 4 months.

Dr. Lancaster also served as president of the American Association of Colleges of Nursing. She has practiced psychiatric nursing and taught both psychiatric and community health nursing. She formerly directed the master's program in community health nursing at the University of Alabama, Birmingham, and served as dean of the School of Nursing at Wright State University in Dayton, Ohio. Her publications and presentations have been largely in the areas of community and public health nursing, leadership and change, and the significance of nurses to effective primary health care. Dr. Lancaster is a graduate of the University of Tennessee Health Sciences Center, College of Nursing. She holds a master's degree in psychiatric nursing from Case Western Reserve University in Cleveland and a doctorate in public health from the University of Oklahoma. Dr. Lancaster is the author of another Mosby/Elsevier publication, *Nursing Issues in Leading and Managing Change,* and co-author (with Dr. Stanhope) of *Public Health Nursing.*

DEDICATION AND ACKNOWLEDGMENTS

DEDICATION

This edition of the text is dedicated to Amber, Bink, G.B., BeBe, Connie, Sam, and Brendy for the joy and fun we have shared for many years.

Marcia Stanhope

ACKNOWLEDGMENTS

We would like to thank our families, friends, and colleagues who supported us in the completion of the fifth edition. Special thanks to those who provided generous support and assistance. We especially thank Jamie Blum, Tina Kaemmerer, Charlene Ketchum, Richard Barber, and staff at Elsevier and the chapter authors for their time and thoughtfulness in assisting us as the revisions were completed. Three very important people who assisted us through their research efforts for this project are Dr. Lisa Turner, Dr. Judy Ponder, and Dr. Erika Metzler Sawin.

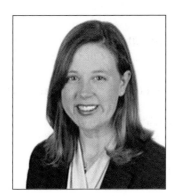 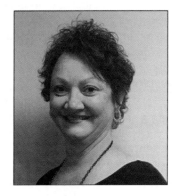 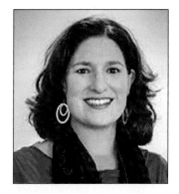

Lisa Pedersen Turner, PhD, RN, PHCNS-BC   Judy L. Ponder, MSN, DNP, RN   Erika Metzler Sawin, PhD, RN

Dr. Lisa Turner served as an assistant to the authors in review and revision of the fifth edition of the text. Dr. Judy Ponder contributed to the revision of select sections of the text. Dr. Erika Metzler Sawin contributed to the revision of several chapters in the text. Thanks to all three of you.

CONTRIBUTORS

We gratefully acknowledge the following individuals who wrote chapters for the ninth edition of *Public Health Nursing*, on which the chapters in this book are based.

Swann Arp Adams, MS, PhD
Associate Professor
College of Nursing and the Department of Epidemiology and Biostatistics
Associate Director
Cancer Prevention and Control Program
University of South Carolina
Columbia, South Carolina

Mollie Aleshire, DNP, FNP-BC, PPCNP-BC
Assistant Professor
College of Nursing
University of Kentucky
Lexington, Kentucky

Jeanne Alhusen, PhD, CRNP, RN
Assistant Professor
Department of Community and Public Health
Johns Hopkins University School of Nursing
Baltimore, Maryland

Debra Gay Anderson, PhD, PHCNS-BC
Associate Professor
College of Nursing
University of Kentucky
Lexington, Kentucky

Dyan A. Aretakis, RN, FNP, MSN
Project Director and APN3
University of Virginia Teen Health Center
Charlottesville, Virginia

Sydney Axson, MPH, RN
Hillman Scholar in Nursing Innovation
University of Pennsylvania
Philadelphia, Pennsylvania

Linda K. Birenbaum, PhD, RN†
Public Health Program Supervisor
Washington County Health & Human Services
Hillsboro, Oregon

Tina Bloom, PhD, MPH, RN
Assistant Professor and Robert Wood Johnson Foundation Nurse Faculty Scholar
Sinclair School of Nursing
Columbia, Missouri

Kathryn H. Bowles, PhD, RN, FAAN
van Ameringen Professor in Nursing Excellence
Director, Center for Integrative Science in Aging
Beatrice Renfield Visiting Scholar, Visiting Nurse Service of New York
Philadelphia, Pennsylvania

Angeline Bushy, PhD, RN, FAAN, PHCNS-BC
Professor and Bert Fish Chair
College of Nursing
University of Central Florida
Daytona Beach, Florida

Jacquelyn C. Campbell, PhD, RN, FAAN
Professor
Anna D. Wolf Chair
National Program Director, Robert Wood Johnson Foundation Nurse Faculty Scholars
The Johns Hopkins University
Baltimore, Maryland

Ann H. Cary, PhD, MPH, RN
Professor and Dean, School of Nursing and Health Studies
University of Missouri-Kansas City
Robert Wood Johnson Foundation Executive Nurse Fellow
Kansas City, Missouri

Ann Connor, DNP, MSN, RN, FNP-BC
Assistant Professor, School of Nursing
Emory University
Atlanta, Georgia

Lois Davis, RN, MSN, MA
Public Health Nursing Manager
Lexington—Fayette County Health Department
Lexington, Kentucky

Cynthia E. Degazon, PhD, RN
Professor Emerita
Hunter College of the City University of New York
New York, New York

---

† = deceased

Janna Dieckmann, PhD, RN
Clinical Associate Professor
School of Nursing
University of North Carolina at Chapel Hill
Chapel Hill, North Carolina

Amanda Fallin, PhD, RN
Postdoctoral Fellow
University of California San Francisco Center for Tobacco
    Control Research and Education
San Francisco, California

Sharon L. Farra, PhD, RN
Assistant Professor of Nursing
Wright State University
Dayton, Ohio

Hartley Feld, RN, MSN, PHCNS-BC
Lecturer/Clinical Instructor, Public and Community Health
    Nursing
College of Nursing
University of Kentucky
Lexington, Kentucky

Mary Gibson, PhD, RN
Associate Professor in Nursing
Assistant Director, Bjoring Center for Nursing Historical
    Inquiry
University of Virginia School of Nursing
Charlottesville, Virginia

Rosa Gonzales-Guarda, PhD, MPH, RN, CPH
Assistant Professor
Robert Wood Johnson Foundation Nurse Faculty Scholar
University of Miami School of Nursing and Health Studies
Coral Gables, Florida

Monty Gross, PhD, RN, CNE, CNL
Clinical Nurse Educator
Veterans Administration
North Las Vegas, Nevada

Patty J. Hale, RN, FNP, PhD, FAAN
Professor and Graduate Program Director
James Madison University
Harrisonburg, Virginia

Susan B. Hassmiller, PhD, RN, FAAN
Robert Wood Johnson Foundation Senior Advisor for Nursing
Director, Future of Nursing: Campaign for Action
Princeton, New Jersey

DeAnne K. Hilfinger Messias, PhD, RN, FAAN
Professor
College of Nursing and Women's and Gender Studies
University of South Carolina
Columbia, South Carolina

Linda Hulton, PhD, RN
Professor of Nursing
Coordinator of Doctor of Nursing Practice Program
James Madison University
Harrisonburg, Virginia

Susan C. Long-Marin, DVM, MPH
Epidemiology Manager
Mecklenburg County Health Department
Charlotte, North Carolina

Karen S. Martin, RN, MSN, FAAN
Health Care Consultant
Martin Associates
Omaha, Nebraska

Mary Lynn Mathre, RN, MSN, CARN
Addictions Nurse Consultant
President, Patients Out of Time
President, American Cannabis Nurses Association
Howardsville, Virginia

Marie Napolitano, PhD, RN, FNP
Director, Doctor of Nursing Practice Program
University of Portland
Portland, Oregon

Bobbie J. Perdue, RN, PhD
Professor, Nursing
South Carolina State University
Orangeburg, South Carolina

Judy L. Ponder, MSN, DNP, RN
Director, Education and Professional Development
Baptist Health Richmond
Richmond, Kentucky

Bonnie Rogers, DrPH, COHN-S, LNCC, FAAN
Director
North Carolina Occupational Safety and Health and
    Education and Research Center
Director
Occupational Health Nursing Program
School of Public Health
University of North Carolina
Chapel Hill, North Carolina

Joanna Rowe Kaakinen, PhD, RN
Professor
School of Nursing
Linfield College-Portland Campus
Portland, Oregon

Cynthia Rubenstein, PhD, RN, CPNP-PC
Undergraduate Program Director
Assistant Professor
Department of Nursing
James Madison University
Harrisonburg, Virginia

Barbara Sattler, RN, DrPH, FAAN
Professor, Masters of Public Health Program
School of Nursing and Health Professions
University of San Francisco
San Francisco, California

Erika Metzler Sawin, PhD, RN
Associate Professor
James Madison University
Harrisonburg, Virginia

George F. Shuster, RN, DNSc
Associate Professor
College of Nursing
University of New Mexico
Albuquerque, New Mexico

Sharon A. R. Stanley, PhD, RN, FAAN
Visiting Professor, Wright State University
Robert Wood Johnson Executive Nurse Fellow, 2011-2014
Dayton, Ohio

Sharon Strang, RN, DNP, APRN, FNP-BC
Associate Professor and Graduate Faculty
Department of Nursing
James Madison University
Harrisonburg, Virginia

Francisco S. Sy, MD, PhD
Editor, *AIDS Education and Prevention—An Interdisciplinary Journal*
Director, Office of Extramural Research Administration
National Institute on Minority Health and Health Disparities (NIMHD)
National Institutes of Health
Bethesda, Maryland

Esther Thatcher, PhD, RN, APHN-BC
Postdoctoral Fellow
School of Nursing
University of North Carolina at Chapel Hill
Chapel Hill, North Carolina

Anita Thompson-Heisterman, MSN, PMHCNS-BC, PMHNP-BC
Assistant Professor
University of Virginia School of Nursing
Charlottesville, Virginia

Lisa Pedersen Turner, PhD, RN, APHN-BC
Assistant Professor
Berea College Nursing Program
Berea, Kentucky

Connie M. Ulrich, PhD, MSN, RN
Lillian S. Brunner Chair in Medical and Surgical Nursing
Professor of Bioethics and Nursing
Secondary Appointment, Department of Medical Ethics and Health Policy
Associate Director, NewCourtland Center for Transitions and Health
University of Pennsylvania Schools of Nursing and Medicine
Philadelphia, Pennsylvania

Lynn Wasserbauer, PhD, FNP, RN
Nurse Practitioner
Strong Memorial Hospital
University of Rochester Medical Center
Rochester, New York

Jackie F. Webb, FNP-BC, MS, RN
Assistant Professor
Linfield College School of Nursing
Portland, Oregon

Carolyn A. Williams, PhD, RN, FAAN
Professor and Dean Emeritus
College of Nursing
University of Kentucky
Lexington, Kentucky

Lisa M. Zerull, PhD, RN
Academic Liaison and Program Manager, Wincester Medical Center, Valley Health System
Adjunct Clinical Faculty, Senandoah University (Wincester, Virginia)
Editor, Perspectives out of the Church Health Center (Memphis, Tennessee)

REVIEWERS

Grace Buttriss DNP, RN, FNP-BC, CNL
Assistant Professor of Nursing
Queens University of Charlotte
Nursing Department
Charlotte, North Carolina

Jennifer Wing MSN, RN
Assistant Professor
Upper Iowa University
Nursing Department
Des Moines, Iowa

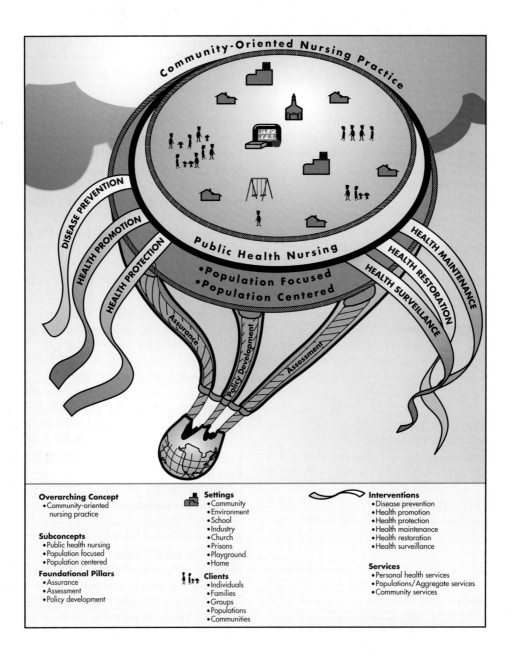

The figure illustrates a conceptual model of Community-Oriented Nursing Practice, with an outer ring labeled "Community-Oriented Nursing Practice" and an inner dome labeled "Public Health Nursing • Population Focused • Population Centered." Ribbon streamers are labeled: Disease Prevention, Health Promotion, Health Protection, Health Maintenance, Health Restoration, Health Surveillance. The three foundational pillars are labeled Assurance, Policy Development, and Assessment.

Overarching Concept
- Community-oriented nursing practice

Subconcepts
- Public health nursing
- Population focused
- Population centered

Foundational Pillars
- Assurance
- Assessment
- Policy development

Settings
- Community
- Environment
- School
- Industry
- Church
- Prisons
- Playground
- Home

Clients
- Individuals
- Families
- Groups
- Populations
- Communities

Interventions
- Disease prevention
- Health promotion
- Health protection
- Health maintenance
- Health restoration
- Health surveillance

Services
- Personal health services
- Populations/Aggregate services
- Community services

COMMUNITY NURSING DEFINITIONS

Community-Oriented Nursing Practice is a philosophy of nursing service delivery that involves the generalist or specialist public health and community health nurse providing "health care" through community diagnosis and investigation of major health and environmental problems, health surveillance, and monitoring and evaluation of community and population health status for the purposes of preventing disease and disability and promoting, protecting, and maintaining "health" to create conditions in which people can be healthy.

Public Health Nursing Practice is the synthesis of nursing theory and public health theory applied to promoting and preserving health of populations. The focus of practice is the community as a whole and the effect of the community's health status (resources) on the health of individuals, families, and groups. Care is provided within the context of preventing disease and disability and promoting and protecting the health of the community as a whole. Public Health Nursing is population focused, which means that the population is the center of interest for the public health nurse. *Community Health Nurse* is a term used interchangeably with *Public Health Nurse.*

Community-Based Nursing Practice is a setting-specific practice whereby care is provided for "sick" individuals and families where they live, work, and go to school. The emphasis of practice is acute and chronic care and the provision of comprehensive, coordinated, and continuous services. Nurses who deliver community-based care are generalists or specialists in maternal-infant, pediatric, adult, or psychiatric-mental health nursing.

Health care is in a rapid state of flux. In the early tenure of a new administration in the United States, health care and the many possible changes are at the forefront of the minds of Americans. As we look back at the preface to the fourth edition of this text, it is clear that many of the concerns at that time about health care still exist. In the United States, an increasing amount of money is spent annually on health care, yet not all people get affordable, accessible, and high-quality care. For 27 years, the United Health Foundation has published *America's Health Rankings Annual Report*. In the 2016 report they said that encouraging progress was being made against selected long-standing public health challenges including reducing the prevalence of smoking and the number of people without health insurance (www.americashealthranking.org). However, several significant challenges remain, including rising rates of cardiovascular- and drug- related deaths and an increasing prevalence of obesity. Clearly, drug-related deaths and obesity are preventable, and the incidence of cardiovascular diseases can often be prevented or postponed by healthy behaviors. The findings of this report, which assesses health status annually by individual states, were confirmed in the reflections of former Surgeon General Everett Koop in an editorial in the *American Journal of Public Health* in late 2006. He commented that in nearly six decades of public health work, he was "awed at what has been achieved and shocked at what has not" (Koop, 2006, p. 2090). He commented on the many medical miracles that have saved lives and led to longer lives but that have often failed to make those added years any freer of disability and discomfort. He went on to talk about preventable health problems, including obesity; orthopedic injury; unintentional pregnancies, many of which lead to abortions; and lack of adequate preparation to deal effectively with potential influenza pandemics, bioterrorism, or HIV/AIDS. His comments still reflect the current issues in health and health care today. However, there have been some improvements over time.

For several years, many of us in public health and public health nursing have thought that some national priorities are misaligned. In recent years, we have spent more money on war than on dealing with poverty. We continue to spend more on complex reparative procedures than to spend money on prevention, including health education and health promotion. Despite the fact that many people across the world know that lifestyle plays a large role in morbidity and mortality, only a portion of the people in each country "walk the talk" in terms of their own personal behavior. It is important to remember that numerous deaths each year are still attributed to tobacco, alcohol, and illicit drug use; diet and activity patterns; microbial agents; toxic agents; firearms; sexual behavior; and motor vehicle accidents. Over the years the most significant improvements in the health of the population have come from advances in public health, such as improvements in motor vehicle safety, mandatory helmet use on cycles, food and water sanitation, food pasteurization and

refrigeration, immunizations, workplace safety, and emphasis on personal lifestyle and environmental factors that affect health. Changes in the public health system are essential if health in the United States is to improve.

The need to focus attention on health promotion, lifestyle factors, and disease prevention led to the development of a healthy public policy in the United States. This policy was designed by a large number of people representing a wide range of groups interested in health. The policy is reflected in the document *Healthy People 2020*, which identifies a comprehensive set of national health-promotion and disease-prevention objectives. Despite the development of these guidelines for health and the acceptance of the goals and objectives set forth, health indicators are simply not measuring up to expectations.

Public health nurses have a unique view of their "clients." They view the community as the client; they focus on prevention strategies to promote **population health** according to population-based data, and they know to organize resources in the community to address the problems. Public health nurses view health from a broad perspective and include the biology of a person, relationship interactions, genetics, community resources, policies, and the environment in which the population lives, to name only a few.

Specifically, to develop healthy populations, individuals, families, and communities, there must be a commitment to **population level** health goals. In addition, society, through the development of health policy, must support better health care, the design of improved health education, the financing of strategies to alter health status, and the support of alliances and coalitions that truly and consistently work together to improve health care. Of most importance, healthy public policy must be evidence based and outcomes of the policies evaluated. Growing interest in health reform is an opportunity for public health workers to find ways to be involved in charting the future of health care in America.

Our message to you, our readers, is to ask, "How are you going to use the knowledge and skills that you have to make a difference in health care?" We ask you to remember that behind every public health decision, there is a political decision. This means that your role in health care is broad and includes care to individuals, families, communities, and the nation. In late 2008, Bill Foege, MD, MPH, former head of the Centers for Disease Control and Prevention and now with the Bill and Melinda Gates Foundation, offered these comments that have direct usefulness to students of public health nursing, "Leadership in the future will require knowing the rules of coalitions. Most coalitions (however) are formed around an idea. The best will be formed around an outcome" (American Academy of Nursing, 2008 meeting). His words emphasize that public health work is not the work of a soloist and that the work should focus on the outcome versus the process. We hope that this text will provide you with some of the tools to accomplish the goal Dr. Foege sets forth. It is our belief that nurses are the backbone of public health in both developed and developing countries.

This text focuses on the processes and practices for promoting health principally by the nurse, who is considered to be an ideal person to demonstrate and teach others how to promote health. To be effective, health promotion requires that people cease focusing on how to "fix" themselves and others only when they detect physical and emotional problems and that they instead assume personal responsibility for health promotion. Such a change in emphasis requires that health care providers incorporate health-promotion techniques into their practice.

Because people do not always know how to improve their health status, the challenge of nursing is to initiate change. **Public health nursing focuses on the health of populations to change the health of individuals, families, and groups living, working, and playing within the community as a whole.** The practice takes place in a variety of public and private settings and includes disease prevention, health promotion, health protection, education, maintenance, restoration, coordination, management, and evaluation of care of those populations, as well as the whole of the communities.

To meet the demands of a constantly changing health care system, nurses must be visionary in designing their roles and identifying their practice areas. To do so effectively, nurses must understand concepts and theories of public health, **population health;** the changing health care system; the actual and potential roles and responsibilities of nurses and other health care providers; the importance of a health-promotion and disease-prevention orientation; and the necessity to involve consumers in the planning, implementation, and evaluation of health care efforts.

This text was written to provide nursing students and practicing nurses with a comprehensive source book that provides a foundation for designing nursing strategies **for populations, including the individuals, families and groups within the communities.** The book integrates health-promotion and disease-prevention concepts into all aspects of practice.

REFERENCES

Koop CE: Health and health care for the 21st century: for all the people, *Am J Public Health* 96:2090-2091, 2006.

America's Health Rankings: *2016 America's health rankings*, Minnetonka, Minn, 2016, United Health Group. Retrieved March 2017 from www.americashealthrankings.org.

ORGANIZATION

The text is divided into seven sections:

- *Part 1,* **Perspectives in Health Care Delivery and Nursing,** describes the historical and current status of the health care delivery system and nursing practice in the community.
- *Part 2,* **Influences on Health Care Delivery and Nursing,** addresses specific issues and societal concerns that affect nursing practice in the community.
- *Part 3,* **Conceptual Frameworks Applied to Nursing Practice in the Community,** provides conceptual models for nursing practice in the community; selected models from nursing and related sciences are also discussed.
- *Part 4,* **Issues and Approaches in Health Care Populations,** examines the management of health care and select community environments, as well as issues related to managing cases, programs, disasters, and groups.
- *Part 5,* **Issues and Approaches in Family and Individual Health Care,** discusses risk factors and health problems for families and individuals throughout the life span.
- *Part 6,* **Vulnerability: Predisposing Factors,** covers specific health care needs and issues of populations at risk.
- *Part 7,* **Nursing Practice in the Community: Roles and Functions,** examines diversity in the role of nurses in the community and describes the rapidly changing roles, functions, and practice settings.

PEDAGOGY

Each chapter is organized for easy use by students and faculty. Chapters begin with Objectives to guide student learning and assist faculty in knowing what students should gain from the content. The Chapter Outline alerts students to the structure and content of the chapter. Key Terms, along with text page references are also provided at the beginning of the chapter to assist the student in understanding unfamiliar terminology. The key terms are in boldface within the text. A full Glossary is available in Appendix E as well as on the student Evolve website at http://evolve.elsevier.com/stanhope/foundations.

The following features are presented in most or all chapters:

HOW TO Provides specific, application-oriented information.

EVIDENCE-BASED PRACTICE

Illustrates the use and application of the latest research findings in public health, community health, and nursing.

LEVELS OF PREVENTION

Applies primary, secondary, and tertiary prevention to the specific chapter content.

HEALTHY PEOPLE 2020

Selected *Healthy People 2020* objectives are integrated into each chapter.

APPLYING CONTENT TO PRACTICE

Provides highlights and links chapter content to nursing practice in the community.

QSEN FOCUS ON QUALITY AND SAFETY EDUCATION FOR NURSES (QSEN)

Gives examples of how quality and safety goals, competencies, objectives, knowledge, skills, and attitudes can be applied in nursing practice in the community.

CASE STUDY

Real-life clinical situations help students develop their assessment and critical thinking skills.

■ PRACTICE APPLICATION

At the end of each chapter, this section provides readers with an understanding of how to apply chapter content in the clinical setting through the presentation of a case situation with questions students will want to think about as they analyze the case.

■ REMEMBER THIS!

Provides a summary in list form of the most important points made in the chapter.

TEACHING AND LEARNING PACKAGE

A website, http://evolve.elsevier.com/stanhope/foundations, includes instructor and student materials.

(a) For The Instructor:

- TEACH for Nurses, which contains:
  - Detailed chapter Lesson Plans containing references to curriculum standards such as QSEN, BSN Essentials and Concepts, BSN Essentials for Public Health, new and unique Case Studies, Critical Thinking Activities, and Critical Analysis Questions and Answers
- Test Bank, with 800 questions
- Image Collection, with all illustrations from the book
- PowerPoint slides

(b) For The Student:

- NCLEX® Review Questions, with answers and rationale provided
- Case Studies, with Questions and Answers
- Answers to Practice Application Questions

CONTENTS

Contributors, v
Preface, ix

PART 1 Perspectives in Health Care Delivery and Nursing

1. Community- and Prevention-Oriented Practice to Improve Population Health, 1
2. The History of Public Health and Public and Community Health Nursing, 15
3. The Changing U.S. Health and Public Health Care Systems, 33

PART 2 Influences on Health Care Delivery and Nursing

4. Ethics in Public and Community Health Nursing Practice, 49
5. Cultural Influences in Nursing in Community Health, 65
6. Environmental Health, 84
7. Government, the Law, and Policy Activism, 105
8. Economic Influences, 125

PART 3 Conceptual Frameworks Applied to Nursing Practice in the Community

9. Epidemiological Applications, 147
10. Evidence-Based Practice, 170
11. Using Health Education and Groups in the Community, 182

PART 4 Issues and Approaches in Health Care Populations

12. Community Assessment and Evaluation, 203
13. Case Management, 221
14. Disaster Management, 236
15. Surveillance and Outbreak Investigation, 255
16. Program Management, 265
17. Managing Quality and Safety, 276

PART 5 Issues and Approaches in Family and Individual Health Care

18. Family Development and Family Nursing Assessment, 294
19. Family Health Risks, 310
20. Health Risks Across the Life Span, 333

PART 6 Vulnerability: Predisposing Factors

21. Vulnerability and Vulnerable Populations: An Overview, 357
22. Rural Health and Migrant Health, 374
23. Poverty, Homelessness, Teen Pregnancy, and Mental Illness, 392
24. Alcohol, Tobacco, and Other Drug Problems in the Community, 415
25. Violence and Human Abuse, 433
26. Infectious Disease Prevention and Control, 455
27. HIV Infection, Hepatitis, Tuberculosis, and Sexually Transmitted Diseases, 478

PART 7 Nursing Practice in the Community: Roles and Functions

28. Nursing Practice at the Local, State, and National Levels in Public Health, 498
29. The Faith Community Nurse, 510
30. The Nurse in Home Health and Hospice, 524
31. The Nurse in the Schools, 540
32. The Nurse in Occupational Health, 560

Appendixes, 579
Appendix A: Guidelines for Practice, 580
Appendix B: Assessment Tools, 583
Appendix C: Essential Elements of Public Health Nursing, 594
Appendix D: Hepatitis Information, 606
Appendix E: Glossary, 610

Index, 623

CHAPTER 1

Community- and Prevention-Oriented Practice to Improve Population Health

Carolyn A. Williams

OBJECTIVES

After reading this chapter, the student should be able to:

1. State the mission and core functions of public health and the services generally provided by practitioners of public health.
2. Discuss the role of the public health nurse specialist and how the role influences nursing practice in the community.
3. Contrast community-based nursing practice with community-oriented nursing practice.
4. Describe the role of public health and nursing in population health.

CHAPTER OUTLINE

What Is Public Health?
Public Health Core Functions
 Defined
Population-Focused Nursing Practice
Practice Focusing on Individuals, Families, and Groups
 Community-Oriented Nursing
 Community-Based Nursing
Challenges for the Future

KEY TERMS

aggregate, 7
assessment, 5
assurance, 5
community, 1
community based, 1
community-based nursing, 1
community health nursing, 1
community-oriented nursing, 1
policy development, 5
population, 7
population focused, 10
population-focused practice, 8
population health, 3
primary health care services, 5
public health, 3
public health core functions, 4
public health mission, 4
public health nursing, 1
secondary health care services, 5
subpopulations, 7
tertiary health care services, 5

Professional nurses must actively participate in developing evidence-based, cost-effective, high-quality, innovative, and useful ways to provide care to citizens. Evidence-based practice is the norm today and simply means that a nurse's practice is based on the use of the best available evidence to provide this care. This evidence may be research, but if research is not available, practice may be based on opinions, case studies, or professional and governmental reports, to name a few examples. Of course it is always the best if research related to a strategy, an intervention, a program, or an application of a model can be found.

Because of the growing costs of hospital care, more services are being provided in community-based settings. Increasingly, nurses will engage in what is called community-based nursing (CBN). In CBN, the nurse focuses on "illness care" of individuals and families across the life span. The aim is to manage acute and chronic health conditions in the community, and the focus of the practice is individual- or family-centered illness care. While providing health care to individuals and families, the nurse maintains an appreciation for the values of the community. CBN is not a specialty in nursing but rather a philosophy that guides care in all nursing specialties when applied in the community.

In contrast, community-oriented nursing has as its primary focus the health care of either the community or populations, as in public health nursing (PHN), or of individuals, families, and groups in a community. Care of individuals, families, and groups is also referred to as community health nursing, although this term was more common in the past. In community-oriented nursing the goal is to preserve, protect,

1

promote, or maintain health. The key difference between CBN and community-oriented nursing is that community-based nurses deal primarily with illness-oriented care, whereas community-oriented nurses provide health care to promote quality of life. They both may deal with individuals and families, and the community-oriented nurse also typically deals with groups in the community. Table 1.1 lists the similarities and differences between community-oriented nursing and CBN.

As mentioned, community-oriented nursing includes PHN. This is a specialty area whose primary focus is on the health care of communities and populations rather than on individuals, groups, and families. The goal of this specialty is to prevent disease and preserve, promote, restore, and protect health for the

TABLE 1.1	Select Examples of Similarities and Differences Between Community-Oriented and Community-Based Nursing	
	Community-Oriented Nursing	**Community-Based Nursing**
Philosophy	Primary focus is on "health care" of individuals, families, groups, and the community or populations within the community	Focus is on "illness care" of individuals and families across the life span
Goal	Preserve, protect, promote, or maintain health and prevent disease	Manage acute or chronic conditions
Service context	Community health care Population health	Family-centered illness care
Community type	Varied; usually local community	Human ecological
Client characteristics	• Individuals at risk • Families at risk • Groups at risk • Communities • Usually healthy • Culturally diverse • Autonomous • Able to define their own problems • Primary decision makers	• Individuals • Families • Usually ill • Culturally diverse • Autonomous • Able to define their own problems • Involved in decision making
Practice setting	• Community agencies • Home • Work • School • Playground • May be organization • May be government	• Community agencies • Home • Work • School
Interaction patterns	• One to one • Groups • May be organizational	• One to one
Type of service	• Direct care of at-risk individuals • Indirect (program management)	• Direct illness care
Emphasis on levels of prevention	• Primary • Secondary (screening) • Tertiary (maintenance and rehabilitation)	• Secondary • Tertiary • May be primary
Roles	**Client and Delivery Oriented: Individual, Family, Group, Population** • Caregiver • Social engineer • Educator • Counselor • Advocate • Case manager	**Client and Delivery Oriented: Individual, Family** • Caregiver
	Group Oriented • Leader (personal health management) • Change agent (screening) • Community advocate/developer • Case finder • Community care agent • Assessment • Policy developer • Assurance • Enforcer of laws/compliance	**Group Oriented** • Leader (disease management) • Change agent (managed-care services)

TABLE 1.1	**Select Examples of Similarities and Differences Between Community-Oriented and Community-Based Nursing—cont'd**	
	Community-Oriented Nursing	**Community-Based Nursing**
Priority of nurse's activities	• Case findings • Client education • Community education • Interdisciplinary practice • Case management (direct care) • Program planning and implementation • Individual, family, and population advocacy	• Case management (direct care) • Client education • Individual and family advocacy • Interdisciplinary practice • Continuity of care providers

community and the population within it. The focus is on the public health ethic of "the greatest good for the greatest number." This specialty is built on the blending of nursing and the discipline of public health (American Nurses Association, 2013).

This chapter examines both CBN and community-oriented nursing. It describes the similarities and differences between these two areas of nursing and also discusses public health and the core functions and services included in public health practice. In addition, the essential services of public health nurses are discussed because nurses working from both a CBN and a community-oriented community health nursing framework may use some of these skills. For nurses to work effectively in the community, regardless of their focus, it is useful to know exactly what public health is and how the functions of that discipline work to improve the health of the people in their communities.

WHAT IS PUBLIC HEALTH?

Public health is a scientific discipline that includes the study of epidemiology, statistics, and assessment—including attention to behavioral, cultural, and economic factors—in addition to program planning and policy development. In recent years, efforts in the United States to change the way in which health care is delivered have focused heavily on looking at ways to change the delivery of medical care and on health insurance. Until recently, limited attention has been focused on looking at population health or the health of a population as a whole, including the distribution of health outcomes and disparities in the population (Nash et al, 2011).

Although people are excited when a new drug is discovered that cures a disease or when a new way to transplant organs is perfected, it is important to know about the significant gains in the health of populations that have come largely from public health accomplishments. For example, public health has influenced the safety and adequacy of food and water, sewage disposal, public safety from biological threats, and changes in personal behaviors such as smoking. There has been a dramatic increase in life expectancy for Americans in the 21st century compared with the 20th century, from less than 50 years in 1900 to 78.8 years in 2013 (National Center for Health Statistics, 2015). The change is credited primarily to improvements in sanitation, the control of infectious diseases through immunizations, and other public health activities. Population-based preventive programs launched in the 1970s were also largely responsible for the more recent changes in tobacco use, blood-pressure control, dietary patterns (except obesity),

automobile safety restraint, and injury-control measures that have fostered declines in adult death rates. A more than 50% decline in stroke and coronary heart disease deaths has occurred (National Center for Health Statistics, 2015, p. 89). Overall death rates for children have declined by approximately 40% (Singh, 2010).

Another way of looking at the benefits of public health practice is to look at how early deaths can be prevented. The US Public Health Service (1994/2008) estimated that medical treatment could prevent only approximately 10% of all early deaths in the United States, whereas population-focused public health approaches could help prevent approximately 70% of early deaths through measures targeted to the factors that contribute to those deaths. Many of these contributing factors are behavioral, such as tobacco use, diet, and sedentary lifestyle. Other factors that affect health are the environment, social conditions, education, culture, economics, working conditions, and housing (US Department of Health and Human Services [USDHHS], 2016).

The passage of the Affordable Care Act of 2010 created the National Prevention, Health Promotion, and Public Health Council and charged it with developing the National Prevention and Health Promotion Strategy to focus on community-oriented approaches to prevention and wellness to "reduce the incidence and burden of the leading causes of death and disability." (prevention.council@hhs.gov.) The strategy identifies the five leading causes of death as heart disease, cancers, stroke, chronic lower respiratory disease, and unintentional injuries. Other noted priorities are behavioral and mental health, substance use, and domestic violence screenings. In addition, the four health-promoting behaviors associated with the underlying causes of death that will be targeted through prevention measures are tobacco use, nutrition, physical activity, and underage and excessive alcohol use (National Prevention Council, 2011).

Public health practice is of great value. In 2014, the Centers for Medicare and Medicaid Services (CMS) reported that only 3% (up from 1.5% in 1960) of all national health expenditures supported population-focused public health functions. Unfortunately, the public is largely unaware of the contributions of public health practice. Federal and private monies were sparse in their support of public health, so public health agencies began to provide personal care services for persons who could not receive care elsewhere. The health departments benefited by receiving Medicaid and Medicare funds. The result was a shift of resources and energy away from public health's traditional and unique population-focused perspective to include a primary-care focus (Levi et al, 2015; Meit et al, 2013). As overall health needs become the focus of care in the United States, a stronger commitment to population-focused services is emerging. In July 2008, the Trust for America's Health released a study that highlighted the effects of preventive services on improving lives and reducing costs in addition to ways to change the health care system. The threats of terrorism and bioterrorism, highlighted by the events of September 11, 2001, and the anthrax scares, increased awareness for public safety. Important to the public health community is the emergence of modern-day epidemics and infectious diseases, such as the mosquito-borne Zika virus, Ebola, new strains of influenza, and other causes of mortality, many of which affect the very young. Most of the causes are preventable (Bauer et al, 2014).

Public health is best described as what society collectively does to ensure that conditions exist in which people can be healthy (Institute of Medicine, 2003). Public health is a community-oriented, population-focused specialty area. The overall public health mission is to organize community efforts that will use scientific and technical knowledge to prevent disease and promote health (Institute of Medicine, 2003). The three public health core functions are *assessment, policy development,* and *assurance.*

PUBLIC HEALTH CORE FUNCTIONS DEFINED

Fig. 1.1 describes public health in the United States. The functions provide a framework for defining the services to be

---

PUBLIC HEALTH IN AMERICA

Vision:
Healthy people in healthy communities

Mission:
Promote physical and mental health and
prevent disease, injury, and disability

Public health
- Prevents epidemics and the spread of disease
- Protects against environmental hazards
- Prevents injuries
- Promotes and encourages healthy behaviors
- Responds to disasters and assists communities in recovery
- Ensures the quality and accessibility of health services

Essential public health services by core function
Assessment
1. Monitor health status to identify community health problems
2. Diagnose and investigate health problems and health hazards in the community

Policy Development
3. Inform, educate, and empower people about health issues
4. Mobilize community partnerships to identify and solve health problems
5. Develop policies and plans that support individual and community health efforts

Assurance
6. Enforce laws and regulations that protect health and ensure safety
7. Link people to needed personal health services and assure the provision of health care when otherwise unavailable
8. Assure a competent public health and personal health care workforce
9. Evaluate effectiveness, accessibility, and quality of personal and population-based health services

Serving All Functions
10. Research for new insights and innovative solutions to health problems

FIG. 1.1 Public health in America. (Modified from Public Health Functions Steering Committee: Public Health in America, 1994, US Public Health Service agencies, and U.S. Public Health Service: The core functions project, Washington, DC, 1994 [update 2008], Office of Disease Prevention and Health Promotion.)

provided by the public health system. The core functions are defined as follows:

- **Assessment** involves systematically collecting data on the population, monitoring the population's health status, and making information available about the health of the community.
- **Policy development** refers to efforts to develop policies that support the health of the population, including using a scientific knowledge base to make policy decisions.
- **Assurance** is making sure that essential community-oriented health services are available. These services might include providing essential personal health services for those who would otherwise not receive them. Assurance also includes making sure that a competent public health and personal health care workforce is available.

A working group within the US Public Health Service developed the Health Services Pyramid (Fig. 1.2). In this pyramid, population-focused public health programs with the goals of disease prevention, health protection, and health promotion provide a foundation for primary, secondary, and tertiary health care services. Each service level in the pyramid is important to the health of the population. The base of the pyramid shows the effective services that support the top tiers and contribute to better health. All tiers of the pyramid need to be adequately financed (US Public Health Service, 1994/2008). The pyramid has been referenced to show how health care services can be offered to specific population groups (Frieden, 2010). In reality, health care in the United States has been organized with the pyramid upside down. That is, more attention, support, and funding are given to tertiary and secondary care than to primary and preventive services, including population-focused care. The How To box on p. 6 lists the 10 essential public health services.

These services need to be implemented to support the base of the pyramid and to support the services offered through the

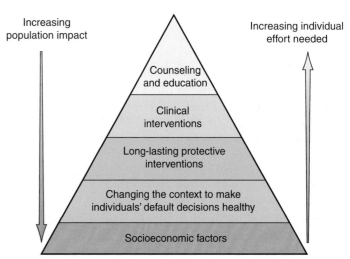

FIG. 1.3 Five-tier health impact pyramid. (From Frieden TR: A framework for public health action: the health impact pyramid, *Am J Public Health*, 100(4): 590–595, 2010.)

top tiers of the pyramid. Together, all services at all levels contribute to better health in the United States.

Another conceptual framework highlighting the effects of public health action on population health and individual health is the five-tier health impact pyramid (Fig. 1.3). The tiers in this pyramid are as follows:

- *Socioeconomic determinants*, the bottom tier of the health impact pyramid, represents changes in socioeconomic factors (e.g., poverty reduction, improved education), often referred to as social determinants of health, that help form the basic foundation of society.
- *Public health interventions* represents interventions that change the context of health, such as clean water and safe roads.
- *Protective interventions with long-term benefits* represents one-time or infrequent protective interventions that do not require ongoing clinical care, such as immunizations, smoking cessation programs, and male circumcision.
- *Direct clinical care* represents ongoing clinical interventions, such as interventions to prevent cardiovascular disease, that have the greatest potential health impact. Evidence-based clinical care can also reduce disability and prolong life.
- *Counseling and education*, the pyramid's top tier, represents health education (education provided during clinical encounters and in other settings), which is perceived by some as the essence of public health action. It is generally the least effective type of intervention. However, educational interventions are often the only ones available, and when applied consistently over time, they may influence individual health.

Interventions at the top tiers are designed to help individuals, whereas interventions at the bottom tiers help entire populations and thus could have a large population impact if universally and effectively applied (Frieden, 2015). As in the Health Services Pyramid, the greater the emphasis given to the bottom tiers, the greater is the impact on population health.

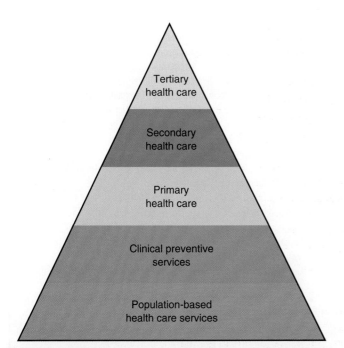

FIG. 1.2 Health services pyramid. (From US Public Health Service: *For a healthy nation: return on investments in public health*, Washington, DC, 1994 [update 2008], USDHHS.)

POPULATION-FOCUSED NURSING PRACTICE

PHN is a specialty with a distinct focus and scope of practice; it requires a special knowledge base. The role of the public health nurse has changed over the years in response to the following:

- Changes in health care
- Priorities for health care funding
- The needs of the population
- The educational preparation of nurses

As noted in Chapter 2, PHN began more than 100 years ago; early public health nurses provided direct care to people, most often in their homes. The Henry Street Settlement, established in New York City in the late 1800s by Lillian Wald, was an early model for PHN. At Henry Street Settlement the nurses took care of the sick in their homes and also looked at the overall population of low-income people in the community from

which their home-care clients came. The primary focus that has differentiated PHN from other specialties is the emphasis on the population rather than on single individuals or families. In the spirit of Lillian Wald, public health nurses have done the following:

- Looked at the community or population as a whole
- Raised questions about the overall population health status and the factors associated with that status, including environmental factors such as physical, biological, social, economic, and cultural aspects
- Worked with the community to improve health status
- Provided health education to individuals, families, and groups to encourage healthier living.

HOW TO Participate as a Public Health Nurse in the Essential Services of Public Health

1. Monitor health status to identify community health problems.
   - Participate in community assessment.
   - Identify subpopulations at risk for disease or disability.
   - Collect information on interventions with special populations.
   - Define and evaluate effective strategies and programs.
   - Identify potential environmental hazards.
2. Diagnose and investigate health problems and hazards in the community.
   - Understand and identify determinants of health and disease.
   - Apply knowledge about environmental influences on health.
   - Recognize multiple causes of or factors in health and illness.
   - Participate in case identification and treatment of persons with communicable diseases.
3. Inform, educate, and empower people about health issues.
   - Develop health and educational plans for individuals and families in multiple settings.
   - Develop and implement community-based health education.
   - Provide regular reports on the health status of special populations within clinic settings, community settings, and groups.
   - Advocate for and with underserved and disadvantaged populations.
   - Ensure health planning, which includes strategies for primary prevention and early intervention.
   - Identify healthy population behaviors, and maintain successful intervention strategies through reinforcement and continued funding.
4. Mobilize community partnerships to identify and solve health problems.
   - Interact regularly with many providers and services within each community.
   - Convene groups and providers who share common concerns and interests in special populations.
   - Provide leadership to prioritize community problems and develop interventions.
   - Explain the significance of health issues to the public, and participate in developing plans of action.
5. Develop policies and plans that support individual and community health efforts.
   - Participate in community and family decision-making processes.
   - Provide information and advocacy for consideration of the interests of special groups in program development.
   - Develop programs and services to meet the needs of high-risk populations as well as other community members.
   - Participate in disaster planning and mobilization of community resources in emergencies.
   - Advocate for appropriate funding for services.
6. Enforce laws and regulations that protect health and ensure safety.
   - Regulate and support safe care and treatment for dependent populations, such as children and frail older adults.

   - Implement ordinances and laws that protect the environment.
   - Establish procedures and processes that ensure competent implementation of treatment schedules for diseases of public health importance.
   - Participate in the development of local regulations that protect communities and the environment from potential hazards and pollution.
7. Link people to needed personal health services and ensure the provision of health care that is otherwise unavailable.
   - Provide clinical preventive services to certain high-risk populations.
   - Establish programs and services to meet special needs.
   - Recommend clinical care and other services to clients and their families in clinics, homes, and the community.
   - Provide referrals through community links to needed care.
   - Participate in community provider coalitions and meetings to educate others and to identify service centers for community populations.
   - Provide clinical surveillance and identification of communicable diseases.
8. Ensure a competent public health and personal health care workforce.
   - Participate in continuing education and preparation to ensure competence.
   - Define and support proper delegation to unlicensed assistive personnel in community settings.
   - Establish standards for performance.
   - Maintain client record systems and community documents.
   - Establish and maintain procedures and protocols for client care.
   - Participate in quality assurance activities, such as record audits, agency evaluation, and adherence to clinical guidelines.
9. Evaluate the effectiveness, accessibility, and quality of personal and population-based health services.
   - Collect data and information related to community interventions.
   - Identify unserved and underserved populations within the community.
   - Review and analyze data on the health status of the community.
   - Participate with the community in the assessment of services and outcomes of care.
   - Identify and define enhanced services required to manage the health status of complex populations and special risk groups.
10. Research for new insights and innovative solutions to health problems.
    - Implement nontraditional interventions and approaches to effect change in special populations.
    - Participate in the collecting of information and data to improve the surveillance and understanding of special problems.
    - Develop collegial relationships with academic institutions to explore new interventions.
    - Participate in the early identification of factors detrimental to the community's health.
    - Formulate and use investigative tools to identify and influence care delivery and program planning.

From the U.S. Public Health Service: `The core functions project,` Washington, DC, 1994/update 2008, Office of Disease Prevention and Health Promotion.

The primary goal of public health—the prevention of disease and disability—is achieved by ensuring that conditions exist in which people can remain healthy. The How To box on the policy-development process describes ways to distinguish what actually makes up the specialty of PHN.

HOW TO Distinguish the Specialty of Public Health Nursing

- **Population focused:** Primary emphasis on populations of individuals who live in the community, as opposed to those who are institutionalized
- **Community oriented:**
  - Concern for the connection between the population's health status and the environment in which the population lives (e.g., physical, biological, sociocultural)
  - An imperative to work with members of the community to carry out core public health functions
- **Health and disease-prevention focused:** Predominant emphasis on strategies for health promotion, health maintenance, and disease prevention, particularly primary and secondary prevention
- **Interventions at the community and population levels:**
  - The use of political processes to affect public policy as a major intervention strategy for achieving goals
  - Concern for the health of all members of the population or community, particularly vulnerable subpopulations

---

In 1981 the PHN section of the American Public Health Association (APHA) defined PHN and described how this role contributes to health care delivery. This statement was reaffirmed in 1996 and again in 2013 (APHA, 1996, 2013). PHN is defined as a specialty that brings together knowledge from the social and public health sciences and nursing to promote and protect the health of populations. It is defined by the Quad Council Coalition of Public Health Nursing Organizations as population-focused, community-oriented nursing practice. The goals of PHN are "the promotion of health, the prevention of disease and disability for all people through the creation of conditions in which people can be healthy" (American Nurses Association, 2013, p. 5). Box 1.1 presents the PHN process from the APHA definition.

Public health nurses, like others in public health, engage in assessment, policy development, and assurance activities. These functions are achieved when nurses work in partnerships with others, including nations, states, communities, organizations, groups, and individuals. Public health nurses carry out this mission by participating in the essential public health services described earlier in the chapter.

Although population-focused practice is the central feature of PHN, many of the skills and activities are used when community-oriented nurses and community-based nurses work in the community. For this reason, these practices are described in detail here. A population or aggregate is a collection of people who share one or more personal or environmental characteristics. Members of a community can be defined in terms of either geography (e.g., a county, a group of counties, or a state) or a special interest (e.g., children attending a particular school). These members make up a population. Generally, there are subpopulations within the larger population. Examples of subpopulations within a population of a county are high-risk infants younger than 1 year old, unmarried pregnant adolescents, and individuals exposed to a particular hazardous event (e.g., a chemical spill).

BOX 1.1   The Public Health Nursing Process

Public health nursing is a systematic process of working with the client as a partner that does the following:

- Assesses the health and health care needs of a population in collaboration with other disciplines to identify subpopulations (aggregates), families, and individuals at increased risk for illness, disability, or premature death.
- Develops and plans interventions to meet these needs. The plan includes resources available and activities that contribute to health and its recovery and the prevention of illness, disability, and premature death.
- Implements the plan effectively, efficiently, and equitably.
- Evaluates progress to determine the extent to which these activities have influenced the health-status outcomes of the population.
- Uses the results to influence and direct the delivery of care, the use of health resources, and the development of local, regional, state, and national health policy and research to promote health and prevent diseases.

Data from American Public Health Association, Public Health Nursing Section: *The definition and practice of public health nursing: a statement of the public health nursing section,* Washington, DC, 2013, American Public Health Association; American Public Health Association: *The definition and role of public health nurses: a statement of the American Public Health Association's Public Health Nursing Section,* Washington, DC, 1996, The Association; American Public Health Association: *The definition and role of public health nursing in the delivery of health care: a statement of the Public Health Nursing section,* Washington, DC, 1981, The Association; and American Nurses Association: *Public health nursing: scope and standards of practice,* 2013, ANA.

EVIDENCE-BASED PRACTICE

Kneipp, Kairalla, and Sheely (2013) conducted a study that used a randomized controlled design to evaluate the effectiveness of a public health nursing case-management intervention to address the needs of 432 American women with chronic health conditions who received Temporary Assistance for Needy Families (TANF). This study explored the effect of the PHN intervention on employment outcomes, particularly during the recent economic recession. Previous studies noted the high prevalence of health conditions among US women receiving TANF, thus impeding this population's employment opportunities. The intervention was developed with input from the community and used community members on the research team. Control-group participants received what would be considered usual care in the local Welfare Transition Program (WTP) in north-central Florida. Referral and case-management activities began for the intervention-group participants at their initial visits and focused on ensuring access to and coordination of care, disease management, health education, and disease prevention. Outcomes were assessed at 3, 6, and 9 months. Study findings indicated that outcomes for employment entry (any employment, $p = 0.05$; time to employment, $p = 0.01$) were significantly improved for women in WTPs with chronic health conditions who received a PHN case-management intervention to address their health needs compared with women receiving standard WTP services.

Nurse Use

The results of this study suggest that public health interventions can improve employment outcomes among women receiving TANF. Such improvements were theorized to have occurred because the PHNs working with the intervention group helped the participants "to better manage chronic health conditions and decrease health-related functional limitations" (p. 138).

Data from Kneipp SM, Kairalla JA, Sheely AL: A randomized controlled trial to improve health among women receiving welfare in the U.S.: the relationship between employment outcomes and the economic recession, *Social Science & Medicine,* 80(1): 130–140, 2013.

In **population-focused practice,** problems are defined (assessments/diagnoses) and solutions (interventions), such as policy development or providing a given preventive service, are implemented for or with a defined population or subpopulation as opposed to diagnoses, interventions, and treatment carried out at the individual level. This contrasts with basic professional education in nursing, medicine, and other clinical disciplines, which emphasizes developing competence in decision making at the level of the individual client by assessing health status, making management decisions (ideally with the client), and evaluating the effects of care. The ways in which nurses provide care to people with high blood pressure can demonstrate how population-focused practice differs from the clinical direct-care practice so often used in nursing. Specifically, in a clinical direct-care situation, a nurse practicing in the community might decide that a person is hypertensive based on certain clinical signs. The nurse would evaluate different interventions to find the best one for this person and implement an appropriate intervention, such as a change in diet.

In contrast to the nurse providing direct clinical care, a public health nurse engaged in population-focused practice would ask the following questions related to the population of the center:

- What is the prevalence rate of hypertension among various age, race, and gender groups?
- Which subpopulations have the highest rates of untreated hypertension?
- What programs could reduce the problem of untreated hypertension and decrease the risk for further cardiovascular morbidity and mortality?
- The public health nurse's approach focuses on improving the health of populations in addition to having an effect on the individual.

Public health nurses are typically concerned with more than one subpopulation, and they often deal with the health of the entire community. *Assessment,* one of the public health core functions, is a logical first step in examining a community setting to determine its health status.

The core public health function of assessment includes the following aspects:

- Engaging in activities that involve the collection, analysis, and dissemination of information on both the health and health-relevant aspects of a community or a specific population
- Questioning whether the health services of the community are available to the population and are adequate to address needs

CHECK YOUR PRACTICE

You have been asked by a local health agency to monitor the health status of the population in a community center that serves older persons living in the area of the center. The problem noted by the center staff is that they would like to know the most prevalent health problem shared by the clients of the center to offer programs based on the primary problem of the total population of the center. What would you do?

- Monitoring the health status of the community or population and the services provided over time
- Evaluating the social, economic, environmental, and lifestyle characteristics and practices of a population and the health services and capacity available within the community to support good health for the population

The How To box provides a general set of questions that can be used or modified to gather assessment data.

HOW TO Assess: Assessment Questions to Ask
- What are the major health problems in this community?
- Which population groups are at greatest risk?
- How are risks distributed geographically?
- What services are available?
- What services need to be provided but are unavailable?
- What is the level of quality of the available and needed services?
- What do citizens think their most pressing health needs are?
- Are the most pressing health needs considered to be the same by both providers and citizens?
- What is the history of agency collaboration and cooperation in this community?

Excellent examples of assessment at the national level are the efforts of the USDHHS to organize the goal setting, data collection and analysis, and monitoring necessary to develop the series of publications describing the health status and health-related aspects of the US population. These efforts began with *Healthy People* in 1980 and continued with *Promoting Health, Preventing Disease: 1990 Health Objectives for the Nation, Healthy People 2000,* and *Healthy People 2010* and are now moving forward into the future with Healthy People 2020 (USDHHS, 1979, 1991, 2000, 2016).

In a local health department, public health nurses would participate in and provide leadership for assessing community needs, the health status of populations within the community, and environmental and behavioral risks. They also look at trends in the factors that determine health in the community, identify priority health needs, and determine the adequacy of existing community resources.

Policy development is a core function of public health and one of the core intervention strategies used by PHN specialists. Policy development relies heavily on planning and begins with the identified needs and priorities set by the people involved. It also includes building constituencies that can bring about policy changes. It is important to know what the powerful people in the community think about a specific public health concern. Health and human services providers and the people who will be served or affected must be included. PHN is an approach to planning characterized as "with the people" rather than "to the people" or "for the people." Historically, health care providers have been accused of providing care for or to people without actually involving the recipients in the decisions. The beneficiaries of services in public health need to be included from the very beginning in identifying the need, planning the intervention, and deciding on the format for the evaluation (Box 1.2).

BOX 1.2   Policy Development Process

The policy development function has the following characteristics:

- It is essentially a planning process that uses the assessment data to define health needs; set priorities; identify alternatives; outline a plan, including the determination of available and needed resources; and determine who needs to be involved to ensure some measure of success.
- It serves as a resource or catalyst to help elected officials or heads of community organizations develop population-based health plans.
- It assists people who make policies to do so in such a way that the needs of many people or groups are met. It also advises these individuals and groups about which needs are most important and should be handled first.
- It consistently advocates for better health conditions for the population as a whole.

The third core public health function, *assurance*, focuses on the responsibility of public health agencies to be sure that activities are appropriately carried out to meet public health goals and plans. Not only does PHN include assessment or investigative functions, but the role also requires skill in collaboration, consultation, and cooperation. The assurance function ensures that the activities designed during the policy-development or planning phase are carried out. This is done through collaboration with people in a variety of health and human service organizations to promote, monitor, and improve both the availability and quality of providers and services. PHN is not a good field for people who like to work alone. Although considerable opportunity exists for autonomy in thinking and planning, effective and consistent collaboration is vital to success. Assurance does not always mean to provide something. Rather, another agency may provide the needed service. Assurance means making certain that the services determined to be needed are provided by some agency within the community. Further, assurance includes assisting communities with implementing and evaluating plans and projects. It includes maintaining the ability of both public health agencies and private providers to manage day-to-day operations and ensuring the capacity to respond to critical situations and emergencies.

In PHN, the nurse often reaches out to those who might benefit from a service or intervention. In other forms of nursing, the client is more likely to seek and request assistance. As is discussed in later chapters, the people or populations most in need of public health services are often the least likely to ask for them, such as people who are homeless, poor, or mentally ill. The dominant needs of the population outweigh the expressed needs of one or a few people. Because resources are often limited, careful assessment to identify key needs is important.

However, the contributions of public health nurse specialists include looking at the community or population as a whole; raising questions about its overall health status and factors associated with that status, including environmental factors (e.g., physical, biological, sociocultural); and working *with the community* to improve the population's health status.

HEALTHY PEOPLE 2020

Overview and Goals

In 1979, the Surgeon General issued a report that began a 20-year focus on promoting health and preventing disease for all Americans. The report, entitled *Healthy People,* used morbidity rates to track the health of individuals through the five major life cycles of infancy, childhood, adolescence, adulthood, and older age.

In 1989, *Healthy People 2000* became a national effort of representatives from government agencies, academia, and health organizations. Their goal was to present a strategy for improving the health of the American people. Their objectives are being used by public and community health organizations to assess current health trends, health programs, and disease-prevention programs.

Throughout the 1990s, all states used *Healthy People 2000* objectives to identify emerging public health issues. The success of the program on a national level was accomplished through state and local efforts. Early in the 1990s, surveys from public health departments indicated that 8% of the national objectives had been met, and progress on an additional 40% of the objectives was noted. In the midcourse review published in 1995, it was noted that significant progress had been made toward meeting 50% of the objectives.

Using the progress made in the past decade, the committee for *Healthy People 2010* proposed the following two goals:

- To increase years of healthy life
- To eliminate health disparities among different populations

The committee hopes to reach these goals through such measures as promoting healthy behaviors, increasing access to quality health care, and strengthening community prevention.

The major premise of *Healthy People 2010* was that the health of the individual can rarely be separated from the health of the larger community. Therefore the vision for *Healthy People 2010* was "Healthy People in Healthy Communities."

The vision for *Healthy People 2020* is "A society in which all people live long, healthy lives." The overarching goals for 2020 are as follows:

- To eliminate preventable disease, disability injury, and premature death
- To achieve health equity, eliminate disparities, and improve the health of all groups
- To create social and physical environments that promote good health for all
- To promote healthy development and healthy behaviors across every stage of life

In contrast to previous years, *Healthy People 2020* has a web-accessible database that is searchable, multilevel, and interactive, enhancing its usefulness. The objectives for 2020 are now available online at https://www.healthypeople.gov/2020/topics-objectives.

Data from US Department of Health and Human Services: *Healthy People 2000: national health promotion and disease prevention objectives,* DHHS Pub. No. 91-50212, Washington, DC, 1991, US Government Printing Office; US Department of Health and Human Services: *Healthy People 2010: understanding and improving health,* ed 2, Washington, DC, 2000, US Government Printing Office; US Department of Health, Education, and Welfare: *Healthy People: the Surgeon General's report on health promotion and disease prevention,* DHEW Pub. No. 79-55071, Washington, DC, 1979, US Government Printing Office; and US Department of Health and Human Services: *Healthy People 2020* [Internet], Washington, DC, 2016, Office of Disease Prevention and Health Promotion. Available from https://www.healthypeople.gov/.

PRACTICE FOCUSING ON INDIVIDUALS, FAMILIES, AND GROUPS

As mentioned, community-based nursing practice, with its focus on the provision or assurance of care to individuals and families in the community, is different from community-oriented practice. The latter is broader in scope and is a form of care in which the nurse provides health care after completing a community diagnosis to determine what conditions need to be altered for individuals, families, and groups in the community to stay healthy. Although it is hoped that all direct-care providers contribute to the community's health in the broadest sense, not all are primarily concerned with a population health focus, or the "big picture." All nurses in a given community, including those working in hospitals, physicians' offices, and health clinics, contribute positively to the health of the community. Examples of community settings for treating individuals include ambulatory surgery clinics, outpatient clinics, physician and advanced-practice nursing offices and clinics, and employment and school sites, in addition to preschool programs, housing projects, and migrant camps. These sites often provide individual-focused health care services in contrasts to population-focused services (i.e., services focused on a large group). A specific example is Head Start, the federally funded program for preschool children. From a community-oriented nursing care perspective, nursing services could be provided to individual children by conducting developmental-level screening tests to evaluate each child's level of cognitive and psychomotor development for comparison with established standards for children of the same age. The community-based nurse could then deliver illness care to the children in the school. In contrast, a public health or population-focused approach would look at the entire group of children being served by the program and the characteristics of the facility and its programs to evaluate whether they are effective in achieving the goals of making the school population healthier.

COMMUNITY-ORIENTED NURSING

Most nurses practicing in the community and many staff public health nurses—both historically and at present—focus on providing direct-care services, including health education, to persons or families outside of institutional settings, either in the home or in a clinic. Historically, the term *community health nurse* applied to all nurses who practiced in the community, regardless of whether they had preparation in PHN. Thus nurses providing secondary or tertiary care in a home, school, or clinic or any nurse who did not practice in an institutional setting could be considered a "community health nurse." To a large extent, the development of what has been called *community health nursing* was influenced by the development of the specialty of community medicine within the medical field. At that time, both community medicine and community health nursing reached out to the community and began doing community assessments to determine more effectively the needs of the people so that disease prevention

and health promotion could be targeted to the specific needs in a given community. Specifically, the community health nurse operated from a health care focus based on an understanding of broader community needs. Today, the term *community health nurse* and *public health nurse* are used interchangeably, and both are referred to as *community-oriented nurses.*

The nurse must continually evaluate the community to see if changes are occurring that will influence the health of the people who live there. The accompanying case study provides an example of community-oriented nursing practice. Work through the case study and answer the questions for a better understanding of this specialty area.

The practice of community-oriented nursing involves health promotion, health maintenance, health education, management, coordination, and continuity of care in the management of the health care of individuals, families, and groups in a community. A holistic approach is used, and the goal of this care is to provide personal health services that promote and preserve the health of the community in which the clients live. The community-oriented nurse uses both nursing and public health theory to guide practice.

Evidence that entry-level nurses are practicing effectively in the community includes the following (Babenko-Mould et al, 2016; Joyce et al, 2014):
- Provide quality services that can control costs.
- Focus on disease prevention and health promotion.
- Organize services where people live, work, play, and learn.
- Provide referrals when clients need them.

CASE STUDY

Community Assessment to Identify Population Health Risks

This is Debbie Brown's first year working as a nurse at the local health department in a rural county. Most of her days are spent in the clinic, seeing clients who usually do not have health insurance.

Over the course of a month, several young Hispanic men, all migrant farm workers, come to the health department, and tuberculosis is diagnosed in all of them. Ms. Brown is concerned about what the outbreak of tuberculosis in the migrant workers could mean for the community. Through a community health assessment, Ms. Brown identifies the group of migrant farm workers to be at the highest risk of contracting tuberculosis.

Ms. Brown brings the tuberculosis outbreak to the attention of the health department's communicable disease control department, which in turn contacts the local school system and makes tuberculosis skin testing a requirement for enrollment in school. Ms. Brown also develops an educational program for the migrant workers, their families, and their employers to teach them about tuberculosis and how to prevent its spread.

1. What indicators should Ms. Brown look at when she performs her community health assessment?
2. What is Ms. Brown's nursing area?
   A. Community-oriented nursing practice
   B. Public health nursing practice
   C. Community-based nursing practice
   D. Home health nursing
3. In this case study, how were the core functions of public health applied?

Answers can be found on the Evolve website.

- Work in partnerships and with coalitions and other health care providers.
- Work across the life span and with culturally diverse populations.
- Work with at-risk populations to promote access to services.
- Participate in epidemiological investigations and disaster services.
- Develop the community's capacity for health.
- Work with policymakers for policy change.
- Work to make the environment healthier.

As can be seen, community-oriented nurses emphasize health protection, maintenance, and promotion; disease prevention; and self-reliance among clients. Regardless of whether the client is a person, a family, or a group, the goal is to promote health through education about prevailing health problems, proper nutrition, beneficial forms of exercise, and environmental factors such as safe food, water, air, and buildings. The nurse is likely to be involved in immunizing individuals and organizing the immunization programs for vaccinating the community for influenza, for example, and educating the community about the value of this service. Other individual and family services include provision of maternal and child health care, treatment of common communicable and infectious diseases and injuries, and provision of basic screening programs for problems such as lice, vision, hearing, and scoliosis.

Nurses have always been involved in providing family-centered care to individuals, families, and groups across the life span; however, they also work to identify high-risk groups in the community. Once such groups are identified, the nurse can work with others to develop appropriate policies and interventions to reduce risk and provide beneficial services. Both community-oriented nurses and community-based nurses must be aware of cultural diversity and provide care that is appropriate to the needs of the recipient. Likewise, both groups of nurses provide care in homes. The Focus on Quality and Safety Education for Nurses box provides the list of competencies a nurse will need to improve the quality and safety of interventions and outcomes in the community. Compare these competencies with the public health nursing competencies noted in Appendix C.3.

COMMUNITY-BASED NURSING

As mentioned, the goal of CBN is to manage acute or chronic conditions while promoting self-care among individuals and families (Kane et al., 2013). In CBN the nursing care is family centered, which means that the nurse works to improve the competencies of families to enable them to take better care of themselves. The nurse pays particular attention to the uniqueness of each family and works to plan the most useful interventions. A "cookbook" approach cannot be used because no single nursing approach will fit each family or individual. Cultural diversity is taken into account, as are the situations and stressors facing the person or the family at a given time. The nurse promotes client autonomy and helps clients learn to do as much as possible for themselves.

FOCUS ON QUALITY AND SAFETY EDUCATION FOR NURSES

Quality and Safety Education for Nurses (QSEN) Competencies

QSEN Competency	Competency Definition
Client-Centered Care	Recognize the client or designee as the source of control and full partner in providing compassionate and coordinated care based on respect for client preferences, values, and needs.
Teamwork and Collaboration	Function effectively within nursing and interprofessional teams, fostering open communication, mutual respect, and shared decision making to achieve quality care.
Evidence-Based Practice	Integrate best current evidence with clinical expertise and client/family preferences and values for delivery of optimal health care.
Quality Improvement	Use data to monitor the outcomes of care processes, and use improvement methods to design and test changes to continuously improve the quality and safety of health care systems.
Safety	Minimizes risk for harm to clients and providers through both system effectiveness and individual performance.
Informatics	Use information and technology to communicate, manage knowledge, mitigate error, and support decision making.

Prepared by Gail Armstrong, DNP, ACNS-BC, CNE, Associate Professor, University of Colorado Denver College of Nursing.

LEVELS OF PREVENTION

Related to Public Health

Primary Prevention
The public health nurse develops a health education program for a population of school-age children that teaches them about the effects of smoking on health.

Secondary Prevention
The public health nurse provides toxin screenings for migrant workers who may be exposed to pesticides.

Tertiary Prevention
The public health nurse provides a diabetes clinic for a defined population of adults in a low-income housing unit in the community.

The nurse practicing CBN is more likely to give direct care to people than are nurses who practice from a community-oriented framework. To plan the most appropriate course of action, the nurse assesses client needs and the services available to meet those needs. Throughout care delivery, the nurse teaches and counsels

BOX 1.3 Definitions of the Three Key Nursing Modes in the Community

Community-Oriented Nursing Practice: A philosophy of nursing care delivery that involves generalist or specialist public health and community health nurses providing "health care" through community diagnosis and investigation of major health and environmental problems, health surveillance, monitoring, and evaluation of community and population health status to prevent disease and disability and promoting, protecting, and maintaining health to create conditions in which people can be healthy.

Public Health Nursing Practice: The synthesis of nursing and public health theory applied to promoting and preserving the health of populations. Practice focuses on the community as a whole and the effect of the community's health status (resources) on the health of individuals, families, and groups. The goal is to prevent disease and disability and promote and protect the health of the community as a whole. *Community health nurse* is a term that is often used interchangeably with *public health nurse*.

Community-Based Nursing Practice: A setting-specific practice in which "illness care" is provided for individuals and families where they live, work, and attend school. The emphasis is on acute and chronic care and the provision of comprehensive, coordinated, and continuous care. These nurses may be generalists or specialists in maternal–infant, pediatric, adult, or psychiatric mental health nursing.

⟩⟩ APPLYING CONTENT TO PRACTICE

In this chapter emphasis is placed on defining and explaining public health nursing practice with populations. As the nurse works in the community, the focus of the practice will involve the three essential functions of public health and public health nursing: assessment, policy development, and assurance. The *Core Competencies for Public Health Professionals* developed by the Council on Linkages and revised in 2014 describes the skills of public health professionals, including nurses. It is these skills that the nurse will need to apply in the community setting. In the assessment function, one skill is the assessment of the health status of populations and the related determinants of health and illness. For policy development, one of the skills is the development of a plan to implement policy and programs. For the assurance function, one skill that public health nurses will need is to incorporate ethical standards of practice as the basis of all interactions with organizations, communities, and individuals. These skills can also be linked to the 10 essential services of public health nursing found on page 6. Assessment of health status is a skill needed for implementing essential service 1, the monitoring of health status to identify community problems. Development of a plan for policy and program implementation is a skill needed for essential service 5, supporting individual and community health efforts. Incorporating ethical standards is done in essential service 3 when informing, educating, and empowering people about health issues.

clients so they can more fully develop their own ways of taking care of themselves. Box 1.3 provides definitions of each of the three key modes of nursing practice seen in the community, with discussion of PHN and community health nursing combined.

CHALLENGES FOR THE FUTURE

Over the past few years, the places in which care is given have changed dramatically. In previous decades the majority of care was given in an inpatient setting. At present, the trend is to move more care into community settings and to reduce the number of hospital days for "sick" clients. A variety of reasons explain the change. First, community care is often much less expensive than hospital care. Because the cost of health care in the United States has risen considerably over the past decade, it is increasingly necessary to find new ways to deliver care that are accessible to the recipients, less expensive, and of adequate quality to meet client needs. Also, care in the community is usually more appealing to people who prefer to remain at home

rather than be treated in a hospital. Currently, care is given in homes, in schools, at the work site, and in a variety of outpatient clinics. This trend is predicted to grow, and it is expected that the role of the nurse in community settings will likewise grow and continue to change. Many factors will affect the changing role of the nurse in the community, such as new and emerging infectious diseases, the need for emergency preparedness, increases in chronic illness, and the continued reduction of numbers of days in the hospital for serious illnesses. As a result of the Affordable Care Act and other changes in health care delivery, massive changes are occurring in how care is delivered and where. The primary focus of the health care system of the future will likely be on community-oriented strategies for health promotion and disease prevention and on community-based strategies for primary and secondary care. With the focus on quality and safety education for nurses, public health nursing education will likely focus more attention toward assisting nurses to develop competencies focused on population health, as noted in the box on the QSEN competencies.

PRACTICE APPLICATION

Debate with classmates where and how PHN specialists practice and how their practice compares with what has been defined as CBN. Be specific about the differences.

Debate with classmates which of the nurses in the following categories are practicing population-focused nursing:

A. School nurses
B. Staff nurses in home care
C. Director of nursing for a home-care agency
D. Nurse practitioners in a health maintenance organization
E. Vice president of nursing in a hospital
F. Staff nurses in a public health clinic or community health center
G. Director of nursing in a health department

Choose three categories from the previous list, then interview at least one nurse in each category.

1. Determine the scope of their practice.
2. Are they carrying out population-focused practice?
3. Could they?
4. How?
5. Ask them if they would change their roles if this were possible.
6. Inquire whether they believe their role is either community-oriented nursing or CBN practice. Compare and contrast their answers with what you have learned about these roles.

Answers can be found on the Evolve website.

REMEMBER THIS!

- Public health is what members of a society do collectively to ensure that conditions exist in which people can be healthy.
- Assessment, policy development, and assurance are the core public health functions at all levels of government.
- Assessment refers to systematically collecting data on the population, monitoring of the population's health status, and making information available on the health of the community.
- Policy development refers to the need to provide leadership in developing policies that support the health of the population, including the use of the scientific knowledge base in decision making about policy.
- Assurance refers to the way public health practice makes sure that essential community-wide health services are available. This may include providing essential personal health services for those who would otherwise not receive them. Assurance also includes making sure that a competent public health and personal health care workforce is available.

- The setting is frequently viewed as the feature that distinguishes PHN from other specialties. A more useful approach is to use characteristics such as the following: a focus on populations of individuals who live in the community, an emphasis on prevention, concern for the interface between the health status of the population and the environment (e.g., physical, biological, sociocultural), and the use of political processes to influence public policy to achieve goals.
- Specialization in PHN is seen as a subset of community-oriented nursing practice.
- Population-focused practice is the focus of specialization in PHN. The focus on populations in the community and the emphasis on health protection, health promotion, and disease prevention are the fundamental factors that distinguish PHN from other nursing specialties.
- *Population* is defined as a collection of individuals who share one or more personal or environmental characteristics. The term *population* may be used interchangeably with the term *aggregate*.

ⓔ EVOLVE WEBSITE

http://evolve.elsevier.com/Stanhope/foundations
- Case Study, with Questions and Answers
- NCLEX® Review Questions
- Practice Application Answers

REFERENCES

American Nurses Association: *Public health nursing: scope and standards of practice*, Silver Spring, MD, 2013, ANA.

American Public Health Association: *The definition and role of public health nursing in the delivery of health care: a statement of the Public Health Nursing Section*, Washington, DC, 1981, The Association.

American Public Health Association: *The definition and role of public health nurses: a statement of the American Public Health Association's Public Health Nursing Section*, Washington, DC, 1996, APHA.

American Public Health Association, Public Health Nursing Section: *The definition and practice of public health nursing: a statement of the Public Health Nursing Section*, Washington, DC, 2013, American Public Health Association.

Babenko-Mould Y, Ferguson K, Atthill S: Neighbourhood as community: a qualitative descriptive study of nursing students' experiences of community health nursing, *Nurse Education in Practice* 17:223–228. doi:10.1016/j.nepr.2016.02.002.

Bauer UE, Briss PA, Goodman RA, Bowman BA: Prevention of chronic disease in the 21st century: elimination of the leading preventable causes of premature death and disability in the USA, *The Lancet* 384(9937):45–52, 2014.

Centers for Medicare and Medicaid Services, Office of the Actuary, National Health Statistics Group: *The nation's health dollar ($3.0 trillion), calendar year 2014, where it went*, Washington, DC, January, 2014, CMS. Retrieved March 2016 from https://www.

cms.gov/Research-Statistics-Data-and-Systems/Statistics-Trends-and-Reports/NationalHealthExpendData/Downloads/PieChart-SourcesExpenditures2014.pdf.

Frieden T: A framework for public health action: the health impact pyramid, *Am J Public Health* 100:590–595, 2010.

Institute of Medicine: *The future of the public's health: the 21st century*, Washington, DC, 2003, National Academies Press.

Joyce BL, O'Brien K, Belew-LaDue B, Dorjee TK, Smith CM: Revealing the voices of public health nurses by exploring their lived experience, *Public Health Nursing* 32(2):151–160, 2014.

Kane RL, Lum TY, Kane RA, Homyak P, Parashuram S, Wysocki A: Does home- and community-based care affect nursing home use? *J of Aging & Social Policy* 25(2):146–160, 2013.

Kneipp SM, Kairalla JA, Sheely AL: A randomized controlled trial to improve health among women receiving welfare in the U.S.: the relationship between employment outcomes and the economic recession, *Social Science and Medicine* 80(1):130–140, 2013.

Levi J, Segal LM, Gougelet R, St. Laurent R: *Investing in America's health: a state-by-state look at public health funding and key health facts*, April 2015, Trust for America's Health, Robert Wood Johnson Foundation. Retrieved March 23, 2016 from http://healthyamericans.org/assets/files/TFAH-2015-InvestIn AmericaRpt-FINAL.pdf.

Meit M, Knudson A, Dickman I, Brown A, Hernandez N, Kronstadt J: *An examination of public health financing in the United States*. (Prepared by NORC at the University of Chicago.) Washington, DC, March 2013, The Office of the Assistant Secretary for Planning and Evaluation.

Nash DB, Reifsnyder J, Fabius RJ, Pracilio VP: *Population health: creating a culture of wellness*, Sudbury, MA, 2011, Jones and Bartlett.

National Center for Health Statistics: *Health, United States, 2014: with special feature on adults aged 55–64*, Hyattsville, MD, 2015, USDHHS. Retrieved from http://www.cdc.gov/nchs/data/hus/hus14.pdf.

National Prevention Council: *National prevention strategy*, Washington, DC, 2011, USDHHS, Office of the Surgeon General.

Public Health Functions Steering Committee: *Public health in America*, Rockville, MD, 1994, US Public Health Service agencies.

Singh GK: *Child mortality in the United States, 1935–2007: large racial and socioeconomic disparities have persisted over time, a 75th anniversary publication*, Rockville, MD, 2010, USDHHS, Health Resources and Services Administration, Maternal and Child Health Bureau.

Trust for America's Health: *Prevention for a healthier America: investments in disease prevention yield significant savings, stronger communities*, July 2008. Retrieved June 2012 from http://healthyamericans.org/reports/prevention08/.

US Department of Health, Education, and Welfare: *Healthy people: the Surgeon General's report on health promotion and disease prevention*, DHEW Pub. No. 79-55071, Washington, DC, 1979, U.S. Government Printing Office.

US Department of Health and Human Services: *Healthy people 2000: National health promotion and disease prevention objectives*, DHHS Pub. No. 91-50212, Washington, DC, 1991, US Government Printing Office.

US Department of Health and Human Services: *Healthy people 2010: Understanding and improving health*, Washington, DC, 2000, US Government Printing Office.

U.S. Department of Health and Human Services: Healthy People 2020 [Internet], Washington, DC, (cited March 22, 2016), Office of Disease Prevention and Health Promotion. Available from https://www.healthypeople.gov/.

U.S. Department of Health and Human Services: *Health US: 2000*, Washington, DC, 2002, National Center for Statistics.

US Department of Health and Human Services: *National Center for Statistics*, Washington, DC, 2010a, USDHHS.

US Department of Health and Human Services: *Healthy people 2020*, Washington, DC, 2016, Office of Disease Prevention and Health Promotion. Retrieved from https://www.healthypeople.gov/.

US Public Health Service: *For a healthy nation: return on investments in public health. The core functions project*, Washington, DC, 1994 (update 2008), Office of Disease Prevention and Health Promotion, USDHHS.

CHAPTER 2

The History of Public Health and Public and Community Health Nursing

Janna Dieckmann

OBJECTIVES

After reading this chapter, the student should be able to:

1. Discuss historical events that have influenced how current health care is delivered in the community.
2. Trace the ongoing interaction between the practice of public health and that of nursing.
3. Explain significant historical trends that have influenced the development of public health nursing.
4. Examine the contributions of Florence Nightingale, Lillian Wald, and Mary Breckinridge and the influence these

three nursing leaders had on current public health and nursing.
5. Examine the ways in which nursing has been provided in the community, including settlement houses, visiting nurse associations, official health organizations, and schools.
6. Discuss the status of public health nursing in the 21st century, including the major organizations that have contributed to the current state of public health nursing.

CHAPTER OUTLINE

Early Public Health
Public Health During America's Colonial Period and the New Republic
Nightingale and the Origins of Trained Nursing
Continued Growth in Public Health Nursing

Public Health Nursing During the Early 20th Century
African American Nurses in Public Health Nursing
Economic Depression and the Impact on Public Health
From World War II until the 1970s
Public Health Nursing from the 1970s to the Present

KEY TERMS

American Association of Colleges of Nursing (AACN), 26
American Nurses Association (ANA), 26
American Public Health Association (APHA), 21
American Red Cross, 20
Breckinridge, Mary, 22
district nursing, 17

district nursing association, 18
Frontier Nursing Service (FNS), 22
instructive district nursing, 18
Metropolitan Life Insurance Company, 21
National League for Nursing (NLN), 26
National Organization for Public Health Nursing (NOPHN), 20

Nightingale, Florence, 17
official health agencies, 24
Rathbone, William, 18
settlement houses, 18
Shattuck Report, 17
Social Security Act of 1935, 24
visiting nurse associations, 18
visiting nurses, 18
Wald, Lillian, 18

One of the best ways to understand today and plan for tomorrow is to examine the past. This is certainly true for public health and public health nursing. Nurses use historical approaches to examine both the profession's present and its future. Questions are asked: What worked in the past? What did not work? What lessons can be learned about health care, nursing, and the communities in which care is provided? During times of rapid social change, it is important to examine history and try to learn from the events of the past and build on the events and actions that were effective. This chapter serves as an introduction to an examination of the past in terms of both public health and nursing.

For nearly 125 years, public health nurses in the United States have worked to develop strategies to respond effectively

to public health problems. Public health is an interdisciplinary specialty that emphasizes prevention. Nurses have worked in communities to improve the health status of individuals, families, and populations, especially those who belong to vulnerable groups. This work has not been easy for many reasons. One reason is that it is more difficult to measure the effects of prevention than it is to measure the effects of treatment. In recent years, as health care costs have grown, it has become increasingly important to emphasize prevention.

Many varied and challenging public health nursing roles originated in the late 1800s, when public health efforts focused on environmental conditions such as sanitation, control of communicable diseases, education for health, prevention of disease and disability, and care of aged and sick persons in their homes.

Although the threats to health have changed over time, the foundational principles and goals of public health nursing have remained the same. Many communicable diseases, such as diphtheria, cholera, and typhoid fever, have been largely controlled in the United States, but others, such as HIV, tuberculosis, and hepatitis, continue to affect many lives around the world. Emerging communicable diseases, such as the varying types of influenza, illustrate the global nature of health threats. Even though environmental pollution in residential areas has been reduced, communities are now threatened by emissions from the many vehicles on their roads, overcrowded garbage dumps, and pollutants in the air, water, and soil. Natural disasters continue to challenge public health systems, and bioterrorism, natural disasters, and the many human-made disasters threaten to overwhelm existing resources. Research has identified means to avoid or postpone chronic disease, and nurses play an important role in helping implement strategies to modify individual and community risk factors and behaviors. Finally, with the increased numbers of older adults in the United States and their preference to remain at home, additional nursing services are required to sustain the frail, the disabled, and the chronically ill in the community.

Nurses who have worked in the community have done so to improve the health status of individuals, families, and populations. They have spent time, energy, and effort working with high-risk or vulnerable groups. Part of the appeal of public health nursing has been its autonomy of practice and independence in problem solving and decision making, in addition to the interdisciplinary nature of the specialty. This chapter describes the beginnings of public health, the role of nursing in the community, the contributions made by nurses to public health, and the influence of nurses on community health.

EARLY PUBLIC HEALTH

People in all cultures have been concerned with the events surrounding birth, illness, and death. They have tried to prevent, understand, and control disease. Their ability to preserve health and treat illness has depended on their knowledge of science, the use and availability of technologies, and the degree of social organization. For example, ancient Babylonians understood the need for hygiene and had some medical skills. The Egyptians in approximately 1000 BCE (before the Common Era) developed a variety of pharmaceutical preparations and constructed earth privies and public drainage systems. In England, the Elizabethan Poor Law of 1601 guaranteed assistance for poor, blind, and "lame" individuals. This minimal care was generally provided in almshouses supported by local government. The goal was to regulate the poor and provide a refuge during illness.

The Industrial Revolution in 19th-century Europe led to social changes while making great advances in technology, transportation, and communication. Previous caregiving structures, which relied on families, neighbors, and friends, became inadequate because of migration, urbanization, and increased demand. During this period, small numbers of Roman Catholic and Protestant religious women provided nursing care in institutions and sometimes in the home. Many lay women who performed nursing functions in almshouses and early hospitals in Great Britain were poorly educated and untrained. As the practice of medicine became more complex in the mid-1800s, hospital work required a more skilled caregiver. Physicians and community advocates wanted to improve the quality of nursing services. Early experiments led to some improvement in care, but it was because of the efforts of Florence Nightingale that health care was revolutionized when she founded the profession of nursing.

PUBLIC HEALTH DURING AMERICA'S COLONIAL PERIOD AND THE NEW REPUBLIC

In the early years of America's settlement, as in Europe, the care of the sick was usually informal and was provided by women. The female head of the household typically supervised care during sickness and childbirth and also grew and gathered healing herbs to use throughout the year. This traditional system of care became insufficient as the number of urban residents grew in the early 1800s.

British settlers in the New World influenced the American ideas of social welfare and care of the sick. Just as American law is based on English common law, colonial Americans established systems of care for the sick, poor, aged, mentally ill, and dependents based on England's Elizabethan Poor Law of 1601. Early county or township government was responsible for the care of all dependent residents but provided almshouse charity carefully, economically, and only for local residents. Travelers and people who lived elsewhere were returned to their native counties for care. Few hospitals existed and then only in the larger cities. Pennsylvania Hospital was founded in Philadelphia in 1751 and was the first hospital in what would become the United States.

Early colonial public health efforts included the collection of vital statistics, improvements to sanitation systems, and control of any communicable diseases brought in at the seaports. The colonists did not have a system to ensure that public health efforts were supported or enforced. Epidemics often occurred and strained the limited local organization for health during the 17th, 18th, and 19th centuries (Rosen, 1958).

After the American Revolution, the threat of disease, especially yellow fever, led to public support for establishing government-sponsored, or official, boards of health. By 1800, New York City, with a population of 75,000, had established public health services, which included monitoring water quality, constructing sewers and a waterfront wall, draining marshes, planting trees and vegetables, and burying the dead (Rosen, 1958).

Industrialization attracted increasing numbers of urban residents, leading to inadequate housing and sanitation complicated by epidemics of smallpox, yellow fever, cholera, typhoid, and typhus. Tuberculosis and malaria were always present, and infant mortality was approximately 200 per 1000 live births (Pickett and Hanlon, 1990). American hospitals in the early 1800s were generally unsanitary and staffed by poorly trained workers. Physicians had limited education, and medical care was scarce. Public dispensaries, similar to outpatient clinics, and private charitable efforts tried to provide some care for the poor.

The federal government focused its early public health work on providing health care for merchant seamen and protecting seacoast cities from epidemics. The Public Health Service, still the most important federal public health agency in the 21st century, was established in 1798 as the Marine Hospital Service. The first Marine Hospital opened in Norfolk, Virginia, in 1800. Additional legislation to establish quarantine regulations for seamen and immigrants was passed in 1878.

In the first half of the 1800s, some agencies began to provide lay nursing care in clients' homes, including the Ladies' Benevolent Society of Charleston, South Carolina (Buhler-Wilkerson, 2001); lay nurses in Philadelphia; and visiting nurses in Cincinnati, Ohio (Rodabaugh and Rodabaugh, 1951). Although these programs provided useful services, they were not adopted elsewhere. Table 2.1 presents milestones of public health efforts that occurred during the 17th, 18th, and 19th centuries.

During the mid-1800s, national interest increased in addressing public health problems and improving urban living conditions. New responsibilities for urban boards of health reflected changing ideas of public health as the boards began to address communicable diseases and environmental hazards. Soon after it was founded in 1847, the American Medical Association (AMA) formed a hygiene committee to conduct sanitary surveys and develop a system to collect vital statistics. The Shattuck Report, published in 1850 by the Massachusetts Sanitary Commission, was the first attempt to describe a model approach to the organization of public health in the United States. This report called for broad changes to improve the public's health: the establishment of a state health department and local health boards in every town; sanitary surveys and collection of vital statistics; environmental sanitation; food, drug, and communicable disease control; well-child care; health education; tobacco and alcohol control; town planning; and the teaching of preventive medicine in medical schools (Kalisch and Kalisch, 1995). It took 19 years for these recommendations to be implemented in Massachusetts, and they were added in other states much later.

TABLE 2.1 Milestones in the History of Community Health and Public Health Nursing: 1600–1865

Year	Milestone
1601	Elizabethan Poor Law written
1617	Sisterhood of the Dames de Charité organized in France by St. Vincent de Paul
1789	Baltimore Health Department established
1798	Marine Hospital Service established; later became Public Health Service
1812	Sisters of Mercy established in Dublin, Ireland, where nuns visited the poor
1813	Ladies Benevolent Society of Charleston, South Carolina, founded
1836	Lutheran deaconesses provided home visits in Kaiserwerth, Germany
1851	Florence Nightingale visited Kaiserwerth, Germany, for 3 months of nurse training
1855	Quarantine Board established in New Orleans; beginning of tuberculosis campaign in the United States
1859	District nursing established in Liverpool, England, by William Rathbone
1860	Florence Nightingale Training School for Nurses established at St. Thomas Hospital in London
1864	Beginning of Red Cross

In some areas, charitable organizations addressed the gap between known communicable disease epidemics and the lack of local government resources. For example, the Howard Association of New Orleans, Louisiana, responded to periodic yellow fever epidemics between 1837 and 1878 by providing physicians, lay nurses, and medicine for the sick. The Howard Association established infirmaries and used sophisticated outreach strategies to locate cases (Hanggi-Myers, 1995).

NIGHTINGALE AND THE ORIGINS OF TRAINED NURSING

Even with the growth of technology during this time, cities lacked important public health systems, such as sewage disposal, and also depended on private enterprise for water supply. Previous caregiving structures, which relied on the assistance of family, neighbors, and friends, became inadequate in the early 19th century because of human migration, urbanization, and changing demand. During this period, a few groups of Roman Catholic and Protestant women provided nursing care for the sick, poor, and neglected in institutions and sometimes in the home. For example, Mary Aikenhead, also known by her religious name Sister Mary Augustine, organized the Irish Sisters of Charity in Dublin, Ireland, in 1815. These sisters visited the poor at home and established hospitals and schools (Kalisch and Kalisch, 1995).

Florence Nightingale's vision of trained nurses and her model of nursing education influenced the development of professional nursing and, indirectly, public health nursing in the United States. In 1850 and 1851, Nightingale studied nursing "system and method" during an extended visit to Pastor Theodor Fliedner at his Kaiserwerth, Germany, School for Deaconesses. Her work with Pastor Fliedner and the Kaiserwerth Lutheran deaconesses, with their systems of district nursing, later led her to promote nursing care for the sick in their homes.

During the Crimean War (1854–1856), the British military established hospitals for sick and wounded soldiers in Scutari in Asia Minor. The care of soldiers was poor, with cramped quarters, poor sanitation, lice and rats, not enough food, and inadequate medical supplies (Kalisch and Kalisch, 1995; Palmer, 1983). When the British public demanded improved conditions, Florence Nightingale asked to work in Scutari. Because of her wealth, social and political connections, and knowledge of hospitals, the British government sent her to Asia Minor with 40 women, 117 hired nurses, and 15 paid servants. In Scutari, Nightingale progressively improved the soldiers' health using a population-based approach that improved both environmental conditions and nursing care. Using simple epidemiology measures, she documented a decreased mortality rate from 415 per 1000 at the beginning of the war to 11.5 per 1000 at the end (Cohen, 1984; Palmer, 1983). Like Nightingale and her efforts in Scutari, public health nurses today identify health care needs that affect the entire population. They then mobilize resources and organize themselves and the community to meet these needs.

After the Crimean War, Nightingale returned to England in 1856. Her fame was established. She organized hospital nursing practices and nursing education in hospitals to replace untrained lay nurses with Nightingale nurses. Nightingale thought that nursing should promote health and prevent illness, and she emphasized proper nutrition, rest, sanitation, and hygiene (Nightingale, 1894, 1946).

In 1859 British philanthropist William Rathbone founded the first district nursing association in Liverpool, England. His wife had received excellent care from a Nightingale nurse during her terminal illness. He wanted to provide similar care to poor and needy people. Together the work of Nightingale and Rathbone led to the organization of district nursing in England (Nutting and Dock, 1935).

During the last quarter of the 1800s, the number of jobs for women rapidly increased. Educated women became teachers, secretaries, or saleswomen, and less-educated women worked in factories. As it became more acceptable to work outside the home, women were more willing to become nurses. The first nursing schools based on the Nightingale model opened in the United States in the 1870s. The early graduate nurses worked as private duty nurses or were hospital administrators or instructors. The private duty nurses often lived with the families for whom they cared. Because it was expensive to hire private duty nurses, only the well-to-do could afford their services. Community nursing began in an effort to meet urban health care needs, especially for the disadvantaged, by providing visiting nurses. In 1877 in New York City, trained nurse Francis Root was hired by a New York City mission to visit and care for the sick poor in their homes.

Visiting nurses took care of several families each day (rather than attending to only one client or family as the private duty nurse did), which made their care more economical. The visiting nurse became the key to communicating the prevention campaign, through home visits and well-baby clinics. Visiting nurses worked with physicians, gave selected treatments, and kept temperature and pulse records. Visiting nurses emphasized education of family members in the care of the sick and in personal and environmental prevention measures, such as hygiene and good nutrition (Fig. 2.1). The movement grew, and visiting

nurse associations were established in Buffalo (1885), Philadelphia (1886), and Boston (1886). Wealthy people interested in charitable activities funded both settlement houses and visiting nurse associations. Wealthy upper-class women who were freed at this time from social restrictions were instrumental in doing charitable work and in supporting the early visiting nurses.

The public wanted to limit disease among all classes of people, partly for religious reasons, partly as a form of charity, but also because the middle and upper classes were afraid of diseases that were prevalent in the large communities of European immigrants. During the 1890s in New York City, about 2,300,000 people were packed into 90,000 tenement houses. The environmental conditions of immigrants in tenement houses and sweatshops were familiar features of urban life across the northeastern United States and upper Midwest. From the beginning, community nursing practice included teaching and prevention (Fig. 2.2). Community interventions led to improved sanitation, economic improvements, and better nutrition. These interventions were credited with reducing the incidence of acute communicable disease by 1901.

In 1886 in Boston, two women, to improve their chances of gaining financial support for their cause, coined the term instructive district nursing to emphasize the relationship of nursing to health education. Support for these nurses was also secured from the Women's Education Association, and the Boston Dispensary provided free outpatient medical care. In February 1886 the first district nurse was hired in Boston, and in 1888 the Instructive District Nursing Association was incorporated as an independent voluntary agency (Brainard, 1922).

Other nurses established settlement houses and neighborhood centers, which became hubs for health care and social welfare programs. For example, in 1893 trained nurses Lillian Wald (Fig. 2.3) and Mary Brewster began visiting the poor on

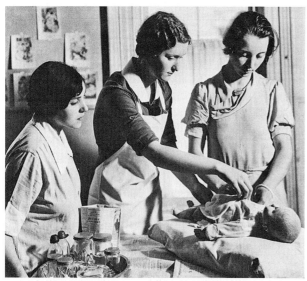

FIG. 2.1 Public health nurse demonstrating well-child care during a home visit. (Courtesy Visiting Nurse Service of New York.)

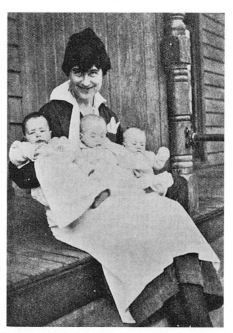

FIG. 2.2 Teaching well-child care was a significant public health nursing role. (Courtesy Instructional Visiting Nurse Association of Richmond, Virginia.)

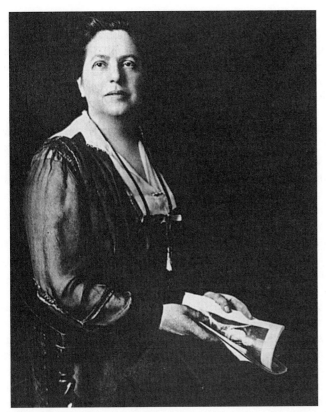

FIG. 2.3 Lillian Wald. (Courtesy Visiting Nurse Service of New York.)

New York's Lower East Side. They established a nurses' settlement that became the Henry Street Settlement and later the Visiting Nurse Service of New York City. By 1905, public health nurses had provided almost 48,000 visits to more than 5000 clients (Kalisch and Kalisch, 1995). Lillian Wald emerged as a prominent leader of public health nursing during these decades (Box 2.1). Lillian Wald demonstrated an exceptional ability to develop approaches and programs to solve the health care and social problems of her times. We can learn much from her that can be applied to today's nursing practice.

Jessie Sleet (Scales), a Canadian graduate of Provident Hospital School of Nursing (Chicago), became the first African American public health nurse when she was hired in 1900 by the New York Charity Organization Society. Although it was hard for her to find an agency willing to hire her as a district nurse, she persevered and was able to provide exceptional care for her clients until she married in 1909. At the Charity Organization Society in 1904 to 1905, she studied health conditions related to tuberculosis among African American people in Manhattan using interviews with families and neighbors, house-to-house canvassing, direct observation, and speeches at neighborhood churches. Sleet reported her research to the Society board, recommending improved employment opportunities for African Americans and better prevention strategies to reduce the excess burden of tuberculosis morbidity and mortality among the African American population (Buhler-Wilkerson, 2001; Hine, 1989; Mosley, 1994; Thoms, 1929).

BOX 2.1   Lillian Wald: First Public Health Nurse in the United States

Public health nursing evolved in the United States in the late 19th and early 20th centuries largely because of the pioneering work of Lillian Wald. Born on March 10, 1867, Lillian Wald decided to become a nurse after Vassar College refused to admit her at 16 years of age. She graduated in 1891 from the New York Hospital Training School for Nurses and spent the next year working at the New York Juvenile Asylum. To supplement what she thought had been inadequate training in the sciences, she enrolled in the Woman's Medical College in New York (Frachel, 1988).

Having grown up in a warm, nurturing family in Rochester, New York, her work in New York City introduced her to an entirely different side of life. In 1893, while conducting a class in home nursing for immigrant families on the Lower East Side of New York, Wald was asked by a small child to visit her sick mother. Wald found the mother in bed after childbirth, having hemorrhaged for 2 days. This home visit confirmed for Wald all of the injustices in society and the differences in health care for poor persons versus those persons able to pay (Frachel, 1988).

She believed poor people should have access to health care. With her friend Mary Brewster and the financial support of two wealthy laypeople, Mrs. Solomon Loeb and Joseph H. Schiff, she moved to the Lower East Side and occupied the top floor of a tenement house on Jefferson Street. This move eventually led to the establishment of the Henry Street Settlement. In the beginning, Wald and Brewster helped individual families. Wald believed that the nurse's visit should be friendly, more like a visit from a friend than from someone paid to visit (Dolan, 1978).

Wald used epidemiological methods to campaign for health-promoting social policies to improve environmental and social conditions that affected health. She

not only wrote *The House on Henry Street* to describe her own public health nursing work, but she also led in the development of payment by life insurance companies for nursing services (Frachel, 1988).

In 1909, along with Lee Frankel, Lillian Wald established the first public health nursing program for life insurance policyholders at the Metropolitan Life Insurance Company. She advocated that nurses at agencies such as the Henry Street Settlement provide complex nursing care. Wald convinced the company that it would be more economical to use the services of public health nurses than to employ its own nurses. She also convinced the company that services could be available to anyone desiring them, with fees scaled according to the ability to pay. This nursing service designed by Wald continued for 44 years and contributed several significant accomplishments to public health nursing, including the following (Frachel, 1988):

1. Providing home nursing care on a fee-for-service basis
2. Establishing an effective cost-accounting system for visiting nurses
3. Using advertisements in newspapers and on radio to recruit nurses
4. Reducing mortality from infectious diseases

Lillian Wald also believed that the nursing efforts at the Henry Street Settlement should be aligned with an official health agency. She therefore arranged for nurses to wear an insignia that indicated that they served under the auspices of the Board of Health. Also, she led the establishment of rural health nursing services through the Red Cross. Her other accomplishments included helping to establish the Children's Bureau and fighting in New York City for better tenement living conditions, city recreation centers, parks, pure food laws, graded classes for mentally handicapped children, and assistance to immigrants (Backer, 1993; Dock, 1922; Frachel, 1988; Zerwekh, 1992).

Data from Backer BA: Lillian Wald: connecting caring with action, *Nurs Health Care* 14:122-128, 1993; Dock LL: The history of public health nursing, *Public Health Nurs* 14:522, 1922; Dolan J: *History of nursing*, ed 14, Philadelphia, 1978, Saunders; Frachel RR: A new profession: the evolution of public health nursing, *Public Health Nurs* 5:86-90, 1988; and Zerwekh JV: Public health nursing legacy: historical practical wisdom, *Nurs Health Care* 13:84-91, 1992.

The American Red Cross, through its Rural Nursing Service (later the Town and Country Nursing Service), initiated home nursing care in areas outside larger cities. Lillian Wald secured the initial donations to support this agency, which provided care to the sick, instruction in sanitation and hygiene in rural homes, and improved living conditions in villages and farms. These nurses dealt with diseases such as tuberculosis, pneumonia, and typhoid fever. By 1920, 1800 Red Cross Town and Country Nursing Services were in operation. This number eventually grew to almost 3000 programs in small towns and rural areas.

The emphasis of community nursing has varied and changed over time. In recent years, federal and state financing has influenced the growth. In addition to visiting nurse associations and settlement houses, a variety of other organizations sponsored visiting nurse work, including boards of education, boards of health, mission boards, clubs, churches, social service agencies, and tuberculosis associations. With tuberculosis then responsible for at least 10% of all mortality, visiting nurses contributed to its control through gaining "the personal cooperation of patients and their families" to modify the environment and individual behavior (Buhler-Wilkerson, 1987, p 45). Most visiting nurse agencies depended financially on the philanthropy and social networks of metropolitan areas. As today, fund-raising and service delivery in less densely populated and rural areas were challenging. Learning about the history of a practice agency, such as a visiting nurse association, can provide important perspectives on current agency values, decision-making structures, funding, clinical priorities and service areas, and obstacles to success.

Occupational health nursing, originally called industrial nursing, grew out of early home visiting efforts. In 1895 Ada Mayo Stewart began work with employees and families of the Vermont Marble Company in Proctor, Vermont. As a free service for the employees, Stewart provided obstetrical care, sickness care (e.g., for typhoid cases), and some postsurgical care in workers' homes. However, she provided few services for work-related injuries. Although her employer provided a horse and buggy, she often made home visits on a bicycle. Before 1900 a few nurses were hired in industry, such as in department stores in Philadelphia and Brooklyn. Between 1914 and 1943, industrial nursing grew from 60 to 11,220 nurses, reflecting increased governmental and employee concerns for health and safety at work (American Association of Industrial Nurses, 1976; Kalisch and Kalisch, 1995).

School nursing was also an extension of home visiting. In New York City in 1902 more than 20% of children might be absent from school on a single day because of conditions such as pediculosis, ringworm, scabies, inflamed eyes, discharging ears, and infected wounds. Physicians began to make limited inspections of school students in 1897. They focused on excluding infectious children from school rather than on providing or obtaining medical treatment to enable children to return to school. Familiar with this community-wide problem from her work with the Henry Street Settlement, Lillian Wald introduced the English practice of providing nurses for the schools. Lina Rogers, a Henry Street Settlement resident, became the first school nurse. She worked with the children in New York City schools and made home visits to teach parents and to follow up on children absent from school. The school nurses found that many of the children were absent because they did not have shoes or clothing; many were hungry, and others had to take care of the younger children in the family (Hawkins, Hayes, and Corliss, 1994). School nursing was a success; New York City soon added 12 more nurses. School nursing was soon implemented in Los Angeles, Philadelphia, Baltimore, Boston, Chicago, and San Francisco. The scope of school nursing remains highly variable in the United States in the 21st century, and most school nurses are employed directly by a board of education.

CONTINUED GROWTH IN PUBLIC HEALTH NURSING

The *Visiting Nurse Quarterly,* begun in 1909 by the Cleveland Visiting Nurse Association, initiated a professional communication medium for clinical and organizational concerns. Also in 1909, the University of Minnesota began the first continuing nursing program given on a university campus. In 1911 a joint committee of existing nurse organizations convened, under the leadership of Wald and Mary Gardner, to standardize nursing services outside the hospital. They recommended the formation of a new organization to address public health nursing concerns. Their committee invited 800 agencies involved in public health nursing activities to send delegates to an organizational meeting in Chicago in June 1912. After a heated debate on its name and purpose, the delegates established the National Organization for Public Health Nursing (NOPHN) and chose Wald as its first president (Dock, 1922). Unlike other professional nursing organizations, the NOPHN membership included both nurses and their lay supporters. The NOPHN, which worked "to improve the educational and services standards of the public health nurse, and promote public understanding of and respect for her work" (Rosen, 1958, p 381), soon became the dominant force in public health (Roberts, 1955).

The NOPHN sought to standardize public health nursing education. At that time, newly graduated nurses often were unprepared for home visitation because the diploma schools emphasized care of hospital clients. Thus public health nurses needed education in how to care for the sick at home and to design population-focused programs. In 1914 Mary Adelaide Nutting, working with the Henry Street Settlement, began the first course for postdiploma school training in public health nursing at Teachers College in New York City (Deloughery, 1977). The American Red Cross provided scholarships for graduates of nursing schools to attend the public health nursing course. Its success encouraged the development of other programs, using curricula that might seem familiar to today's nurses. During the 1920s and 1930s, many newly hired public health nurses had to verify completion or promptly enroll in a certificate program in public health nursing. Others took leave for a year to travel to an urban center to obtain this further education. Correspondence courses (distance education) were even acceptable in some areas, for example, for public health nurses in upstate New York.

Public health nurses were also active in the American Public Health Association (APHA), which was established in 1872 to facilitate interprofessional efforts and promote the "practical application of public hygiene" (Scutchfield and Keck, 1997, p 12). The APHA focused on important public health issues, including sewage and garbage disposal, occupational injuries, and sexually transmitted diseases. In 1923 the Public Health Nursing Section (PHNS) was formed within the APHA to provide nurses with a national forum to discuss their concerns and strategies within the larger context of the major public health organization. The PHNS continues to serve as a focus of leadership and policy development for public health nursing.

Public health nursing in voluntary agencies and through the Red Cross grew more quickly than public health nursing supported by local, state, and national government. In the late 1800s, local health departments were formed in urban areas to target environmental hazards associated with crowded living conditions and dirty streets and to regulate public baths, slaughterhouses, and pigsties (Pickett and Hanlon, 1990). By 1900, 38 states had established state health departments, following the lead of Massachusetts in 1869; however, these early state boards of health had limited impact because only three states—Massachusetts, Rhode Island, and Florida—annually spent more than 2 cents per capita for public health services (Scutchfield and Keck, 1997).

The federal role in public health gradually expanded. In 1912 the federal government redefined the role of the US Public Health Service, empowering it to "investigate the causes and spread of diseases and the pollution and sanitation of navigable streams and lakes" (Scutchfield and Keck, 1997, p 15). The NOPHN loaned a nurse to the US Public Health Service during World War I to establish a public health nursing program for military outposts. This led to the first federal government sponsorship of nurses (Shyrock, 1959; Wilner, Walkey, and O'Neill, 1978).

During the 1910s public health organizations began to target infectious and parasitic diseases in rural areas. The Rockefeller Sanitary Commission, a philanthropic organization active in hookworm control in the southeastern United States, concluded that concurrent efforts for all phases of public health were necessary to successfully address any individual public health problem (Pickett and Hanlon, 1990). For example, in 1911 efforts to control typhoid fever in Yakima County, Washington, and to improve health status in Guilford County, North Carolina, led to the establishment of local health units to serve local populations. Public health nurses were the primary staff members of local health departments. These nurses assumed a leadership role on health care issues through collaboration with local residents, nurses, and other health care providers.

The experience of Orange County, California, during the 1920s and 1930s illustrates the growing importance of the nurse in the community. Based on the work of a private physician, social welfare agencies, and a Red Cross nurse, the county board created the public health nurse's position in 1922. Presented with a shining new Model T car sporting the bright orange seal

of the county, the nurse began her work by dealing with the serious communicable disease problems of diphtheria and scarlet fever. Typhoid became epidemic when a drainage pipe overflowed into a well, infecting those who drank the water and those who drank raw milk from an infected dairy. Almost 3000 residents were immunized against typhoid. At weekly well-baby conferences, the nurse weighed infants and gave them immunizations and taught mothers how to care for the infants. Also, children with orthopedic disorders and other disabilities were identified and referred for medical care in Los Angeles. The first year of this public health nursing work was so successful that the Rockefeller Foundation and the California Health Department provided funds for more public health professionals.

PUBLIC HEALTH NURSING DURING THE EARLY 20TH CENTURY

The personnel needs of World War I in Europe depleted the ranks of public health nurses, even as the NOPHN identified a need for second and third lines of defense within the United States. Jane Delano in 1909 was appointed both as superintendent of the Army Nurse Corps and chairman of the National Committee on Red Cross Nursing services. She was instrumental in preparing nurses to serve in the military, and she also supported the need for public health nurses to stay at home and serve the needs of those not serving in the military. Over 3 weeks in 1918 the worldwide influenza pandemic swept across the United States. A coalition of the NOPHN and the Red Cross worked to turn houses, churches, and social halls into hospitals for the immense numbers of sick and dying. Some of the nurse volunteers died of influenza.

Limited funding during the early 20th century was the major obstacle to extending nursing services in the community. Most early visiting nurse associations relied on contributions from wealthy and middle-class supporters. Consistent with the goal of encouraging economic independence, poor families were asked to pay a small fee for nursing services. In 1909 with encouragement from Lillian Wald in collaboration with Dr. Lee Frankel, the Metropolitan Life Insurance Company began a program using visiting nurse organizations to provide care for sick policyholders. The nurses assessed illness, taught health practices, and collected data from policyholders. By 1912, 589 Metropolitan Life nursing centers provided care through existing agencies or visiting nurses hired directly by the company. In 1918 Metropolitan Life calculated an average decline of 7% in the mortality rate of policyholders and almost a 20% decline in the mortality rate of policyholders' children under the age of 3 years. The insurance company attributed this improvement and its reduced costs to the work of visiting nurses.

Nurses also influenced public policy by advocating for the Children's Bureau and the Sheppard-Towner Program. Wald and other nursing leaders urged that the Children's Bureau be established in 1912 to address national problems of maternal and child welfare. Children's Bureau experts conducted extensive scientific research on the effects of income, housing, employment, and other factors on infant and maternal mortality. Their research led to federal child labor laws and the 1919

BOX 2.2   Mary Breckinridge and the Frontier Nursing Service

Born in 1881 into the fifth generation of a well-to-do Kentucky family, Mary Breckinridge devoted her life to the establishment of the Frontier Nursing Service (FNS). Learning from her grandmother, who used a large part of her fortune to improve the education of Southern children, Breckinridge later used money left to her by her grandmother to start the FNS (Browne, 1966).

Tutored in childhood and later attending private schools, Mary Breckinridge did not consider becoming a nurse until her husband died. At that time she wanted to have more adventure in her life and to find opportunities to do something useful for others (Hostutler et al, 2000). In 1907 she enrolled at St. Luke's Hospital School of Nursing in New York. She later married for a second time and had two children. Her second marriage ended after her daughter died at birth and her son died at age 4. From the time of her son's death in 1918, she devoted her energy to promoting the health care of disadvantaged women and children (Browne, 1966).

After World War I and work in postwar France, she returned to the United States, passionate about helping the neglected children of rural America. To prepare herself for what would become her life's work, she studied for a year at Teacher's College, Columbia University, to learn more about public health nursing (Browne, 1966).

Early in 1925 she returned to Kentucky. She decided that the mountains of Kentucky were an excellent place to demonstrate the value of community health nursing to remote, disadvantaged families. She thought that if she could establish a nursing center in rural Kentucky, this effort could then be duplicated anywhere. The first health center was established in a five-room cabin in Hyden, Kentucky. Establishing the center took not only nursing skills but also the construction of the center and later the hospital and other buildings; it required extensive knowledge about developing a water supply, disposing of sewage, getting electric power, and securing a mountain area in which landslides occurred (Browne, 1966). Despite many obstacles inherent in building in the mountains, six outpost nursing centers were established between 1927 and 1930. The FNS hospital was built in Hyden, Kentucky, and physicians began entering service. Payment of fees ranged from labor and supplies to funds raised through annual family dues, philanthropy, and the fund-raising efforts of Mary Breckinridge (Holloway, 1975).

The FNS established medical, surgical, and dental clinics; provided nursing and midwifery services 24 hours a day; and served nearly 10,000 people spread over 700 square miles. Baseline data were obtained on infant and maternal mortality before beginning services. FNS services are especially remarkable considering the environmental conditions in which rural Kentuckians lived. Many homes had no heat, electricity, or running water. Often physicians were located more than 40 miles from their patients (Tirpak, 1975).

During the 1930s, nurses lived in one of the six outposts, from which they traveled to see clients; they often had to make their visits on horseback. Like her nurses, Mary Breckinridge traveled many miles through the mountains of Kentucky on her horse, Babette, providing food, supplies, and health care to mountain families (Browne, 1966).

Over the years, several hundred nurses have worked for the FNS. Although Mary Breckinridge died in 1965, the FNS has continued to grow and provide needed services to people in the mountains of Kentucky. This service continues today as a vital and creative way to deliver community health services to rural families.

Data from Browne H: A tribute to Mary Breckinridge, *Nurs Outlook* 14:54-55, 1966; Goan MB: *Mary Breckinridge: the frontier nursing service and rural health in Appalachia,* Chapel Hill, NC, 2008, The University of North Carolina Press; Holloway JB: Frontier Nursing Service 1925-1975, *J Ky Med Assoc* 73:491-492, 1975; Hostutler J, Kennedy MS, Mason D, et al: Nurses: then and now and models of practice, *Am J Nurs* 100:82-83, 2000; Tirpak H: The Frontier Nursing Service: fifty years in the mountains, *Nurs Outlook* 33:308-310, 1975.

White House Conference on Child Health. The Sheppard-Towner Act of 1921, which focused on maternal and infant health, was credited with saving many lives. This act provided federal matching funds to establish maternal and child health divisions in state health departments. Education during home visits by public health nurses emphasized promoting the health of the mother and child and encouraged mothers to seek prompt medical care during pregnancy. Although credited with saving many lives, the program ended in 1929 in response to charges by the AMA and others that the legislation gave too much power to the federal government and too closely resembled socialized medicine (Pickett and Hanlon, 1990). Just as we see today, there has long been an inability to provide public health services because of the lack of funds.

Some nursing innovations were the result of individual commitment and private financial support. In 1925 Mary Breckinridge established the Frontier Nursing Service (FNS). This creative service was based on systems of care in Scotland (Box 2.2 and Fig. 2.4). The pioneering spirit of the FNS influenced the development of public health programs to improve the health care of the rural and often inaccessible populations in the Appalachian region of southeastern Kentucky (Browne, 1966; Tirpak, 1975). Breckinridge introduced the first nurse-midwives into the United States when she deployed FNS nurses trained in nursing, public health, and midwifery. Their efforts

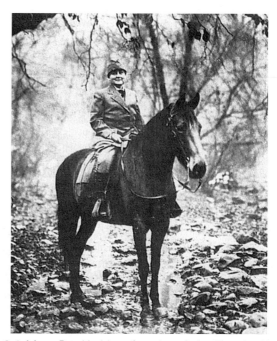

FIG. 2.4 Mary Breckinridge, founder of the Frontier Nursing Service. (Courtesy Frontier Nursing Service of Wendover, Kentucky.)

led to reduced pregnancy complications and maternal mortality and to one-third fewer stillbirths and infant deaths in an area of 700 square miles (Kalisch and Kalisch, 1995). Today the FNS continues to provide comprehensive health and nursing services to the people of that area and sponsors the Frontier Nursing University.

AFRICAN AMERICAN NURSES IN PUBLIC HEALTH NURSING

African American nurses seeking to work in public health nursing faced many challenges. Nursing education was absolutely segregated in the South until at least the 1960s and elsewhere was also generally segregated or rationed until the mid-20th century. Even public health nursing certificate and graduate education programs were segregated in the South; study outside the South for Southern nurses was difficult to afford, and study leaves from the workplace were rarely granted. The situation improved somewhat in 1936 when collaboration between the US Public Health Service and the Medical College of Virginia (Richmond) established a certificate program in public health nursing for African American nurses for which the federal government paid nurses' tuition. Discrimination continued during nurses' employment: African American nurses in the American South were paid lower salaries than their white counterparts for the same work. In 1925 only 435 African American public health nurses were employed in the United States, and in 1930 only six African American nurses held supervisory positions in public health nursing organizations (Buhler-Wilkerson, 2001; Hine, 1989; Thoms, 1929).

African American public health nurses significantly influenced the communities they served (Fig. 2.5). The National Health Circle for Colored People was organized in 1919 to promote public health work in African American communities in the South. One strategy adopted was providing scholarships to assist African American nurses in pursuing university-level public health nursing education. Bessie M. Hawes, the first

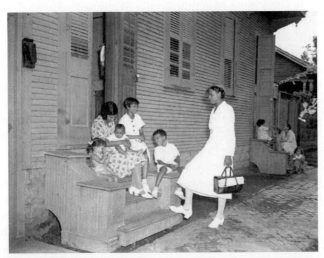

FIG. 2.5 A New Orleans nurse visiting a family on the doorstep of their home. (Courtesy New Orleans Public Library WPA Photograph Collection.)

recipient of the scholarship, completed the program at Columbia University (New York) and was then sent by the Circle to Palatka, Florida. In this small, isolated lumber town, Hawes's first project was to recruit schoolgirls to promote health by dressing as nurses and marching in a parade while singing community songs. She conducted mass meetings, led clubs for mothers, provided school health education, and visited the homes of the sick. Eventually she gained the community's trust, overcame opposition, and built a health center for nursing care and treatment (Thoms, 1929).

ECONOMIC DEPRESSION AND THE IMPACT ON PUBLIC HEALTH

The economic depression of the 1930s affected the development of nursing. Not only were agencies and communities unprepared to address the increased needs and numbers of the impoverished, but decreased funding for nursing services reduced the number of employed nurses in hospitals and in community agencies. Federal funding led to a wide variety of programs administered at the state level, including new public health nursing programs; as a result of NOPHN's enormous efforts, public health nursing was included in federal relief programs.

The Federal Emergency Relief Administration (FERA) supported nurse employment through increased grants-in-aid for state programs of home medical care. FERA often purchased nursing care from existing visiting nurse agencies, thus supporting more nurses and preventing agency closures. The FERA program focus varied among states; the state FERA program in New York emphasized bedside nursing care, whereas in North Carolina, the state FERA prioritized maternal and child health and school nursing services. The public health nursing programs of the FERA and its successor, the Works Progress Administration (WPA), were sometimes later incorporated into state health departments.

In another Depression-era initiative, more than 10,000 nurses were employed by the Civil Works Administration (CWA) programs and assigned to official health agencies. "While this facilitated rapid program expansion by recipient agencies and gave the nurses a taste of public health, the nurses' lack of field experience created major problems of training and supervision for the regular staff" (Roberts and Heinrich, 1985, p 1162).

A 1932 survey of public health agencies found that only 7% of nurses employed in public health were adequately prepared for that role (Roberts and Heinrich, 1985). Basic nursing education emphasized the care of individuals, and students received little information on groups and the community as a unit of service. Thus in the 1930s and early 1940s, new graduates required considerable remedial education when they were hired into public health work (NOPHN, 1944).

During this period the tension persisted between preventive care and care of the sick and the related question of whether nursing interventions should be directed toward groups and communities or toward individuals and their families. Although each nursing agency was unique and services varied from region to region, voluntary visiting nurse associations tended to emphasize care of the sick, and official public health agencies provided more preventive services. Not surprisingly, this splintering of services led to a rivalry between "visiting," or community, and "public health" nurses and interfered with the development of comprehensive community nursing services (Roberts and Heinrich, 1985). For example, one household could receive services from several community nurses representing different agencies, with separate visits for a postpartum woman and new baby, for a child sick with scarlet fever, and for an elderly bedridden person. This was confusing and costly, with duplicated services.

One solution was to establish the "combination service," which merged sick-care services and preventive services into one comprehensive agency by combining visiting nurse and official public health agencies. However, in contrast to visiting nurse organizations, public health nurses in official health agencies often had less control of the program because physicians and politicians determined services and the assignment of personnel. The "ideal program" of the combination agency was hard to administer, and many of the combination services implemented between 1930 and 1965 later reverted to their former, divided structures of visiting nurse agencies and official health departments.

Expansion of federal government programs during the 1930s affected the structure of community health resources and led to "the beginning of a new era in public nursing" (Roberts and Heinrich, 1985, p 1162). In 1933 Pearl McIver became the first nurse employed by the US Public Health Service. In providing consultation services to state health departments, McIver was convinced that the strengths and ability of each state's director of public health nursing would determine the scope and quality of local health services. Together with Naomi Deutsch, director of nursing for the federal Children's Bureau, and with the support of nursing organizations, McIver and her staff of nurse consultants influenced the direction of public health nursing. Between 1931 and 1938 over 40% of the increase in public health nurse employment was in local health agencies. Even so, nationally, more than one-third of all counties still lacked local public health nursing services (Fig. 2.6).

The Social Security Act of 1935 was designed to prevent reoccurrence of the problems of the Depression. Title VI of this act provided funding for expanded opportunities for health protection and promotion through education and employment of public health nurses. In 1936 more than 1000 nurses completed educational programs in public health. Title VI also provided $8 million to assist states, counties, and medical districts to establish and maintain adequate health services, as well as $2 million for research and investigation of disease (Buhler-Wilkerson, 1985, 1989; Kalisch and Kalisch, 1995).

In the late 1930s and especially in the late 1940s, Congress supported categorical funding to provide federal money for priority diseases or groups rather than for a comprehensive community health program. In response, local health departments designed programs to fit the funding priorities. This included maternal and child health services and crippled children (1935), venereal disease control (1938), tuberculosis (1944), mental health (1947), industrial hygiene (1947), and dental health (1947) (Scutchfield and Keck, 1997). This pattern of funding continues today.

World War II increased the need for nurses both for the war effort and at home. Many nurses joined the US Army and Navy

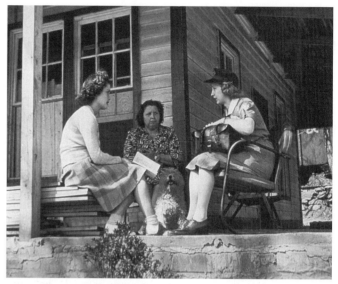

FIG. 2.6 A public health nurse talks with a young woman and her mother about childbirth as they sit on a porch. (US Public Health Service photo by Perry. Images from the History of Medicine, National Library of Medicine, Image ID 157037.)

Nurse Corps. US Representative Frances Payne Bolton of Ohio led Congress to pass the Bolton Act of 1943, which established the Cadet Nurses Corps. This legislation supported increased undergraduate and graduate enrollment in schools of nursing. Funding became more available to educate nurses by providing financial support for them to go to school, with many focusing on public health.

Because of the number of nurses involved in the war, civilian hospitals and visiting nurse agencies shifted care to families and nonnursing personnel. "By the end of 1942, over 500,000 women had completed the American Red Cross home nursing course, and nearly 17,000 nurse's aides had been certified" (Roberts and Heinrich, 1985, p 1165). By the end of 1946, more than 215,000 volunteer nurse's aides had received certificates. During this time, community health nursing expanded its scope of practice. For example, more community health nurses practiced in rural areas, and many official agencies began to provide bedside nursing care (Buhler-Wilkerson, 1985; Kalisch and Kalisch, 1995).

After the war the need increased for services from local health departments to respond to sudden increases in demand for care of emotional problems, accidents, alcoholism, and other responsibilities new to official health agencies. Changes in medical technology improved the ability to screen and treat infectious and communicable diseases. Penicillin, which was developed during the war, became available to treat civilians with rheumatic fever, venereal diseases, and other infections. Job opportunities for public health nurses increased, and nurses were a major portion of health department staff. More than 20,000 nurses worked in health departments, visiting nurse associations, industry, and schools. Table 2.2 highlights significant milestones in community and public health nursing from the mid-1800s to the mid-1900s.

TABLE 2.2	Milestones in the History of Community Health and Public Health Nursing: 1866–1944
Year	**Milestone**
1866	New York Metropolitan Board of Health established
1872	American Public Health Association established
1873	New York Training School opened at Bellevue Hospital, New York City, as first Nightingale-model nursing school in the United States
1877	Women's Board of the New York Mission hired Frances Root to visit the sick poor
1885	Visiting Nurse Association established in Buffalo
1886	Visiting nurse agencies established in Philadelphia and Boston
1893	Lillian Wald and Mary Brewster organized a visiting nursing service for the poor of New York, which later became the Henry Street Settlement; Society of Superintendents of Training Schools of Nurses in the United States and Canada was established (in 1912 it became known as the National League for Nursing Education)
1896	Associated Alumnae of Training Schools for Nurses established (in 1911 it became the American Nurses Association)
1902	School nursing started in New York; Lina Rogers was the first school nurse
1903	First nurse practice acts
1909	Metropolitan Life Insurance Company initiated the first insurance reimbursement for nursing care
1910	Public health nursing program instituted at Teachers College, Columbia University, in New York City
1912	National Organization for Public Health Nursing formed, with Lillian Wald as the first president
1914	First undergraduate nursing education course in public health offered by Adelaide Nutting at Teachers College
1918	Vassar Camp School for Nurses organized; US Public Health Service (USPHS) established division of public health nursing to work in the war effort; worldwide influenza epidemic began
1919	Textbook *Public Health Nursing* written by Mary S. Gardner
1921	Maternity and Infancy Act (Sheppard-Towner Act)
1925	Frontier Nursing Service using nurse-midwives established
1934	Pearl McIver becomes the first nurse employed by USPHS
1935	Passage of the Social Security Act
1941	Beginning of World War II
1943	Passage of the Bolton-Bailey Act for nursing education; Cadet Nurse Program established; Division of Nursing begun at USPHS; Lucille Petry appointed chief of the Cadet Nurse Corps
1944	First basic program in nursing accredited as including sufficient public health content

FROM WORLD WAR II UNTIL THE 1970s

Between 1900 and 1955, the national crude mortality rate decreased by 47%. Many more Americans survived childhood and early adulthood to live into middle and older ages. Although in 1900 the leading causes of mortality were pneumonia, tuberculosis, diarrhea, and enteritis, by midcentury the leading causes had become heart disease, cancer, and cerebrovascular disease. Nurses helped reduce communicable disease mortality through immunization campaigns, nutrition education, and provision of better hygiene and sanitation. Additional factors included improved medications, better housing, and innovative emergency and critical care services.

Increasing numbers of older adults also increased the population at risk for increasing prevalence of chronic diseases. Nurses now dealt with challenges related to chronic illness care, long-term illness and disability, and chronic disease prevention. In official health agencies, categorical programs focusing on a single chronic disease emphasized narrowly defined services, which might be poorly coordinated with other community programs. Screening for chronic illness was a popular method of both detecting undiagnosed disease and providing individual and community education.

Some visiting nurse associations adopted coordinated home-care programs to provide complex, long-term care to the chronically ill, often after long-term hospitalization. These home-care programs established a multidisciplinary approach to complex client care. For example, beginning in 1949, the Visiting Nurse Society of Philadelphia provided care to clients with stroke, arthritis, cancer, and fractures using a wide range of services, including physical and occupational therapy, nutrition consultation, social services, laboratory and radiographic procedures, and transportation. During the 1950s, often in response to family demands and the shortage of nurses, many visiting nurse agencies began experimenting with auxiliary nursing personnel, variously called housekeepers, homemakers, or home health aides. These innovative programs provided a substantial basis for an approach to bedside nursing care that would be reimbursable by commercial health insurance (such as Blue Cross) and later by Medicare and Medicaid.

During the 1930s and 1940s, more Americans chose to obtain care in hospitals because this was where physicians worked and where technology was readily available to diagnose and treat illness. Health insurance programs now allowed middle-class people to pay for care in hospitals. In 1952 the Metropolitan Life Insurance Company and the John Hancock Life Insurance Company ended their support of visiting nurse services (Fig. 2.7) for their policyholders, and the American Red Cross ended its programs of direct nursing service.

Nursing organizations also continued to change. The functions of the NOPHN, the National League for Nursing Education, and the Association of Collegiate Schools of Nursing were

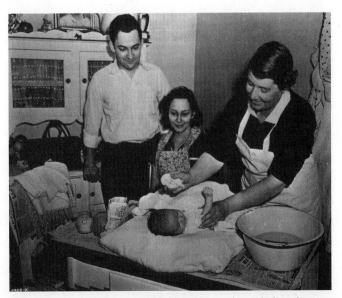

FIG. 2.7 A nurse from the Visiting Nurse Association demonstrates proper infant care and bathing techniques to the parents.

distributed to the new National League for Nursing (NLN) in 1952. The American Nurses Association (ANA) continued as the second national nursing organization, after merging with the National Association for Colored Graduate Nurses in 1951.

In 1948 the NLN adopted the recommendations of Esther Lucile Brown's study of nursing education, *Nursing for the Future,* and this considerably influenced how nurses were prepared. She recommended that basic nursing education take place in colleges and universities. In the 1950s, public health nursing became a required part of most baccalaureate nursing education programs. In 1952 nursing education programs began in junior and community colleges. Louise McManus, a director of the Division of Nursing Education at Teachers College, Columbia University, wanted to see if bedside nurses could be prepared in a 2-year program. The intent was to prepare nurses more quickly than in the past to ease the prevailing nursing shortage (Kalisch and Kalisch, 1995). This would also move more nursing education into American higher education. Mildred Montag, an assistant professor of nursing education at Teacher's College, became the project coordinator. In 1958, when the 5-year study was completed, this experiment was determined to be a success.

EVIDENCE-BASED PRACTICE

Nursing has a long and rich past, yet this is rarely conveyed to undergraduate nursing students; as a result, nurses devalue the achievements of earlier nurses. This chapter argues that studying the history of nursing has benefits for undergraduate students and the profession at large. It provides students with a realistic understanding of nursing and what has influenced past developments to bring us to the present situation. Thus it provides students with the context of nursing practice and a firm foundation on which other nursing courses can build. Introducing students to the history of nursing introduces them to a heritage of working in the community and in institutions; of working independently and interdependently; and of ongoing struggles to forge a professional status based on philanthropy, ethics, and, later, education. Studying the history of nursing, especially at the beginning of the undergraduate program, allows students to understand the factors that have influenced past events and how these factors continue to have an impact on nursing today and into the future.

In addition to the contextual benefits gleaned from the study of the history of nursing, fundamental critical thinking skills can be developed by encouraging students to question the evidence before them and seek influencing factors or the "bigger picture." Additional benefits include the ability to debunk some well-known myths that have affected nursing over the years, the ability to explore gender roles in nursing and discuss how gender affects today's practice, and the ability to understand the unwritten rules of the clinical environment.

Nurse Use

The influence of nursing should be valued and understood within the context of the time it was being practiced. Students who have an appreciation of nursing's past have a better understanding of nursing and who nurses are. With knowledge of the history of nursing, students can better understand that they are entering a profession with a rich and diverse past and that this can provide a firm platform on which to base their other studies. By studying the history of nursing, they also develop their critical thinking skills, which allows them to question and evaluate information that is presented to them on a daily basis.

From Madsen W: Teaching history to nurses: will this make me a better nurse? *Nurs Educ Today* 28:524-529, 2008.

Currently, associate degree nursing (ADN) programs educate the largest percentage of nurses. Both health care and ADN education have changed; both have moved away from a heavy focus on inpatient care to community-based care. Curricula in ADN programs often include content and clinical experiences in management, community health, home health, and gerontology. These clinical areas have typically been key components of baccalaureate education. The American Association of Colleges of Nursing (AACN) was founded in 1969 to respond to the need for an organization that would further nursing education in American universities and 4-year colleges, including establishing essentials of nursing education for baccalaureate and higher-degree programs.

New personnel also added to the flexibility of the public health nurse to address the needs of communities. Beginning in 1965 at the University of Colorado, the nurse practitioner movement opened a new era for nursing involvement in primary care that affected the delivery of services in community health clinics. Initially, the nurse practitioner was often a public health nurse with additional skills in the diagnosis and treatment of common illnesses. Although some nurse practitioners chose to practice in other clinical areas, those who continued in public health settings made sustained contributions to improving access and providing primary care to people in rural areas, inner cities, and other medically underserved areas (Roberts and Heinrich, 1985). As evidence of the effectiveness of their services grew, nurse practitioners became increasingly accepted as cost-effective providers of a variety of primary care services.

PUBLIC HEALTH NURSING FROM THE 1970s TO THE PRESENT

During the 1970s, nurses made many contributions to improving the health care of communities, including participation in the new hospice movement and through the development of birthing centers, daycare for elderly and disabled persons, drug-abuse treatment programs, and rehabilitation services in long-term care. Adequate funding for population health remained difficult to secure. Health care costs grew during the 1980s. Growing costs of acute hospital care, medical procedures, and institutional long-term care reduced funding for health promotion and disease prevention programs. The use of ambulatory services, including health maintenance organizations, was encouraged, and utilization of nurse practitioners (advanced-practice nurses) increased. Despite unstable reimbursement, home health care increased its role in the care of the sick at home. By the 1980s, individuals and families assumed more responsibility for their own health, and health education—always a part of community health nursing—became more popular. Consumer and professional advocacy groups urged the passage of laws to prohibit unhealthy practices in public, such as smoking and driving under the influence of alcohol. However, reduced federal and state funds led to decreases in the number of nurses in official public health agencies.

The Division of Nursing of the US Public Health Service conducted and sponsored nursing research beginning in the late 1930s. This expanded in the late 1940s (Uhl, 1965).

The National Center for Nursing Research (NCNR) was established in 1985 within the federal National Institutes of Health. The NCNR focused attention on the value of nursing research and promoted the work of nurses. With the effort of many nurses the NCNR attained institute (rather than center) status in 1993 and became the National Institute of Nursing Research (NINR), reflecting the continued growth in nursing research.

By the late 1980s the public health initiative had declined in its ability to implement its mission and influence the health of the public. The disarray resulting from reduced political support, financing, and effectiveness was clearly described by the Institute of Medicine (IOM) in *The Future of Public Health* (IOM, 1988). Although many people agreed about what the mission of public health should be, there was much less agreement about how to turn the mission of public health into action and effective programs. The IOM report emphasized the core functions of public health as assessment, policy development, and assurance.

The *Healthy People* initiative has influenced goals and priority setting in public health and in public health nursing. In 1979 *Healthy People* proposed a national strategy to improve the health of Americans significantly by preventing or delaying the onset of major chronic illnesses, injuries, and infectious diseases. Specific goals and objectives were established, and the goals were to be evaluated at the end of each decade. Implementation of these strategies has considerably influenced the work of nurses, through their employment in health agencies and through participation in state or local *Healthy People* coalitions (*Healthy People 2020* box). The most recent initiative, the development of *Healthy People 2020* (US Department of Health and Human Services, 2010) objectives, has built on the work of *Healthy People 2010* (US Department of Health and Human Services, 2000). Some objectives in *Healthy People 2010* have been met; others are being retained in *Healthy People 2020,* and new ones have been added. *Healthy People 2020* objectives and intervention strategies are included in each chapter of this text.

Since the 1990s, public concerns about health have focused on cost, quality, and access to services. Despite widespread interest in universal health insurance coverage, neither individuals nor employers are willing to pay for this level of service. The core debate of the economics of health care—who should pay for what—has emphasized the need for reform of medical care rather than comprehensive reform of health care. In 1993 a blue-ribbon group assembled by President Clinton, with First Lady Hillary Rodham Clinton serving as chair, proposed the American Health Security Act. This proposal led to broad discussion of the key issues and concerns in health care, especially the organization and delivery of medical care, with an emphasis on managed care. When Congress failed to pass the American Health Security Act, considerable change followed in health care financing, and the private sector assumed even greater control. As managed care grew, costs were contained, but constraints increased in terms of how to access care and how much and what kind of care would be reimbursed. Throughout these debates, public health was generally ignored. Little attention was given to ensuring that populations and the communities in which they lived were healthy. This omission reflected the large gap between the proposal and actual comprehensive health care reform.

In 1991 the ANA, AACN, NLN, and more than 60 other specialty nursing organizations joined to support health care reform. The coalitions of organizations emphasized the key health care issues of access, quality, and cost. Improved primary care and public health efforts would help build a healthy nation. Professional nursing continues to support revisions in health care delivery and extension of public health services to prevent illness, promote health, and protect the public (Table 2.3). Chapters 3 (The Changing US Health and Public Health Care Systems) and 8 (Economic Influences) describe the current work to change the way health is provided and who pays for the care.

TABLE 2.3   Milestones in the History of Community Health and Public Health Nursing: 1946–2013

Year	Milestone
1946	Nurses classified as professionals by US Civil Service Commission; Hill-Burton Act approved, providing funds for hospital construction in underserved areas and requiring these hospitals to provide care to poor people; passage of National Mental Health Act
1950	25,091 nurses employed in public health
1951	National nursing organizations recommended that college-based nursing education programs include public health content
1952	National Organization for Public Health Nursing merged into the new National League for Nursing; Metropolitan Life Insurance Nursing Program closed
1964	Passage of the Economic Opportunity Act; public health nurse defined by the American Nurses Association (ANA) as a graduate of a bachelor of science in nursing (BSN) program
1965	ANA position paper recommended that nursing education take place in institutions of higher learning; Congress amended the Social Security Act to include Medicare and Medicaid
1977	Passage of the Rural Health Clinic Services Act, which provided indirect reimbursement for nurse practitioners in rural health clinics
1978	Association of Graduate Faculty in Community Health Nursing/Public Health Nursing (later renamed Association of Community Health Nursing Educators)
1980	Medicaid amendment to the Social Security Act to provide direct reimbursement for nurse practitioners in rural health clinics; both ANA and the American Public Health Association (APHA) developed statements on the role and conceptual foundations of community and public health nursing, respectively
1983	Beginning of Medicare prospective payments
1985	National Center for Nursing Research (NCNR) established within the National Institutes of Health (NIH)
1988	Institute of Medicine published *The Future of Public Health*

Continued

TABLE 2.3	Milestones in the History of Community Health and Public Health Nursing: 1946–2013—cont'd
Year	**Milestone**
1990	Association of Community Health Nursing Educators published *Essentials of Baccalaureate Nursing Education*
1991	More than 60 nursing organizations joined forces to support health care reform and published a document entitled *Nursing's Agenda for Health Care Reform*
1993	American Health Security Act of 1993 was published as a blueprint for national health care reform; the national effort, however, failed, leaving states and the private sector to design their own programs
1993	NCNR became the National Institute for Nursing Research, as part of the National Institutes of Health
1993	Public Health Nursing section of the American Public Health Association updated the definition and role of public health nursing
1996	Passage of the Health Insurance Portability and Accountability Act
2001	Significant interest in public health ensues from concerns about biological and other forms of terrorism in the wake of the intentional destruction of buildings in New York City and Washington, D.C., on September 11
2002	Office of Homeland Security established to provide leadership to protect against intentional threats to the health of the public
2003–2005	Multiple natural disasters, including earthquakes, tsunamis, and hurricanes, demonstrated the weak infrastructure for managing disasters in the United States and other countries and emphasized the need for strong public health programs that included disaster management
2007	An entirely new *Public Health Nursing Scope and Standards of Practice* released through the ANA, reflecting the efforts of the Quad Council of Public Health Nursing Organizations
2010	Patient Protection and Affordable Care Act signed by President Barack Obama; *Healthy People 2020* realized by the US Department of Health and Human Services
2011	The Quad Council of Public Health Nursing Organizations published *Competencies for Public Health Nursing*
2013	The American Nurses Association published the second edition of *Public Health Nursing: Scope and Standards of Practice*
2013	The Quad Council of Public Health Nursing Organizations updated *Competencies for Public Health Nursing Practice*

❤ HEALTHY PEOPLE 2020

History of the Development of Healthy People

In 1979 the groundbreaking *Healthy People: The Surgeon General's Report on Health Promotion and Disease Prevention* noted "the health of the American people has never been better" (US Department of Health, Education and Welfare, 1979, p 3). But this was only the prologue to deep criticism of the status of American health care delivery. Between 1960 and 1978, health care spending increased 700%—without striking improvements in mortality or morbidity. During the 1950s and 1960s, evidence accumulated about chronic disease risk factors, particularly cigarette smoking, alcohol and drug use, occupational risks, and injuries. But these new research findings were not systematically applied to health planning and to improving population health.

In 1974 the Canadian government published *A New Perspective on the Health of Canadians* (Lalonde, 1974), which found death and disease to have four contributing factors: inadequacies in the existing health care system, behavioral factors, environmental hazards, and human biological factors. Applying the Canadian approach, in 1976, US experts analyzed the 10 leading causes of US mortality and found that 50% of American deaths were the result of unhealthy behaviors, and only 10% were the result of inadequacies in health care. Rather than just spending more to improve hospital care, clearly, prevention was the key to saving lives, improving the quality of life, and saving health care dollars.

A multidisciplinary group of analysts conducted a comprehensive review of prevention activities. These analysts verified that the health of Americans could be significantly improved through "actions individuals can take for themselves" and through actions that public and private decision makers could take to

"promote a safer and healthier environment" (p 9). Like Canada's *New Perspectives,* in the United States Healthy People (1979) identified priorities and measurable goals. *Healthy People* grouped 15 key priorities into three categories: key preventive services that could be delivered to individuals by health providers, such as timely prenatal care; measures that could be used by governmental agencies, organizations, and industry to protect people from harm, such as reduced exposure to toxic agents; and activities that individuals and communities could use to promote healthy lifestyles, such as improved nutrition.

In the late 1980s, success in addressing these priorities and goals was evaluated, new scientific findings were analyzed, and new goals and objectives were set for the period from 1990 to 2000 through *Healthy People 2000: National Health Promotion and Disease Prevention Objectives* (US Public Health Service, 1991). This process was repeated 10 years later to develop goals and objectives for the period from 2000 to 2010 and for 2010 to 2020. Recognizing the continuing challenge of the use of emerging scientific research to encourage modification of health behaviors and practices, *Healthy People 2020* (US Department of Health and Human Services, 2010) addresses health equity, elimination of disparities, and improved health for all groups across the life span through disease prevention, improved social and physical environments, and healthy development and health behaviors.

Like the nurse in the early 20th century who spread the gospel of public health to reduce communicable diseases, today's population-centered nurse uses *Healthy People* to reduce chronic and infectious diseases and injuries through health education, environmental modification, and policy development.

During the late 20th and early 21st centuries, challenges continued to trigger growth and change in nursing in the community. Nurse-managed centers now provide a diversity of nursing services, including health promotion and disease and injury prevention, in areas where existing organizations have been unable to meet community and neighborhood needs. These centers provide valuable services but typically face many challenges in securing

adequate funding. As population needs also continue to grow and change, schools of nursing, health departments, rural health clinics, migrant health centers, and other community agencies are challenged to provide the range of services necessary to meet specific needs. Transfer of official health services to private control has sometimes reduced professional flexibility and service delivery. A nursing shortage reduces staffing when community nurses look to employment in acute-care facilities that often pay higher salaries. The Association of Community Health Nurse Educators recommends increased graduate programs to educate public health nurse leaders, educators, and researchers. Natural disasters (e.g., floods, hurricanes, and tornados) and human-made disasters (including explosions, building collapses, airplane crashes, and toxic ingredients added to food) have required rapid, innovative, and time-consuming responses. Preparation for future disasters and possible bioterrorism requires well-prepared nurses. Some states hear new calls to deploy school nurses in every school; a new recognition of the link between school success and health is making the school nurse as essential as in Lillian Wald's era. Many of these topics are detailed in the chapters that follow.

The Affordable Care Act of 2010 has been controversial, and many compromises have been made between the House of Representatives and the Senate in the final crafting of this health care act. Much of the Affordable Care Act deals with changes in insurance plans and coverage. See http://www.healthcare.gov/news/factsheets/index.html for details about the Affordable Care Act.

Public health nursing, historically and at present, is characterized by reaching out to care for the health of people in need and providing safe and high-quality care where needed. Currently, many nurses work in the community. Some bring a public health population-based approach and have as their goal preventing illness and protecting health. Other nurses have a community-oriented approach and deal primarily with the health care of individuals, families, and groups in a community. Still other nurses bring a community-based approach that focuses on "illness care" of individuals and families in the community. Each type of nurse is needed in today's communities. It is important that we learn from the past and use time and resources carefully and effectively. Regardless of the level of education of the nurse who provides care in the community, including population-based care, all nurses need to provide care that is safe and of high quality. The accompanying box below describes the history of the Quality and Safety Education for Nurses (QSEN) initiative, which aims to include quality and safety knowledge, skills, and attitudes in all levels of nursing education.

QSEN FOCUS ON QUALITY AND SAFETY EDUCATION FOR NURSES

Although the scope and responsibilities of public health nurses have changed over time, the commitment to quality and safety has remained constant. Since the beginning of population-centered nursing in the United States, the nurses involved in this specialty have been committed to preserving health and preventing disease. They have focused on environmental conditions such as sanitation and control of communicable diseases, education for health, prevention of disease and disability, and, at times, care of the sick and aged in their homes. This long-standing commitment to quality and safety is consistent with the work of the QSEN, a national initiative designed to transform nursing education by including in the curriculum content and experiences related to building knowledge, skills, and attitudes for six quality and safety initiatives (Cronenwett, Sherwood, and Gelmon, 2009). The QSEN work, led by Drs. Linda Cronenwett and Gwen Sherwood at the University of North Carolina, has made great progress in bridging the gap between quality and safety in both practice and academic settings (Brown, Feller, and Benedict, 2010). The six QSEN competencies for nursing are as follows:

1. **Patient-centered care:** Recognizes the client or designee as the source of control and as a full partner in providing compassionate and coordinated care that is based on the preferences, values, and needs of the client.
2. **Teamwork and collaboration:** Refers to the ability to function effectively with nursing and interprofessional teams and to foster open communication, mutual respect, and shared decision making to provide quality client care.
3. **Evidence-based practice:** Integrates the best current clinical evidence with client and family preferences and values to provide optimal client care.
4. **Quality improvement:** Uses data to monitor the outcomes of the care processes and uses improvement methods to design and test changes to continually improve the quality and safety of health care systems.
5. **Safety:** Minimizes the risk of harm to clients and providers through both system effectiveness and individual performance.
6. **Informatics:** Uses information and technology to communicate, manage knowledge, mitigate error, and support decision making (Brown et al, 2010, p 116).

Of the six QSEN competencies, all but safety were derived from the IOM report *Health Professions Education* (2003). The QSEN team added safety because this competency is central to the work of nurses. Articles have been published to teach educators about QSEN, and national forums have been held. In addition, the AACN has hosted faculty-development institutes for faculty and academic administrators using a train-the-trainer model, and safety and quality objectives have been built in the AACN essentials for nursing education. Similarly, the NLN

has incorporated the "NLN Educational Competencies Model" into its educational summits. The six QSEN competencies are integrated throughout the text to emphasize the importance of quality and safety in public health nursing today. *Note:* The terms *patient* and *care* will be changed to *client* and *intervention* to reflect a public health nursing approach.

Specifically related to the history of nursing, the following targeted competency can be applied:

Targeted Competency: Safety—Minimizes the risk of harm to clients and providers through both system effectiveness and individual performance. Important aspects of safety include the following:

- **Knowledge:** Discuss potential and actual impact of national client safety resources initiatives and regulations
- **Skills:** Participate in analyzing errors and designing system improvements
- **Attitudes:** Value vigilance and monitoring by clients, families, and other members of the health care team

Safety Question

Updated definitions around client safety include addressing safety at the individual level and at the systems level. The history of public health nursing demonstrates the myriad ways that public health nurses have addressed client safety in their evolving practice. Public health nurses support safety by caring for individuals and providing care for communities and groups. Historically, how have public health nurses addressed safety at the individual client level? How have public health nurses addressed client safety at the systems level? How have public health nurses been involved in system improvements?

Answer: *Individual level: A rich part of public health nursing's history has been the development of home visitation, in which clients are cared for in their own environment. Similarly, public health nurses have improved client outcomes by pioneering new models of interventions for maternal–child health and individuals in rural communities.*

Systems level: *Through their work with communities, public health nurses were an integral part of reducing the incidence of communicable diseases by the mid-20th century. More recently, public health nursing has contributed to health care system improvements through the development of the hospice movement, birthing centers, daycare for elderly and disabled persons, and drug-abuse and rehabilitation services. These initiatives have updated the health care system to provide targeted care for previously overlooked populations.*

Prepared by Gail Armstrong, PhD, DNP, ACNS-BC, CNE, Associate Professor, University of Colorado College of Nursing.

Today, nurses look to their history for inspiration, explanations, and predictions. Information and advocacy are used to promote a comprehensive approach to addressing the multiple needs of the diverse populations served. Nurses will seek to learn from the past and to avoid known pitfalls, even as they seek successful strategies to meet the complex needs of today's vulnerable populations. The How To box describes how to conduct an oral history interview. This is one effective way to learn from the successes and failures of our predecessors.

HOW TO Conduct an Oral History Interview
1. Identify an issue or event of interest.
2. Gather information from written materials.
3. Find a person to interview.
4. Get permission from the person to do the interview, and make an appointment to do so.
5. Gather information about the person's background and the period of interest.
6. Write an outline of your questions. Use open-ended questions because they usually give you more information.
7. Meet with the person being interviewed; use a recording device.
8. Conduct the interview by asking only one question at a time and allowing adequate time for the reply.
9. Clarify points when needed; ask for examples; remember, most people like to talk about themselves.
10. After the interview, write it up as soon as possible when your recall is best.
11. Compare your written report with the audio recording. There may be times when you can ask the person interviewed to read your report for accuracy.

As plans for the future are made, as the public health challenges that remain unmet are acknowledged, it is the vision of what nursing can accomplish that sustains these nurses. Nurses continue to rely on both nursing and public health standards and competency guides to help chart their practice.

The ANA's (2013) *Scope and Standards of Public Health Nursing Practice*, the Council on Linkages' (2010) *Domains and Core Competencies*, and the Quad Council's (Swider et al, 2013) *Competencies of Public Health Nurses* each include the processes of assessment, analysis, and planning. Each also incorporates the importance of communication, cultural competency, policy, and public health skills in its recommendations for effective public health nurse practice. Specific to this chapter, the Council on Linkages (2014, p. 17) features a core competency under the domain of public health sciences skills: "Identifies prominent events in the history of public health." Moreover, the Quad Council (Swider et al, 2013) builds on this competency with an application to nursing under Domain 6 that a public health nurse "Describes the historical foundation of public health and public health nursing" (p 533).

▶▶ APPLYING CONTENT TO PRACTICE

Public Health Nursing, a major journal in the field of public health nursing, publishes articles that broadly reflect contemporary research, practice, education, and public policy for population-based nurses. Begun in 1984, *Public Health Nursing* was published quarterly through 1993 and has been a bimonthly journal since 1994.

More than any other journal, *Public Health Nursing* has assumed responsibility for preserving the history of public health nursing and for publishing new historical research on the field. The contemporary *Public Health Nursing* shares its name with the official journal of the NOPHN in the period 1931 to 1952 (earlier names were used for the official journal from 1913 to 1931, which built on the *Visiting Nurse Quarterly*, published 1909 to 1913).

Public Health Nursing presents a wide variety of articles, including both new historical research and reprints of classic journal articles that deserve to be read and reapplied by modern public health nurses. For example, one historical article reprinted in *Public Health Nursing* addressed a nurse's 1931 work on county drought relief that underscores continuing professional themes of case-finding, collaboration, and partnership (Wharton, 1999). Original historical research presented in *Public Health Nursing* is extremely varied, from public health nursing education, to public health nurse practice in Alaska's Yukon, to excerpts from the oral histories of public health nurses. Contemporary nurses find inspiration and possibilities for modern innovations in reading the history of public health nursing in the pages of *Public Health Nursing*.

▌ PRACTICE APPLICATION

Mary Lipsky has worked for a visiting nurse association in a large urban area for 2 years. She is responsible for a wide variety of services, including caring for older and chronically ill clients recently discharged from hospitals, new mothers and babies, mental health clients, and clients with long-term health problems, such as chronic wounds.

Daily when she leaves the field to go home, she finds that she continues to think about her clients. She keeps going over these and other questions in her mind: Why is it so difficult for mothers and new babies to qualify for and receive Special Supplemental Nutrition Program for Women, Infants, and Children (WIC) services? Why must she limit the number of visits and length of service for clients with chronic wounds? Why are so few services available for clients with behavioral health problems? In particular, she thinks about the burdens and challenges that families and friends face in caring for the sick at home.

A. Why might it be difficult to solve these problems at the individual level, on a case-by-case basis?

B. What information would you need to build an understanding of the policy background for each of these various populations?

Answers can be found on the Evolve website.

REMEMBER THIS!

- A historical approach can be used to increase the understanding of public and community health nursing in the past and its contemporary dilemmas and future challenges.
- Public health and community health nursing are products of various social, economic, and political forces and incorporate public health science in addition to nursing science and practice.
- Federal responsibility for health care was limited until the 1930s, when the economic challenges of the Depression highlighted the need for and led to the expansion of federal assistance for health care.
- Florence Nightingale designed and implemented the first program of trained nursing, and her contemporary, William Rathbone, founded the first district nursing association in England.
- Urbanization, industrialization, and immigration in the United States increased the need for trained nurses, especially in public and community health nursing.
- The increasing acceptance of public roles for women permitted public and community health nursing employment for nurses and public leadership roles for their wealthy supporters.
- Frances Root was the first trained nurse in the United States who was salaried as a visiting nurse. She was hired in 1887 by the Women's Board of the New York City Mission to provide care to sick persons at home.
- The first visiting nurse associations were founded in 1885 and 1886 in Buffalo, Philadelphia, and Boston.
- Lillian Wald established the Henry Street Settlement, which became the Visiting Nurse Service of New York City, in 1893. She played a key role in innovations that shaped public and community health nursing in its first decades, including school nursing, insurance payment for nursing, national organizations for public health nurses, and the US Children's Bureau.
- Founded in 1902, with the vision and support of Lillian Wald, school nursing tried to keep children in school so that they could learn.
- The Metropolitan Life Insurance Company established the first insurance-based program in 1909 to support community health nursing services.
- The National Organization for Public Health Nursing (founded in 1912) provided essential leadership and coordination of diverse public and community health nursing efforts; the organization merged into the new National League for Nursing in 1952.
- Official health agencies slowly grew in numbers between 1900 and 1940, accompanied by a steady increase in public health nursing positions.

- The innovative Sheppard-Towner Act of 1921 expanded community health nursing roles for maternal and child health during the 1920s.
- Mary Breckinridge established the Frontier Nursing Service in 1925 to provide rural health care.
- The tension between the nursing roles of caring for the sick and of providing preventive care and the related tension between intervening for individuals and for groups have characterized the specialty since at least the 1910s.
- The challenges of World War II sometimes resulted in extension of community health nursing care and sometimes in retrenchment and decreased public health nursing services.
- By the mid-20th century, the reduced incidence of communicable diseases and the increased prevalence of chronic illness, accompanied by large increases in the population older than 65 years of age, led to a reexamination of the goals and organization of community health nursing services.
- From the 1930s to 1965, organized nursing and community health nursing agencies sought to establish health insurance reimbursement for nursing care at home.
- Implementation of Medicare and Medicaid programs in 1966 established new possibilities for supporting community-based nursing care but encouraged agencies to focus on postacute-care services rather than prevention.
- Efforts to reform health care organization, pushed by increased health care costs during the past 40 years, have focused on reforming acute medical care rather than on designing a comprehensive preventive approach.
- The 1988 *Future of Public Health* report documented the reduced political support, financing, and impact of increasingly limited public health services at the national, state, and local levels.
- In the late 1990s federal policy changes dangerously reduced financial support for home health care services, threatening the long-term survival of visiting nurse agencies.
- The *Healthy People* program has brought a renewed emphasis on prevention to public and community health nursing.
- In 2011 the Quad Council, an alliance of four national nursing organizations that addresses public health nursing issues, finalized its own set of public health nursing competencies. These competencies were revised in 2013.
- The 2000, 2010, and 2020 versions of *Healthy People;* recent disasters and acts of terrorism; and, most recently, the Patient Protection and Affordable Care Act of 2010 have brought a renewed emphasis on the benefits of both public health and nursing.

Ⓔ **EVOLVE WEBSITE**

http://evolve.elsevier.com/Stanhope/foundations
- NCLEX® Review Questions
- Practice Application Answers

REFERENCES

American Association of Industrial Nurses: *The nurse in industry: a history of the American Association of Industrial Nurses, Inc,* New York, 1976, AAIN.

American Nurses Association: *Public health nursing: scope and standards of practice,* Silver Spring, MD, 2013, ANA.

Backer BA: Lillian Wald: connecting caring with action, *Nurs Health Care* 14:122–128, 1993.

Brainard A: *Evolution of public health nursing,* Philadelphia, 1922, Saunders.

Brown R, Feller L, Benedict L: Reframing nursing education: the Quality and Safety Education for Nurses Initiative, *Teach Learn Nurs* 5:115–118, 2010.

Browne H: A tribute to Mary Breckinridge, *Nurs Outlook* 14:54–55, 1966.

Buhler-Wilkerson K: Public health nursing: in sickness or in health? *Am J Pub Health* 75:1155–1161, 1985.

Buhler-Wilkerson K: Left carrying the bag: experiments in visiting nursing. 1977-1909, *Nurs Res* 36:42–45, 1987.

Buhler-Wilkerson K: *False dawn: the rise and decline of public health nursing, 1900-1930,* New York, 1989, Garland Publishing.

Buhler-Wilkerson K: *No place like home: a history of nursing and home care in the United States,* Baltimore, 2001, Johns Hopkins.

Cohen IB: Florence Nightingale, *Sci Am* 3:128–137, 1984.

Council on Linkages between Academic and Public Health Practice: *Core competencies for public health professionals,* Washington DC, 2014, Public Health Foundation, Health Resources and Services Administration.

Cronenwett, L, Sherwood, G, Gelmon, SB: Improving quality and safety education: the QSEN learning collaborative, *Nurs Outlook* 57:304–312, 2009.

Deloughery GL: *History and trends of professional nursing,* ed 8, St. Louis, 1977, Mosby.

Dock LL: The history of public health nursing, *Public Health Nurs* 1922. (Reprinted by the American Public Health Association).

Dolan J: *History of nursing,* ed 14, Philadelphia, 1978, Saunders.

Frachel RR: A new profession: the evolution of public health nursing, *Public Health Nurs* 5:86–90, 1988.

Goan MB: Mary Breckinridge: *The frontier nursing service and rural health in Appalachia,* Chapel Hill, NC, 2008, The University of North Carolina.

Hanggi-Myers L: The Howard Association of New Orleans: precursor to district nursing, *Public Health Nurs* 12:78, 1995.

Hawkins JW, Hayes ER, Corliss CP: School nursing in America: 1902–1994—a return to public health nursing, *Public Health Nurs* 11:416–425, 1994.

Hine DC: *Black women in white: racial conflict and cooperation in the nursing profession, 1890-1950,* Bloomington, 1989, Indiana University Press.

Holloway JB: Frontier nursing service 1925–1975, *J Ky Med Assoc* 73:491–492, 1975.

Hostutler J, Kennedy MS, Mason D, et al: Nurses: then and now and models of practice, *Am J Nurs* 100:82–83, 2000.

Institute of Medicine: *The future of public health,* Washington, DC, 1988, National Academy of Science.

Institute of Medicine: *Health Professions Education,* Washington, DC, 2003, National Academy of Science.

Kalisch PA, Kalisch BJ: *The advance of American nursing,* ed 3, Philadelphia, 1995, Lippincott.

Lalonde M: *New perspective on the health of Canadians,* Ottawa, ON, 1974, Government of Canada.

Madsen W: Teaching history to nurses: will this make me a better nurse? *Nurse Educ Today* 28:524–529, 2008.

Mosley MOP: Jessie Sleet Scales: first black public health nurse, *ABNF J* 5:45, 1994.

National Organization for Public Health Nursing: Approval of Skidmore College of Nursing as preparing students for public health nursing, *Public Health Nurs* 36:371, 1944.

Nightingale F: Sick nursing and health nursing. In Billings JS, Hurd HM, editors: *Hospitals, dispensaries, and nursing,* Baltimore, 1894, Johns Hopkins. (Reprinted New York, 1984, Garland.)

Nightingale F: *Notes on nursing: what it is, and what it is not,* Philadelphia, 1946, Lippincott.

Nutting MA, Dock LL: *A history of nursing,* New York, 1935, GP Putnam's Sons.

Palmer IS: *Florence Nightingale and the first organized delivery of nursing services,* Washington, DC, 1983, American Association of Colleges of Nursing.

Pickett G, Hanlon JJ: *Public health: administration and practice,* St. Louis, 1990, Mosby.

Quad Council of Public Health Nursing Organizations: *Quad Council: competencies for public health nurses,* Washington, DC, 2011, ASTDN.

Roberts DE, Heinrich J: Public health nursing comes of age, *Am J Public Health* 75:1162–1172, 1985.

Roberts M: *American nursing: history and interpretation,* New York, 1955, Macmillan.

Rodabaugh JH, Rodabaugh MJ: *Nursing in Ohio: a history,* Columbus, Ohio, 1951, Ohio State Nurses Association.

Rosen G: *A history of public health,* New York, 1958, MD Publications.

Scutchfield FD, Keck CW: *Principles of public health practice,* Albany, NY, 1997, Delmar.

Shyrock H: *The history of nursing,* Philadelphia, 1959, Saunders.

Swider SM, Krothe J, Reyes D, and Cravetz M: The Quad Council Practice Competencies for Public Health Nursing, *Public Health Nursing* 30(6):519–536, 2013.

Thoms AB: *Pathfinders: a history of the progress of colored graduate nurses,* New York, 1929, Kay Printing House.

Tirpak H: The Frontier Nursing Service: fifty years in the mountains, *Nurs Outlook* 33:308–310, 1975.

Uhl G: The Division of Nursing: USPHS, *Am J Nurs* 65:82–85, 1965.

US Department of Health, Education and Welfare: *Healthy People: the Surgeon General's report on health promotion and disease prevention,* DHEW Pub no. 79-55071, Washington, DC, 1979, US Government Printing Office.

US Department of Health and Human Services: *Healthy People 2010: understanding and improving health,* Washington, DC, 2000, US Government Printing Office.

US Department of Health and Human Services: *Healthy People 2020: a roadmap to improve America's Health,* Washington, DC, 2010, USDHHS, Public Health Service.

US Public Health Service: *Healthy People 2000: national health promotion and disease prevention objectives,* Washington, DC, 1991, US Government Printing Office.

Wharton AL: Country drought relief: a public health nurse's problem, *Public Health Nurs* 16:307–308, 1999; reprinted from *Public Health Nurs* 23, 1931.

Wilner DM, Walkey RP, O'Neill EJ: *Introduction to public health,* ed 7, New York, 1978, Macmillan.

Zerwekh JV: Public health nursing legacy: historical practical wisdom, *Nurs Health Care* 13:84–91, 1992.

CHAPTER 3

The Changing U.S. Health and Public Health Care Systems

Marcia Stanhope

OBJECTIVES

After reading this chapter, the student should be able to do the following:

1. Describe the events and trends that influence the status of the health care system.
2. Discuss key aspects of the private health care system.
3. Define public health and the nurse's role.
4. Compare and contrast the current public health system with the model of primary health care.
5. Assess the effects of health care and insurance reform on population health care.

CHAPTER OUTLINE

Health Care in the United States
Forces Stimulating Change in the Demand for Health Care
  Demographic Trends
  Social and Economic Trends
  Health Workforce Trends
  Technological Trends
Current Health Care System in the United States
  Cost
  Access
  Quality
Organization of the Current Health Care System
  Primary Care System

Public Health System
The Federal System
The State System
The Local System
Forces Influencing Changes in the Health Care System
Integration of Public Health and the Primary Care System
  Potential Barriers to Integration
  Primary Health Care
  Promoting Health/Preventing Disease: Year 2020 Objectives for the Nation

KEY TERMS

advanced-practice nursing (APN), 36
Affordable Care Act, 38
community participation, 44
Declaration of Alma-Ata, 33
disease prevention, 33
electronic health record (EHR), 37
health, 33
health promotion, 33
managed care, 39
primary care, 39
primary health care (PHC), 44
public health, 39
US Department of Health and Human Services (USDHHS), 39

In September 1978, an international conference was held in the city of Alma-Ata, which at that time was the capital of the Soviet Republic of Kazakhstan. During this conference, the Declaration of Alma-Ata and a new concept in health care delivery emerged: the primary health care model. This declaration states that health is a human right and that the health of its people should be the primary goal of every government. One of the main themes of this declaration was the involvement of community health workers and traditional healers in a new health system (World Health Organization [WHO], 1978).

Primary health care (PHC) was introduced, defined, and described. In 2008 WHO renewed its call for health care improvements and reemphasized the need for public policymakers, public health officials, primary care providers, and leadership within countries to improve health care delivery. WHO said, "Globalization is putting the social cohesion of many countries under stress, and health systems . . . are clearly not performing as well as they could and should" (WHO, 2008).

As defined by WHO, PHC, which is defined differently than primary care or public health, promotes the integration of all health care systems within a community to come together to improve the health of the community, including primary care and public health.

Therefore PHC provides for the integration of health promotion, disease prevention, and curative and rehabilitative

BOX 3.1　Definitions of Selected Terms

- **Disease prevention:** Activities whose goal is to protect people from becoming ill as a result of actual or potential health threats
- **Disparities:** Racial or ethnic differences in the quality of health care, not based on access or clinical needs, preferences, or appropriateness of an intervention
- **Electronic medical record:** A computer-based client medical record
- **Globalization:** A trend toward an increased flow of goods, services, money, and disease across national borders
- **Health:** A state of complete physical, mental, and social well-being, not merely the absence of disease or infirmity (WHO, 1986a)
- **Health promotion:** Activities that have as their goal the development of human attitudes and behaviors that maintain or enhance well-being
- **Institute of Medicine:** A part of the National Academy of Sciences and an organization whose purpose is to provide national advice on issues relating to biomedical science, medicine, and health
- **Primary care:** The providing of integrated, accessible health care services by clinicians who are accountable for addressing a large majority of personal health care needs, developing a sustained partnership with clients, and practicing in the context of family and community
- **Primary health care:** A combination of primary care and public health care made universally accessible to individuals and families in a community, with their full participation, and provided at a cost that the community and country can afford (WHO, 1978)
- **Public health:** Organized community and multidisciplinary efforts, based on epidemiology, aimed at preventing disease and promoting health (Institute of Medicine, 1988, p 4)

services (WHO, 1978). Because of the changing environment in health care delivery in the United States, the work by WHO in 1978 is becoming increasingly important. Box 3.1 lists selected definitions that will help explain the concepts introduced in this chapter.

HEALTH CARE IN THE UNITED STATES

Despite the fact that health care costs in the United States are the highest in the world and comprise the greatest percentage of the gross domestic product, the indicators of what constitutes good health do not document that Americans are really getting their money's worth. In the first decade of the 21st century there have been massive and unexpected changes in health, economic, and social conditions as a result of terrorist attacks, hurricanes, fires, floods, infectious diseases, and an economic turndown in 2008. New systems have been developed to prevent and/or deal with the onslaught of these horrendous events. Not all of the systems have worked, and many are regularly criticized for their inefficiency and costliness. Simultaneously, new and nearly miraculous advances have been made in treating health-related conditions. Organs and joints are being replaced, and medicines are keeping people alive who only a few years ago would have suffered and died. These advances and "wonder drugs" save and prolong lives, and a number of deadly and debilitating diseases have been eliminated through effective immunizations and treatments. In addition, sanitation, water

supplies, and nutrition have been improved, and animal cloning has begun.

However, attention to all of these advances may overshadow the lack of attention to public health and prevention. Several of the most destructive health conditions can be prevented either through changes in lifestyle or interventions such as immunizations. The increasing rates of obesity, especially among children; substance use; lack of exercise; violence; and accidents have alarming repercussions, particularly when they lead to disruptions in health.

This chapter describes a health care system in transition as it struggles to meet evolving global and domestic challenges. The overall health care and public health systems in the United States are described and differentiated, and the changing priorities are identified, with emphasis on integrating public health and primary care. Nurses play a pivotal role in meeting these needs, and the role of the nurse is described.

FORCES STIMULATING CHANGE IN THE DEMAND FOR HEALTH CARE

In recent years, enormous changes have occurred in society, both in the United States and most other countries of the world. The extent of interaction among countries is stronger than ever, and the economy of each country depends on the stability of other countries. The United States has felt the effects of rising labor costs as many companies have shifted their production to other countries with lower labor costs. It is often less expensive to assemble clothes, automobile parts, and appliances and to have call distribution centers and call service centers in a less industrialized country and pay the shipping and other charges involved than to have the items fully assembled in the United States. In recent years the vacillating cost of fuel has affected almost every area of the economy, leading to both higher costs of products and layoffs as some industries have struggled to stay solvent. This has affected the employment rate in the United States. The economic downturn of 2008 left many people unemployed, and many lost their homes because they could not pay their mortgages. When the unemployment rate is high, more people lack comprehensive insurance coverage because in the United States this has been typically provided by employers. In late November 2008, the US unemployment rate was 6.7%. This represented an increase from 4.6% in 2007. In July 2012 the unemployment rate had increased to 8.2%, close to double the rate in 2007. In recent years the economy has begun to recover. In 2014, for example, the unemployment rate decreased to 6.1%—down 2.1 percentage points from 2012 (Bureau of Labor Statistics [BLS], 2014a). Also, health care services and the ways in which they are financed are changing with the continuing implementation of the Patient Protection and Affordable Care Act (ACA), enacted in 2010. Many of the planned changes were implemented by 2016. However, in 2016, with the election of a new president, there were many threats related to the future of the ACA.

EVIDENCE-BASED PRACTICE

It is often said that the states are the laboratories of democracy. One state, Massachusetts, began an experiment in health reform in 2006. Two years after health reform legislation became effective, only 2.6% of Massachusetts's residents were uninsured, the lowest percentage ever recorded in any state (Dorn et al, 2009). However, the program became one of the most successful and a model for the Affordable Care Act. After 5 years approximately 98% to 99% of all of the commonwealth's citizens were covered by the plan.

Although other states have experimented with various programs to decrease the number of uninsured individuals, the Massachusetts plan has had the most success. The health reform plan rests on an individual mandate that requires everyone who can afford insurance to purchase coverage. Those unable to afford insurance receive subsidies that allow low-income individuals and families to purchase coverage. A new state-run program, Commonwealth Care (CommCare), provides benefits to adults who are not eligible for Medicaid but whose incomes fall below 300% of the federal poverty level.

To understand how the state has achieved such success in this effort toward universal coverage, a group of evaluators met with 15 key informants representing hospitals, community health centers, insurance companies, Medicaid, and CommCare. Several factors, it was found, have contributed to the historic level of coverage seen in the state. Rather than requiring consumers to complete separate applications for programs such as Medicaid, the Children's Health Insurance Program (CHIP), or CommCare, a single application system provides entry to all the state programs. If an uninsured client is admitted to a hospital or visits a community health center, his or her eligibility is automatically evaluated; if eligible, the client is automatically converted to CommCare coverage, even without completing an application. A "Virtual Gateway" has been developed through which staff members of community-based organizations have been trained to complete online applications on behalf of consumers and to provide education and counseling about insurance options to underserved communities. Because reimbursement is held back from providers that do not offer staff to help consumers sign up for one of the available insurance options, hospitals and health centers are motivated to dedicate staff to provide education and counseling to the formerly uninsured. The result is that at least half of the new enrollees in Medicaid and CommCare have been enrolled without filling out any forms on their own. In addition to these efforts, shortly after the reform legislation was enacted, the state financed a massive public education effort to inform consumers about their new options.

Nurse Use

As health reform is implemented on the national level, nurses can play a crucial role in driving down the number of uninsured individuals. Nurses should educate themselves so that they can encourage clients to apply and take advantage of all available coverage options. Taking an active role in consumer educational programs is a natural extension of a nurse's role as a client advocate. Nurses can promote legislation to simplify enrollment processes and encourage the development of shared databases for community health care providers, thus preventing consumers from falling through the cracks in our fragmented health care system.

From Dorn S, Hill I, Hogan S: The secrets of Massachusetts' success: why 97 percent of state residents have health coverage: state health access reform evaluation, Romneycare-The truth about Massachusetts health care. 2014, accessed at mittromneycentral.com. 9/25/2014, Robert Wood Johnson Foundation. Available at http://www.urban.org Accessed September 19, 2012.

DEMOGRAPHIC TRENDS

The population of the world is growing as a result of increased fertility and decreased mortality rates. The greatest growth is occurring in underdeveloped countries, and this is accompanied by decreased growth in the United States and other developed countries. The year 2000, however, marked the first time in more than 30 years that the total fertility rate in the United States was above the replacement level. *Replacement* means that for every person who dies, another is born (Hamilton et al, 2010). Both the size and the characteristics of the population contribute to the changing demography.

Seventy-seven million babies were born between the years of 1946 and 1963, giving rise to the often-discussed baby-boomer generation (Office for National Statistics [ONS], 2014) The oldest of these boomers reached 65 years of age in 2011, and they are expected to live longer than people born in earlier times. The impact on the federal government's insurance program for people 65 years of age and older, Medicare, is expected to be enormous, and this population is predicted to double between the years 2000 and 2030, representing 20% of the total population (Centers for Disease Control and Prevention [CDC], 2013a).

In 2016, the US population totaled more than 322 million people, representing the third most populated country in the world. From 1990 to 2012, the US foreign-born immigrant population grew from about 19 million to approximately 41 million, and it is continuing to increase every year (US Census Bureau, 2016).

At the time of the 1990 census, African Americans were the largest minority group in the United States (US Census Bureau, 1996). However, in 2014, the US Census Bureau announced that Hispanic persons outnumbered African Americans, with non-Hispanic whites being the largest single ethnic group in the United States (ONS, 2014). The nation's foreign-born population is growing, and it is projected that from now until 2050 the largest population growth will be attributable to immigrants and their children. The states with the largest percentage of foreign-born populations are California, New York, Texas, and Florida (Migration Policy Institute, 2015).

The composition of the US household is also changing. From 1935 to 2010, mortality for both genders in all age groups and races declined (Hoyert, 2012) as a result of progress in public health initiatives, such as antismoking campaigns, AIDS prevention programs, and cancer screening programs. The leading causes of death have changed from infectious diseases to chronic and degenerative diseases (National Center for Health Statistics [NCHS], 2014). New infectious diseases are emerging, such as the Ebola virus, which affected the United States in 2014, with the first case occurring in Dallas, Texas (CDC, 2014a), and now the Zika virus, which is spread by infected mosquitoes. This virus, which can result in birth defects and Guillain–Barré syndrome, has created a public health emergency throughout the world. All but four states reported cases in 2016 (CDC, 2016).

New treatments for infectious diseases have resulted in steady declines in mortality among children, but such declines depend on parents' participation in immunization programs. A recent measles outbreak in Orange County, California, shows that continuous focus on control of infectious diseases is essential (Orange County Health Care Agency, 2014). The mortality for older Americans has also declined. However, people 50 years of age and older have higher rates of chronic and degenerative illness than other age groups, and they use a larger portion of health care services.

SOCIAL AND ECONOMIC TRENDS

In addition to the size and changing age distribution of the population, other factors also affect the health care system. Several social trends that influence health care include changing lifestyles, a growing appreciation for the quality of life, the changing composition of families and living patterns, changing household incomes, and a revised definition of quality health care.

Americans spend considerable money on health care, nutrition, and fitness (BLS, 2012) because health is seen as an irreplaceable commodity. To be healthy, people must take care of themselves. Many people combine traditional medical and health care practices with complementary and alternative therapies to achieve the highest level of health. Complementary therapies are those that are used in addition to traditional health care, and alternative therapies are those that are used instead of traditional care. Examples include acupuncture and herbal medications, among others (National Center for Complementary and Alternative Medicine [NCCAM], 2014). People often spend a considerable amount of their own money for these types of therapies because few are covered by insurance. In recent years, some insurance plans have recognized the value of complementary therapies and have reimbursed for them. State offices of insurance are good sources to determine whether these services are covered and by which health insurance plans.

Approximately 65 years ago, income was distributed in such a way that a relatively small portion of households earned high incomes; families in the middle-income range made up a somewhat larger proportion, and households at the lower end of the income scale made up the largest proportion. By the 1970s, household income had risen, and income was more evenly distributed, largely as a result of dual-income families.

From 1970 through 2011, several trends in income distribution emerged. The economic downturn now known as the Great Recession, which began in 2008, resulted in layoffs, outsourcing, and other economic changes, with many families seeing decreases in wages. From 2011 through 2015, the average per-person income in the United States increased. The income of households in the top 1% of earners grew by 200%, compared with growth of 67% for the next 18%, growth of 40% for 60% of middle-income households, and 48% growth for the bottom 20% of households (Congressional Budget Office [CBO], 2016). It is obvious that the gap between the richest and the poorest is widening because of the evident differences in the wage-increase percentages of the higher-income levels. Chapter 8 provides a detailed discussion of the economics of health care and how financial constraints influence decisions about public health services.

HEALTH WORKFORCE TRENDS

The health care workforce ebbs and flows. The early years of the 21st century saw the beginning of what is expected to be a long-term and sizable nursing shortage. Similarly, most other health professionals are documenting current and anticipated future shortages. Historically, nursing care has been provided in a variety of settings, primarily in the hospital. Approximately 63% of all registered nurses (RNs) continue to be employed in hospitals (National Center for Health Workforce Analysis, 2013). A few years ago hospitals began reducing their bed capacities as care became more community based. Now they are expanding, including the construction of new facilities for both acute and longer-term chronic care. This growth is attributable to the factors previously discussed: the ability to treat and perhaps cure more diseases, the complexity of the care and the need for inpatient services, and the growth of the older age group.

The nursing shortage has been discussed in recent years, yet new graduates often have difficulty finding positions when they graduate (American Association of Colleges of Nursing [AACN], 2014a, 2014b, 2014c). Participating in a nurse internship program and holding a bachelor of science in nursing (BSN) degree or higher will provide more opportunities for the new graduate. In 2014, the BLS predicted there would be 527,000 new nursing positions by 2016 (BLS, 2014b). In addition, 55% of nurses reported in a recent survey that they intended to retire between 2011 and 2020, which will open positions for others (National Council of State Boards of Nursing [NCSBN], 2013).

Periodic shortages are especially common in the primary-care workforce in the United States, and nurse practitioners (NPs), clinical nurse specialists (CNSs), and certified nurse-midwives (CNMs), who are considered to be practitioners of advanced-practice nursing (APN) specialties, are vital members of primary-care teams. However, as the baby boomers age, there are projections for increasing RN needs in the workforce through 2022 (AACN, 2016)

In terms of the nursing workforce, increasing the number of minority nurses remains a priority and a strategy for addressing the current nursing shortage. In 2013 minority nurses represented approximately 22% of the RN population. It is thought that increasing the minority population will help close the health-disparity gap for minority populations (AACN, 2014b). For example, persons from minority groups, especially when language is a barrier, often are more comfortable with and more likely to access care from a provider from their own minority group.

TECHNOLOGICAL TRENDS

The development and refinement of new technologies such as telehealth have opened up new clinical opportunities for nurses and their clients, especially in the areas of managing chronic conditions, assisting persons who live in rural areas, and providing home health care, rehabilitation, and long-term care. On the positive side, technological advances promise improved health care services, reduced costs, and more convenience in terms of time and travel for consumers. Reduced costs result from a more efficient means of delivering care and from replacement of people with machines. Advanced technology also reduces paperwork; enables providers, clients, and agencies to access accurate information; facilitates care coordination and safety; and provides direct access to health records between agencies and to clients (Health Information Technology, 2013). Contradictory as it may seem, cost is also the most significant negative aspect of advanced health care technology. The more high-technology equipment and computer programs become available, the more

QSEN FOCUS ON QUALITY AND SAFETY EDUCATION FOR NURSES

Targeted Competency: Informatics—Use information and technology to communicate, manage knowledge, mitigate error, and support decision making. Important aspects of informatics include the following:

Knowledge: Identify essential information that must be available in a common database to support interventions in the health care system.

Skills: Use information management tools to monitor outcomes of intervention processes.

Attitudes: Value technologies that support decision making, error prevention, and case coordination.

Informatics Question: Updated informatics definitions focus on having access to the necessary client and system information at the right time, to make the best clinical decision. In the *Strategic Plan for 2010 to 2015* of the US Department of Health and Human Services (USDHHS), there are five overarching goals. *Goal 1, Objective C* focuses on "Emphasizing primary and preventive care linked with community prevention services." Which community data would a public health nurse assess to determine the work that needs to be done in a community related to this USDHHS strategic goal?

Answer: To assess future work that could be done to effectively address Goal 1, Objective C, public health nurses might gather data in the following areas:

- How informed are members of the community about existing community services that support health promotion (e.g., exercise classes, educational classes, self-management training, and nutrition counseling)?
- How relevant are the services offered by health centers to the needs of a community?
- Do payment or insurance barriers exist for individuals to access preventive health services?
- How accessible is entry to care for vulnerable populations such as pregnant women and infants?
- What community-based prevention programs exist for individuals with and at risk for chronic diseases and conditions?
- How available are substance-abuse screening and intervention programs?
- How linked are primary care and health promotions and wellness programs in a community?

Prepared by Gail Armstrong, PhD(c), DNP, ACNS-BC, CNE, Associate Professor, University of Colorado Denver College of Nursing.

they are used. High-technology equipment is expensive, quickly becomes outdated when newer developments occur, and often requires highly trained personnel. There are other drawbacks to new technology, particularly in the area of home health care. These include increased legal liability, the potential for decreased privacy, too much reliance on technological advances, and the inconsistent quality of resources available on the Internet and other sources, like magazines and newspapers (Palma, 2014).

Advances in health care technology will continue. One example of an effective use of technology is the funding provided to health centers by the Health Resources and Services Administration (HRSA) of the US Department of Health and Human Services so that they can adopt and implement electronic health records (EHRs) and other health information technology (HIT) (HRSA, 2008). The HRSA's Office of Health Information Technology was created in 2005 to promote the effective use of HIT as a mechanism for responding to the needs of the uninsured, underinsured, and special-needs populations (HRSA, 2014). Specifically, in December 2012, an award of more than $18 million made available through the Affordable Care Act was announced to expand HIT in 600 health centers (HRSA, 2012). One innovative use of the EHR in public health is to embed reminders or guidelines into the system. For example, the CDC published health guidelines that contain clinical recommendations for screening, prevention, diagnosis, and treatment. To find and keep current on these guidelines, clinicians must visit the CDC website. The availability of an EHR system allows the embedding of reminders so that the clinician can have access to practice guidelines at the point of care. Some additional benefits in public health (and these are some of the uses health centers make of such records) include the following:

- 24-hour availability of records, with downloadable laboratory results and up-to-date assessments
- Coordination of referrals and facilitation of interprofessional care in chronic disease management
- Incorporation of protocol reminders for prevention, screening, and management of chronic disease
- Improvement of quality measurement and monitoring
- Increased client safety and decline in medication errors

Two federal programs, Medicaid and the State Children's Health Insurance Program (SCHIP), have effectively used HIT in several key functions, including outreach and enrollment, service delivery, and care management, in addition to communications with families and the broader goals of program planning and improvement. In early 2009, the Surgeon General's Office reopened a website that had been tried first in 2004 but then closed: My Family Health Portrait, which helps the user to create an electronic family tree (National Institutes of Health [NIH], 2010). This is described as an easy-to-use computer application that allows the user to keep a personal record of family health history (https://familyhistory.hhs.gov/FHH/html/index.html). In addition, the CDC recently began a family history public health initiative through the Office of Public Health Genomics to increase awareness of family history as an important risk factor for common chronic diseases. This initiative had four main activities:

1. Research to define, measure, and assess family history in populations and individuals
2. Development and evaluation of tools for collecting family history
3. Evaluation of the effectiveness of strategies based on family history
4. Promotion of evidence-based applications of family history to health professionals and the public (CDC, 2013b)

CURRENT HEALTH CARE SYSTEM IN THE UNITED STATES

Despite the many advances and the sophistication of the US health care system, the system has been plagued with problems related to cost, access, and quality. These problems are different for each person and are affected by the ability of individuals to obtain health insurance. Most industrialized countries want the same things from their health care system; several give their government a greater role in health care delivery and eliminate or reduce the use of market forces to control cost, access, and quality. Seemingly, there is no one perfect health care system in the world.

COST

Beginning in 2008, a historic weakening of the national and global economy—the Great Recession—led to the loss of 7 million jobs in the United States (Economic Report, 2010). Even as the gross domestic product (GDP), an indicator of the economic health of a country, declined in 2009, health care spending continued to grow and reached $2.5 trillion in the same year (Truffer et al, 2010). In the years between 2010 and 2019, national health spending is expected to grow at an average annual rate of 6.1%, reaching $4.5 trillion by 2019, for a share of approximately 19.3% of the GDP. This translates into a projected increase in per-capita spending.

In Chapter 8, additional discussion illustrates how health care dollars are spent. The largest share of health care expenditures goes to pay for hospital care, with physician services being the next largest item. The amount of money that has gone to pay for public health services is much lower than that for the other categories of expenditures. Other significant drivers of the increasingly high cost of health care include prescription drugs, technology, and chronic and degenerative diseases.

The economic rebound following the Great Recession will likely continue with the increasing Medicare enrollment of the aging baby-boomer population. It is projected that these new Medicare enrollees will increase Medicare expenditures for the foreseeable future. The number of Medicaid recipients can be expected to decline as jobs are added to the economy, and the percentage of workers covered by employer-sponsored insurance rises to reflect that growth. For the first time since 2008, unemployment rates in 2016 dropped to less than 5% of the working population (BLS, 2016).

Although workers' salaries have not kept pace, employer-sponsored insurance premiums have grown 119% since 1999 (Kaiser Family Foundation, 2015a), and the inability of workers to pay this increased cost has led to a rise in the percentage of working families who are uninsured. It will be essential for nurses to keep abreast of any changes in these facts as the Affordable Care Act undergoes reevaluation in the years ahead (Cox et al, 2015).

ACCESS

Another significant problem is poor access to health care. The American health care system is described as a two-class system: private and public. People with insurance or those who can personally pay for health care are viewed as receiving superior care; those who receive lower-quality care are (1) those whose only source of care depends on public funds or (2) the working poor, who do not qualify for public funds either because they make too much money to qualify or because they are illegal immigrants. Employment-provided health care is tied to both the economy and to changes in health insurance premiums. One study found that in 2009, 61% of the nonelderly population obtained employer-sponsored health insurance as a benefit; however, employment did not guarantee insurance (Rowland et al, 2009). This became clear when considering that 9 in 10 (91%) of the middle-class uninsured came from families with at least one full-time worker in jobs that did not offer health insurance or where coverage was unaffordable (Rowland et al, 2009).

Issues with Childhood Dental Caries

Public health nurses who worked with local Head Start programs noted that many children had untreated dental caries. Although these children qualified for Medicaid, only two dentists in the area would accept appointments from Medicaid patients. Dentists asserted that Medicaid patients frequently did not show up for their appointments and that reimbursement was too low compared with that from other third-party payers. They also said the children's behavior made it difficult to work with them. So, the waiting list for local dental care was approximately 6 years long. Although some nurses found ways to transport clients to dentists in a city 70 miles away, it was very time consuming and was feasible for only a small fraction of the clients. When decayed teeth abscessed, it was possible to get extractions from the local medical center. The health department dentist also saw children, but he, too, was booked for years in advance.

Created by Deborah C. Conway, Assistant Professor, University of Virginia School of Nursing.

In 2012, the total number of uninsured persons in the United States was 48 million. As discussed, there is a strong relationship between health insurance coverage and access to health care services. Insurance status determines the amount and kind of health care people are able to afford and where they can receive care. As a result of the Affordable Care Act, by 2014, the uninsured nonelderly population had dropped to 32 million people, approximately 16% of the total population. During this same time period, 58% of the total population was covered by employer health insurance. Others, such as the elderly and the Medicaid-eligible populations, were covered by government insurance programs (Kaiser Family Foundation, 2015b).

The uninsured receive less preventive care and are diagnosed at more advanced disease states; once diagnosed, they tend to receive less therapeutic care in terms of surgery and treatment options. There is a safety net for the uninsured or underinsured. As discussed later in this chapter, there are more than 1300 federally funded community health centers throughout the country. Federally funded community health centers provide a broad range of health and social services, which are delivered by NPs, RNs, physician assistants, physicians, social workers, and dentists. Community health centers are primarily located in medically underserved areas, which can be rural or urban. These centers serve people of all ages, races, and ethnicities, with or without health insurance.

QUALITY

The quality of health care leaped to the forefront of concern following the 1999 release of the Institute of Medicine (IOM) report *To Err Is Human: Building a Safer Health System* (IOM, 2000). As indicated in this groundbreaking report, as many as 98,000 deaths a year could be attributed to preventable medical errors. Some of the untoward events categorized in this report included adverse drug events and improper transfusions, surgical injuries and wrong-site surgery, suicides, restraint-related injuries or death, falls, burns, pressure ulcers, and mistaken client identities. It was further determined that high rates of errors with serious consequences were most likely to occur in intensive care units, operating rooms, and emergency departments. Beyond the cost in human lives, preventable medical errors result in the loss of several billions of dollars annually in hospitals nationwide. Categories of error include diagnostic, treatment, and prevention errors and communication, equipment, and other system failures. Significant to nurses, the IOM estimated that the number of lives lost to preventable errors in medication alone represented more than 7000 deaths annually, with a cost of about $2 billion nationwide.

Although the IOM report made it clear that the majority of medical errors were not produced by provider negligence, lack of education, or lack of training, questions were raised about the nurse's role and workload and their effects on client safety. In a follow-up report, *Keeping Patients Safe: Transforming the Work Environment of Nurses,* the IOM (2003) stated that nurses' long work hours pose a serious threat to patient safety because fatigue slows reaction time, saps energy, and diminishes attention to detail. The group called for state regulators to pass laws barring nurses from working more than 12 hours a day and 60 hours a week—even if by choice (IOM, 2003). Although this information is largely related to acute care, many of the patients who survive medical errors are later cared for in the community.

The culture of quality improvement and safety has made providers and consumers more conscious of safety, but medical errors and untoward events continue to occur. As a means to improve consumer awareness of hospital quality, the Centers for Medicare and Medicaid Services (CMS) began publishing a database of hospital quality measures, Hospital Compare, in 2005. Hospital Compare, a consumer-oriented website that provides information on how well hospitals provide recommended care in such areas as heart attack, heart failure, and pneumonia, is available through the CMS website (www.cms.gov). In a further effort, the CMS announced in 2008 that it would no longer reimburse hospitals, under Medicare guidelines, for care provided for "preventable complications," such as hospital-acquired infections. This reimbursement policy was extended to Medicaid reimbursement in 2011 (CMS, 2009; Galewitz, 2011).

The accreditation process for public health is new, and the impact of quality and safety monitoring has not yet been determined. The ability of a public health agency or a community to respond to community disasters is one event that will be monitored in the accreditation process. In May 2016, 135 of 303 local, tribal, and state centralized integration systems and multijurisdictional health departments had received accreditation in this new process. The accredited health departments served 167 million people, amounting to 54% of the total population base. The aims of this process are as follows:
- To assist and identify quality health departments to improve performance and quality and to develop leadership
- To improve management
- To improve community relationships (Public Health Accreditation Board [PHAB], 2016)

ORGANIZATION OF THE CURRENT HEALTH CARE SYSTEM

An enormous number and range of facilities and providers make up the health care system. These include physicians' and dentists' offices, hospitals, nursing homes, mental health facilities, ambulatory care centers, freestanding clinics and clinics inside stores such as drugstores, free clinics, public health agencies, and home health agencies. Providers include nurses, advanced-practice nurses, physicians and physician assistants, dentists and dental hygienists, pharmacists, and a wide array of essential allied health providers, such as physical, occupational, and recreational therapists; nutritionists; social workers; and a range of technicians. In general, however, the American health care system is divided into the following two, somewhat distinct, components: a private or personal care component and a public health component. These components have some overlap, as discussed in the following sections. It is important to discuss primary health care and examine the interest in developing a primary-care system.

PRIMARY-CARE SYSTEM

Primary care, the first level of the private health care system, is delivered in a variety of community settings, such as physicians' offices, urgent-care centers, in-store clinics, community health centers, and community nursing centers. Near the end of the past century, in an attempt to contain costs, the number of managed-care organizations grew. Managed care is defined as a system in which care is delivered by a specific network of providers that agree to comply with the care approaches established through a case-management approach. The key factors are a specified network of providers and the use of a gatekeeper to control access to providers and services. This form of care has not become as prominent as the original concept outlined.

The government tried to reap the benefits of cost savings by introducing the managed-care model into Medicare and Medicaid, with varying levels of success. The traditional Medicare plan involves Parts A and B. Part C, the Medicare Advantage program, incorporates private insurance plans into the Medicare program, including health maintenance organization (HMO) and preferred provider organization (PPO) managed-care models and private fee-for-service plans. In addition, Medicare Part D has been added to cover prescriptions (see Chapter 8).

PUBLIC HEALTH SYSTEM

The public health system is mandated through laws that are developed at the national, state, or local level. Examples of public health laws instituted to protect the health of the community include a law mandating immunizations for all children entering kindergarten and a law requiring constant monitoring of the local water supply. The public health system is organized into many levels in the federal, state, and local systems. At the local level, health departments provide care that is mandated by state and federal regulations.

THE FEDERAL SYSTEM

The US Department of Health and Human Services (USDHHS, or simply HHS) is the agency most heavily involved with the health and welfare concerns of US citizens. The organizational chart of the HHS (Fig. 3.1) shows the office of the secretary, 11

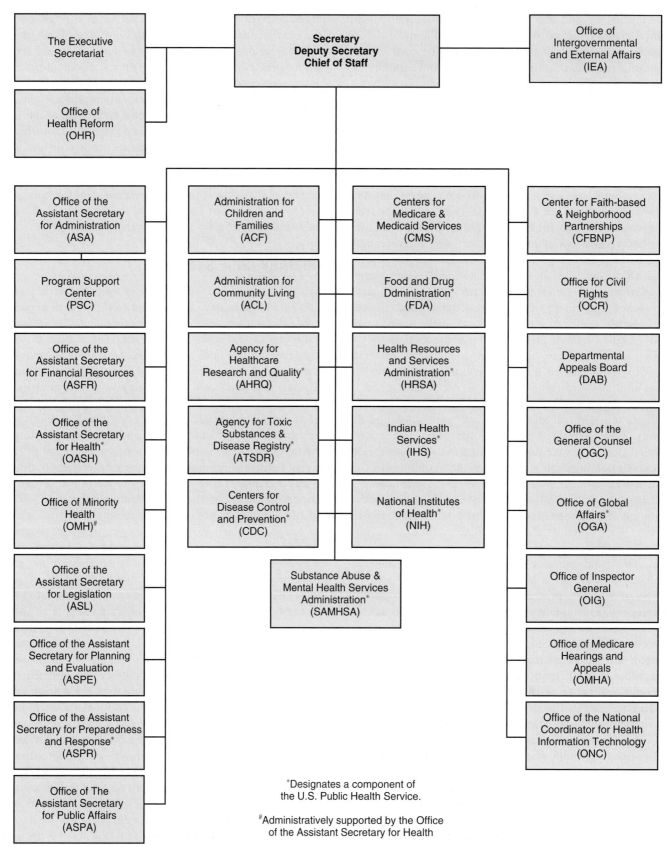

FIG. 3.1 Organization of the US Department of Health and Human Services. (From US Department of Health and Human Services, HHS Organizational Chart, http://www.hhs.gov/about/orgchart/.)

BOX 3.2   USDHHS Strategic Plan Goals and Objectives—Fiscal Years 2010 to 2015*

GOAL 1: Strengthen Health Care

Objective A	Make coverage more secure for those who have insurance, and extend affordable coverage to the uninsured.
Objective B	Improve health care quality and patient safety.
Objective C	Emphasize primary and preventive care linked with community prevention services.
Objective D	Reduce the growth of health care costs while promoting high-value, effective care.
Objective E	Ensure access to quality, culturally competent care for vulnerable populations.
Objective F	Promote the adoption and meaningful use of health information technology.

GOAL 2: Advance Scientific Knowledge and Innovation

Objective A	Accelerate the process of scientific discovery to improve patient care.
Objective B	Foster innovation to create shared solutions.
Objective C	Invest in the regulatory sciences to improve food and medical product safety.
Objective D	Increase our understanding of what works in public health and human service practice.

GOAL 3: Advance the Health, Safety, and Well-Being of the American People

Objective A	Promote the safety, well-being, resilience, and healthy development of children and youth.
Objective B	Promote economic and social well-being for individuals, families, and communities.
Objective C	Improve the accessibility and quality of supportive services for people with disabilities and older adults.
Objective D	Promote prevention and wellness.
Objective E	Reduce the occurrence of infectious diseases.
Objective F	Protect Americans' health and safety during emergencies, and foster resilience in response to emergencies.

GOAL 4: Increase Efficiency, Transparency, Accountability and Effectiveness of HHS Programs

Objective A	Ensure program integrity and responsible stewardship of resources.
Objective B	Fight fraud and work to eliminate improper payments.
Objective C	Use HHS data to improve the health and well-being of the American people.
Objective D	Improve HHS environmental, energy, and economic performance to promote sustainability.

GOAL 5: Strengthen the Nation's Health and Human Service Infrastructure and Workforce

Objective A	Invest in the HHS workforce to meet America's health and human service needs today and tomorrow.
Objective B	Ensure that the Nation's health care workforce can meet increased demands.
Objective C	Enhance the ability of the public health workforce to improve public health at home and abroad.
Objective D	Strengthen the Nation's human service workforce.
Objective E	Improve national, state, local, and tribal surveillance and epidemiology capacity.

From the US Department of Health and Human Services, 2014. USDHHS Strategic Plan Goals and Objectives—Fiscal Years 2010 to 2015. Retrieved July 2, 2014, from www.hhs.gov.
*In the process of being updated for 2014–2018.

agencies, and a program support center (USDHHS, 2014a). Ten regional offices are maintained to provide more direct assistance to the states. Their locations are shown in Table 3.1. The HHS is charged with regulating health care and overseeing the health status of Americans. See Box 3.2 for the goals and objectives of the HHS strategic plan for fiscal years 2010 to 2015. Newer areas in the HHS are the Office of Public Health Preparedness, the Center for Faith-Based and Neighborhood Partnerships, and the Office of Global Affairs. The Office of Public Health Preparedness was added to assist the nation and states to prepare for bioterrorism after September 11, 2001. The Faith-Based Initiative Center was developed by President George W. Bush to allow faith communities to compete for federal money to support their community activities. The goal of the Office of Global Affairs is to promote global health by coordinating HHS strategies and programs with other governments and international organizations (USDHHS, 2014a). The activities of several key agencies include the following:

1. The US Public Health Service (USPHS, or simply PHS) is a major component of the DHHS. The PHS consists of eight agencies: Agency for Healthcare Research and Quality,

Agency for Toxic Substances and Diseases Registry, Centers for Disease Control and Prevention, Food and Drug Administration, Health Resources and Services Administration, Indian Health Service, National Institutes of Health, and Substance Abuse and Mental Health Services Administration. Each has a specific purpose (see Chapter 8 for a discussion of the relevancy of the agencies to policy and the provision of health care). The PHS also has a Commissioned Corps, the National Health Services Corp (NHSC), which is a uniformed service of more than 6500 health professionals who serve in many HHS and other federal agencies. The surgeon general of the United States is the head of the Commissioned Corps. The corps fills essential services for public health clinics and provides leadership within the federal government departments and agencies to support the care of underserved and vulnerable populations (USPHS, 2014).

2. An important agency and a recent addition to the federal government, the US Department of Homeland Security (USDHS, or simply DHS), was created in 2003 (USDHS, 2014). The

TABLE 3.1   Regional Offices of the U.S. Department of Health and Human Services

Region	Location	Territory
1	Boston	Connecticut, Maine, Massachusetts, New Hampshire, Rhode Island, Vermont
2	New York	New Jersey, New York, Puerto Rico, Virgin Islands
3	Philadelphia	Delaware, District of Columbia, Maryland, Pennsylvania, Virginia, West Virginia
4	Atlanta	Alabama, Florida, Georgia, Kentucky, Mississippi, North Carolina, South Carolina, Tennessee
5	Chicago	Illinois, Indiana, Michigan, Minnesota, Ohio, Wisconsin
6	Dallas	Arkansas, Louisiana, New Mexico, Oklahoma, Texas
7	Kansas City	Iowa, Kansas, Missouri, Nebraska
8	Denver	Colorado, Montana, North Dakota, South Dakota, Utah, Wyoming
9	San Francisco	Arizona, California, Hawaii, Nevada, American Samoa, Commonwealth of the Northern Mariana Islands, Federated States of Micronesia, Guam, Republic of the Marshall Islands, Republic of Palau
10	Seattle	Alaska, Idaho, Oregon, Washington

Data from US Department of Health and Human Services: *HHS Regional Offices,* Retrieved December 2014 from http://www.hhs.gov/about/regions/

 LEVELS OF PREVENTION

Related to the Public Health Care System

Primary Prevention

Implement a community-level program, such as walking for exercise, to assist citizens in improving health behaviors related to lifestyle.

Secondary Prevention

Implement a family-planning program to prevent unintended pregnancies among young couples who attend the local community health center.

Tertiary Prevention

Provide a self-management asthma program for children with chronic asthma to reduce their need for hospitalization.

---

mission of the DHS is to prevent and deter terrorist attacks and protect against and respond to threats and hazards to the nation. The goals for the department include awareness, prevention, protection, response, and recovery. The DHS works with first responders throughout the United States, and through the development of programs such as the Community Emergency Response Team (CERT), it trains people to be better prepared to respond to emergency situations in their communities. Nurses working in state and local public health departments and those employed in hospitals and other health facilities may be called on to respond to acts of terrorism or natural disasters in the course of their careers, and the DHS, along with the Food and Drug Administration (FDA) and CDC, is developing programs to ready nurses and other health care providers for an uncertain future (USDHS, 2014).

THE STATE SYSTEM

When the United States faced a pandemic H1N1 flu outbreak in 2009, the federal government and the public health community quickly prepared to meet the challenge of educating the public and health professionals about the flu and making vaccinations available. In 2014 public health efforts within the states were responding to an enterovirus affecting large numbers of children with symptoms of upper respiratory disease and weakness in the arms and legs. The virus was considered life-threatening (CDC, 2014b). In addition to standing ready for disaster prevention or response, state health departments have other equally

important functions, such as providing health care financing and administration for programs such as Medicaid, providing mental health and professional education, establishing health codes, licensing facilities and personnel, and regulating the insurance industry. State systems also have an important role in direct assistance to local health departments, including ongoing assessment of health needs.

Nurses serve in many capacities in state health departments; they are consultants, direct-service providers, researchers, teachers, and supervisors. They also participate in program development, planning, and the evaluation of health programs.

THE LOCAL SYSTEM

The local health department has direct responsibility to the citizens in its community or jurisdiction. Services and programs offered by local health departments vary depending on the state and local health codes that must be followed, the needs of the community, and available funding and other resources. For example, one health department might be more involved with public health education programs and environmental issues, whereas another health department might emphasize direct client care. Local health departments vary in providing sick care or even primary care. More often than at other levels of government, public health nurses at the local level provide population health and direct services. Some of these nurses deliver special or selected services, such as following up on contacts in cases of tuberculosis or venereal disease or providing child immunization clinics. Others provide more general care, delivering services to families in certain geographical areas. This method of delivery of nursing services involves broader needs and a wider variety of nursing interventions. The local level often provides an opportunity for nurses to take on significant leadership roles, with many nurses serving as directors or managers.

Since the tragedy of September 11, 2001, state and local health departments have increasingly focused on emergency preparedness and response. In case of an event, state and local health departments in the affected area will be expected to collect data and accurately report the situation, to respond appropriately to any type of emergency, and to ensure the safety of the residents of the immediate area while protecting those just outside the danger zone. This level of knowledge—to enable public health agencies to anticipate, prepare for, recognize, and respond to terrorist threats or natural disasters such as hurricanes or floods—has required a level of interstate and federal–local planning and cooperation that is unprecedented for these agencies. Whether participating in disaster drills or preparing a local high school for use as a shelter, nurses play a major role in meeting the challenge of an uncertain future.

FORCES INFLUENCING CHANGES IN THE HEALTH CARE SYSTEM

Although most people are personally satisfied with their own physicians or nurse practitioners, at present, few people are satisfied with the health care system in general. Costs have been high and have continued to rise while quality and access have been uneven across the country and within communities, depending on the ability to pay. What, then, are some of the factors that might influence health care to change? First, as a nation, citizens must decide what has to be provided for all people, who will be in charge of the system, and who will pay for what. In recent years, federal and state services have been reduced, and more responsibility for health care delivery has been moved to the private sector. Health care has become big business. Health care company stocks are now traded on major stock exchanges, directors receive benefits when profits are high, and the locus of control has shifted from the provider to the payer. Many competing forces have influenced the changing design of the health care system, some of which are consumers, employers (purchasers), care delivery systems, and state and federal legislation.

First, consumers want lower costs and high-quality health care without limits and with an improved ability to choose the providers of their choice. Second, employers (purchasers of health care) want to be able to obtain basic health care plans at reasonable costs for their employees. Many employers have seen their profits diminish as they put more money into providing adequate health care coverage for employees. Third, health care systems want a better balance between consumer and purchaser demands. Thus they continually watch their own budgets and expenses. To maintain a profit while providing quality care, many health care delivery groups have downsized and created alliances, mergers, and other joint ventures. Finally, legislation, especially concerning access and quality, continues to be enacted, thus creating one more force helping to shape the health care system. The goal of "evidence-based care" is to ensure quality.

Many have said that solving the health care crisis requires the institution of a rational health care system that balances equity, cost, and quality. The fact that millions of people have been uninsured, that wide disparities have existed in access, and that a large proportion of deaths each year seem attributable to preventable causes (e.g., errors, tobacco use, alcohol abuse, preventable injuries, and obesity), has indicated that the American system is currently not serving the best interests of the American population. WHO has suggested that integrating primary care and public health into a primary health care system will be the basis for better health for all world citizens (WHO, 1986a).

INTEGRATION OF PUBLIC HEALTH AND THE PRIMARY-CARE SYSTEM

Although primary care and public health share the goal of promoting the health and well-being of all people, these two disciplines historically have operated independently of each other. Problems that stem from this separation have long been recognized, but new opportunities are emerging for bringing these systems together to promote lasting improvements in the health of individuals, communities, and populations (IOM, 2012).

In recognition of this potential, the CDC and the HRSA, both agencies of the DHHS, asked the IOM to convene a committee of experts, including input from nursing, to examine the integration of primary care and public health (IOM, 2012).

To recognize the differences in these two systems, definitions were used to guide the work of the experts. Primary care was defined as "the providing of integrated, accessible health care services by clinicians who are accountable for addressing a large majority of personal health care needs, while developing partnerships with patients and practicing in the context of family and community" (IOM, 1996, p. 1). Public health was defined as "fulfilling society's interest in assuring conditions in which people can be healthy" (IOM, 1988, p. 140). The purpose of the integration is to achieve the WHO goal of primary health care.

❓ CHECK YOUR PRACTICE

You are working in a community health center, which is designed to offer both primary care and public health services to improve the health of the population in the geographical location of the center. Identify barriers to your practice as a nurse as you work to integrate these services in your practice.

POTENTIAL BARRIERS TO INTEGRATION

Contrasting the two systems, primary care, which can be either a public or a private entity, is person focused, provides a point of first contact for individuals to address health problems, is considered comprehensive, and provides coordination of individual care; public health can also be delivered through public and private entities to contribute to the health of society, but government plays a major role in public health. Health departments are legally bound to provide essential public health services and to work with the total community and multiple stakeholders to address community-level health problems. Public health also has specific functions of assurance, assessment, and policy development to address community-level health issues and has a charge to create healthy communities (see Chapter 1).

In addition to differing roles and functions and issues related to funding, different clients and different foci will need to be addressed to form a solid foundation for a partnership. Primary care is largely funded through individual client payments, health insurance, and sometimes through federal grants. Public health is largely funded through tax dollars, federal and state grants, and sometimes health insurance payments through Medicare and Medicaid. Primary care serves the individuals who present to the practice, while public health serves to assess population health problems. Both focus on meeting the most prevalent health needs of the population. Primary care focuses more on the curative aspect of care, while public health focuses more on the prevention of health problems (Levesque et al, 2013).

The common goal of both public health and primary care, although these systems operate independently, is to ensure a healthier population. The committee of experts convened by the IOM (2012) noted that integration of these two systems has the potential to produce a greater impact on the health of populations than either could have when working alone.

The *Healthy People* initiatives, beginning with the US Surgeon General's 1979 report, indicate the long-standing desire to improve population health in the United States.

PRIMARY HEALTH CARE

Primary health care (PHC), the goal of the integration of public health and primary care, includes a comprehensive range of services, including public health and preventive, diagnostic, therapeutic, and rehabilitative services. This system is composed of public health agencies, community-based agencies and primary-care clinics, and health care providers. From a conceptual point of view, PHC is essential care made universally accessible to individuals, families, and the community. Health care is made available to them with their full participation and is provided at a cost that the community and country can afford. This care is not uniformly available and accessible to all people in many countries, including the United States. Full community participation means that individuals within the community help in defining health problems and in developing approaches to address the problems. The setting for primary health care is within all communities of a country, and it involves all aspects of society (WHO, 1978).

The primary health care movement officially began in 1977 when the 30th WHO Health Assembly adopted a resolution accepting the goal of attaining a level of health that permitted all citizens of the world to live socially and economically productive lives. At the international conference in 1978 in Alma-Ata, in the former Soviet Union (currently Almaty, in Kazakhstan), it was determined that this goal was to be met through PHC. This resolution, the Declaration of Alma-Ata, became known by the slogan "Health for All [HFA] by the Year 2000," which captured the official health target for all the member nations of WHO. In 1998 the program was adapted to meet the needs of the new century and was deemed "Health for All in the 21st Century."

In 1981 WHO established global indicators for monitoring and evaluating the achievement of HFA. In the *World Health Statistics Annual* (WHO, 1986b), these indicators are grouped into the following four categories:
- Health policies
- Social and economic development
- Provision of health care
- Health status

The indicators suggest that health improvements are a result of efforts in many areas, including agriculture, industry, education, housing, communications, and health care. Because PHC is as much a political statement as a system of care, each United Nations member country interprets PHC according to its own culture, health needs, resources, and system of government. Clearly, the goal of PHC has not been met in most countries, including the United States.

PROMOTING HEALTH/PREVENTING DISEASE: YEAR 2020 OBJECTIVES FOR THE NATION

As a WHO member nation, the United States has endorsed primary health care as a strategy for achieving the goal of "Health for All in the 21st Century." However, the PHC emphasis on broad strategies, community participation, self-reliance, and a multidisciplinary health care delivery team is not the primary strategy for improving the health of the American people. The national health plan for the United States identifies disease prevention and health promotion as the areas of most concern in the nation. Each decade since the 1980s has been measured and tracked according to health objectives set at the beginning of the decade. The PHS of the DHHS publishes the objectives after gathering data from health professionals and organizations throughout the country.

Healthy People 2020, which was officially launched in December 2010 (USDHHS, 2010a), is composed of a large number of objectives related to 42 topic areas. These objectives are designed to serve as a road map for improving the health of all people in the United States during the second decade of the 21st century. These objectives are described by four main goals (USDHHS, 2010b):
- Attain high-quality, longer lives free of preventable disease, disability, injury, and premature death.
- Achieve health equity, eliminate disparities, and improve the health of all groups.
- Create social and physical environments that promote good health for all.
- Promote quality of life, healthy development, and healthy behaviors across all life stages.

These goals provide the framework with which measurable health indicators can be tracked. The emphasis on the social and physical environment moves *Healthy People 2020* from the traditional disease-specific focus to a more holistic view of health consistent with a public health frame of reference (*Healthy People 2020*, 2012). This in turn will encourage public health nurses to broaden their scope to all aspects of their clients' lives that may need assessment and intervention, including where they live, the condition of their homes, and how the appropriateness of the home environment may change as clients age. The *Healthy People 2020* box presents indicators of *Healthy People 2020* related to the strengthening of the public health infrastructure. These objectives will assist nurses in having data to show that their assessments and interventions are changing practice.

♥ HEALTHY PEOPLE 2020

Selected Objectives That Pertain to Strengthening the Public Health Infrastructure

- **PHI-7** (Developmental): Increase the proportion of population-based *Healthy People 2020* objectives for which national data are available for all major population groups.
- **PHI-8**: Increase the proportion of *Healthy People 2020* objectives that are tracked regularly at the national level.

From US Department of Health and Human Services. Healthy People 2020. Available at http://www.healthypeople.gov Accessed December 27, 2010.

⟩ APPLYING CONTENT TO PRACTICE

Discussions and debates will continue about the impact of the ACA and the IOM's discussions of integrating public health and primary care, reducing cost, and increasing quality and access for all Americans. It is important not to lose sight of the goal: to protect and improve the health of all populations. After spending 18 months in a public policy fellowship and working with the Ways and Means Committee in Congress, Nancy Ridenour, PhD, RN, and dean of the College of Nursing at the University of New Mexico, described her opportunity to work with others as the ACA was being developed. At a board of nursing celebration in Kentucky in the summer of 2014, Dr. Ridenour

explained to the audience that it would be important for nurses to be involved in the implementation of the ACA to promote the success of the health care changes proposed. It is all about the influence of nurses and the nursing profession (Kentucky Board of Nursing, 2014). Focus efforts on the implementation of the key features of the ACA (Table 3.2) in work with individual clients and populations in your community. An example of this application would be working with families to encourage enrolling children in the state child health insurance programs to assure that the family's children will receive preventive and primary care as needed.

TABLE 3.2 Overview of Key Features of the Affordable Care Act by Year

2010

New Consumer Protections
- Putting information for consumers online
- Prohibiting denial of coverage of children based on preexisting conditions
- Prohibiting insurance companies from rescinding coverage
- Eliminating lifetime limits on insurance coverage
- Regulating annual limits on insurance coverage
- Establishing consumer assistance programs in the states

Improving Quality and Lowering Costs
- Providing small business health insurance tax credits
- Offering relief for 4 million seniors who hit the Medicare prescription drug "donut hole"
- Providing free preventive care
- Preventing disease and illness
- Cracking down on health care fraud

Increasing Access to Affordable Care
- Providing access to insurance for uninsured Americans with preexisting conditions
- Extending coverage for young adults
- Expanding coverage for early retirees
- Rebuilding the primary-care workforce
- Holding insurance companies accountable for unreasonable rate hikes
- Allowing states to cover more people on Medicaid
- Increasing payments for rural health care providers
- Strengthening community health centers

2011

Improving Quality and Lowering Costs
- Offering prescription drug discounts
- Providing free preventive care for seniors
- Improving health care quality and efficiency
- Improving care for seniors after they leave the hospital
- Introducing new innovations to bring down costs

Increasing Access to Affordable Care
- Increasing access to services at home and in the community

Holding Insurance Companies Accountable
- Bringing down health care premiums
- Addressing overpayments to big insurance companies and strengthening Medicare Advantage

2012

Improving Quality and Lowering Costs
- Linking payment to quality outcomes
- Encouraging integrated health systems
- Reducing paperwork and administrative costs
- Understanding and fighting health disparities

Increasing Access to Affordable Care
- Providing new, voluntary options for long-term care insurance

2013

Improving Quality and Lowering Costs
- Improving preventive health coverage
- Expanding authority to bundle payments

Increasing Access to Affordable Care
- Increasing Medicaid payments for primary care doctors
- Open enrollment in the health insurance marketplace begins.

2014

New Consumer Protections
- Prohibiting discrimination due to preexisting conditions or gender
- Eliminating annual limits on insurance coverage
- Ensuring coverage for individuals participating in clinical trials

Improving Quality and Lowering Costs
- Making care more affordable
- Establishing the health insurance marketplace
- Increasing the small business tax credit

Increasing Access to Affordable Care
- Increasing access to Medicaid
- Promoting individual responsibility

2015

Improving Quality and Lowering Costs
- Paying physicians based on value, not volume

For more detail about each of the bulleted statements, please refer to HHS.gov/HealthCare (Key Features of the Affordable Care Act, 2014: http://www.hhs.gov/healthcare/facts/timeline/).

PRACTICE APPLICATION

During a well-child clinic visit, Jenna Wells, RN, met Sandra Farr and her 24-month-old daughter, Jessica. The Farrs had recently moved to the community. Mrs. Farr stated that she knew that Jessica needed the last in a series of immunizations, and because they did not have health insurance, she brought her daughter to the public health clinic. On initial assessment, Mrs. Farr told the nurse that her husband would soon be employed, but the family would have no health care coverage for the next 30 days. She also said that they needed to decide which health care package they wanted. Mr. Farr's company offers a PPO, an HMO, and a community nursing clinic plan to all employees. Neither Mr. nor Mrs. Farr has ever used an HMO or a community nursing clinic, and they are not sure what services are provided.

Mrs. Farr asks Nurse Wells what she should do.

Nurse Wells should do which of the following?

A. Encourage Mrs. Farr to choose the HMO because it will pay more attention to the family's preventive needs, and direct Mrs. Farr to other sources of health care should the family need to see a provider while they are uninsured.

B. Encourage Mrs. Farr to choose the PPO because it will have a greater number of qualified providers from which to choose, and direct Mrs. Farr to other sources of health care should the family need to see a provider while they are uninsured.

C. Encourage Mrs. Farr to choose the local community nursing center because it is staffed with nurse practitioners who are well qualified to provide comprehensive health care with an emphasis on health education, and direct Mrs. Farr to other sources of health care should the family need to see a provider while they are uninsured.

D. Explain the differences between a PPO, HMO, and community nursing clinic; encourage Mrs. Farr to discuss the options with her husband about signing up for a health insurance plan under the ACA plans; and direct Mrs. Farr to other sources of health care should the family need to see a provider while they are uninsured.

Answers can be found on the Evolve website.

REMEMBER THIS!

- Health care in the United States is made up of a personal care system and a public health system, with overlap between the two systems.
- Primary care is a personal health care system that provides for first contact and continuous, comprehensive, and coordinated care.
- Primary health care is essential care made universally accessible to individuals and families in a community. Health care is made available to them through their full participation and is provided at a cost that the community and country can afford.
- Primary care and the public health systems are part of primary health care.
- Public health refers to organized community efforts designed to prevent disease and promote health.
- Important trends that affect the health care system include demographic, social, economic, political, and technological trends.
- More than 48 million people in the United States were uninsured in 2012, and many more simply lacked access to adequate health care.
- With the implementation of the Affordable Care Act (ACA), by 2014 the numbers of uninsured dropped to 32 million people.

- Many federal agencies are involved in government health care functions. The agency most directly involved with the health and welfare of Americans is the US Department of Health and Human Services (USDHHS).
- Most state and local jurisdictions have government activities that affect the health care field.
- Health care and insurance reform measures seek to make changes in the cost and quality of and access to the present system, such as the ACA passed in 2010.
- To achieve the specific health goals of programs such as *Healthy People 2020*, primary care and public health must work within the community for community-based care.
- The most sustainable individual and system changes come when people who live in the community have actively participated.
- Nurses are more than able to fill the gap between personal care and public health because they have skills in assessment, health promotion, and disease and injury prevention; knowledge of community resources; and the ability to develop relationships with community members and leaders.
- Nurses are important to the success of the ACA.

EVOLVE WEBSITE

http://evolve.elsevier.com/Stanhope/foundations
- Case Study, with Questions and Answers
- NCLEX® Review Questions
- Practice Application Answers

REFERENCES

American Association of Colleges of Nursing (AACN): *Employment of new nurse graduates and employer preference for baccalaureate-prepared nurses*, Washington, DC, 2014a, AACN. Retrieved June 2016 from http://www.aacn.nche.edu.

American Association of Colleges of Nursing (AACN): *Enhancing diversity in the workforce*, Washington, DC, 2014b, AACN. Retrieved June 2016 from http://www.aacn.nche.edu.

American Association of Colleges of Nursing (AACN): *Nursing shortage*, Washington, DC, 2014c, AACN. Retrieved June 2016 from http://www.aacn.nche.edu.

American Association of Colleges of Nursing (AACN): *Fact Sheet*, Washington, DC, 2016, AACN. Retrieved June 2016 from http://www.aacn.nche.edu.

Bureau of Labor Statistics (BLS), US Department of Labor: *Consumer Price Index—May 2012*, 2012. Retrieved December 2014a from www.bls.gov/cpi/.

Bureau of Labor Statistics (BLS), US Department of Labor: *Employment Situation News Release*, 2014b. Retrieved May 2016 from http://www.bls.gov/news.release.

Bureau of Labor Statistics (BLS), US Department of Labor: *Employment Situation News Release*, 2016. Retrieved May 2016 from http://www.bls.gov/news.release.

Centers for Disease Control and Prevention (CDC): *The state of aging and health in America, 2013*, Atlanta, GA, 2013a, CDC, US Department of Health and Human Services. Retrieved December 2014 from http://www.cdc.gov.

Centers for Disease Control and Prevention (CDC): *Public health genomics: family history public health initiative*, Atlanta, GA, 2013b, CDC, US Department of Health and Human Services.

Centers for Disease Control and Prevention (CDC): *Ebola update, 2014*, Atlanta, GA, 2014a, CDC, US Department of Health and Human Services.

Centers for Disease Control and Prevention (CDC): *Non-polio enterovirus: enterovirus D68*, Atlanta, GA, 2014b, CDC, US Department of Health and Human Services. Retrieved December 2014 from http://www.cdc.gov.

Centers for Disease Control and Prevention (CDC): *Zika virus update in US 2015-16*, Atlanta, GA, 2016, CDC, US Department of Health and Human Services.

Centers for Medicare and Medicaid Services (CMS): *National health expenditure data*, 2008. Retrieved December 2009 from http://www.cms.gov.

Congressional Budget Office (CBO): *Trends in the distribution of household income 2011-2015*, Washington, DC, 2016, CBO. Retrieved June, 2016 from https://www.cbo.gov.

Cox C, Gonzales S, et al: *Analysis of 2016 premium changes in ACA health insurance markets*, Menlo park, CA, 2015, Kaiser Family Foundation. Retrieved May 2016 from http://KaiserFamilyFoundation.org.

Dorn S, Hill I, Hogan S: *The secrets of Massachusetts' success: why 97 percent of state residents have health coverage: state health access reform evaluation, Rommneycare—The truth about Massachusetts health care*, New Jersey, 2014, accessed at mittromneycentral.com, Robert Wood Johnson Foundation. http://www.urban.org. Accessed September 19, 2015.

Economic Report of the President: Washington, DC, 2010, US Government Printing Office. Retrieved December 2014 from http://www.whitehouse.gov.

Galewitz P: *Medicaid to stop paying hospitals for mistakes*, Menlo Park, CA, 2011, Kaiser Health News. Retrieved December 2014 from http://kaiserhealthnews.org.

Hamilton BE, Martin JA, Ventura SJ: Births: preliminary data for 2009, *Natl Vital Stat Rep* 59(3):2010. Atlanta Georgia, Center for Disease Control and prevention. Retrieved December 2014 from www.cdc.gov/nchs.

Health Information Technology: *Information technology in health care. The next consumer revolution*, Rockville MD, 2013, USDHHS. Retrieved Oct 2014 from www.HIT.gov.

Health Resources and Services Administration (HRSA): *HRSA awards $18.9 million to expand use of health information technology at health centers*, Washington, DC, 2008, HRSA, US Department of Health and Human Services. Retrieved December 2014 from http://archive.hrsa.gov.

Health Resources and Services Administration (HRSA): *Affordable Care Act helps expand the use of health information technology*, Washington, DC, 2012, HRSA, US Department of Health and Human Services. Retrieved December 2014 from http://www.hrsa.gov.

Health Resources and Services Administration (HRSA): *What is a health center?* Washington, DC, 2014, HRSA, US Department of Health and Human Services. Retrieved December 2014 from http://bphc.hrsa.gov.

Healthy People 2020: *Brochure with leading health indicators*, 2012. Retrieved at http://www.healthypeople.gov/2020.

Hoyert DL: *75 Years of mortality in the United States, 1935-2010*. National Center for Health Statistics (NCHS) Data Brief No. 88, 2012. Hyattsville, MD, 2012, NCHS. Retrieved December 2014 from http://www.cdc.gov/nchs.

Institute of Medicine (IOM): *The future of public health*, Washington, DC, 1988, National Academies Press.

Institute of Medicine (IOM): *Primary care: America's health in a new era*, Washington, DC, 1996, National Academies Press. Retrieved December 2014 from http://www.nap.edu.

Institute of Medicine (IOM): *To err is human: building a safer health system*, Washington, DC, 2000, National Academies Press. Retrieved December 2014 from http://www.iom.edu.

Institute of Medicine (IOM): *Keeping patients safe: transforming the work environment of nurses*, Washington, DC, 2003, National Academies Press. Retrieved December 2014 from http://www.iom.edu/Reports.

Institute of Medicine (IOM): *Primary care and public health: exploring integration to improve population health*, Washington, DC, 2012, National Academies Press.

Kaiser Family Foundation: *Kaiser/HRET Survey of employer-sponsored health benefits*, 2015a. Retrieved May 2016 from http://facts.kff.org.

Kaiser Family Foundation: *Key facts about the uninsured population*, 2015b. Retrieved May 2016 from http://kaiser Family Foundation.org.

Kentucky Board of Nursing: *100th anniversary celebration keynote by N. Ridenour*, 2014, Kaiser Family Foundation

Levesque JF, Breton M, Senn N, et al: The interaction of public health and primary care: functional roles and organizational models that bridge individual and population perspectives, *Public Health Rev* 35:1–27, 2013.

Migration Policy Institute: *American community survey and census data on the foreign born by state*, Washington, DC, 2015, Migration Policy Institute. Retrieved May 2016 from www.migrationinformation.org.

National Center for Complementary and Alternative Medicine (NCCAM), National Institutes of Health: Complementary, Alternative or Integrative Health: *What's in a name*, Bethesda, MD, 2014, NCCAM. Retrieved December 2014 from http://nccam.nih.gov.

National Center for Health Statistics (NCHS): *Indicators of success of public health initiatives to improve health*, Hyattsville, MD, 2014, NCHS. Retrieved December 2014 from www.healthindicators.gov.

National Center for Health Workforce Analysis: *Registered nurse employment*, Rockville Md, 2013, Health Resources and Services Administration.

National Council of State Boards of Nursing (NCSBN): *2013 National nursing workforce survey of registered nurses*, July 2013. Retrieved from https: www.ncsbn.org.

National Institutes of Health (NIH): *My family health portrait: a tool from the surgeon general*, NIH MedlinePlus Winter 5(1):4, 2010. Retrieved December 2014 from http://www.nlm.nih.gov.

Office for National Statistics (ONS): *Vital statistics: population and health reference tables, annual time series data*, Newport, England, 2014, Office for National Statistics.

Orange County Health Care Agency: *Confirmed measles outbreak in Orange County, California*, 2014 Retrieved December 2014 from http://ochealthinfo.com.

Palma G: Electronic Health Records: *The good, the bad and the ugly* [Becker's HealthIT and CIO review], Chicago, 2014, Becker's Healthcare. Retrieved December 2014 from http://www.beckershospitalreview.com.

Public Health Accreditation Board (PHAB): *Accredited health departments*, Alexandria, VA, 2016, PHAB. Retrieved May 2016 from http://www.phaboard.org.

Rowland D, Hoffman C, McGinn-Shapiro M: *Health care and the middle class: more costs and less coverage*, Menlo Park, CA, 2009, Kaiser Family Foundation.

Truffer CJ, Keehan S, Smith S, et al: Health spending projections through 2019: the recession's impact continues, *Health Aff (Millwood)* 29:522–529, 2010. Retrieved December 2014 from http://content.healthaffairs.org.

US Census Bureau: *Statistical files*, Washington, DC, 1996, US Department of Commerce. Retrieved May 1996 from http://www.census.gov.

US Census Bureau: *Statistical files*, Washington, DC, 2016, US Department of Commerce. Retrieved May 2016 from http://www.census.gov.

US Department of Health and Human Services (USDHHS): *Healthy People 2020: improving the health of Americans*, 2010a. Retrieved November 2014 from http://www.healthypeople.gov.

US Department of Health and Human Services (USDHHS): *Healthy People 2020* [brochure updated with the leading health indicators]. 2010b. Retrieved December 2014 from https://www.healthypeople.gov.

US Department of Health and Human Services (USDHHS): *HHS organizational chart*, 2014a. Retrieved December 2014 from http://www.hhs.gov/about/orgchart/.

US Department of Health and Human Services (USDHHS): *Strategic plan: fiscal years 2010-2015*, 2014b. Retrieved December 2014 from http://www.hhs.gov/strategic-plan/stratplan.

US Department of Homeland Security (USDHS): *Homeland Security*, 2014. Retrieved December 2014 from http://www.dhs.gov/.

US Public Health Service (USPHS): *The Commissioned Corps of the PHS, Office of the Assistant Secretary for Health*, 2014. Retrieved December 2014 from http://www.usphs.gov.

World Health Organization (WHO): *Primary health care: report of the International Conference on Primary Health Care, Alma-Ata, USSR, September 6-12, 1978* [Health for All Series No. 1], Geneva, 1978, WHO.

World Health Organization (WHO): *Basic Documents*, ed 36, Geneva, 1986a, WHO.

World Health Organization (WHO): *World Health Statistics Annual*, Geneva, 1986b, WHO.

World Health Organization (WHO): *The World Health Report 2008: primary health care (now more than ever)*, Geneva, 2008, WHO. Retrieved December 2014 from http://www.who.int.

CHAPTER 4

Ethics in Public and Community Health Nursing Practice

Sydney Axson and Connie M. Ulrich[1]

OBJECTIVES

After reading this chapter, the student should be able to do the following:

1. Describe a brief history of the ethics of nursing in public and community health.
2. Discuss ethical decision-making processes.
3. Compare and contrast ethical theories and principles, virtue ethics, caring ethics, and feminist ethics.
4. Describe how ethics is part of the core functions of nursing in public health.
5. Analyze codes of ethics for nursing and for public health.
6. Apply the ethics of advocacy to nursing in public health.

CHAPTER OUTLINE

Introduction
Brief History of Ethics and Bioethics: Relationship to Nursing and Public Health
   Foundations of Nursing and Public Health's Codes of Ethics
Ethical Decision Making
   Ethical Principles and Theories as Guides to Ethical Decision Making

Ethics and the Core Functions of Public Health Nursing
Nursing Code of Ethics
Public Health Code of Ethics
Advocacy and Ethics
   Definitions, Codes, Standards
Advocacy and Health Care Reform

KEY TERMS

advocacy, 61
beneficence, 50
bioethics, 50
code of ethics, 51
consequentialism, 53
deontology, 54
distributive justice, 54

ethic of care, 56
ethical decision making, 52
ethical dilemmas, 51
ethical issues, 50
ethics, 50
feminist ethics, 56
feminists, 57

moral distress, 50
nonmaleficence, 50
principlism, 54
utilitarianism, 53
values, 52
virtue ethics, 56
virtues, 56

INTRODUCTION

Public health and community health nurses focus on prevention, protecting, promoting, preserving, and maintaining health. Working within public health settings, however, can challenge

nurses in many ways. First, public health nurses may be the first point of contact for patients and their families within the local community. Therefore these nurses are in a unique position as they work to establish trusting relationships not only with their patients and families but also with a broad array of community groups that represent local interests. As health care providers, nurses navigate personal beliefs, patient and/or family wishes, and community values. They must do so within the parameters of community resources and organizational policy and within the guidelines of their professional codes of conduct. This

[1]We acknowledge Mary Cipriano Silva, Jeanne Merkle Sorrell, and James J. Fletcher for their previous work on this chapter. We have kept their original thoughts in the majority of this chapter and added additional information pertinent to thinking about ethics in public health nursing practice.

complex and challenging process has tangible ramifications. One such possible effect is moral distress, that is, knowing (or thinking one knows) the morally right course of action but not being able to act accordingly (Corely et al, 2005; Jameton, 1984; Epstein and Hamric, 2009; Raines, 2000; Ulrich, O'Donnell, Taylor et al, 2007; Ulrich, Hamric, and Grady, 2010). In more recent commentary, Hamric (2014) has defined moral distress as a serious violation of one's moral integrity based on a failure to act or where attempted actions failed. Experiencing moral distress has negative consequences; it affects job satisfaction and can lead to nurses leaving the profession altogether (Hamric and Blackhall, 2007; Ulrich, O'Donnell, Taylor et al, 2007). Unsurprisingly, the supply of nurses able to appropriately engage with the challenges of their jobs directly affects the health of any community.

Second, public health or community nurses must also be prepared for any emerging or reemerging infectious disease that might arise within their communities. Here, they have to weigh or balance the potential benefits and risks to individuals as well as the risks and harms to the broader community. Most recently, an outbreak of the Zika virus (a mosquito-borne virus) is presenting a significant public health threat to communities across the United States as well as globally. Lucey and Gostin (2016) suggests that "training health workers to observe and report Zika-related disease and robust systems for collecting and analyzing surveillance data will complement public health strategies" (p 865). This raises important questions about the ethics preparedness of public health nurses and the ethical issues that they might face. The lead levels in the water supply in a largely minority and poor population in Flint, Michigan, is another example of a public and community health crisis and highlights ethical issues associated with concepts of inclusion, diversity, participation, empowerment, social justice, advocacy, and interdependence (Racher, 2007). This chapter applies core knowledge of ethics to public health nursing to help nurses develop effective coping strategies for ethical issues, including moral distress and other issues of import. Further, characteristics unique to community health practice are explored.

BRIEF HISTORY OF ETHICS AND BIOETHICS: RELATIONSHIP TO NURSING AND PUBLIC HEALTH

Ethics is both a process for reflection and a body of knowledge that focuses on the study of morality or the moral life (Beauchamp and Childress, 2013). Stated differently, Chaloner says "Ethics is a branch of philosophy concerned with determining right and wrong in relation to people's decisions and actions" (2007, p 42). Ethics-related questions often ask the following: How should I behave? What actions should I perform? What kind of person should I be? What are my obligations to myself and to others? Ethics is important in all aspects of life and is inherent in nursing; basing actions on ethical principles supports clinical decision making and the practice of nursing. For example, the ethical principles of beneficence (doing good) and nonmaleficence (do no harm) can be traced back to the

Hippocratic Oath for health care professionals and provides a framework for patient–clinician relationships (Racher, 2007).

Bioethics, a multidisciplinary subfield of ethics, is the systematic study of ethical issues in research, clinical care, or other areas in the life sciences, using both normative and empirical methodological approaches (Jonsen, 1998; Reich, 1995). Several sentinel historical events have shaped the field of bioethics, including the well-known Nuremberg Tribunal that followed World War II. The Nuremberg Tribunal reviewed the egregious human rights abuses performed under the guise of scientific experimentation by Nazi leaders, including physicians (Easley and Allen, 2007). These abuses, and the prosecution of their perpetrators, led to the development of the Nuremberg Code of 1947, "which provides the foundation for the protection of human subjects in research" (Easley and Allen, 2007, p 367). Major social movements of the 1960s and 1970s in the United States facilitated further development of the field of bioethics. Examples include the campaign for nuclear disarmament, the civil rights and peace movements, the protests against the war in Vietnam, and new medical technologies that raised challenging ethical questions about life and death (Easley and Allen, 2007). In addition, the first institution in the United States devoted to the study of bioethics was the Hastings Center, founded by Daniel Callahan, PhD, and Willard Gaylin, MD, in 1970. The Hastings Center (2017) addresses core ethical issues that arise in all areas of the life sciences and that affect the health and well-being of individuals, communities, and societies. It remains an excellent resource for nurses and other health care practitioners in the rapidly changing health care landscape.

Despite the atrocities of Nuremberg, violation of human rights in the name of research continued, including the Tuskegee syphilis study sanctioned by the US Public Service. From this, the 1974 National Research Act established the National Commission for the Protection of Human Subjects of Biomedical and Behavioral Research; this commission created the seminal Belmont Report (1979). A set of guidelines differentiating clinical practice from research, the Belmont Report also outlines the ethical principles of respect for persons (informed consent and respecting autonomous decisions), beneficence (maximizing the benefits and minimizing the harms), and justice (fair subject selection in research) in the protection of human subjects who participate in research (Belmont Report, 1979).

The field of bioethics continues to evolve as ethical issues remain prevalent in clinical practice and research and as new questions arise in the care of the most vulnerable in our communities. For example, questions abound on how to allocate scarce resources in a just manner both at the micro and macro levels and the benefits and harms of health technologies and research, including renal dialysis, organs for transplants, precision science, genetics and genomics, and emerging and reemerging infectious diseases, among others.

FOUNDATIONS OF NURSING AND PUBLIC HEALTH'S CODES OF ETHICS

Modern nursing also has a rich heritage of ethics and morality. Florence Nightingale (1820–1910) is often seen as nursing's first moral leader and nurse in community health. Nightingale saw nursing as a call to service and thought nurses should be people of good moral character. She was a champion of primary prevention, passionate about the need to provide care to the disenfranchised, and committed to the importance of a sanitary environment, as seen in her work with soldiers in the Crimean War (1854–1856). The ethical foundations of clinical practice that Nightingale contributed to nursing have endured. Chapter 2 provides details about the many contributions of Nightingale to the development of the nursing profession.

In the 1960s, two seminal events that changed the course of nursing practice occurred. First, the American Nurses Association (ANA) recommended all nursing education occur in institutions of higher education. Before this time, many of the schools of nursing were offered by religious institutions and had ethics included in their curricula. As the process of moving nursing into higher education took place, ethics as a course was removed from many schools of nursing. Often the decision to omit ethics courses was influenced by the need to include more general education courses in the nursing curriculum. Second, because of major advances in science and technology, the field of bioethics began to emerge and was also developing in nursing curricula. Today, although many nursing programs integrate bioethical content into their courses or have separate courses on this topic, research suggests that approximately 23% of nurses still have no ethics education (Grady et al., 2008).

Nurses' codes of ethics are important in the history of nursing practice in the community. The Nightingale Pledge is generally considered to be nursing's first code of ethics (ANA, 2001). After the Nightingale Pledge, a "suggested" code and a "tentative" code were published in the *American Journal of Nursing* but were not formally adopted. The *Code for Professional Nurses* was formally adopted by the ANA House of Delegates in 1950. It was amended and revised five more times, until in 2001 the ANA House of Delegates adopted the *Code of Ethics for Nurses with Interpretive Statements*. Most recently, the *Code of Ethics for Nurses* underwent another significant revision with approval in 2014. As stated by Marsha Fowler (2015), "the *Code of Ethics for Nurses with Interpretive Statements* is remarkable in its breadth and compass. It retains nursing's historical and ethical values, obligations, ideals, and commitments while extending them into the ever-growing art, science, and practice of nursing in 2015" (pp viii–ix).

The first known international code of ethics was adopted by the International Council of Nurses in 1953. Like the *Code of Ethics for Nurses with Interpretive Statements,* it has undergone various revisions and adoptions. The most recent revision of the *ICN Code of Ethics for Nurses* was adopted in 2005, copyrighted in 2006, and revised in 2012 (International Council of Nurses, 2012).

As mentioned earlier in the chapter, the bioethics movement of the late 1960s influenced both nursing ethics and public health ethics. The relationship between public health and ethics has also been made explicit through the development of a Code of Ethics (Public Health Leadership Society, 2002). After input from many public health professionals and associations, the Code of Ethics for Public Health was approved in 2002 (Olick, 2005). This code, entitled *Principles of the Ethical Practice of Public Health,* defines public health in the following way: "public health not only seeks to assure the health of whole communities but also recognizes that the health of individuals is tied to their life in the community" (Public Health Leadership Society, 2002, p 1). It also identifies 12 guiding principles, including, but not limited to, respect for individuals within their communities, community engagement in policies and procedures that affect the community's overall health and well-being, community consent, collaborative practices that support trust within diverse communities, and upholding ethical principles of confidentiality and justice. (For clarity in this chapter, this document is referred to as the Code of Ethics for Public Health unless the official title is used.)

Professional codes provide a foundation from which nurses and other public health advocates can meet their professional and moral obligations to their patients and communities. Nurses in public health have to honor their professional duties in ways that extend beyond one-on-one care, and this can present unique ethical challenges. Indeed, in public health nursing, the role of prevention is increasingly being informed by genomics as well as other factors. Here, nurses must become more skilled in learning how to reduce the potential influence of genetic risk factors by teaching clients how to live healthier lives, or address the individual health effects of environmental risks within communities, such as drinking water, lead levels, air pollutants, or radiation exposure. Questions that arise in regard to genomics and how this and other factors may affect public health nursing include the following: Should people be held accountable for making unhealthy life choices? To whom should you give information about a genetic predisposition to an environmental health problem? Should society's resources be used for people who knowingly engage in risky behavior given their genetic makeup (Easley and Allen, 2007; Sharp et al, 2003)?

ETHICAL DECISION MAKING

Ethical issues are moral challenges facing all health care practitioners, and are particularly common in community or public health nursing. Ulrich, Taylor, Soeken, et al (2010) state that "ethical issues can occur in any situation where profound moral questions of 'rightness' or 'wrongness' underlie professional decision-making and the beneficent care of patients" (p 251). A good example of an ethical issue in community or public health nursing at both the individual and community level is Ebola. One of the central ethical issues surrounding Ebola was informed consent of health care providers as well as the community regarding the risks of contracting the virus and its implications for individual and community health and well-being. From a public health perspective, other ethical issues included concerns about surveillance and tracking measures, availability of personal protective equipment, and quarantine and isolation procedures for hospitalized patients as well as American and foreign citizens who entered or reentered the country. In contrast, ethical dilemmas are human dilemmas and puzzling moral problems in which a person, group, or community can envision morally justified reasons for both taking and not taking a certain course of action

(Purtilo and Doherty, 2016; Barrett, 2012). With Ebola, arguments on who should receive the experimental drug (ZMapp)—the American health care workers who became infected or the African citizens who were dying on the front lines of the virus outbreak in Africa—was a classic example of an ethical dilemma. Here, various stakeholders presented sound arguments regarding the allocation and testing of ZMapp for each respective group.

Making ethical decisions on allocation priorities of a scarce and untested resource such as ZMapp required a systematic analysis and evaluation of the ethical issue or dilemma. Thus ethical decision making is the part of ethics that focuses on the process of how ethical decisions are made. Ethical theories, principles, and decision-making frameworks help nurses and others think through these issues and dilemmas. Often, ethical content is abstract, which makes decision making more difficult.

Ethical decision-making frameworks use problem-solving processes. They provide guides for making sound ethical decisions that can be morally justified. Some of these frameworks are discussed in this chapter. It is important to remember that, when all is said and done, we each make our own decisions. Weston (2002) said, "Whether we admit it or not, we do make our own decisions. We cannot pretend that we are simply obeying some rules (or authorities) that settle matters—ours only to obey. Choosing is inescapable" (p 28). Because we make our own decisions, the following generic ethical decision-making framework may be useful:

1. Identify the ethical issues and dilemmas.
2. Place the ethical issues and dilemmas within a meaningful context.
3. Obtain all relevant facts.
4. Reformulate ethical issues and dilemmas, if needed.
5. Consider appropriate *approaches* to actions or options (i.e., utilitarianism, deontology, principlism, virtue ethics, care ethics, feminist ethics).
6. Make the decision and take action.
7. Evaluate the decision and the action.

The steps of a generic ethics framework are often nonlinear, and with the exception of the ethical approach, they do not change substantially. Their rationales are presented in Table 4.1. Step 5 (the one exception) lists six approaches to the ethical decision-making process; these approaches are outlined throughout the chapter in the How To boxes.

Several factors can affect the ethical decision-making process. First, we live in a multicultural society in which nurses might face ethical issues and dilemmas related to the diverse cultures, values, and beliefs of their patients, families, and communities. This, at times, can create conflict. Callahan (2000), cofounder of the Hastings Center, helps explain these conflicts and describes the following four situations for reflection and consideration when working with diverse individuals and communities:

1. Situations that place persons at direct risk for harm, whether psychological or physical
2. Situations in which cultural standards conflict with professional standards

TABLE 4.1 Rationale for Steps of an Ethical Decision-Making Framework

Steps	Rationale
1. Identify the ethical issues and dilemmas.	Persons cannot make sound ethical decisions if they cannot identify ethical issues and dilemmas.
2. Place them within a meaningful context.	The historical, sociological, cultural, psychological, economic, political, communal, environmental, and demographic contexts affect the way ethical issues and dilemmas are formulated and justified.
3. Obtain all relevant facts.	Facts affect the way ethical issues and dilemmas are formulated and justified.
4. Reformulate ethical issues or dilemmas if needed.	The initial ethical issues and dilemmas may need to be modified or changed on the basis of context and facts.
5. Consider appropriate approaches to actions or options.	The nature of the ethical issues and dilemmas determines the specific ethical approaches used.
6. Make decisions and take action.	Professional persons cannot avoid choice and action in applied ethics.
7. Evaluate decisions and action.	Evaluation determines whether the ethical decision-making framework used resulted in morally justified actions related to the ethical issues and dilemmas.

3. Situations in which the greater community's values are jeopardized by values of a smaller culture within that community.
4. Situations in which community customs may cause mild offense or annoyance to other communities, but no major problems.

Chapter 5 further discusses cultural influences on public health nursing. Applying Callahan's four standards to content in that chapter will be helpful. Callahan (2000) discusses how to consider diversity in the four situations. In situation 1, he says that "we in America imposed some standards on ourselves for important moral reasons; and there is no good reason to exempt subgroups from those standards" (p 43). Regarding situations 2 and 3, Callahan recognizes a challenge between cultural standards of individuals and communities and health care providers' professional standards. Within this scenario, health care providers have to recognize that some groups hold values different from those generally accepted as normative in society. Callahan notes "in the absence of grievous harm, there is no clear moral mandate to interfere with those values" (p 43). However, sometimes there is some degree of moral pressure (not coercion) to intervene with differing values for the sake of community consensus. This often requires compromise and negotiation between differing parties. Finally, regarding situation 4, he notes there is no moral mandate to intervene in nonthreatening cultural traditions and values even if they create some degree of burden on others. Intervention only becomes necessary when the imposed burdens cause harm or undue hardship to other groups.

Because decision making is central to the practice of nursing, and many decisions are difficult to make, it is useful to consider the experience of moral distress. As noted earlier, moral distress occurs when one is unable to act in a way that he or she thinks is right (consistent with their own personal or professional values, cultural expectations, and/or religious beliefs) due to internal or external constraints. Moral distress is different from what we may consider emotional distress because there is not only an ethical component associated with this phenomenon but also the threat to an individual's moral integrity (Epstein and Delgado, 2010; Hamric, 2014; Ulrich, Hamric, and Grady, 2010; Varcoe et al, 2012). Nurses, as well as other types of health care providers, have experienced moral distress (Epstein and Delgado, 2010; Austin et al, 2008; Chen, 2009; Forde and Aasland, 2008; Hamric and Blackhall, 2007; Lomis, Carpenter, and Miller, 2009). In a national survey, Ulrich et al (2007) reported that nurses identified feeling powerless, overwhelmed, frustrated, and fatigued when they cannot resolve ethical issues experienced while working. These reported feelings are psychosocial consequences of moral distress. When this conflict occurs, it can lead to a sense of personal failure in the kind of care nurses give and to subsequent performance issues and may lead to work or career dissatisfaction. However, moral distress may be addressed in some of the following ways:

1. Identifying the type(s) of situation that leads to distress
2. Communicating that concern to your manager and examining ways to work toward addressing the stressor
3. Seeking support from colleagues
4. Seeking support from ethics committees, social workers, and pastoral care, among others
5. Being proactive and expressing one's voice on matters that are ethically concerning

It is often useful to talk with colleagues. You may learn that they have similar concerns or that they have found ways to interrupt the stressful situation(s) (Carlock and Spader, 2007). Additionally, open dialogue with those in leadership positions such as nurse managers can be helpful. Collaboration like this can lead nurses to connect with other services such as ethics committees and social work, both of which have important roles in ethical practice.

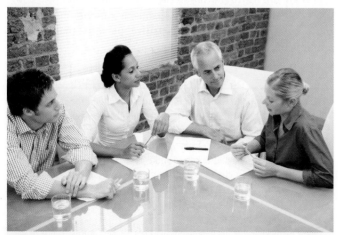

Colleagues participate in ethical decision making. (© 2012 Photos.com, a division of Getty Images. All rights reserved. Image #92202428.)

Three cases will be presented in the following chapter sections. Each one should be examined using the ethical decision-making processes outlined in the How To boxes and the different codes of ethics provided in the chapter. These cases provide an excellent opportunity to debate your personal beliefs about the application of ethical processes with classmates and to assess your own thoughts, feelings, and possible actions. The cases deal with what the nursing response should be (1) when a client will not assume responsibility for his or her health, (2) when the question arises about whether a parent can adequately care for a young child, and (3) when a client is not able or willing to take personal responsibility and does not want the nurse to report the situation.

ETHICAL PRINCIPLES AND THEORIES AS GUIDES TO ETHICAL DECISION MAKING

The remainder of this section of the chapter summarizes content about ethical theories and principles. As you read these sections, remember that the ways ethical theories and principles are applied in the community may differ from how they are applied with individuals. As Racher (2007, p 68) aptly says, "Community practice is traditionally based on utilitarianism, adheres to the axiom 'the greatest good for the greatest number,' and supports the position that maximizing benefits to socially disadvantaged groups ultimately benefits society as a whole." Community practitioners work to increase participation in health promotion and manage chronic diseases; they see these actions as benefiting the individual and the community. Public health is concerned with collective action that benefits the greatest number of people, such as having clean water, public safety, or the societal regulation of shared risks, for example, reporting of some communicable diseases (Easley and Allen, 2007). The public health perspective of care may require that individuals forfeit some of their self-interests for the benefits of a safe and healthy society. For example, prohibiting people from smoking in restaurants, to benefit the other people in the restaurant, may inconvenience the smoker while providing a healthier environment for all people, including the smoker. Similarly, at times a person's right to privacy and confidentiality may be usurped by the public benefit of disclosure. This might take place during epidemics or other national events when contact tracing and surveillance epidemiological measures are warranted (Gostin, Bayer, and Fairchild, 2003).

Utilitarianism and Deontology

At times, decisions are based on outcomes or consequences. In this approach, referred to as consequentialism, the right action is the one that produces the greatest amount of good or the least amount of harm in a given situation. Utilitarianism is a well-known consequentialist ethical theory associated with outcomes or consequences in determining which choice to make. In utilitarianism, "the moral value of an action is determined by its overall benefit" (Chaloner, 2007, p 43). Stated differently, because the outcome is the key factor, the end justifies the means.

*Moral rules of action that produce the greatest good for the greatest number of communities or populations affected by or most affected by the rules.

In other situations, nurses may conclude that the action is right or wrong in itself, regardless of the amount of good that might come from it. This is the ethical theory known as deontology, or adhering to moral rules or duty rather than to the consequences of the actions (Munson, 2014). This view is based on the premise that persons should always be treated as ends in themselves and never as mere means to the ends of others.

Each theory maintains that there is a universal first principle, the principle of utility for utilitarianism and the categorical imperative for deontology, which serves as a rational norm for behavior and allows us to calculate the rightness or wrongness of each individual action. According to both utilitarianism and deontology, the individual is the special center of moral concern (Steinbock, Arras, and London, 2008). Deontology comes from the Greek roots *deon*, meaning "duty," and *logos*, meaning "study of." Giving priority to individual rights and needs refers to the concept that a person's rights and dignity should never (or rarely) be sacrificed to the interests of society (Steinbock, Arras, and London, 2008).

Health professionals have specific obligations that exist because of the practices and goals of the profession. These health care obligations can be interpreted in terms of a set of principles in bioethics as outlined by Beauchamp and Childress (2009): respect for autonomy, nonmaleficence, beneficence, and justice (as shown in Box 4.1). Principlism relies on these ethical principles to guide decision making. As such, the principle of autonomy refers to self-governance. Respecting autonomy requires health care providers to understand a client's ability to decide and act with his or her own plan (Beauchamp and Childress, 2009). Nonmaleficence is the noninfliction of harm, and is often closely linked to the principle of beneficence or the duty to act in ways that will benefit others. Distributive justice or social justice refers to the allocation of benefits and burdens to members of society. Benefit refers to basic needs, including material and social goods, liberties, rights, and entitlements. Some benefits of society are wealth, education, and public services. Among the burdens to

be shared are items such as taxes, military service, and the location of incinerators and power plants. Justice requires that the distribution of benefits and burdens in a society be fair. Although it is recognized that distribution should be based on what one needs and deserves, considerable disagreement exists when considering what these terms mean in the context of fairness. The three primary theories of distributive justice are egalitarian, libertarian, and liberal democratic (see Box 4.2).

Although principlism has been used effectively to analyze ethics-related situations in bioethics, it also has its critics (Callahan, 2000, 2003; Walker, 2009). First, some argue that the principles are too abstract and narrow to serve as guides for action. Second, the principles themselves can conflict in a given situation, and there is no independent basis for prioritizing them (Walker, 2009). Third, Walker (2009) contends that there are more than four principles that reflect the "common morality." And, fourth, ethical judgments may depend more on the judgment of sensitive persons than on the application of abstract principles.

BOX 4.2 Three Primary Theories of Distributive Justice

Distributive Justice Theory	Principles
Egalitarian	This view advocates that everyone is entitled to equal rights and equal treatment in society. Ideally, each person has an equal share of the goods of society, and it is the role of government to ensure that this happens. The government has the authority to redistribute wealth if necessary to ensure equal treatment. Thus egalitarians support welfare rights—that is, the right to receive certain social goods necessary to satisfy basic needs. These include adequate food, housing, education, and police and fire protection. Both practical and theoretical weaknesses are inherent in egalitarianism (Beauchamp and Childress, 2009).
Libertarian	The libertarian view of justice advocates for social and economic liberty. Whereas egalitarianism lacks incentives for individuals, libertarianism emphasizes the contribution and merit of the individual (Beauchamp and Childress, 2009). Government has a limited role.
Liberal Democratic	This view values both liberty and equality.
	It is based on Rawls's theory of justice and the "veil of ignorance." Behind this veil, people (or their representatives) are unaware of social position, race, culture, doctrine, sex, endowments, or any other distinguishing circumstances (Rawls, 2001). This is known as the original position and is an exercise to address the inequalities and bargaining advantages that result from birth, natural endowments, and historical circumstances. Without these inequalities, all people are free and equal and can work together as citizens to decide what is fair and therefore just. Once impartiality is guaranteed, Rawls suggests all rational people will choose a system of justice containing the following two basic principles (Rawls, 2001, p 42):
	Each person has the same claim to a fully adequate scheme of equal basic liberties, and this scheme is compatible with the same scheme of liberties for all.
	Social and economic inequalities are to satisfy two conditions: first, they are to be attached to offices and positions open to all under conditions of fair equality of opportunity; and second, they are to be to the greatest benefit to the least-advantaged members of society (the difference principle).

CASE STUDY 1

Applying the Principlism Ethics Decision Process

Jeff Williams, team leader in Home Health Care Services at the county health department, was preparing to visit Mr. Chisholm, a 59-year-old client recently diagnosed as having emphysema. Mr. Chisholm, who was unemployed because of a farming accident several years earlier, was well known to the health department. Hypertensive and overweight, he was also a heavy, long-term cigarette smoker despite his decreased lung function. Mr. Williams visited Mr. Chisholm to find out why the client had missed his latest chest clinic appointment. He also wanted to determine whether the client was continuing his medications as ordered.

As Mr. Williams parked his car in front of his client's house, he could see Mr. Chisholm sitting on the front porch smoking a cigarette. A flash of anger made him wonder why he continued trying to encourage Mr. Chisholm to stop smoking and why he took the time from his busy home-care schedule to follow up on Mr. Chisholm's missed clinic appointments. This client certainly did not seem to care enough about his own health to give up smoking.

During the home visit, Mr. Williams determined that Mr. Chisholm had discontinued the use of his prophylactic antibiotic and was not taking his expectorant and bronchodilator medication on a regular basis. Mr. Chisholm's blood pressure was 210/114 mm Hg, and he coughed almost continuously. Although he listened politely to Mr. Williams's concerns about his respiratory function and the continued use of his medications, Mr. Chisholm simply made no effort to take responsibility for his health care. Even so, another clinic appointment was made, and Mr. Williams encouraged the client to attend.

As he drove to his next home visit, Mr. Williams wondered to what extent he was obligated as a nurse to spend time on clients who took no personal responsibility for their health. He also wondered if there was a limit to the amount of nursing care a noncooperative client could expect from a service provided in the community.

Consider this case using the principlism ethics decision process:

1. If the nurse wants to respect Mr. Chisholm's right to autonomy, should he try to explain the need for compliance with the treatment plan and urge the client to comply? Or should the nurse tell Mr. Chisholm that he will be given a clinic appointment when he begins to follow the treatment plan? Or should the nurse schedule the next appointment and hope Mr. Chisholm will soon understand why he should follow the care plan? Or is there an action you would choose that is not listed here?
2. What are Mr. Williams's professional responsibilities for Mr. Chisholm's rights to health care?
3. Is there a limit to the amount of care nurses should be expected to give to clients?
4. What authority defines the moral requirements and moral limits of nursing care to clients?
5. Using content in at least one of the How To boxes, apply one of the ethical processes to this case. For example, debate with a classmate whether the deontological ethics decision process is useful in determining the nursing action with Mr. Chisholm. Specifically, examine your motives for being reluctant to continue providing care to this client who seemingly has no desire to promote his own health.
6. What ethical principles are causing distress for the nurse?

Modified from: Fry ST, Veatch RM, Taylor C: *Case studies in nursing ethics,* Boston, 2011, Jones and Bartlett Learning, pp 28-29.

HOW TO **Apply the Principlism Ethics Decision Process**

1. Determine the ethical principles (i.e., respect for autonomy, nonmalefi-cence, beneficence, justice) that are relevant to an ethical issue or dilemma.
2. Analyze the relevant principles within a meaningful context of accurate facts and other pertinent circumstances.
3. Act on the principle that provides, within the meaningful context, the stron-gest guide to action that can be morally justified by the tenets foundational to the principle.

NOTE: Remember that using principlism in the ethics decision process is one of the approaches in step 5 of the general ethical decision-making framework.

EVIDENCE-BASED PRACTICE

Smoking, drinking, and poor nutrition are costly habits. They are costly to the health of the person, to the family, and to society. As nations look at ways to contain their health care costs and pay for their many obligations, many are looking at taxing items considered to not be essential to health and well-being of their citizens. Sin taxes are taxes on commodities and activities that society thinks are nonessential and potentially harmful. Ethical questions arise in the consideration of the use of sin taxes—for example, the question of whose good will benefit: the good of the person or the good of the com-munity? Green (2011) uses a public health nursing model based on the Public Health Code of Ethics, the American Nurses Association Code of Ethics, and other relevant ethical theories to examine the arguments for and against the use of sin taxes. She determines that a position advocating the limited use of sin taxes can be supported as a reasonable approach for a public health professional to take.

Nurse Use

Two of the core functions of public health are considered to be advocacy and policy development; therefore, it is important for nurses to understand the pros and cons of issues such as sin taxes. Understanding the issues involved will help nurses determine their own personal stance and provide them with information to both be an advocate for a position and take part in policy development.

Green R: The ethics of sin taxes, *Public Health Nurs* 28:68-77, 2011.

Virtue, Feminist, and Care Ethic Theories

Several other ethical theories are important to consider in rela-tionship to public health. For example, virtue ethics, one of the oldest ethical theories, dates back to the ancient Greek philoso-phers Plato and Aristotle. Rather than being concerned with actions as seen in utilitarianism and deontology, virtue ethics asks: What kind of person should I be? Virtue ethics seeks to enable persons to flourish as human beings. Not to be confused with principles, Aristotle defines virtues as acquired, excellent traits of character that dispose humans to act in accord with their natural good. Examples of virtues include benevolence, compassion, discernment, trustworthiness, integrity, and con-scientiousness (Beauchamp and Childress, 2009). Virtue ethics emphasizes practical reasoning applied to character develop-ment rather than focusing on moral justification by relying on theories and principles. In practice, virtues in nursing shape job responsibilities and patient care. For example, the virtues listed previously contribute to a nurse's role as one of the most trusted health professions.

HOW TO **Apply the Virtue Ethics Decision Process**

1. Identify communities that are relevant to the ethical dilemmas or issues.
2. Identify moral considerations that arise from a communal perspective, and apply the consideration to specific communities.
3. Identify and apply virtues that facilitate a communal perspective.
4. Modify moral considerations as needed to apply to the specific ethical dilemmas or issues.
5. Seek ethical community support to enhance character development.
6. Evaluate and modify the individuals or community character traits that impede communal living.

NOTE: Remember that the virtue ethics decision process is one of the approaches in step 5 of the generic ethical decision-making framework.

Modified from Volbrecht RM: *Nursing ethics: communities in dialogue,* Upper Saddle River, NJ, 2002, Prentice Hall, p 138.

Care Ethics

Caring in nursing, the ethic of care, and feminist ethics are in-terrelated and converged between the mid-1980s and early 1990s. Nurses have written about caring as the essence of, or the moral ideal, of nursing for many years (Leininger, 1984; Watson, 2007). Caring and the ethic of care are core values of public health nursing and address the importance of the fidu-ciary relationship between the patient and the care provider.

Carol Gilligan (1982) and Nel Noddings (1984) are often associated with the ethic of care. Gilligan's study of the psycho-logical and moral development of women was novel. Her work emerged at a time when abilities associated with autonomous and effective decision making were considered masculine. This perpetuated a devaluing of the stereotypical feminine charac-teristics. Through her work, Gilligan was able to accentuate the feminine experience as distinctive rather than less valuable. She formulated basic premises of responsibility, care, and relation-ships. In doing so, the link between caring and relationships continued to grow more explicit. From this, it was posited that women not only judge themselves within the context of their relationships, but they also accept and are defined by the re-sponsibility to care for others. Noddings echoed this sentiment and stated an obligation to enhance caring. The commitment that is inherent with caring facilitates ethical ideals. Gilligan and Noddings have in common a feminine ethic because they believe in the morality of responsibility in relationships that emphasize connection and caring. To them, caring is a moral imperative.

Feminist Ethics

Like virtue ethics and other communitarian views (i.e., the relationship and responsibility between the individual and the community), feminist ethics rejects abstract rules and princi-ples. According to Rogers (2006), feminist ethics is pertinent to public health because it recognizes the role of political and social structures in health. Issues of equity present major chal-lenges in public health. Inequalities in gender, historically af-fecting females, gave rise to the feminist stance that devaluing and systematic oppression of women are morally wrong. To-day, feminism encompasses more than just issues unique to women. Rogers says that the feminist perspective leads people to think critically about the connections among gender, disadvantage, and health, as well as the distribution of power in public health processes. Feminists advocate economic, social, and political equity. They pay attention to power relations that constitute a community, the rules that regulate it, and who pays and who benefits from membership in the community (Rogers, 2006).

HOW TO Apply the Care Ethics Decision Process
1. Recognize that caring is a moral imperative.
2. Identify personally lived caring experiences as a basis for relating to self and others.
3. Assume responsibility and obligation to promote and enhance caring in relationships.
   NOTE: Remember that the care ethics decision process is one of the approaches in step 5 of the generic ethical decision-making framework.

HOW TO Apply the Feminist Ethics Decision Process
1. Identify the social, cultural, political, economic, environmental, and professional contexts that contribute to the identified problem (e.g., underrepresentation of women in clinical trials).
2. Evaluate how the preceding contexts contribute to the oppression of women.
3. Consider how women's lives are defined by their status in subordinate social groups.
4. Analyze how social practices marginalize women.
5. Plan ways to restructure those social practices that oppress women.
6. Implement the plan.
7. Evaluate the plan, and restructure it as needed.
   NOTE: Remember that the feminist ethics decision process is one of the approaches in step 5 of the generic ethical decision-making framework.

Modified from Volbrecht RM: *Nursing ethics: communities in dialogue,* Upper Saddle River, NJ, 2002, Prentice Hall, p 219.

ETHICS AND THE CORE FUNCTIONS OF PUBLIC HEALTH NURSING

In Chapter 1, the three core functions of public health nursing (i.e., assessment, policy development, and assurance) were discussed. The following discussion links these three core functions to ethics.

Assessment

"*Assessment* refers to systematically collecting data on the population, monitoring the population's health status, and making information available about the health of the community" (Williams, 2012, p 7). Two ethical tenets support these core functions: beneficence and nonmaleficence. The first is beneficence. "Doing good" or maximizing the benefits and minimizing the harms requires clinicians' competency related to knowledge development, analysis, and dissemination. Here one can ask the following: Are the persons assigned to develop community knowledge adequately prepared to collect data on groups and populations? This question is important because the research, measurement, and analysis techniques used to gather information about groups and populations usually differ from the techniques used to assess individuals. Wrong research techniques can lead to wrong assessments, which in turn may hurt rather than help the intended group or population.

Additionally, do the persons selected to develop, assess, and disseminate community knowledge possess integrity? Beauchamp and Childress (2009) define integrity as the holistic integration of moral character. It requires conscientious thought during which people reflect on the rightness or wrongness of actions. The previous discussion of virtue ethics is helpful in exploring this tenet. The importance of integrity is clear: without integrity, the core function of assessment is endangered. Providers lacking integrity pose a risk for misconduct and are a

---

QSEN FOCUS ON QUALITY AND SAFETY EDUCATION FOR NURSES

One of the six tenets of Quality and Safety Education for Nurses (QSEN) is client-centered intervention (Sherwood and Drenkard, 2007). This chapter discusses many ways in which an understanding of basic principles of ethics can guide safe and effective nursing practice. Some key aspects of client-centered interventions in public health nursing include being certain that the information provided to individuals, families, and communities is accurate and reflects the most current evidence and that it is presented in a timely fashion. Community health education should take into account the age, gender, and cultural and religious backgrounds of those who receive the information. Giving health information that does not meet these criteria can be unsafe and clearly does not reflect attention to quality nursing care. One of the QSEN competencies related to client-centered care states: Recognize the client or designee as the source of control and full partner in providing compassionate and coordinated care (intervention) based on respect for client preferences, values, and needs. Specific aspects of client-centered care related to communication are as follows:
- **Knowledge:** Integrate understanding of multiple dimensions of client-centered intervention: information, communication, and education.
- **Skills:** Communicate client values, preferences, and expressed needs to other members of the health care team.

- **Attitudes:** Respect and encourage individual expression of client values, preferences, and expressed needs.
   A second set of knowledge, skills, and attitudes included in this competency helps us understand the public health dilemma of serving the good of the population versus the good of the individual.
Consider this:
- **Knowledge:** Explore ethical and legal implications of client-centered interventions.
- **Skills:** Recognize the boundaries of therapeutic relationships.
- **Attitudes:** Acknowledge the tension that may exist between client rights and the organizational responsibility for professional, ethical interventions. (Cronenwett et al, 2007)
   Client-centered ethical activity: Public health is more concerned about the good of the collective group than of the individual. Debate with a classmate whether children should be required to have all of the Centers for Disease Control and Prevention vaccines before they can enter school or remain in school. Some parents are choosing not to give their children all the recommended immunizations because of fear of side effects of the vaccine. To support your argument, see http://www.cdc.gov/vaccines/schedules/index.html for what is required. See web articles, such as those at http://www.responsibility-project.libertymutual.com.

threat to public health. The role of assessment is to provide information to the benefit of public health; any action that deters from this mission is troubling. The second ethical tenet relates to "do no harm." In any public health situation, balancing the benefits and risks is essential. As discussed in the Ebola case, minimizing harm to both individuals and communities required thoughtful dialogue on personal protective equipment as well as community surveillance and monitoring measures.

Policy Development

Public health nurses are critical to the development of policies that reflect the preferences and goals of their constituents. They are in key positions to provide leadership on the ethical issues that might arise within their communities and can use their unique training and skills to make policy decisions (Williams, 2012). In fact, an important goal of both policy and ethics is to achieve the public good (Silva, 2002), which is a part of the concept of citizenship (Denhardt and Denhardt, 2000; Rogers, 2006; Ruger, 2008). To be an effective citizen, people must be both informed about policy and able and willing to do what is in the best interests of the community (Denhardt and Denhardt, 2000). Here, the voice of the community is the foundation on which policy is developed. Silva (2002) also argues that service to others over self is a necessary condition of what is "good" or "right" policy (Silva, 2002). Denhardt and Denhardt (2000) provide three perspectives on this belief:

1. **Serve rather than steer.** An increasingly important role of the public servant (e.g., nurses and administrators) is to help citizens articulate and meet their shared interests rather than to attempt to control or steer society in new directions (p 553).
2. **Serve citizens, not customers.** The public interest results from a dialogue about shared values rather than the aggregation of individual self-interests. Therefore public servants do not merely respond to the demands of "customers" but focus

on building relationships of trust and collaboration with and among citizens (p 555).

3. **Value citizenship and public service above entrepreneurship.** The public interest is better advanced by public servants and citizens committed to making meaningful contributions to society rather than by entrepreneurial managers acting as if public money were their own (p 556).

Service, an enduring nursing value, is at the core of these three perspectives. Service requires ethical action and what is ethical is also good policy (Silva, 2002). Therefore moral leadership from nurses is critical to the development of ethical health care policies.

Assurance

"*Assurance* refers to the role of public health in making sure that essential community health services are available including essential personal health services for those who would otherwise not receive them, and that there is a competent public health and personal health care workforce." (Williams, 2012, p 7). The ethical principle of justice can apply to this core function as follows:

1. All persons should receive essential personal health services. Put in terms of justice, "to each person a fair share" or, "to all groups or populations a fair share." This does not necessarily mean that all persons in a society should share all of society's benefits equally but that they should share at least essential benefits. Many people think that basic health care for all is essential for social justice.
2. Providers of public health services should be competent and available. Although the Code of Ethics for Public Health does not speak directly to workforce availability, it does speak directly to ensuring professional competency of public health employees. *Healthy People 2020* discusses both competencies and workforce, as seen in the *Healthy People 2020* box.

CASE STUDY 2

Autonomy and Distributive Justice

Amelia Lewis, a 31-year-old African American woman with multiple diagnoses, has been followed by the local mental health system for over 10 years. Four years ago, while a client at the local day hospital, she met and married another client, James Wood. She became pregnant and now has Tyesha, who is 3 years old. Multiple agencies have followed Ms. Lewis and her little girl, who live in a sparsely furnished apartment in subsidized housing. Mr. Wood lives separately, and he and his family welcome contact with Tyesha, but the relationship between Ms. Lewis and Mr. Wood has deteriorated. A guardian handles all of Ms. Lewis's financial affairs.

Ms. Lewis has issues of trust, and she is often suspicious of the care providers who come to her home. She does rely on some of the professionals with whom she interacts on a weekly or biweekly basis. Her developmental level places her at a stage at which her own needs are her primary focus, and this is not expected to change; her interaction with Tyesha is perfunctory, involving little outward affection. She is unable to understand that Tyesha is not capable of self-care and that her 3-year-old child will not always obey when Ms. Lewis instructs her to do something. Tyesha's needs, level of functioning, and cognitive development are quickly surpassing her mother's ability to cope. Frustration and misunderstanding ensue when Ms. Lewis thinks that Tyesha does not listen to her, and

encouragement and parent education have done little to improve the situation as Tyesha gets older and more assertive. This has made toilet training, provision of an appropriate diet, and other aspects of normal child care problematic.

Many services besides those for mental health are involved to help this family of two cope. There is concern about abuse or neglect because of Ms. Lewis's lack of understanding of how to be a parent. Supplemental Security Income provides monetary support because of her mental disability, and they have Medicaid coverage for their health care needs, as well as food stamps and modest financial assistance through Temporary Assistance for Needy Families (TANF). Ms. Lewis cannot currently work and take care of her child because of her mental disability. Before Tyesha's birth, Ms. Lewis held a job and maintained self-care, but the care of Tyesha has precluded her managing employment at this time. Child Protective Services are also monitoring Ms. Lewis's situation. Ms. Lewis attends a local program to complete her General Education Development (GED), which provides child care during the day. Although Ms. Lewis is not expected to complete her GED, this program provides structured time for Tyesha three times per week. The child is considered developmentally normal at this time. Tyesha is being followed by an infant development program that monitors her progress on developmental issues. The Child Health Partnership, an agency

CASE STUDY 2—cont'd

Autonomy and Distributive Justice

that addresses the needs of challenged families, provides regular visits, family support, and parenting education, and the GED teachers make regular home visits to check on Ms. Lewis and Tyesha. Ms. Lewis thinks things are going just fine.

The Child Health Partnership nurse is concerned about this family and thinks that some permanent resolution of the situation is inevitable. There is minimal coordination of services and no "lead agency" in the family's care. Choose one of the ethical decision processes or one set of code of ethics discussed in the chapter and discuss and debate these questions:

1. Should the nurse involved in the Child Health Partnership program initiate any action to try to coordinate the work of the many agencies involved with this family?
2. Who has a professional responsibility to determine when the mother can no longer cope with the developing child?

3. Whose needs, Ms. Lewis's or Tyesha's, should take precedence?
4. Using one of the ethics decision processes, analyze the role of the nurse in this situation. For example, considering the utilitarian ethics decision process, decide if it is morally right for you to take the child away from the mother. If you do this, what are the implications for the mother, the child, and the community? What would be the possible consequences of removing the child? Of not removing the child? What principles can best guide your decision making? What possible moral dilemmas will you experience?
5. Safety is a core concept of public health nursing. Using two of the six quality and safety competencies (client-centered care and safety) for nurses identified in the Quality and Safety Education for Nurses (QSEN) work, develop a plan of action for the nurse who is caring for this family (Sherwood and Drenkard, 2007).

Created by Mary E. Gibson, PhD, RN Assistant Professor, School of Nursing, University of Virginia.

 HEALTHY PEOPLE 2020

Objectives Related to Access to Health Services

- **AHS-2:** Increase the proportion of insured persons with coverage for clinical preventive services.
- **AHS-4:** Increase the proportion of practicing primary care providers.

Both of these areas that relate to access to care reflect important ethical considerations for nurses.

From U.S. Department of Health and Human Services: *Healthy People 2020*, 2010. Retrieved October 15, 2016. http://www.healthypeople.gov

NURSING CODE OF ETHICS

As noted in the discussion of history earlier in this chapter, the *Code of Ethics for Nurses with Interpretive Statements* was adopted by the ANA House of Delegates in 2001 and most recently revised in 2015. This code serves three broad purposes, as follows (ANA, 2015):

1. "It is a succinct statement of the ethical values, obligations, duties, and professional ideals of nurses individually and collectively" (p viii).
2. "It is the profession's nonnegotiable ethical standard" (p viii).
3. "It is an expression of nursing's own understanding of its commitment to society" (p viii).

These purposes are reflected in nine provisional statements of the code. The *Code of Ethics for Nurses* and its interpretive statements apply to nurses in community health, although the emphasis for each type of nursing sometimes varies. For example, provision 1 and its interpretive statement primarily address the individual when discussing how the nurse practices with compassion and respect for the person being cared for regardless of the person's status, the person's attributes, or the nature of the health problem. However, it is also recognized under provision 1 that there are times when individual rights may be limited because of public health concerns (p 3). The interpretive statements of provisions 2 and 8 are pertinent to public health nurses, including those who identify as community health nurses. Provision 2 states "the nurse's primary commitment is to the patient whether an individual, family, group, community, or population" (p 5). Provision 8 highlights the need for collaborative practice with other disciplines as well as the public to mitigate health disparities and promote human rights. All nurses have a responsibility to meet the obligations highlighting professional standards, active involvement in nursing, and the integrity of the profession as outlined in the Code (see the *Code of Ethics for Nurses with Interpretative Statements* for all provisions at http://www.nursingworld.org).

CASE STUDY 3

Using the Deontological Decision-Making Process

Because finding affordable housing was difficult, 26-year-old Terry White lived with her 6-month-old son, Tommy, and his father, Billy Smith, in one room of the landlord's own house. Ms. White was morbidly obese and was diagnosed with bipolar disease. Mr. Smith had served time for drug dealing and was out on parole and staying straight. Neither had finished high school. Mr. Smith's past drug use had rendered him unable to do much manual labor because of heart damage, but on occasion, he would work in construction to support the family.

Public health nurse Jim Lewis had received a referral on Tommy when he was diagnosed with failure to thrive (FTT) 2 months earlier. Ms. White (who had had two children removed from her custody by Child Protective Services [CPS] in the past) and Mr. Smith seemed to adore their baby, so much so that Ms. White

would hold the baby all day long. In the past 2 months, the nurse had taught Ms. White about infant nutrition and gotten her enrolled in the Women, Infants, and Children (WIC) nutrition program; as a result, Tommy had increased his rate of physical growth and was above the 5% level of his growth percentile. Yet he was not meeting his gross motor milestones per Denver Developmental Screening Test II (DDST II) testing. Mr. Lewis thought that Tommy was not allowed to play on the floor enough to progress in sitting, pushing his shoulders up, or crawling. Most of their small room was taken up with the bed and the boxes that stored their belongings. There wasn't really space for "tummy time" or play. When not in the room, the family would take the bus to a discount store and spend the day walking around to get a change of scene.

Continued

CASE STUDY 3—cont'd

Using the Deontological Decision-Making Process

One week Ms. White told the nurse she was not taking her medications for bipolar disease anymore because they caused her to gain weight. The next week she confided that Mr. Smith had had a "dirty" urine specimen check and would have to return to prison in the near future. The following week Mr. Lewis found the family living in a run-down motel because they were evicted after a disagreement with the landlord. Ms. White was agitated, and she told the nurse that they had only $100, Mr. Smith was going to have to return to prison that week, and the motel bill was already $240. Ms. White knew she would be homeless soon without Mr. Smith's support but refused to talk with her social worker about her needs. She asked the nurse not to tell anyone about her situation because she was afraid CPS would take Tommy from her. It was clear to Mr. Lewis that he might not know where Tommy was after they left this motel.

1. Considering the principle of telling the truth, what are Mr. Lewis's professional responsibilities to Ms. White, to Tommy, and to the social worker assigned to this family?

2. Using the generic ethical decision-making framework discussed earlier in the chapter and considering the deontological ethical decision-making process, how should Mr. Lewis respond to Ms. White's request to not tell anyone about their situation? What communication, if any, should the nurse initiate with the social worker? With others?

3. Using virtue ethics, what actions would you take to resolve any moral dilemmas you have about the safety of Tommy in this family situation? If you do not tell anyone about the possible dangers to the child, what moral principles come into play? If you do tell the social worker about the situation and the child is removed from the mother, what moral principles come into play for you?

4. What ethical dilemmas may you experience if you are the nurse in this case? How can you deal effectively with these potential dilemmas?

Created by Deborah C. Conway, Assistant Professor of Nursing, School of Nursing, University of Virginia.

PUBLIC HEALTH CODE OF ETHICS

The Code of Ethics for Public Health (Public Health Leadership Society, 2002) was noted in the discussion of history earlier in this chapter. Created with the assumption that all humans have the right to adequate health resources, this code consists of 12 principles related to the ethical practice of public health (Box 4.3); this includes those values and beliefs that focus on health, community, and action and a commentary on each of the 12 principles. The preamble describes the collective and societal nature of public health to keep people healthy. In doing so, it reaffirms the World Health Organization's (WHO) definition of health as "a state of complete physical, mental, and social well-being, and not merely the absence of disease" (WHO, 2006). Similar to other Codes of Ethics, the 12 value statements incorporate the ethical tenets of preventing harm; doing no harm; promoting good; respecting both individual and community rights; respecting autonomy, diversity, and confidentiality when possible; ensuring professional competency; trustworthiness; and promoting advocacy for disenfranchised persons within a community. The Code also lists values and beliefs regarding community and public health. These include the belief that collaboration is a key element of public health, that each person should have opportunities to contribute to public discourse, and that identifying and promoting requirements for health is a primary public health concern.

BOX 4.3 Principles of the Ethical Practice of Public Health

1. Public health should principally address the fundamental causes of disease and requirements for health, aiming to prevent adverse health outcomes.
2. Public health should achieve community health in a way that respects the rights of individuals in the community.
3. Public health policies, programs, and priorities should be developed and evaluated through processes that ensure an opportunity for input from community members.
4. Public health should advocate and work for the empowerment of disenfranchised community members, aiming to ensure that the basic resources and conditions necessary for health are accessible to all.
5. Public health should seek the information needed to implement effective policies and programs that protect and promote health.
6. Public health institutions should provide communities with the information they have that is needed for decisions on policies or programs and should obtain the community's consent for their implementation.
7. Public health institutions should act in a timely manner on the information they have within the resources and the mandate given to them by the public.
8. Public health programs and policies should incorporate a variety of approaches that anticipate and respect diverse values, beliefs, and cultures in the community.
9. Public health programs and policies should be implemented in a manner that most enhances the physical and social environment.
10. Public health institutions should protect the confidentiality of information that can bring harm to an individual or community if made public. Exceptions must be justified on the basis of the high likelihood of significant harm to the individual or others.
11. Public health institutions should ensure the professional competencies of their employees.
12. Public health institutions and their employees should engage in collaborations and affiliations in ways that build the public's trust and the institution's effectiveness.

From the Public Health Leadership Society (PHLS): *Code of ethics for public health,* New Orleans, La, 2002, Louisiana Public Health Institute. The ethics project was funded in part by the Centers for Disease Control and Prevention.
*Officially titled *Principles of the Ethical Practice of Public Health,* as noted by Thomas (2002).

LEVELS OF PREVENTION
Related to Ethics

Primary Prevention
Use the *Code of Ethics for Nurses* to guide your nursing practice.

Secondary Prevention
If you are unable to behave in accordance with the *Code of Ethics for Nurses* (e.g., you speak in a way that does not communicate respect for a client), take steps to correct your behavior. You could explain to the client your error and apologize.

Tertiary Prevention
If you have treated a client or staff member in a way that is inconsistent with ethics practices, seek guidance on other choices you could have made.

Commonalities exist between the *Code of Ethics for Nurses with Interpretative Statements* and the Code of Ethics for Public Health. Both Codes provide general ethical principles and approaches that are enduring and dynamic. They require nurses to think and act in accordance with the underlying ethics of their profession. Of note, they each encourage evidence-based and collaborative approaches for the betterment of health. Although the two codes do not specify (nor should they specify) details for every ethical issue, other mechanisms such as standards of practice, ethical decision-making frameworks, and ethics committees provide further guidance. Nevertheless, these two codes address most approaches to ethical justification, including traditional and emerging ethical theories and principles, humanist and feminist ethics, virtue ethics, professional–individual or community relationships, and advocacy.

ADVOCACY AND ETHICS
DEFINITIONS, CODES, STANDARDS

Advocacy is a powerful ethical concept in nursing. But what does *advocacy* mean? "Advocacy is the application of information and resources (including finances, effort, and votes) to effect systemic changes that shape the way people in a community live" (Christoffel, 2000, p 722). Bateman (2000) suggests that advocacy includes acting in the client's best interest, maintaining confidentiality, addressing informational needs, acting impartially, and carrying out the preferences and goals of the patient with diligence and competence. *Public health advocacy* is intended "to reduce death or disability in groups of people and that is not confined to clinical settings" (p 722). As mentioned, public health includes aggregates or populations. It also encompasses both preventative and reactionary measures. Thus the problems addressed with public health advocacy affect, or have the potential to affect, a sizeable portion of a community. Several codes and standards of practice address advocacy and the various roles of nursing. Three are

noted here. Advocacy is addressed in the ANA and the Public Health Leadership Society's codes of ethics, as well as the ANA's *Public Health Nursing: Scope and Standards of Practice* (ANA, 2013).

According to the ANA's *Code of Ethics for Nurses with Interpretive Statements,* "The nurse promotes, advocates for, and protects the rights, health, and safety of the patient" (ANA, 2015, p 9). The focus of the interpretive statements regarding advocacy is the nurse's responsibility to take action when the client's best interests are jeopardized by questionable practice on the part of any member of the health team, the health care system, or others. However, Shannon argues that nursing does not bear the "advocacy" label alone. Working with communities as a public health nurse requires collaborative leadership and a team-based approach to address the needs of vulnerable patients (Shannon, 2016).

According to the Public Health Leadership Society's Code of Ethics for Public Health, "Public health should advocate and work for the empowerment of disenfranchised community members, aiming to ensure that the basic resources and conditions necessary for health are accessible to all" (Public Health Leadership Society, 2002, p. 1). The Public Health Leadership Society's code elaborates on the preceding principle by addressing the following two issues: that the voice of the community should be heard and that the marginalized or underserved in a community should receive "a decent minimum" (p 4) of health resources.

According to the ANA's *Public Health Nursing: Scope and Standards of Practice* (ANA, 2013), public health nurses have a moral mandate to establish ethical standards when advocating for health care policy. The preceding standards extend the prior two concepts of advocacy by moving advocacy into the policy arena, particularly health and social policy as applied to populations.

ADVOCACY AND HEALTH CARE REFORM

The signing of the 2010 Affordable Care Act by President Obama, after many years of controversial attempts at health care reform, provides an excellent opportunity for nurses to advocate for tying health care for all to ethics and social justice. Dr. Mary Wakefield, at that time acting deputy secretary of the Department of Health and Human Services (HHS), noted that not only should nurses participate in implementing new directions for health care, but that it is important that they help to envision these new directions (Wakefield, 2008). Nurses can advocate for access to consistent, effective, efficient health care for all people. Wakefield notes that educating the public can be a unique challenge because clever sound bites and attack ads in the media can lure consumers into thinking the status quo is the best option. Nurses are an important part of the health care industry and are respected by the public; they can make meaningful contributions toward health care reform through advocating for clients and families.

⟫ **APPLYING CONTENT TO PRACTICE**

Throughout this chapter, there has been application of the content related to ethics in public health nursing and the many documents that influence the role of public health nurses. These include the ANA's *Scope and Standards of Public Health Nursing*, the ANA's *Code of Ethics*, the core functions of public health as outlined by the Institute of Medicine, and the *Healthy People 2020* objectives. Ethics is also an integral part of the Core Competencies for Public Health

Professionals. Skill 8 in the section on analytic and assessment skills states that a public health professional uses "ethical principles in the collection, maintenance, use, and dissemination of data and information," and skill 2 under leadership and systems thinking says a professional "incorporates ethical standards of practice as the basis of all interactions with organization, communities, and individuals."

Council on Linkages Between Academia and Public Health Practice: *Core competencies for public health professionals,* Washington, DC, 2010, Public Health Foundation, Health Resources and Services Administration.

PRACTICE APPLICATION

The retiring director of the division of primary care in a state health department had recently hired Ann Jones, a 34-year-old nurse with a master's degree in public health, to be director of the division. Ms. Jones was responsible for monitoring of millions of dollars of state and federal money and supervising the funded programs within her division.

She received many requests for funding from a particular state agency that served a large, poor district. The poor people of the district consisted primarily of young families with children and homebound older adults with chronic illnesses. Over the past 3 years, the federal government had allocated considerable money to the state agency to subsidize pediatric primary-care programs, but no formal evaluation of these programs had occurred.

The director of the state agency was a physician who had been in this position for more than 20 years. He was good at obtaining funding for primary-care needs in his district, but the statistics related to the pediatric primary-care program

seemed implausible—that is, few physical examinations were performed on the children, which had resulted in extra money in the budget. This unspent federal money was being used to supplement home health care services for the indigent homebound older adults in his district. The thinking of the physician was that he was doing good by providing some needed services to both indigent groups in his district. Ms. Jones experienced moral discomfort because she did not have either the money or the personnel to provide both services.

What should she do?

A. What facts are the most relevant in this scenario?
B. What are the ethical issues?
C. How can Ms. Jones resolve the issues?

NOTE: The preceding case and answers are adapted and paraphrased from a real practice application shared by J. L. Chapin (Chapin, 1990).

Answers can be found on the Evolve website.

REMEMBER THIS!

- Nursing has a rich heritage of ethics and morality.
- The field of bioethics began to emerge and influence nursing in the late 1960s.
- Ethical decision making is the component of ethics that focuses on the process of how ethical decisions are made.
- Many different ethical decision-making frameworks exist; however, the problem-solving process underlies each of them.
- Ethical decision making applies to all approaches to ethics—utilitarianism, deontology, principlism, virtue ethics, the ethic of care, and feminist ethics.
- Cultural diversity and moral distress make ethical decision making more challenging.
- Classic ethical theories are utilitarianism and deontology.
- Principlism consists of respect for autonomy, nonmaleficence, beneficence, and justice.
- The core functions of nursing in public health (i.e., assessment, policy development, assurance) are all grounded in ethics.

- *Healthy People 2020* discusses access to care.
- The 2015 *Code of Ethics for Nurses* contains nine statements that address the moral standards that delineate nursing's values, goals, and obligations.
- The 2002 Code of Ethics for Public Health contains 12 statements that address the moral standards that delineate public health's values, goals, and obligations.
- Advocacy is the act of pleading for or supporting a course of action on behalf of a person, group, or community.
- The *Code of Ethics for Nurses with Interpretive Statements*, the *Principles of the Ethical Practice of Public Health*, and *Public Health Nursing: Scope and Standards of Practice* all address advocacy.
- The processes of public health advocacy include, but are not limited to, identifying problems, collecting data, developing and endorsing regulations and legislation, enforcing policies, and assessing the policy process.

EVOLVE WEBSITE

http://evolve.elsevier.com/Stanhope/foundations
- Case Study, with Questions and Answers
- NCLEX® Review Questions
- Practice Application Answers

REFERENCES

American Nurses Association: *Code of ethics for nurses with interpretive statements*, Washington, DC, 2001, ANA.

American Nurses Association: *Public health nursing: the scope and standards of practice*, Silver Spring, MD, 2013, ANA.

American Nurses Association: *Code of ethics for nurses with interpretive statements*, Washington, DC, 2015, ANA.

Austin W, Kagan L, Rankel M, Bergum V: The balancing act: psychiatrists' experience of moral distress, Medicine, *Health Care and Philosophy* 11(1):89–97, 2008.

Barrett MS: Ethical decision-making: a framework for understanding and resolving mental health dilemma. In Ulrich C, editor: *Nursing ethics in everyday practice*, Indianapolis, 2012, Sigma Theta Tau International.

Bateman N: *Advocacy skills for health and social care professionals*, Philadelphia, PA, 2000, Jessica Kingsley.

Beauchamp TL, Childress JF: *Principles of biomedical ethics*, ed 6, New York, 2009, Oxford.

Beauchamp TL, Childress JF: *Principles of biomedical ethics*, ed 7, New York, 2013, Oxford.

Belmont Report: *Ethical principles and guidelines for the protection of human subjects of research*, Washington DC, 1979, Government Printing Office.

Callahan D: Universalism and particularism fighting to a draw, *Hastings Center Report* 30(1):37–44, 2000.

Callahan D: Principlism and communitarianism, *Journal of Medical Ethics* 29:287–291, 2003.

Carlock C, Spader C: *Communication and understanding relieve distress*, Hoffman Estates, IL, 2012, Nursing Spectrum. Retrieved July 2012 from http://news.nurse.com/article/20071008/NATIONAL02/310080026.

Chaloner C: An introduction to ethics in nursing, *Nursing Standard* 21:42–46, 2007.

Chapin JL: The inappropriate distribution of primary health care funds. In Silva M, editor: *Ethical decision making in nursing administration*, Norwalk, Conn, 1990, Appleton and Lange.

Chen P: *When nurses and doctors can't do the right thing*, February 5, 2009. Retrieved October 14, 2016 from http://www.nytimes.com/2009/02/06/health/05chen.html.

Christoffel KK: Public health advocacy: process and product, *American Journal of Public Health* 90:722–726, 2000.

Corley M, Minick P, Elswick RK, Jacobs M: Nurse moral distress and ethical work environment, *Nursing Ethics* 12(4):381–390, 2005.

Council on Linkages Between Academia and Public Health Practice: *Core competencies for public health professionals*, Washington DC, 2010, Public Health Foundation, Health Resource and Services Administration.

Cronenwett L, Sherwood G, Barnsteiner J, et al: Quality and safety education for nurses, *Nursing Outlook* 55:122–131, 2007.

Denhardt RB, Denhardt JV: The new public service: serving rather than steering, *Public Administrative Review* 60:549–552, 2000.

Easley CE, Allen CE: A critical intersection: human rights, public health nursing, and nursing ethics, *Advances in Nursing Science* 30:367–382, 2007.

Epstein EG, Hamric AB: Moral distress, moral residue, and the crescendo effect, *J Clinical Ethics* 20(4):330–342, 2009.

Epstein G, Delgado S: *Understanding and addressing moral distress, The Online Journal of Issues in Nursing*, 2010. Retrieved October 14, 2016, from http://www.nursingworld.org/MainMenuCategories/EthicsStandards/Courage-and-Distress/Understanding-Moral-Distress.html.

Forde R, Aasland OG: Moral distress among Norwegian doctors, *J Medical Ethics* 34(7):521–525, 2008.

Fowler MDM: *Guide to the Code of Ethics for nurses with interpretive statements: Development, interpretation, and application*, ed 2, Silver Spring, MD, 2015, ANA.

Fry ST, Veatch RM, Taylor C: *Case studies in nursing ethics*, ed 4, Sudbury Mass, 2011, Jones and Bartlett Learning.

Gilligan C: *In a different voice: psychological theory and women's development*, Cambridge, MA, 1982, Harvard University.

Gostin LO, Bayer R, Fairchild AL: Ethical and legal challenges posed by severe acute respiratory syndrome: implications for the control of severe infectious disease threats, *JAMA* 290(24):3229–3237, 2003.

Grady C, Danis M, Soeken K, O'Donnell P, Taylor C, Farrar A, Ulrich, C: Does ethics education influence the moral action of practicing nurses and social workers, *The American Journal of Bioethics* 8(4):4–11, 2008.

Green R: The ethics of sin taxes, *Public Health Nursing* 28:68–77, 2011.

Hamric AB: A case study of moral distress, *Journal of Hospice and Palliative Nursing* 16(8):457–463, 2014.

Hamric AB, Blackhall J: Nurse-physician perspectives on the care of dying patients in intensive care units: collaboration, moral distress, and ethical climate, *Critical Care Medicine* 35(2):422–429, 2007.

Hastings Center: *Our Mission*, 2017. Retrieved from http://www.thehastingscenter.org/who-we-are/our-mission/.

International Council of Nurses: *ICN code of ethics for nurses*, Geneva, 2012, ICN.

Jameton A: *Nursing practice: the ethical issues*, Englewood Cliffs NJ, 1984, Prentice Hall.

Jonsen A: *The birth of bioethics*, New York, NY, 1998, Oxford.

Leininger M: *Care: the essence of nursing and health*, Thorofare, NJ, 1984, Slack.

Lomis KD, Carpenter RO, Miller BM: Moral distress in the third year of medical school; a descriptive review of student case reflections, *American Journal of Surgery* 197(1):107–112, 2009.

Lucey DR, Gostin LO: The emerging Zika pandemic: enhancing preparedness, *JAMA* 315(9):865–866, 2016.

Munson R: *Intervention and reflection: basic issues in medical ethics*, ed 8, Belmont CA, 2014, Thomson Wadsworth.

Noddings N: *Caring: a feminine approach to ethics and moral education*, Berkeley CA, 1942, University of California.

Olick RS: From the column editor: ethics in public health, *Journal of Public Health Management Practice* 11:258–259, 2005.

Public Health Leadership Society: *Public Health Code of Ethics*, Washington DC, 2002, American Public Health Association.

Purtilo R, Doherty RF: *Ethical dimensions in the health professions*, ed 6, St. Louis MO, 2016, Elsevier.

Racher FE: The evolution of ethics for community practice, *J Community Health Nursing* 24:65–76, 2007.

Raines ML: Ethical decision making in nurses: relationships among moral reasoning, coping style, and ethics stress, *JONA'S healthcare law, ethics and regulation* 2(1):29–41, 2000.

Rawls J: Justice as fairness: a restatement. In Kelly E, editor: Cambridge, MA, 2001, Harvard University.

Reich WT: *Encyclopedia of bioethics*, New York, 1995, Macmillan.

Rogers WA: Feminism and public health ethics, *J Med Ethics* 32:351–354, 2006.

Ruger JP: Ethics in American health 2: an ethical framework for health system reform, *Am J of Public Health* 98:1756–1763, 2008.

Shannon SE: The nurse as the patient's advocate: A contrarian view. In Ulrich CM, Grady C, Hamric AB, Berlinger N, editors: *Nurses at the table: nursing, ethics, and health policy*, New York, 2016, Hastings Center, pp S43–S47.

Sharp RR, de Serres F, Newman L, Sandhaus RA, Walsh JW, Hood E, Harry GJ: Environmental, occupational, and genetic risk factors for alpha-1 antitrypsin deficiency, *Environ Health Perspect* 111(14):1749–1752, 2003.

Sherwood G, Drenkard K: Quality and safety curricula in nursing education: matching practice realities, *Nurs Outlook* 55:151–155, 2007.

Silva MC: Ethical issues in health care, public policy, and politics. In Mason D, Leavitt J, Chaffee M, editors: *Policy and politics in nursing and health care*, ed 4, Philadelphia, 2002, Saunders.

Steinbock B, Arras JD, London AJ: *Ethical issues in modern medicine*, ed 7, New York, 2008, McGraw-Hill.

Ulrich C, O'Donnell P, Taylor C, Farrar A, Danis M, Grady C: Ethical climate, ethics stress, and the job satisfaction of nurses and social workers in the United States, *Social Science and Medicine* 65:1708–1719, 2007.

Ulrich CM, Hamric A, Grady C: Moral distress: a growing problem in the health professions? *Hastings Center Report* 40(1):20–22, 2010.

Ulrich CM, Taylor C, Soeken K, O'Donnell P, Farrar A, Danis M, Grady C: Everyday ethics: ethical issues and stress in nursing practice, *J of Advanced Nursing* 66(11):2510–2519, 2010.

US Department of Health and Human Services: *Healthy People 2020: a roadmap to improve America's health*, Washington, DC, 2010, US Government Printing Office.

Varcoe C, Pauly B, Webster G, Storch J: Moral distress: tensions as springboards for action, *HEC Forum* 24(1):51–62, 2012.

Volbrecht RM: *Nursing ethics: communities in dialogue*, Upper Saddle River, NJ, 2002, Prentice Hall.

Wakefield MK: Envisioning and implementing new directions for health care, *Nursing Economics* 26:49–51, 2008.

Walker T: What principlism misses, *J of Medical Ethics* 35:229–231, 2009.

Watson J: *Nursing: human science and human care—a theory of nursing*, Burlington, MA, 2007, Jones and Bartlett.

Weston A: *A practical companion to ethics*, ed 2, New York, 2002, Oxford University.

Williams CA: Population-focused practice: the foundation of specialization in public health nursing. In Stanhope M, Lancaster J, editors: *Public health nursing: population-centered health care in the community*, ed 8, St. Louis, 2012, Mosby.

World Health Organization: *Constitution of the World Health Organization*, October 2006. http://www.who.int/governance/eb/who_constitution_en.pdf.

CHAPTER 5

Cultural Influences in Nursing in Community Health

Cynthia E. Degazon and Bobbie J. Perdue

OBJECTIVES

After reading this chapter, the student should be able to:

1. Discuss ways in which culture can affect nursing practice.
2. Describe methods for developing cultural competence to meet the health needs of culturally diverse individuals, communities, and organizations.
3. Evaluate the effects of cultural organizational factors on health and illness.
4. Conduct a cultural assessment of a person from a cultural group other than yours.
5. Develop culturally competent nursing interventions to promote positive health outcomes for clients.

CHAPTER OUTLINE

Immigrant Health Issues
Culture, Race, and Ethnicity
  Culture
  Race
  Ethnicity
Cultural Diversity
  Communication
  Space
  Social Organization
  Time Perception
  Environmental Control
  Biological Variations
  Nutrition

Culture, Diversity, and Social Determinants of Health
  Cultural Competence
Culturally Competent Nursing Interventions
  Cultural Preservation
  Cultural Accommodation
  Cultural Repatterning
  Cultural Brokering
Inhibitors to Developing Cultural Competence
Cultural Nursing Assessment
Building Culturally Competent Organizations

KEY TERMS

biological variations, 72
cultural accommodation, 77
cultural awareness, 75
cultural blindness, 79
cultural brokering, 78
cultural competence, 74
cultural conflict, 79
cultural desire, 77
cultural diversity, 70
cultural encounter, 76
cultural imposition, 79

cultural knowledge, 75
cultural nursing assessment, 80
cultural preservation, 77
cultural relativism, 79
cultural repatterning, 78
cultural shock, 80
cultural skill, 76
cultural variations, 70
culture, 68
environmental control, 72
ethnicity, 70

ethnocentrism, 79
immigrants, 66
nonverbal communication, 71
prejudice, 79
race, 69
racism, 79
social organization, 71
space, 71
stereotyping, 78
time, 71
verbal communication, 70

Nurses have cared for culturally diverse groups since the beginning of the discipline. As early as 1893, nurses in New York City started public health nursing under the leadership of Lillian Wald and provided home care to people who lived in the inner city, particularly immigrants who were recent arrivals (Anderson and McFarlane, 2011). When nurses were not from the same cultural background as the immigrants, they had to deal with the cultural differences between themselves and the persons in their care. Often the same situation still exists; that is, the nurse and client come from different cultural groups and may not recognize or understand their differences.

These first migrants were largely English-speaking white Protestants who thought of themselves as founders and settlers in a new country rather than as immigrants. The first blacks to arrive in America were free men who brought their own slaves with them. Another early group of people who came to America were Africans brought on slave ships. These Africans were instrumental in developing much of early America with their skills, including farming. They also brought their unique culture with them, and much of that culture has lasted over time.

The next wave was from the 1820s to the 1920s and was made up of immigrants who were different in color, language, place of origin, and religion. This group brought their own foreign cultures. At present, another increase in immigration is occurring. There were an estimated 13.1 million lawful permanent residents, often called "green card" holders, living in the United States in 2013, and 8.8 million were thought to be eligible to become naturalized citizens (Baker and Rytina, 2014). Data from the US Census Bureau (2010, 2011) showed that (72.4%) of the US population defined themselves as a member of a non-Hispanic white ethnic group followed by African Americans (12.6%), Asian Americans (4.8%), American Indians/Alaskan Natives (0.9%), Native Hawaiian and other Pacific Islanders (0.2%), some other race (6.2%), and two or more races (2.9%). Hispanic origin was considered to be a separate concept from race but accounted for 16.4% of the population with those predominantly identified as white or as some other race. These changes reflect a society that is becoming more diverse with regard to racial and ethnic groups. As a result, significant differences in beliefs about health and illness are becoming apparent among the various groups. Nurses who provide care to clients of diverse cultures face many challenges, and this is especially true when the nurse comes from a different cultural group than the clients.

This chapter discusses strategies to assist nurses in providing culturally competent care. The special concerns of immigrants are discussed, and the following four groups are emphasized: African Americans, Asian Americans, Latinos and Hispanics, and Native Americans. There is also discussion of selected religious beliefs of people who practice Islam and how these beliefs need to be taken into account in providing nursing care.

IMMIGRANT HEALTH ISSUES

Immigration has a large effect on many aspects of life in the United States from the workplace to the classroom and throughout communities. Immigration and the laws that pertain to it have become increasingly controversial in recent years. Ambivalence among people in the United States about immigrants and the policies pertaining to them has grown due to the turmoil in the world with the relocation of people from any different countries. Some misunderstanding also

exists about what distinguishes an immigrant. Some states are passing laws to reduce the number of illegal immigrants who work in their state. The Refugee Act of 1980 provided a uniform procedure for refugees (based on the United Nations definition) to be admitted to the United States (US Census Bureau, 2001). People come to the United States for religious and political freedom and for economic opportunities. The 1986 Immigration Reform and Control Act permitted illegal aliens already living in the United States to apply for legal status if they met certain requirements. In 2014, about 41.2 million people in the United States were immigrants, making this an all-time high for the country (Artiga et al, 2016). Foreign-born residents are those who are not US citizens at birth, regardless of their current legal or citizen status. About one-half of the noncitizens were people without authorization to live or work in the United States (Congress of the United States, 2012). Immigrants in the United States and their US-born children represent one-quarter of the population or approximately 80 million people. In 2013 Mexican-born immigrants made up nearly 28% of the 41.3 million foreign-born persons. India accounted for the second largest with 5%, closely trailed by China (including Hong Kong but not Taiwan) (Zong and Batalova, 2015). Approximately 51% of the immigrant population was female, and the immigrant population had a median age of 43.1 compared with 35.9 for native-born citizens. In 2013 the following five states had the largest number of immigrants: California (10.3 million), New York and Texas (4.3 million each), Florida (3.8 million), and New Jersey (1.9 million). An especially difficult problem in public health nursing is that in 2013 there were 25.1 million individuals ages 5 and older who were limited English proficient (LEP), accounting for more than 8% of the population. The complex issues involved with immigrants and their health are beyond the scope of this discussion, but several are discussed, and suggestions are made for nursing actions.

There are four categories of foreign-born persons. First are the *legal immigrants,* who are also known as *lawful permanent residents* or *green-card holders.* These people are not citizens, but they are by law allowed to both live and work in the United States, often because they have useful job skills or family ties. Nonelderly noncitizens are as likely as citizens to have a full-time worker in the family; however, they are more likely to be a low-income worker who works in low-wage, blue-collar jobs and industries (Artiga et al, 2016). In regard to health care, noncitizens are significantly more likely than citizens to be uninsured. Noncitizens can obtain private coverage as an individual, through an employer, or as a dependent. Noncitizens are lawfully in the United States can enroll in Medicaid and the Children's Health Insurance Program (CHIP), but they are subject to eligibility restrictions. Since 1966, most lawfully present immigrants must wait 5 years after being considered "qualified" before they can enroll in Medicaid and CHIP. The Children's Health Program Reauthorization Act of 2009 gave states the option of eliminating the 5-year waiting period for "lawfully residing children and pregnant women who are otherwise eligible for Medicaid or CHIP" (Artiga et al, 2016, p. 5).

The second category of foreign-born immigrants consists of refugees and people seeking asylum. *Refugees* are admitted outside the usual quota restrictions based on fear of persecution in their homeland. The grounds for seeking asylum or refugee status must be at least one of five that include the person's race, religion, nationality, social group, political opinion, or national origin (National Immigration Forum, 2010). These are people seeking protection because they fear harm if they return to their home country. A person who receives refugee status is considered to be in the country lawfully and can receive the benefits described for lawful immigrants. The Centers for Disease Control and Prevention (CDC) provides "Refugee Health Guidelines" designed to promote and improve the health of the refugee, prevent disease, and familiarize refuges with the US health care system (CDC, 2012). The third category of foreign-born people, *nonimmigrants,* includes those who are admitted to the United States for a limited time and for a specific purpose. Examples include students, tourists, temporary workers, business executives, diplomats, artists, entertainers, and reporters. The fourth category consists of *unauthorized immigrants,* or undocumented or illegal aliens. They may have crossed a border into the United States illegally, or their legal permission to stay may have expired. They are eligible only for emergency medical services, immunizations, treatment for the symptoms of communicable diseases, and access to school lunches. Undocumented immigrants are ineligible for coverage under the Affordable Care Act (ACA), and they may not purchase coverage through the marketplace or receive tax credits (Artiga et al, 2016). Some states have state-funded health programs to provide coverage to some groups of immigrants regardless of their immigration status.

Although these numbers may change as changes occur in health care coverage, approximately one-third of immigrants are uninsured. Noncitizens are more likely to be uninsured than are citizens because of lower rates of both public and private coverage. Similarly, noncitizen children and citizen children in families with mixed citizenship status are more likely to be uninsured than are children of citizens (Artiga et al, 2016).

Several misperceptions exist about the economic value of allowing immigrants to enter or to stay in the United States. In 2013 immigrants made up nearly 17% (26.2 million) of the 158.6 million workers in the civilian workforce. The 24.2 million employed foreign-born workers were engaged in the following types of work: management, professional, and related (29.8); service (25.1); sales and office (17.1); production, transportation, and material moving (15.2); and natural resources, construction, and maintenance (12.9) (the numbers may not total to 100% due to rounding) (Zong and Batalova, 2015). Even though noncitizens are as likely as citizens to work, they may be in jobs that do not provide health coverage to employees.

The opinions about immigrants and the national debate about them have changed since the events of September 11,

2001, and subsequent acts of terrorism around the world. Since these attacks began, various immigration laws have been enacted that reflect more difficulty for people seeking visas, and there is more scrutiny of both visa and entry documents (*Changes in Immigration Law,* 2008).

Carlock (2007) has compiled useful material on how to find and access information that is culturally suited to the nation's increasingly diverse population, including culturally and linguistically appropriate client education. In addition to financial constraints on providing health care for immigrants, the following factors need to be considered:

- Language barriers
- Differences in social, religious, and cultural backgrounds between the immigrant and the health care provider
- Providers' lack of knowledge about high-risk diseases in the specific immigrant groups for whom they care
- The fact that many immigrants rely on traditional healing or folk health care practices that may be unfamiliar to their US health care providers

When working with immigrant populations, consider how your own background, beliefs, and knowledge may be significantly different from those of the people receiving care. *Language barriers* may interfere with efforts to provide assistance. Community members may be excellent resources as translators, not only of the actual words but also of the cultural beliefs, expectations, and use of nontraditional health practices.

The inability to speak English interferes with an immigrant's ability to access health care or even to seek health care (Douglas et al, 2014). Nurses need to know whether there are *specific risk factors* for a given immigrant population. For example, Southeast Asians are often at risk for hepatitis B (with its attendant effects on the liver), tuberculosis, intestinal parasites, and visual, hearing, and dental problems. Most of these conditions are either preventable or treatable if managed correctly (Office of Minority Health, 2008).

Nurses need to understand the *nontraditional healing practices* that their clients use. Many of these treatments have proved effective and can be blended with traditional Western medicine. The key is to know what practices are being used so the blending can be knowledgeably done. Community members are excellent sources for this information, and nurses working with immigrant populations should use the community assessment, group work, and family techniques described in other chapters. They can help clients and providers with communication, explanation, crisis intervention, emotional and other forms of support and housing. It is important to learn the strengths of the community and its members.

Often children and adolescents adjust to the new culture more easily than their elders. This can lead to *family conflict* and, at times, violence. Be alert for warning signs of family stress and tension. On the other hand, family members can help translate their culture, religion, beliefs, practices, support systems, and risk factors for the health care provider. They also can assist with decision making and provide support to enable the person or group seeking care to change behaviors to become more health conscious. Nurses need to understand the role of the family in immigrant populations and to treat individuals in the context of the families from which the immigrants come.

The following skills are useful when working with immigrant populations:

- Know yourself and how culture influences you.
- Get to know the families and their health-seeking behaviors. Ask who the family members are, where they live, and who is missing or dead. Ask about holidays and who attends and who does not attend.
- Get to know the communities that you serve. Read about them, volunteer, take a course, hold a forum with two-way communication, attend festivals and other key event such as religious meetings, and identify both formal and informal resources and leaders.
- Learn how the community deals with common illnesses or events.
- Try to see things from the viewpoint of the client, family, or community.

HOW TO   Guidelines for Selecting and Using an Interpreter

1. The interpreter must interpret everything that is said by all the people in the interaction and inform the public health nurse if the content might be perceived as insensitive or harmful to the dignity of the client.
2. The interpreter conveys the content and the spirit of what is said without omitting or adding.
3. The educational level and the socioeconomic status of the interpreter are important. The nurse should know that the interpreter understands the community's interpretation of the disease, and the nurse should understand the community's health care practices regarding the disease.
4. The nurse needs to evaluate the interpreter's style, approach to clients, and ability to develop a relationship of trust and respect.
5. The gender and/or age of the interpreter may be of concern; in some cultures, women may prefer a female interpreter and men may prefer a male, and older clients may want a more mature interpreter. Avoid using children as interpreters, particularly when the client is an adult. If possible, avoid family members as interpreters.
6. Identify the client's country of origin and language or dialect spoken before selecting the interpreter. For example, Chinese clients speak different dialects depending on the region in which they were born.
7. Observe the client for nonverbal messages such as facial expressions, gestures, and other forms of body language. If the client's responses do not fit with the question, the nurse should check to be sure that the interpreter understood the question.
8. Make phrase charts and picture cards available.
9. Increase accuracy in the transmission of information by asking the interpreter to translate the client's own words, and ask the client to repeat the information that was communicated.
10. The interpreter must maintain the confidentiality of all information and interactions. At the end of the interview, review the material with the client and the interpreter to ensure that nothing has been missed or misunderstood.

Data from Giger JN: *Transcultural nursing: assessment and intervention,* ed 7, St. Louis, 2016, Mosby; and Randall-David E: *Culturally competent HIV counseling and education,* McLean, Va, 1994, Maternal and Child Health Clearinghouse

---

Special note should be made about refugees. Unlike many of immigrants, refugees may have left their homes as a result of a disaster, and this might have led to physical or psychological consequences. Some may have been tortured; others may have lost family members in horrible ways. Still others may have lived in camps and lost all or most of their possessions. Some will have come from poor countries, and much of American culture will be alien to them. Nurses need to be sensitive and be skilled in finding resources to both help understand clients and their needs and then meet those needs (Plumb, 2003). Non-English-speaking refugees face challenges and barriers in accessing health care. Some of the barriers, in addition to those related to language, may include lack of transportation and not understanding how to use any public transportation in their area. Applying for Medicaid may be a barrier because of the complexity of the process. A nurse-led clinical program in Boise, Idaho, provides a useful exemplar of how nurses in the community can help refugees. This program, Culturally Appropriate Resources and Education Clinic (C.A.R.E.), provides a "convenient, one-stop access to a seamless continuum of health care services and education provided in a group setting" (Reavy et al, 2012). The clinic is located at the Family Center, an outpatient resource at the regional medical center. Two-hour group sessions are held at the clinic for about 10 clients. Peer health advisors and certified medical interpreters provide the teaching.

CULTURE, RACE, AND ETHNICITY

The concepts of culture, race, and ethnicity influence our understanding of human behavior. These three terms are often used incorrectly. Nurses need to understand the meaning of each when providing culturally competent health care to clients of diverse cultures.

CULTURE

Culture is a set of beliefs, values, and assumptions about life that is widely held among a group of people and that is transmitted across generations (Leininger, 2002a). Culture is an individual concept, a group phenomenon, and an organizational reality. It develops over time and is resistant to change. It takes many years for individuals to become familiar enough with a new value for it to become part of their culture. In response to the needs of its members and their environment, culture provides tested solutions to life's problems.

Individuals learn about their culture during the processes of learning language and becoming socialized, usually as children. Parents and family, the most important sources for the transfer of traditions, teach both explicit and implicit behaviors of the culture. The explicit behaviors, such as language, interpersonal distance, and kissing in public, can be observed and allow the individual to identify with other persons of the culture. In this way, people share traditions, customs, and lifestyles with others. The implicit behaviors are less visible and include the way individuals perceive health and illness, body language, difference in language expressions, and the use of titles. These behaviors are subtle and may be difficult for persons to describe, yet they are a part of the culture. For example, deferring to older adults, standing when they enter the room, or offering them a seat suggests a cultural value related to older adults.

Another example of an implicit aspect of culture is the use of language to communicate. For instance, in one culture a sign might read "No smoking is permitted." In another culture the sign might read "Thank you for not smoking." The former statement represents a culture that values directness, whereas the latter values indirectness. Each culture has an organizational structure that distinguishes it from others and provides the structure for what members of the cultural group determine to be appropriate or inappropriate behavior (Figs. 5.1 and 5.2).

Andrews and Boyle (2012), Giger (2017), Leininger (2002b), Purnell and Paulanka (2008), and Spector (2008) describe the organizational elements of culture. These elements include childrearing practices, religious practices, family structure, space, and communication. In the case of language, each language has unique characteristic expressions. Nurses need to know these organizational elements to provide appropriate care to persons of diverse cultures. This does not mean, however, that you should overlook or fail to incorporate the individuality of any person within any culture when developing a plan of care. Just as all cultures are not alike, all individuals within a culture are not alike. Within a culture, often people speak different dialects, have different religions and religious practices, represent widely divergent ages, and have different socioeconomic and educational status. Also, in many countries, people who live there may be native to that country or may have immigrated there. If an immigrant, the person may continue to adhere to customs, language, and religion from the native country. Each person should be viewed as a unique human being with differences that are respected. People in some cultures consider diseases such as cancer, mental illness, and HIV to carry a stigma.

RACE

Race is a biological variation within population groups based on physical markers derived from genetic ancestry such as skin color, physical features, and hair texture. Individuals may be of the same race but of different cultures. For example, African Americans, who may have been born in Africa, the Caribbean, North America, or elsewhere, are a heterogeneous group, but they are often viewed as culturally and racially homogeneous. This perception can cause providers to be unaware of cultural differences among individuals who come from different countries but who share similar racial characteristics. This often blurs an understanding of this culturally diverse group.

It is important to understand the growing numbers of interracial families. Physical changes in biracial and multiracial generations lead to changes in the physical appearance of individuals and make race less important in ethnic identity. Before 1989, biracial babies who had one white parent were assigned the race of the nonwhite parent. Currently the US Census Bureau allows people to choose more than one race (Fig. 5.3).

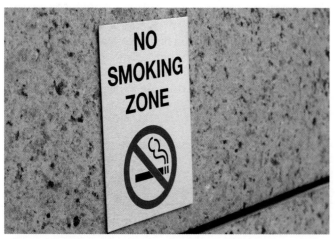

FIG. 5.1 This sign is from a culture that values directness in communication. (© 2012 Photos.com, a division of Getty Images. All rights reserved. Image #122153579.)

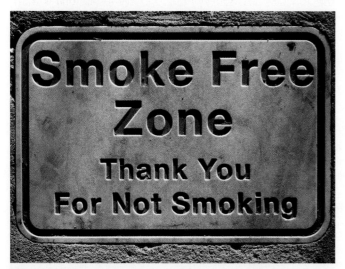

FIG. 5.2 This sign is from a culture that values an indirect approach to communication. (© 2012 Photos.com, a division of Getty Images. All rights reserved. Image #91883504.)

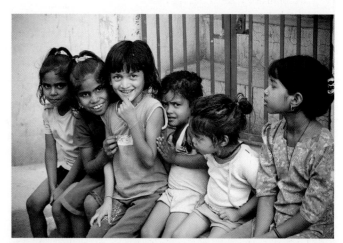

FIG. 5.3 In countries around the world, there are distinct differences in people who represent the same cultural group. (Copyright © 2013 Thinkstock. All rights reserved. Image # 117003112).

ETHNICITY

Ethnicity is the shared feeling of peoplehood among a group of individuals and relates to cultural factors such as nationality, geographical region, culture, ancestry, language, beliefs, and traditions (Giger, 2017). It reflects cultural membership and is based on individuals sharing similar cultural patterns (e.g., beliefs, values, customs, behaviors, traditions) that, over time, create a common history that is resistant to change. Ethnicity represents the identifying characteristics of culture (e.g., race, religion, national origin) and is influenced by education, income level, geographical location, and association with people from other ethnic groups. Therefore a reciprocal relationship exists between the individual and society. Members of an ethnic group give up aspects of their identity and society when they adopt characteristics of the group's identity. However, when the ethnic identity is strong, the group maintains its values, beliefs, behaviors, practices, and ways of thinking.

CULTURAL DIVERSITY

Cultural diversity refers to the degree of variation that is represented among populations based on lifestyle, ethnicity, race, and interest across place and place of origin across time. It also includes social class, gender identity, sexual orientation, and physical abilities/disabilities as well as the changing populations of the world. Although all cultures are not the same, all cultures have the same basic organizing factors (Giger, 2017). These factors should be explored in a cultural assessment because of the potential for differences among groups. Some of these differences among cultural groups are presented in Table 5.1. See the Levels of Prevention box for preventions related to cultural differences. Cultural diversity also includes the awareness of the presence of differences among the members of a social group or unit (Darnell and Hickson, 2015).

COMMUNICATION

Effective cross-cultural communication is a core competency for public health professionals (Swider et al, 2013), and is the fourth domain of the Guidelines for Implementing Culturally Competent Nursing Care (Douglas et al, 2014). Communication with the client or family is required for a cultural assessment. It is important to understand variations in patterns of verbal communication and nonverbal communication and to use words that a layperson can understand. Verbal communication is words used to express ideas and feelings; cultural variations are found, for example, in pronunciation, word meaning, voice quality, use of humor, and speed of talking. For example, many people from the United States and the United Kingdom have English as their first language. However, the word *boot* has different meanings for them. In the United States

TABLE 5.1 Cultural Variations Among Selected Groups				
	African Americans	**Asian-Americans**	**Hispanics**	**Native Americans**
Verbal communication	Asking personal questions of someone you have met is seen as improper and intrusive	High level of respect is shown for others, especially those in positions of authority	Expression of negative feelings is considered impolite	Low tone of voice is used, and the listener is expected to be attentive
Nonverbal communication	Direct eye contact in conversation is often considered rude	Direct eye contact with superiors may be considered disrespectful	Avoidance of eye contact is usually a sign of attentiveness and respect	Direct eye contact is often considered disrespectful
Touch	Touching someone else's hair is often considered offensive	It is not customary to shake hands with persons of the opposite sex	Touching is often observed between two persons in conversation	A light touch of the person's hand instead of a firm handshake is often used as a greeting
Family organization	Usually have close extended family networks; women play key roles in health care decisions	Usually have close extended family ties; emphasis may be on family needs rather than individual needs	Usually have close extended family ties; all members of the family may be involved in health care decisions	Usually have a close extended family; emphasis tends to be on the needs of the family rather than on individual needs
Time	Often present oriented	Often present oriented	Often present oriented	Often past oriented
Perception of health	Harmony of mind, health, body, and spirit with nature	When the "yin" and "yang" energy forces are balanced	Balance and harmony among mind, body, spirit, and nature	Harmony of mind, body, spirit, and emotions with nature
Alternative healers	"Granny," "root doctor," voodoo priest, spiritualist	Acupuncturist, acupressurist, herbalist	*Curandero, espiritualista, yerbero*	Medicine man, shaman
Self-care practices	Poultices, herbs, oils, roots	"Hot" and "cold" foods, herbs, teas, soups, cupping, burning, rubbing, pinching	"Hot" and "cold" foods, herbs	Herbs, cornmeal, medicine bundle
Biological variations	Sickle cell anemia, mongolian spots, keloid formation, inverted "T" waves, lactose intolerance, skin color	Thalassemia, drug interactions, mongolian spots, lactose intolerance, skin color	Mongolian spots, lactose intolerance, skin color	Cleft uvula, lactose intolerance, skin color

LEVELS OF PREVENTION

Related to Cultural Differences (Hypertension, Stroke, and Heart Disease)

Primary Prevention
Provide health teaching about a balanced diet and exercise.

Secondary Prevention
Teach clients and/or family to monitor blood pressure. Teach about diet, keeping in mind the client's cultural preferences. Talk about health beliefs and cultural implications, such as the use of alternative therapies; make sure alternative therapies are compatible with any medications that may be prescribed.

Tertiary Prevention
If blood pressure cannot be controlled by diet, refer the client to a physician or nurse practitioner for medication; advise the client to engage in a cardiac program that will oversee diet and exercise.

a boot typically refers to something one puts on one's feet; in the United Kingdom the boot may refer to what Americans call the trunk of the car. Just as understanding verbal communication is important, so is the understanding of nonverbal communication. Nonverbal communication is the use of body language or gestures to convey a message. Aspects of nonverbal language include eye contact, gestures, body posture, facial expressions, and silence. For example, some Hispanic women are reluctant to make direct eye contact or answer questions, and this behavior should not be seen as rudeness. Also, different cultures have their own perspective of how close they should stand to another person. In the United States, for many people, standing close when talking to someone other than a friend or family member may be seen as threatening or as invading one's personal space. In some cultures, standing close when speaking to another person is a usual way to communicate, whereas in other cultures, standing close seems intrusive and people may be uncomfortable. Culturally appropriate verbal and nonverbal communication helps nurses identify client's values, beliefs, practices, perceptions, and unique health care needs (Douglas et al, 2014).

An example of misunderstood nonverbal communication occurred when a nurse gave instructions to Asian American clients about taking antituberculin drugs. The clients smilingly responded with "yes, yes." The nurse interpreted this response to mean that the clients understood the instructions and accepted the treatment protocol. A week later, when the clients returned for a follow-up visit, the nurse discovered that the medications had not been taken. The nurse knew that acceptance by and avoidance of confrontation or disagreement with those in authority are important behaviors in the Asian American culture; interventions were therefore adjusted accordingly. The nurse repeated the medication instructions and gave the clients an opportunity to raise questions and concerns and to repeat the instructions that were given. The nurse also discussed the cultural meaning and treatment of tuberculosis. It is important to respect all information that a client shares with you, even when the information is in conflict with your own value system.

SPACE

Personal space is the physical area individuals need between themselves and others to feel comfortable. When this space is violated, the client may become uncomfortable. Nurses should take cues from clients to place themselves in the appropriate spatial zone and avoid misinterpretation of clients' behavior as they handle their spatial needs. Most cultural groups have spatial preferences. Some groups typically stand close to one another. However, one group may be comfortable with only a 9-inch distance between faces, whereas another group might find that small distance threatening and overly aggressive. It is important to understand the space preferences of the groups with whom you work because you may offend the client by placing yourself at a distance when his or her culture values close proximity to those with whom they speak and vice versa.

SOCIAL ORGANIZATION

Social organization refers to the way in which a cultural group structures itself around the family to carry out role functions. In some cultures, family may include people who are not actually related to one another. Find out who is considered to be in the family, who the key decision makers are, and if the needs of the family supersede those of an individual in the family. Nurses should be aware that some Hispanic and Asian cultures place the needs of the family above those of the individual. In the American Indian/Alaskan Native family, members honor and respect their elders. Nurses should advocate for the individual, so that when families make decisions, the individual's needs are also considered. However, members of the family may need to be included in the decision making.

TIME PERCEPTION

Regarding time, cultures are considered to be future, past, or present oriented. Historically, the American middle-class culture has tended to be future oriented, and individuals were willing to delay immediate gratification until future goals are accomplished. Recently this has changed as some people have become less future oriented and more focused on the present. In contrast, African American and Hispanic families may place greater value on quality of life and view present time as being more important than future time. The future is unknown, but the present is known. When nurses discuss health promotion and disease prevention strategies with persons from a present orientation, they should focus on the immediate benefits these clients would gain rather than emphasizing future outcomes.

In cultures that focus on a past orientation (e.g., the Vietnamese culture), individuals may focus on wishes and memories of their ancestors and look to them to provide direction for current situations (Giger, 2017). In a past-oriented culture, time is viewed as being more flexible than in a present-oriented culture. Nurses socialized in the Western culture may view time as money and equate punctuality with goodness and being responsible. Working with clients who have a different perception of time than the nurse can be problematic. Nurses should clarify the clients' perception to avoid misunderstanding. It is not realistic to expect clients to change their behavior and adopt the nurse's schedule.

ENVIRONMENTAL CONTROL

Environmental control refers to the relationships between humans and nature. Cultural groups might perceive humans as having mastery over nature, being dominated by nature, or having a harmonious relationship with nature. Those who view nature as dominant (e.g., African Americans and Hispanics) believe they have little or no control over what happens to them. They may not adhere to a cancer treatment protocol because of the belief that nothing will change the outcome because it is their destiny. These individuals are less likely to engage in illness prevention activities than those who have other worldviews.

Persons who view a human harmony with nature (e.g., African Americans, Asians, and Native Americans) may perceive that illness such as cancer is disharmony with other forces and that medicine can relieve the symptoms but cannot cure the disease. They would seek treatment for the malignancy from the mind, body, and spirit connection because they believe that healing comes from within. These groups are likely to look to naturalistic solutions, such as herbs, acupuncture, and hot and cold treatments, to resolve or cure a cancerous condition. Some clients may view their illness as punishment for misdeeds and may have difficulty accepting care from nurses who do not share their belief. Individuals from cultures that view the environment as being dominant over nature (e.g., Hispanics) may believe that they have little or no control over a serious illness for which they have been diagnosed. These individuals are less likely to engage in illness management interventions that are harsh and that they cannot trust to lead to a positive health outcome.

BIOLOGICAL VARIATIONS

Biological variations are the physical, biological, and physiological differences that distinguish one racial group from another. They occur in areas of growth and development, skin color, enzymatic differences, and susceptibility to disease (Andrews and Boyle, 2012; Giger, 2017). Other common and obvious variations include eye shape, hair texture, adipose tissue deposits, shape of earlobes, thickness of lips, and body configuration. There are also genetic differences that differentially affect some groups. Lactose intolerance is much more common in African blacks and African Americans than in the general population. Also, Western-born neonates are slightly heavier at birth than those born in non-Western cultures. Mongolian spots are bluish discolorations that are sometimes present on the skin of African American, Asian, Hispanic, and Native American/Alaskan Native babies. These discolorations may be mistaken for bruises. When nurses are exposed to situations involving biological variations of which they are unfamiliar, they may create embarrassing situations. Consider the following scenario: The school nurse observes a bluish discoloration on the thigh of a Filipino child that she mistook for a bruise. The nurse reported her observation to the child

protective agency in her state. When the child's mother arrived to pick her child up at the end of the school day, she was accused of child abuse. The mother had to disprove the allegation before her child could be released into her care.

NUTRITION

Nutritional practices are an integral part of the assessment process for all families, especially because they play a prominent role in the health problems of some groups. For many cultures, the preparation and eating of food are a social activity, and members of the group come together to celebrate life events and family rituals with food as a focus of the event. Efforts to understand dietary patterns of clients should go beyond relying on membership in a defined group. Knowing clients' nutrition practices makes it possible to develop treatment regimens that will not conflict with their cultural food practices. Box 5.1 identifies several questions that nurses should ask when conducting a nutritional assessment. Table 5.2

BOX 5.1 Assessment of Dietary Practices and Food Consumption Patterns

- What is the social significance of food in the family?
- What foods are most frequently bought for family consumption?
- What foods, if any, are taboo (prohibited) for the family?
- Does religion play a significant role in food selection?
- Who prepares the food? How is it prepared?
- How much food is eaten? When is it eaten, and with whom?
- Where does the client live, and what types of restaurants does he or she frequent?
- Has the family adopted foods of other cultural groups?
- What are the family's favorite recipes?

TABLE 5.2 Food Preferences and Associated Risk Factors in Selected Cultural Groups

Cultural Group	Food Preferences	Nutritional Excess	Risk Factors
African Americans	Fried foods, greens, bread, lard, pork, rice, foods with high sodium and starch content	Cholesterol, fat, sodium, carbohydrates, calories	Coronary artery disease, obesity
Asians	Soy sauce, rice, pickled dishes, raw fish, teas, balance between yin (cold) and yang (hot) concepts	Cholesterol, fat, sodium, carbohydrates, calories	Heart disease, liver disease, cancer of the stomach, ulcers
Hispanics	Fried foods, beans and rice, chili, carbonated beverages, high-fat and high-sodium foods	Cholesterol, fat, sodium, carbohydrates, calories	Heart disease, obesity

Data from Andrews MM, Boyle JS: *Transcultural concepts in nursing care*, ed 6, Philadelphia, 2012, Lippincott Williams and Wilkins; and Giger JN: *Transcultural nursing: assessment and intervention*, ed 7, St. Louis, 2017, Mosby.

>> **APPLYING CONTENT TO PRACTICE**

As has been discussed throughout the chapter, culturally competent nursing care uses many of the standards, guidelines, and competencies from key nursing and public health documents. For example, the Council on Linkages (2010) has a set of skills related to cultural competency and a set related to communication that is consistent with the information in this chapter. Likewise, the Quad Council further develops and applies the skills of the Council on Linkages related to both cultural competency and communication to public health nursing practice. As an example, the Council on Linkages states that a necessary skill in public health is to consider "the role of cultural, social, and behavioral factors in the accessibility, availability, acceptability and delivery of public health services." The Quad Council says that "public health nurses should consider the role of cultural, social, and behavioral factors in the accessibility, availability, acceptability and delivery of public health nursing services." Swider et al (2013) apply each of the Council on Linkages core competencies to public health nursing practice.

identifies the nutritional disadvantages to health of selected food preferences associated with four cultural groups. In working with clients of different cultures, the nurse might need to consult culturally oriented magazines. For example, some popular magazines such as *Essence, Ebony,* and *Latina* have altered old family recipes using healthier ingredients. These dishes taste good and allow those who use them to continue their old traditions related to food. As another example, many people who subscribe to the Buddhist religion are vegetarian. Their faith teaches self-control as a means to search for happiness. The Buddhist code of morality is in their Five Moral Precepts, and eating meat would conflict with both the first and the fifth (i.e., meat is seen as an intoxicant). These precepts are as follows: Do not harm or kill living things, steal, engage in sexual misconduct, lie, or consume intoxicants, such as alcohol, tobacco, or mind-altering drugs (ElGindy, 2013). Also, Muslims avoid pork and foods cooked with alcohol.

CULTURE, DIVERSITY, AND SOCIAL DETERMINANTS OF HEALTH

Socioeconomic factors contribute greatly to understanding perceptions of health and illness among minority groups. These groups may not have opportunities for education, occupation, income earning, and property ownership similar to those of the dominant group. Socioeconomic status, which is a measure often based on income, education, or occupation, is a critical factor in determining access to health care and the development of some chronic health problems and in health outcomes (Mohammed, 2011; Sims, Sims, and Bruce, 2008). According to the US Census Bureau (2011), in 2010 more white families than minorities lived below the poverty level. However, the proportion of poor families in a minority group is greater. For example, white families represent 9.3% of those in poverty, whereas African Americans represent 22.7% and Hispanics represent 22.7%. Consequently, minority families are disproportionately represented on the lower tiers of the socioeconomic ladder. Poor economic achievement is also a common characteristic among at-risk populations, such as those in poverty, the homeless, migrant workers, and refugees. Data suggest that when

nurses and clients come from the same social class, it is more likely that they operate from the same health belief model and consequently there is less opportunity for misinterpretation and problems in communication.

Social determinants of health are thought to have a major impact on health. These are the determinants and conditions in which people are born, live, work, and age and include such factors as education, racial segregation, social supports, and poverty. For example, "children born to parents who have not completed high school are more likely to live in an environment that poses barriers to health" (Heiman and Artiga, 2015, p 1). The neighborhoods of these children are less likely to have parks in which they can play, sidewalks, recreation centers, or a library. They are more likely to be unsafe, have exposed garbage or litter, have poor or run-down housing, and be plagued by vandalism (Heiman and Artiga, 2015). As will be discussed in Chapter 23, Poverty, Homelessness, Mental Illness, and Teen Pregnancy, more minority families than white families live below the poverty level. Poor economic achievement is also a common characteristic among at-risk populations, such as those in poverty, the homeless, migrant workers, and refugees. Data suggest that when nurses and clients come from the same social class, it is more likely that they operate from the same health belief model, and consequently, there is less opportunity for misinterpretation and problems in communication.

A danger also exists in believing that certain cultural behaviors, such as folk practices, are restricted to lower socioeconomic classes. For example, health professionals, such as nurses and physicians, may also use folk systems in conjunction with the biomedical system to promote their health and prevent disease. Therefore nurses must conduct a cultural assessment for all individuals when they first come in contact with them. Nurses should be able to distinguish between issues of culture and socioeconomic class and not misinterpret behavior as having a cultural origin when, in fact, it should be attributed to socioeconomic class.

CULTURAL COMPETENCE

Many people are taught by and have knowledge of a dominant culture. As long as the person operates within that culture, responses occur without thought to a variety of situations and do not require examination of the cultural context. However, as multiculturalism grows, it becomes increasingly important for health care providers, including nurses and organizations, to provide quality and effective care. For example, consider the situation of a recent Mexican immigrant who speaks little English and goes to a community health center because of a urinary tract infection. The nurse understands that she must use strategies that will allow her to effectively communicate with the client; the client has the right to receive effective care, to judge whether she received the care she wanted, and to follow up with appropriate action if she did not receive the expected care. Culturally competent care is provided not only to individuals of racial or ethnic minority groups but also to individuals belonging to groups held together by factors such as age, religion, sexual orientation, and socioeconomic status. Nurses must be culturally competent to provide nursing care that meets the needs of these persons. Such nursing actions can decrease racial and health disparities and improve health outcomes (Brondolo, Gallo, and Myers, 2009).

Cultural competence in nurses is a combination of culturally congruent behaviors, practice attitudes, and policies that allow nurses to work effectively in cross-cultural situations. The term *competence* refers to performance that is sufficient and adequate. Culturally competent nurses function effectively when caring for clients of other cultures. Culturally competent nurses learn about the cultures of the clients whom they serve and they respect people from other cultures and value diversity; this helps them provide more responsive care. Cultural competence includes acknowledging the fundamental differences in the ways clients and families respond to illness and treatment from what might be your response or a more typical Western health care response. It is important for nurses to continuously engage in critical reflection to examine their own values, beliefs, and cultural heritage in order to increase their awareness of how these qualities can influence their care (Douglas et al, 2014). This can include paying attention to dietary practices, pain, death and dying, modesty, eye contact, closeness, and touching others. YouTube offers many videos that address cultural competence. Use key words such as "cultural competence in nursing" and see what you can find.

Ten guidelines, formerly referred to as standards, have been developed by a collaborative task force of members of the American Academy of Nursing (AAN) Expert Panel on Global Nursing and Health and the Transcultural Nursing society. These standards were developed to serve as a guide for providing culturally competent care. The authors of the standards say that due to the migration of both nurses and clients, it is important to have a set of universally applicable guidelines for providing culturally competent care. The recipient of the nursing care can be an individual, a family, a community, or a population. The standards are based on the principles of social justice and human rights. These concepts are discussed in Chapter 4, Ethics in Community Health Nursing Practice. The 10 standards are (1) knowledge of cultures, (2) education and training in culturally competent care, (3) critical reflection, (4) cross-cultural communication, (5) culturally competent practice, (6) cultural competence in health care systems and organizations, (7) patient advocacy and empowerment, (8) multicultural workforce, (9) cross-cultural leadership, and (10) evidence-based practice and research (Douglas et al, 2014). These guidelines are important because both health care professionals and organizations are responsible for providing the infrastructure needed to deliver safe, culturally congruent, and compassionate care (Douglas et al, 2014).

Nurses must be culturally competent for several key reasons, including the following:

- First, the nurse's culture often differs from that of the client, leading to different understandings of communication, behaviors, and plans for care.
- Second, care that is not culturally competent may increase the cost of health care and decrease the opportunity for positive client outcomes. Clients who do not feel understood may

 HEALTHY PEOPLE 2020

Objectives Related to Cultural Issues

Goal
To eliminate health disparities among different segments of the population as defined by gender, race or ethnicity, education, income, disability, geographic location, and sexual orientation.

Selected Objectives
- **AHS-3:** Increase the proportion of persons with a usual primary-care provider.
- **AHS-7:** Reduce the proportion of individuals who are unable to obtain or delay in obtaining necessary care, dental care, or prescription medicine.

From U.S. Department of Health and Human Services: *Healthy People 2020: understanding and improving health,* Washington, DC, 2010, US Government Printing Office.

delay seeking care or may withhold key information. For example, if a person is afraid of disapproval, he may not tell the nurse that he is using both folk medicine and Western medicine. The two medicines may have cumulative or contradictory effects that could be dangerous to the client.
- Third, to meet some of the objectives for persons of different cultures as outlined in *Healthy People 2020* (see the *Healthy People 2020* box) (US Department of Health and Human Services, 2010), lifestyle, background, traditions, values, practices, and personal choices must be considered.
- Fourth, legal regulations and accreditation mandates specify that culturally competent health care must be provided so that health disparities can be reduced and ultimately eliminated. A goal of *Healthy People 2020* deals with eliminating health disparities among people that occur as a result of gender, race or ethnicity, education or income, disability, geographical location, or sexual orientation. Diabetes is discussed in this context because its prevalence is associated with disparities of income and education, and it is more prevalent among Hispanics living in the United States than among non-Hispanic whites. Diabetes is more prevalent among American Indians and Alaska Natives than among whites, demonstrating the need to look at culture when working with these populations.

Developing Cultural Competence

Developing cultural competence is one of the core competencies for public health nurses (Swider et al, 2013). It is an ongoing life process that involves every aspect of client care. It is challenging and at times painful as nurses struggle to adopt new ways of thinking and performing. Leininger (2002a) suggests that the following two principles are useful in developing cultural competence:

1. Maintain a broad, objective, and open attitude toward individuals and their cultures.
2. Avoid seeing all individuals as alike.

Nurses develop cultural competence in different ways, but the key elements are experience with clients of other cultures, an awareness of this experience, and the promotion of mutual respect for differences. Because degrees of cultural competence vary, not all nurses may reach the same level of development. Also, developing cultural competence is a life-long process.

TABLE 5.3 The Cultural Competence Framework: Stages of Competence Development

	Culturally Incompetent	Culturally Sensitive	Culturally Competent
Cognitive dimension	Oblivious	Aware	Knowledgeable
Affective dimension	Apathetic	Sympathetic	Committed to change
Skills dimension	Unskilled	Lacking some skills	Highly skilled

From Orlandi MA: Defining cultural competence: an organizing framework. In Orlandi MA, editor: *Cultural competence for evaluators*, Washington, DC, 1992, US Department of Health and Human Services.

BOX 5.2 Early Cultural Awareness

- Think about the first time you had contact with someone you realized was culturally different from you.
- Briefly describe the situation or event. How old were you? What were your feelings? What were your thoughts?
- What did your parents and other significant adults say about those who were culturally different from your family? What adjectives were used? What attitudes were conveyed?
- As you got older, what messages did you get about minority groups from the larger community or culture?
- As an adult, how do you see others in the community talk about culturally different people? What adjectives are used? What attitudes are conveyed? How does this reinforce or contradict your earlier experience?
- What parts of this cultural baggage make it difficult to work with clients from different cultural groups?
- What parts of this cultural baggage facilitate your work with clients?

From Randall-David E: *Culturally competent HIV counseling and education*, McLean, VA, 1994, Maternal and Child Health Clearinghouse.

Orlandi (1992) suggests that there are three stages in the development of cultural competence: culturally incompetent, culturally sensitive, and culturally competent (Table 5.3). Each stage has three dimensions—cognitive (thinking), affective (feeling), and psychomotor (doing)—that together have an overall effect on nursing care.

A widely used model to explain the process of cultural competence is that of Campinha-Bacote (2011). This model has the following five elements of cultural competence: (1) cultural awareness, (2) cultural knowledge, (3) cultural skill, (4) cultural encounter, and (5) cultural desire.

Cultural Awareness

Cultural awareness is the self-examination and in-depth exploration of one's own biases, stereotypes, and prejudices that influence behavior (Campinha-Bacote, 2011). Nurses who have developed cultural awareness are able to do the following:

- Learn about the cultural dimensions of clients.
- Understand their own behavior and how it helps or hinders the delivery of competent care to persons from cultures other than their own.
- Recognize that health is expressed differently across cultures and that culture influences an individual's responses to health, illness, disease, and death.

For example, at a community outreach program, a nurse was teaching a racially mixed group the screening protocol for the detection of breast and cervical cancer. An African American woman in the group refused to give the return demonstration for breast self-examination. When encouraged to do so, she said, "My breasts are much larger than those on the model. Besides, the models are not like me. They are all white." After hearing the client's comments, the nurse realized that she had made no reference in her talk to the influence of culture or race on screening for breast and cervical cancer.

The nurse talked with the client, asked for her recommendations, and encouraged her to return to the demonstration. The nurse coached the client through the self-examination process while pointing out that regardless of breast size, shape, and color, the technique is the same for feeling the tissue and squeezing the nipple to make certain that there is no discharge. Because this nurse was culturally aware, she neither became

angry with herself or the client nor imposed her own values on the client. Rather, the client talked about her beliefs, attitudes, and feelings about screening for cancer that may be influenced by her culture. Subsequently, the nurse purchased a model of an African American woman's breast to use in future health education programs with African American women. A nurse who was not culturally aware may have misunderstood the client's concerns and acted in a defensive manner. This might have led to lack of information being provided or a confrontation between the nurse and client. Cultural awareness is consistent with guideline 3, critical reflection, of the Guidelines for Implementing Culturally Competent Nursing Care (Douglas et al, 2014). Critical reflection implies that nurses examine their own values, beliefs, and cultural heritage in order to provide effective care to patients of different cultures. See Box 5.2 for questions to ask yourself about your development of cultural awareness.

Cultural Knowledge

Cultural knowledge is information about organizational elements of diverse cultures and ethnic groups. Emphasis is on learning about the client's worldview from an emic (native) perspective. An understanding of the client's culture decreases misinterpretations and misapplication of scientific knowledge and facilitates the client's cooperation with the health care regimen (Campinha-Bacote, 2011). For example, cultural knowledge informs us that Middle Eastern women may not attend prenatal classes without encouragement and support from the nurse (Meleis, 2005). The reason for this is that attending the classes is about the future of the baby, whereas the mother's main concern may be on the present and what is happening now. If nurses understand the cultural difference in this example, they can select strategies to help the mother understand the value of the classes. In contrast, knowledge about Nigerian culture would allow the nurse to understand that the mother might begin prenatal classes but not continue because Nigerian women view birth as a natural process and not a process they need to attend a class to understand (Ogbu, 2005). Nurses who lack cultural knowledge may develop feelings of inadequacy

EVIDENCE-BASED PRACTICE

The purpose of this descriptive correlation study was to assess personal beliefs about the causes and meaning of having diabetes among members of the Lumbee Indian tribe living in rural southeastern North Carolina. The sample consisted of 40 adult men and women. A mixed-method approach using qualitative and quantitative data was used to conduct this study.

The participant responses indicated a moderate belief in the efficacy of diabetes treatment, a moderate belief in their ability to understand a coherent model of diabetes, and a low level of emotional distress related to having diabetes. Two major themes emerged from the open-ended questions about the causes of diabetes: (1) genetic predetermination and (2) lifestyle practices. Although participants believed that their prescribed diabetes medications were a necessary part of controlling their illness, several expressed fatigue and "felt worn out" with having to persist with their treatment expectations. Limitations were that the sample only included persons who were seeking health care treatment for diabetes and did not include those who were not scheduled for an appointment at the clinic during the data-collection period or those who did not have access to health care.

Nurse Use

Nurses should be aware that their Lumbee Indian clients may not always have a high degree of confidence in conventional treatment regimens or an understanding of the unpredictable course of diabetes. Nurses should work with these clients to provide culturally congruent education using appropriate communication to increase clients' knowledge about current treatment regimens. Nurses should incorporate culturally specific strategies that will assist clients to take a more active role in their illness management, dispel the attitude that a diagnosis of diabetes is genetically predetermined, link concrete behaviors to disease progression and outcomes, and demonstrate to clients how attainable decreases in blood sugar can reduce the risk of long-term consequences. Such strategies would help eliminate negative perceptions that may interfere with the health care delivery process. The researchers suggested that by using a broad systems approach, nurses will increase the availability of Native American health care providers who can serve as role models for the community as well as become activists for developing community infrastructure to support healthy lifestyles.

From Jacobs A, Kemppainen JK, Taylor JS, et al: Beliefs about diabetes and medication adherence among Lumbee Indians living in rural southeastern North Carolina. *J Transcult Nurs* 25:167–175, 2014.

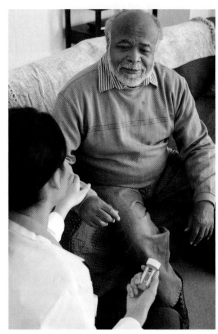

FIG. 5.4 An Asian American nurse interacts with an African American man in his home. (© 2012 Photos.com, a division of Getty Images. All rights reserved. Image #86497393.)

and helplessness when they cannot effectively help their clients. Studies have shown that when students are not exposed to a variety of cultures, they may have gaps in their cultural knowledge and ability to care for diverse clients (Jones, Cason, and Bond, 2004). Although it is unrealistic to expect that nurses will have knowledge of all cultures, they should be aware of and know how to obtain knowledge of cultural influences that affect groups with whom they most frequently interact. Cultural knowledge is consistent with guideline 1, knowledge of cultures, in the Guidelines for Implementing Culturally Competent Nursing Care (Douglas et al, 2014).

The Evidence-Based Practice box provides an example of learning how to meet the needs of a cultural group that is different from that of the nurse.

Cultural Skill

Cultural skill refers to the effective integration of cultural awareness and cultural knowledge to obtain relevant cultural data and meet the needs of culturally diverse clients. Culturally skillful nurses use appropriate touch during conversation, modify the physical distance between themselves and others, and use strategies to avoid cultural misunderstandings while meeting mutually agreed-upon goals. Cultural skill is consistent with guideline 5, culturally competent practice, of the Guidelines for Implementing Culturally Competent Nursing Care (Douglas et al, 2014) (Fig. 5.4).

Cultural Encounter

A cultural encounter is the fourth construct essential to becoming culturally competent. Cultural encounter is the process that permits nurses to seek opportunities to engage in cross-cultural interactions with clients of diverse cultures to modify existing beliefs about a specific cultural group and possibly avoid stereotyping (Campinha-Bacote, 2011). Culture encounters are part of the interpersonal nurse–patient relationship and focus on caring, compassion, presence, caring consciousness, and empathy. There are both direct (face-to-face) and indirect types of cultural encounters. Aspects of cultural encounter include effective communication, use of appropriate language and literacy level, and learning directly from clients about their life experiences and the significance of these experiences for health (Leininger, 2002a).

An example of a direct cultural encounter is when nurses learn directly from their Puerto Rican American clients about spicy food they avoid when breastfeeding. Indirect cultural encounters occur when nurses share this information about the effect of spicy food on breastfeeding with other nurses. When nurses come into contact with persons who are culturally different from themselves, they should adapt general cultural concepts to the situation until they are able to learn directly from the clients about their culture (Fig. 5.5). Nurses can develop cultural competence by reading about, taking courses on, and discussing different cultures within multicultural settings.

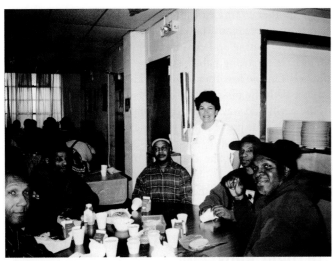

FIG. 5.5 A Hispanic nursing student interacting with African American men at a nutrition center. To interact in a culturally competent manner, the nurse needs to have an awareness of and knowledge about the differences between her culture and the men's culture and the skill to portray this in her behavior toward them.

Cultural Desire

Cultural desire is the fifth construct in the development of cultural competence. It refers to the nurse's intrinsic motivation to provide culturally competent care (Campinha-Bacote, 2012). Nurses who desire to become culturally competent do so because they want to rather than because they are directed to do so. They are energetic, enthusiastic, and goal directed in providing culturally competent care. Unlike the other constructs, cultural desire cannot be directly taught in the classroom or other educational settings. However, nurses are more likely to demonstrate cultural desire when their work environment reflects a philosophy that values cultural competence at all levels of the organization and for all its clients. Campinha-Bacote (2011) encourages nurses not to be afraid of making mistakes but to enthusiastically try to learn about other people. Box 5.3 lists several important points to remember when trying to increase your cultural competence.

CULTURALLY COMPETENT NURSING INTERVENTIONS

Nurses integrate their professional knowledge with the client's knowledge and practices to negotiate and promote culturally relevant care. Leininger (2002a) suggests that the following three modes of action, based on negotiation between the client and nurse, can guide the nurse in providing culturally competent care: cultural preservation, cultural accommodation, and cultural repatterning. When these decisions and actions are used with cultural brokering, the nurse is able to fulfill the various roles vital to providing holistic care for culturally diverse clients.

CULTURAL PRESERVATION

Cultural preservation means that the nurse supports and facilitates the use of scientifically supported cultural practices from a person's culture along with those from the biomedical health care system. Examples are acupressure and acupuncture. Acupuncture is an ancient Chinese practice of inserting needles at specific points in the skin to cure disease or relieve pain. These practices are being accepted by increasing numbers of Western practitioners as a legitimate method of health care. It is important to know when clients are blending traditional health practices with those prescribed by the health care provider to make certain they support rather than interfere with one another.

CULTURAL ACCOMMODATION

Cultural accommodation means that the nurse supports and facilitates clients in their use of cultural practices when such cultural practices are not harmful to clients. For example, consider the practice of home burial of the placenta. In this

---

BOX 5.3 Developing Cultural Competency: Points to Remember

- Culture is applicable to groups of whites, such as Italians or Irish Americans, as well as to racial and ethnic minorities.
- During each interaction with clients, be sensitive to the cultural implications of the encounter.
- Ask questions to stimulate learning about how clients identify and express their cultural background.
- Much diversity exists within groups, and not all persons of the same racial or ethnic group may share the same culture. Assess both cultural group patterns and individual variations within a cultural group to avoid stereotyping.
- When misunderstandings arise, acknowledge the problem, and take responsibility for your own errors.
- Be knowledgeable about your own cultural heritage, biases, beliefs, values, and practices when providing care.
- Avoid making assumptions about nonverbal cues when interacting with clients from unfamiliar cultures.
- Use a variety of sources, including clients, to develop cultural knowledge.
- Understand that developing cultural competence is an ongoing journey and an evolving process.

❓ CHECK YOUR PRACTICE

Ms. Lin, a 73-year-old Chinese American woman, is discharged to home care after surgery for cancer of the large intestine. The nurse found her at home alone with her 76-year-old husband. After the physical assessment, the nurse discussed making a referral for Ms. Lin to have a home health aide to assist her with physical care and light housekeeping chores. The family was gracious but seemed hesitant to accept the referral. The nurse knew that Chinese people often value the extended family network and family decision making. She asked the couple if they would like to discuss the situation with their daughters. Both the client and her husband seemed pleased with the idea, and the nurse promised to return the next day. When the nurse returned for her visit, one of Ms. Lin's daughters was present and told the nurse that the family could manage without additional help. The three daughters had made a schedule to take turns caring for their parents.

Which of the following should the nurse do? (1) Try to persuade Ms. Lin's daughters to accept help. (2) Accept and support the family's decision and tell them that if they decide at a later time to have the home health aide, they should call the agency, and give them the telephone number. (3) Schedule the next follow-up visit with them.

example, the delivery room nurse was helpful when Ms. Sanchez asked her not to discard a piece of the amniotic sac that was present on her grandbaby's face immediately after birth. Ms. Sanchez asked the nurse to give it to her instead. The grandmother believed that being born with a piece of the amniotic sac on the face was a visible sign that something special was going to happen in the person's life. The grandmother explained that after she dried the piece of the amniotic sac, she would keep it in a safe place. She would also spend extra time protecting the baby to prevent her from being harmed. Although the delivery room nurse did not know about this practice, she gave the grandmother the piece of the sac as she requested. As another example, using cultural accommodation, a nurse can assist older Chinese American clients to more effectively manage their hypertension by modifying their use of high-sodium soy sauce by substituting low-sodium soy sauce in their cooking. Similarly, African Americans can be guided to use more broiled and boiled foods and eat fewer fried foods.

In providing care to clients who practice the Islamic faith, it is important to understand some of the key tenets of their faith. The Five Pillars of Islam define the duties that each Muslim should practice to be consistent with their faith. The second pillar, Salat, can have implications for nurses caring for these patients. Salat says that a Muslim must pray five times a day while facing Mecca, which is in an easterly direction in the United States (Charles and Daroszewski, 2012). The prayers are given in a kneeling position on a prayer mat or carpet. It is important for the agency and the health care professionals to make it possible for these clients to pray at the appointed times. The Qur'an also dictates various health care choices related to contraception and birth, sanitary practices, dietary practices, and medical care concerns, to name a few (Charles and Daroszewski, 2012). In providing culturally appropriate care to Muslim clients, it is important to take into account the tenets of their religion. Cultural accommodation is consistent with guideline 4, cross-cultural communication, of the Guidelines for Implementing Culturally Competent Nursing Care (Douglas et al, 2014).

CULTURAL REPATTERNING

Cultural repatterning means that the nurse works with clients to help them reorder, change, or modify their cultural practices when these practices are harmful to them. For example, a culturally competent nurse knows of the high incidence of obesity among Mexican American women 20 years of age and older. A school nurse was invited to develop a health education program for Mexican teenagers in the local high school. While respecting their cultural traditions, the nurse discussed weight management strategies with the teenagers. The nurse understood the teenagers' cultural issues pertaining to food and knew how to negotiate with them. She discouraged the use of fried foods (such as tortillas), sour cream, and regular cheese and encouraged and demonstrated the use of baked tortillas and of salsa as dip and topping.

In another example, a nurse who was giving prenatal instructions to pregnant Haitian women discovered that many of them were visiting an herbalist to obtain teas that would help them have a "strong baby." The nurse asked for the names of the herbs in the teas they were drinking and scheduled a conference with the pharmacist to discuss the specific ingredients in the herbs and ways they might help the client meet her cultural needs. The nurse found that one of the herbs contributed to high blood pressure, a problem that many of the women were experiencing. She explained to the women why they should not drink the tea with the specific herb. The nurse enlisted the aid of the herbalist because she understood the importance of supernatural causes of illness in the Haitian culture (Miller, 2000).

CULTURAL BROKERING

Cultural brokering is advocating, mediating, negotiating, and intervening between the client's culture and the biomedical health care culture on behalf of clients. Cultural brokering is similar to guideline 6, patient advocacy and empowerment, of the Guidelines for Implementing Culturally Competent Nursing Care (Douglas et al, 2014). It is important to understand both your culture and that of the client and to resolve or decrease problems that result from individuals in either culture not understanding the other person's values. To illustrate, migrant workers tend to have high occupational mobility; many are poor and have limited formal education. They may seek health care only when they are ill and cannot work. Whenever a nurse interacts with them, it is important to teach them about prevention, health maintenance, environmental sanitation and pesticides, and nutrition because it may be the only opportunity that the nurse will have to treat a particular migrant worker. Nurses also should advocate for the rights of the migrant worker to receive quality health care. For example, the nurse may contact the migrant health services for follow-up or referral care for the migrant worker. Advocacy is consistent with guideline 6 of the Guidelines for Implementing Culturally Competent Nursing Care (Douglas et al, 2014).

INHIBITORS TO DEVELOPING CULTURAL COMPETENCE

Nurses may fail to provide culturally competent nursing care if they do not understand transcultural nursing, their supervisors are pressuring them to increase productivity by increasing their caseloads, or they are pressured by colleagues who are not knowledgeable about other cultures and who are critical or offended when others use these concepts. These and similar issues can inhibit delivery of culturally competent care and may result in nurse behaviors such as stereotyping, prejudice and racism, ethnocentrism, cultural imposition, cultural conflict, and cultural shock.

- Stereotyping means attributing certain beliefs and behaviors about a group to an individual without giving adequate attention to individual differences. Examples of stereotypes are "All Asian people are hardworking" and "All Chinese people are good at math."

- **Prejudice** refers to having a deeply held reaction, often negative, about another group or person. For example, a person may be viewed negatively because of skin color, race, religion, or social standing, with no regard for the worth of the person as an individual.

- **Racism** is a form of prejudice and refers to the belief that persons who are born into a particular group are inferior, for example, in intelligence, morals, beauty, or self-worth. Because of their race, individuals may be denied opportunities that are available to people of other races. Racism can be one of three forms: individual because of the characteristics of the group of which the person is a member, such as skin color, hair texture, or facial features; institutional, such as discriminatory policies, priorities, and resource allocation pertaining to certain groups; or cultural, in which a culture is viewed in derogatory or stereotypical ways because of, for example, how a group dresses or the language the group uses. See Box 5.4 for examples of prejudice and racist behaviors.

- **Ethnocentrism,** a type of cultural prejudice at the population level, is the belief that one's own group determines the standards for behavior by which all other groups are to be judged. Ethnocentric nurses are unfamiliar and uncomfortable with anything that is different from their culture. Their inability to accept different worldviews often leads them to devalue the experiences of others, judge them to be inferior, and treat people who are different with suspicion or hostility (Andrews and Boyle, 2012). Some American nurses may think that the way we do something is the best (or only) way to provide this care. Ethnocentrism contrasts with **cultural blindness,** which is the tendency to ignore all differences among cultures, to act as though these differences do not exist, and as a result, to treat all people the same (when in truth, each person is an individual with unique needs). Nurses who say that they treat all clients the same, regardless of cultural orientation, are demonstrating cultural blindness.

- **Cultural imposition** involves the belief in one's own superiority, or ethnocentrism, and the act of imposing one's values on others. Nurses impose their values on clients when they forcefully promote Western medical traditions while ignoring the clients' value of non-Western treatments such as acupuncture, herbal therapy, or spiritual remedies. A goal for nurses is to develop the approach of **cultural relativism,** in which they recognize that clients have different approaches to their health, and that each culture should be judged on its own merit and not on the nurse's personal beliefs.

- **Cultural conflict** is a perceived threat that may arise from a misunderstanding of expectations between clients and

---

BOX 5.4 Types of Prejudice and Racist Behaviors

Overt Intentional Prejudice and Racism

Two homeless women, one African American and the other Irish American, are clients at the neighborhood health care center. Both women are having financial difficulty. The African American client's husband was laid off 4 years ago after his company merged with another company. The Irish American client is undergoing radiation treatment for metastatic cancer and has lost her job as a result of her prolonged illness. Both women are without health insurance. A nurse referred the Irish American client to social services but did not refer the African American woman. The nurse believed that minority clients have direct experience with some local and national government programs; therefore these clients know about available resources and can negotiate the social system for themselves and their families. In contrast, the nurse believed that the Irish American woman had a catastrophic illness and had no experience negotiating government programs, and therefore the nurse needed to advocate for her. The nurse, not knowing the health-seeking behaviors of either client, stereotyped both women and intentionally used her informational power to help one client while denying assistance to the other client.

Overt Unintentional Prejudice and Racism

A nurse was assigned to make an initial visit to two clients recently discharged from the hospital with a diagnosis of hypertension. The nurse performed physical assessments on both clients. He developed an extensive culturally relevant teaching plan with the Filipino American client that included information on sodium restriction and the effect on kidney functioning, ways to integrate cultural foods into the diet, and support in lifestyle changes. With the Puerto Rican American client, the nurse performed a routine physical assessment and did not discuss the client's culturally special dietary requirements. The nurse believed that the Puerto Rican American client was not capable of understanding such complex information and was going to continue to seek help from her *curandera* (a folk practitioner) to manage the hypertension.

At the end of his visit, the nurse said to this client, "Take care of yourself. See you next time." This nurse did not realize that he had stereotyped the client and that his actions were hurtful. He believed that he was providing quality care on the basis of the client's needs.

Covert Intentional Prejudice and Racism

A Native American nurse works in a home health agency that serves an ethnically diverse community. The nurse has observed that the clients are always among the poorest and live in the unsafe areas of the community, and she is very concerned about her client care assignment. Her nonminority colleagues are not assigned to those sections of the community. In a recent staff meeting, she raised the concerns with her nursing supervisors. On hearing her observations, the supervisors looked at her in a skeptical manner and asked what she was talking about. This is covert racism because the nursing supervisors were aware of the informal policy dictating that they assign minority nurses to clients in a particular area of the community. They had discussed the practice among themselves but would never admit to it. The supervisors believed that the best way to ensure that minority clients would be the recipients of culturally competent care was to assign a minority nurse to care for them.

Covert Unintentional Prejudice and Racism

A lesbian middle-class couple legally adopted a physically challenged child. Their insurance refuses to pay for the child's medical care. The nurse, who has been working for the agency for many years, is aware but failed to tell the parents that the baby can qualify for Medicaid through the handicapped insurance program, even though both parents work and their income is above the Medicaid guidelines limit. This nurse was unaware that her dislike for the parents' sexual lifestyle influenced her thinking (she had in the past provided heterosexual couples with information on how to apply for Medicaid).

nurses when either group is not aware of cultural differences (Andrews and Boyle, 2012). Although cultural conflict is unavoidable, it is important to know how to manage it while delivering culturally competent care.

- Cultural shock is the feeling of helplessness, discomfort, and disorientation experienced by an individual attempting to understand or effectively adapt to another cultural group that differs in practices, values, and beliefs. It results from the anxiety caused by losing familiar sights, sounds, and behaviors.

Being aware of clients' cultural beliefs and knowing about other cultures may help nurses be less judgmental, more accepting of cultural differences, and less likely to engage in the behaviors just listed that inhibit cultural competence.

CULTURAL NURSING ASSESSMENT

A cultural nursing assessment is a systematic way to identify the beliefs, values, meanings, and behaviors of people while considering their history, life experiences, and the social and physical environments in which they live.

Skills such as listening, explaining, acknowledging, recommending, understanding, and negotiating help the nurse be nonjudgmental. It is vital that nurses listen to clients' perceptions of their problems and, in turn, that nurses explain to clients the nurses' perceptions of the problems. Nurses and clients should acknowledge and discuss similarities and differences between the two perceptions to develop suggestions and recommendations for managing problems. Nurses also negotiate with clients on nursing care actions to meet the needs of the clients.

Numerous tools are available to assist nurses in conducting cultural assessments (Andrews and Boyle, 2012; Leininger, 2002b). The focus of such tools varies, and selection is determined by the dimensions of culture to be assessed.

During an initial contact with clients, nurses should perform a general cultural assessment to obtain an overview of the clients' characteristics. Nurses ask clients about their ethnic background, language, education, religious affiliation, dietary practices, family relationships, hospital experiences, occupation and socioeconomic status, cultural beliefs, and language. Nurses also want to know about clients' distinctive features, perceptions of the health issue, causation, treatment, anticipated results, and the impact the issue might have on the client. This basic data can help nurses understand the clients from the clients' points of view and recognize their uniqueness, thus avoiding stereotyping. Data for an in-depth cultural assessment should be gathered over a period of time and not restricted to the first encounter with the client. This gives both the client and the nurse time to get to know each other, and it helps the client see the nurse in a helping relationship. An in-depth cultural assessment should be conducted in two phases: a data-collection phase and an organization phase.

The data-collection phase consists of three steps:
1. The nurse collects self-identifying data similar to those collected in the brief assessment.
2. The nurse raises a variety of questions that seek information on the clients' perception of what brings them to the health care system, the illness, and previous and anticipated treatments.
3. After the nursing diagnosis is made, the nurse identifies cultural factors that may influence the effectiveness of nursing care actions.

QSEN FOCUS ON QUALITY AND SAFETY EDUCATION FOR NURSES

The six quality and safety competencies for nurses that were identified in the Quality and Safety Education for Nurses (QSEN) project are client-centered care, teamwork and collaboration, evidence-based practice, quality improvement, safety, and informatics. Although each of these is important and pertinent to the nursing actions taken with people from cultural groups other than that of the nurse, perhaps the most significant is client-centered care. The chapter presents many guidelines and principles for aiding nurses in providing culturally competent care. Client-centered care is often less than effective when the nurse and client do not communicate effectively with one another. The lack of communication may occur when they speak different languages, when they have different cultural practices and expectations that lead them to hear messages differently, or when clients simply do not understand what the nurse is saying and are reluctant to acknowledge it. Nurses must observe for both verbal and nonverbal cues that a message is either understood or not understood. When the latter occurs, the nurse should take action to clarify the message, and this may include asking someone from that cultural group to assist or to enlist the aid of an interpreter (Issel and Bekemeier, 2010).

The following targeted competency applies the QSEN competency of client-centered interventions that reflect cultural competence:

Targeted Competency: Client-Centered Intervention—Recognize the client or designee as the source of control and full partner in providing compassionate and coordinated interventions based on respect for client's preferences, values, and needs.

Important aspects of client-centered intervention include:

Knowledge: Describe strategies to empower clients or families in all aspects of the health care process.

Skills: Communicate client values, preferences, and expressed needs to other members of health care team.

Attitudes: Willingly support client-centered care for individuals and groups whose values differ from own.

Client-centered care question: Competence in providing client-centered interventions involves not only effective interviewing of individual clients but developing an awareness of their context. As a community-based clinician, it is helpful to familiarize yourself with the cultural context of your clients. Learning about community resources can sometimes be helpful in learning about the cultural context. You have just been hired as a visiting nurse in a Hispanic community. What community resources could you explore to assist you in providing effective client-centered care?

Answer:

- You might explore community centers. Where are they? How well frequented are the community centers? Which programs are most popular? Which community center programs are health oriented?
- Are community members very involved with one or more churches? You might familiarize yourself with elements of this faith tradition.
- Are there community elders who are publicly recognized as leaders in the community? Can you meet with them to understand how the community has changed and evolved over time?

Prepared by Gail Armstrong, PhD, DNP, ACNS-BC, CNE, Associate Professor, University of Colorado College of Nursing.

In the organization phase, data related to the client's and family's views on optimal treatment choices are examined, and areas of difference between the client's cultural needs and the goals of Western medicine are identified. Nurses may use Leininger's (2002a) three actions (discussed previously in this chapter) to guide them in selecting and discussing culturally appropriate interventions with clients.

The key to a successful cultural assessment lies in nurses being aware of their own culture. The nurse should consider the following suggestions when eliciting cultural information:

- Be sensitive to the cues in the environment and be in tune with the verbal and nonverbal communications before taking action.
- Know about the resources in the community such as schools, churches, clubs and other groups, hospitals, tribal councils, restaurants, taverns, and bars.
- Know the specific areas to focus on before beginning the cultural assessment.
- Select a strategy for gathering cultural data. Possible strategies include in-depth interviews, informal conversations, observations of the client's everyday activities or specific events, survey research, and a case-method approach to study certain aspects of a client.
- Identify a confidante who will help "bridge the gap" between cultures. Be aware that in some cultures the woman's husband or a close male family friend may be the person from whom the nurse may need to obtain the cultural information.
- Know the appropriate questions to ask without offending the client.
- Interview other nurses or health care professionals who have worked with the specific individual, family, or community to get their input.
- Use a trained interpreter if the client has limited proficiency with English.
- Talk with formal and informal community leaders to gain a comprehensive understanding about significant aspects of community life.
- Be aware that all information has both subjective and objective aspects, and verify and cross-check the information that is collected before acting on it.
- Avoid the pitfalls that may occur when making premature generalizations.
- Be sincere, open, and honest with yourself and the client.

BUILDING CULTURALLY COMPETENT ORGANIZATIONS

Although many of the same guidelines that apply to providing culturally competent care also apply to building culturally competent organizations, there are some areas that should be emphasized at the organizational level. In considering how to build a more culturally competent organization, it is useful to ask these questions:

1. Who lives in the community right now?
2. What kinds of diversity exists?
3. What kinds of relationships are established between cultural groups?
4. Are the different cultural groups well organized?
5. What struggles exist between cultures?
6. What struggles exist within cultural groups?
7. Are these struggles openly recognized and talked about?
8. Are there efforts to build alliances and coalitions between groups?
9. What issues do different cultural groups have in common (Axner, 2015)?

Organizations have a culture that includes policies, procedures, programs, and processes and that incorporates certain values, beliefs, assumptions, and customs (Brownlee and Lee, 2015). Researchers at the University of Kansas have developed a toolbox to help organizations become culturally competent. They note that a culturally competent organizational model has five essential principles: (1) valuing diversity, (2) conducting cultural assessment, (3) understanding the dynamics of difference, (4) institutionalizing cultural knowledge, and (5) adapting to diversity (Brownlee and Lee, 2015). These researchers posit that diversity is reality and that changes in one part of the world affect people everywhere. They cite the following steps as key to building a multicultural organization that recognizes diversity and aims to enable cultural differences to strengthen rather than weaken the organization (Brownlee and Lee, 2015):

- Form a cultural competence committee.
- Write a mission statement.
- Find out what similar organizations have done, and develop partnerships.
- Use free resources.
- Complete a comprehensive cultural competence assessment of your organization.
- Find out which cultural groups exist in your community and whether they access community services.
- Have a brown-bag lunch to get staff involved in discussion and activities about cultural competence.
- Ask your personnel about their staff development needs.
- Assign part of your budget to staff development programming in cultural competence.
- Include cultural competency requirement in job descriptions.
- Be sure your facility's location is accessible and respectful of difference.
- Collect resource materials on culturally diverse groups for your staff to use.
- Build a network of natural helpers, community "informants" and other "experts."

PRACTICE APPLICATION

Shu Ping was concerned about her father's deteriorating health and contacted her church friend, Ms. Johnson, a registered nurse, for advice. A public health nurse had been visiting the father since his recent discharge from the hospital, but the father had asked this nurse not to discuss his diagnosis with his family. After several weeks with the family, Ms. Johnson was able to establish a close enough relationship with the father so that she could talk with him privately about his health. He told

Ms. Johnson that he was diagnosed with cancer of the small intestine, and he feared he was dying. He did not want the family to know the "bad news." He refused treatment because his view was that people never got better after they were diagnosed with cancer; they always died.

Which of the following actions by the public health nurse would best demonstrate culturally competent care to the family?

A. Discussing the medical treatment and surgical intervention for cancer of the small intestine

B. Discussing with Shu Ping's father the prognosis for a person diagnosed with cancer of the small intestine in the United States

C. With the father's consent, requesting a conference involving the primary physician, the father, and the family to discuss the diagnosis and treatment options

D. Contacting the public health agency and discussing the problem with them

Answers can be found on the Evolve website.

REMEMBER THIS!

- The population of the United States is increasingly diverse. Changes in immigration laws and policies have increased migration, contributed to changes in community demographics, and heightened the need to recognize the impact of culture on health care and the need for nurses to learn about the culture of the individuals to whom they give care.
- Nurses who do not speak or understand the client's language should use an interpreter. In selecting an interpreter, nurses should consider the clients' cultural needs and respect their right to privacy.
- Culture is a learned set of behaviors that is widely shared among a group of people; the culture of people helps guide individuals in problem solving and decision making.
- Members of minority groups are overrepresented on the lower tiers of the socioeconomic ladder. Poor economic achievement is also a common characteristic among populations at risk, such as those in poverty, the homeless, migrant workers, and refugees. Nurses should be able to distinguish between cultural issues and socioeconomic class issues and not interpret behavior as having a cultural origin when, in fact, it is based on socioeconomic class.
- Culturally competent nursing care is designed for a specific client, reflects the individual's beliefs and values, and is provided with sensitivity. Such nursing care helps improve health outcomes and reduce health care costs.

- Nurses who are culturally competent use cultural knowledge and specific skills, such as intracultural communication and cultural assessment, in selecting interventions to care for clients.
- Four modes of action that nurses may use to negotiate with clients and give culturally competent care are cultural preservation, cultural accommodation, cultural repatterning, and cultural brokering.
- Barriers to providing culturally competent care are stereotyping, prejudice and racism, ethnocentrism, cultural imposition, cultural conflict, and cultural shock.
- Nurses should perform a cultural assessment on every client with whom they interact. Cultural assessments help nurses understand clients' perspectives of health and illness and thereby guide them in discussing culturally appropriate interventions. The needs of clients vary with their age, education, religion, and socioeconomic status.
- Dietary practices are an integral part of the assessment data. Efforts to understand dietary practices should go beyond relying on membership in a defined group and should include individual nutritional practices and religious requirements.
- A variety of steps can be taken to develop culturally competent organizations, and nurses can play a leading role in doing so.

ⓔ EVOLVE WEBSITE

http://evolve.elsevier.com/Stanhope/foundations
- NCLEX® Review Questions
- Practice Application Answers

REFERENCES

Anderson ET, McFarlane J: *Community as partner: theory in practice in nursing*, ed 6, Philadelphia, 2011, Lippincott Williams and Wilkins.

Andrews MM, Boyle JS: *Transcultural concepts in nursing care*, ed 6, Philadelphia, 2012, Lippincott Williams and Wilkins.

Artiga S, Damico A, Young K, et al: *Health coverage and care for immigrants*, Issue Brief, Menlo Park, CA, January 2016, The Henry J. Kaiser Family Foundation. http://www.kff.org. Accessed January 20, 2016.

Axner M: *Understanding culture and diversity in building communities*, Lawrence, KS, 2015, Community Tool Box. University of Kansas. See ctb.ku.edu. Accessed January 22, 2016.

Baker B, Rytina N: *Estimates of the lawful permanent resident population in the United States: January 2013*, September 2014, Office of Immigration Statistics. Policy Directorates. Population Estimates, Office of Immigration Statistics, Washington, DC. See http://www.dhs.gov/sites/default/files/publications/ois-1pr-pe-2013-0.pdf.

Brondolo E, Gallo LC, Myers HF: Race, racism and health interventions, *J Behav Med* 32:1–8, 2009.

Brownlee T, Lee K: *Building culturally competent organizations*, Lawrence, KS, 2015, Community Tool Box. University of Kansas. See ctb.ku.edu. Accessed January 22, 2016.

Campinha-Bacote J: Coming to know cultural competence in evolutionary process, *Internl J Human Caring* 15:42–48, 2011.

Campinha-Bacote J: People of African heritage. In Purnell L, Paulanka BJ, editors. *Transcultural health care: a culturally competent approach*, ed 4, Philadelphia, 2012, FA Davis, pp 91–114.

Carlock DM: Finding information on immigrant and refugee health, *J of Transcult Nurs* 18:373–379, 2007.

Centers for Disease Control and Prevention. *Refugee health guidelines*, 2012. http://www.cdc.gov/immigrantrefugeehealth/guidelines/refugee-guidelines.html. Accessed January 21, 2016.

Changes in immigration law, 2008. Retrieved December 2010 from http://www.lawcom.com/immigration/chngs.shtml.

Charles CE, Daroszewski EB: Culturally competent nursing care of the Muslim patient, *Issues in Mental Health Nursing* 33:61–63, 2012.

Congress of the United States: *A description of the immigrant population: an update*, Washington, DC, June 2012, Congressional Budget Office, US Government Printing Office.

Council on Linkages between Academia and Public Health Practice: *Core competencies for public health professionals*, Washington DC, 2010, Public Health Foundation, Health Resource and Services Administration.

Darnell LK, Hickson SV: Cultural competent patient-centered nursing care, *Nurs Clin N Am* 50:99–108, 2015.

Douglas MK, Rosenkoetter M, Pacquiao DF, et al: Guidelines for implementing culturally competent nursing care, *J Transcult Nurse* 25:109–121, 2014.

ElGindy G: www.minoritynurse.com. Accessed March 30, 2013.

Giger JN: *Transcultural nursing: assessment and intervention*, ed 7, St Louis, 2017, Elsevier.

Heiman HJ, Artiga S: *Beyond health care: the role of social determinants in promoting health and health equity*, Issue Brief, Menlo Park, CA, November 2015, The Henry J. Kaiser Family Foundation. http://www.kff.org. Accessed January 20, 2016.

Issel LM, Bekemeier B: Safe practice of population-focused nursing care: development of a public health nursing concept, *Nurs Outlook* 58:226–232, 2010.

Jacobs A, Kemppainen JK, Taylor JS, et al: Beliefs about diabetes and medication adherence among Lumbee Indians living in rural southeastern North Carolina. *J transcult Nurs* 25:167–175, 2014.

Jones ME, Cason CL, Bond ML: Cultural attitudes, knowledge, and skills of a health workforce, *J Transcult Nurs* 158:283–290, 2004.

Leininger M: Essential transcultural nursing care concepts, principles, examples, and policy statements. In Leininger MM, McFarland M, editors: *Transcultural nursing: concepts, theories, research, and practices*, ed 3, New York, 2002a, McGraw-Hill, pp 45–69.

Leininger M: The theory of culture care and the ethnonursing research method. In Leininger MM, McFarland M, editors: *Transcultural nursing: concepts, theories, research, and practices*, ed 3, New York, 2002b, McGraw-Hill, pp 71–98.

Meleis AI: Arabs. In Lipson JG, Dibble SL, editors: *Providing culturally appropriate care in culture and clinical care*, San Francisco, 2005, UCSF Nursing Press, pp 42–57.

Miller NK: Haitian ethnomedical systems and biomedical practitioners: directions for clinicians, *J Transcult Nurs* 11:204, 2000.

Mohammed S: The dynamic interplay between low socioeconomic status and diabetes for urban American Indians, *Family Community Health* 34:211–220, 2011.

National Immigration Forum: *Immigration basics 2010*, Washington, DC, 2010, National Immigration Forum. Retrieved January 2016, from http://www.immigrationforum.org/images/uploads/2010/ImmigrationBasics2010.pdf.

Office of Minority Health: *Asian American/Pacific Islander profile*, 2008. Retrieved August 2012 from http://www.minorityhealth.hhs.gov/templates/browse.aspx?lvl 2andlvlid 53.

Ogbu M: Nigerians. In Lipson JG, Dibble SL, editors: *Providing culturally appropriate care in culture and critical care*, San Francisco, 2005, UCSF Nursing Press, pp 243–259.

Orlandi MA, editor: *Cultural competence for evaluators*, Washington, DC, 1992, US Department of Health and Human Services.

Plumb AL: Refuges for refugees and their caregivers, *Am J Nurs* 103:98–99, 2003.

Purnell LD, Paulanka BJ: *Transcultural health care*, ed 3, Philadelphia, 2008, FA Davis.

Randall-David E: *Strategies for working with culturally diverse communities and clients*, Bethesda, MD, 1989, Washington, DC, US Department of Health and Human Services.

Reavy K, Hobbs J, Hereford M, Crosby K: A new clinic model for refugee health care: adaptation of cultural safety, *Rural Remote Health* 12:1826, 2012.

Sims M, Sims TL, Bruce MA: Race, ethnicity, concentrated poverty and low weight disparities, *J Black Nurses Assoc* 19:12–18, 2008.

Spector RE: *Cultural diversity in health and illness*, ed 7, Upper Saddle River, NJ, 2008, Prentice Hall.

Swider Sm, Krothe J, Reyes D and Cravetz M: The Quad Council practice competencies for public health nursing, *Public Health Nursing* 30(6):519–536, 2013.

US Census Bureau: *Statistical abstract of the United States 2001*, Washington, DC, 2001, US Government Printing Office.

US Census Bureau: *Income, poverty and health insurance in the United States*, 2010. Available at http://www.census.gov/hhes/www/poverty/data/threshld/index/html. Accessed April 24, 2014.

US Census Bureau: *Statistical abstract of the United States 2012*, ed 131, Washington, DC, 2011. Retrieved March 2012 from http://www.census.gov/compendia/statab/.

US Department of Health and Human Services: *Healthy People 2020*, Washington, DC, 2010, US Government Printing Office.

Zong J, Batalova J: Frequently requested statistics on immigrants and immigration in the United States, *Migration Policy Institute* February 26, 2015. http://www.migrationpolicy.gov/article/frequently-requested-statistics-immigrants-and-immigration-united-states/. Accessed January 8, 2016.

6 | CHAPTER

Environmental Health

Barbara Sattler

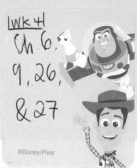

©Disney/Pixar

OBJECTIVES

After reading this chapter, the student should be able to:

1. Explain how the environment influences human health and disease.
2. Know which disciplines work most closely with nurses in environmental health.
3. Describe legislative and regulatory policies that have influenced the effect of the environment on health and disease patterns.
4. Describe the skills needed by nurses practicing in environmental health, and apply the nursing process to the practice of environmental health.

CHAPTER OUTLINE

Historical Context
Environmental Health Sciences
  Toxicology
  Epidemiology
  Multidisciplinary Approaches
Climate Change
Environmental Health Assessment
  Air
  Water
  Land
  Food
  The Right to Know

Risk Assessment
  Assessing Environmental Health Risks in Children
Reducing Environmental Health Risks
  Risk Communication
  Ethics
  Government Environmental Protection
Advocacy
  Environmental Justice and Environmental Health Disparities
  Unique Environmental Health Threats in the Health Care Industry: New Opportunities for Advocacy
Referral Resources
Roles for Nurses in Environmental Health

KEY TERMS

agent, 88
bioaccumulated, 101
climate change, 89
compliance, 100
consumer confidence report (CCR), 94
enforcement, 99
environment, 84
environmental epidemiology, 88
environmental justice, 101

environmental standards, 100
epidemiological triangle, 88
epidemiology, 88
fracking, 93
host, 88
indoor air quality, 92
methylmercury, 101
monitoring, 100
nonpoint sources, 92
permitting, 99

persistent bioaccumulative toxins (PBTs), 101
persistent organic pollutants (POPs), 101
point sources, 92
right to know, 94
risk assessment, 94
risk communication, 98
toxicology, 87

"Environmental hazards influence over 80% of the communicable and noncommunicable diseases and injuries monitored by WHO [World Health Organization]" and overall are responsible for over one-half of the total burden of disease in the world (WHO, 2011, p 1). Nurses can define environment in a variety of ways, including homes, schools, workplaces, and communities. The environment is everything around us. Each location holds potential health risks. It is both important for and a responsibility of nurses to understand as much as possible about these risks—how to assess them, how to eliminate or reduce them, how to communicate and educate about them, and how to advocate for policies that support healthy environments. We often take the environment for granted and may fail to see the hazards in front of us. For example, how many of us know for certain that our drinking water is safe, or that the air we breathe is free from pollutants that aggravate our individual respiratory functions? Environmental health risks come in the form of poor air and water quality, the use of pesticides, and paint containing lead. Environmental hazards come in the forms of biological, chemical, and radiological hazards. The Environmental Protection Agency (EPA) lists six common air pollutants. They are: ozone, particulate matter, carbon monoxide, nitrogen oxides, sulfur dioxide, and lead (EPA, 2015b). As will be discussed later, the EPA also provides information about safe drinking water and many of the other environmental hazards.

A variety of factors, including genetics, socioeconomic status, and environmental exposure, affect environmental health. In evaluating environmental exposures in a home, nurses' assessments can begin with a set of questions: What exposures can you identify in your own home? Do you use pesticides? Does your home have lead-based paint? (The age of a home is a good proxy for identifying the presence of lead-based paint because it is most likely found in homes built before 1978 when the use of lead was banned in household paint.) Is the paint chipping or peeling? Are any of your appliances or heat sources producing unhealthy levels of carbon monoxide? Have you checked your home for radon, the second largest cause of lung cancer in the United States? How about your workplace? Do you eat fish on a regular basis? (Some fish can have unhealthy levels of mercury.)

The American Nurses Association (ANA) recommends that all nurses understand basic environmental health concepts, including knowledge about environmental health and its effect on nursing practice, the Precautionary Principle, and nurses' rights to work in a safe workplace and use materials, products, technology, and practices that reflect an evidence-based approach. Other principles relate to quality assessment of the environment, interdisciplinary work in environmental health, involvement in research, and support of nurses who advocate for a safe environment (ANA, 2007).

If children are in the home, are all the toxic cleaning materials and insecticides out of reach? Does the home or apartment have lead in its paint? Many homes and apartments built before 1978 have lead in the paint. Beginning in April 2010, any contractor performing renovation or painting in a home, child-care facility, or school built before 1978 and disturbing more than 6 square feet must be trained and certified in how to prevent lead contamination (EPA, 2015a). We know that exposure to lead can cause premature birth, learning disabilities in children, hypertension in adults, and other health problems (Fig. 6.1). The levels of the six common pollutants measured by the EPA have been declining in recent years. (EPA, 2015b). Thirty million Americans drink water that exceeds one or more of the EPA's safe drinking water standards, and 50% of Americans live in areas that exceed current national ambient air quality standards. Given such reported exposures, what is the role of nurses in community health? Insecticides used in the home increase the risk of childhood leukemia (Turner et al, 2010). Childhood leukemia is also

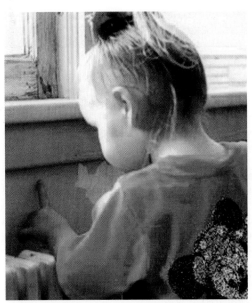

FIG. 6.1 Child in home with lead-based paint. (From State of Hawaii Department of Public Health. Retrieved September 2012 from http://hawaii.gov/health/environmental/noise/asbestoslead/images2/child.jpg.)

associated with prenatal exposures by parents who are exposed to insecticides at work (Wigle et al, 2009). Exposure to pesticides is especially problematic for children. Pesticides are often found in lawn sprays and household bug sprays, and they can also be found in foods such as strawberries, blueberries, and apples (Gilden et al, 2010). Considering this snapshot of the extent of environmental health issues, it is clear why nurses need to be informed about the health of the environment and its effect on people.

▶▶ APPLYING CONTENT TO PRACTICE

Key documents that guide practice in both nursing and public health help practitioners learn how to apply environmental health principles at home and work. Specifically, the core competencies of the Council on Linkages (2010) have, within the domain of public health science skills, a competency that says practitioners will apply "the basic public health sciences (including, but not limited to, environmental health sciences, health services administration, and social and behavioral health sciences) to public health policies and programs." The Quad Council of Nursing (Swider et al, 2013) updated the competences in 2013. The most explicit set of principles was developed by the ANA (2007) in its Principles of Environmental Health for Nursing Practice.

The ANA (2007) lists 10 principles of environmental health. Although all 10 are essential, 4 are mentioned here: Nurses should know about environmental health concepts; participate in assessing the quality of the environment in which they practice; live and use the Precautionary Principle, which refers to using products and practices that do not harm human health or the environment; and take preventive action when uncertain. Another principle points out that healthy environments are sustained through multidisciplinary collaboration, which is a key concept discussed throughout the chapter.

BOX 6.1   General Environmental Health Competencies for Nurses

Basic Knowledge and Concepts

All nurses should understand the scientific principles and underpinnings of the relationship between individuals or populations and the environment (including the work environment). This understanding includes the basic mechanisms and pathways of exposure to environmental health hazards, basic prevention and control strategies, the interdisciplinary nature of effective interventions, and the role of research.

Assessment and Referral

All nurses should be able to successfully complete an environmental health history, recognize potential environmental hazards and sentinel illnesses, and make appropriate referrals for conditions with probable environmental causes. An essential component is the ability to locate referral sources, access them, and provide information to clients and communities.

Advocacy, Ethics, and Risk Communication

All nurses should be able to demonstrate knowledge of the role of advocacy (case and class), ethics, and risk communication in client care and community intervention with respect to potential adverse effects of the environment on health.

Legislation and Regulation

All nurses should understand the policy framework and major pieces of legislation and regulations related to environmental health.

From Pope AM, Snyder MA, Mood LH, editors: *Nursing, health, and environment,* Washington, DC, 1995, Institute of Medicine, National Academies Press.

Chemical, biological, and radiological exposures that affect our health come from the air we breathe, the water we drink, the food we eat, and the products we use. Nurses need to know how to assess for environmental health risks and develop educational and other preventive interventions to help individuals, families, and communities understand and, where possible, decrease the risks. The National Academy of Science's Institute of Medicine (IOM) recommends that all nurses have a basic understanding of environmental health principles and that these principles be integrated into all aspects of practice, education, advocacy, policies, and research (Pope, Snyder, and Mood, 1995). This chapter explores the basic competencies recommended by the IOM (Box 6.1) and integrates them with the ANA (2007) Principles of Environmental Health. Although developed many years ago, the IOM principles remain useful for today's integration of environmental health into the Standards for Environmental Health Nursing practice. Since 2008 the development of the first environmental health nursing organization, the Alliance of Nurses for Healthy Environments (ANHE), and collaboration with other nursing organizations, has been able to advance the recommendations of the 1995 IOM report (Leffers et al, 2014). The federal government, like important nursing and public health associations, has long recognized the importance of the relationship between environmental risks and diseases. Consistent with this recognition, environmental health is one of the priority areas

HEALTHY PEOPLE 2020

Selected Objectives Related to Environmental Health

EH-8.1: Eliminate elevated blood lead levels in children.

EH-8.9: Minimize the risks to human health and the environment posed by hazardous sites.

EH-8.10: Reduce pesticide exposures that result in visits to a health care facility.

EH-8.11: Reduce the amount of toxic pollutants released into the environment.

EH-8.13: Reduce indoor allergen levels.

EH-8.18: Decrease the number of US homes that are found to have lead-based paint or related hazards.

From US Department of Health and Human Services: *Healthy People 2020,* Washington, DC, 2010, US Government Printing Office.

of the *Healthy People 2020* objectives (see the *Healthy People 2020* box).

HISTORICAL CONTEXT

Nurses, like physicians, have been taught little about the environment and environmental threats to health. This recognition led the IOM to evaluate the current state of environmental health knowledge and skills applied in nursing. The IOM report *Nursing, Health, and Environment* (Pope et al, 1995), written nearly two decades ago, noted that the environment, as a determinant of health, is deeply rooted in nursing's heritage. As mentioned in Chapter 2, Florence Nightingale, well known for her work in the Crimean War, practiced and wrote about how the quality of the environment influenced health and recovery from illness. She talked about the importance to the patient's health of fresh air, pure water, adequate food, good drainage, cleanliness, and light, especially good sunlight. Early in the 20th century, Lillian Wald, who coined the term *public health nurses,* and her colleague Mary Brewster worked tirelessly to improve the environment of the Henry Street neighborhood and used their network of influential contacts to make changes in the physical environment and social conditions that affected health (Wright, 2003). The need to pay close attention to the environment and its effect on health is as crucial today as it was in earlier times. The environment is different than it was a century ago, and people have made many of the detrimental changes. In addition to environmental contamination, many of the human-made chemicals can now also be found in our bodies (including in breast milk) in measurable amounts. To understand the relationship between the environment and health, some knowledge about toxicology and other environmental sciences is necessary.

It is also important to know that people who live in poverty are more likely to be exposed to environmental hazards in situations such as crowded living conditions, living closer to hazardous wastes, having poorer-quality foods available to them, and being exposed to hazards such as lead in paint, pollution in the air or water, or hazardous jobs.

ENVIRONMENTAL HEALTH SCIENCES

TOXICOLOGY

Toxicology is the basic science that studies the health effects associated with chemical exposures. Its corollary in health care is pharmacology, which studies the human health effects, both desirable and undesirable, associated with drugs. In toxicology, only the negative effects of chemical exposures are studied. However, the key principles of pharmacology and toxicology are the same. Just as the dose of a drug influences its effectiveness and its toxicity, the quantity of an air or water pollutant to which we may be exposed will determine the risk for experiencing a negative health effect. Also, the timing of exposure affects the risk for an untoward health effect. For example, during embryonic and fetal development, exposure to toxic chemicals can create immediate harm or create a critical pathway for future disease. Very young children are especially susceptible to exposures because of the immature development of their systems.

Both drugs and pollutants can enter the body by a variety of routes. Most drugs are given orally and are absorbed via the gastrointestinal tract. Water- and food-associated pollutants, including pesticides and heavy metals, enter the body via the digestive tract. Some drugs are administered as inhalants, and some pollutants in the air (including indoor air) enter the body via the lungs. Some drugs are applied topically. In work settings, employees can receive dermal exposures from toxic chemicals when they immerse unprotected hands in chemical solutions. Pollution can enter the body via the lungs (inhalation), gastrointestinal tract (ingestion), and skin and mucous membranes (dermal absorption). Some chemicals can cross the placental barrier and affect the fetus. In addition to direct damage to cells, tissues, organs, and organ systems, changes to the DNA can occur from chemical exposures that can change gene expression, which in turn, can predict disease. This latter effect is the focus of a relatively new field of biological study—epigenetics. Scientists now understand that many variables predict disease outcomes, including environmental exposures.

When we administer medications to patients, we consider age, weight, other drugs taken, and the underlying health status of the person. We should also make it clear to clients that taking the prescription or over-the-counter drug more often than recommended can have a toxic effect. Likewise, we must also consider how environmental exposures affect community members. For example, children are more vulnerable to almost all pollutants. More vulnerable to foodborne and waterborne pathogens are immunocompromised people, such as (1) those infected with the human immunodeficiency virus (HIV), (2) those who have acquired immunodeficiency syndrome (AIDS), (3) those who are taking chemotherapeutic drugs, or (4) those who are organ recipients. When assessing a community's environmental health status, be sure to review the general health status of the community to identify members who

Drug Enforcement Administration: DEA Announces 10th National Drug Take-Back. 2015. http://www.dea.gov/divisions/hq/2015/hq072815.shtml; US Food and Drug Administration: "Disposal of unused medicines: what should you know?" http://www.fda.gov/drug disposal. Washington, DC, 2015, FDA. Retrieved February 2016.

CHECK YOUR PRACTICE:

Many cities and counties sponsor medicine take-back programs during which residents can drop off unused medicines. These community events may be sponsored by the US Drug Enforcement Administration (DEA) or by local law enforcement agencies. You can contact a city or county government's trash and recycling service to learn what is available in the local area. Pharmacists are also a good source of information about disposing of unused medicines. If no take-back program is available, follow these steps:

- Mix medicines (do not crush tablets or capsules) with an unpalatable substance such as kitty litter, dirt, or used coffee grounds.
- Place the mixture in a container, such as a sealed bag.
- Throw the container in your household trash.
- Scratch out all personal information on the prescription label of your empty container or packaging, then dispose of the container.
- In 2015, the national take-back initiative was held on September 26, except in Pennsylvania and Delaware, which chose September 12, 2015, and it was discussed on the radio, on television, and in newspapers in many local areas. At this time communities teamed up with local law enforcement agencies. Since this program began in 2010, 2411 tons of unwanted, unneeded, or expired medications have been taken back.
- There are a small number of drugs that that are especially harmful, and possibly fatal, if only one dose is used by someone other than the person for whom the medication was prescribed.
- The DEA provides a list of medications that can be disposed of by flushing down the sink or toilet (see the DEA citation in the source note).

may have higher risk factors as well as to assess the environmental exposures. It is also important to teach community residents how to effectively dispose of medications they no longer need.

Knowing about chemicals and using that information in practice can seem like a huge task. Fortunately, chemicals can be grouped into families so that it is possible to understand the actions and risks associated with these groups. The following are examples:

1. Metals and metallic compounds, such as arsenic, cadmium, chromium, lead, and mercury
2. Hydrocarbons, such as benzene, toluene, ketones, formaldehyde, and trichloroethylene
3. Irritant gases, such as ammonia, hydrochloric acid, sulfur dioxide, and chlorine
4. Chemical asphyxiants, including carbon monoxide, hydrogen sulfide, and cyanides
5. Pesticides, such as organophosphates, carbamates, and chlorinated hydrocarbons

Technology helps us understand environmental threats. The National Library of Medicine (NLM) has a set of user-friendly online databases that focus on environmental health and toxicology called TOXNET (see http://www.toxnet.nlm.nih.gov). Using chemical name search terms and display options of health effects, some potential environmental threats to health can be understood or ruled out. It is important to remember that all nursing assessments, whether of individuals or communities, must consider environmental exposures that may contribute to illness. Once you identify potential health risks, you can then develop a risk reduction plan.

EPIDEMIOLOGY

Whereas toxicology is the science that studies the poisonous effects of chemicals, epidemiology is the science that helps us understand the strength of the association between exposures and health effects in human populations. Chapter 9 discusses epidemiology in detail. However, a few points are relevant here because epidemiology is an applied science used in environmental health. Epidemiological studies have helped explain the association between learning disabilities and exposure to lead-based paint dust, as well as asthma exacerbation and air pollution (Smargiasssi et al, 2014; Habre et al, 2014) and gastrointestinal disease and exposure to *Cryptosporidium* in contaminated water (Yoder et al, 2012). Epidemiology also helps in the examination of occupation-related illnesses. Environmental surveillance efforts, such as childhood lead registries, use epidemiological methods to track and analyze incidence, prevalence, and health outcomes.

As discussed in Chapter 9, three major concepts—agent, host, and environment—form the classic epidemiological triangle. This simple model helps explain the often-complex relationships among agent, which may include chemical mixtures (i.e., more than one agent); host, which may refer to a community spanning different ages, both sexes, ethnicities, cultures, and disease states; and environment, which may include dynamic factors such as air, water, soil, and food, as well as temperature, humidity, and wind. Limitations of environmental epidemiology include a reliance on occupational health studies to characterize certain toxic exposures. Studies are usually performed on healthy adults whose biological systems are different from those of neonates, pregnant women, children, the immunosuppressed, and older adults. Geographic information systems (GIS) are used in environmental health studies to code data so that they can be related spatially to a place on Earth. For example, a nurse could combine geographically related data to develop maps to note where the data can be related. Specifically, by taking a data set that geographically notes where children under 10 years of age live and overlaying another data set that notes geographic areas designated by the age of housing stock, a public health nurse could determine locations with the largest number of children who live in areas with older housing stock. Using this information, the nurse could target a lead surveillance and educational program (Fig. 6.2).

MULTIDISCIPLINARY APPROACHES

In addition to toxicology and epidemiology, some earth sciences help explain how pollutants travel in air, water, and soil. Geologists, meteorologists, and chemists all contribute

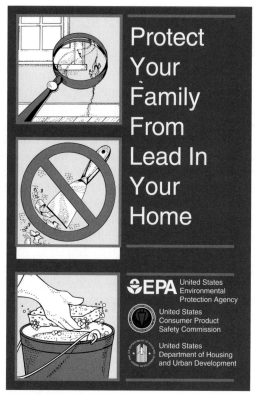

FIG. 6.2 Lead paint warning. (From US Environmental Protection Agency.)

information to help understand how and when humans may be exposed to hazardous chemicals, radiation (such as radon), and biological contaminants. The public health field also depends on food safety specialists, sanitarians, radiation specialists, and industrial hygienists.

The nature of environmental health requires a multidisciplinary approach to assess and decrease environmental health risks. For instance, to assess and address a case of lead-based paint poisoning, the team might include a housing inspector with expertise in lead-based paint or a sanitarian to assess the lead-associated health risks in the home; clinical specialists to manage the clients' health needs; laboratory workers to assess lead levels in the clients' blood as well as in the paint, house dust, and drinking water; and lead-based paint remediation specialists to reduce the lead-based paint risk in the home. This approach could potentially involve the local health department, the state department of environmental protection, the housing department, a tertiary care setting, and public or private sector laboratories. It is important that nurses understand the roles of each respective agency and organization, know the public health laws (particularly as they pertain to lead-based paint poisoning), and work with the community to coordinate services to address the community's needs. The nurse also might set up a blood-lead screening program through the local health department, educate local health providers to encourage them to systematically test children for lead poisoning, or work with local landlords to improve the condition of their housing stock. Factors contributing to

Targeted Competency: Function effectively within nursing and interprofessional teams, fostering open communication, mutual respect, and shared decision making to achieve quality client care.

Important aspects of safety include the following:

- **Knowledge:** Describe scopes of practice and roles of health care team members.
- **Skills:** Assume role of team member or leader based on the situation.
- **Attitudes:** Value the perspectives and expertise of all health team members.

Safety Question: One of the objectives in *Healthy People 2020* related to environmental health is as follows: "Reduce pesticide exposures that result in visits to a health care facility" (ED: 8-10). The public health nurse who is working on a project to help mothers develop parenting skills visits a new mother who lives and works on a large farm. When the nurse drives into the farm on her way to the housing where workers live, she sees that the fields are being sprayed with pesticides from a truck and that two young children are riding in the back of the truck. What action should she take?

Answer: At the individual level, she should talk with the owner or manager of the farm and remind him or her of the toxicity of pesticides and the danger to those who are in the vicinity of the spraying. She should recommend that he or she not allow anyone to ride in the open portion of the vehicle and that the driver should leave the window closed and wear a mask to protect his or her nose and mouth.

At the systems level, she should identify areas where the workers on the area farms congregate, such as churches, social halls, and so forth. Then she should ask if she could provide an educational program on the dangers of coming into contact with pesticides. She could distribute pamphlets about this hazard in local venues where both farm managers and workers will be able to access them. What else might the nurse do?

---

the reduction of lead levels in the United States include elimination of lead in paint, reduction of lead in gasoline, reduction in the number of manufactured food and drink cans and household plumbing components containing lead solder, lead screening laws, and lead paint–abatement programs in communities.

CLIMATE CHANGE

According to the WHO, climate change "is a significant and emerging threat to public health, and changes the way we must look at protecting vulnerable populations" (WHO, 2015). The 2014 report of the Intergovernmental Program on Climate Change (IPCC), a WHO-related group of scientists, concludes that "climate change will act mainly, at least until the middle of this century, by exacerbating health problems that already exist, and the largest risks will apply to populations that are currently most affected by climate-related diseases" (IPCC, 2014). Between 2030 and 2050 climate change is expected to cause approximately 250,000 additional deaths annually as a result of malnutrition, malaria, diarrhea, and heat stress (WHO, 2015). Climate change affects social and environmental determinants of health, including clean air, safe drinking water, adequate food, and secure shelter (WHO, 2015). In the United States we have seen some of the earlier climate change predictions materialize: long-term warming trends, extreme weather conditions leading to dangerous traffic conditions, as well as disruption in water supplies, agriculture, ecosystems, and coastal communities. Children; the elderly; the sick, especially those with chronic health conditions; the poor; and some minority communities, especially those with language barriers, mental health issues, and lack of access to comprehensive health care, are among the most vulnerable to these health effects (Allen, 2015).

Climate changes around the world lead to global warming. The greenhouse effect is influencing the prevalence of global warming. The greenhouse effect refers to the rise in temperature that occurs when the Earth experiences certain gases in the atmosphere, such as water vapor, carbon dioxide, nitrous oxide, and methane, which trap incoming solar radiation from the sun (Afzal, 2007). A certain amount of the greenhouse effect is essential for human life; however, an excess is dangerous. The goal is to reduce the amount of heat in the environment, because high temperatures in the presence of sunlight and certain air pollutants can lead to the formation of ground-level ozone. Increased exposure to ozone is associated with increased risk of premature mortality. This risk supports the growing trend toward actions such as walking not driving, recycling, and purchasing energy-efficient cars, appliances, and lightbulbs. Remember, electricity is wasted each day when lights are left on, so teach clients to turn off lights when not using them to decrease the amount of carbon dioxide (CO_2) greenhouse gas emissions (Fig. 6.3).

There are two concurrent categories of roles for nurses: mitigation and response. There is still much we can do to mitigate the steep upward slope that we are now observing for temperatures, CO_2 levels, desertification, and sea water levels. Working at the individual, community, institutional (school, hospital, etc.), and governmental levels, there is much work to be done to ensure energy-conserving policies and practices, rational transportation practices, and changes in our consumption patterns.

Regarding response preparation, public health nurses must lead the development of contingencies for long-term, high-heat weather conditions, as well as increased storm activities (that include more severe storm patterns), more extensive fires in areas prone to fires, and the associated disaster preparedness. Often, the recovery from extreme climate change is long and complicated when people lose homes and their possessions and when the community infrastructure, including schools and hospitals, is damaged (Allen, 2015). Standing water and warm temperatures are breeding grounds for mosquitos, and this can increase the disease burden for humans. Other climate-change events that affect health are extreme heat events, air pollution, airborne allergens, and the mental health risks associated with changes in climate that lead to significant community and health disruption (Allen, 2015). For more on disaster preparedness, see Chapter 23 on nurses' roles in disaster management.

The National Environmental Public Health Tracking Network, known as the Tracking Network, is a surveillance system

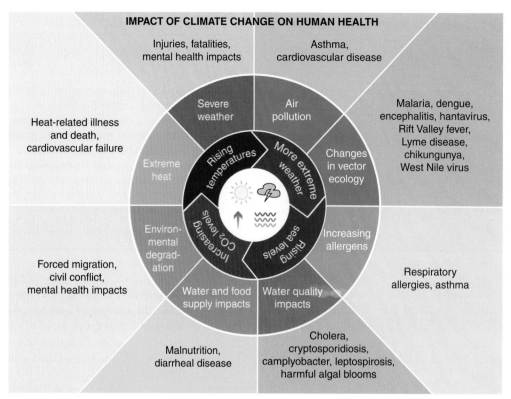

FIG. 6.3 Climate effects on health. (From CDC, Climate and Health, 2015, www.cdc.gov/climateandhealth/effects/default.htm. Retrieved February 2016.)

EVIDENCE-BASED PRACTICE

Hurricanes pose enormous challenges for public health nurses in many ways, including their effects on the environment. Reifsnider et al (2014) used a community-based study that was in effect when Hurricane Ike struck the Texas coast. Their purpose was to detail the challenges faced by public health nurse researchers when a costly hurricane interrupts their ongoing study. Hurricane Ike was a Category 2 storm that was the fourth most destructive hurricane to make landfall in the United States as of 2008. The hurricane affected the physical, environmental, economic, and health and social service subsystems of the community. A year later about 20% of the population had failed to return to Galveston, Texas. The hurricane disproportionally affected low-income residents. Also, all nonessential personnel were not allowed to return to Galveston, an island, for weeks following the hurricane, and this included researchers.

The researchers in this National Institutes of Health (NIH)–funded study, titled "Reducing Overweight Among Galveston WIC Participants," had significant problems due to damage to clinic sites and their subsequent closure and the inability to reach

residents due to lack of telephones and electricity. The WIC clinics in Galveston County did resume operations after 2 months, but many participants could not be located. The researchers creatively found ways to adapt or modify their study to accomplish their goals despite the disruption to their original plan and patient population.

Nurse Use

These researchers learned firsthand the importance of storing their research documentation away from potential flooding and having multiple ways to reach the research team. They learned how important it is to create emergency contact cards and have an emergency contact procedure. The article clearly describes what can go wrong when a disaster hits a community and interrupts the usual environment, including the technological systems as well as water, air, soil, and so forth. The authors identify many lessons they learned from this disaster that can be transferred to other environmental disasters.

Reifsnider E, Bishop, SL, An, K, Mendias, E, Welker-Hood, K, Moramarco ME and Davila YR: 2014. We stop for no storm: coping with an environmental disaster and public health research, *Public Health Nursing* 31(6):500-507.

---

coordinated by the Centers for Disease Control and Prevention (CD) that collects, integrates, analyzes, interprets, and disseminates data from environmental hazard monitoring and from human exposure and health effects surveillance. At present the CDC is funding 23 states and New York City to build local tracking networks. On the Tracking Network website, you can view maps, tables, and charts about the following:

- Chemicals and other substances found in the environment
- Selected chronic diseases and conditions
- Conditions or issues in the area where you live
- Pesticide exposure and pesticide-related illnesses (Anderko et al, 2014; CDC, 2014).

ENVIRONMENTAL HEALTH ASSESSMENT

Environmental health risks can be assessed in various ways. You might assess by environmental factors such as air, water, soil, or food. Or you could assess by setting, such as urban, rural, or suburban. You can also divide the environment into functional locations, such as home, school, workplace, and community. Each of these locations may provide unique environmental exposures and overlapping exposures. For instance, ethylene oxide, the toxic gas used to sterilize equipment in hospitals, is typically found only in a workplace. However, pesticides might be found in all four areas. When assessing environments, determine whether an exposure is in the air, water, soil, or food (or a combination) and whether it is a chemical, biological, or radiological exposure. In any form of assessment, be sure to cover past and present conditions in work, home, and community environments. The How To box demonstrates how to apply the nursing process to environmental health.

HOW TO Apply the Nursing Process to Environmental Health

If you suspect that a client's health problem is influenced by environmental factors, use the nursing process, noting the environmental aspects of the problem in every step of the process as follows:

1. **Assessment:** Include inventories and history questions that cover environmental issues as a part of the general assessment.
2. **Diagnosis:** Relate the disease and the environmental factors in the diagnosis.
3. **Goal setting:** Include outcome measures that mitigate and eliminate the environmental factors.
4. **Planning:** Look at community policy and laws as methods to facilitate the care needs for the client; include environmental health personnel in the planning.
5. **Intervention:** Coordinate medical, nursing, and public health actions to meet the client's needs.
6. **Evaluation:** Examine criteria that include the immediate and long-term responses of the client, as well as the recidivism of the problem for the client.

A mnemonic was developed to help health professionals remember the questions to ask when taking an environmental history and determine the environmental exposure history. Exposures may occur in any setting in which people spend time; be sure to assess them all. The "I PREPARE" mnemonic can be used when assessing an individual, family, or community (Box 6.2).

A windshield survey is a helpful first step to understanding the potential environmental health risks in a community. If the community is urban, the age and condition of the housing and potential trash problems (and the associated pest problems) can be easily determined by driving around the neighborhood. Note also the proximity to factories, dumpsites, major transportation routes, and other sources of pollution.

In rural communities, pay attention to the use of aerial and other types of pesticide and herbicide spraying. Do people use wood-burning stoves? Do you see or suspect contaminated waterways, and are there industrial-type agricultural practices that might contribute to pollution?

BOX 6.2 The "I PREPARE" Mnemonic

An exposure history should identify current and past exposures, have a preliminary goal of reducing or eliminating current exposures, and have a long-term goal of reducing adverse health effects. The "I PREPARE" mnemonic consigns the important questions to categories that can be easily remembered.

I Investigate Potential Exposures
Investigate potential exposures by asking,
- Have you ever felt sick after coming in contact with a chemical, pesticide, or other substance?
- Do you have any symptoms that improve when you are away from your home or work?

P Present Work
At your present work,
- Are you exposed to solvents, dust, fumes, radiation, loud noise, pesticides, or other chemicals?
- Do you know where to find material data safety sheets on the chemicals with which you work?
- Do you wear personal protective equipment?
- Are work clothes worn home?
- Do coworkers have similar health problems?

R Residence
At your place of residence,
- When was your residence built?
- What type of heating do you have?
- Have you recently remodeled your home?
- What chemicals are stored on your property?
- Where does your drinking water come from?

E Environmental Concerns
In your living environment,
- Are there environmental concerns in your neighborhood (i.e., air, water, soil)?
- What types of industries or farms are near your home?
- Do you live near a hazardous waste site or landfill?

P Past Work
About your past work,
- What are your past work experiences?
- What is the longest job you held?
- Have you ever been in the military, worked on a farm, or done volunteer or seasonal work?

A Activities
About your activities,
- What activities and hobbies do you and your family engage in?
- Do you burn, solder, or melt any products?
- Do you garden, fish, or hunt?
- Do you eat what you catch or grow?
- Do you use pesticides?
- Do you engage in any alternative healing or cultural practices?

R Referrals and Resources
Use these key referrals and resources:
- Environmental Protection Agency (http://www.epa.gov)
- National Library of Medicine, TOXNET programs (http://www.nlm.nih.gov)
- Agency for Toxic Substances and Disease Registry (http://www.atsdr.cdc.gov)
- Association of Occupational and Environmental Clinics (http://www.aoec.org)
- Material safety data sheets (http://www.hazard.com/msds)
- Occupational Safety and Health Administration (http://www.osha.gov)
- Local health department, environmental agency, poison control center

E Educate
Use this checklist of educational materials:
- Are materials available to educate the client?
- Are alternatives available to minimize the risk for exposure?
- Have prevention strategies been discussed?
- What is the plan for follow-up?

Prepared by Grace Paranzino, RN, MPH, for the Agency for Toxic Substances and Disease Registry (ATSDR). For more information, contact ATSDR at 1-888-42-ATSDR, or visit the ATSDR's website at http://www.atsdr.cdc.gov.

In addition to the tools used for a general community assessment, some specific tools are available to detect the environmental health risks within a community. The Right to Know section of the chapter describes the types of information available to the public about air and water emissions, drinking water quality, and other environmental sources. In addition, Appendix B.3 is a community health assessment tool that provides an example of an environmental health assessment form. Observe also for positive environmental factors such as green spaces in parks and gardens, bike and walking paths, and water features.

AIR

Air pollution is a significant contributor to health problems. Air pollution is divided into two major categories: point sources, often called fixed sites, which are individual, identifiable sites, such as smokestacks, and nonpoint sources, which include vehicles, such as cars, trucks, and buses. The Clean Air Act, passed in 1970, regulates air pollution from both point sources and nonpoint sources. Motor vehicles are the greatest single source of air pollution in the United States. The burning of fossil fuels (diesel, industrial boilers, and power plants) and waste incineration are two other major contributors. The single greatest source of mercury in our air is coal-fired power plants. Health effects associated with air pollution include asthma and other respiratory diseases, cardiovascular diseases (including heart disease and hypertension), cancer, immunological effects, reproductive health problems (including birth defects), infant deaths, and neurological problems (Smargiassi et al, 2014).

According to WHO (2013), approximately 235 million people suffer from asthma; it is common among children, and the strongest risk factors are genetic factors and inhaled substances and particles that provoke an allergic response or irritate the airways. Also, many people do not know that a pea-sized amount of mercury is sufficient to contaminate a 25-acre lake and make its fish unfit to eat. Mercury, like lead, is an element, and it persists in the fresh waterways and oceans from which we continue to get our fish. We cannot readily take these elements out once they have been released into the environment; our job is to focus on policies that prevent them from being released.

You can learn the major pollutants being released in your zip code area and other geographically related environmental information by accessing http://www.epa.gov/enviro/.

Indoor air quality in the workplace, schools, and homes is a growing concern because of the alarming rise in the incidence of asthma in the United States, particularly among children. Both the EPA and the American Lung Association provide excellent materials on indoor air quality. The EPA has a free kit called Indoor Air Quality: Tools for Schools, which includes a video and materials to help people improve the air quality in a school building. The major culprits contributing to poor indoor air are carbon monoxide, dust, molds, dust mites, cockroaches, pests and pets, cleaning and personal care products (particularly aerosols), lead, and, of course, environmental tobacco smoke (Fig. 6.4). It is important to assess both the environmental exposures and the human health status in a community. Health status is assessed using local, state, and national health data; by collecting our own data; or by a combination of

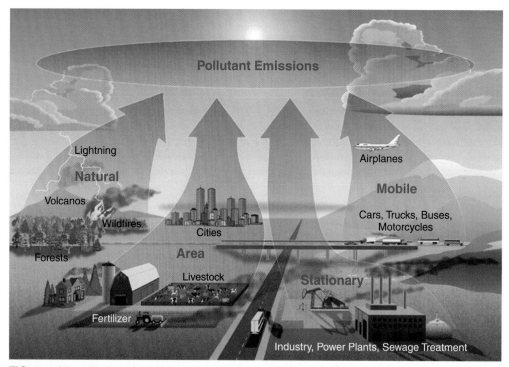

FIG. 6.4 Air pollution. Air pollution comes from a wide range of sources. The EPA's Envirofacts site (http:www.epa.gov/enviro/) allows you to check the air and other pollutants in your zip code. (From National Park Service. Sources of air pollution, www.nature.nps.gov. Accessed May 7, 2017.)

BOX 6.3 Environmental Health Resources

Resources for Environmental Assessments

- American Nurses Association (http://www.nursingworld.org): provides information on workplace health and safety and environmental health as it pertains to nursing.
- US Environmental Protection Agency (EPA) (http://www.epa.gov): provides a range of timely information. For example, in January 2016, the website had a feature related to storm preparedness. Other EPA resources include the following:
  - Envirofacts (http://www3.epa.gov/enviro/): search by location and find the environmental concerns related to air, water, toxic emissions, and compliance.
  - IAQ Tool for Schools (http://www.epa.gov/iaq-schools): for a free copy of the EPA's IAQ Tools for Schools.
  - Safe water (https://www.epa.gov/ground-water-and-drinking-water)
  - "Surf Your Watershed" database (https://cfpub.epa.gov/surf/locate/index.cfm)
  - Office of Pesticides (http://www.epa.gov/pesticides)
  - Children's page (http://www.epa.gov/children)
  - EPA lead programs (http://www.epa.gov/lead)
  - Advisories and technical resources for fish and shellfish consumption (https://www.epa.gov/fish-tech)
- Local Poison Control: call 1-800-222-1222
- Housing and Urban Development lead programs (https://portal.hud.gov/hudportal/HUD?src=/program_offices/healthy_homes/leadinfo)
- The National Lead Information Center: 1-800-424-LEAD
- National Pesticide Telecommunications Network: 1-800-858-7378
- Health Care Without Harm (http://www.noharm.org): a resource for the health care sector to play a leading role in promoting the health of people and the environment. Resources include safer chemicals, healthy food systems, green building and energy, pharmaceuticals, and green purchasing.
- Toxtown (http://toxtown.nlm.nih.gov): an NLM site where a visitor can travel to different locations, including farms, towns, cities, ports, and border regions, and learn about environmental health issues in each area.
- EnviRN (www.envirn.org): this site from the Alliance of Nurses for Healthy Environments (ANHE) is an active learning environment for all nurses in the area of environmental health. There were four featured topics in January 2016: fracking and public health, climate change and health, vulnerable populations, and nursing and environmental health.

Resources on Environmental Health Risks Associated with the Health Care Industry

- Children's Environmental Health Network (http://www.CEHN.org): a great online resource guide, as well as a manual for health professionals on children's environmental health basics.
- Healthy Schools Network (http://www.healthyschools.org): great resources on school-based environmental health risk.
- Center for Health, Environment, and Justice (http://www.chej.org): excellent resources for communities that are experiencing environmental challenges.
- Centers for Disease Control and Prevention (CDC) National Center for Environmental Health (NCEH) (http://www.cdc.gov/nceh): provides expertise in environmental pesticide surveillance and disease outbreak investigations.
- Agency for Toxic Substances and Disease Registry (ATSDR) (http://atsdr.cdc.gov): offers hazardous chemical fact sheets and an A–Z list of toxic substances and their characteristics, risks, and health effects.
- American Lung Association (http://www.lungusa.org): good resources on reducing environmental asthma triggers (1-800-LUNG-USA, which is 800-586-4872).
- Consumer Product Safety Commission (http://www.cpsc.gov)

---

the two. Box 6.3 provides governmental, nongovernmental professional, and other online resources.

Carbon monoxide is a particularly dangerous gas that can be emitted into the air. It is an odorless, colorless, tasteless gas that is produced when carbon-containing fuels, such as oil, kerosene, coal, or wood, are not completely combusted; it can also build up as a result of inadequate natural gas ventilation. Poisoning by carbon monoxide occurs most often in the fall and winter when buildings are being heated. When teaching clients how to avoid exposure to carbon monoxide, be sure to advise them to be aware of the possibility of faulty furnaces, motor vehicles, stoves and gas ranges, and vented gas heaters, which are common sources of carbon monoxide poisoning (Rosenthal, 2006). Because carbon monoxide is so difficult to detect, it is the leading cause of death attributable to poisoning in industrialized nations.

Fracking presents a number of public health issues because of its effects on both water and air. It is the process of drilling down into the earth and then directing a pressurized mixture of water, sand, and chemicals into the shale to allow the gas to flow out of the head of the well. Up to 600 chemicals are used in fracking, and many are known to be carcinogens and toxic. See http://www.dangersoffracking.com for details. The ANHE has an excellent fact sheet on public health and fracking. It provides a list of select pollutants associated with fracking that have known health effects. In general, public health issues related to fracking relate to the chemicals that pollute the water and air. Air pollution from drilling and fracking operations comes from shale drilling, gas processing, gas escapes, and diesel exhaust, which have a negative effect on air quality. There is a range of hazardous air emissions associated with a range of diseases, including asthma, chronic obstructive pulmonary disease, and cancer, to name a few. In addition, the chemicals often get into drinking water, especially water from private wells. Specifically, drinking water can be contaminated through methane migration, spills and leaks of fracking chemicals and fluids, radiation, and mismanagement of fracking water. Additionally, the process of fracking consumes huge amounts of water (ANHE, 2013).

WATER

Water is necessary for all forms of life. Human bodies are 70% water. Only 2.5% of the water on this planet is freshwater, and saltwater comprises the rest. Much of the freshwater is in the ice of the polar icecaps; groundwater makes up most of what remains, leaving only 0.01% in lakes, creeks, streams, rivers, and rainfall. People's lives are tied to a safe and adequate water supply. Water is necessary for the production of food—another essential to life. The quality of the soil is affected by its water supply, the chemicals that are intentionally added by humans, and the deposition of pollutants from the air. Soil that is free from harmful contaminants and pathogens is basic to life and health.

Discharges into water bodies from industries and from wastewater treatment systems can contribute to the degradation of water quality. Water quality is also affected by nonpoint sources of pollution, such as stormwater runoff from paved roads and parking lots, erosion from clear-cut tracts of land (after timbering and mining), and runoff from chemicals added to soil, such as fertilizers. The chain of potential damage continues with the additives to farm produce and animal diets, such as antibiotics and growth hormones (which are then consumed by humans).

LAND

Past and present use of land can affect a community's health. Local governments determine land use through their zoning laws. For example, a zoning law would prevent a housing development from being built on top of a previously used landfill that is now filled in and may look attractive. Agricultural soil is affected by its water supply, the chemicals that are added by people, and the pollutants that are deposited in the land from the air. A growing source of concern is what is referred to as "urban sprawl and the built community." The built environment includes "building conditions, neighborhood design, recreational area safety and accessibility, and transportation infrastructure" (Lopez and Welker-Hood, 2007, p 56). Lead also can get into the soil. When lead-containing paint chips are scraped from a wall, they become airborne in the breathing space for a brief time and then end up in nearby soil. Children play in the soil, where their hand-to-mouth activity results in exposure to lead, which has developmental and behavioral effects on them, both known and being discovered through research.

There is beginning to be a correlation between the way in which communities are configured and obesity. That is, does the community encourage and support walking or bike riding? Can people shop without needing to do so via a motor vehicle? How long is the average commute time? Is the environment totally built up, and concrete, not grass, covers much of the area?

FOOD

Food and food production are a source of concern. In recent years, foodborne illnesses have been associated with *Salmonella* and *Escherichia coli* O157:H7 in foods such as chicken, eggs, spinach, and hamburger. Good food preparation practices, such as washing and adequate cooking temperature and time, can prevent foodborne illnesses associated with most pathogens. Local health departments are responsible for monitoring food establishments (restaurants, food trucks, etc.) in the community, and the US Department of Agriculture is responsible for oversight of meat, poultry, fish, and produce production.

However, there are also environmental health risks posed by the presence of pesticide residues in our food; the use of recombinant bovine growth hormone (rBGH), which is given to many dairy cows; the administration of antibiotics to beef cattle, pigs,

and chickens at nontherapeutic doses that are given to promote growth; and the use of genetically modified organisms (GMOs) for genetically engineered crops.

When assessing a community's environmental health risks, a nurse must consider air, water, soil, and food. It is important that nurses understand the term "organic" regarding food labeling. If a food is labeled "Certified Organic," this is a meaningful term that has a legal US Department of Agriculture (USDA) definition. For foods to carry the Certified Organic label, they must have been produced without the use of pesticides, GMOs, or unnecessary (nontherapeutic) antibiotics. If a food is merely labeled "organic," the consumer does not have the same guarantee regarding what chemicals or farming practices have been used. When purchasing foods directly from farmers through farm stands or farmers' markets, consumers can directly ask about the chemicals and farm practices.

THE RIGHT TO KNOW

Several environmental statutes give the public the right to know about hazardous chemicals in the environment. One of the right-to-know laws allows health professionals and community members to access, by zip code, information regarding major sources of pollution being emitted into the air or water in their community. The EPA has an "Envirofacts" section on its website that provides data on sources of exposure by typing in a zip code.

Water suppliers that provide drinking water to consumers are responsible for testing the water according to EPA standards. The results of the testing must be reported to those who purchase the water, in the form of a consumer confidence report (CCR). Nurses should review CCRs, sometimes referred to as *right-to-know reports,* to learn what pollutants have been found in the drinking water. If the drinking water poses an immediate health threat, the water provider must send emergency warnings to the community via the local newspapers, radio, and television. The Freedom of Information Act is a federal law that allows citizens to request public documents.

Employees have the right to know, through the federal Hazard Communication Standard, about the hazardous chemicals with which they work. This standard requires employers (including hospitals) to maintain a list of all hazardous chemicals used on-site. Each of these chemicals should have an associated chemical information sheet, known as a *material safety data sheet* (MSDS), written by the chemical manufacturer. These safety sheets, available to any employee or his or her representative, should provide information about the chemical makeup, the health risks, and any special guidance on safe use and handling (e.g., requirements for protective gloves or respiratory protection). For more information on workplace health and safety, see http://www.osha.gov.

RISK ASSESSMENT

Currently, the EPA uses the process of risk assessment when it develops health-based standards. The term risk assessment refers to a process to determine the probability of a health threat associated with an exposure. The following discussion describes the four phases of a risk assessment related to chemical exposures.

First, by accessing toxicological or epidemiological data, determine whether a chemical is known to be associated with negative health effects (in animals or humans). Remember, the available toxicological data will probably be based on animal studies (from which the potential effects on humans are estimated), whereas the results of the epidemiological studies will be for human health effects.

Second, determine whether the chemical has been released into the environment via the air, water, soil, or food. Environmental professionals, such as sanitarians, food inspectors, air and water pollution scientists, meteorologists, environmental engineers, and others, can test for the presence of the suspected chemical in the various media (air, water, soil, food). In performing a risk assessment, determine whether multiple sources of the questionable chemical are present. For example, is lead found in the drinking water, in the ambient air, and in the paint in houses in a given community? If so, the lead will have a cumulative effect and be more of a danger.

In the third phase, estimate how much of the chemical might enter the human body and by which route. This estimate can be based on a one-time exposure, a short-term exposure, or a projected lifetime exposure. Federal standards created for air, water, and other pollutants are based on an estimation of a lifetime exposure. However, in workplace settings, the chemical exposure standards are based on an average exposure during a typical work shift or are set for a maximum exposure at any given time.

The final stage of the risk assessment process takes into account all three of the previous steps and *asks* the following questions:

- Is the chemical toxic?
- What are the source and amount of the exposure?
- What are the route and duration of the exposure for humans?

The goal is to try to predict the potential for harm on the basis of the estimated exposure. Like all science, risk assessment is subject to interpretation, and there may be more than one interpretation for each step, which could lead to different recommendations. Also, environmental laws are often contentious not only because of public or ecological health concerns but also because economic interests are at stake. Remember that for persons to be harmed by something in the environment, the following factors must be in place and connected:

1. A source of harm that has chemical and/or physical properties
2. An environmental medium for transport—air, water (i.e., surface water or groundwater), or soil
3. A receptor population within the exposure pathway for harm to human health
4. A route of exposure (for humans, these are inhalation, ingestion, and skin absorption)
5. An adequate amount (dose) of the chemical to result in human harm

ASSESSING ENVIRONMENTAL HEALTH RISKS IN CHILDREN

Toxic chemicals can have different effects depending on the timing of exposure. During fetal development, there are periods of heightened sensitivity to the effects of toxic chemicals. During such times, even extraordinarily small exposures can prevent or change a process that may permanently affect normal development. The brain undergoes rapid structural and functional changes during late pregnancy and in the neonatal period. Therefore it is extremely important to safeguard women's environments when they are pregnant (Table 6.1).

Fish are a lean, low-calorie source of protein. However, some fish may contain chemicals that could pose health risks. When the level of contaminants is unsafe, people may be advised to reduce or avoid eating certain fish caught in specific locations. The EPA provides specific information to inform people about the recommended level of consumption of fish in their local waters (EPA, 2016). Advisories are available for all 50 states and some US territories and tribes.

Nurses need to understand the implications that the fish advisories have for their clients and communities while at the same time counseling on the positive contribution of fish to a nutritionally balanced diet. Because more than 100,000 chemicals are used in the world, it is important to understand the possible effects on health.

Companies are not required to divulge all of the results of their private testing. A full battery of neurotoxicity tests is not required even for pesticides that may be sprayed in nurseries and labor and delivery areas, not to mention in homes. To make things even more complicated, risks from multiple chemical exposures are rarely considered when regulations are drafted. Such an omission ignores the reality that both children and adults are exposed to many toxic chemicals, often concurrently. The only exception to this rule is in the case of regulations regarding pesticides that are used on food (Fig. 6.5). This exception was created

TABLE 6.1 Environmental Agents Implicated in Adverse Reproductive Outcomes

Exposure	Known/Suspected Effect
Anesthetic compounds	Infertility, spontaneous abortion, fetal malformations, low birthweight
Antineoplastics	Infertility, spontaneous abortion
Dibromochloropropane	Sperm abnormalities, infertility
Ionizing radiation	Infertility, microcephaly, chromosomal abnormalities, childhood malignancies
Lead	Infertility, spontaneous abortion, developmental disabilities
Manganese	Infertility
Organic mercury	Developmental disabilities, neurological abnormalities
Organic solvents	Congenital malformations, childhood malignancies
Chlorinated biphenyls, polybrominated biphenyls	Fetal mortality, low birthweight, congenital abnormalities, developmental disabilities

From Aldrich T, Griffith J: *Environmental epidemiology and risk assessment*, New York, 1993, Van Nostrand Reinhold.

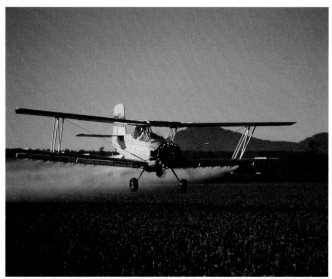

FIG. 6.5 Aerial application of agricultural pesticides makes it very difficult to control exposures. The chemicals get tracked into homes of farming communities. (Copyright 2011 Photos.com, a division of Getty Images. All rights reserved. Photo #87531230.)

by the 1996 Food Quality Protection Act, in which Congress acknowledged that children eat foods that may be contaminated by more than one pesticide residue. See Box 6.4 for the provisions under the Food Quality Protection Act.

Children are especially at risk for environmental hazards because of factors such as poverty, lack of access to health care, and the dangerous environmental situations in which they may live. Children are also at risk because of their size and the immaturity of their systems, such as the respiratory system. Infants and young children breathe more rapidly than adults, and this increase in respiratory rate leads to a proportionately greater exposure to air pollutants. While infants' lungs are developing, they are particularly susceptible to environmental toxicants. Although full function of the lungs is attained at approximately age 6, changes continue to occur in the lungs through adolescence (Dietert et al, 2000). Children are short, and thus their breathing zones are lower than those of adults, causing them to have closer contact with the chemical and biological agents on floors, carpeting, and the ground. Children are also at risk during disasters. For example, after Hurricane Katrina, a risk for children was inhaling the dangerous toxins from tar balls. Because children are shorter than adults, they were thus closer to the ground and subsequently closer to tar balls than were adults, with greater risk of inhalation. Brief exposure to the crude oil in tar balls can lead to contact dermatitis and skin rashes; longer exposure can lead to erythema, edema, and burning. Gastrointestinal and respiratory effects of this exposure also can occur (Murray, 2011). Children of color and poor children in America are disproportionately affected by a range of environmental health threats, including lead exposure, air pollution, pesticides, incinerator emissions, industrial and agricultural chemicals, and exposures from hazardous-waste sites (Suk and Davis, 2008).

BOX 6.4 Food Quality Protection Act of 1996

New provisions under the Food Quality Protection Act are related to protection of infants and children from pesticide exposure from multiple sources:

• **Health-based standard:** A new standard of a reasonable certainty of "no harm" that prohibits taking into account economic considerations when children are at risk.
• **Additional margin of safety:** Requires that the Environmental Protection Agency (EPA) to use an additional 10-fold margin of safety when adequate data exist to assess prenatal and postnatal developmental risks.
• **Account for children's diet:** Requires the use of age-appropriate estimates of dietary consumption in establishing allowable levels of pesticides on food to account for children's unique dietary patterns.
• **Account for all exposures:** In establishing acceptable levels of a pesticide on food, the EPA must account for exposures that may occur through other routes, such as drinking water and residential application of the pesticide.
• **Cumulative impact:** The EPA must consider the cumulative impacts of all pesticides that may share a common mechanism of action.
• **Tolerance reassessments:** All existing pesticide food standards must be reassessed over a 10-year period to ensure that they meet the new standards to protect children.
• **Endocrine disruption testing:** The EPA must screen and test all pesticides and pesticide ingredients for estrogen effects and other endocrine disruptor activity.
• **Registration renewal:** Establishes a 15-year renewal process for all pesticides to ensure that they have up-to-date scientific evaluations over time.

From the Environmental Protection Agency: *Summary of the Food Quality Protection Act,* n.d. Retrieved July 25, 2016 from https://www.epa.gov/laws-regulations/summary-food-quality-protection-act

Some of the health conditions in children that are associated with environmental factors include autism spectrum disorder; cancer; respiratory diseases, including asthma; obesity; and problems in neurodevelopment (American Cancer Society [ACS], 2016; CDC, 2016). In regard to cancer, only a small percentage of childhood cancers are associated with heredity. However, exposure to ionizing radiation increases the risk of childhood leukemia and possibly other cancers. All of the causes of autism spectrum disorder are not currently known. Environmental factors are thought to be a possible cause, as are biologic and genetic factors. The NIH has identified that understanding the effects of environmental exposures on child health and development is a priority. It has launched a 7-year initiative called the Environmental Influences on Child Health Outcomes (ECHO) program. The program supports studies that focus on four key pediatric outcomes that are public health priorities: (1) upper and lower airway; (2) obesity; (3) pre-, peri-, and postnatal outcomes; and (4) neurodevelopment (US Department of Health and Human Services, 2015). Clearly, the environment plays an important role in children's health. Think about this question: When building a school, should the government require the same environmental assessment of the land as it would if a commercial enterprise, like a hotel, was being placed on the same site? Currently, it requires less stringent environmental assessments.

Children's bodies also operate differently. Some of the protective mechanisms that are well developed in adults, like the blood–brain barrier, are immature in young children, thereby increasing their vulnerability to the effects of toxic chemicals. Finally, the kidneys of young children are less effective at filtering out undesirable toxic chemicals, and these chemicals then continue to circulate and accumulate.

Infants and young children drink more fluids per body weight than adults do, and this increases the dose of contaminants in their drinking water, milk (hormones and antibiotics), and juices (particularly pesticides). If an adult were to drink an amount of water proportionate to the amount an infant drinks, the adult would have to drink about 50 glasses of water a day. Children also eat more per body weight, eat different proportions of food, and absorb food differently from adults. Children consume much greater quantities of fruits and fruit juices than adults do, once again adding exposure to doses of pesticide residues.

REDUCING ENVIRONMENTAL HEALTH RISKS

Preventing problems is less costly, whether the cost is measured in resources consumed or health effects. Education is a primary preventive strategy. When examining the sources of environmental health risks in communities and planning intervention strategies, it is important to apply the basic principles of disease prevention. For a home with lead-based paint, apply the primary prevention strategy of removing that specific source of lead. Good surveillance, a secondary prevention strategy, will not prevent lead exposure, but it may help with early identification of rising blood lead levels. For a symptomatic child brought to a health care provider, a system should be in place for specialists familiar with lead poisoning to provide immediate care; swift medical interventions to reduce blood levels of lead can reduce the risk of further harm. This might be a tertiary prevention response.

For workplace exposures, industrial hygienists have developed a list of precautions for avoiding or minimizing employee exposures to potentially hazardous chemicals. Industrial hygienists are public health professionals who specialize in workplace exposures to hazards—physical, chemical, and biological—that create conditions of health risk (Box 6.5). Once it is established that a human health threat exists, develop a plan of action to eliminate or manage (reduce) the risk. Risk management, which should be informed by the risk assessment

process, involves the selection and implementation of a strategy to reduce risks, which can take many forms. For example, the "Three R's for Reducing Environmental Pollution" are as follows:

1. **Reduce:** Reducing consumption reduces waste and unnecessary packaging and nonessentials.
2. **Reuse:** Choosing reusable rather than disposable products creates less waste (e.g., using glass dishes rather than paper ones).
3. **Recycle:** Recycling paper, glass, cans, and plastic decreases pollution.

Risk assessment includes considering ways to dispose of materials. Once waste products are generated, they must be disposed of in one of the following three ways:

1. **Incineration:** Burning can change the chemical composition through heat, but the products of burning, such as ash and air emissions, must be controlled and disposed of using one of the following two options.
2. **Water discharge:** When products are disposed of in water, the water must be treated to ensure that the dose in the water is not great enough to do harm.
3. **Landfilling or burying in soil:** When using landfills or burying products, protections must be put in place, such as liners and leachate pumps and monitors, to avoid seepage of harmful doses into the groundwater or air.

Each of the options for waste disposal is intended to provide a way either to alter the waste product to a less toxic form through chemical intervention (biodegradation) or to store the product in a bio-unavailable form or place. Because all of the options for disposal can be a problem, prevention is desirable.

Remember that human effects are intensified in the most sensitive, vulnerable environments, such as estuaries, the nurseries for much of sea and coastal plant and animal life. Some of the most valued food sources are also the most sensitive to pollution. Shellfish are efficient filters of contaminants in the water in which they live. For example, oysters filter and retain almost all contaminants from the water in which they grow. It is impossible to rid them of contaminants after harvesting. The only protection for humans is to grow oysters in environments free from harmful contamination. Safe seafood depends on clean water.

Another form of risk reduction is to reduce the risk from exposure to ultraviolet rays. People need to avoid being outside during peak sun hours and need to wear protective clothing and/or sunblock. To reduce exposure to dangerous heavy metals, special processes can be used at the water filtration plant that supplies the public water. In the home, running the cold water tap for 1 or 2 minutes each morning before collecting water for coffee or drinking will reduce the presence of lead that may have leached from old pipes (or the solder used on them) overnight. In communities that report to the media the local pollution levels, it is important to encourage residents to not exercise or walk excessively outside when the air pollution index is high. Individuals, communities, and nations can reduce risks. In recent years, there have been global agreements to reduce persistent pollutants and decrease global warming. However, not all nations are subscribing to this goal. The national and international news provide many examples of extreme pollution around the world.

BOX 6.5 Industrial Hygiene Controls

- Substitute less hazardous or nonhazardous substances for hazardous ones (e.g., use water-based instead of solvent-based products).
- Isolate the hazardous chemicals from human exposure (closed systems).
- Apply engineering controls (e.g., ventilation systems, including exhausts).
- Reduce the exposures through administrative controls (rotating employees).
- Use personal protective equipment (gloves, respirators, protective clothing).
- Educate employees about controls.

From Levy B, Wegman D: *Occupational health: recognizing and preventing work-related disease and injury,* ed 5, Philadelphia, 2006, Lippincott Williams & Wilkins.

📋 LEVELS OF PREVENTION

Related to the Environment: Lead Exposure

Primary Prevention
Use only non–lead-based paint

Secondary Prevention
If lead is found in paint, remove this paint and replace with nonlead paint.

Tertiary Prevention
At the first sign of symptoms of lead exposure, take steps to reduce blood lead levels.

Nursing interventions to reduce environmental health risks can also take many forms. Education is a key nursing action. By working with a variety of community members, nurses can explain the relationship between harmful environmental exposures and human health and guide the community toward risk reduction based on both changes in individual behavior and community-wide approaches. For example, a nurse could help clients know how important it is to purchase a carbon monoxide detector. The detectors are designed to measure carbon monoxide levels over time and sound an alarm when the levels reach a specific point. These devices are sold in many stores in the United States.

RISK COMMUNICATION

Risk is a familiar term in nursing practice. We counsel people about risks of pregnancy, communicable disease (especially sexually transmitted disease), intentional and unintentional injury, and personal health-related choices (e.g., smoking, alcohol consumption, diet). Risk assessment in environmental health has focused on characterizing the hazard (i.e., the source), its physical and chemical properties, its toxicity, and the presence of (or potential for) other elements in the exposure pathway—mode of transmission, route of exposure, receptor population, and dose. Risk is typically viewed as the process of estimating the likelihood of an unwanted, adverse effect and the probable magnitude and intensity of that effect (Fairbrother and Turnley, 2005). For example, an environmental risk assessment of a contaminated site includes a calculation of the dose that might be received through all routes of exposure, the toxicity of the chemical, the size and vulnerability (e.g., age, health) of the population potentially exposed (e.g., resident, future resident, transient), and the likelihood of exposure.

Communication of risk is both an area of practice and a skill. It involves understanding the outrage factors relevant to the risk being addressed so that both can be incorporated in the message, with the result that either action is taken to ensure safety or unnecessary fear is reduced. Outrage factors are those things that cause people to feel a sense of outrage toward a behavior. An example of raising outrage to produce action can be seen in the way people respond to smokers who smoke in public. Because of the fear of secondhand or involuntary, passive smoking, people have advocated to stimulate public policy that limits or bans smoking in public places. When the emphasis on risk went from a voluntary choice of smokers to an involuntary exposure of nonsmokers, the outrage level of the nonsmoking public became high enough to result in legislation guaranteeing smoke-free public spaces (e.g., public buildings, airplanes, restaurants). On the other hand, outrage diminishes when people obtain information about a situation from a trusted source, and nurses are often cited in surveys as trusted sources of information on environmental risks.

Risk communication includes general principles of good communication. It is a combination of the following:

- *The right information:* Accurate, relevant, and in a language that audiences can understand. A good risk assessment is essential information for shaping the message.
- *To the right people:* Those affected and those who may not be affected but are worried. Information about the community is essential and includes geographic boundaries, who lives there (demographics), how they get information (i.e., flyers, newspapers, radio, television, the Internet, text messages, word of mouth), where they get together (i.e., school, church, community center), and who within the community can help plan the communication.
- *At the right time:* For timely action or to allay fear.

ETHICS

Public health has been defined as "what we, as a society, do collectively to assure the conditions for people to be healthy" (Public Health Leadership Society, 2002, p 22). Public health is concerned with public goods that can be achieved through collective action such as clean water, safe and adequate housing, and public safety with societal regulation of shared risks (Easley and Allen, 2007). The public health goal would likely ask individuals to sacrifice some of their self-interests to benefit the greater good of more people. This could be seen when companies are asked to reduce air or water pollution, even though it might be expensive for them to do so to protect the health of the people who might be affected. As discussed in Chapter 4, understanding ethics is essential for nurses making their own choices, in describing issues and options within groups, and in advocating for ethical choices. When the sticking points are around competing commodities (e.g., jobs versus environmental protection, production versus conservation, economic development versus the health of the environment), the skillful nurse can change the discussion from "either/or" to "both" by opening new possibilities for ethical and mutually satisfactory outcomes. The following ethical issues may arise in environmental health decisions:

- Who has access to information and when?
- How complete and accurate is the available information?
- Who is included in decision making and when?
- What and whose values and priorities are given weight in decisions?
- How are short-term and long-term consequences considered?

A review of ethical issues in Chapter 4 may help nurses decide what actions they could and should take in regard to environmental health issues.

GOVERNMENT ENVIRONMENTAL PROTECTION

The federal government is involved with many major pieces of environmental legislation (Box 6.6). The government manages environmental exposures through the development and enforcement of standards and regulations that limit a polluter's ability to put hazardous chemicals into our food, water, air, or soil. The government may also be involved in educating the public about risks and risk reduction. Several federal agencies are involved in environmental health regulation, including the EPA, the Food and Drug Administration, and the Department of Agriculture. In every state, an equivalent state agency exists as well. The local health department may manage environmental health issues at the city or county level. However, environmental protection issues are typically directed by the state using both federal and state laws. The organization and approach to environmental protection vary somewhat among states, but the common

essential strategies of prevention and control via the permitting process, establishment of environmental standards, and monitoring, as well as compliance and enforcement, are found in every state.

Potentially harmful pollution that cannot be prevented must be controlled. The first step in the process of controlling pollution is permitting, a process by which the government places limits on the amount of pollution emitted into the air or water. Industries and businesses whose processes will result in releases (i.e., discharges, emissions) that have the potential for harm are required to obtain environmental permits to construct and operate. A range of permits may be required (e.g., storm water control, construction, operations for air and wastewater discharges, waste management). It is in the permitting process that maximum opportunities to incorporate prevention strategies can be exercised. For example, waste minimization can be included as a permit condition, with the agreement of the industry even if it is not required by law or

BOX 6.6 Environmental Laws

National Environmental Policy Act (NEPA)
The NEPA established the Environmental Protection Agency (EPA) and a national policy for the environment and provides for the establishment of a Council on Environmental Policy. All policies, regulations, and public laws shall be interpreted and administered in accordance with the policies set forth in this act.

Federal Insecticide, Fungicide, and Rodenticide Act (FIFRA)
FIFRA provides federal control of pesticide distribution, sale, and use. The EPA was given the authority to study the consequences of pesticide usage and requires users such as farmers and utility companies to register when using pesticides. Later amendments to the law required applicators to take certification examinations, registration of all pesticides used in the United States, and proper labeling of pesticides that, if in accordance with specifications, will cause no harm to the environment (summary from FIFRA, 1972).

Clean Water Act (CWA)
The CWA sets basic structure for regulating pollutants to US waters. The law gave the EPA the authority to set effluent standards on an industry basis and continued the requirements to set water quality standards for all contaminants in surface water. The 1977 amendments focused on toxic pollutants. In 1987 the CWA was reauthorized and again focused on toxic pollutants, authorized citizen suit provisions, and funded sewage treatment plants.

Clean Air Act
The Clean Air Act regulates air emissions from area, stationary, and mobile sources. The EPA was authorized to establish National Ambient Air Quality Standards (NAAQSs) to protect public health and the environment. The goal was to set and achieve the NAAQSs by 1975. The law was amended in 1977 when many areas of the country failed to meet the standards. The 1990 amendments to the Clean Air Act intended to meet unaddressed or insufficiently addressed problems, such as acid rain, ground-level ozone, stratospheric ozone depletion, and air toxins. Also in the 1990 reauthorization, a mandate for Chemical Risk Management Plans was included. This mandate requires industry to identify "worst-case scenarios" regarding the hazardous chemicals that they transport, use, or discard (summary from Clean Air Act, 1970).

Occupational Safety and Health Act (OSHA)
The OSHA was passed to ensure worker and workplace safety. The goal was to make sure employers provide an employment place free of hazards to health and

safety, such as chemicals, excessive noise, mechanical dangers, heat or cold extremes, or unsanitary conditions. To establish standards for the workplace, the act also created the National Institute for Occupational Safety and Health (NIOSH) as the research institution for OSHA.

Safe Drinking Water Act (SDWA)
The SDWA was established to protect the quality of drinking water in the United States. The SDWA authorized the EPA to establish safe standards of purity and required all owners or operators of public water systems to comply with primary (health-related) standards.

Resource Conservation and Recovery Act (RCRA)
The RCRA gave the EPA the authority to control the generation, transportation, treatment, storage, and disposal of hazardous waste. The RCRA also proposed a framework to manage nonhazardous waste. The 1984 Federal Hazardous and Solid Waste Amendments to this act required phasing out land disposal of hazardous waste. The 1986 amendments enabled the EPA to address problems from underground tanks storing petroleum and other hazardous substances.

Toxic Substances Control Act (TSCA)
The TSCA gives the EPA the ability to track the 75,000 industrial chemicals currently produced or imported into the United States. The EPA can require reporting or testing of chemicals that may pose environmental health risks and can ban the manufacture and import of those chemicals that pose an unreasonable risk. TSCA supplements the Clean Air Act and the Toxic Release Inventory.

Comprehensive Environmental Response, Compensation, and Liability Act (CERCLA or Superfund)
This law created a tax on the chemical and petroleum industries and provided broad federal authority to respond directly to releases or threatened releases of hazardous substances that may endanger public health or the environment.

Superfund Amendments and Reauthorization Act (SARA)
SARA amended the CERCLA with several changes and additions. These changes included increased size of the trust fund, encouragement of greater citizen participation in decision making on how sites should be cleaned up, increased state

Continued

BOX 6.6 **Environmental Laws—cont'd**

involvement in every phase of the Superfund program, increased focus on human health problems related to hazardous waste sites, new enforcement authorities and settlement tools, emphasis on the importance of permanent remedies and innovative treatment technologies in cleanup of hazardous waste sites, and Superfund actions to consider standards in other federal and state regulations. (Under Superfund legislation, the Federal Agency for Toxic Substances and Disease Registry was established.)

Emergency Planning and Community Right to Know Act (EPCRA)

The EPCRA, also known as Title III of SARA, was enacted to help local communities protect public health safety and the environment from chemical hazards. Each state was required to appoint a State Emergency Response Commission that was required to divide the state into Emergency Planning Districts and establish a Local Emergency Planning Committee (LEPC) for each district.

National Environmental Education Act

The National Environmental Education Act created a new and better coordinated environmental education emphasis at the EPA. It created the National Environmental Education and Training Foundation.

Pollution Prevention Act (PPA)

The PPA focused industry, government, and public attention on reduction of the amount of pollution through cost-effective changes in production, operation, and use of raw materials. Pollution prevention also includes other practices that increase efficient use of energy, water, and other water resources, such as recycling, source reduction, and sustainable agriculture.

Food Quality Protection Act (FQPA)

The FQPA amended the Federal Insecticide, Fungicide, and Rodenticide Act and the Federal Food, Drug, and Cosmetic Act. FQPA changed the way the EPA regulates pesticides. The requirements included a new safety standard of reasonable certainty of no harm to be applied to all pesticides used on foods.

Chemical Safety Information, Site Security, and Fuels Regulatory Act (Amendment to Section 112 of the Clean Air Act)

This act removed from coverage by the Risk Management Plan (RMP) any flammable fuel when used as fuel or held for sale as fuel by a retail facility (flammable fuels used as a feedstock or held for sale as a fuel at a wholesale facility are still covered). The law also limits access to off-site consequence analyses, which are reported in RMPs by covered facilities.

---

regulation. Once a condition exists in the permit, it has the force of law.

The permitting process includes submission of an application, which requires details on the proposed operation. Plans are studied, engineering processes are modeled, validated, and technical requirements are reviewed by appropriate regulatory experts. Usually some form of public participation is required or included voluntarily. The public involvement can include public notice, public comment, and public meetings and hearings initiated by the regulatory agency. Public involvement also can take the form of voluntary agreements and dispute resolution between the industry and the community, which may or may not involve a government entity. Limits on what an industry or business can release or emit lawfully are based on environmental standards.

Environmental standards may be expressed as a permitted level of emissions, a maximum contaminant level allowed, an action level for environmental cleanup, or a risk-based calculation. A standard often reflects the level of pollution that will limit a number of excess deaths at a given level of exposure over a specified period. It is the responsibility of the polluters to operate within the standards. Compliance and enforcement are the next steps for controlling pollutions. Compliance refers to the processes for ensuring that permit and standard requirements are met. Cleanup or remediation of environmental damage is another control step. Public information and involvement processes, such as citizen advisory panels or community forums, are integral to the development of standards, ongoing monitoring, and remediation. Monitoring procedures, which must use methods approved by the EPA or scientific consensus, must follow accepted protocols (e.g., maintaining a documented chain of custody of samples to ensure accuracy and protection from contamination at the laboratory after sampling).

ADVOCACY

The more than 3 million nurses in the United States today can and should be a strong voice for change. As informed citizens, nurses can work to protect the environmental health of clients, families, and communities. Nurses are seen as trusted sources of information, and they need to serve as reliable sources of environmental health information. They can act in the best interest of public health and use their abilities as educators, advocates, and communicators to affect public policy, laws, and regulations that protect public health. Nurses can serve as a resource for state and federal legislators and their staff. Often, legislators are asked to vote on environmental legislation without a sound understanding of how the legislation may affect public health. Although not every nurse can be an expert in all aspects of environmental health, every nurse has a basic education in human health and can identify people who may be most vulnerable to environmental insult. Nurses' thoughts about the potential effects of new laws on the health of individuals and communities are valuable to legislators. As communicators and educators, nurses can do the following:

- Write letters to local newspapers responding to environmental health issues affecting the community.
- Participate in blogs or other web mediums that capture the attention of people about the environment and threats to it.
- Serve as a credible source of information at community gatherings, formal governmental hearings, and professional nursing forums.
- Volunteer to serve on local, state, or federal commissions; know the zoning and permit laws that regulate the effects of industry and land use on the community.
- Read, listen, and ask questions. As informed citizens, nurses can lead in fostering community action to address threats to environmental health.

ENVIRONMENTAL JUSTICE AND ENVIRONMENTAL HEALTH DISPARITIES

Some diseases differentially affect different populations. Certain environmental health risks disproportionately affect poor people and people of color in the United States. A poor person of color is more likely to (1) live near a hazardous waste site or an incinerator, (2) have children who are exposed to lead, and (3) have children with asthma, which has a strong association with environmental exposures. Campaigns in communities of color and poor communities to improve the unequal burden of environmental risks strive to achieve environmental justice or environmental equity.

In 1993 the Environmental Justice Act was passed, and in 1994 Executive Order 12898, Federal Actions to Address Environmental Justice in Minority Populations, was signed. These created policies to more comprehensively reduce the incidence of environmental inequity by mandating that every federal agency act in a manner to address and prevent illnesses and injuries. Nursing interventions and involvement in environmental health policies can have a significant effect on the health disparities experienced by our most challenged communities.

UNIQUE ENVIRONMENTAL HEALTH THREATS IN THE HEALTH CARE INDUSTRY: NEW OPPORTUNITIES FOR ADVOCACY

We rarely think of health care facilities as sources of environmental harm. Nurses often lead in reducing the use of mercury-containing products in hospitals. The use of mercury-containing thermometers and sphygmomanometers leads to a risk of breakage, which releases a highly toxic substance into the workplace. Further, when a hospital uses incineration to dispose of its waste, the mercury-containing products will create significant releases of mercury into the air, thus contaminating communities. This airborne mercury will be present in raindrops. When airborne mercury lands on water bodies (e.g., lakes, rivers, or oceans), it is converted by the microorganisms in the water to methylmercury, which is highly toxic to humans. The methylmercury is then bioaccumulated in fish: as larger fish eat smaller fish, the body burden of methylmercury increases significantly.

Many synthetic chemicals that contaminate the environment are referred to as persistent bioaccumulative toxins (PBTs) or persistent organic pollutants (POPs). These are chemicals that do not break down in air, water, or soil, or in the plant, animal, and human bodies to which they may be passed. Ultimately, because humans are at the top of the food chain, these chemicals may come to reside in our bodies. For instance, lead, which should not be found in the human body, can be found in the long bones of almost any human in the world because of its ubiquitous use and presence in our environment.

Dioxin, another pollutant that contaminates communities, is created, in part, by the health care industry. Dioxins are created when we manufacture or burn (incinerate) products that contain chlorine, such as bleached white paper or polyvinyl chloride (PVC) plastics. When dioxins are released into the environment, they are consumed by agricultural animals and by fish. The dioxins are stored in fat cells as they work their way up the food chain. This phenomenon has resulted in dioxin deposition in breast tissue, and dioxin has been found in both cow and human milk. Virtually all women now have dioxin in their breast tissue. Dioxin, an endocrine-disrupting chemical and a strong carcinogen, is associated with several neurodevelopmental problems, including learning disabilities and is now in every human's body. The solution to this problem is to stop releasing dioxins into the environment. In the health care setting, one way to eliminate the creation and release of dioxins is to stop using products like PVC plastics and select safer alternatives by employing environmentally preferable purchasing policies and practices.

An international campaign called Health Care Without Harm is working to reduce and eliminate the use of mercury and PVC plastic in the health care industry and to eliminate incineration of medical waste. The ANA was a founding member of the Health Care Without Harm campaign, and nurses have taken many leadership roles in the activities in the United States and around the world. The Health Care Without Harm website (http://www.noharm.org) provides outstanding information on greening hospitals and resources about pollution prevention in the health care sector.

REFERRAL RESOURCES

No single source of information about environmental health is available, nor is there a single resource to which individuals or a community can be referred if they suspect an environmental problem. Information is widely accessible on the Internet, but finding an actual person to assist you or the communities you serve may not be as easy. One starting point may be the environmental epidemiology unit or toxicology unit of your state health department or environmental agency. Another local or state resource may be environmental health experts in nursing or medical schools or schools of public health. The Association of Occupational and Environmental Clinics (http://www.AOEC.org) is a national network of specialty clinics and individual practitioners available for consultation and sometimes for the provision of educational programs for health professionals.

Local resources include local health and environmental protection agencies, poison control centers, agricultural extension offices, and occupational and environmental departments in schools of medicine, nursing, and public health. Some local and state agencies have developed topical directories to assist in accessing the appropriate staff for specific questions. Many resources have websites that allow ready access through the Internet and can be located by using any of the popular search methods (see Box 6.3).

ROLES FOR NURSES IN ENVIRONMENTAL HEALTH

Nurses are involved in many ways in environmental health, whether in full-time work, as an adjunct to existing roles, or as informed and involved citizens. Two of these nursing roles are assessment and referral. Assessment and referral are familiar parts of nursing practice, but they have specific meaning in environmental health. Assessment activities of nurses can range from individual health assessments to being full participants in community assessment or partners in a specific environmental site assessment. Referral resources may vary in communities. One starting point may be the environmental epidemiology or toxicology unit of the state health department or environmental agency. Box 6.3 lists several good referral sources. Some of the key nursing functions that are discussed throughout the chapter include the following:

- **Community involvement and public participation:** Organizing, facilitating, and moderating. Making public notices effective, making public forums accessible, and welcoming input. Making information exchange understandable and problem solving acceptable to culturally diverse communities are valuable contributions made by nurses. Skills in community organizing and mobilizing can help communities have a meaningful voice in decisions that affect it.
- **Individual and population risk assessment:** Using nursing assessment skills to detect potential and actual exposure pathways and outcomes for clients cared for in the acute, chronic, and healthy communities of practice.

- **Risk communication:** Interpreting and applying principles to practice. Nurses may serve as skilled risk communicators within agencies, working for industries, or working as independent practitioners. Amendments to the Clean Air Act require major industrial sources of air emissions to have risk management plans and to inform their neighbors of specifics of the risks and plans (Clean Air Act, 1996).
- **Epidemiological investigations:** Having the skills to respond in scientifically sound and humanly sensitive ways to community concerns about cancer, birth defects, and stillbirths that citizens fear may have environmental causes.
- **Policy development:** Proposing, informing, and monitoring action from agencies, communities, and organization perspectives.

The assimilation of the concepts of environmental health into a nurse's daily practice gives new life to the traditional public health values of prevention, building community, and social justice. There is great congruence with many personal, religious, and spiritual values of stewardship of creation, preserving the gifts of nature, and decision making that provides for quality of life for present and future generations. It is a context for practice in which nurses are welcomed and valued for their contribution.

As nurses learn more about the environment, opportunities for integration into their practice, educational programs, research, advocacy, and policy work will become evident. Opportunities abound for those pioneering spirits within the nursing profession who are dedicated to creating healthier environments for their clients and communities.

PRACTICE APPLICATION

Two case scenarios related to exposure pathways are presented here. The first involves lead poisoning, and the second involves gasoline contamination of groundwater.

At the county health department, a 3-year-old boy presents with gastric upset and behavior changes that have persisted for several weeks. Billy's parents report that they have been renovating their home to remove lead paint. They had been discouraged from routinely testing their child because their insurance does not cover testing, and they could not find information on where to have the tests done. Their concern has heightened with Billy's persistent symptoms.

You test the level of lead in Billy's blood and find it to be 45 µg/dL. You research lead poisoning and discover that children are at great risk because they absorb lead into the central nervous system. You also find that chronic lead poisoning may have long-term effects, such as developmental delays and impaired learning ability. You refer Billy to his primary-care physician. On further investigation, you find that Billy's home was built before 1950 and is still under renovation. The sanitarian tests the interior paint and finds a high lead content. Ample amounts of sawdust from sanding are noted in various rooms of the home.

You determine that a completed exposure pathway exists.
A. What would you include in an assessment of this situation?
B. What prevention strategies would you use to resolve this issue?
   1. At the individual level?
   2. At the population level?

A citizen calls the local health department to report that his drinking water, from a private well, "smells like gasoline." A water sample is collected, and analysis reveals the presence of petroleum products. A nearby rural store with a service station has removed its old underground gasoline storage tanks and replaced them, as required by law. Contaminated soil from the old leaking tank has been removed, and a well to monitor groundwater contamination is scheduled for installation. However, sandy soil has allowed rapid movement of the contamination through the groundwater, and the plume has reached the neighbor's drinking-water well at levels that exceed the drinking-water standard.

What are some possible responses?
Answers can be found on the Evolve website.

REMEMBER THIS!

- Nurses have responsibilities to be informed consumers and to be advocates for citizens in their community regarding environmental health issues.
- Models describing the determinants of health acknowledge the role of the environment in health and disease.
- For many chemical compounds, whether new or familiar, scientific evidence of possible health effects is lacking.
- Prevention activities include education, waste minimizing, and land-use planning. Control activities include environmental permitting, environmental standards, monitoring, compliance and enforcement, and cleanup and remediation.
- Each nursing assessment should include questions and observations about intended and unintended environmental exposures.
- Environmental databases facilitate the easy and immediate access to environmental data useful in assessment, diagnosis, intervention, and evaluation.

- Risk communication is an important skill and must acknowledge the outrage factor experienced by communities with environmental hazards.
- Federal, state, and local laws and regulations exist to protect citizens from environmental hazards.
- Environmental health practice engages multiple disciplines, and nurses are important members of the environmental health team.
- Environmental health practice includes principles of health promotion, disease prevention, and health protection.
- The objectives of *Healthy People 2020* address targets for the reduction of risk factors and diseases related to environmental causes.

Ⓔ EVOLVE WEBSITE

http://evolve.elsevier.com/Stanhope/foundations

- NCLEX® Review Questions
- Practice Application Answers

REFERENCES

Afzal, BM: Global warming: a public health concern, *Online J Issues Nurs* 12:5, 2007.

Aldrich T, Griffith J: *Environmental epidemiology and risk assessment*, New York, 1993, Van Nostrand Reinhold.

Allen, PJ: Climate change: it's our problem, *Pediatric Nursing* 41(1):42–46, 2015.

Alliance of Nurses for Healthy Environments: *Public health and fracking*, 2013. Available at http://envirn.org/pg/pages/view/79720/public-health-and-fracking? Retrieved January 2016.

American Cancer Society: *Cancer facts and figures*, Atlanta GA, 2016, American Cancer Society.

American Nurses Association: *Principles of environmental health for nursing practice*, Silver Spring, MD, 2007, ANA.

Anderko, L, Davies-Cole J, Strunk, A: Identifying populations at risk: interdisciplinary environmental climate change tracking, *Public Health Nursing* 31(6):484–491, 2014.

Centers for Disease Control and Prevention: *Facts about ASD*, 2016. Retrieved February 2016 from http://www.cdc.gov.autism/facts.

Centers for Disease Control and Prevention: *National environmental public health tracking*, 2014. Retrieved February 2016 from http://www.cdc.gov/nceh/tracking.

Centers for Disease Control and Prevention: *Climate effects on health*, 2015. Retrieved February 2016 from http://www.cdc.gov/climateand health/effects/default.htm.

Clean Air Act: Risk Management Programs, Section 112(7), Fed Reg Part III EPA, 40 CFR, Part 68, June 20, 1996.

Council on Linkages between Academic and Public Health Practice: *Core competencies for public health professionals*, Washington DC, 2010, Public Health Foundation, Health Resources and Services Administration.

Drug Enforcement Administration: *DEA Announces 10th National Drug Take-Back*, 2015. Retrieved February 2016 from http://www.dea/gov/divisions/hq/2015/hq072815.shtml.

Dietert RR, Etzel RA, Chen D, et al: Workshop to identify critical windows exposure for children's health: immune and respiratory systems work group summary, *Environ Health Perspect* 108(Suppl 3):483–490, 2000.

Easley CE, Allen CE: A critical intersection: human rights, Standards for Environmental Health Nursing, and nursing ethics, *Adv Nurs Sci* 30:367–382, 2007.

Environmental Protection Agency: *Lead poisoning is preventable*, Washington DC, 2015a. Retrieved July 25, 2016 from Environmental Protection Agency.

Environmental Protection Agency: *What are the six common air pollutants?* Washington DC, 2015b. Retrieved July 25, 2016 from http://www.epa.gov/airquality/urbanair/.

Environmental Protection Agency: *Fish and shellfish advisories and safe eating guidelines*, 2016. http://www.cdc.gov/choose-fish-and-shellfish-wisely/fish-and-shellfish-advisories-and-safe-eating-guidelines.

Environmental Protection Agency: *Summary of the food quality protection act*, n.d. Retrieved July 25, 2016 from https://www.epa.gov/laws-regulations/summary-food-quality-protection-act.

Environmental Protection Agency: *Lead in paint, dust, and soil*, Washington, DC, n.d., EPA. Retrieved February 1, 2013 from http://www.epa.gov/lead/pubs/leadpdfe.pdf.

Fairbrother A, Turnley JG: Predicting risks of uncharacteristic wildfires: application of the risk assessment process, *Forest Ecol Manae* 211:28–35, 2005.

Federal Insecticide, Fungicide, and Rodenticide Act (FIFRA), 1972. http://www.epa.law . . . /summary-federal-insecticide-fungicide-rodenticide-act-ffra-amd-federalfacilities. Accessed May 7, 2017.

Gilden RC, Huffling K, Sattler B: Pesticides and health risks, *J Obstet Gynecol Neonatal Nurs* 39:103–110, 2010.

Habre R, Moshier E, Castro W, et al: The effect of PM 2.5 and its components from indoor and outdoor sources on cough and wheeze symptoms in asthmatic children, *J Expo Sci Environ Epidemiol* 2014. doi: 10.1038/jes.2014.21.

Intergovernmental Program on Climate Change: *Climate Change 2014: impacts, adaptation, and vulnerability*, 2014, Cambridge University Press, IPCC Working Group II Contribution to the 5th assessment report. Retrived June 10, 2014 from http://www.who.int/globalchange/environment/climatechange-2014-report/en/. Accessed May 7, 2017.

Leffers JM, McDermott-Levy R, Smith CM, et al: Nursing's education's response to the 1995 Institute of Medicine Report: Nursing, Health and the Environment, *Nurs Forum* 40(4):214–224, 2014.

Levy B, Wegman D: *Occupational health: recognizing and preventing work-related disease and injury*, ed 5, Philadelphia, 2006, Lippincott Williams & Wilkins.

Lopez R, Welker-Hood K: Urban sprawl and the built environment, *Am Nurse Today* 2:56, 2007.

Murray JS: The effects of the gulf oil spill on children, *J Spec Pediatr Nurs* 16:70–74, 2011.

Paranzino G: *Agency for Toxic Substances and Disease Registry:* I PREPARE: development and clinical utility of an environmental exposure history mnemonic, *AAOHN J* 53(1):37–42, 2005. Retrieved from http://www.atsdr.cdc.gov.

Pope AM, Snyder MA, Mood LH, editors: *Nursing, health, and the environment*, Washington, DC, 1995, Institute of Medicine, National Academies Press.

Public Health Leadership Society: *Principles of the ethical practice of public health, version 2.2*, New Orleans, La, 2002, Public Health Leadership Society.

Reifsnider F, Bishop, SL, An, K, et al: We stop for no storm: coping with an environmental disaster and public health research, *Public Health Nursing* 31(6):500–507, 2014.

Rosenthal LD: Carbon monoxide poisoning, *Am J Nurs* 106:40–46, 2006.

Smargiassi A, Goldberg MS, Wheeler AJ, et al: Associations between personal exposure to air pollutants an lung function tests and cardiovascular indicates among children with asthma living near an industrial complex and petroleum refineries. *Environ Res* 132C:38–45, 2014.

Suk WA, Davis EA: Strategies for addressing global environmental health concerns, *Ann N Y Acad Sci* 1140:40–44, 2008.

Swider SM, Krothe J, Reyes D, et al: The Quad Council Practice Competencies for Public Health Nursing, *Public Health Nursing* 30(6):519–536, 2013.

Turner MC, Wigle DT, Krewski D: Residential pesticides and childhood leukemia: a systematic review and meta-analysis, *Environ Health Perspect* 118:33–41, 2010.

US Department of Health and Human Services: *Healthy People 2020*, Washington, DC, 2010, US Government Printing Office.

US Department of Health and Human Services: *Environmental influences on child health outcomes (ECHO) program*, 2015. Retrieved February 1, 2016 from http://www.nih.gov.environmental.

US Food and Drug Administration: *"Disposal of unused medicines: what should you know?"* Washington, DC, 2015, FDA. Retrieved February 2016 from http://www.fda.gov/drug disposal.

Wigle DT, Turner MC, Krewski D: A systematic review and meta-analysis of childhood leukemia and parental occupational pesticide exposure, *Environ Health Perspect* 117:1505–1513, 2009.

World Health Organization: *Public health and environment global strategy overview*, 2011. Retrieved July 25, 2016 from http://www.who.int/phe/publications/PHE_2011_global_strategy_overview_2011.pdf?ua=1.

World Health Organization: *Asthma*, 2013. Retrieved June 2016 from http://www.who/int/entity/mediacentre/factsheets/fs307/en/.

World Health Organization: *Climate change and human health*, 2015. Retrieved July 2016 from http://www.who.int/entity.mediacentre/factsheets/fs266/en/.

Wright DJ: Collaborative learning experiences for nursing students in environmental health, *Nurs Educ Perspect* 24:189–191, 2003.

Yoder JS, Wallace RM, Collier SA, et al. Cryptosporidiosis surveillance—United States, 2009-2010, Centers for Disease Control and Prevention (CDC), *MMWR Surveill Summ* 61(5):1–12, 2012.

CHAPTER 7

Government, the Law, and Policy Activism

Marcia Stanhope

OBJECTIVES

After reading this chapter, the student should be able to:

1. Discuss the structure of the US government and health care roles.
2. Identify the functions of key governmental and quasi-governmental agencies that affect public health systems and nursing, both around the world and in the United States.
3. Contrast the primary bodies of law that affect nursing and health care.
4. Define key terms related to policy and politics.
5. State the relationships among nursing practice, health policy, and politics.
6. Develop and implement a plan to communicate with policymakers on a chosen public health issue.

CHAPTER OUTLINE

Definitions
Governmental Role in US Health Care
  Trends and Shifts in Governmental Roles
  Government Health Care Functions
  Healthy People 2020: An Example of National Health Policy
    Guidance
Organizations and Agencies that Influence Health
  International Organizations
  Federal Health Agencies
  Federal Nonhealth Agencies
  State and Local Health Departments
Impact of Government Health Functions and Structures
  on Nursing
The Law and Health Care
  Constitutional Law

Legislation and Regulation
Judicial and Common Law
Laws Specific to Nursing Practice
  Scope of Practice
  Professional Negligence
Legal Issues Affecting Health Care Practices
  School and Family Health
  Occupational Health
  Home Care and Hospice
  Correctional Health
The Nurse's Role in the Policy Process
  Legislative Action
  Regulatory Action
  The Process of Regulation
  Nursing Advocacy

KEY TERMS

advanced-practice nurses, 120
Agency for Healthcare Research and
  Quality (AHRQ), 112
American Nurses Association
  (ANA), 118
block grants, 107
board of nursing, 115
categorical programs and
  funding, 114
constitutional law, 115
devolution, 107

health policy, 106
judicial law, 115
legislation, 115
legislative staff, 119
licensure, 115
National Institute of Nursing
  Research (NINR), 108
nurse practice act, 115
Occupational Safety and Health
  Administration (OSHA), 110
Office of Homeland Security, 114

police power, 106
policy, 106
politics, 106
regulations, 115
US Department of Health and Human
  Services (USDHHS), 106
World Health Organization
  (WHO), 110

Nurses are an important part of the health care system and are greatly affected by governmental and legal systems. Nurses who select the community as their area of practice must be especially aware of the impact of government, law, and health policy on nursing, health, and the communities in which they practice. Knowing how government, law, and political action have changed over time is necessary to understand how the health care system has been shaped by these factors. Also, understanding how these factors have influenced the current and future roles for nurses and the public health system is critical for establishing a better health policy for the nation.

Nurses have historically viewed themselves as advocates for the health of the population. It is this heritage that has moved the discipline into the policy and political arenas. To secure a more positive health care system, nurse professionals must develop a working knowledge of government, key governmental and quasi-governmental organizations and agencies, health care law, the policy process, and the political forces that are shaping the future of health care. This knowledge and the motivation to be an agent of change in the discipline and in the community are necessary ingredients for success as a nurse working in the community.

DEFINITIONS

To understand the relationships among health policy, politics, and laws, it is first necessary to understand the definitions of the terms.

1. **Policy** is a specific course of action to be followed by a government or institution to obtain a desired end.
2. **Health policy** is a set course of action to obtain a desired health outcome for an individual, family, group, community, or society.

Policies are made not only by governments but also by institutions such as a health department or other health care agency, a family, or a professional organization.

Politics plays a role in the development of such policies. It is found in families, professional and employing agencies, and governments. Politics is the art of influencing others to accept a specific course of action. Therefore political activities are used to arrive at a course of action (the policy). *Law* is a system of privileges and processes by which people solve problems based on a set of established rules.

Laws govern the relationships of individuals and organizations to other individuals and to government. Through political action, a policy becomes a law. After a law is established, regulations further define the course of action (policy) to be taken by organizations or individuals in reaching an outcome. Government is the ultimate authority in society and is designated to enforce the policy—whether it is related to health, education, economics, social welfare, or any other society issue. The following discussion explains the role of government in health policy.

GOVERNMENTAL ROLE IN US HEALTH CARE

In the United States the federal and most state and local governments are comprised of three branches, each of which has separate and important functions. The executive branch is composed of the president (or governor or mayor) along with the staff and cabinet appointed by this executive, various administrative and regulatory departments, and agencies such as the US Department of Health and Human Services (USDHHS). The legislative branch (i.e., Congress at the federal level) is made up of two bodies, the Senate and the House of Representatives, whose members are elected by the citizens of particular geographic areas. The judicial branch is comprised of a system of federal, state, and local courts guided by the opinions of the Supreme Court.

- The executive branch suggests, administers, and regulates policy.
- The legislative branch identifies problems and proposes, debates, passes, and modifies laws to address those problems.
- The judicial branch interprets laws and their meaning and interprets states' rights to provide health services to citizens of the states.

One of the first constitutional challenges to a federal law passed by Congress was in the area of health and welfare in 1937, after the 74th Congress had established unemployment compensation and old-age benefits for US citizens (US Law, 1937b). Although Congress had created other health programs previously, its legal basis for doing so had never been challenged. In *Steward Machine Co. v Davis* (US Law, 1937a), the Supreme Court (judicial branch) reviewed this legislation and determined, through interpretation of the Constitution, that such federal governmental action was within the powers of Congress to promote the general welfare.

Most legal bases for the actions of Congress in health care are found in Article I, Section 8, of the US Constitution, including the following:

1. Provide for the general welfare
2. Regulate commerce among the states
3. Raise funds to support the military
4. Provide spending power

Through a continuing number and variety of cases and controversies, these Section 8 provisions have been interpreted by the courts to appropriately include a wide variety of federal powers and activities. State power concerning health care is called **police power**. This power allows states to act to protect the health, safety, and welfare of their citizens. Such police power must be used fairly, and the state must show that it has a compelling interest in taking actions, especially actions that might infringe on individual rights. Examples of a state using its police powers include requiring immunization of children before being admitted to school and requiring case finding, reporting, treating, and follow-up care of persons with tuberculosis. These activities protect the health, safety, and welfare of state citizens.

TRENDS AND SHIFTS IN GOVERNMENTAL ROLES

The government's role in health care at both the state and federal level began gradually. Wars, economic instability, and political differences between parties all shaped the government's role. The first major federal governmental action relating to health was the creation in 1798 of the Public Health Service (PHS). In 1934 Senator Wagner of New York initiated the first national health insurance bill. The Social Security Act of 1935 was passed to provide assistance to older adults and the unemployed; it also offered survivors' insurance for widows and children. In addition, it provided for child welfare, health department grants, and maternal and child health projects. In 1948 Congress created the National Institutes of Health (NIH). In 1965 it passed the most important health legislation to date—creating Medicare and Medicaid to provide health care service payments for older adults, the disabled, and the categorically poor. These legislative acts by Congress created programs that were implemented by the executive branch. In March 2010 the most recent legislation passed and signed by President Obama to improve the health of the nation and access to care was the health reform law, the Patient Protection and Affordable Care Act (US Law, 2010). The legislation was designed to do the following:

- "Rein in the worst excesses and abuses of the insurance industry with some of the toughest consumer protections this country has ever known."
- "Hold insurance companies accountable to keep premiums down and prevent denials of care and coverage, including for pre-existing conditions."
- "Make health insurance affordable for middle class families and small businesses with one of the largest tax cuts for health care in history—reducing premiums and out-of-pocket costs."
- "Provide the security of knowing that if a job is lost, changed, or a new business started, there will always be the ability to purchase quality, affordable care in a new competitive health insurance market that keeps costs down."
- "Strengthen Medicare benefits with lower prescription drug costs for those in the 'donut hole,' chronic care, free preventive care, and nearly a decade more of solvency for Medicare."
- "Improve the nation's fiscal health by reducing the federal deficit by more than $100 billion over the next decade, and more than $1 trillion in the decade after that."

By 2012 the law was simply referred to as the Affordable Care Act (ACA). (See http://kff.org for updated outcomes of the ACA implementation.)

The USDHHS (known first as the Department of Health, Education, and Welfare [DHEW]) was created in 1953. The Health Care Financing Administration (HCFA) was created in 1977 as the key agency within the USDHHS to provide direction for Medicare and Medicaid. In 2002 the HCFA was renamed the Centers for Medicare and Medicaid Services (CMS). During the 1980s, a major effort of the administration was to shift federal government activities, including federal programs for health care, to the states. The process of shifting the responsibility for planning, delivering, and financing programs from the federal level to the states level is called devolution. From 1980 until the present, Congress has increasingly funded health

programs by giving block grants to the states. Devolution processes, including block granting, should alert professional nurses that state and local policy is growing in importance in the health care arena. With the new health reform law, stimulus grants are being provided to state and local areas to improve health care access (Health Resources and Services Administration [HRSA], 2015).

The role of government in health care is shaped both by the needs and demands of its citizens and by the citizens' beliefs and values about personal responsibility and self-sufficiency. These beliefs and values often clash with society's sense of responsibility and need for equality for all citizens. A recent federal example of this ideological debate occurred in the 1990s over health care reform. The Democrats proposed the Health Security Act of 1993, which failed to gain Congress's approval. In an effort to make some incremental health care changes, both the Democrats and the Republicans in Congress passed two new laws.

The Health Insurance Portability and Accountability Act (HIPAA) allows working persons to keep their employee group health insurance for up to 16 months after they leave a job (US Law, 1996).

The State Child Health Improvement Act (SCHIP) of 1997 provides insurance for children and families who cannot otherwise afford health insurance (US Law, 1997a).

This discussion has focused primarily on trends in and shifts between different levels of government. An additional aspect of governmental action is the relationship between government and individuals. Freedom of individuals must be balanced with governmental powers. Since the terrorist attacks on the United States in September (World Trade Center attack) and October (anthrax outbreak) of 2001, much government activity has been conducted in the name of protecting the safety of US citizens. Government has a great deal of influence on the way health care services are delivered and on who receives care.

It is interesting to note that before September 11, 2001, the Congress and president, recognizing that the public health system infrastructure needed help, passed the Public Health Threats and Emergencies Act (US Law, 2000) in 2000. This law "addresses emerging threats to the public's health and authorizes the Secretary of HHS to take appropriate response actions during a public health emergency, including investigations, treatment, and prevention" (Katz et al, 2014, p 133). In June 2002 the Public Health Security and Bioterrorism Preparedness and Response Act was signed into law (US Law, 2002), with $3 billion appropriated by Congress in December 2002 to implement the following antibioterrorism activities:

- Improving public health capacity
- Upgrading of the ability of health professionals to recognize and treat diseases caused by bioterrorism
- Speeding the development of new vaccines and other countermeasures
- Improving water and food supply protection
- Tracking and regulating the use of dangerous pathogens within the United States (Katz et al, 2014)

Yet there is considerable debate on just how much governmental intervention is necessary and effective and how much will be tolerated by citizens. For example, in 2010 approximately 49% of citizens were against the new health care reform acts, and Republicans were seen as being obstructionists. In 2014, 50% of citizens were for government intervention and 50% against (Debate.org, 2013).

GOVERNMENT HEALTH CARE FUNCTIONS

Federal, state, and local governments carry out five health care functions, which fall into the general categories of direct services, financing, information, policy setting, and public protection.

Direct Services

Federal, state, and local governments provide direct health services to certain individuals and groups. For example, the federal government provides health care to members and dependents of the military, certain veterans, and federal prisoners. State and local governments employ nurses to deliver a variety of services to individuals and families, frequently on the basis of factors such as financial need or the need for a particular service, such as screening for hypertension or tuberculosis, immunizations for children and older adults, and primary care for inmates in local jails or state prisons.

Financing

Governments pay for some health care services; the 2012 percentage of the bill paid by the government was about 45.3%, and this was projected to increase to 47.6% by the year 2015. The government also pays for training some health personnel and for biomedical and health care research (National Center for Health Statistics [NCHS], 2014). However, as a result of the ACA, the government's share of health expenses dropped to 43.2% (NCHS, 2015). Support in the following areas has greatly affected both consumers and health care providers. Federal government finances the direct care of clients through the Medicare, Medicaid, Social Security, and SCHIP programs. State governments contribute to the costs of Medicaid and SCHIP programs. Many nurses have been educated with government funds through grants and loans, and schools of nursing in the past have been built and equipped using federal funds. Governments also have financially supported other health care providers, such as physicians, most significantly through the program of Graduate Medical Education funds.

The federal government invests in research and new program demonstration projects, with the NIH receiving a large portion of the monies. The National Institute of Nursing Research (NINR) is a part of the NIH and, as such, provides a substantial sum of money to the discipline of nursing for the purpose of developing the knowledge base of nursing and promoting nursing services in health care (NINR, 2014). See the Evidence-Based Practice box for an example of developing the knowledge base of nursing through funded research.

EVIDENCE-BASED PRACTICE

Chronic obstructive pulmonary disease (COPD) is a serious, chronic, progressive lower respiratory disorder that negatively affects several health indicators, such as quality of life and functional status. The primary risk factor for COPD is cigarette smoke, by exposure both directly (firsthand smoking) and indirectly (secondhand smoke). Previous studies have shown a decrease in hospitalization and mortality rates for respiratory diseases after implementation of smoke-free legislation. The purpose of this study was to determine the impact of smoke-free municipal public policies on hospitalizations for COPD. The researchers conducted a secondary analysis of hospital discharges with primary diagnosis of COPD over an 8-year period (2003–2011). Controlling for several factors, such as gender, age, and length of stay, researchers found that those living in a community with comprehensive smoke-free laws or regulations were 22% less likely to experience COPD hospitalizations than those living in a community with weak to moderate laws or no laws.

Nurse Use

This study indicates that strong smoke-free public policies may protect against COPD hospitalizations, thus having the potential to save lives and decrease health care costs. This study supports the value of health policy, the benefits of funding for research, and the need to evaluate the effectiveness of the policy in accomplishing its purposes.

Data from Hahn EJ, Rayens, MK, Adkins S, et al: Fewer hospitalizations for chronic obstructive pulmonary disease in communities with smoke-free public policies, *American Journal of Public Health, 104*(6): 1059-1065, 2014.

Information

All branches and levels of government collect, analyze, and disseminate data about health care and the health status of citizens. An example is the annual report *Health, United States,* compiled each year by the USDHHS (NCHS, 2016). Collecting vital statistics, including mortality and morbidity data; gathering census data; and conducting health care status surveys are all government activities. Table 7.1 lists examples of available federal and international data sources on the health status of populations in the United States and around the world. These sources are available on the Internet and in the governmental documents section of most large libraries. This information is especially important because it can help nurses understand the major health problems in the United States and those in their own states and local communities.

Policy Setting

Policy setting is a primary government function. Governments at all levels and within all branches make policy decisions about health care. These health policy decisions have broad implications for financial expenses, resource use, delivery system change, and innovation in the health care field. One law that has played a very important role in the development of public health policy, public health nursing, and social welfare policy in the United States is the Sheppard-Towner Act of 1921. Box 7.1 lists excerpts from this act (Brown and Fee, 2013; US Law, 1921).

Public Protection

The US Constitution gives the federal government the authority to provide for the protection of the public's health. This

TABLE 7.1 International and National Sources of Data on the Health Status of the US Population

Organization	Data Sources
International	
United Nations	http://www.un.org/ *Demographic Yearbook*
World Health Organization	http://www.who.int/en/ *World Health Statistics Annual*
Federal	
Department of Health and Human Services	http://www.DHHS.gov
	National Vital Statistics System
	National Survey of Family Growth
	National Health Interview Survey
	National Health Examination Survey
	National Health and Nutrition Examination Survey
	National Master Facility Inventory
	National Hospital Discharge Survey
	National Nursing Home Survey
	National Ambulatory Medical Care Survey
	National Morbidity Reporting System
	US Immunization Survey
	Surveys of Mental Health Facilities
	Estimates of National Health Expenditures
	AIDS Surveillance
	Nurse Supply Estimates
Department of Commerce	http://www.commerce.gov
	US Census of Population
	Current Population Survey
	Population Estimates and Projections
Department of Labor	http://www.dol.gov
	Consumer Price Index
	Employment and Earnings

BOX 7.1 The Sheppard-Towner Act

The Sheppard-Towner Act did the following:
- Made nurses available to provide health services for women and children, including well-child and child-development services
- Provided adequate hospital services and facilities for women and children
- Provided grants-in-aid for establishing maternal and child welfare programs
- Set precedents and patterns for the growth of modern-day public health policy
- Defined the role of the federal government in creating standards to be followed by states in conducting categorical programs, such as today's Special Supplemental Nutrition Program for Women, Infants, and Children (WIC) and Early Periodic Screening and Developmental Testing (EPSDT) programs
- Defined how the consumer could influence, formulate, and shape public policy
- Defined the government's role in research
- Developed a system for collecting national health statistics
- Explained how health and social services could be integrated
- Established the importance of prenatal care, anticipatory guidance, client education, and nurse–client conferences, all of which are viewed today as essential nursing responsibilities

to reproductive privacy (*Roe v Wade*), requiring vaccinations, and setting conditions for states to receive public funds for highway construction and repair by requiring a minimum drinking age.

HEALTHY PEOPLE 2020: AN EXAMPLE OF NATIONAL HEALTH POLICY GUIDANCE

In 1979 the Surgeon General issued a report that began a 20-year focus on promoting health and preventing disease for all Americans (DHEW, 1979). In 1989 *Healthy People 2000* became a national effort, with many stakeholders representing the perspectives of government, state, and local agencies; advocacy groups; academia; and health organizations (USDHHS, 1991).

Throughout the 1990s, states used *Healthy People 2000* objectives to identify emerging public health issues. The success of this national program was accomplished and measured through state and local efforts. The *Healthy People 2010* document focused on a vision of healthy people living in healthy communities. *Healthy People 2020* has four overarching goals, found in the *Healthy People 2020* box, which compares the goals of *Healthy People* documents from 2000 to 2020 (USDHHS, 1991, 2000, 2010).

♥ HEALTHY PEOPLE 2020

A Comparison of the Goals of Healthy People 2000, Healthy People 2010, and Healthy People 2020

1. *Healthy People 2000* Goals	2. *Healthy People 2010* Goals	3. *Healthy People 2020* Goals
Increase the years of healthy life for Americans	Increase quality and years of healthy life	Attain high-quality, longer lives free of preventable disease, disability, injury, and premature death
Reduce health disparities among Americans	Eliminate health disparities	Achieve health equity, eliminate disparities, and improve the health of all groups
Achieve access to preventive services for all Americans		Create social and physical environments that promote good health for all
		Promote quality of life, healthy development, and healthy behaviors across all life stages

From the US Department of Health and Human Services: *Healthy People 2000: national health promotion and disease prevention objectives,* Washington, DC, 1991, US Government Printing Office. Retrieved Dec 2010 from http://www.health.gov/healthypeople; US Department of Health and Human Services: *Healthy People 2010: understanding and improving health,* ed 2, Washington, DC, 2000, US Government Printing Office; US Department of Health and Human Services: *Healthy People 2020,* Washington, DC, 2010, US Government Printing Office.

function is carried out in numerous ways, such as by regulating air and water quality and by protecting the borders from an influx of diseases by controlling food, drugs, and animal transportation. The Supreme Court interprets and makes decisions related to public health, for example, affirming a woman's rights

ORGANIZATIONS AND AGENCIES THAT INFLUENCE HEALTH

INTERNATIONAL ORGANIZATIONS

In June 1945, after World War II, many national governments joined together to create the United Nations. By charter, the aims and goals of the United Nations deal with human rights, world peace, international security, and the promotion of the economic and social advancement of all the world's peoples. The United Nations, headquartered in New York City, is made up of six principal divisions, several subgroups, and many specialized agencies and autonomous organizations.

With the approval and support of the UN Commission on the Status of Women, four world conferences on women have been held. Others are being planned. At these conferences, the health of women and children and their rights to personal, educational, and economic security as well as initiatives to achieve these goals at the country level are debated and explored, and policies are formulated (United Nations, 1975, 1980, 1985, 1995, 2000, 2010).

One of the special autonomous organizations growing out of the United Nations is the World Health Organization (WHO). Established in 1946, the WHO works with the United Nations to achieve its goal to attain the highest possible level of health for all persons. "Health for All" is the creed of the WHO. Headquartered in Geneva, Switzerland, the WHO has six regional offices. The office for the Americas, in Washington, DC, is known as the Pan American Health Organization. The WHO provides services worldwide with the following aims (United Nations, 2014):

- Promoting health
- Cooperating with member countries in promoting their health efforts
- Coordinating the collaboration efforts among countries
- Disseminating biomedical research
  Its services, which benefit all countries, include the following:
- Providing day-to-day information service on the occurrence of internationally important diseases
- Publishing the international list of causes of disease, injury, and death
- Monitoring adverse reactions to drugs
- Establishing world standards for antibiotics and vaccines
  Assistance available to individual countries includes the following:
- Supporting national programs to fight disease
- Training health workers
- Strengthening the delivery of health services
  The World Health Assembly (WHA) is the WHO's policy-making body, and it meets annually. The WHA's health policy work provides policy options for many countries of the world in their development of in-country initiatives and priorities; however, although important everywhere, WHA policy statements are guides and not law. The WHA's latest policy statement on nursing and midwifery was released in 2003, and in 2010 the WHO provided a document outlining strategic directions for

2011–2015 on implementing the WHA policy statement (WHA, 2003; WHO, 2010).

The current worldwide shortage of professional nurses is a continuing concern on the WHO agenda and is being addressed by country. The World Health Report, first published in 1995, is WHO's leading publication. Each year the report combines an expert assessment of global health, including statistics relating to all countries, with a focus on a specific subject. The main purpose of the report was to provide countries, donor agencies, international organizations, and others with the information they need to help them make policy and funding decisions (WHO, 2016).

The presence of nursing in international health is increasing to include the following:
- Direct health services in every country in the world
- Consultants
- Educators
- Program planners
- Evaluators
  Nurses focus their work on a variety of public health issues:
- Health care workforce and education
- Environment
- Sanitation
- Infectious diseases
- Wellness promotion
- Maternal and child health
- Primary care
  Dr. Naeema Al-Gasseer of Bahrain has served as the scientist for nursing and midwifery at the WHO; Marla Salmon, former dean of nursing at the University of Washington, chaired a Global Advisory Group on Nursing and Midwifery; and Linda Tarr Whelan served as the US ambassador to the UN Commission on the Status of Women. Virginia Trotter Betts, past president of the American Nurses Association (ANA), served as a US delegate to both the WHA and the Fourth World Conference on Women in Beijing in 1995, where she participated on the negotiating team of the conference to develop a platform on the health of women across the life span. Many US nurse leaders, such as Dr. Carolyn Williams, current author in this book, have been WHO consultants. These examples show the impact that nurses have on international public health policy.

FEDERAL HEALTH AGENCIES

Laws passed by Congress may be assigned to any administrative agency within the executive branch of government for implementing, supervising, regulating, and enforcing. Congress decides which agency will monitor specific laws. For example, most health care legislation is delegated to the USDHHS. However, legislation concerning the environment would most likely be implemented and monitored by the Environmental Protection Agency (EPA), and legislation concerning occupational health is monitored by the Occupational Safety and Health Administration (OSHA) in the US Department of Labor.

US Department of Health and Human Services

The USDHHS is the agency most heavily involved with the health and welfare of US citizens. It touches more lives than any other federal agency. The organizational chart of the USDHHS (see Chapter 3, Fig. 3.1) shows and provides more discussion for the key agencies within the organization. The following agencies have been selected for their relevance to this chapter.

Health Resources and Services Administration

The Health Resources and Services Administration (HRSA) has been a long-standing contributor to the improved health status of Americans through the programs of services and health professions education that it funds. The HRSA contains the Bureau of Health Professions (BHPr), which includes the Division of Nursing as well as the Divisions of Medicine, Dentistry, and Allied Health Professions. The Division of Nursing is the key federal focus for nursing education and practice, and it provides national leadership to ensure an adequate supply and distribution of qualified nursing personnel to meet the health needs of the nation.

In 2013 the Division of Nursing had the following strategic goals (USDHHS, 2013a):

- Increase access to quality care through improved composition, distribution, and retention of the nursing workforce through financial assistance.
- Identify and use data, program performance measures, and outcomes to make informed decisions on nursing workforce issues.
- Increase cultural competence in the nursing workforce.
- Increase diversity in the nursing workforce.

At the 122nd meeting of the Division of Nursing's National Advisory Council for Nursing Education and Practice (NACNEP), the participants discussed the role of public health nurses in participating in primary care in their communities (NACNEP, 2010). The speaker indicated several factors that need to be in place to support the public health nurse role:

- Baccalaureate standard for entry into practice
- Ongoing stable funding for health departments
- Competitive salaries commensurate with responsibilities
- Interventions grounded in and responsive to community needs
- Consideration of health determinants
- Experience in health promotion and prevention
- Long-term trusting relationships in the community (i.e., with clients)
- Established network of community partners
- Commitment to social justice and eliminating health disparities

Through the input of the NACNEP, the Division of Nursing sets policy for nursing nationally. At the 133rd meeting of the NACNEP, the discussion had progressed to population health and aimed to identify how nurses could best contribute and lead population health initiatives and to identify the training and skills that nurses would need in population health (USDHHS, 2016).

Centers for Disease Control and Prevention

The Centers for Disease Control and Prevention (CDC) serves as the national focus for developing and applying disease prevention and control, environmental health, and health promotion and education activities designed to improve the health of the people of the United States. The mission of the CDC is to promote health and quality of life by preventing and controlling disease, injury, and disability. The CDC seeks to accomplish its mission by working with partners throughout the nation and the world in the following ways:

- Monitoring health
- Detecting and investigating health problems
- Conducting research that will enhance prevention
- Developing and advocating sound public health policies
- Implementing prevention strategies
- Promoting healthy behaviors
- Fostering safe and healthful environments
- Providing leadership and training

The disease outbreak that occurred in the summer of 2014 provides an example of how the CDC fulfills its mission. The Shiga toxin–producing *Escherichia coli* outbreak linked to raw clover sprouts affected six states and 19 people, and 44% of those affected were hospitalized. Idaho was determined to be the most likely source of the outbreak. The CDC regularly collects data from states about foodborne illnesses through the National Notifiable Disease Surveillance System and on a weekly basis through the Morbidity and Mortality Weekly Report (MMWR). Because of the recognized increase in cases, states were asked to report aggregate numbers of cases twice a week along with foodborne-related hospitalizations and complications. The CDC implemented an investigation to track the cases and worked with state and local health departments to perform the following:

- Detect the possible outbreak.
- Define and find cases.
- Generate hypotheses about the likely source.
- Test the hypothesis.
- Find the point of contamination.
- Control the outbreak from further spread.
- Decide when the outbreak is over.

In the 3 months from June 2014 to August 2014, 19 cases occurred in 6 states (CDC, 2014a). The six states involved and number of cases were as follows: California (1), Idaho (3), Michigan (1), Montana (2), Utah (1), and Washington (11). By August 2014 the CDC determined the outbreak to be over. Although few people were involved in this outbreak, the outcome could have been deadly for the persons who ate the sprouts.

While the Ebola virus of West Africa continues to spread, the CDC is monitoring the effects of the virus as part of its global monitoring system. The CDC has information and training materials ready for those who may need them (CDC, 2014b). The CDC took an active role in the recent outbreak of measles that resulted from exposure to the virus at Disneyland in California. This outbreak resulted in 140 people from seven states being infected. On January 23, 2015, the CDC issued a health advisory to all public health and health care facilities nationwide (Zipprich et al, 2015). In addition, the CDC took active roles in monitoring and tracking the Zika virus outbreaks in the United States. By 2016, over 800 cases involving the virus were reported in 45 states. At that point, all cases were caused by travel to countries whose mosquitoes harbored the virus (CDC, 2016). Fig. 7.1 shows the location of the US Zika virus cases.

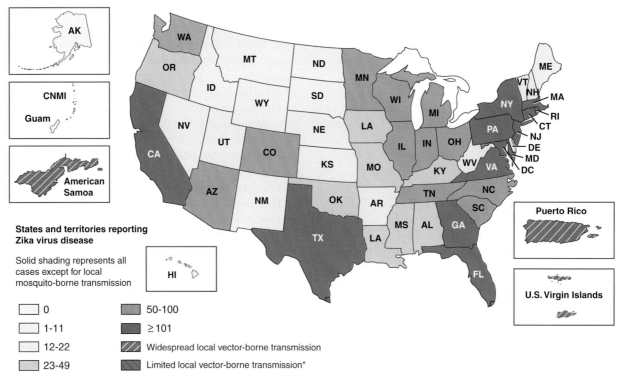

FIG. 7.1 Laboratory-confirmed Zika virus disease cases reported to ArboNET by state or territory, United States, 2015–2016, National Center for Emerging and Zoonotic Diseases (NCEZID), Atlanta, Georgia.

National Institutes of Health

Founded in 1887, the NIH today is one of the world's foremost biomedical research centers and the federal focus point for biomedical research in the United States. The NIH comprises 27 separate institutes and centers. The goal of NIH research is to acquire new knowledge to help prevent, detect, diagnose, and treat disease and disability, from the rarest genetic disorder to the common cold, to lead to better health for everyone. The NIH mission is to uncover new knowledge that will lead to better health for everyone. The NIH works toward that mission by conducting research in its own laboratories; supporting the research of nonfederal scientists in universities, medical schools, hospitals, and research institutions throughout the country and abroad; helping in the training of research investigators; and fostering communication of medical and health sciences information (NIH, n.d.).

In late 1985 Congress overrode a presidential veto, allowing the creation of the National Center for Nursing Research within the NIH. In 1993 the center became one of the divisions of the NIH and was renamed the National Institute of Nursing Research (NINR).

The research and research-related training activities previously supported by the Division of Nursing were transferred to the new institute. The NINR is the focal point of the nation's nursing research activities. It promotes the growth and quality of research in nursing and client care, provides important leadership, expands the pool of experienced nurse researchers, and serves as a point of interaction with other bases of health care research. The mission of NINR is to promote and improve the health of individuals, families, communities, and populations. NINR supports and conducts clinical and basic research and research training on health and illness across the life span. The research focus encompasses health promotion and disease prevention, quality of life, health disparities, and end of life. NINR seeks to extend nursing science by integrating the biological and behavioral sciences, using new technologies to research questions, improving research methods, and developing the scientists of the future (NINR, n.d.).

Agency for Healthcare Research and Quality

The Agency for Healthcare Research and Quality (AHRQ) is the lead federal agency charged with improving the quality, safety, efficiency, and effectiveness of health care for all Americans. As one of the 12 agencies within the USDHHS, AHRQ supports health services research that will improve the quality of health care and promote evidence-based decision making. AHRQ is committed to improving care safety and quality by developing successful partnerships and generating the knowledge and tools required for long-term improvement. The goal of AHRQ research is to promote measurable improvements in health care in America. AHRQ organizes their measures of health care quality into four Quality Indicator modules: Prevention Quality Indicators, Inpatient Quality Indicators, Patient Safety Indicators, and Pediatric Quality Indicators (AHRQ, n.d.).

By examining what works and what does not work in health care, the AHRQ fulfills its missions of translating research findings into better patient care and providing consumers,

QSEN FOCUS ON QUALITY AND SAFETY EDUCATION FOR NURSES

- **Targeted competency:** Quality improvement
- **Knowledge:** Describe strategies for learning about the outcomes of care in the public setting.
- **Skills:** Seek information about outcomes of care for populations served in care settings.
- **Attitudes:** Appreciate that continuous quality improvement is an essential part of the daily work of all professionals.

QI Question

The Quad Council competency of policy development and program planning skills indicates that the beginning public health nurse collects information that will inform policy decisions. Also, the public health nurse describes the legislative policy development process and identifies outcomes of current health policy relevant to public health nursing practice. The 2014 outbreak of the Ebola virus in the United States brought quick recognition that there was a need for improvement in policies related to infectious disease control. What were the indicators that the infection control policies in place were not sufficient to prevent the spread of disease? Describe the continuous quality improvement (CQI) data-collection processes that determined the need for policy change. What role did nurses and organized nursing play in improving the infection control policy and guidelines nationally? What has been the outcome of the new policy, and how were populations affected both locally and nationally?

policymakers, and other health care leaders with information needed to make critical health care decisions. In 1999 Congress, through legislation, specifically directed the AHRQ to focus on measuring and improving health care quality; promoting client safety and reducing medical errors; advancing the use of information technology for coordinating client care and conducting quality and outcomes research; and seeking to eliminate disparities in health care delivery for the priority populations of low-income groups, minorities, women, children, older adults, and individuals with special health care needs.

The AHRQ has published protocols for care of clients with a variety of health problems. These protocols have become the standards of health care delivery. The agency maintains a clinical practice guidelines clearinghouse for use by clinicians and others. In addition, the AHRQ has a project called "Put Prevention into Practice" to promote the use of standardized protocols for primary care delivery for clients across the age span (see **Resource Tool 7A** for the Schedule of Clinical Preventive Services). These protocols can be used by nurses in planning disease prevention and health promotion activities for their clients.

Centers for Medicare and Medicaid Services

One of the most powerful agencies within the USDHHS is the Centers for Medicare and Medicaid Services (CMS), which administers Medicare and Medicaid accounts and guides payment policy and delivery rules for services for the poor, elderly, disabled, and unemployed. In addition to providing health insurance, the CMS also performs various quality-focused health care or health-related activities, including regulating laboratory testing, developing coverage policies, and improving quality of care. CMS maintains oversight of the surveying and certifying of nursing homes and continuing care providers (including

home health agencies, intermediate care facilities for the mentally retarded, and hospitals). It makes available to beneficiaries, providers, researchers, and state surveyors information about these activities and nursing home quality.

FEDERAL NONHEALTH AGENCIES

Although the USDHHS has the primary responsibility for federal health functions, several other departments of the executive branch carry out important health functions for the nation. Among these are the Departments of Defense, Labor, Agriculture, and Justice.

- **Department of Defense:** The Department of Defense delivers health care to members of the military and their dependents. In each branch of the uniformed services, nurses of high military rank are part of the administration of these health services (see www.defense.gov for more information).
- **Department of Labor:** The Department of Labor has two agencies with health functions: OSHA and the Mine Safety and Health Administration. Both are charged with writing safety and health standards and ensuring compliance in the workplace.
- **Department of Agriculture:** The Department of Agriculture is involved in health care primarily by administering the Food and Nutrition Service. This service collaborates with state and local government welfare agencies to provide food stamps to needy persons to increase their food purchasing power. Other programs include school breakfast and lunch programs; the Special Supplemental Nutrition Program for Women, Infants, and Children (WIC); and grants to states for nutrition education and training.
- **Department of Justice:** Health services to federal prisoners are administered within the Department of Justice. The Federal Bureau of Prisons is responsible for the custody and care of approximately 214,000 federal offenders (Bureau of Federal Prisons, 2014). The Medical and Services Division of the Bureau of Prisons includes medical, psychiatric, dental, and health support services.

STATE AND LOCAL HEALTH DEPARTMENTS

Depending on funding, public commitment and interest, and access to other resources, programs offered by state and local health departments vary greatly. Many state and local health officials report that employees in public health agencies lack skills in the core sciences of public health and that this has hindered their effectiveness. The lack of specialized education and skill is a significant barrier to population-based preventive care and the delivery of quality health care to the public. Public health workforce specialists report that the number of retirees expected in this decade will result in a major shortage of public health workers, including nurses. More often than at other levels of government, nurses at the local level provide direct services. Some nurses deliver special or selected services, such as follow-up of contacts in cases of tuberculosis or venereal disease or providing child immunization clinics. Other nurses have a more generalized practice, delivering services to families in certain geographic areas (University of Michigan Center of Excellence in Public Health Workforce Studies, 2013).

CASE STUDY

Child Immunization Policies

Tammy Jones is the school nurse at Caseyville Middle School. The state requires all entering sixth-grade students to have a current immunization certificate on file before the student's enrollment. It is now 6 months into the school year, and Ms. Jones is reviewing the students' records. Ms. Jones finds that several students do not have current immunization certificates on file. Although the state law requires immunization certificates, it does not specify the course of action in cases of noncompliance.

Ms. Jones goes to her supervisor to discuss possible resolutions to the situation. Should they suspend the noncompliant students because the law states the certificate for immunization is required for enrollment? This solution could mean many missed days of valuable lessons for the students. What implications for the students and the community could arise if the students continue to go without immunizations?

Ms. Jones and her supervisor decide to contact each student and meet with his or her family individually. The meetings reveal that many of the parents have tried to get their child immunized but have not been able to do so because of the costs of the shots or the inability to make an appointment at the busy doctor's office. Ms. Jones works with these families to make appointments at the local health department to fulfill the immunization requirement.

At the local and state levels, coordinating health efforts between health departments and other county or city departments is essential. Gaps in community coordination are showing up in glaring ways as states and communities scramble to address bioterrorism preparedness since September 11, 2001, and since such natural disasters as Hurricane Katrina.

IMPACT OF GOVERNMENT HEALTH FUNCTIONS AND STRUCTURES ON NURSING

The variety and range of functions of governmental agencies have had a major impact on the practice of nursing. Funding, in particular, has shaped roles and tasks of population-centered nurses. The designation of money for specific needs, or categorical programs and funding, has led to special and more narrowly focused nursing roles. Examples are in emergency preparedness, school nursing, and family planning. Funds assigned to antibioterrorism cannot be used to support unrelated communicable disease programs or family planning.

Since the events of September 11, 2001, the public and the profession of nursing have been concerned about the ability of the present public health system and its workforce to deal with bioterrorism, especially outbreaks of deadly and serious communicable diseases. For example, smallpox vaccinations stopped in 1972, but immunity lasts for only 10 years; as a result, although there have been no reported cases of smallpox since the early 1970s, almost no one in the United States has immunity. Thus the population is vulnerable to an outbreak of smallpox because it could be used as a weapon of bioterrorism. Two laboratories in the world retain a small amount of the smallpox virus. Because of these potential threats, the US government has begun to increase production of the smallpox vaccine and has enough vaccine to inoculate every person in the United States, if necessary (see http://www.emergency.cde.gov for smallpox vaccination facts). Few public health professionals are knowledgeable about

the symptoms, treatment, or mode of transmission of this disease. Most health professionals, including registered nurses (RNs), currently working in the United States have never seen a case of anthrax, smallpox, or plague, the three major biological weapons of concern in the world today. The USDHHS and the new federal Office of Homeland Security have provided funds to address this serious threat to the people of the United States. One of the first things being done is the rebuilding of the crumbling public health infrastructures of each state to provide surveillance, intervention, and communication in the face of future bioterrorism events. On December 19, 2006, President George W. Bush signed the Pandemic and All-Hazards Preparedness Act (PAHPA), which was intended to improve the organization, direction, and utility of preparedness efforts. PAHPA, which was reauthorized by President Obama in 2013, centralizes federal responsibilities, requires state-based accountability, proposes new national surveillance methods, addresses surge capacity, facilitates the development of vaccines and other scarce resources, and enables communities to build systems to support populations during and after disasters (Morhard and Franco, 2013; USDHHS 2013b).

THE LAW AND HEALTH CARE

The United States is a nation of laws, which are subject to the US Constitution. The law is a system of privileges and processes by which people solve problems on the basis of a set of established rules. It is intended to minimize the use of force. Laws govern the relationships of individuals and organizations to other individuals and to government. After a law is established, regulations further define the course of actions to be taken by the government, organizations, or individuals in reaching an agreed-on outcome. Government and its laws are the ultimate authority in society and are designed to enforce official policy, whether it is related to health, education, economic, social welfare, or any other societal issue. The number and types of laws influencing health care are ever increasing. Definitions of law include, but are not limited to, the following (Merriam-Webster at http://www.merriam-webster.com/dictionary/law):

- A rule established by authority, society, or custom
- The body of rules governing the affairs of people, communities, states, corporations, and nations
- A set of rules or customs governing a discrete field or activity (e.g., criminal law, contract law)

These definitions reflect the close relationship of law to the community and to society's customs and beliefs. The law has had a major impact on nursing practice. Although nursing emerged from individual voluntary activities, society passed laws to give formality to public health, and, through legal mandates (i.e., laws), positions and functions for nurses in community settings were created. These functions in many instances carry the force of law. For example, if the nurse discovers a person with smallpox, the law directs the nurse and others in the public health community to take specific actions. In a mumps outbreak, nurses and other health professionals are required to report cases of mumps. This requirement for reporting helps locate and treat cases as they occur, thus preventing further spread of disease. Three types of laws in the United States have particular importance to the nurse. They are constitutional law, legislation and regulation, and judicial or common law.

CONSTITUTIONAL LAW

Constitutional law derives from federal and state constitutions. It provides overall guidance for selected practice situations. For example, on what basis can the state require quarantine or isolation of individuals with tuberculosis? The US Constitution specifies the explicit and limited functions of the federal government. All other powers and functions are left to the individual states. The major constitutional power of the states relating to population-centered nursing practice is the state's right to intervene in a reasonable manner to protect the health, safety, and welfare of its citizens. The state has police power to act through its public health system, but it has limits. First, it must be a "reasonable" exercise of power. Second, if the power interferes with or infringes on individual rights, the state must demonstrate that there is a "compelling state interest" in exercising its power. Isolating an individual or separating someone from a community because that person has a communicable disease has been deemed an appropriate exercise of state powers. The state can isolate an individual, such as someone who has tuberculosis and is noncompliant with treatment, even though it infringes on individual rights (such as freedom and autonomy), under the following conditions (Cole, 2014):

1. A compelling state interest exists in preventing an epidemic.
2. The isolation is necessary to protect the health, safety, and welfare of individuals in the community or the public as a whole.
3. The isolation is done in a reasonable manner.

In such circumstances the community's rights are more important than the individual's rights when there is a threat to the health of the public.

LEGISLATION AND REGULATION

Legislation is law that comes from the legislative branches of the federal, state, or local government. This is referred to as *statute law* because it becomes coded in the statutes of a government (Birkland, 2015). Much legislation has an effect on nursing. Regulations are specific statements of law related to defining or implanting individual pieces of legislation. For example, state legislatures enact laws (statutes) establishing boards of nursing and defining terms such as *registered nurse* and *nursing practice*. Every state has a board of nursing. The board may be found either in the department of licensing boards of the health department or in an administrative agency of the governor's office. Created by legislation known as a state nurse practice act, the board of nursing is made up of nurses and consumers. The functions of this board are described in the nurse practice act of each state and generally include licensing and examination of registered nurses and licensed practical nurses; approval of schools of nursing in the state; revocation, suspension, or denying of licenses; and writing of regulations about nursing practice and education. The state boards of nursing operationalize, implement, and enforce the statutory law by writing explicit statements (called rules) on what it means to be a registered nurse, and on the nurse's rights and responsibilities in delegating work to others and in meeting continuing education requirements.

All nurses employed in community settings are subject to legislation and regulations. For example, home health care nurses employed by private agencies must deliver care according to federal Medicare or state Medicaid legislation and regulations, so the agency can be reimbursed for those services. Private and public health care services rendered by nurses are subject to many governmental regulations for quality of care, standards of documentation, and confidentiality of client records and communications. All state health departments have a public health practice reference that governs the practice of nurses and others and state public health laws that define the essential public health services that must be offered in the state, as well as the optional services that may also be offered.

JUDICIAL AND COMMON LAW

Both judicial law and common law have a great impact on nursing. Judicial law is based on court or jury decisions. The opinions of the courts are referred to as *case law* (Birkland, 2015). The court uses other types of laws to make its decisions, including previous court decisions or cases. Precedent, one principle of common law, means that judges are bound by previous decisions unless they are convinced that the older law is no longer relevant or valid. This process is called *distinguishing*, and it usually involves a demonstration of how the current situation in dispute differs from the previously decided situation. Other principles of common law, such as justice, fairness, respect for an individual's autonomy, and self-determination, are part of a court's rationale and the basis on which to make a decision.

LAWS SPECIFIC TO NURSING PRACTICE

Despite the broad nature and varied roles of nurses in practice, two legal areas are most applicable to nurse practice situations. The first is the statutory authority for the profession and its scope of practice, and the second is professional negligence or malpractice.

SCOPE OF PRACTICE

The issue of scope of practice involves defining nursing, setting its credentials, and then distinguishing among the practices of nurses, physicians, and other health care providers. The issue is especially important to nurses in community settings, who have traditionally practiced with much autonomy.

Health care practitioners are subject to the laws of the state in which they practice, and they can practice only with a license. The states' nurse practice acts differ somewhat, but they are the most important statutory law affecting nurses. The nurse practice act of each state accomplishes at least four functions: (1) defining the practice of professional nursing, (2) identifying the scope of nursing practice, (3) setting educational qualifications and other requirements for licensure, and (4) determining the legal titles nurses may use to identify themselves. The usual and customary practice of nursing can be determined through a variety of sources, including the following:

1. Content of nursing educational programs, both general and special

2. Experience of other practicing nurses (peers)
3. Statements and standards of nursing professional organizations
4. Policies and procedures of agencies employing nurses
5. Needs and interests of the community
6. Updated literature, including research, books, texts, and journals

All of these sources can describe, determine, and refine the scope of practice of a professional nurse. Every nurse should know and follow closely any proposed changes in the practice acts of nursing, medicine, pharmacy, and other related professions. The nurse should always examine all legislation, rules, and regulations related to nursing practice. For example, a review of the Pharmacy Act will let the nurse know whether to question the right to dispense medications in a family planning clinic in a local health department. Defining the scope of practice makes it necessary to clarify independent, interdependent, and dependent nursing functions.

Just as practice acts vary by state, so do the evolving issues and tensions of scopes of practice among the health professions. In the past few years, several state legislatures (working closely with the National Council of State Boards of Nursing) have embarked on a legislative effort to develop the Interstate Nurse Licensure Compact. The compact allows mutual recognition of generalist nursing licensure across state lines in the compact states. By 2015, 25 states had adopted the compact (National Council of State Boards of Nursing, 2015.)

PROFESSIONAL NEGLIGENCE

Professional negligence, or malpractice, is defined as an act (or a failure to act) that leads to injury of a client. To recover money damages in a malpractice action, the client must prove all of the following:

1. The nurse owed a duty to the client or was responsible for the client's care.
2. The duty to act the way a reasonable, prudent nurse would act in the same circumstances was not fulfilled.
3. The failure to act reasonably under the circumstances led to the alleged injuries.
4. The injuries provided the basis for a monetary claim from the nurse as compensation for the injury.

Reported cases involving negligence and population-centered nurses are very few in number.

🄠 CHECK YOUR PRACTICE

As a student, you are working as a school health nurse along with an employee of the health department in your community. The state law requires that upon entry into the school system, all children must be vaccinated for childhood communicable diseases. The nurses in the schools may administer the vaccines if a child needs any or all of the required immunizations. A family has recently moved into your school district, and the parents cannot find the immunization record from the prior school system or from the physician in the previous community. The mother insists that the vaccinations are not up to date and wants the child to be able to enter school immediately. You are aware that it only takes one sick child for a major outbreak. To reduce the risk and protect the school population from communicable disease outbreaks, what should you do?

The author of this chapter has known of some cases in the community that related to serious side effects from child vaccinations. In one instance, the family was new to the community, and the child was enrolling in school. By state law the child had to be vaccinated for childhood communicable disease before entering school. The public health nurse asked the mother of the child about the child's history of vaccinations and the family physician's certificate of immunizations. The mother indicated that they had recently moved to the community and that she could not find the record. The mother assured the nurse that immunizations were needed. In an attempt to be accommodating, the nurse accepted the mother's knowledge regarding the need for vaccination and proceeded to vaccinate the child. In a brief time period the child developed complications from the immunizations, specifically, a severe neurological disorder. The family sued the nurse and the health department for negligence.

An integral part of all negligence actions is the question of who should be sued. *In the eyes of the law, the "prudent nurse" practicing anywhere in the United States is used as the example, or standard, by which to judge the competency of a nurse's practice.* When a nurse is employed and functioning within the scope of employment, the employer is responsible for the nurse's negligent actions. This is referred to as the doctrine of *respondeat superior.* By directing a nurse to carry out a particular function, the employer becomes responsible for negligence, along with the individual nurse. Because employers are usually better able to pay for the injuries suffered by clients, they are sued more often than the nurses themselves, although an increasing number of judgments include the professional nurse by name as a codefendant.

Thus it is imperative that all nurses engaged in clinical practice carry their own professional liability insurance. Nurses may have personal immunity for particular practice areas, such as giving immunizations. In some states, the legislature has granted personal immunity to nurses employed by public agencies to cover all aspects of their practice under the legal theory of *sovereign immunity* (Cherry and Jacobs, 2013).

In the immunization case described previously, the nurse was judged to be negligent and was held liable for the injury to the child because she did not follow the protocol of the health department or the school system. She neglected to obtain the necessary documents from the previous school system or the physician to determine the actual status of the child's immunizations. Both the health department and the school system had sovereign immunity and were not held liable and could show the protocol the nurse was directed to follow.

Nursing students need to be aware that the same laws and rules that govern the professional nurse govern them. Students are expected to meet the same standard of care as that met by any licensed nurse practicing under the same or similar circumstances. Students are expected to be able to perform all tasks and make clinical decisions on the basis of the knowledge they have gained or been offered, according to their progress in their educational programs and along with adequate educational supervision.

LEGAL ISSUES AFFECTING HEALTH CARE PRACTICES

Specific legal issues of nursing vary depending on the setting in which care is delivered, the clinical arena, and the nurse's functional role. The law, including legislation and judicial opinions, significantly affects each of the following areas of nursing practice. Nurses responsible for setting and implementing program priorities need to identify and monitor laws related to each special area of practice.

SCHOOL AND FAMILY HEALTH

Nurses employed by health departments or boards of education may deliver school and family health nursing. School health legislation establishes a minimum of services that must be provided to children in public and private schools. For example, most states require that children be immunized against certain communicable diseases before entering school. Children must have had a physical examination by that time, and most states require at least one physical at a later time in their schooling. Legislation also specifies when and what type of health screening will be conducted in schools (e.g., vision and hearing testing). These requirements are found in statutory laws of states. Some states are now requiring a simple dental examination in schools for the purpose of referring children to a dental health professional if needed.

Statutes addressing child abuse and neglect make a large impact on nursing practice within schools and families. Most states require nurses to notify police and/or a social service agency of any situation in which they suspect a child is being abused or neglected. This is one instance in which the law mandates that a health professional breach client confidentiality to protect someone who may be in a helpless or vulnerable position. There is *civil immunity* for such reporting, and the nurse may be called as a witness in a court hearing of the case.

OCCUPATIONAL HEALTH

Occupational health is another special area of practice that has specific legal requirements as a result of state and federal statutes. Of special concern are the state workers' compensation statutes, which provide the legal foundation for claims of workers injured on the job. Access to records, confidentiality, and the use of standing orders are legal issues that have great practice significance to nurses employed in industries.

HOME CARE AND HOSPICE

Home care and hospice services rendered by nurses are shaped through state statutes and have specific nursing requirements for licensure and certification. Compliance with these laws is directly linked to the method of payment for the services. For example, a service must be licensed and certified to obtain payment for services through Medicare. Federal regulations implementing Medicare and Medicaid have an enormous effect on much of nursing practice, including how nurses record details of their visits, record time spent in care activities, and document client care and the client's status and progress.

In addition, many states have passed laws requiring nurses to report elder abuse to the proper authorities, as is done with children and youth. Laws affecting home care and hospice services have focused on issues such as the right to death with dignity, rights of residents of long-term facilities and home health clients, definitions of death, and the use of living wills and advance directives. The legal and ethical dimensions of nursing practice are particularly important. Individual rights, such as the right to refuse treatment, and nursing responsibilities, such as the legal duty to render reasonable and prudent care, may appear to be in conflict in delivering home and hospice services. Much case discussion (sometimes including outside ethics consultation) may be needed to resolve such conflicts.

CORRECTIONAL HEALTH

Correctional health nursing practice is significantly shaped by federal and state laws and regulations and by recent Supreme Court decisions. The laws and decisions primarily relate to the type and amount of services that must be provided for incarcerated individuals. For example, physical examinations are required for all prisoners after they are sentenced. Regulations specify basic levels of care that must be provided for prisoners, and access to care during illness is a particular focus. Court decisions requiring adequate health services are based on constitutional law. If minimal services are not provided, it is a violation of a prisoner's right to freedom from cruel and unusual punishment. Such decisions provide a framework that strongly influences the setting of nursing priorities. For example, providing care to the sick would take priority over wellness or health education classes.

THE NURSE'S ROLE IN THE POLICY PROCESS

The number and types of laws influencing health care are increasing. Because of this, nurses need to be involved in the policy process and understand the importance of involvement of nursing to the clients they serve.

For nurses to effectively care for their client populations and their communities in the complex US health care system, professional advocacy for logical health policy that considers equality is essential. Professional nurses working in the community know all too well about the health care problems they and their clients encounter daily, and it is through policy and political activism that both big-picture and long-term solutions can be developed.

Although the term *policy* may sound rather lofty, health policy is quite simply the process of turning health problems into workable action solutions. Health policy is developed on the three-legged stool of access, cost, and quality.

The policy process, which is very familiar to professional nurses, includes the following:

- Statement of a health care problem
- Statement of policy options to address the health problem
- Adoption of a particular policy option
- Implementation of the policy product
- Evaluation of the policy's intended and unintended consequences in solving the original health problem

Thus the policy process is very similar to the nursing process, but the focus is on the level of the larger society, and the adoption strategies require political action. For most professional nurses, action in the policy arena comes most easily and naturally through participation in nursing organizations such as the American Nurses Association (ANA) at the state level, the Association of Community Health Nursing Educators (ACHNE) or the Association of Public Health Nurses at the national or state level, and certain specialty organizations such as the American Public Health Association (APHA).

The nurse's basic understanding of the political process should include knowing who the lawmakers are, how bills become laws (see Fig. 7.2), the process of writing regulations (see Fig. 7.3), and methods of influencing the process and

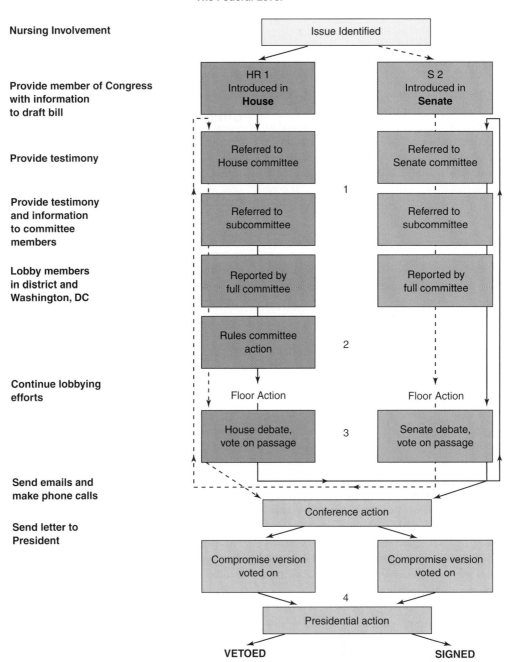

FIG. 7.2 How a bill becomes a law. (From Mason DJ, Leavitt JK, Chaffee MW: *Policy and politics in nursing and health care,* ed 7, St Louis, 2016, Elsevier.)

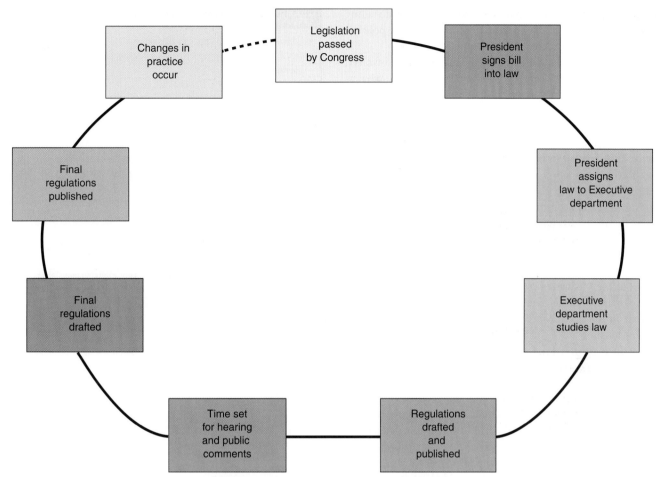

FIG. 7.3 The process of writing regulations.

shaping of health policy. With this knowledge, nurses can influence nursing practice at local, state, and national levels.

LEGISLATIVE ACTION

It is often helpful to review the legislative and political processes that may have been a part of high school education. It becomes important material to remember as a professional career is embarked upon.

The people within geographic jurisdictions elect their legislative representatives and senators. An important part of the legislative process is the work of the legislative staff. These individuals do the legwork, research, paperwork, and other activities that move policy ideas into bills and then into law. In addition to the individual legislator's office, the congressional committee staffs are also important. They are usually experts in the content of the work of a committee, such as a health and welfare committee. Frequently, developing a working relationship with key legislative staffers can be as important to achieving a policy objective as the relationship with the policymaker (i.e., the legislator).

The legislative process begins with ideas (policy options) that are developed into bills. After a bill is drafted, it is introduced to the legislature, given a number, read, and assigned to a committee. Hearings, testimony, lobbying, education, research, and

informal discussions follow. If the bill is passed from the legislative committee, the entire House hears the bill, amends it as necessary, and votes on it. A majority vote moves the bill to the other House, where it is read and amended, and then a vote is taken. Fig. 7.2 shows the necessary formal process of the legislative pathway.

Nurses can be involved in the legislative process at any point. Many professional nursing associations have legislative committees made up of volunteers, governmental relations staff professionals, and sometimes political action committees (PACs), all engaged in efforts to monitor, analyze, and shape health policy.

Common methods of influencing health policy outcomes include face-to-face encounters, personal letters, mail-grams, electronic mail, telephone calls, testimony, petitions, reports, position papers, fact sheets, letters to the editor, news releases, speeches, coalition building, demonstrations, and lawsuits. Depending on the issue, any of these can be effective. Although most business, including politics and the policy agendas, depends on the Internet today for instant communication and quick response, all of these methods continue to be of great importance in influencing policy agendas. For example, if a face-to-face encounter is used with a legislator or a staffer, these persons can put a "face on the policy agenda," and the reality that the policy affects real persons is an important consideration when the legislator or staff pushes the policy agenda forward. Tips on communication and visiting legislators and their staffs, as well as general tips on political action, are presented in Boxes 7.2, 7.3, and 7.4.

Political activities in which nurses can and should be involved are varied and include being informed voters (*a must!*), participating in a political party, registering others to vote, getting out the vote, fund-raising for candidates, building networks or communication links for issues (e.g., a phone tree or Internet distribution list), and participating in organizations to ensure their effective involvement in health policy and politics. To communicate effectively, present a simple argument with examples; consider the culture, age, and educational backgrounds of the person with whom you are communicating; target your communication toward the issue; do not use jargon; indicate the expertise you bring to the table; use data to support your argument; and show the relevance to nursing and to the legislator. *Above all, be polite!*

The direct reimbursement of advanced-practice nurses (APNs) in the Medicare program is one example of how nurses can use their influence. The inclusion of amendments to Medicare that authorized APN reimbursement regardless of specialty or client location in the Balanced Budget Act of 1997 required the sustained efforts of the ANA and other national nursing organizations over a long period (Nursing World, Legislative Branch, 2000; USDHHS, Centers for Medicare and Medicaid Services, 2015). During that time, individual nurses provided testimony to Congress and to MEDPAC (the physicians' political action committee) on the importance of direct reimbursement to APNs. Many APNs worked closely and vigorously with their congressional representatives to lobby for this Medicare amendment. Even more wrote letters and provided position papers and fact sheets to help legislators understand the value of APNs. Although the process took more than 10 years to be fully

---

BOX 7.3 Tips for Writing to Legislators

- Communicate in writing to express opinions.
- Acknowledge the Congress member's work as positive or negative, but be courteous.
- Follow up on meetings or phone calls with a letter or e-mail message.
- Share knowledge about a particular problem.
- Recommend policy solutions.
- The letter should be typed, a maximum of two pages, and focused on one or two issues at most.
- The purpose of the letter should be stated at the beginning.
- Present clear and compelling rationales for your concern or position on an issue.
- If the purpose of the letter is to express disappointment regarding a stance on an issue or a vote that has been cast, the letter should be as positive as possible.
- Write letters thanking a Congress member for taking a particular position on an issue.
- A letter to the editor of the local newspaper or a nursing newsletter praising a legislator's position (with a copy forwarded to the legislator) is welcome publicity, especially during an election year.
- Review the major points covered in person and answer any questions that were raised during conversation.
- Have business cards for yourself and include them with letters.
- Address written correspondence as follows (the same general format applies to state and local officials):

US Senator	US Representative
Honorable Jane Doe	Honorable Jane Doe
United States Senate	House of Representatives
Washington, DC 20510	Washington, DC 20515
Dear Senator Doe:	Dear Representative Doe:

Modified from Mason DJ, Leavitt JK, Chaffee MW: *Policy and politics in nursing and health care,* ed 5, St Louis, 2007, Elsevier.

BOX 7.2 Tips for Visits With Legislators

- Call ahead and ask how much time the staff or legislator is able to give you.
- When you arrive, ask if the appointment time is the same or if a scheduled vote on the House or Senate floor is going to need the legislator's attention and you will need to reschedule your appointment.
- Engage in small talk at the beginning of the conversation only if the staff or legislator has time.
- Structure time so that the issue can be presented briefly.
- Allow an opportunity for the staff or Congress member to seek clarity or ask questions.
- Do not assume that the legislator or the legislator's staff is well informed on the issue.
- Numbers count. If the views you express are shared by a local nurses' organization or by nurses employed at a health care facility, let the legislator know.
- Invite Congress members and their staffs to conferences or meetings of nurses' organizations or to tour nursing education facilities to meet others interested in the same policy issues.
- If appropriate, invite the media and let the legislator know.
- Send future invitations.
- Provide a one-page summary that gives key points at the conclusion of every meeting.

Modified from Mason DJ, Leavitt JK, Chaffee MW: *Policy and politics in nursing and health care,* ed 5, St Louis, 2007, Elsevier.

BOX 7.4 Tips for Action

- Become involved in the state nurses' association.
- Build communication and leadership skills.
- Increase your knowledge about a range of professional issues.
- Expand and strengthen your professional network.
- Serve on committees and in elected positions.
- Build relationships within the profession and with representatives of public- and private-sector organizations with an interest in health care.
- Participate in political activities.
- Be aware of what is taking place in health care beyond the environment and the practice in which you work.
- Be well informed across a range of health-related issues.
- Identify yourself as a nurse with associated education and expertise.
- Let people know that nurses are capable of functioning in many different roles and making substantial contributions.
- Be confident.
- Do not burn bridges behind you. On another occasion, they may provide the only route to your destination.
- Be friendly.
- Lend a hand to other nurses. It benefits all of us.
- If you are new to the policy arena, seek support from many people of diverse backgrounds. Accomplished people, whether nurses or not, often value mentoring others.

Modified from Mason DJ, Leavitt JK, Chaffee MW: *Policy and politics in nursing and health care,* ed 5, St Louis, 2007, Elsevier.

achieved, APN reimbursement in Medicare became a reality. Both the nursing profession and clients benefit from this change The ANA was likewise a strong supporter of the Patient Safety Act of 1997 (ANA, 1997). This law requires health care agencies to make public some information on nursing staff levels, staff mix, and outcomes, and it requires the USDHHS to review and approve all health care acquisitions and mergers. All of these requirements are intended to determine any long-term effect on the health and safety of clients, communities, and staff.

On the state legislative level, all 50 states have passed title protection for registered nurses; this was achieved by individual nurses, state nurses associations, and various nursing specialty groups participating in the legislative process with the 50 state legislators. Title protection means that only certain nurses who meet state criteria can call themselves advanced-practice nurses.

REGULATORY ACTION

The regulatory process, although it may not be as visible a process as legislation, also can be used to shape laws and dramatically affect health policy. This process should be on the radar screen of professional nurses who wish to successfully participate in policy activity.

At each level of government, the executive branch can and, in most cases, must prepare regulations for implementing policy and new programs. These regulations are detailed, and they establish, fix, and control standards and criteria for carrying out certain laws. Fig. 7.3 shows the steps in the typical process of writing regulations. When the legislature passes a law and delegates its oversight to an agency, it gives that agency the power to make regulations. Because regulations flow from legislation, they have the force of law.

THE PROCESS OF REGULATION

After a law is passed, the appropriate executive department begins the process of regulation by studying the topic or issue. Advisory groups or special taskforces are sometimes formed to provide the content for the regulations. Nurses can influence these regulations by writing letters to the regulatory agency in charge or by speaking at open public hearings. Many letters are now accepted via the Internet.

After rewriting, the proposed regulations are put into final draft form and printed in the legally required publication (e.g., at the federal level, the *Federal Register*). Similar registers exist in most states, in which regulations from state executive departments, including state health departments, are published. Public comment is called for in written form within a given period.

Revisions made to proposed regulations are based on public comment and public hearing. Depending on the amount and content of the public reaction, final regulations are prepared, or the area and issues are studied further. Final published regulations carry the force of law. When regulations become effective, health care practice is changed to conform to the new regulations. Monitoring administrative regulations is essential for the professional nurse, who can influence regulations by attending

the hearings, providing comments, testifying, and engaging in lobbying aimed at individuals involved in the writing. Concrete, written suggestions for revision submitted to these individuals are frequently persuasive and must be acknowledged by the government in publishing the final rules. An excellent example of how nurses must continue to influence health policy outcomes, even after positive legislation has passed, occurred after the passage of the Balanced Budget Act (BBA) of 1997 (US Law, 1997b). The HCFA began to implement the BBA through the publication of draft regulations seeking to define APN practice and Medicare reimbursement. The nursing community responded vigorously with negative opinions about the initial restrictive definitions and requirements. Their reactions were effective and reshaped the final regulations to recognize the state definitions for APN practice autonomy.

Final regulations, published in a *code of regulations* (both federal and state), usually lead to changes in practice. For example, Medicare regulations setting standards for nursing homes and home health are incorporated into these agencies' manuals. In the case of APN reimbursement, some Medicare fiscal intermediaries have had difficulty in recognizing APNs as appropriate providers, but professional nursing organization advocates have forcefully addressed these implementation barriers.

NURSING ADVOCACY

Advocacy begins with the art of influencing others (politics) to adopt a specific course of action (policy) to solve a societal problem. This is accomplished by building relationships with the appropriate policymakers—the individuals or groups that determine a specific course of action to be followed by a government or institution to achieve a desired end (policy outcome). Relationships for effective advocacy can be built in various ways. In January 2006, Medicare Part D—the prescription drug benefit policy—became effective. Public health professionals were needed to assist vulnerable persons to understand the value of enrolling in Part D, to educate them on how to use the benefits, and to ensure that the populations who are "dually" enrolled in both Medicare and Medicaid are registered. Coordinating efforts among civic, religious, and health care agencies to provide health education is a necessity.

Likewise, when the Affordable Care Act was passed it was essential to get the word out to communities and to Medicaid recipients, the unserved, the working poor, and others who could receive both preventive and other sources of health care through the programs established by this act (US Law, 2010).

A letter or visit to the district, state, or national office of a legislator to discuss a particular policy or health care issue can be interesting, educational, and effective. Contributions of money, labor, expertise, or influence also may be welcomed by the policymakers involved in setting a course of action to obtain a desired health outcome for an individual, a family, a group, a community, or society (health policy). Additionally, it is possible to develop a grassroots network of community and professional friends with a mutual interest in health policy advocacy. The network may be able to promote health policy initiatives for the community. During the Obama presidential campaign, many advocacy networks were established via the Internet, and money was solicited using this process.

Many special interest groups in health care have the potential, desire, and resources to influence the health policy process. A tremendous advantage that nursing has in advocating for issues and in influencing policymakers is the force of its numbers because nursing is the largest of the health professions. However, nursing must organize its numbers in such a way that each nurse joins with others to speak with one voice. The greatest effect will be had when all nurses make similar demands for policy outcomes (see the Applying Content to Practice box at the end of chapter for an example of nurses' input into the Affordable Care Act).

Advocacy by expert and committed health professionals works; it can bring about positive change for the profession, the community, and the clients that nurses serve. Keeping up to date on issues within government, professional organizations, law, and public policy is vitally important. Informed activism directed toward a professional role, image, and value for professional nurses and toward a health care system in the United States that provides universal access to health care that is of high quality and is affordable should be a lifelong commitment for all professional nurses.

▶▶ APPLYING CONTENT TO PRACTICE

The information here gives an example of how the policy process works and how the reader can use the content in this chapter. This example involves a nursing organization and its individual members. Whether you are a member of a group or working on your own to influence health policy, the steps described here apply.

Over a 15-month time frame, the American Nurses Association (ANA) was involved in advocating for health care reform. During the presidential campaign, candidates were educated about the nursing profession and the ANA's Agenda for Health System Reform. The ANA and its members participated in national media interviews and local media events. The message was that the association and its members believed that health care is a basic right. The ANA collaborated with the nursing community to outline the profession's priorities as proposals were developed in Congress. Testimony was given before three key congressional committees. ANA representatives met with White House and congressional health care reform staff and took part in two presidential press conferences at the White House.

As reported by the ANA, thousands of nurses joined the ANA's health care reform team, sending letters to representatives of Congress, sharing their stories, and meeting with members of Congress. They also participated in rallies and events.

For more information on ANA's health care reform work, visit http://www.rnaction.org/toolkit.

■ PRACTICE APPLICATION

Larry was in his final rotation in the Bachelor of Science in Nursing program at State University. He was anxious to complete his final nursing course because on graduation he would begin a position as a staff nurse specializing in school health at the local health department. His wife was expecting their first child, and she had been receiving prenatal care at the health department.

Larry was aware that a few years ago, the federal government had, by law, provided block grants to states for primary care, maternal–child health programs, and other health care needs of states. He had read the *Federal Register* and knew that the regulations for these grants had been written through USDHHS departments. He was aware that these regulations did not require states to fund specific programs.

Larry read in the local newspaper that the health department was closing its prenatal clinic at the end of the month. When his state had received its block grant, the state decided to spend the money for programs other than prenatal care. Larry found that a 3-year study in his own state showed improved pregnancy outcomes as a result of prenatal care. The results were further improved when the care was delivered by population-centered nurses.

Larry was concerned that as a student, he would have little influence. However, he decided to call his classmates together to plan a course of action.

What would such an action plan include?
Answers can be found on the Evolve website.

■ REMEMBER THIS!

- The legal basis for most congressional action in health care can be found in Article I, Section 8, of the US Constitution.
- The four major health care functions of the federal government are direct service, financing, information, and policy setting.
- The goal of the World Health Organization is the attainment by all people of the highest possible level of health.
- Many federal agencies are involved in government health care functions. The agency most directly involved with the health and welfare of Americans is the US Department of Health and Human Services.
- Most state and local governments have activities that affect nursing practice.

- The variety and range of functions of governmental agencies have had a major impact on nursing. Funding, in particular, has shaped the role and tasks of nurses.
- The private sector (of which nurses are a part) can influence legislation in many ways, especially through the process of writing regulations.
- The number and types of laws influencing health care are increasing. Because of this, involvement in the political process is important to nurses.
- Professional negligence and the scope of practice are two legal aspects particularly relevant to nursing practice.
- Nurses must consider the legal implications of their own practice in each clinical encounter.

- The federal and most state governments comprise three branches—the executive, the legislative, and the judicial.
- Each branch of government plays a significant role in health policy.
- The US Public Health Service was created in 1798.
- The first national health insurance legislation was challenged in the Supreme Court in 1937.
- *Health, United States* (NCHS, 2016) is an important source of data about the nation's health care problems.
- In 1921 the Sheppard-Towner Act was passed, and it had an important influence on child health programs and community-oriented nursing practice.
- The Division of Nursing, the National Institute of Nursing Research, and the Agency for Healthcare Policy and Research are governmental agencies important to nursing.

- Nurses, through state and local health departments, function as consultants, direct-care providers, researchers, teachers, supervisors, and program managers.
- The state governments are responsible for regulating nursing practice within the state.
- Federal and state social welfare programs have been developed to provide monetary benefits to the poor, older adults, the disabled, and the unemployed.
- Social welfare programs affect nursing practice. These programs improve the quality of life for special populations, thus making the nurse's job easier in assisting the client with health needs.
- The nurse's scope of practice is defined by legislation and by standards of practice within a specialty.

EVOLVE WEBSITE

http://evolve.elsevier.com/Stanhope/foundations
- Case Study, with Questions and Answers
- NCLEX® Review Questions
- Practice Application Answers

REFERENCES

Agency for Healthcare Research and Quality: *AHRQuality Indicators: Introduction*, Bethesda, MD, n.d., USDHHS. http://www.qualityindicators.ahrq.gov/. Accessed June 22, 2016.

American Nurses Association: *Press Release, ANA Applauds Introduction of Patient Safety Act of 1997*, March 1997. Available at http://www.nursingworld.org. Accessed December 10, 2010.

Birkland T: *An introduction to the policy process: theories, concepts, and models of public policy making*, ed 4, New York, NY, 2015, Routledge.

Brown TM, Fee E: Social movements in health, *Annual Review of Public Health*, 35:385–398, 2013. DOI:10.1146/annurev-publhealth-031912-114356.

Bureau of Federal Prisons: *Weekly population report*, 2014. Available at http://www.bop.gov. Accessed September 15, 2014.

Cherry B, Jacobs SR: *Contemporary nursing issues, trends and management*, ed 6, St Louis, 2013, Elsevier.

Debate.Org: *Is government intervention ruining health care in America*, 2013. http://www.debate.org. Accessed September 15, 2014.

Centers for Disease Control and Prevention: *Epidemiology of Escherichia coli outbreak*, United States, Atlanta, 2014a, USDHHS.

Centers for Disease Control and Prevention: *Ebola outbreak*, Atlanta, 2014b. http://www.cdc.gov. Accessed September 16, 2014.

Centers for Disease Control and Prevention: *Laboratory-confirmed Zika virus disease cases reported to ArboNET by state or territory-United States, 2015-2016*, Atlanta, Georgia, 2016, National Center for Emerging and Zoonotic Diseases (NCEZID).

Cole James: *Federal and State Quarantine and Isolation Authority-CRS Report; Congressional Research Service*, Washington, DC, Oct, 9, 2014.

Department of Health, Education and Welfare: Improving health. In *Healthy People: the Surgeon General's report on health promotion and disease prevention, Pub. no. 79-55-71*, Washington, DC, 1979, US Government Printing Office. Retrieved July 2002 from http://www.census.gov/statab/www.

Hahn EJ, Rayens MK, Adkins S, et al: Fewer hospitalizations for chronic obstructive pulmonary disease in communities with smoke-free public policies, *American Journal of Public Health* 104(6):1059–1065, 2014.

Health Resources and Services Administration: *HHS awards nearly $500 million in Affordable Care Act funding to health centers to expand primary care services*, September 15, 2015, HHS Press Office, USDHHS. Retrieved June 21, 2016 from http://www.hhs.gov/about/news/2015/09/15/hhs-awards-nearly-500-million-affordable-care-act-funding-health-centers-expand-primary-care.html.

Katz R, Macintyre A, Barbera J: Emergency public health. In Pines JM, Abualenain J, Scott J, et al: editors: *Emergency care and the public's health*, Hoboken, NJ, 2014, John Wiley and Sons, Ltd.

Mason DJ, Keavitt JK, Chaffee MW: *Policy and politics in nursing and health care*, ed 5, St Louis, 2007, Elsevier.

Mason DJ, Keavitt JK, Chaffee MW: *Policy and politics in nursing and health care*, ed 6, St Louis, 2012, Elsevier.

Morhard R, Franco C: The Pandemic and All-Hazards Preparedness Act: its contributions and new potential to increase public health preparedness, *Biosecur Bioterror* 11(2):145–152, 2013. Available at http://online.liebertpub.com/doi/pdf/10.1089/bsp.2013.0042. Accessed May 7, 2014.

National Advisory Council on Nursing Education and Practice: *The eighth report to the Secretary of HHS and Congress*, Rockville, MD, 2010, The Department of Health and Human Services (DHHS).

National Center for Health Statistics: *Health, United States, 2013: with special feature on prescription drugs*, Hyattsville, MD, 2014, US Government Printing Office.

National Center for Health Statistics: *Health, United States, 2014: with special feature on adults aged 55-64*, Hyattsville, MD, 2015, US Government Printing Office.

National Center for Health Statistics: *Health, United States, 2015: with special feature on racial and ethnic health disparities*, Hyattsville, MD, 2016, US Government Printing Office.

National Council of State Boards of Nursing: *Map and implementation dates of NLC member states*, 2015. https://www.ncsbn.org. Retrieved June 22, 2016 from https://www.ncsbn.org/nurse-licensure-compact.htm.

National Institute of Nursing Research: *National Institutes of Health: funding opportunities*, Bethesda, Md, 2014, US Department of Health and Human Services.

National Institute of Nursing Research: *About NINR*, Bethesda, MD, n.d., USDHHS. Retrieved June 21, 2016 from http://www.ninr.nih.gov/aboutninr#.V2oBr9IrK00.

National Institutes of Health: *About NIH*, Bethesda, Md, n.d., US Department of Health and Human Services. Retrieved June 21, 2016 from https://www.nih.gov/about-nih.

Nursing World, Legislative Branch: *State government relations: advanced practice recognition with Medicaid reimbursement*, 2000. Retrieved December 2010 from http://www.nursingworld.org.

United Nations: *Report of the World Conference of the International Women's Year, Mexico City, June 19 to July 2, Chapter I, Section A.2, Pub. no. E.76.IV.1*, New York, 1975, UN.

United Nations: *Report of the World Conference of the United Nations Decade for Women: equality, development and peace, Copenhagen, July 24-30, Chapter I, Section A, Pub. no. E.80.IV.3*, New York, 1980, UN.

United Nations: *Report of the World Conference to Review and Appraise Achievements of the United Nations Decade for Women: Equality, Development and Peace, Nairobi, July 15-26*, New York, 1985, UN.

United Nations: *Report of the Fourth World Conference on Women, Beijing, September 4-15, Chapter I, Resolution 1, Annex I, Publication No. E.96.IV.13*, New York, 1995, UN.

United Nations: *Women 2000: Gender Equality, Development and Peace for the 21st Century, Beijing, 23rd session of the United Nations General Assembly*, New York, 2000, UN.

United Nations: *Report of the World Conference to Review and Appraise Achievements of the United Nations Decade for Women: management activity: the military health system*, Falls Church, Va, 2010, UN. Retrieved December 2010 from http://www.tricare.com.

United Nations: *Report of Future World Conferences*, New York, 2014, UN.

University of Michigan Center of Excellence in Public Health Workforce Studies: *Enumeration and characteristics of the public health nurse workforce: findings of the 2012 public health nurse workforce surveys*, Ann Arbor, MI, 2013, University of Michigan.

US Department of Health and Human Services: *Healthy People 2000: national health promotion and disease prevention objectives*, Washington, DC, 1991, US Government Printing Office. Retrieved Dec 2010 from http://www.health.gov/healthypeople.

US Department of Health and Human Services: *Healthy People 2010: understanding and improving health*, ed 2, Washington, DC, 2000, US Government Printing Office.

US Department of Health and Human Services: *Healthy People 2020*, Washington, DC, 2010, US Government Printing Office.

US Department of Health and Human Services: *The Division of Nursing's National Advisory Committee on Nursing Education and Practice*, Rockville, MD, 2013a, Division of Nursing.

US Department of Health and Human Services: *Assistant Secretary Nicole Lurie statement on the Pandemic and All Hazards Preparedness Reauthorization Act*, Rockville, MD, March 13, 2013b, HHS Press Office. Available at http://www.hhs.gov/news/press/2013pres/03/20130313a.html. Accessed May 7, 2014.

US Department of Health and Human Services: *The Division of Nursing's National Advisory Committee on Nursing Education and Practice*, Rockville, MD, 2016, Division of Nursing.

US Department of Health and Human Services, Centers for Medicare and Medicaid Services: *Medicare information for advanced practice registered nurses, anesthesiologist assistants, and physician assistants*, 2015. ICN 901623. Retrieved June 22, 2016 from https://www.cms.gov/Outreach-and-Education/Medicare-Learning-Network-MLN/MLNProducts/Downloads/Medicare-Information-for-APRNs-AAs-PAs-Booklet-ICN-901623.pdf.

US Law: 42 SC 301, Stewart Machine Co. v Davis, 1937a.

US Law: 49 Stat 622, Title II, 1937b.

US Law (Public Law 67-97): 1921-1929 Maternity and Infancy (Sheppard-Towner) Act, 1921.

US Law (Public Law 104-191): Health Insurance Portability and Accountability Act (HIPAA), 1996.

US Law (Public Law 105-33): Title XXI of the Social Security Act, Balanced Budget Act - State Child Health Improvement Act (SCHIP), 1997a.

US Law (Public Law 105-33): Title XXL of the Social Security Act, Balanced Budget Act, 1997b.

US Law (Public Law 106-505): Public Health Threats and Emergencies Act, 2002.

US Law (Public Law 107-188): Public Health Security and Bioterrorism Preparedness and Response Act, 2002.

US Law (Public Law 111-148): Patient Protection and Affordable Care Act (PPACA), 2010.

World Health Assembly: *Strengthening nursing and midwifery, 56th session*, Geneva, 2003, WHA. Retrieved December 2010 from http://www.who.org.

World Health Organization: *Health systems financing: the path to universal coverage-the world health report*, Geneva, 2010, WHO. Retrieved December 2010 from http:/www.who.org.

World Health Organization: *World Health Report*, Geneva, 2016, WHO. Retrieved June 2016 from http://www.who.int/whr/en/.

Zipprich J, Winter K, Hacker J, et al: Measles outbreak – California, December 2014 – February 2015, *Morbidity and Mortality Weekly Report* 64(06):153–154, 2015.

CHAPTER **8**

Economic Influences

Marcia Stanhope

OBJECTIVES

After reading this chapter, the student should be able to:

1. Relate public health and economic principles to nursing and health care.
2. Identify major factors influencing national health care spending.
3. Describe the role of government and other third-party payers in health care financing.
4. Identify mechanisms for public health financing of services.
5. Discuss the implications of health care rationing from an economic perspective.
6. Evaluate levels of prevention as they relate to public health economics.

CHAPTER OUTLINE

Public Health and Economics
Factors Affecting Resource Allocation in Health Care
  The Uninsured
  The Poor
  Access to Health Services
  Rationing Health Care
  Healthy People 2020
Primary Prevention
The Context of the US Health System
  First Phase
  Second Phase
  Third Phase
  Fourth Phase
  Challenges for the 21st Century

Trends in Health Care Spending
Factors Influencing Health Care Costs
  Demographics Affecting Health Care
  Technology and Intensity
  Chronic Illness
Financing of Health Care
  Public Support
  Public Health
  Other Public Support
  Private Support
Health Care Payment Systems
  Paying Health Care Organizations
  Paying Health Care Practitioners
Economics and the Future of Nursing Practice

KEY TERMS

capitation, 143
covered lives, 143
diagnosis-related groups (DRGs), 133
economics, 126
effectiveness, 143
efficiency, 143
enabling, 141
fee-for-service, 143
gross domestic product (GDP), 135
health care rationing, 127
health economics, 126
human capital, 130
inflation, 126
intensity, 130
managed care, 141
means testing, 136
Medicaid, 128
medical technology, 131
Medicare, 136
prospective payment system (PPS), 139
public health economics, 126
retrospective reimbursement, 142
return on investment, 130
safety net providers, 129
third-party payers, 130

Strong evidence suggests that poverty can be directly related to poorer health outcomes. Poorer health outcomes lead to reduced educational outcomes for children, poor nutrition, low productivity in the adult workforce, and unstable economic growth in a population, community, or nation. However, improving health status and economic health depends on the "degree of equality" in policies that improve living standards for all members of a population, including the poor. To move toward improving a population's health there must be an "investment in public health" by all levels of government (Robert Wood Johnson Foundation [RWJF], 2013).

Estimates indicate that public spending on health care makes a difference but needs the support of increased private health care spending to improve the overall health status of populations (Trust for America's Health, 2013a, 2013b, 2014). The following facts are known from the literature (Kaiser Family Foundation [KFF], 2013; RWJF, 2013; DeNavas-Walt et al., 2013; US Department of Health and Human Services [USDHHS], 2016c):

- In 2012, approximately 48 million (15.4%) of the estimated 311.1 million people in the United States were without health insurance (DeNavas-Walt et al., 2013). Over the past decade, the number of uninsured individuals had increased, largely due to the struggling economy and weak job market (KFF, 2013). As the Affordable Care Act (ACA) was implemented, the uninsured rate dropped to 10.7% in 2015, and new and affordable options became available. This reduced the number of uninsured individuals and families by 8.8 million people by 2014, the year the ACA was fully implemented (The Commonwealth Fund, 2016; KFF 2015a).
- The rate of uninsured remains higher among people with lower incomes and lower among those with higher incomes. Households of three with less than $20,000 in annual income are at the highest risk for being uninsured (KFF, 2015a).
- Adults are more likely to be uninsured than children (KFF, 2015a).
- Young adults (ages 19–25 years) account for a disproportionately large share of the uninsured, largely due to their low incomes (KFF, 2015; USDHHS, 2016c).
- The uninsured rate for all children was 8.9% in 2012. For children living in poverty the uninsured rate was 12.9%, which was higher than the rate for children not in poverty (7.7%) (DeNavas-Walt et al, 2013). This rate has declined since 2014 but is still higher for children in poverty than those not in poverty (KFF, 2015a).
- Nonwhites are more likely to be uninsured than whites (KFF, 2015a).
- Most of the uninsured are in low-income working families (KFF, 2015a).
  - About 80% are from families with one or more workers (full or part time).
  - About 50% are from families who are at 200% of the poverty level. This percentage has improved and dropped from 400% in 2012.
- Individuals without health insurance continue to have worse access to care than those with insurance coverage (KFF, 2015a).
- Those without health insurance are more likely to be hospitalized for preventable problems, and when hospitalized, they receive fewer diagnostic and therapeutic services; they also have higher mortality rates than those with insurance (KFF, 2015a).
- Adults without insurance are nearly twice as likely to report being in fair or poor health than those with private insurance (KFF, 2012a).
- Studies indicate that gaining health insurance restores access to health care considerably and reduces the adverse effects of having been uninsured (KFF, 2012a).

- The poor have been more likely to receive health care through publicly funded agencies. The rates of low-income/no-income persons receiving health care have dropped in those states that have participated in the Medicaid expansion program offered through the ACA (The Commonwealth Fund, 2016).
- Some persons who are eligible for insurance coverage under the ACA do not sign up due to lack of information or enrollment barriers, and some simply do not believe in the ACA (KFF, 2015a).
- An emphasis on individual health care will not guarantee improvement of a population or a community's health (see Chapter 3 for more discussion).

Approximately 97% of all health care dollars are spent for individual care, whereas only 3% is spent on population-level health care. The 3% includes monies spent by the government on public health, as well as the preventive health care dollars spent by private sources. The conclusion from these figures is that there is not a large investment in the public's health or population health in the United States (National Center for Health Statistics [NCHS], 2016).

The United States spends more on health care than any other nation. The cost of health care has been rising more than the rate of inflation since the mid-1960s. Yet the US population does not enjoy better health than nations that spend far less than the United States. To highlight this point, the majority (79%) of the uninsured are citizens of the United States, with the remaining being lawfully present and undocumented noncitizens (KFF, 2012a). The current health care system is at a point at which it is not affordable (Turnock, 2016; Trust for America's Health, 2013b). Knowledge about health economics is particularly important to community-oriented nurses because they are the ones who are often in a position to allocate resources to solve a problem or to design, plan, coordinate, and evaluate community-based health services and programs.

PUBLIC HEALTH AND ECONOMICS

Economics is the science concerned with the use of resources, including the production, distribution, and consumption of goods and services. Health economics is concerned with how scarce resources affect the health care industry (McPake et al, 2013; Phelps, 2012). Public health economics then focuses on the production, distribution, and consumption of goods and services as related to public health (Centers for Disease Control and Prevention [CDC], 2015). Economics provides the means to evaluate society's attainment of its wants and needs in relation to limited resources. In addition to the day-to-day decision making about the use of resources, focus is on evaluating economics in health care (McPake et al, 2013; Phelps, 2012). Although in the past, focus on evaluation of public health economics has been limited, it is becoming more obvious what evaluating public health and preventive care can do in terms of cost savings and, more importantly, quality of life (Trust for America's Health, 2013b). This type of evaluation will help present challenges to public policymakers (legislators). Public health financing often causes conflict because the views and priorities of individuals and groups in society may differ from those of the public health care industry. If money is spent on public health care, money for other public needs, such as education, transportation, recreation, and defense, may be limited. When trying to argue that more money should be spent for population-level health care or prevention, data must be available from this report and more reports like it to show the investment is worthwhile. Public health finance is a growing field of science and practice that involves the acquisition, management, and use of monies to improve the health of populations through disease prevention and health promotion strategies. This field of study also focuses on evaluating the use of the money and the impact on the public health system (Honoré, 2012).

Although the public health system had been considered for many years to involve only government public health agencies, such as health departments, today the public health system is known to be much broader and includes schools, industry, media, environmental protection agencies, voluntary organizations, civic groups, local police and fire departments, religious organizations, industry and business, and private-sector health care systems, including the insurance industry. All can play a key role in improving population health (Institute of Medicine, 2003; Trust for America's Health, 2013a).

The goal of public health finance is "to support population focused preventive health services" (Honoré, 2012). Four principles are suggested that explain how public health financing may occur.

- The source and use of monies are controlled solely by the government.
- The government controls the money, but the private sector controls how the money is used.
- The private sector controls the money, but the government controls how the money is used.
- The private sector controls the money and controls how it is used. (Sturchi and Goel, 2012)

When the government provides the funding and controls the use, the monies come from taxes, user fees (e.g., license fees, purchase of alcohol and cigarettes), and charges to consumers of the services. Services offered at the federal government level include the following:

- Policymaking
- Public health protection
- Collecting and sharing information about US health care and delivery systems
- Building capacity for population health
- Direct-care services

Select examples of services offered at the state and local levels include the following:

- Maternal and child health
- Family planning
- Counseling
- Preventing communicable and infectious diseases (see Chapters 7 and 28 for more examples)

When the government provides the money but the private sector decides how it is used, the money comes from business and individual tax savings related to private spending for illness prevention care. When a business provides disease prevention and health promotion services to their employees and sometimes families, such as immunizations, health screening, and counseling, the business taxes owed to the government are reduced. This is considered a means by which the government provides money through tax savings to businesses to use for population health care.

When the private sector provides the money but the government decides how it is used, either voluntarily or involuntarily, the money is used for preventive care services for specific populations.

- A voluntary example is the private contributions made to reaching *Healthy People 2010* goals.
- An involuntary example is the Occupational Safety and Health Administration's requirement that industry adhere to certain safety standards for the use of machinery, air quality, ventilation, and eyewear protection to reduce disease and injury. This has the effect of reducing occupation-related injuries in the population as a whole.

When the private sector is responsible for both the money and its use of resources, the benefits incurred are many. For example, an industry may offer influenza vaccine clinics for workers and families that may lead to "herd immunity" in the community (see Chapter 9). A business or community may institute a "no smoking" policy that reduces the risk for smoking-related illnesses to workers, family, and the consumers of the business's services. A voluntary philanthropic organization may partner with a local school system to improve school-linked clinical services, such as immunizations, preventive dental care, mental health coverage, and laboratory tests (Minyard et al, 2016).

These are but a few examples of how public health services and the ensuring of a healthy population are not only government related. The partnerships between government and the private sector are necessary to improve the overall health status of populations.

FACTORS AFFECTING RESOURCE ALLOCATION IN HEALTH CARE

The distribution of health care is affected largely by the way in which health care is financed in the United States. Third-party coverage, whether public or private, greatly affects the distribution of health care. Also, socioeconomic status affects health care consumption because it determines the ability to purchase insurance or to pay directly out-of-pocket expenses. The effects of barriers to health care access and the effects of health care rationing on the distribution of health care follow. Although the barriers are still issues, changes to the barriers to access and distribution are improving.

THE UNINSURED

In 1996, 68% of the total US population had private health insurance. An additional 15% received insurance through public programs, and 17% (37 million people) were uninsured. In 2008 the number of uninsured persons had increased to 47 million.

By 2012 the number had grown to 48 million persons (DeNavas-Walt et al, 2013). The typical uninsured person was a member of the workforce or a dependent of this worker. Uninsured workers are likely to be in low-paying jobs, part-time or temporary jobs, or jobs at small businesses (KFF, 2015a). These uninsured workers cannot afford to purchase health insurance, or their employers may not offer health insurance as a benefit. Others who are typically uninsured are young adults (especially young men), nonwhites, persons younger than 65 years of age in good or fair health, and the poor or near poor. The following may be the case for these individuals:

- May be unable to afford insurance
- May lack access to job-based coverage
- Because of their age or good health status, may not perceive the need for insurance

Because of the eligibility requirements for Medicaid, the near poor are actually more likely to be uninsured than the poor because they cannot afford even the cost of health care through the national or state health care marketplaces and are not eligible for tax credits (KFF, 2015b).

The ACA passed in 2010 was a result of a promise to the American public by President Obama that health care reform would occur as part of his presidential agenda to address the issues affecting the uninsured and underinsured. Basically, this law addresses the following:

- Quality, affordable health care for all Americans
- A defined role of public programs
- Improving the quality and efficiency of health care
- Prevention of chronic disease and improving public health
- Health care workforce
- Transparency and program integrity
- Improving access to innovative medical therapies
- Community living assistance services and supports
- Revenue provisions

Before this act was passed, the following situations were the case:

- Twenty-five states were considering making it mandatory for employers to provide coverage.
- Seven states were looking at approaches to universal coverage.
- Six states were considering the development of universal health care plan commissions.

Only three states had passed comprehensive health care reform by 2008—Massachusetts, Maine, and Vermont. State fiscal capacity, structural deficits, and then a worsening economy and severe state budget shortfalls had limited states' ability to further advance coverage initiatives. The experiences of pace-setting states informed the federal action, with the ACA which was attempting to address the fiscal crisis, because it was difficult for many states to achieve health care reform on their own. By 2015 only 29 states had participated in the Medicaid expansion program to increase the numbers of eligible persons for health insurance in their states (KFF, 2015b).

As the health care reform debate continues, the impact of federal reform on states will have differential effects. In general, states will be greatly affected (some positive/some negative) if they are states with the following (KFF, 2015b):

- More extensive poverty
- Higher budget shortfalls

- Lower eligibility levels for public programs
- Higher rates of uninsured
- Greater shortages in primary-care direct-services providers

Those states that have accepted the opportunity for Medicaid expansion have experienced increased numbers of enrollees in health care, thereby reducing the numbers of uninsured; improved budgets overall but some tax increases; and increased administrative costs initially, with drops in the second year. There have been improvements in preventive care to the low-income populations as well. Those states that have budget shortfalls, more extensive poverty levels, and fewer health care providers to meet the demands may not see overall benefit from the ACA (KFF, 2015c).

THE POOR

Socioeconomic status is inversely related to mortality and morbidity for almost every disease. Poor Americans with an income below the poverty level have a mortality rate nearly three times that of middle-income Americans, even after accounting for age, sex, race, education, and risky health behaviors (such as smoking, drinking, overeating, and lack of exercise) (RWJF, 2013). Historically, the link between poor health and socioeconomic status resulted from poor housing, malnutrition, inadequate sanitation, and hazardous occupations. Today, explanations include the cumulative effects of various characteristics that explain the concept of poverty. These characteristics include low educational levels, unemployment or low occupational status (blue collar or unskilled laborer), low wages, being a child or being older than 65 years, and being a member of a minority group (NCHS, 2016).

ACCESS TO HEALTH SERVICES

Access to health services is a public health issue (USDHHS, 2016a). Medicaid is intended to improve access to health care for the poor. Although persons with Medicaid have improved access (approximately twofold) in contrast to the uninsured, Medicaid recipients are only about half as likely to obtain needed health services (e.g., medical-surgical care, dental care, prescription drugs, eyeglasses) as the privately insured. Specifically, the poorest Americans have Medicaid insurance, yet they also have had the worst health (KFF, 2015b).

The primary reasons for delay, difficulty, or failure to access care have included the inability to afford health care and a variety of insurance-related reasons, such as the following:

- The insurer not approving, covering, or paying for care
- The client having preexisting conditions
- Physicians refusing to accept the insurance plan

The ACA addresses these reasons, with those enrolled in the marketplaces knowing what their plans will cover and including preexisting conditions. There may still be providers who will not accept the health plans.

Other barriers to seeking health care may include lack of transportation, physical barriers, communication problems, childcare needs, lack of time or information, or refusal of services by providers. Additionally, lack of after-hours care, long office waits, and long travel distance are cited as access barriers. Community characteristics contribute to the ability of individuals to access care. For example, the prevalence of managed care and the number of safety net providers, for those who are not eligible or have not enrolled in the marketplaces, as well as the wealth and size of the community, affect accessibility. It should be noted that by 2014, unless an individual reported approximately $10,500 on income tax forms or was a member of a family of four with income of less than $20,300, all persons were required to have health insurance coverage or pay a penalty (KFF, 2012b).

Because reimbursement for services provided to Medicaid recipients has been low, physicians were discouraged from serving this population. Thus people on Medicaid frequently had no primary-care provider and often relied on the emergency department for primary-care services. Although physicians have been able to choose clients based on their ability to pay, emergency departments have been required by law to evaluate all clients regardless of their ability to pay. Emergency department copayments were usually modest and were frequently waived if the client was unable to pay. Thus low out-of-pocket costs provided incentives for Medicaid clients and the uninsured to use emergency departments for primary-care services.

With the ACA (PL 111-148), some of the issues and barriers that have previously existed may disappear. Continuation of the issues and barriers depends on whether Congress decides to repeal all or part of the ACA or change some of the mandates in the law. By 2014, Medicaid recipients benefited from the law in its current structure as follows:

1. Expansion of Medicaid to include all non–Medicare eligible persons under age 65 with incomes up to 133% of federal poverty level.
2. All Medicaid-eligible persons were guaranteed a benchmark benefit package.
3. States were given the option to develop a basic health plan for uninsured individuals who did not qualify for the Medicaid program, at 133% to 200% of poverty level. As indicated, only 29 states chose to participate by 2016.

Poverty-level income is adjusted annually for each state by the federal government to indicate how much money an individual or families may earn to qualify for subsidies such as food stamps, Medicaid, and the Children's Health Insurance Program. In 2016 the federal poverty level for an individual was $11,880; for a family of four, the poverty level was $24,300 (USDHHS, 2016c). If an individual's income was at 133% of the poverty level, then the individual earned no more than $15,800 (USDHHS, 2016c).

RATIONING HEALTH CARE

Rationing health care in any form implies reduced access to care and potential decreases in the acceptable quality of services offered. For example, a health provider's refusal to accept Medicare or Medicaid clients is a form of rationing. As with access to care, rationing health care is a public health issue. Where care is not provided, the public health system and nurses must ensure that essential clinical services are available. Managed care was

thought to offer the possibility of more appropriate health care access and better-organized care to meet the basic health care needs of the total population. A shift in the general approach to health care from a reactionary, acute-care orientation toward a proactive, primary prevention orientation is necessary to achieve not only a more cost-effective but also a more equitable health care system in the United States. The ACA, despite providing coverage to more people, will not do away with rationing because the new law provides for a four-tiered plan (bronze, silver, gold, platinum) by creating state-based American Health Benefit Exchanges. Persons at differing levels of poverty will have reductions in out-of-pocket expenses based on income up to 400% of the poverty level and may receive tax credits and subsidies to assist with out-of-pocket expenses (US Law, PL 111-148, 2010).

HEALTHY PEOPLE 2020

Healthy People 2020 (USDHHS, 2010) goals are examples of strategies to provide better access for all people. The Levels of Prevention box shows the levels of economic prevention strategies.

 HEALTHY PEOPLE 2020

Objectives Related to Access to Care

- **AHS-1:** Increase the proportion of persons with health insurance.
- **AHS-6:** Reduce the proportion of individuals who experience difficulties or delays in obtaining necessary medical care, dental care, or prescription medicines.

 LEVELS OF PREVENTION

Economic Prevention Strategies

Primary Prevention
Work with legislators and insurance companies to provide coverage for health promotion to reduce the risk for diseases.

Secondary Prevention
Encourage clients who are pregnant to participate in prenatal care and the Special Supplemental Nutrition Program for Women, Infants, and Children (WIC) to increase the number of healthy babies and reduce the costs related to preterm baby care.

Tertiary Prevention
Participate in home visits to mothers who are at risk for neglecting babies, to reduce the costs related to abuse.

CHECK YOUR PRACTICE

At the local nurse-managed clinic for mothers and new babies, you are assigned to assist mothers in understanding the benefits of primary prevention. You are focusing on the Special Supplemental Nutrition Program for Women, Infants, and Children (WIC) program and are encouraging mothers to participate in this program to help their babies have a good start toward a healthy life. Why do you think such a program is important, and why is primary prevention even a focus in health care delivery?

PRIMARY PREVENTION

Society's investment in the health care system has been based on the premise that more health services will result in better health, but factors not related to health care also have an effect. Of the four major factors that affect health—personal behavior (or lifestyle), environmental factors (including physical, social, and economic environments), human biology, and the health care system—medical services are said to have the least effect. Behavior and lifestyle have been shown to have the greatest effect, with the environment and biology accounting for the greatest effect on the development of all illnesses (NCHS, 2016).

Despite the significant impact of behavior and environment on health, estimates indicate that most of the health care dollars are spent on secondary and tertiary care. Such a reactionary, secondary-care system results in high-cost, high-technology, and disease-specific care and is consistent with the US system's traditional emphasis on "sickness care." A more proactive investment in disease prevention and health promotion targeted at improving health behaviors, lifestyle, and the environment has the potential to improve the health status of populations, thereby improving the quality of life while reducing health care costs. The USDHHS has argued that a higher value should be placed on primary prevention. The goal of this approach is to preserve and maximize human capital by providing health promotion and social practices that result in less disease. An emphasis on primary prevention has the goal of reducing dollars spent and increasing the quality of life.

The return on investment in primary prevention through gains in human capital has, unfortunately, not been acknowledged in the past. The ACA is designed to acknowledge and improve primary prevention access and improve the return on investment of dollars in health care. In the past, large investments in primary prevention and public health care were not made. Reasons given for this lack of emphasis on prevention in clinical practice and lack of financial investment in prevention included the following:

- Provider uncertainty about which clients should receive services and at what intervals
- Lack of information about preventive services
- Negative attitudes about the importance of preventive care
- Lack of time for delivery of preventive services
- Delayed or absent feedback regarding the success of preventive measures
- Less reimbursement for these services than for curative services
- Lack of organization to deliver preventive services
- Lack of use of services by the poor and the elderly
- More out-of-pocket expenses for the poor and those who lack health insurance

A focus on prevention could mean reducing the need for and use of medical, dental, hospital, and health provider services as they are delivered today. With the increasing costs of health care and consumer demand and the changes in financing mechanisms, there is a new trend toward financing more preventive care services and offering some of these services free (US Law, 2010).

Today, third-party payers are beginning to cover preventive services, recognizing that the growth of the health care system can no longer be supported. Under capitated health plans, health care providers stand to make money by keeping clients healthy and reducing health care use. Through combining client interests with financial interests of the health care industry, primary prevention and public health can be raised to the status and priority of acute care and chronic care. Support for an increasing national investment in primary prevention is sound and long-standing. Despite difficulties, methods for determining prevention effectiveness, such as cost-effectiveness analysis (CEAs) and cost/benefit analysis (CBAs), are becoming standard and used more widely. Two agendas for preventive services are published that promote the preventive agenda:

- The US Preventive Services Task Force's *Guide to Clinical Preventive Services* (Agency for Healthcare Research and Quality [AHRQ], 2014) is for clinicians in primary care and outlines the regular screening and risk factors to look for at various ages.
- The Community Preventive Services Task Force's (2015) publication *The Community Guide* emphasizes population-level interventions to promote primary prevention.

Regardless of the method, prevention effectiveness analyses (PEAs) are outcome oriented. This area of research seeks to link interventions with health outcomes and economic outcomes and to reveal the tradeoffs between the two. Since the public health movement of the mid-19th century, public health officials, epidemiologists, and nurses have been working to advance the agenda of primary prevention to the forefront of the health care industry. Today these efforts continue across various disciplines and in both the public and the private sectors, and through the efforts for health care reform (US Law, 2010).

THE CONTEXT OF THE US HEALTH SYSTEM

The US health care system is a diverse collection of industries involved directly or indirectly in providing health care services. The major players in the industry are the health professionals who provide health care services, pharmacy and equipment suppliers, insurers (public, government, private), managed care organizations (health maintenance organizations, preferred provider organizations), and other groups, such as educational institutions, consulting and research firms, professional associations, and trade unions. Today the health care industry is large, and its characteristics and operations differ between rural and urban geographic areas.

In the 21st century, health policy and national politics reflect the importance of health care delivery in the general economy. Conflicts arise between competing special-interest groups that have different goals and objectives when it comes to the producing and consuming of health services. To some degree this is caused by federal and state policy changes about how health services are financed (public and private).

Fig. 8.1 illustrates the four basic components that make up the framework of health services delivery: service needs and intensity, facilities, technology, and labor. Intensity is the extent of use of technologies, supplies, and health care services by or

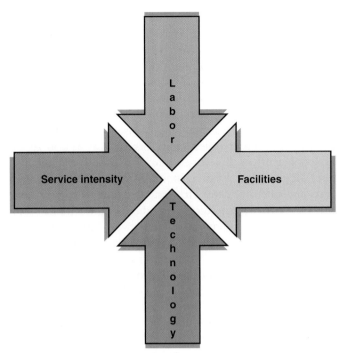

FIG. 8.1 Components of health services development.

for the client. Intensity includes and is a partial measure of the use of technology (NCHS, 2016). **Medical technology** refers to the set of techniques, drugs, equipment, and procedures used by health care professionals in delivering medical care to individuals. It also includes information technology and the system within which such care is delivered (NCHS, 2016).

Health care systems have developed in four phases from the 1800s to today. These developmental stages correspond to different economic conditions. Developmentally, the four components of the health services delivery framework have changed over time, reflecting changes in morbidity and mortality, national health policy, and economics (Fig. 8.2).

FIRST PHASE

The first developmental stage (1800–1900) was characterized by epidemics of infectious diseases, such as cholera, typhoid, smallpox, influenza, malaria, and yellow fever. Health concerns of the time related to social and public health issues, including contaminated food and water supplies, inadequate sewage disposal, and poor housing conditions (Shi and Singh, 2014). Family and friends provided most health care in the home. Hospitals were few in number and suffered from overcrowding, disease, and unsanitary conditions. Sick persons who were cared for in hospitals often died as a result of these conditions. Most people avoided being cared for in a hospital unless there was no alternative. In this first developmental phase, health care was paid for by individuals who could afford it, through bartering with physicians, or through charity from individuals or organizations. The first county health departments were established in 1908.

Technology to aid in disease control was very basic and practical but in keeping with the knowledge of the time. The physician's "black bag" contained the few medicines and tools available for treatment. The economics of health care was influenced by the types of health care providers and the number of practitioners, with the labor force composed mostly of physicians and nurses who attained their skills through apprenticeships or on-the-job training. Nurses in the United States were predominantly female, and education was linked to religious orders that expected service, dedication, and charity (Knickman and Kovner, 2015). The focus of nursing was primarily to support physicians and assist clients with activities of daily living.

SECOND PHASE

The second developmental stage (1900–1945) of US health care delivery was focused on the control of acute infectious diseases. Environmental conditions influencing health began

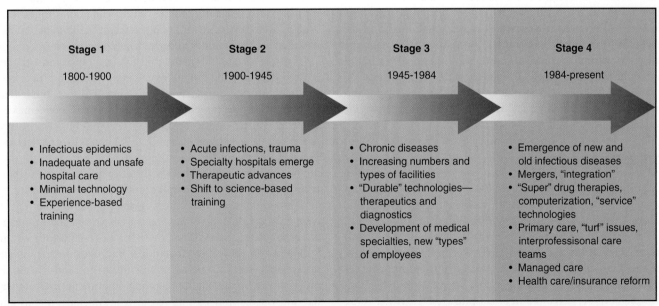

FIG. 8.2 Developmental framework for health service needs and intensity, facilities, technology, and labor.

to improve, with major advances in water purity, sanitary sewage disposal, milk and water quality, and urban housing quality. The health problems of this era were no longer mass epidemics, but rather individual acute infections or traumatic episodes (Shi and Singh, 2014).

Hospitals and health departments experienced rapid growth during the late 1800s and early 1900s as technological advances in science were made (Knickman and Kovner, 2015). In addition to private and charitable financing of health care, city, county, and state governments were beginning to contribute by providing services for poor persons, state mental institutions, and other specialty hospitals, such as tuberculosis hospitals. Public health departments were emphasizing case finding and quarantine. Although health care was paid for primarily by individuals, the Social Security Act of 1935 signaled the federal government's increasing interest in addressing social welfare problems.

Clinical medicine entered its golden age during this period. Major technological advances in surgery and childbirth and the identification of disease processes, such as the cause of pernicious anemia, increased the ability to diagnose and treat diseases. The first serological tests used as a tool for diagnosis and control of infectious diseases were developed in 1910 to detect syphilis and gonorrhea (Shi and Singh, 2014). The first virus isolation techniques were developed to filter yellow fever virus, for example. The discovery and development of pharmacological agents, such as insulin in 1922 for the control of diabetes, sulfa drugs in 1932 for the treatment of infectious diseases, and antibiotics such as penicillin in the 1940s, eradicated certain infectious diseases, increased treatment options, and decreased morbidity and mortality (Shi and Singh, 2014).

Advances in technology and knowledge shifted physician education away from apprenticeships to scientifically based college education, which occurred as a result of the Flexner Report in 1910. Nurses were trained primarily in hospital schools of nursing, with an emphasis on following and executing physicians' orders. Nurses in training were unmarried and under the age of 30. They provided the bulk of care in hospitals (Knickman and Kovner, 2015). Public health nurses, who tracked infectious diseases and implemented quarantine procedures, worked more collegially with physicians (Knickman and Kovner, 2015). In this period the university-based nursing programs were established to accommodate the expanding practice base of nursing. Client education became a nursing function early in the development of the health care delivery system.

THIRD PHASE

The third developmental stage (1945–1984) included a shift away from acute infectious health problems of previous stages toward chronic health problems such as heart disease, cancer, and stroke. These illnesses resulted from increasing wealth and lifestyle changes in the United States. To meet society's needs, the number and types of facilities expanded to include, for example, hospital clinics and long-term care facilities. The Joint Commission on Accreditation of Hospitals, established in 1951 and later renamed The Joint Commission on Accreditation of

Healthcare Organizations (and now called The Joint Commission [TJC]), focused on the safety and protection of the public and the delivery of quality care.

Changes in the overall health of the American society also shifted the focus of technology, research, and development. Major technological advances included developments in the realms of chemotherapeutic agents; immunizations; anesthesia; electrolyte and cardiopulmonary physiology; diagnostic laboratories with complex modalities such as computed tomography; organ and tissue transplants; radiation therapy; laser surgery; and specialty units for critical care, coronary care, and intensive care. The first "test-tube baby" was born through in vitro fertilization, and other fertility advances soon emerged. Negative staining techniques for screening viruses with the electron microscope became available in the 1960s (Shi and Singh, 2014).

Health care providers constituted more than 5% of the total US workforce during this period. The three largest health care employers were hospitals, convalescent institutions, and physicians' offices. Between 1970 and 1984 alone, the number of persons employed in the health care industry grew by 90%. The number of personnel employed in the community also increased. The expansion of care delivery into other sites, such as community-based clinics, increased not only the number but also the types of health care employees.

Technological advances brought about increased special training for physicians and nurses, and care was organized around these specialties. The ongoing shortage of nurses throughout the century was being seen in the 1970s and early 1980s. Nursing education expanded from hospital-based diploma and university-based baccalaureate education to include associate degree programs at the entry level. As the diploma schools of nursing began closing in the early to mid-1980s, the number of baccalaureate and associate degree programs began to increase. Graduate nursing education expanded to include the nurse practitioner (NP) and clinical nurse specialist (CNS) to meet increasing demands for the education of nurses in a specialty such as public health. The first doctoral programs in nursing were instituted to build the scientific base for nursing and increase the number of nurse faculty members.

The role of the commercial health insurance industry increased, and a strong link between employment and the provision of health care benefits emerged. Furthermore, the federal government's role expanded through landmark policymaking that would affect health care delivery well into the 21st century. Specifically, the passage of Titles XVIII and XIX of the Social Security Act (1965) created the Medicare and Medicaid programs, respectively. The health care system appeared to have access to unlimited resources for growing and expanding.

Throughout the 20th century, many public health advances were achieved. The life expectancy of US citizens increased and has been related to public health activities. The most important achievements were in vaccinations, improved motor vehicle safety, safer workplaces, safer and healthier foods, healthier mothers and babies, family planning, fluoride in drinking water, and recognition of tobacco as a health hazard (Shi and Singh, 2014).

FOURTH PHASE

The fourth developmental stage (1984 to the present) has been a period of limited resources, with an emphasis on containing costs, restricting growth in the health care industry, and reorganizing care delivery. For example, amendments were made to the Social Security Act in 1983 that created diagnosis-related groups (DRGs) and a prospective system of paying for health care provided to Medicare recipients. The 1997 Balanced Budget Act legislated additional federal changes in Medicare and Medicaid. Private-sector employer concerns about the rising costs of health care for employees and fear of profit losses spurred a major change in the delivery and financing of health care. Managed care systems were developed during this time.

This period has included drastic change in the settings and organization of health care delivery. Transforming health care organizations became commonplace, and buzz words of the period were *reorganization, reengineering, restructuring,* and *downsizing.* Organization mergers occurred at an increased rate to consolidate care, save money, and coordinate care across the continuum (i.e., from "cradle to grave"). Merger discussions focused on horizontal integration, which indicated the union of similar agencies (e.g., a merger of hospitals) and vertical integration between different types of organizations (e.g., an acute care hospital, a long-term care institution, and a home health facility).

Initially these pressures brought about hospital closings and a shifting of care to other settings, such as ambulatory and community-based clinics and specialty diagnostic centers that offer technologies such as magnetic resonance imaging (MRI) and sonography. Rehabilitative, restorative, and palliative care, once delivered in the hospitals, was shifted to other settings, such as subacute care hospitals, specialty rehabilitation hospitals, long-term care institutions, and even individual homes. Although the basis of care delivery was no longer the traditional acute care hospital, the nature of the care delivered in hospitals changed remarkably, as evidenced by the following:

- Patients admitted to hospitals were more acutely ill.
- The length of stay for patients admitted to hospitals became shorter.
- Care delivery became more intense as a result of the first two items.

The widespread use of computers and the Internet has enabled society to become increasingly sophisticated about health. The public's increasing knowledge about health care and their awareness of health care advances have influenced the demand for health care, such as diagnostic and therapeutic services for treatment. Furthermore, pharmaceutical companies and other technological suppliers actively marketed their products through television, printed advertisements, the Internet, and other sources, so clients rapidly become aware of the new technologies.

Health professionals depend on technology to care for clients. Distance, as a barrier to the diagnosis and treatment of disease, has been overcome through the use of telehealth. The insurance industry has become the principal buyer of technology for the client. They often make decisions about when and whether a certain technology will be used for a client problem.

Nurses have become dependent on technologies to monitor client progress, make decisions about care, and deliver care in innovative ways.

The shift away from traditional hospital-based care to the community, together with the need to consider new models of care, brought about an increased emphasis on providing primary care, on developing care delivery teams, and on collaborating in practice and education. The substitution of one type of health personnel for another was occurring to control care delivery costs. As examples, the NPs were replacing physicians as primary-care providers and unlicensed personnel were replacing staff nurses in hospitals and long-term care facilities. These replacements caused much debate, with territorial, or "turf," battles, for example, between physicians and nurses.

The increase in specialization by health professionals has led to changes in certification, qualifications, education, and standards of care in health professions. These factors, in turn, have caused an increase in the number and kinds of providers to meet the demands of the health care system (Lockard and Wolf, 2012). The Bureau of Labor Statistics (BLS) predicted that health care employment would be among the top eight professional and related industries, with significant employment growth of 16% from 2014 to 2024 (BLS, 2015).

In the last part of the 20th century, molecular tools were developed that provide a means of detecting and characterizing infectious disease pathogens and a new capacity to track the transmission of new threats, such as bioterrorism, and determine new ways to treat them.

CHALLENGES FOR THE 21ST CENTURY

In the 21st century the emergence of new and the reemergence of old communicable and infectious diseases are occurring, as well as larger foodborne disease outbreaks and acts of terrorism. In 2010, 70% of all deaths were related to chronic disease (CDC, 2016). In 2012 approximately half of all adults had one or more chronic conditions, with arthritis being the most common cause of disability (CDC, 2016). There is some concern that certain chronic diseases may be caused or intensified by infectious disease processes. Often, complications occur as a result of infectious disease, such as with human immunodeficiency virus/acquired immunodeficiency syndrome (HIV/AIDS) and tuberculosis, which can result in chronic lung disease and certain types of cancer, because of the compromised immune system. Health behaviors and economics related to poverty are also continuing to build the path to acute and chronic health problems (e.g., the global obesity epidemic) (Chaufan et al, 2015). Although some people choose to ignore behavioral factors related to obesity, such as physical activity and eating, those with insufficient income choose foods high in fat and sugar because those are the cheaper foods to obtain. The chronic disease burden is concentrated among the poor. Poor people are more vulnerable for several reasons, including increased exposure to risks and decreased access to health services. Chronic diseases can cause poverty in individuals and families and draw them into a downward spiral of worsening disease and poverty.

Investment in chronic disease prevention programs is going to be essential for many low- and middle-income countries struggling to reduce poverty. For the United States, this issue is addressed in the new health care reform program of 2010. Health promotion and protection, disease surveillance, emergency preparedness, new laboratory and epidemiological methods, continued antimicrobial and vaccine development, and environmental health research are continuing challenges for this century. The role of technology has also intensified during this century. Technology is now defined as the application of science to develop solutions to health problems or issues such as the prevention or delay of onset of diseases or the promotion and monitoring of good health. The labor force is changing to include radiology oncologists, geneticists, and surgical subspecialists, as well as allied and support professions such as medical sonographers, radiation technologists, and laboratory technicians. These have all been created to support the use of specific types of technology.

The infrastructure necessary to support more complex technologies is also considered to be a part of health care technology. Use of electronic medical records and electronic prescribing are methods for coordinating the increasingly complex array of services provided, as well as allowing for electronic checks of quality to reduce medical errors for things such as drug interactions. Because technologies have become a part of standard medical practice, there are concerns about whether they are consistently being used properly and about the quality of the information provided by tests, imaging, and other technological outputs (Kvedar et al, 2014).

In addition to the labor force changes just described, physicians are increasingly moving away from solo practice to group practices, selling primary-care practices to hospitals, working as hospital or corporation employees. The emerging role of hospital intensivists is growing, with hospitals employing physicians and sometimes nurse practitioners to be in house and available to patients and to their community physicians to cover nonurgent, urgent, and emergent care while the patient is hospitalized. More nurse practitioners and physician assistants can be found working side by side with the physician in the community as a member of the office or clinic team.

Public health nurses are more involved with population-centered care, assessment of community needs, and the development or implementation of programs that meet the needs of certain populations. A move is underway to provide more care to clients in the home, such as the programs to provide care to new mothers and babies who are defined as being at risk. Public health nurses play key roles in developing and implementing plans for bioterrorism and natural disasters in the community.

Nursing education is seeing a dramatic change in this century. There is a recommendation to move all advanced practice nursing to the level of the new doctoral program, begun in 2000, titled the Doctorate of Nursing Practice. This has the potential for closing specialists masters programs in nursing. This means the new bachelor of science in nursing (BSN) graduate, for example, can go into a doctoral program at graduation and become an advanced public health nurse or a nurse practitioner working in the community. The health care industry is one of the largest employers in the United States and, despite the economic downturn in 2008, has continued to grow. In addition, the largest number of employees in the health care industry are registered nurses (RNs) (BLS, 2016; Lockard and Wolf, 2012).

Along with other changes in health care delivery and health insurance plans, the ACA (US Law, 2010) proposed an emphasis on prevention and wellness by establishing the National Prevention, Health Promotion, and Public Health Council to coordinate health promotion and public health activities, as well as the creation of a prevention and public health fund to expand and sustain these activities. The council was established in the Office of the US Surgeon General, and every year, the council submits a report describing national progress in meeting specific prevention, health promotion, and public health goals defined in the National Prevention Strategy to the president and the relevant committees of Congress. The National Prevention Strategy developed through the council "aims to guide our nation in the most effective and achievable means for improving health and well-being. This Strategy envisions a prevention-oriented society where all sectors recognize the value of health for individuals, families, and society and work together to achieve better health for all Americans" (USDHHS, 2016b). The council activities were to assist in the development

QSEN FOCUS ON QUALITY AND SAFETY EDUCATION FOR NURSES

Teamwork and Collaboration

Both teamwork and collaboration refer to the ability to function effectively with nursing and interprofessional teams and to foster communication, mutual respect, and shared decision making to provide quality client care.

- **Knowledge:** Identify system barriers and facilitators of effective team functioning.
- **Skill:** Participate in designing systems that support effective teamwork.
- **Attitudes:** Values the influences of systems solutions in achieving effective functioning.

Teamwork and Collaboration Question

As a strategy set forth by the Affordable Care Act, a fund was established to support prevention and wellness activities within states to reduce risks. Among the options for spending the funds was the establishment of programs and processes to reduce the rate of chronic disease.

Monies have been distributed to states to promote prevention and wellness. Find out through your state government how the money is to be used.

The Quad Council public health nursing competency "community dimensions of practice" indicates that beginning public health nurses will collaborate with community partners to promote the health of their clients.

Have public health nurse at the state level or locally in your state been involved in collaborations to determine how chronic disease rates might be reduced in your area? If yes, how? If not, can you suggest how they might be?

Also, the public health nursing competency that addresses financial management and planning suggests that public health nurses may provide input into the fiscal planning and narrative components of proposals submitted for external funding. Determine what the process will be for obtaining local funds for chronic disease and whether public health nurses have had or will have the opportunity to provide input into the proposals.

of the national strategy to improve health, reduce chronic disease rates, and address health disparities. With these developments, it seems that we are moving toward a fifth developmental phase in health care delivery.

TRENDS IN HEALTH CARE SPENDING

Much has been written in the popular and scientific literature about the costs of US health care and how society makes decisions about using available and scarce resources. Given that economics in general and health care economics in particular are concerned with resource use and decision making, any discussion of the economics of health care must consider past and current health care spending. The trends shown here reflect public and private decisions about health care and health care delivery in the past. Spending from that time reflects past decision making; likewise, past decisions reflect the values and beliefs held by society and policymakers that underlie policymaking at any given point in time.

According to the NCHS (2016), national health expenditures reached $3 trillion in 2014. This is in contrast to the $700 billion spent on health care in 1990 (NCHS, 2016). The increase in health spending, from $1.6 trillion in 2001 to $1.8 trillion in 2002, was the largest single-year jump in US history (Centers for Medicare [CMS], 2014a). The CMS (2014b) predicts total US health spending in 2024 will be $5.4 trillion. Health spending has outpaced increases in the gross domestic product (GDP), accounting for 17.5% of the GDP by 2014 (NCHS, 2016). This means that $17.50 of every $100 spent in 2014 was for health care. The CMS (2015a) relates the spending growth to major coverage expansions under the ACA, particularly for Medicaid and private health insurance. The effect of this economic growth represents a large increase in contrast to the approximately 13% GDP spent on health care between 1992 and 2001.

Fig. 8.3 shows a breakdown of the distribution of health care expenses for 2014, and Table 8.1 shows the growth in US health care expenditures between 1960 and 2014 (NCHS, 2016). Spending for health care increased from approximately $27 billion in 1960 to over $3 trillion in 2014. These numbers reflect per-person spending amounts of $143 in 1960 and over $9000 in 2014. In 2014 approximately $248 was spent per person for public health activities (NCHS, 2016).

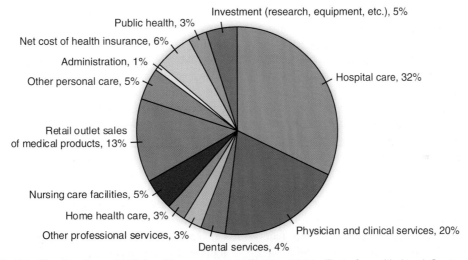

FIG. 8.3 Distribution of US health care expenditures, 2014. (Data from National Center for Health Statistics: *Health, United States, 2015, with special feature on racial and ethnic health disparities,* Hyattsville, MD, 2016, US Government Printing Office. Table 94, p. 295.)

TABLE 8.1 Health Care Expenditures: 1960 to 2014

Calendar Year	Total Health Expenditures (in billions of dollars)	Total Health Expenditures per Capita per Person (in dollars)	Percent of Gross Domestic Product
1960	$26.7	$146	5.0
1970	$74.6	$355	6.9
1980	$255.3	$1108	8.9
1990	$721.4	$2843	12.1
2000	$1369.7	$4857	13.3
2009	$2496.4	$8147	17.3
2012	$2799.0	$8927	17.3
2013	$2879.9	$9115	17.3
2014	$3031.3	$9523	17.5

Data from National Center for Health Statistics: *Health, United States, 2015, with special feature on racial and ethnic health disparities,* Hyattsville, MD, 2016, US Government Printing Office. Table 93, p. 293-294.

The largest portions of health care expenses were for hospital care and physician/clinical services, respectively, in 2014 (NCHS, 2016). Only a small fraction of total health care dollars was spent on home health, public health, and research and construction in 2014. The trends over time indicate that this is an ongoing pattern of spending.

FACTORS INFLUENCING HEALTH CARE COSTS

Health economists, providers, payers, and politicians have explored a variety of explanations for the rapid rate of increase in health expenses in contrast to population growth. That individuals have, over time, consumed more health care is not an adequate explanation. The following factors are frequently cited as having caused the increases in total and per capita health care spending since 1960: inflation, changes in population demographics, technology and intensity of services, and increased health coverage for individuals from the ACA (CMS, 2015b; NCHS, 2012).

DEMOGRAPHICS AFFECTING HEALTH CARE

A major demographic change under way in the United States is the aging of the population. Population changes are also affected by illnesses such as acquired immunodeficiency syndrome and by chemical dependency epidemics. These changes have implications for providers' health services, and they affect the overall costs of health care. Because the majority of older adults and other special populations receive services through publicly funded programs, the growing health needs among these populations have a great impact on costs, payments, and providers associated with Medicaid and Medicare programs. As the population ages and the Baby Boom generation ages and retires, federal expenses for Social Security will increase (Congressional Budget Office [CBO], 2015). At 78 million strong, the oldest of the Boomers—born between 1946 and 1964—are already making unsustainable demands on federal entitlement programs such as Medicare and Medicaid.

In its *Long-Term Outlook for Major Federal Health Care Programs,* the CBO reports that spending for those programs will account for about 8% each of GDP in 2040 (CBO, 2015).

By 2035, in the absence of change, spending for Medicare alone (which is more likely to be affected by aging Boomers) will have more than doubled to 8%, and by 2080 it will have grown to 15% unless changes are implemented.

The aging population is expected to affect health services more than any other demographic factor. In 1950 more than half of the US population was under 30 years of age; in 1994, half of the population was 34 years of age or older. In 1990 individuals 65 and older made up 4.1% of the population; in 2011, they accounted for 13.3% of the population, or more than 1 in 8 Americans. By 2050, it is estimated that they will account for up to 20% of the population. In addition, the number of individuals 85 and older is expected to double between 1990 and 2050 because the population is living longer, healthier lives (USDHHS, 2012).

Although many older adults are independent and active, they are likely to experience multiple chronic conditions that may become disabling. They are admitted to hospitals three times more often than the general population, and their average length of stay is more than 3 days longer than the overall average. They visit physicians more often and make up a larger percentage of nursing home residents than the general population (CDC, 2013; NCHS, 2012).

Life expectancy and health status have been increasing in the United States. However, older adults continue to consume a large portion of financial resources. Health care providers are concerned about the growth in the older adult population because public funding sources, such as Medicare, have not been increasing their reimbursement rates sufficiently to cover inflation, and thus, providers collect a smaller amount for visits by older adult clients each year.

The aging of the population also spurs concerns about funding their health care because of changes in the proportion of employed individuals to retired individuals. Persons in the workforce pay the majority of income taxes and all Social Security payroll taxes. The funding base for Medicare decreases as the population ages, as retirement rates increase, and as the numbers in the workforce decrease. As a result, some policymakers believe that Medicare and system reforms are needed to ensure adequate financing and delivery of health care services to an aging population (US Law, 2010).

Health policy reform options being considered include increased age limits to become eligible for Medicare, means testing (i.e., determining a lack of financial resources) for Medicare eligibility, increased coverage for long-term care insurance, increased incentives for prevention, and less expensive and more efficient delivery arrangements and care settings (e.g., managed care arrangements). Meanwhile, the debate continues over how to best handle the future funding of the growing Medicare program. One example of a policy change to reduce the Medicare program burden is the prescription plan (Medicare D) passed by Congress in 2005 and effective in January 2006. This plan, although complicated, requires most Medicare recipients to provide a copayment for prescription medications. Although controversial, the plan is thought to provide a positive impact for the elderly who could not afford to pay for their prescriptions while reducing the cost burden for those who had to pay full price for prescriptions (US Law, 2003).

TECHNOLOGY AND INTENSITY

The introduction of new technology enhances the delivery of care, but it also has the potential to increase the costs of care. As new and more complex technology is introduced into the system, the cost is typically high. However, clients often demand access to the technology, and providers want to use it. In an effort to keep health care costs down, however, payers have attempted to restrict the use of certain technologies. For example, the drug Viagra, developed for the treatment of impotence by Pfizer Pharmaceuticals, is an example of a controversial technological advance that, as soon as it was available to the public, was in high demand and prescribed by providers. Initially, use was restricted by payers because of cost. It is now covered by health insurance plans.

The adoption of new technology demands investment in personnel, equipment, and facilities. Furthermore, new technology adds to administrative costs, especially if the federal government provides financial coverage for the service or is involved in regulating the technology. Table 8.2 outlines federal policy that has had an impact on technology and the cost of health care over time.

CHRONIC ILLNESS

Chronic illness is a new factor affecting health care spending. Chronic disease accounted for 70% of deaths in 2010 (CDC, 2016). Using Medical Expenditure Panel Survey (MEPS) data, chronic medical conditions are identified by those costing the most, the number of bed days, work-loss days, and activity impairments. The most chronic medical condition was stroke.

TABLE 8.2 Federal Regulations Contributing to Technology and Cost Controls

Year	Federal Regulation
1906	Prescription drug regulation (PL 59-384): Pure Food and Drugs Act , now the Food, Drug, and Cosmetic Act
1935	Social Security Act (PL 74-271): Provides grants-in-aid to states for maternal and child care, aid to dependent and crippled children, and aid to the blind and aged
1938	Food, Drug, and Cosmetic Act (PL 75-540): Establishes federal FDA protections for drug safety and protections for misbranded goods, drugs, and cosmetics
1946	Hill-Burton Act (PL 79-725): Enacts Hospital Survey and Construction Act, providing national direct support for community hospitals; establishes rudimentary standards for construction and planning; establishes community service obligation
1954	Hill-Burton Act amended (PL 83-482): Expands the scope of the program for nursing homes, rehabilitation facilities, chronic disease hospitals, and diagnostic or treatment centers
1963	Community Mental Health and Mental Retardation Center Construction Act (PL 88-164)
1965	Medicare Title 18; Medicaid Title 19 (PL 89-97): Amendments to Social Security Act provide Medicare and Medicaid to support health care services for certain groups
1966	Comprehensive Health Planning Act (PL 89-749): For health services, personnel, and facilities in federal, state, and local partnerships
1971	President Nixon introduces the concept of health maintenance organizations (HMOs) as the cornerstone of his administration's national health insurance proposal
1972	Social Security Act amendments (PL 92-603): Extend coverage to include new treatment technologies for end-stage renal disease; provide for professional standards review organizations to review the appropriateness of hospital care for Medicare and Medicaid recipients
1973	Health Maintenance Organization Act (PL 93-222): Provides assistance and expansion for HMOs
1975	National Health Planning and Resources Development Act (PL 93-641): Designates local health system areas and establishes a national certificate-of-need (CON) program to limit major health care expansion at local and state levels
1978	Medicare End-Stage Renal Disease Amendment: Provides payment for home dialysis and kidney transplantation; Health Services Research, Health Statistics, and Health Care Technology Act establishes a national council on health care technology to develop standards for use
1981	Omnibus Budget Reconciliation Act of 1981 (PL 97-351): Consolidates 26 health programs into four block grants (preventives, health services, primary care, and maternal and child health)
1982	Tax Equity and Fiscal Responsibilities Act (PL 97-248): Seeks to control costs by limiting hospital costs per discharge adjusted to hospital case mix
1983	Amended Social Security Act (PL 98-21): Establishes a new Medicare hospital prospective payment system based on diagnosis-related groups (DRGs)
1986	1974 Health Planning and Resource Development Act (PL 93-641): Moves CON program to states
1989	Omnibus Reconciliation Act of 1989 (PL 101-239): Creates a physician resource-based fee schedule to be implemented by 1992, with emphasis on high-tech specialties of surgery; creates the Agency for Health Care Policy and Research to research the effectiveness of medical and nursing services, interventions, and technologies
1990	Ryan White Care Act (PL 101-381): Authorizes formula-based and competitive supplemental grants to cities and states for HIV-related outpatient medical services
1990	Safe Medical Devices Act (PL 101-629): Gives the FDA authority to regulate medical devices and diagnostic products
1993	Omnibus Budget Reconciliation Act (OBRA 93) (PL 103-66): Cuts Medicare funding and reduces payments to skilled nursing facilities; provides support for immunizations for children on Medicaid
1996	Health Insurance Portability and Accountability Act: Protects health insurance coverage for laid-off or displaced workers
1997	Balanced Budget Act of 1997: Creates a new program for states to offer health insurance to children in low-income and uninsured families
1998	PL 105-33: Authorizes third-party reimbursement for Medicare Part B services for nurse practitioners and clinical nurse specialists
2003	Medicaid Nursing Incentive Act (HR 2295): Expands direct reimbursement to all nurse practitioners and clinical nurse specialists and recognizes specialized services offered by advanced practice registered nurses, such as primary-care case management, pain management, and mental health services
2006	Medicare Part D: Provides a plan for prescription payments
2010	Patient Protection and Affordable Care Act passed and signed into law on March 23, 2010

FINANCING OF HEALTH CARE

Against the backdrop of today's chronic conditions, it must be appreciated that financing for health care has evolved through the 20th century from a system supported primarily by consumers to a system financed by third-party payers (public and private). From 1960 to 2014, the percentage of third-party public insurance payments increased, and the percentage of out-of-pocket payments declined (NCHS, 2016). Combined state and federal governments paid the most in 2014 (NCHS, 2016).

PUBLIC SUPPORT

The US federal government became involved in health care financing for population groups early in its history. In 1798 the federal government created the Marine Hospital Service to provide medical care for sick and disabled sailors and protect the nation's borders against the importing of disease through seaports. The Marine Hospital Service is considered the first national health insurance plan in the United States. The National Health Board was established in 1879 and was later renamed the US Public Health Service (PHS). Within the PHS, the federal government developed a public health liaison with state and local health departments for the purpose of controlling communicable diseases and improving sanitation. Additional health programs were also developed to meet obligations to federal workers and their families within the PHS, the Department of Defense, and the Veterans Administration.

Medicare and Medicaid, two federal programs administered by the CMS, account for the majority of public health care spending. Table 8.3 compares these programs. The CMS is the federal regulatory agency within the USDHHS that is responsible for overseeing and monitoring Medicare and Medicaid spending. This agency routinely collects and reports actual health care use and spending and projects future spending trends. Through these programs, the federal government purchases health care services for population groups through independent health care systems, such as managed care organizations, private practice physicians, and hospitals.

Medicare

The Medicare program, established in Title XVIII of the Social Security Act of 1965, provides hospital insurance and medical insurance to persons aged 65 years and older, to permanently disabled persons, and to persons with end-stage renal disease—altogether approximately 46 million people in 2013 (CMS, 2014b). Medicare has two parts: Part A (hospital insurance) covers hospital care, home care, and skilled nursing care (limited); Part B (noninstitutional care insurance) covers "medically necessary" services, such as health care provider services, outpatient care, home health, and other medical services, such as diagnostic services and physiotherapy. In 1999 a program titled Medicare Advantage was added to the program (Part C). This is an option that can be chosen for additional coverage. This option includes both Part A and Part B services. The Part C plans are coordinated care plans that include health maintenance organizations (HMOs), private fee-for-service plans, and medical savings accounts (MSAs). Part C provides for all health care coverage costs after a high deductible (CMS, 2014b). Medicare Part D was added to the program in 2006 to provide prescription drug coverage.

Medicare Part A is primarily financed by a federal payroll tax that is paid by employers and employees. The proceeds from this tax go to the Hospital Insurance Trust Fund, which is managed by the CMS. Part A coverage is available to all persons who are eligible to receive Medicare. Older adults account for the majority of individuals eligible. There is concern about the future of the Medicare Trust Fund, because projected expenses may be more than the resources of the trust fund. Payments to hospitals for covered services have been and continue to be

TABLE 8.3 Comparison of Medicare and Medicaid Program Features		
Feature	Medicare	Medicaid
Where to obtain information	Local Social Security Administration office	State welfare office
Recipients	Client is 65 years of age or older, is disabled, or has end-stage renal disease	Specified low-income and needy, children, aged, blind, and/or disabled; those eligible to receive federally assisted income
Type of program	Insurance	Insurance
Government affiliation	Federal	All states
Availability	All states	All states
Financing of hospital insurance	Medicare Trust Fund, mandatory payroll deduction, recipient deductibles, trust fund interest	Federal and state governments
Financing of medical insurance	Recipient premium payments; general revenue, US Treasury	Federal and state governments
Types of coverage	Inpatient and outpatient hospital services, skilled nursing facilities (SNFs), limited home health services	Inpatient and outpatient hospital services; prenatal care; vaccines for children; physician, dental, nurse practitioner, and nurse-midwife services; SNF services for persons 21 years of age or older; family services; rural health clinic

From US Department of Health and Human Services, Centers for Medicare and Medicaid Services: Medicare and you, Baltimore, MD, 2016, USDHHS.

higher than fund growth. Thus the Medicare reimbursement policy has been changing in an attempt to control increasing hospital costs. Part A requires a deductible from recipients for the first 60 days of services with a reduced deductible for 61 to 90 days of service, based on a rate equal to a 1-day stay in the hospital. The deductible has increased as daily hospital costs have increased. For skilled nursing facility care, persons pay nothing for the first 20 days and a cost per day for days 21 through 100. After 100 days, persons must pay the total cost for care (CMS, n.d.a). The person pays zero for hospice care and home health.

The medical insurance package, Part B, is a supplemental (voluntary) program available to all Medicare-eligible persons for a monthly premium ($104.90 minimum in 2016) (CMS, n.d.b). The majority of Medicare-covered persons elect this coverage. Part B provides coverage for services (other than hospital, physician care, outpatient hospital care, outpatient physical therapy, and home health care) that are not covered by Part A, such as laboratory services, ambulance transportation, prostheses, equipment, and some supplies. After a deductible, up to 80% of reasonable charges are paid for these services. For mental health services, generally, 80% of the costs are paid (CMS, n.d.b). Part B resembles the major medical insurance coverage of private insurance carriers. Fig. 8.4 shows the total expenses of the Medicare program from 1970 to 2014.

Since the passing of the Medicare amendments to the Social Security Act in 1965, the cost of Medicare has increased dramatically. Hospital care continues to be the major factor contributing to Medicare costs. However, because of shorter hospital stays, home health and nursing home costs have increased dramatically. As a result of rising health costs, Congress passed a law in 1983 that radically changed Medicare's method of payment for hospital services. In 1983 federal legislation (PL 98-21) mandated an end to cost-plus reimbursement by Medicare and instituted a 3-year transition to a prospective payment system (PPS) for inpatient hospital services. The purpose of the new hospital payment scheme was to shift the cost incentives away from provision of more care and toward more efficient services. The basis for prospective reimbursement is the 468 diagnosis-related groups (DRGs). Also, the Balanced Budget Act of 1997

determined that payments to Medicare skilled nursing facilities would be made on the basis of the PPS, effective July 1, 1998. The PPS payment rates cover skilled nursing facility services, including routine, ancillary, and capital-related costs (CMS, 2013). In 2001 CMS developed PPS DRGs for home health with Health Insurance Prospective Payment System (HIPPS) codes.

In 2010 the average out-of-pocket amount spent for services for Medicare beneficiaries was approximately $4700 (KFF, 2014). The average out-of-pocket spending is skewed to beneficiaries who are older or have declining health. This is because of the limits in Medicare coverage, including certain preventive care, and the limited number of physicians and agencies that accept Medicare and Medicaid payment. Older adults who do not have supplemental insurance must cover the difference between the Medicare payment and the additional costs for services.

Medicaid

The Medicaid program, Title XIX of the Social Security Act of 1965, provides financial assistance to states and counties to pay for medical services for poor older adults, the blind, the disabled, and families with dependent children. The Medicaid program is jointly sponsored and financed with matching funds from the federal and state governments. In 2015 more than 58 million people were enrolled in Medicaid (CMS, 2016a). Medicaid expenditures from 1987 to 2014 are shown in Fig. 8.5. Since the institution of Medicaid, full payment has been provided for five types of services (NCHS, 2016):

1. Inpatient and outpatient hospital care
2. Laboratory and radiology services
3. Physician services
4. Skilled nursing care at home or in a nursing home for people older than 21 years of age
5. Early periodic screening, diagnosis, and treatment (EPS-DT) for people younger than 21 years of age

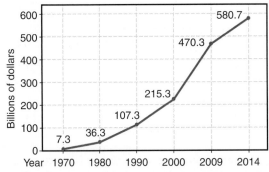

FIG. 8.4 Medicare expenditures for selected years from 1970 to 2014. (Data from National Center for Health Statistics: *Health, United States, 2015, with special feature on racial and ethnic health disparities,* Hyattsville, MD, 2016, US Government Printing Office. Table 95, p. 297.)

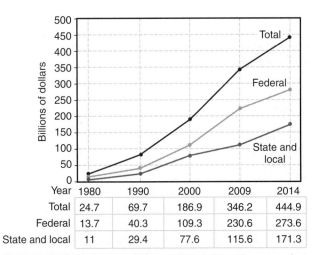

Year	1980	1990	2000	2009	2014
Total	24.7	69.7	186.9	346.2	444.9
Federal	13.7	40.3	109.3	230.6	273.6
State and local	11	29.4	77.6	115.6	171.3

FIG. 8.5 Medicaid expenditures for selected years from 1980 to 2014. (Data from National Center for Health Statistics: *Health, United States, 2015, with special feature on racial and ethnic health disparities,* Hyattsville, MD, 2016, US Government Printing Office. Table 95, p. 297.)

The 1972 Social Security amendments added family planning to the list of full-pay services. States can choose to add prescriptions, dental services, eyeglasses, intermediate care facilities, and coverage for the medically indigent as program options. By law, the medically indigent are required to pay a monthly premium.

Any state participating in the Medicaid program is required to provide the six basic services to persons who are below state poverty income levels. Optional programs are provided at the discretion of each state. In 1989 changes in Medicaid required states to provide care for children younger than 6 years of age and to pregnant women under 133% of the poverty level. For example, if the poverty level were $12,000, a pregnant woman could have a household income as high as $16,000 and still be eligible to receive care under Medicaid. These changes also provided for pediatric and family nurse practitioner reimbursement. In the 1990s, states were allowed to petition the federal government for a waiver. If the waiver was approved, the states could use their Medicaid monies for programs other than the six basic services. The first waiver to be approved was given to Oregon for their health care reform plan. Other states have received waivers to develop Medicaid-managed care programs for special populations. The 2010 health care reform plan provides for new approaches to offering Medicaid services and incentives for states to offer Medicaid services rather than through the waiver option as described previously (US Law, 2010).

The major expense categories for the Medicaid program have historically been long-term care and acute care. When combined, these two categories account today for 96% of all costs to the program (KFF, 2015b).

PUBLIC HEALTH

Most public government agencies operate on an annual budget, and they plan for costs by estimating salaries, expenses, and costs of services for a year. Public health agencies, such as health departments and the Special Supplemental Nutrition Program for Women, Infants, and Children (WIC), receive primary funding from taxes, with additional money for select goods and services through private third-party payers. Selected public health programs receive reimbursement for services through grants given by the federal government to states for prenatal and child health; through Medicare and Medicaid for home health, nursing homes, WIC programs, and EPS-DT; and through collecting of fees on a sliding scale for select client services, such as immunizations (Trust for America's Health, 2014).

In 2014, only 3% of all health care–related federal funds were expended for federal health programs such as WIC, in contrast to 97% for other types of health and illness care (such as hospital and physician services) (NCHS, 2016). In addition to this 3% allotment, public health funds also come through states and territorial health agencies. State and local governments contributed 31% to public and general assistance, maternal and child health, public health activities, and other related services in 2013 (Pew Charitable Trust, 2015).

OTHER PUBLIC SUPPORT

The federal government finances health services for military persons and dependents through TRICARE, the Veterans Administration, and the Indian Health Service (IHS). These programs are very important in providing needed health care services to these populations (see additional information in Chapters 3 and 7). TRICARE is the Department of Defense's health care program for members of the uniformed services, their families, and their survivors. TRICARE also offers health care programs for retired service members, including TRICARE Pharmacy, TRICARE Dental (United Concordia), and TRICARE for Life.

PRIVATE SUPPORT

Private health care payer sources include insurance, employers, managed care, and individuals. Although insurance and consumers have been prominent health care payment sources for some time, the role of employers, managed care, and consumers became increasingly prominent and powerful during the first decade of the 21st century, particularly as concerns grew about the use and changing nature of health insurance.

Evolution of Health Insurance

Insurance for health care was first offered for the private sector in 1847 by a commercial insurance company. The purpose of the insurance was to provide security and protection when health care services were needed by individuals. The idea behind insurance was that it provided security, guaranteeing (within certain limits) monies to pay for health care services to

---

EVIDENCE-BASED PRACTICE

This retrospective study examined the incidence, costs, and factors associated with potentially avoidable hospitalizations (PAHs) in dually eligible Medicare and Medicaid beneficiaries. This population was selected due to their complex clinical needs and high costs of care. PAHs were defined by an expert panel that identified conditions and associated diagnostic related groups (DRGs) that can often be prevented or safely and effectively managed in a skilled nursing facility or home- and community-based services. Seventy-eight percent of the PAHs resulted from five conditions: pneumonia, congestive heart failure, urinary tract infections, dehydration, and chronic obstructive pulmonary disease. The total costs of these hospitalizations were $3 billion for Medicare beneficiaries and $463 million for Medicaid beneficiaries. A sensitivity analysis found that between 77,000 and 260,000 hospitalizations and between $625 million and $1.9 billion in expenditures could be avoided each year in this population.

Nurse Use

Community health nursing initiatives, such as health education and case management, could significantly reduce the number of hospital admissions in this population. Such interventions could greatly reduce the negative health effects and quality of life for this population, as well as reduce the high health care costs for this group.

Modified from Walsh EG, Wiener JM, Haber S, et al: Potentially avoidable hospitalizations of dually eligible Medicare and Medicaid beneficiaries from nursing facility and home- and community-based services waiver program. *J Am Geriatr Soc* 60:821–829, 2012.

offset potential financial losses from unexpected illness or injury related to accidents, catastrophic communicable diseases (such as smallpox and scarlet fever), and recurring (but unexpected) chronic illnesses.

The economic depression of the 1930s, rising medical costs, and the need to spread financial risk across communities spurred the development of the third-party payment system. The system began as a major industry in the 1930s with the Blue Cross system, which initially provided prepayment for hospital care. In 1939 Blue Shield created plans to provide physician payment. The Blue Cross plans began as tax-free, nonprofit organizations established under special enabling legislation in various states.

In the 1940s and 1950s, hospital and medical-surgical coverage increased. Employee group coverage appeared, and profit-making commercial insurance underwriters began offering health insurance packages with competitive premiums. Premium competition, the offering of health insurance as a fringe benefit, and the use of health insurance as a negotiable collective bargaining item led to an increase in covered benefits, first-dollar coverage for medical care expenses, and increased employer-paid premiums. In turn, these factors pushed up insurance premium costs and health care costs and enabled insurance plans to cover high-cost segments of the population (the aged, poor, or disabled).

The health needs of high-risk populations led to the passage of Medicare and Medicaid legislation. These and other national health programs targeted health care coverage for specific population groups. Because these programs directed additional money into the health care system to subsidize care, there were financial incentives to encourage the provision of services (i.e., the more services that were ordered, the greater the amount of money that would be received). Other incentives were related to the use of services by clients (i.e., the more available the payment was for services that might otherwise have gone unused, the more services that were requested).

Employers

Since the beginning of Blue Cross and Blue Shield, health insurance has been tied to employment and the business sector. This tie was strengthened during World War II to compensate, attract, and retain employees. Since that time, employers have played the major role in determining health insurance benefits. However, with the economic downturn in 2008, employers began to reduce their health insurance benefits or return the cost of insurance premiums to the employee.

Before the growth of insurance (i.e., before 1930 and the beginning of Blue Cross), the health care consumer had more influence over health care costs because payment was out of pocket. Consumers made decisions about how they would spend their money, making certain tradeoffs—for example, about the type of health care they were willing to buy and how much they would pay. Entering the system was restricted in large part to those who could afford to pay for care or who could find care financed through charitable and philanthropic organizations. With the beginning of the insurance (or third-party payer) system, health care costs were set by payers, and

they determined the type of care or service that would be offered and its price. This began to change somewhat in the 1980s with the increased use of managed care.

As the cost of health insurance has increased, some employers, in an effort to bypass the costs established by insurers, have found it less costly to self-insure. The employer does this by contracting directly with providers to obtain health care services for employees rather than going through health insurance companies. Some large businesses directly employ onsite providers for care delivery or offer onsite wellness programs. These programs within the private sector offer opportunities for nurses to provide wellness programs and health assessments to screen and monitor employees and their families. This move to self-insure has resulted in savings to companies and has reduced overall sick care costs (Knickman and Kovner, 2015).

Individuals

In 2014, individuals paid only approximately 13% of total health expenditures out of pocket (NCHS, 2016). However, these figures do not reflect the amount of money the consumer pays in taxes to finance government-supported programs such as Medicare and Medicaid, insurance premiums, and money paid for supplemental insurance to cover the gaps in a primary health insurance policy or Medicare.

The average monthly cost for private health insurance has increased greatly through the years. Premiums reflect a shift of the health care cost burden from employers to employees as the percent of employer contributions to health care declines. The decrease in employer contribution to health insurance premiums parallels the economic downturn of 2008, the move away from traditional insurance plans, and the move toward managed care plans or self-insurance plans by both small and large employers or toward dropping health insurance as a benefit. In 2008, 2 million people lost employer health insurance coverage (KFF, 2009).

Managed Care Arrangements

Managed care is the term used for a variety of health care arrangements that integrate the financing and the delivery of health care. Managed care offers an array of services to purchasers, such as employers or Medicare, for a set fee. This fee, in turn, is used to pay providers through preset arrangements for services delivered to individuals who are covered (NCHS, 2016). The concept of managed care is based on the notion that the use of costly care could be reduced if consumers had access to care and services that would prevent illness through consumer education and health maintenance. Therefore managed care uses disease prevention, health promotion, wellness, and consumer education (Knickman and Kovner, 2015).

Two common types of managed care organizations are health maintenance organizations (HMOs) and preferred provider organizations (PPOs). Box 8.1 provides an overview of HMOs and PPOs. Although they seem relatively new to many clients of care, HMOs have actually been around since the 1940s. The Health Maintenance Organization Act

---

BOX 8.1 Types of Managed Care Organizations

Health Maintenance Organization (HMO)

An HMO is a provider arrangement whereby comprehensive care is provided to plan members for a fixed, "per member per month" fee. Common features include the following:

- Capitation
- Use of designated providers
- Point-of-service care, or receiving care from nondesignated plan providers
- One of the following models:
  - Staff model, in which physicians are HMO employees
  - Group model, in which a physician group practice contracts with the HMO to provide care
  - Individual practice association (IPA), in which the HMO contracts with physicians in solo, small group practices, or physician networks to provide care
  - Mixed model, in which the HMO uses a combination group or IPA arrangement

Preferred Provider Organization (PPO)

A PPO is a provider arrangement in which predetermined rates are established for services to be delivered to members. Common features include the following:

- Hospital and physician providers
- Discounted rate setting
- Financial incentives to encourage plan members to select PPO providers
- Expedited claims payment to providers

From Folland S, Goodman AC, Stano M: *The economics of health and health care: Pearson International Edition,* New York, 2016, Routledge; and National Center for Health Statistics: *Health, United States, 2015, with special feature on racial and ethnic health disparities,* Hyattsville, MD, 2016, US Government Printing Office.

was enacted in 1972, and since that time the number of individuals receiving care through HMOs and other types of managed care organizations has increased considerably. Managed care is based, in part, on the principles of managed competition. Managed competition was introduced in health care in the late 1980s and early 1990s to address the increasing costs of health care and to introduce quality into the forefront of discussions. Managed competition simply means that clients make decisions and choose the health care services they want on the basis of the quality or reputation of the service. To make decisions, they use knowledge and information about health care problems, care, and providers, and they look at the costs of care. However, health care is a complex market and not one in which information about health care, health problems, and the costs of care is easy to obtain.

Medical Savings Accounts

Another insurance reform discussion at the political level concerns MSAs. MSAs are touted as a way of turning health care decision-making control over to the individuals receiving care. MSAs are tax-exempt accounts available to individuals who work for small companies, usually established through a bank or insurance company, that enable the individuals to save money for future medical needs and expenses (Internal

Revenue Service, 2016). Money is contributed to an MSA by the employer, and the initial money put into an MSA does not come out of taxable income. Also, interest earned in MSAs is tax-free, and unused MSA money can be held in the account from year to year until the money is used. MSAs, in theory, would allow individuals to make tradeoffs between cost and quality and would require that individuals become knowledgeable about health care, become involved in health care decision making, and take responsibility for the decisions made. Providers, in turn, must be willing to provide and disclose information to individuals and give up control of health care decision making. The Health Insurance and Portability and Accountability Act (HIPAA) and MSAs are examples of health insurance reform efforts, and these efforts will very likely remain at the forefront of political discussions for some time to come.

HEALTH CARE PAYMENT SYSTEMS

Several methods have been used by public and private sources to pay health care providers for health care services. These include retrospective reimbursement and prospective reimbursement for paying health care organizations and fee-for-service and capitation for paying health care practitioners (Knickman and Kovner, 2015).

PAYING HEALTH CARE ORGANIZATIONS

Retrospective reimbursement is the traditional reimbursement method. Fees for the delivery of health care services in an organization are set after services are delivered (Knickman and Kovner, 2015).

Prospective reimbursement, or payment, is a more recent method of paying an organization, in which the third-party payer establishes the amount of money that will be paid for the delivery of a particular service before offering the services to the client (Knickman and Kovner, 2015). Since the establishment of prospective payment in Medicare in 1983, private insurance has followed by requiring preapprovals before clients can receive certain services, such as hospital admission or mammograms, more than once per year (Knickman and Kovner, 2015).

Similarly, ambulatory care services received by Medicare recipients are classified into ambulatory payment classes, which reflect the type of ambulatory clinical services received and resources required (CMS, 2016b). Prospective payment to skilled nursing facilities is also adjusted for case mix and geographic variations (CMS, 2013).

Growth in contracting, or competitive bidding, for health care services, intended to create incentives for providers to compete on price, has occurred as managed care has increased in health care markets. For example, contracting has been used by states to provide Medicaid services to eligible persons. Hospitals and other health care providers who do not have a contract with the state to provide services are not eligible to receive Medicaid payments for client care. Managed care organizations also use this approach to negotiate with health care organizations, such as hospitals, for coverage of services to be provided to covered enrollees, often called covered lives.

PAYING HEALTH CARE PRACTITIONERS

The traditional method of paying health care practitioners is known as fee-for-service payment (Knickman and Kovner, 2015) and is like the retrospective method just described. The practitioner determines the costs of providing a service, delivers the service to a client, submits a bill for the delivered service to a third-party payer, and is paid by the third-party payer. Historically, Medicare, Medicaid, and private insurance companies have used this method of reimbursing physicians.

Capitation is similar to prospective reimbursement for health care organizations. Specifically, third-party payers determine the amount that practitioners will be paid for a unit of care, such as a client visit, before the delivery of the service, thereby placing a limit on the amount of reimbursement received per patient (Knickman and Kovner, 2015). In contrast to a fee-for-service arrangement, in which the practitioner determines both the services that will be provided to clients and the charges for those services, practitioners being paid through capitation are given the rate they will be paid for a client's care, regardless of specific services provided. Therefore, for example, physicians and nurse practitioners are aware, in advance, of the payment they will receive to perform a routine, uncomplicated physical examination or a more complex, detailed physical examination, diagnosis, and treatment (Knickman and Kovner, 2015).

In capitated arrangements, physicians and other practitioners are paid a set amount to provide care to a given client or group of clients for a set period and amount of money. This arrangement, typically used by managed care organizations, is one in which the practitioner contracts with the managed care organization to provide health care services to plan members for a preset and negotiated fee. The agreed-on fee is negotiated between the practitioner and the managed care organization before the delivery of services and is set at a discounted rate, and the practitioner and managed care organization come to a legal agreement, or contract, for the delivery and payment of services. The managed care organization pays the predetermined fee to the practitioner, often before the delivery of services, to provide care to plan members for a set period (Knickman and Kovner, 2015).

Reimbursement for Nursing Services

Historically, practitioners eligible to receive reimbursement for health care services included physicians only. However, nurses who function in certain capacities, such as NPs, CNSs, and midwives, also provide primary care to clients and receive reimbursement for their services. Being recognized as primary-care providers and eligible to receive reimbursement has not been an easy achievement.

Hospital nursing care costs have traditionally been included as part of the overall patient room charge and reimbursed as such. Other agencies, such as home health care agencies, include nursing care costs with administrative costs, supplies, and equipment costs. Nursing organizations, such as the American Nurses Association, have long advocated that nursing care should become a separate budget item in all organizations so that cost studies can show the efficiency and effectiveness of the nursing profession.

Spurred by efforts to control the costs of medical care, effective January 1, 1998, NPs and CNSs were granted third-party reimbursement for Medicare Part B services only, under Public Law 105-33 (American Nurses Association [ANA], 1999). This new law set reimbursement for NPs and CNSs at 85% of physician rates for the same service, an extension of previous legislation that allowed the same reimbursement rate to NPs and CNSs practicing in rural areas (Buppert, 1999). This law was passed after years of work in this area, including research documenting NP and CNS contributions to health care delivery and client outcomes, and after active lobbying efforts by professional nursing organizations. Reimbursement for these nurses has not changed to any extent since the 1990s.

In addition, data about the cost/benefit ratio, efficiency, and effectiveness of nursing care in general have been collected. In about 2012, more than 250 nurse-managed clinics provide health care services to individuals in the United States who might not otherwise have access to health care, such as older adults, the homeless, and schoolchildren (Esperat et al, 2012).

All of these events have moved the discipline toward more autonomy in nursing practice and are serving as a means for evaluating and documenting nurses' contributions to health care delivery. In 2014 it was reported that the number of nurse-managed clinics had grown to 500, largely due to the passing of the ACA (Toner, 2014).

ECONOMICS AND THE FUTURE OF NURSING PRACTICE

Nurses must plan for future changes in health care financing by becoming aware of the costs of nursing services, identifying aspects of care in which cost savings can be safely achieved, and developing knowledge on how nursing practice affects and is affected by the principles of economics. Nursing must continue to focus on improving the overall health of the nation, defining its contribution to the health of the nation, deriving the value of nursing care, and ensuring its economic viability within the health care marketplace. Nurses must effect changes in the health care system by providing leadership in developing new models of care delivery that provide effective, high-quality care and by assuming a greater role in evaluating client care and nurse performance. It is through their leadership that nurses will contribute to improved decision making about allocating scarce health care resources and will promote primary prevention as an answer to improve many of the current population-level health outcomes.

▶ APPLYING CONTENT TO PRACTICE

This chapter focuses on examining the balance of interest within society and health care, which will continue to shift toward a focus on quality, safety, and elimination of health disparities through public- and private-sector partnerships. Health care system concerns of the 21st century are expected to focus on examining the quality of health care relative to the costs of care delivered, reduction in disparities, access to care, and health care reform. These changes will result from continued efforts of both the public and private sectors to reform the US health care system. The current era of health care delivery will be noted as a time of vast changes in all sectors of health care delivery.

Nurses will want to plan for future changes in health care financing by becoming aware of the costs of nursing services and identifying aspects of care where cost savings can be safely achieved. Nursing must continue to focus on improving the overall health of the nation, defining its contribution to the health of the nation, deriving the value of nursing care, and ensuring its economic viability within the health care marketplace. Nurses must effect changes in the health care system by providing leadership in developing new models of care delivery that provide effective, high-quality care and by assuming a greater role in evaluating client care and nurse performance. This chapter will assist the reader in identifying how, through their leadership, nurses will contribute to improved decision making about allocating scarce health care resources and promoting primary prevention as an answer to improve many of the current population-level health outcomes.

▮ PRACTICE APPLICATION

Connie, a nursing student, has identified a caseload of five families in a chronic disease program offered by the local public health department. She is interested in assessing the costs of care to her clients and to the agency. Connie approaches the public health nurse administrator and asks the following questions:

A. How is the agency reimbursed for chronic disease management?

B. Does the client have a responsibility to pay for services?
C. Are nursing care costs known?
D. Are services rationed to clients?
E. What effect will the chronic disease management program have on the community population?

Answers can be found on the Evolve website.

▮ REMEMBER THIS!

- From 1800 to the 1980s, the US health care delivery system experienced three developmental stages, with different emphases on health care economics. In 1985 the health care delivery system entered a fourth developmental stage.
- Four basic components provide the framework for the development of the delivery of health care services: service needs and intensity, facilities, technology, and labor (workforce).
- Three major factors have been associated with the growth of the health care delivery system: price inflation, changes in population demographics, and technology and service intensity.
- Chronic disease is becoming a major health factor affecting health care spending.
- Health care financing has evolved through the 20th century from a system financed primarily by the consumer to a system financed primarily by third-party payers. In the 21st century, the consumer is being asked to pay more.
- To solve the problems of rising health care costs, various plans for future payment of health care are being considered; all include some form of rationing.
- Excessive and inefficient use of goods and services in health care delivery has been viewed as the major cause of rising health care costs.
- Economics is concerned with the use of resources, including money, to fulfill society's needs and wants.
- Health economics is concerned with the problems of producing services and programs and distributing them to clients.
- The goal of public health economics is maximum benefits from services of public health providers, leading to health and wellness of the population.

- The goal of public health is providing the most good for the most people.
- Nurses need to understand basic economic principles to avoid contributing to rising health care costs.
- The gross domestic product (GDP) reflects the market value of goods and services produced by the United States.
- The GDP reflects the market value of the output of labor and property located in the United States.
- Social issues, economic issues, and communicable disease epidemics mark the problems of the 21st century.
- Medicare and Medicaid are two government-funded programs that help meet the needs of high-risk populations in the United States.
- A majority of the US population has health insurance. The remaining uninsured segment represents millions of people, mostly the working poor, older adults, and children.
- Poverty has a detrimental effect on health.
- Health care rationing has always been a part of the US health care system.
- Nurses are cost-effective providers and must be an integral part of health care delivery.
- *Healthy People 2020* is a document that has established US health objectives.
- Human life is valued in health economics, as is money. An emphasis on changing lifestyles and preventive care will reduce the unnecessary years of life lost to early and preventable death.

EVOLVE WEBSITE

http://evolve.elsevier.com/Stanhope/foundations
- NCLEX® Review Questions
- Practice Application Answers

REFERENCES

Agency for Healthcare Research and Quality: *Guide to clinical preventive services, 2014*, Rockville, MD, 2014, AHRQ. Available at http://www.ahrq.gov/professionals/clinicians-providers/guidelines-recommendations/guide/index.html.

American Nurses Association: *Medicare reimbursement for NPs and CNSs*, Silver Spring, MD, 1999, ANA.

Balanced Budget Act: State Children's Health Insurance Program, Title XXI, Social Security Act, 1997, Section 210(a).

Buppert C: HEDIS for the primary care provider: getting an "A" on the managed care report card, *Nurse Pract* 24:84–94, 1999.

Bureau of Labor Statistics (BLS): *Occupational Employment and Wages – May 2015, News Release USDL-16-0661*, Washington, DC, 2016, US Department of Labor. Retrieved June 2016 from http://www.bls.gov/news.release/pdf/ocwage.pdf.

Centers for Disease Control and Prevention: *The state of aging and health in America, 2013*, Atlanta, GA, 2013, CDC, US Department of Health and Human Services. Available at http://www.cdc.gov/aging/pdf/state-aging-health-in-america-2013.pdf.

Centers for Disease Control and Prevention: *Public health economics and methods*, Atlanta, GA, 2015, CDC. Retrieved June 2016 from http://www.cdc.gov/stltpublichealth/pheconomics/.

Centers for Disease Control and Prevention: *Chronic disease overview*, Atlanta, GA, 2016, CDC. Retrieved June 2016 from http://www.cdc.gov/chronicdisease/overview/.

Centers for Medicare and Medicaid Services: *Your medical coverage – skilled nursing facility (SNF) care*, n.d.a. Retrieved June 2016 from https://www.medicare.gov/coverage/skilled-nursing-facility-care.html.

Centers for Medicare and Medicaid Services: *Medicare 2016 costs at a glance*, n.d.b. Retrieved June 2016 from https://www.medicare.gov/your-medicare-costs/costs-at-a-glance/costs-at-glance.html.

Centers for Medicaid and Medicare Services (CMS): *Skilled nursing facility PPS*, Baltimore, MD, 2013, US Department of Health and Human Services. Retrieved June 2016 from https://www.cms.gov/Medicare/Medicare-Fee-for-Service-Payment/SNFPPS/index.html?redirect=/snfpps/.

Centers for Medicaid and Medicare Services (CMS): *NHE Historical and Projections 1960-2024 – Tables*, Baltimore, MD, 2014a, US Department of Health and Human Services. Retrieved June 2016 from https://www.cms.gov/research-statistics-data-and-systems/statistics-trends-and-reports/nationalhealthexpenddata/nationalhealthaccountsprojected.html.

Centers for Medicaid and Medicare Services (CMS): *CMS Fast Facts Overview*, Baltimore, MD, 2014b, US Department of Health and Human Services. Retrieved December 2014 from http://www.cms.gov/Research-Statistics-Data-and-Systems/Statistics-Trends-and-Reports/CMS-Fast-Facts/index.html.

Centers for Medicare and Medicaid Services (CMS): *MA Payment Guide for Out of Network Payments, 4/15/2015 Update*, Baltimore, MD, 2015a, US Department of Health and Human Services. Retrieved December 2015 from http://www.cms.gov/Medicare/Health-Plans/MedicareAdvtgSpecRateStats/Downloads/OONPayments.pdf.

Centers for Medicaid and Medicare Services (CMS): *National Health Expenditures 2014 Highlights*, Baltimore, MD, 2015b, US Department of Health and Human Services. Retrieved June 2016 from https://www.cms.gov/Research-Statistics-Data-and-Systems/Statistics-Trends-and-Reports/NationalHealthExpendData/Downloads/highlights.pdf.

Centers for Medicaid and Medicare Services (CMS): *Total Medicaid enrollees – VIII group break out report*, Baltimore, MD, 2016a, US Department of Health and Human Services. Retrieved June 2016 from https://www.medicaid.gov/medicaid-chip-program-information/program-information/downloads/cms-64-enrollment-report-oct-dec-2015.pdf.

Centers for Medicare and Medicaid Services: *Hospital outpatient PPS*, Baltimore, MD, 2016b, US Department of Health and Human Services. Retrieved June 2016 from https://www.cms.gov/Medicare/Medicare-Fee-for-Service-Payment/HospitalOutpatientPPS/index.html?redirect=/HospitalOutpatientPPS/. http://www.cms.gov/Medicare/Medicare-Fee-for-Service-Payment/HospitalOutpatientPPS/index.html?redirect5/HospitalOutpatientPPS/.

Chaufan C, Yeh J, Ross L, Fox P: You can't walk or bike yourself out of the health effects of poverty: active school transport, child obesity, and blind spots in the public health literature, *Critical Public Health* 25(2):32–47, 2015.

Community Preventive Services Task Force: *What is the Community Guide?* Atlanta, GA, 2015, CPSTF. Retrieved June 2015 from http://www.thecommunityguide.org/about/index.html.

Congressional Budget Office (CBO): *The 2015 long-term outlook*, Washington, DC, 2015, US Government Printing Office. Available at http://www.cbo.gov/sites/default/files/114th-congress-2015-2016/reports/50250/50250-breakout-Chapter2-2.pdf.

DeNavas-Walt C, Proctor BD, Smith JC: *Income, Poverty, and Health Insurance Coverage in the United States, 2012. US Census Bureau, Current Population Reports*, Washington, DC, 2013, US Government Printing Office, pp P60–P245.

Esperat MC, Hanson-Turton T, Richardson M, Debisette AT, Rupinta C: Nurse-managed health centers: safety-net care through advanced nursing practice, *J Am Acad Nurse Pract* 24:24–31, 2012.

Folland S, Goodman AC, Stano M: *The economics of health and health care: Pearson International Edition*, New York, 2016, Routledge.

Honoré PA: Measuring progress in public health finance, *J Public Health Manag Prat* 18:306–308, 2012.

Institute of Medicine: *The future of the public's health in the 21st century*, Washington, DC, 2003, National Academies Press.

Internal Revenue Service: *Health savings accounts and other tax-favored health plans. Pub. no. 969, Cat. No. 24216S*, Washington, DC, 2016, IRS. Retrieved June 2016 from https://www.irs.gov/pub/irs-pdf/p969.pdf.

Kaiser Family Foundation: *The uninsured: a primer key facts about americans without health insurance*, Menlo Park, CA, 2009, Kaiser Family Foundation.

Kaiser Family Foundation: *The uninsured: a primer: key facts about americans without health insurance*, Menlo Park, CA, 2012a, Kaiser Commission on Medicaid and the Uninsured. Retrieved June 2016 from http://kaiserfamilyfoundation.files.wordpress.com/2013/01/7451-08.pdf.

Kaiser Family Foundation: *The uninsured: a primer: key facts about americans without health insurance*, Menlo Park, CA, 2015a, Kaiser Commission on Medicaid and the Uninsured. Retrieved June 2016 from http://kaiserfamilyfoundation.files.wordpress.com/2013/01/7451-08.pdf.

Kaiser Family Foundation: *The reprint of the coverage under the Affordable Care Act*, Menlo Park CA, 2012b, Kaiser Family Foundation.

Kaiser Family Foundation: *Employer Health Benefits Survey*, Menlo Park, CA, 2013, Kaiser Family Foundation.

Kaiser Family Foundation: *How much is enough? Out-of-pocket spending among Medicare beneficiaries: a chartbook*, Menlo Park, CA, 2014a, Kaiser Family Foundation. Available at http://kff.org/medicare/report/how-much-is-enough-out-of-pocket-spending-among-medicare-beneficiaries-a-chartbook/.

Kaiser Family Foundation: *Issue brief: the effect of the Medicaid expansion on state budgets: an early look at select states*, Menlo Park CA, 2015b, Kaiser Family Foundation.

Kaiser Family Foundation: *Medicaid moving forward*, Menlo Park, CA, 2015c, Kaiser Family Foundation. Available at http://files.kff.org/attachment/issue-brief-medicaid-moving-forward.

Kaiser Family Foundation: *The facts on Medicare spending and financing*, Menlo Park, CA, 2015d, Kaiser Family Foundation. Retrieved June 2016 from http://kff.org/medicare/fact-sheet/medicare-spending-and-financing-fact-sheet/.

Knickman JR, Kovner AR: *Jonas and Kovner's health care delivery in the United States*, ed 11, New York, 2015, Springer Publishing Company.

Kvedar J, Coye MJ, Everett W: Connected health: a review of technologies and strategies to improve patient care with telemedicine and telehealth, *Health Affairs* 33(2):194–199, 2014.

Lockard CB, Wolf M: *Occupational Employment Projections to 2020*, Washington, DC, 2012, Bureau of Labor Statistics. Monthly Labor Review. Retrieved December 2014 from http://www.bls.gov/opub/mlr/2012/01/art5full.pdf.

McPake B, Normand C, Smith S: *Health economics: an international perspective*, ed 3, New York, 2013, Routledge.

Minyard K, Phillips MA, Baker S: The philanthropic collaborative for a healthy Georgia: building a public-private partnership with pooled funding, *The Foundation Review* 8(1):74–87, 2016.

National Center for Health Statistics: *Health, United States, 2011: with special feature on socioeconomic status and health*, Hyattsville, MD, 2012, US Government Printing Office.

National Center for Health Statistics: *Health, United States, 2015: with special feature on racial and ethnic health disparities*, Hyattsville, MD, 2016, US Government Printing Office.

Patient Protection and Affordable Care Act (PL 111-148). Retrieved 2010 from http://healthcare.org.

Pew Charitable Trusts: *State and local government spending on health care slowed in 2013*, February 2015. Retrieved June 2016 from http://www.pewtrusts.org/en/research-and-analysis/analysis/2015/02/09/state-and-local-government-spending-on-health-care-slowed-in-2013.

Phelps CE: *Health economics*, ed 5, Upper Saddle River, NJ, 2012, Prentice Hall.

Robert Wood Johnson Foundation (RWJF): *Overcoming obstacles to health in 2013 and beyond*, Princeton, NJ, 2013, RWJF. Retrieved June 2016 from http://www.rwjf.org/content/dam/farm/reports/reports/2013/rwjf406474.

Shi L, Singh DA: *Delivering health care in America*, ed 6, Burlington, MA, 2014, Jones and Bartlett Learning.

Sturgi, JL, Goel, A: *The private sector role in public health*, Washington, DC, 2012, Center for Strategic and International Studies.

The Commonwealth Fund: *To the Point*, Sept. 16, 2015. Retrieved June 2016 from info@cmwf.org.

Toner, Erin: *Nurse led clinics, no doctors required*, St. Paul, MN, 2014, American Public Media. Retrieved at June 2016 http://www.marketplace.org.

Trust for America's Health: *Investing in America's health: a state-by-state look at public health funding and key health facts*, Washington, DC, 2013a, Trust for America's Health. Retrieved June 2016 from http://healthyamericans.org/assets/files/TFAH2013InvstgAmrcsHlth05%20FINAL.pdf.

Trust for America's Health: *A healthier America 2013: Strategies to move from sick care to health care in the next four years*, Washington, DC, 2013b, Trust for America's Health. Retrieved June 2016 from http://healthyamericans.org/assets/files/TFAH2013HealthierAmericaFnlRv.pdf.

Trust for America's Health: *Key health data (by state): public health funding indicators*, 2014. Retrieved June 2016 from http://healthyamericans.org/states/.

Turnock BJ: *Public health: what it is and how it works*, ed 6, Boston, 2016, Jones and Bartlett.

US Department of Health and Human Services: *Healthy People 2000: national health promotion and disease prevention objectives*, Washington, DC, 1990, USDHHS, Public Health Service.

US Department of Health and Human Services: *Healthy People 2010: understanding and improving health*, Washington, DC, 2000, Public Health Service.

US Department of Health and Human Services: *Healthy People 2020: a roadmap to improve all Americans' health*, Washington, DC, 2010, Public Health Service.

US Department of Health and Human Services: *A profile of older Americans*, Washington, DC, 2012, The Administration on Aging.

US Department of Health and Human Services: *Centers for Medicare and Medicaid Services: Medicare and you*, Washington, DC, 2016a, USDHHS.

US Department of Health and Human Services: *Surgeon General— the national prevention council*, Washington, DC, July 2016b, US Department of Health and Human Services (DHHS).

US Department of Health and Human Services: *US Federal Poverty Guidelines, Office of the Assistant Secretary for Planning and Evaluation*, January 25, 2016c. Retrieved June 24, 2016 from https://aspe.hhs.gov/poverty-guidelines.

US Law: *Medicare prescription drug improvement and modernization act of 2003*, Washington, DC, 2003, US Law. Retrieved July 2016 from http://www.govtrak.us.

CHAPTER 9

Epidemiological Applications

DeAnne K. Hilfinger Messias and Swan Arp Adams

OBJECTIVES

After reading this chapter, the student should be able to:

1. Define epidemiology and describe how it has developed over time.
2. Describe the essential elements of epidemiology and an epidemiological approach.
3. Discuss the steps in the epidemiological process.
4. Explain the basic epidemiological concepts of population at risk, natural history of disease, levels of prevention,
host-agent-environment relationships, and the web-of-causation model.
5. Differentiate between descriptive and analytic epidemiology.
6. Explain how nurses use epidemiology in public health practice.

CHAPTER OUTLINE

Definitions
History
How Nurses Use Epidemiology
Basic Concepts in Epidemiology
  Measures of Morbidity and Mortality
  Epidemiologic Triangle: Agent, Host, and Environment
  Levels of Preventive Interventions
Screening
  Reliability and Validity
Basic Methods in Epidemiology
  Sources of Data
  Rate Adjustment
  Comparison Groups
Descriptive Epidemiology
  Person

Place
Time
Analytic Epidemiology
  Cohort Studies
  Prospective Cohort Studies
  Case-Control Studies
  Cross-Sectional Studies
  Ecological Studies
Experimental Studies
  Clinical Trials
  Community Trials
Causality
  Statistical Associations
  Bias
  Assessing for Causality
Applications of Epidemiology in Nursing

KEY TERMS

agent, 155
analytic epidemiology, 148
attack rate, 153
bias, 166
case-control study, 164
case fatality rate (CFR), 154
causal inference, 167
cohort study, 163
confounding, 166

cross-sectional study, 165
descriptive epidemiology, 148
determinants, 148
distribution, 148
ecological fallacy, 165
ecological model, 156
environment, 155
epidemic, 152
epidemiology, 148

host, 155
incidence proportion, 152
incidence rate, 152
levels of prevention, 156
natural history of disease, 156
negative predictive value, 159
point epidemic, 161
positive predictive value, 159
prevalence proportion, 152

Continued

KEY TERMS—cont'd

primary prevention, 156
proportionate mortality ratio
    (PMR), 155
reliability, 158
risk, 151

screening, 157
secondary prevention, 157
secular trends, 161
sensitivity, 158
specificity, 158

surveillance, 159
tertiary prevention, 157
validity, 158
web of causality, 156

The term *epidemiology* comes from the Greek terms *logos* ("study"), *demos* ("people"), and *epi* ("upon"). Literally this would be "the study of what is upon the people." Epidemiology is the study of the distribution and determinants of disease in populations. For example, you would use epidemiology to see if a disease is more common among men or women or if the disease is seen more in older versus younger people. The term originally referred to the spread of infectious epidemics such as cholera or tuberculosis (TB). Now the term is more inclusive and involves infectious diseases and chronic diseases, such as cancer and cardiovascular disease, as well as mental health and other health-related events, such as intentional injuries (accidents), violence, occupational and environmental exposures and their effects, and positive health states. The public health science of epidemiology has made major contributions to (1) the understanding of factors that contribute to health and disease, (2) the development of health promotion and disease-prevention measures, (3) the detection and characterization of emerging infectious agents, (4) the evaluation of health services and policies, and (5) the practice of nursing in public health.

DEFINITIONS

Epidemiology investigates the distribution or the patterns of health events in populations and the determinants or the factors that influence those patterns. When using descriptive epidemiology, health outcomes are considered in terms of what, who, where, and when. That is: What is the outcome? Who is affected? Where are they? When do events occur? Descriptive epidemiology discusses a disease in terms of person, place, and time. The how and why, or determinants of health events, are those factors, exposures, characteristics, behaviors, and contexts that determine (or influence) the patterns: How does it occur? Why are some people affected more than others? Determinants may be individual, relational or social, communal, or environmental. This focus on investigation of causes and associations is called analytic epidemiology.

Epidemiology, like both the research process and nursing process, consists of a set of steps. The first step is to answer the "what" question by defining the outcome. The health outcome can be a disease, or it can refer to injuries, accidents, or even wellness (Koepsell and Weiss, 2003). The aim in epidemiology is to describe the distribution (i.e., determine how, where, and when the disease occurs) and to look for factors that explain the pattern of the disease or the risk for occurrence (i.e., answer the questions of why and how the disease occurs).

Like nursing, epidemiology builds on and draws from other disciplines and methods, including clinical medicine and laboratory sciences, social sciences, quantitative methods (especially biostatistics), and public health policy and goals. Epidemiology focuses on populations, whereas clinical medicine focuses on the diagnosis and treatment of disease in individuals. Epidemiology studies populations to determine the causes of health and disease in communities and to investigate and evaluate interventions that will prevent disease and maintain health. Epidemiological methods are used extensively to determine to what extent the goals of *Healthy People 2020* (US Department of Health and Human Services, 2010) have been met and to monitor the progress of those objectives not fully met at present.

Epidemiology is true detective work. For example, consider a man who visited a country other than where he lived. Within 3 days, he was experiencing nausea and diarrhea. The epidemiological process could help determine what action should be taken. Specifically, what did he eat or drink? Did others eat or drink the same things? Are other people with him experiencing the same symptoms? After a thorough review of the "what, who, where, and when," he realizes that the only thing he did differently from others with him was use water from the bathroom faucet to brush his teeth. Others in his group had used bottled water. Although he knew that people often react negatively to water that is different from their own, he was so accustomed to using tap water to brush his teeth that he did so in this new location without thinking about the effects it might have for him. Similarly, three women shared a meal, and all ate everything, except for one person who did not eat any green peppers. Thirty minutes after eating, the two women who ate the green peppers had painful gastrointestinal symptoms. The only thing different in what they had to eat and drink that day was the peppers. One can conclude that the peppers may not have been washed carefully or had some other way of having bacteria attached to them.

♥ HEALTHY PEOPLE 2020

Examples of Epidemiologic Objectives in Healthy People 2020

- **AH-2:** Increase the percentage of adolescents who participate in extracurricular and out-of-school activities.
- **AOCBC-4:** Reduce the proportion of adults with doctor-diagnosed arthritis who find it "very difficult" to perform specific joint-related activities.
- **D-16:** Increase prevention behaviors in persons at high risk for diabetes with prediabetes.
- **HAI-2:** Reduce invasive methicillin-resistant *Staphylococcus aureus* (MRSA) infections.

From US Department of Health and Human Services: *Healthy People 2020*, Washington, DC, 2010, US Government Printing Office.

HISTORY

Hippocrates, in the 4th century BCE, was one of the first people to use the ideas that are now part of epidemiology (Merrill and Timmreck, 2006). He examined health and disease in a community by looking at geography, climate, the seasons of the year, the food and water consumed, and the habits and behaviors of the people. His approach, like descriptive epidemiology, looked at how health is influenced by personal characteristics, place, and time.

In the 18th and 19th centuries, comparison groups began to be used to measure change or the effects of some action or treatment on an experimental group. Also at this time, quantitative methods (i.e., numeric measurements or counts) were beginning to be used. One of the most famous studies using a comparison group is the mid-19th-century investigation of cholera by John Snow, whom some call the "father of epidemiology" (Merrill and Timmreck, 2006). By mapping cases that clustered around one public water pump during a London cholera outbreak, Snow was able to show how the water supply and cholera were associated. He observed that cholera rates were higher among households supplied by water companies whose water came from downstream than among households whose water came from farther upstream, where it was subject to less contamination. Snow conducted a "natural experiment," as seen in Table 9.1, and documented that foul water was the vehicle for transmission of the agent that caused cholera (Rothman, 2012).

In nursing, Florence Nightingale contributed to the development of epidemiology in her work with British soldiers during the Crimean War (1854 to 1856). At this time, sick soldiers were cared for in cramped quarters that had poor sanitation, were overrun with lice and rats, and had insufficient food and medical supplies. She looked at the relationship between the conditions of the environment and the recovery of the soldiers. Using simple epidemiological measures of rates of illness per 1000 soldiers, she was able to show that improving environmental conditions and adding nursing care decreased the mortality rates of the soldiers (Cohen, 1984; Palmer, 1983). These same principles can be applied today in the many countries that experience war leading to poor food, water, and sanitary conditions. That is, if the environment could be improved and better care provided, the rate of illnesses and death would be reduced.

During the 20th century, several changes in society influenced the further development of epidemiology. Some of these were the Great Depression of the 1920s in the United States; World War II; a rising standard of living for many but poverty for others; improved nutrition; better sanitation; the development of antibiotics, vaccines, and cancer chemotherapies; decreased birth rates in some countries; and decreases in infant and child mortality in

many nations. People began to live longer, and the rates of several chronic diseases such as coronary heart disease (CHD), stroke, cancer, and senile dementia increased. In 1900 the leading causes of death were (1) pneumonia and influenza, followed by (2) tuberculosis and (3) gastritis, enteritis, and colitis; then came (4) heart diseases, (5) symptoms of senility, (6) vascular lesions affecting the central nervous system (CNS), (7) chronic nephritis and renal sclerosis, (8) unintentional injuries, (9) malignant neoplasms, and (10) diphtheria. That contrasts with the changes in patterns that were seen in the 1950s and continue today, with the following leading causes of death in 2013:

1. Diseases of the heart (heart disease)
2. Malignant neoplasms (cancer)
3. Chronic lower respiratory diseases
4. Accidents (unintentional injuries)
5. Cerebrovascular disease (stroke)
6. Alzheimer's disease
7. Diabetes mellitus
8. Influenza and pneumonia
9. Nephritis, nephrotic syndrome, and nephrosis (kidney disease)
10. Intentional self-harm (suicide)

These were followed by septicemia, chronic liver disease and cirrhosis, essential hypertension and hypertensive renal disease, Parkinson's disease, and pneumonitis due to solids and liquids (Xu et al, 2016).

During the 20th century a shift occurred from looking for single agents, such as the infectious agent that causes cholera, to determining the multifactorial etiology or the many factors or combinations of factors that contribute to disease. An example of multifactorial etiology can be found in the complex number and type of factors that cause cardiovascular disease. People began to realize that not all of the diseases of older people were the result of the degenerative processes of aging. Rather, it became clear that many behavioral and environmental factors supported or encouraged the development of diseases. This information led to the belief that some diseases could be prevented and other diseases could at least be delayed.

In addition, the development of genetic and molecular techniques increased the ability of the epidemiologist to classify persons in terms of exposures or inherent susceptibility to disease. Examples included the identification of genetic traits that indicated an increased risk for breast cancer and markers that identified exposures to environmental toxins such as lead or pesticides. These developments are of particular interest to nurses who work with people in their living and work environments and understand the interaction of the environment(s) on health and well-being. Furthermore, nurses in the community can assess a broad range of health outcomes, as well as factors that contribute to wellness and illness.

TABLE 9.1 Household Cholera Death Rates by Source of Water Supply in John Snow's 1853 Investigation			
Company	Number of Houses	Deaths from Cholera	Deaths per 10,000 Households
Southwark and Vauxhall	40,046	1263	315
Lambeth	26,107	98	37

From Snow J: On the mode of communication of cholera. In *Snow on cholera,* New York, 1855, The Commonwealth Fund.

Unfortunately, in recent years new infectious diseases (e.g., Ebola, the Zika virus, Lyme disease, methicillin-resistant *Staphylococcus aureus* [MRSA], the H1N1 and H3N2 viruses) and new forms of old diseases (e.g., drug-resistant strains of tuberculosis [TB], new forms of *Escherichia coli*) have emphasized the dangers that can occur with these diseases. Also, potential threats from terrorist use of infectious agents (e.g., anthrax, smallpox) have once again placed the epidemiology of infectious diseases in the spotlight. Epidemiological methods also have been applied to a broader spectrum of health-related outcomes, including accidents, injuries and violence, occupational and environmental exposures, psychiatric and sociological phenomena, health-related behaviors, and health services research.

HOW NURSES USE EPIDEMIOLOGY

Nurses play a key role in the community's interdisciplinary team looking at health, disease causation, and how to both prevent and treat illness. Nurses use epidemiology in the community to examine factors that affect the individual, family, and population group because it is more difficult to control these factors in the community than in the hospital. Specifically, it is difficult to control the environment, including water and food supplies; air quality conditions, including pollutants; disposal of garbage and trash; insects and animals that carry infectious diseases; quality of paint used to ensure it contains no lead; or what comes in the mail. Therefore community residents are often exposed to many factors affecting their health.

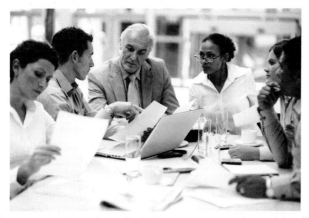

Nurses work in an interdisciplinary team to solve epidemiological problems. (© 2012 Photos.com, a division of Getty Images. All rights reserved. Image #121198999.)

Nurses are involved in the surveillance and monitoring of disease trends. In settings such as homes, schools, workplaces, clinics, and health care organizations, nurses can identify patterns of disease in a group. For example, if several children in a school become sick with abdominal problems within a short period (e.g., a 24-hour period), the nurse would try to determine what these children had in common. For instance, did they eat the same food, drink from the same source of water, or swim in the same pool? Likewise, if workers in a plant displayed a similar pattern of symptoms, the nurse would look for factors in the workplace to locate the cause. The reason for looking at the workplace first is that it is the setting the individuals have in common.

Care of clients, families, and population groups in the community uses the following steps of the nursing process: (1) assessment, (2) diagnosis, (3) planning, (4) implementation, and (5) evaluation. When using the nursing process, epidemiology provides baseline information for assessing needs, identifying problems, designing appropriate strategies to evaluate the problems, setting priorities to develop a plan of care, and evaluating how effective the care was. The information learned from the Human Genome Project completed in 2003 will continue to be the basis of new discoveries about the consequences of genetic variations and the outcomes of the interaction between genes and the environment. Nurses, in their focus on health, can use the information that is now available and will increasingly become available as a result of further research. The "Essential Nursing Competencies and Curricula Guidelines for Genetics" will help nurses care for individuals, families, communities, and populations by including genetic and genomic information in their practice. For example, this information could assist a nurse to recognize whether a newborn is at risk for morbidity or mortality resulting from errors in genetic metabolism and when there is a history of a genetic mutation in the family (American Nurses Association, 2006).

GENETICS IN PRACTICE

A 40-year-old woman returns from a cancer center after learning that she has an ATM gene mutation and that this may cause her to have a higher risk of developing certain types of cancers. There is a likely increased risk for breast, ovarian, and pancreatic cancer. One of her options is a prophylactic mastectomy, which has been shown to significantly reduce the risk of breast cancer. That will be a difficult decision for her to make. However, the other difficult decision will be whether she will inform members of her family of this information because they could also be affected. Consider the following questions:

1. Would you do nothing until she decides whether she will have the mastectomy or not and learns more about the ATM gene?
2. Would you suggest that she think carefully about whether she should tell her siblings and other family members who may also be at increased risk?
3. If she decides to tell her family, should she encourage them to have genetic testing?
4. Would you recommend that she meet with a genetic counselor before she tells her family members?
5. How can you be assured that she is aware of the Genetic Information Nondiscrimination Act (GINA), which prohibits health insurers and most employers from discriminating against individuals based on genetic information (including the results of genetic tests and family history information)?
6. You might encourage her to visit http://www.ginahelp.org; what other steps would you take to advise and counsel her effectively?

The sections that follow discuss the "tools of epidemiology" that are needed by nurses who work in community settings.

CASE STUDY

Church Picnic

Mary Miles is the nurse epidemiologist for the Warren County Health Department. A local church contacted Ms. Miles when several church members became sick after the annual church picnic. Of the 200 people who attended the picnic, 100 were ill with diarrhea, nausea, or vomiting. Ten people required emergency

Church Picnic

medical treatment or hospitalization. Incubation periods ranged from 1.5 to 30 hours, with a mean of 6 hours and a median of 3.5 hours. Duration of illness ranged from 1 to 80 hours, with a mean of 30 hours and a median of 15 hours.

The annual church picnic is a potluck lunch buffet. The menu included macaroni casserole (brought by the Joneses), turkey with gravy and stuffing (brought by the Smiths), potato salad (brought by the Changs), green bean casserole (brought by the Champs), chili (brought by the Turners), homemade bread (brought by Granny Ivy), chocolate cake (brought by the Bushes), and cookies (brought by the Beckmans). Ms. Miles interviewed the church members who were ill and found that three food items were significantly associated with illness: turkey, gravy, and stuffing.

Ms. Miles interviewed the Smiths, who brought the turkey, gravy, and stuffing to the picnic. Review of food-handling procedures indicated that the turkey had cooled for 4 hours at room temperature after cooking—a time and temperature sufficient for bacterial growth and toxin production. Furthermore, the same utensils were used for both the turkey and other foods before and after cooking.

Ms. Miles talked with the Smiths about proper food-handling practices, emphasizing hand washing, proper cooling and preserving methods, and better equipment and utensil sanitation. Ms. Miles also offered a similar class to the church congregation.

1. For the nurse to evaluate why people at the picnic became sick, what questions should she ask the people who brought the food?
    A. Cooking time and how they cooked the food
    B. Hygiene of their equipment
    C. Sources of the water used in cooking the food
    D. All of the above
2. Identify the agent, host, and environment in this.
3. Is Ms. Miles performing descriptive epidemiology or analytic epidemiology?
4. Which level of prevention is Ms. Miles exemplifying?
    A. Primary prevention
    B. Secondary prevention
    C. Tertiary prevention
    D. Combination of the above
    E. None of the above

Answers can be found on the Evolve website.

 APPLYING CONTENT TO PRACTICE

It is important that nurses understand the relationship between population health concepts and clinical practice. Within the field of epidemiology, the definition of *population* is not necessarily confined to large groups of people, such as a population of the United States. Population health concepts also apply to other types of groups, such as the collective group of clients at one clinical practice site. In this case, the clinical epidemiologic application of population health concepts is evident in questions such as: What are the factors that contribute to the health and illness of issues among clients that I see in my clinic? Why do some of my clients fare better than others with the same disease conditions? Are there alternative clinical practices that might help my clients? All of these clinical questions incorporate epidemiologic concepts of describing the *burden of disease* in a population, identifying and understanding *determinants of health*, and examining possible *root causes* of health outcomes. Two important documents highlight ways in which epidemiologic knowledge and skills are essential in nursing practice. The Council on Linkages between Academia and Public Health Practice (2010) outlined essential analytic/assessment and public health science skills, and the Quad Council of Public Health Nursing Competencies (Swider et al, 2013) provided details and examples of ways to implement these skill sets in nursing practice.

BASIC CONCEPTS IN EPIDEMIOLOGY

MEASURES OF MORBIDITY AND MORTALITY

Rates, Proportions, and Risk

Epidemiology looks at the distribution of health states and events. Because people differ in their probability or risk for disease, the primary concern is how they differ. Today epidemiologists use tools such as geographic information systems to study health-related events to identify disease distribution patterns, similar to how John Snow mapped cases of cholera in one area of London. However, mapping of cases is limited in what it can reveal. A larger number of cases may simply be the result of a larger population with more potential cases or the result of a longer period of observation. Any description of disease patterns should take into account the size of the population at risk for the disease. That is, we should look not only at the numerator (the number of cases) but also at the denominator (the number of people in the population at risk) and at the amount of time each was observed. For example, 50 cases of influenza might be seen as a serious epidemic in a population of 250 but would be a low rate in a population of 250,000. Using rates and proportions instead of simple counts of cases takes the size of the population at risk into account.

Epidemiological studies rely on rates and proportions. A *proportion* is a type of ratio in which the denominator includes the numerator. For example, if there were 2,426,264 deaths recorded in the United States, of which 631,636 were reported to have been caused by heart disease, the proportion of deaths attributed to heart disease at a given time was 631,636/2,426,264 = 0.260, or 26.0. Because the numerator must be included in the denominator, proportions can range from 0 to 1. Proportions are often multiplied by 100 and expressed as a percent, literally meaning "per 100." In public health statistics, however, if the proportion is very small, we use a larger multiplier to avoid small fractions, so the proportion may be expressed as a number per 1000 or per 100,000.

A *rate* is a measure of the frequency of a health event in different populations at certain periods (Porta, 2008). A rate is a ratio, but it is not a proportion because the denominator is a function of both the population size and the dimension of time, whereas the numerator is the number of events. Furthermore, depending on the units of time and the frequency of events, a rate may exceed 1. As its name suggests, a rate is a measure of how quickly something is happening: how rapidly a disease is developing in a population or how rapidly people are dying. Rates deal with change: moving from one state of being to another, from well to ill, from alive to dead, or from ill to cured. Because they deal with events (i.e., moving from one state of being to another), time is involved. We must follow a population over time to observe the changes in state, and we typically exclude from the population being followed those persons who have already experienced the event.

Risk refers to the probability that an event will occur within a specified period. A population at risk is the population of persons for whom there is some finite probability (even if small) of that event occurring. For example, although the risk for breast cancer in men is small, a few men do develop breast cancer and therefore are part of the population at risk. There are some outcomes for which certain people would never be at risk (e.g., men cannot be at risk for ovarian cancer, nor can women be at risk of testicular cancer). A high-risk population, on the other hand, would include those persons who, because of exposure, lifestyle, family history, or other factors, are at greater risk for disease than the population at large. For example, although everyone in the population is at risk for human immunodeficiency virus (HIV) infection and acquired immunodeficiency syndrome (AIDS), persons who have multiple sexual partners without adequate protection or who use intravenous drugs are in the high-risk population for HIV infection. However, others may unknowingly be at high risk, such as women who think they are in monogamous relationships and do not know that their partners have sexual relations with other women or men. Genetic testing is becoming more common, but most tests for disease indicate only susceptibility to disease, not certainty. Similarly, screening tests are never perfect, so there is always some probability of misclassifying a person.

Epidemiologists and other health professionals examine measures of morbidity, especially incidence proportions, incidence rates, and prevalence proportions, to learn about the risk for disease, the rate of disease development, and the levels of existing disease in a population, respectively.

Measures of Incidence

Measures of incidence reflect the number of new cases or events in a population at risk during a specified time. An incidence rate quantifies the rate of development of new cases in a population at risk, whereas an incidence proportion indicates the proportion of the population at risk that experiences the event over some period of time (Rothman, 2012). The population at risk is considered to be persons without the event or outcome of interest but who are at risk for experiencing it. People who already have the disease or outcome of interest are excluded from the population at risk for this calculation because they already have the condition and are no longer at risk for developing it. The incidence proportion is also referred to as the *cumulative incidence rate* because it reflects the cumulative effect of the incidence rate over the time period. The risk for disease is a function of both the rate of new disease development and the length of time the population is at risk. The interpretation can be for an individual (i.e., the probability that the person will become ill) or for a population (i.e., the proportion of a population expected to become ill over that period). In epidemiology, we often calculate proportions on the basis of population frequencies. These frequencies are then translated into personal risk statements for people representative of the population on which the estimates are based.

For example, suppose a health department and hospital partner want to develop an intensive, broad-based screening program in an area with overcrowded housing, limited access to

services, and underuse of preventive health practices. They might include physical examinations; tuberculin skin tests with follow-up chest radiography where indicated; cardiovascular, glaucoma, and diabetes screening; and mammography for women and prostate screening for men older than 45 years of age. Of the 8000 women screened, 35 were previously diagnosed with breast cancer; by screening and follow-up, 20 with no history of breast cancer were found to have cancer of the breast. We could follow the 7945 women in whom no breast cancer was detected and note the number of new cases of breast cancer detected over the following 5 years. Assuming no losses to follow-up (i.e., moved away or died from other causes), if 44 women were diagnosed over the 5-year period, the 5-year incidence proportion of breast cancer in this population would be as follows:

$$\frac{44}{7945} = 0.005538, \text{ or } 553.8 \text{ per } 100,000$$

Note the multiplication by 100,000, so that the number of cases is expressed as per 100,000 women. A cumulative incidence rate estimates the risk for developing the disease in that population during that time. Also, as a proportion, each event in the numerator must be represented in the denominator, and only those persons at risk for the event counted in the numerator may be included in the denominator.

A ratio can be used as an approximation of a risk. For example, the infant mortality "rate" is the number of infant deaths (infants are defined as being younger than 1 year of age) in a given year divided by the number of live births in that same year. It approximates the risk for death in the first year of life for live-born infants in a specific year. Some of the infants who die that year were born in the previous year, and some of the infants born that year may die in the following year before their first birthday. However, because about two-thirds of infant deaths occur within the first 28 days of life, the number of infants in the numerator (i.e., deaths in a given year) but not in the denominator (i.e., live births in that same year) will be small. It can be assumed that current year's deaths from the previous year's cohort approximately equal the deaths from the current year's cohort occurring in the following year. Although technically a ratio, this is an approximation to the true proportion and, therefore, an estimate of the risk.

An epidemic occurs when the rate of disease, injury, or other condition exceeds the usual (i.e., endemic) level of that condition. No specific threshold of incidence indicates that an epidemic exists. Because smallpox has been eradicated, any occurrence of smallpox might be considered an epidemic by this definition. In contrast, given the high rates of ischemic heart disease in the United States, an increase of many cases would be needed before an epidemic was noted, although some might argue that the current high rates in contrast to earlier periods already indicate an epidemic.

Prevalence Proportion

The prevalence proportion is a measure of existing disease in a population at a particular time (i.e., the number of existing cases divided by the current population). It is also possible to calculate the prevalence of a specific risk factor or exposure. In the breast cancer example given earlier, the screening program discovered 35 of the 8000 women screened had previously been diagnosed with breast cancer and 20 women with no history of breast cancer were diagnosed as a result of the screening. The prevalence proportion of current and past breast cancer events in this population of women would be as follows:

$$\frac{55}{8000} = 0.006875, \text{ or } 687.5 \text{ per } 100{,}000$$

A prevalence proportion is not an estimate of the risk for developing disease because it is a function of both the rate at which new cases of the disease develop and how long those cases remain in the population. In this example, the prevalence of breast cancer in this population of women is a function of how many new cases develop and how long women live after the diagnosis of breast cancer. A fairly constant prevalence might be seen, for example, if improved survival after diagnosis were offset by an increasing incidence rate. The duration of a disease is affected by case fatality and cure. (For simplicity, in this example, women with a history of the disease are counted in the prevalence proportion even though they may have been cured.) A disease with a short duration (e.g., an intestinal virus) may not have a high prevalence proportion even if the rate of new cases is high because cases do not accumulate (see the discussion of point epidemic). A disease with a long course will have a higher prevalence proportion than a rapidly fatal disease that has the same rate of new cases.

Incidence and Prevalence Compared

The prevalence proportion measures existing cases of disease. The prevalence odds ($P[1 - P]$) are roughly proportional to the incidence rate multiplied by the average duration of disease. The prevalence proportion is therefore affected by factors that influence risk (i.e., incidence) and factors that influence survival or recovery (i.e., duration). For that reason, prevalence measures are less useful when looking for factors related to disease etiology. Because prevalence proportions reflect duration in addition to the risk for getting the disease, it is difficult to sort out what factors are related to risk and what factors are related to survival or recovery. In mathematical notation,

$$p / (1 - P) \cong I \times D,$$
or, when P is small (< 0.1), the $P \cong I \times D,$

where P = prevalence, I = incidence rate, and D = average duration.

For example, the 5-year survival rate for breast cancer is approximately 85%, but the 5-year survival rate for lung cancer in women is only about 15%. Even if the incidence rates of breast and lung cancer were the same in women (and they are not), the prevalence proportions would differ because, on average, women live longer with breast cancer (i.e., it has a longer duration). Incidence rates and incidence proportions, on the other hand, are the measure of choice to study etiology because incidence is affected only by factors related to the risk for developing disease and not to survival or cure. Prevalence is useful in planning health care services because it is an indication of the level of disease existing in the population and therefore of the size of the population in need of services. In the previous example about screening, the health department would want to know both the existing level of TB in the area (the prevalence), to plan services and direct prevention and control measures, and the rate at which new cases are developing (the incidence), to study risk factors and evaluate the effectiveness of prevention and control programs (see the "How To" box).

HOW TO Determine If a Health Problem Exists in the Community

Planning for resources and personnel often requires quantifying the level of a problem in a community. For example, to know how different districts compare in the rates of infants with very low birth weight, you would calculate the prevalence of births of infants with very low birth weight in each district:

1. Determine the number of live births in each district from birth certificate data obtained from the vital records division of the health department.
2. Use the birth weight information from the birth certificate data to determine the number of infants born weighing less than 1500 g in each district.
3. Calculate the prevalence of births of infants with very low birth weight by district as the number of infants weighing less than 1500 g at birth divided by the total number of live births.
4. If the number of births of infants with very low birth weight in each district is small, use several recent years of data to obtain a more stable estimate.

Attack Rate

One final measure of morbidity, often used in infectious disease investigations, is the attack rate, or the proportion of persons who are exposed to an agent and develop the disease. Attack rates are often specific to an exposure; food-specific attack rates, for example, are the proportion of persons becoming ill after eating a specific food item.

Mortality Rates

Several key mortality rates are shown in Table 9.2. Many commonly used mortality rates are not true rates but are proportions, because the population changes throughout the year. Although measures of mortality reflect serious health problems and changing patterns of disease, they have limited usefulness. They provide information only about fatal diseases and do not provide direct information about either the level of existing disease in the population or the risk for getting a particular disease. Also, a person may have one disease (e.g., prostate cancer) yet die of a different cause (e.g., stroke).

Note than many commonly used mortality rates listed in Table 9.2 are in fact proportions, not true rates (Rothman, 2012; Gordis, 2013). Because the population changes during the course of a year, we typically take an estimate of the population at mid-year as the denominator for annual rates because the mid-year populations approximate the amount of person-time contributed by the population during a given year.

TABLE 9.2   Common Mortality Rates

Rate/Ratio	Definition and Example*
Crude mortality (death) rate	$$\dfrac{\text{Number of deaths from any cause during time interval}}{\text{Estimated mid-interval population (mid-year population)}}$$ *Example:* In 2010 there were 2,465,932 deaths in a total population of 275,264,999, or 873.1 per 100,000.
Age-specific rate	$$\dfrac{\text{Number of deaths among persons of a given age group per mid-year population of that age group}}{\text{Estimated population in that age group at mid-interval}} = \text{rate per } 100,000$$ $$\dfrac{17,744}{18,484,615} = 96 \text{ per } 100,000 \text{ persons ages 20 to 24 years}$$
Cause-specific rate	$$\dfrac{\text{Number of deaths from a specific cause per mid-year population}}{\text{Estimated mid-interval populaiton}} = \text{rate per } 100,000$$ $$\dfrac{97,900 \text{ accidental deaths}}{275,264,999 \text{ mid-year population}} = 35.6 \text{ per } 100,000$$
Case fatality rate	$$\dfrac{\text{Number of deaths from a specific disease in a given period}}{\text{Number of persons diagnosed}}$$ *Example:* If 87 of every 100 persons diagnosed with lung cancer die within 5 years, the 5-year case fatality rate is 87%; the 5-year survival rate is 13%.
Proportionate mortality ratio	Number of deaths from a specific disease per total number of deaths in the same period *Example:* If there were 710,760 deaths from diseases of the heart and 2,403,351 deaths from all causes: $$\dfrac{710,760}{2,403,351} = 0.296 \text{ or } 29.6\% \text{ of all deaths were due to heart disease}$$
Infant mortality ratio	Number of deaths of infants under 1 year of age in a year per number of live births in the same year *Example:* If there were 28,035 infant deaths and 4,058,814 live births: $$\dfrac{28,035}{4,058,814} = 0.0069 \text{ or } 6.9 \text{ per } 1000 \text{ live births}$$
Neonatal mortality rate	Number of deaths of infants under 28 days of age in a year per number of live births in the same year *Example:* If there were 18,776 neonatal deaths and 4,058,814 live births: $$\dfrac{18,776}{4,058,814} = 4.63 \text{ per } 1000 \text{ live births}$$
Postneonatal mortality rate	Number of deaths of infants from 28 days to 1 year of age in a year per number of live births in the same year *Example:* If there were 9259 postneonatal deaths and 4,058,814 live births: $$\dfrac{9296}{4,058,814} = 2.28 \text{ per } 1000 \text{ live births}$$

See Murphy SL, Xu JQ, Kochanek KD: Deaths: preliminary data for 2010, *Natl Vital Stat Rep* 60; 2012 for actual 2010 data. Time interval used for the denominator is usually mid-year data.

The crude annual mortality rate is an estimate of the risk for death for a person in a given population for that year. These rates are multiplied by a scaling factor, usually 100,000, to avoid small fractions. The result is then expressed as the number of deaths per 100,000 persons. Although a crude mortality rate is calculated easily and represents the actual death rate for the total population, it has certain limitations. It does not reveal specific causes of death, which change in relative importance over time. Also, the mortality rate is affected by the population's age distribution, because older people are at much greater risk for death than younger people.

Mortality rates are also calculated for specific groups (e.g., age-specific, gender-specific, race-specific rates). In these instances, the number of deaths occurring in the specified group is divided by the population at risk, now restricted to the number of persons in that group. This rate is then viewed as the risk for death for persons in the specified group during the period of observation.

The cause-specific mortality rate is an estimate of the risk for death from some specific disease in a population. It is the number of deaths from a specific cause divided by the total population at risk, usually multiplied by 100,000. Two related measures should be distinguished from the cause-specific mortality rate. The case fatality rate (CFR) is the proportion of persons diagnosed with a particular disorder (i.e., cases) who die within a specified period. It is considered an estimate of the risk for death within that period for a person newly diagnosed with the disease (e.g., the proportion of persons with a disease who die during the natural history of the disease). Because the CFR is the proportion of diagnosed persons who die within the period,

1 minus the CFR yields the survival rate. For example, if the 5-year CFR for lung cancer is 86%, then the 5-year survival rate is only 14% (Remington et al, 2010).

The second measure to be distinguished from the cause-specific mortality rate is the proportionate mortality ratio (PMR), the proportion of all deaths resulting from a specific cause. Some sources, especially those used in occupational health, say it is the proportion of all deaths resulting from a specific cause divided by the same proportion in a standard population. The denominator is not the population at risk for death, but the total number of deaths in the population; therefore the PMR is not a rate, nor does it estimate the risk for death. The magnitude of the PMR is a function of both the number of deaths from the cause of interest and the number of deaths from other causes. If deaths from certain causes decline over time, deaths from other causes that remain fairly constant may have increasing PMRs. For example, the leading cause of death for individuals between the ages of 1 and 44 years was unintentional accidents, with the relative burden of mortality being greater at young ages, accounting for 31.7% of all deaths in the age group of 19 years and under; 39.5% of deaths for persons 10 to 24 years of age, and 27.4% for those in the age group of 25 to 44 years (Heron, 2016). In contrast, for those between 45 and 64 years of age, cancer was the leading cause of death, accounting for 30.9% of deaths. For the population over 65 years of age, heart disease was the leading cause of death (21.4%).

Infant mortality is used around the world as an indicator of overall health and availability of health care services. The most common measure, the infant mortality rate, is the number of deaths to infants in the first year of life divided by the total number of live births. Because the risk for death declines considerably during the first year of life, neonatal (i.e., newborn), and postneonatal mortality rates are also of interest.

EPIDEMIOLOGIC TRIANGLE: AGENT, HOST, AND ENVIRONMENT

Epidemiologists understand that disease results from complex relationships among causal agents, susceptible persons, and environmental factors. These three elements—agent, host, and environment—are called the *epidemiologic triangle* (Fig. 9.1A). Changes in one of the elements of the triangle can influence the occurrence of disease by increasing or decreasing a person's risk for disease. Fig. 9.1B shows that agent and host, as well as their interaction, are influenced by the environment in which they exist. They also may influence the environment. Specifically, these elements or variables are defined as follows:

- Agent: An animate or inanimate factor that must be present or lacking for a disease or condition to develop
- Host: A living species (human or animal) capable of being infected or affected by an agent
- Environment: All that is internal or external to a given host or agent and that is influenced and influences the host and/or agent

Examples of these three components are listed in Box 9.1.

Causal relationships (one thing or event causes another) are often more complex than the epidemiological triangle conveys.

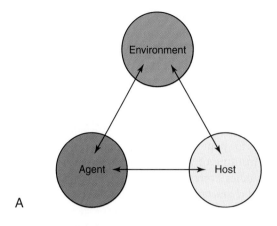

A

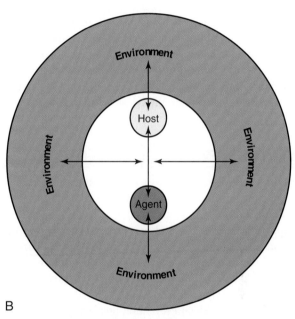

B

FIG. 9.1 (**A** and **B**) Two models of the agent-host-environment interaction (the epidemiologic triangle).

BOX 9.1 Examples of Agent, Host, and Environmental Factors in the Epidemiologic Triangle

Agent
- Infectious agents (bacteria, viruses, fungi, parasites)
- Chemical agents (heavy metals, toxic chemicals, pesticides)
- Physical agents (radiation, heat, cold, machinery)

Host
- Genetic susceptibility
- Immutable characteristics (age, sex)
- Acquired characteristics (immunological status)
- Lifestyle factors (diet, exercise)

Environment
- Climate (temperature, rainfall)
- Plant and animal life (agents, reservoirs or habitats for agents)
- Human population distribution (crowding, social support)
- Socioeconomic factors (education, resources, access to care)
- Working conditions (levels of stress, noise, satisfaction)

The term web of causality recognizes the complex interrelationships of many factors interacting, sometimes in subtle ways, to increase (or decrease) the risk for disease. Also, associations are sometimes mutual, with lines of causality going in both directions. Recently, some researchers advocated for a new paradigm that goes beyond the two-dimensional causal web and considers multiple levels of factors that affect health and disease (Macintyre and Ellaway, 2000). This is consistent with the ecological model for population health supported by the 2002 report of the Institute of Medicine (IOM) that expands epidemiological studies both upward to broader contexts such as neighborhood characteristics and social context and downward to the genetic and molecular level. The ecological model treats the multiple determinants of health as interrelated and acting synergistically (or antagonistically), rather than as discrete factors. This model encompasses determinants at many levels: biological, mental, behavioral, social, and environmental factors, including policy, culture, and economic environments, and includes a life span perspective. The IOM's vision of "healthy people in healthy communities" requires a model that recognizes that healthy communities are more than a collection of healthy individuals and that the characteristics of communities affect the health of people who live in them (IOM, 2002).

LEVELS OF PREVENTIVE INTERVENTIONS

The goal of epidemiology is to identify and understand the causal factors and mechanisms of disease, disability, and injuries so that effective interventions can be implemented to prevent the occurrence of these adverse processes before they begin or before they progress. The natural history of disease is the course of the disease process from onset to resolution (Porta et al, 2008). The three levels of prevention—primary, secondary, and tertiary—provide a framework often used in public health practice. See the Levels of Prevention box later in the chapter.

Primary prevention refers to interventions that promote health and prevent the occurrence of disease, injury, Or disability. Primary prevention is aimed at individuals and groups who are susceptible to disease but have no discernible pathological process (i.e., they are in a state of pre-pathogenesis). An example of primary prevention is when a nurse provides health education and training for daycare workers about issues of health and hygiene, such as proper hand hygiene, diapering, and food preparation and storage. Immunizations are another example of primary prevention, as are teaching about the importance of wearing seat belts and about taking folic acid supplementation at preconception to prevent neural tube defects, fluoridation of water supplies to prevent dental caries, and actions taken to reduce human exposure to agents that may cause cancer.

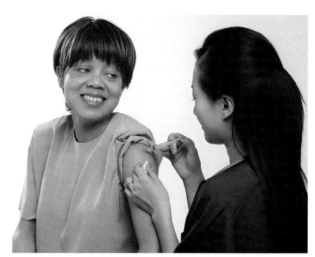

Immunizations are an integral part of primary prevention. (© 2012 Photos.com, a division of Getty Images. All rights reserved. Image #147673258).

EVIDENCE-BASED PRACTICE

Sexual health and well-being affect people of all cultures regardless of race, social class, education, age, or country of origin. Also, sexually transmitted infections (STIs) can affect people of all ages, even though the rates are highest among people under 25 years of age. Wiehe et al (2015) sought to estimate the rates of STIs among criminal offenders in the first year after arrest or release from incarceration. They conducted a retrospective study of risk for having a positive STI (chlamydia, gonorrhea, or syphilis) or positive HIV test in the first year following arrest or incarceration in Marion County, Indiana. They had 247,211 individuals with arrests or incarceration in jail, juvenile detention, or prison in a 5-year period. What they found were that rates of STI and HIV in the year after arrest or incarceration were higher among their sample than for nonoffenders, but rates varied by demographic characteristics and type of detention facility. Specifically, rates were highest for chlamydia and gonorrhea and lower for syphilis and HIV. The rates were 1.5–2.8 times higher among women than men and 2.7–6.9 times higher among blacks than whites. The highest rates of chlamydia and gonorrhea were among persons between ages 15 and 19 years, and syphilis was highest among those ages 45–54 years. HIV was highest among the 20- to 44-year-olds.

Nurse Use

It is important that public health nurses who work with individuals in the community who have been arrested or incarcerated work closely with the local justice system. These individuals need health education and follow-up in locales that are convenient and economical for them. Follow-up can be via appointments at community clinics or telemedicine using texts or e-mail messages to stay in touch and encourage safe sex and immediate follow-up if signs of an STI appear.

Data from Wiehe SE, Rosenman MC, Aalsma MC, Scanlon ML, Fortenberry JD: Epidemiology of sexually transmitted infections among offenders following arrest or incarceration, *American Journal of Public Health* 105(12):26-33, 2015.

CASE STUDY

Inmates at the Local Jail

An infection preventionist (IP) at a local hospital contacted the nurse epidemiologist at the local health department to report that the hospital had received three laboratory reports of *Acinetobacter baumannii* infection from inmates at the local jail. The IP stated that the jail typically sends all of its laboratory specimens to the hospital for processing. The IP stated that the specimens were obtained from wounds and collected within a 2-month period.

1. The nurse epidemiologist suspects an outbreak and launches an investigation for which reason?
   A. This is an unusual problem

B. There is a potential risk to the public

C. There is a casual pathway

D. All the above

2. The nurse epidemiologist decided to visit the jail. Based on what she knows about the transmission of *A. baumannii*, she should collect which of the following information?

   A. Underlying infections and chronic diseases of inmates

   B. Medical procedures performed in the jail

   C. The number of air exchanges in the jail

   D. All of the above

   E. A and B only

3. The nurse epidemiologist discovers that all of the infected inmates have their wound dressings changed on the same day of the week in the same treatment room. She notices there is no sink or evidence of hand sanitizer in the treatment room. She recommends all of the following strategies *except*:

   A. Installing hand-hygiene stations in convenient locations in treatment rooms

   B. Cleaning and disinfecting examination tables after each inmate is seen

   C. Educating staff on proper wound care and hand hygiene

   D. Antibiotics for all inmates and staff

4. The nurse epidemiologist decides to educate all staff about the organism, including how it is transmitted and prevention strategies. This level of prevention is

   A. Primary

   B. Secondary

   C. Tertiary

Case prepared by Mary Beth White-Comstock, MSN, RN, CIC.

Answers can be found on the Evolve website.

Secondary prevention refers to interventions designed to increase the probability that a person with a disease will have that condition diagnosed early enough that treatment is likely to result in a cure. Health screenings are at the core of secondary prevention. Early and periodic screenings are critical for diseases, such as breast cancer, for which there are few specific primary prevention strategies. Screening programs are discussed in the section on screening that follows.

Interventions at the secondary level of prevention often take place in community settings. For example, a nurse may teach an asthmatic client to recognize and avoid exposure to asthma triggers and assist the family to implement specific protection strategies such as replacing carpets, keeping air systems clean and free of mold, staying inside when the pollution level is high, and avoiding pets. A nurse also might ask a family about their history of cancer, heart disease, diabetes, and mental illness as part of a client's health history and then follow up with education about appropriate screening procedures. Other secondary prevention interventions include mammography to detect breast cancer, Papanicolaou (Pap) smears to detect cervical cancer, colonoscopy for early detection of colon cancer, and prenatal screening of pregnant women to screen for gestational diabetes. In developing countries, oral rehydrating therapy (ORT) is an excellent example of secondary prevention. If safe water is available, ORT can be used to treat infant diarrheal disease. To do so you would prepare a homemade ORT solution of water, sugar, and salt to give to infants.

Tertiary prevention includes interventions aimed at limiting disability and interventions that enhance rehabilitation from disease, injury, or disability. Interventions for tertiary prevention occur most often at secondary and tertiary levels of care (e.g., specialized clinics, hospitals, rehabilitation centers) but also may occur in community and primary care settings. Examples of tertiary prevention are medical treatment, physical and occupational therapy, and rehabilitation. With the emergence of new drug-resistant strains of TB, nurses now face the challenge of designing and implementing programs to increase long-term compliance and provide aftercare for clients in a variety of community settings. An example of tertiary prevention for persons diagnosed with active TB is directly observed therapy (DOT) discussed in Chapter 27.

SCREENING

Screening, a key component of many secondary prevention interventions, involves the testing of groups of individuals who are at risk for a specific condition but do not have symptoms. The goal is to determine the likelihood that these individuals will develop the disease. From a clinical perspective, the aim of screening is early detection and treatment when these result in a more favorable prognosis. From a public health perspective, the objective is to sort out efficiently and effectively those who probably have the disease from those who probably do not, again to detect early cases for treatment or begin public health prevention and control programs. A screening test is not a diagnostic test. Effective screening programs must include referrals for diagnostic evaluation for those who have positive findings on screening, to determine if they actually have the disease and need treatment.

Nurses must stay current about screening guidelines because these are regularly reviewed and revised on the basis of epidemiological research results. For example, the US Preventive Services Task Force (USPSTF) recommends screening for high blood pressure in adults 18 years and older (Siu, 2015). "The USPSTF found good evidence that screening for and treatment of high blood pressure in adults substantially reduces the incidence of cardiovascular events" (Siu, 2015, p 779), and that there are few harms associated with the screening. In terms of risk assessment, the USPSTF reported that "Persons at increased risk for high blood pressure are those who have high-normal blood pressure (130–139/85–89 Hg), those who are overweight or obese, and African Americans" (Siu, 2015, p. 779). The net benefit of screening is substantial and outweighs the cost. Adults over age 40 years and those at increased risk should be screened annually, whereas adults from ages 18 to 39 years should be screened every 3 to 5 years (Siu, 2015).

As community health advocates and educators, nurses plan and implement screening and prevention programs for high-risk populations, such as prostate-screening programs among

> ### BOX 9.2 Characteristics of A Successful Screening Program
>
> 1. **Valid (accurate):** A high probability of correct classification of persons tested
> 2. **Reliable (precise):** Results are consistent from place to place, time to time, and person to person
> 3. **Capable of large group administration:**
>   a. Fast in both the administration of the test and the obtaining of results
>   b. Inexpensive in both personnel required and the materials and procedures used
> 4. **Innocuous:** Few if any side effects, and the test is minimally invasive
> 5. **High yield:** Able to detect enough new cases to warrant the effort and expense (yield defined as the amount of previously unrecognized disease that is diagnosed and treated as a result of screening)

African American men. Examples of recent screening recommendations include the following:

- Abnormal blood glucose and Type 2 diabetes mellitus screening was recommended in 2015 for adults between the ages of 40 and 70 years.
- Breast cancer screening with mammography was recommended in 2015 for women between 50 and 74 years of age every 2 years.
- Autism spectrum disorder screening was not recommended routinely due to the lack of scientific evidence to support this practice.

See http://www.uspreventiveservicestaskforce.org for details on recommendations, the year the recommendation was published, and analyses still in progress.

Occupational health nurses and nurses in community health may work together to target populations on the basis of occupational risk. Men with questionable prostate-specific antigen (PSA) levels need to be referred, especially if they have increased risk factors for prostate cancer, such as African American heritage or a family history of prostate cancer. Successful screening programs have several characteristics that depend on the tests and on the population screened (Box 9.2). Criteria for evaluating the usefulness of a screening test include cost-effectiveness, ease and safety of administration, availability of treatment, ethics of administration, or widespread implementation, sensitivity, specificity, validity, and reliability (Gordis, 2013; McKeown and Learner, 2009).

RELIABILITY AND VALIDITY

Reliability

It is important to pay attention to the precision, or reliability, of the measure (i.e., its consistency or repeatability) and the accuracy of the measure, its validity (i.e., whether it is really measuring what we think it is and how exactly). Suppose you want to screen for blood pressure in a community. You will take blood pressure readings on a large number of people, perhaps following up with repeated measures for individuals with higher pressures. If the readings of the sphygmomanometer used for the screening vary so that two consecutive readings are not the same for the same person,

the sphygmomanometer lacks reliability. The instrument would be unreliable even if the overall mean of repeated measurements were close to the true overall mean for the persons measured. The problem would be that the readings would not be reliable for any individual, which is what a screening program requires.

On the other hand, suppose the readings are reliably reproducible, but, unknown to you, they tend to be about 10 mm Hg too high. This instrument is producing precise readings, but the uncorrected (or uncalibrated) instrument lacks accuracy. In short, a measure can be consistent without producing valid results.

The following three major sources of error can affect the reliability of tests:

1. Variation inherent in the trait being measured (e.g., blood pressure changes with time of day, activity, level of stress, and other factors)
2. Observer variation, which can be divided into intraobserver reliability (i.e., consistency by the same observer) and interobserver reliability (i.e., level of consistency from one observer to another)
3. Consistency in the instrument, which includes the level of internal consistency of the instrument (e.g., whether all items in a questionnaire measure the same thing) and the stability (i.e., or test-retest reliability) of the instrument over time

Validity: Sensitivity and Specificity

Validity in a screening test is typically measured by sensitivity and specificity. Sensitivity quantifies how accurately the test identifies those with the condition or trait. Sensitivity represents the proportion of persons with the disease whom the test correctly identifies as positive (true positives). High sensitivity is needed when early treatment is important and when identification of every case is important.

Specificity indicates how accurately the test identifies those *without* the condition or trait (i.e., the proportion of persons whom the test correctly identifies as negative for the disease [true negatives]). High specificity is needed when rescreening is impractical and when it is important to reduce false-positive results. The sensitivity and specificity of a test are determined by comparing the test results with results from a definitive diagnostic procedure (sometimes called the *gold standard*). For example, the Pap smear is used frequently to screen for cervical dysplasia and carcinoma. The definitive diagnosis of cervical cancer requires a biopsy with histological confirmation of malignant cells.

The ideal for a screening test is 100% sensitivity and 100% specificity. That is, the test is positive for 100% of those who actually have the disease, and it is negative for all those who do not have the disease. In practice, sensitivity and specificity are often inversely related. That is, if the test results are such that it is possible to choose some point beyond which a person is considered positive (a "cutpoint"), as in a blood pressure reading to screen for hypertension or a serum glucose reading to screen for diabetes, then moving that critical point to improve the sensitivity of the test will result in a decrease in specificity, or an improvement in specificity can be made only at the expense of sensitivity.

A third measure associated with sensitivity and specificity is the predictive value of the test. The positive predictive value (also called *predictive value positive*) is the proportion of persons with a positive test who actually have the disease, interpreted as the probability that an individual with a positive test has the disease. The negative predictive value (or *predictive value negative*) is the proportion of persons with a negative test who are actually disease-free.

Two or more tests can be combined, in series or in parallel, to enhance sensitivity or specificity. In series testing, the final result is considered positive only if all tests in the series were positive, and it is considered negative if any test was negative. For example, if a blood sample were screened for HIV, a positive enzyme-linked immunosorbent assay (ELISA) might be followed with a Western blot test, and the sample would be considered positive only if both tests were positive. Series testing enhances specificity, producing fewer false positives, but sensitivity will be lower. In series testing, sequence is important; a very sensitive test is often used first to pick up all cases, including false positives, and then a second, very specific test is used to eliminate the false positives. In parallel testing, the final result is considered positive if any test was positive and is considered negative only if *all* tests were negative. To return to the example of a blood sample being tested for HIV, a blood bank might consider a sample positive if a positive result was found on either the ELISA or the Western blot. Parallel testing enhances sensitivity, leaving fewer false negatives, but specificity will be lower.

BASIC METHODS IN EPIDEMIOLOGY

SOURCES OF DATA

It is important to know early in any epidemiological study how the data will be obtained (Gordis, 2013; Koepsell and Weiss, 2003). The following three major categories of data sources are commonly used in epidemiological investigations:

1. Routinely collected data: census data, vital records (i.e., birth and death certificates), and surveillance data (i.e., systematic collection of data concerning disease occurrence) as carried out by the Centers for Disease Control and Prevention (CDC)
2. Data collected for other purposes but useful for epidemiological research: medical, health department, and insurance records
3. Original data collected for specific epidemiological studies

Routinely Collected Data

The US census is conducted every 10 years and provides population data, including demographic distribution (i.e., age, race, sex), geographic distribution, and additional information about economic status, housing, and education. These data provide denominators for various rates. The American Community Survey is an ongoing survey conducted by the US Census Bureau. Data from these surveys provide information about the

status of the population and for public health planning and evaluation.

Vital records are the primary source of birth and mortality statistics. Registration of births and deaths is mandated in most countries and provides one of the most complete sources of health-related data. However, the quality of specific information varies. For example, on birth certificates, sex and date of birth are fairly reliable, whereas reports of gestational age, level of prenatal care, and smoking habits of the mother during pregnancy are less reliable. On death certificates, the quality of the cause-of-death information varies over time and from place to place, depending on diagnostic capabilities and custom. Vital records are readily available in most areas; they are inexpensive and convenient and allow study of long-term trends. Mortality data, however, are informative only for fatal diseases.

Data Collected for Other Purposes

Hospital, physician, health department, and insurance records provide information on morbidity, as do surveillance systems, such as cancer registries and health department reporting systems, which solicit reports of all cases of a particular disease within a geographic region. Other information, such as occupational exposures, may be available from employer records.

Epidemiological Data

The National Center for Health Statistics sponsors periodic health surveys and examinations in carefully drawn samples of the US population. Examples are the National Health and Nutrition Examination Survey (NHANES), the National Health Interview Survey (NHIS), and the National Hospital Discharge Survey (NHDS). The CDC also conducts or contracts for conduct of surveys such as the survey for the Youth Risk Behavior Surveillance System (YRBSS), Pregnancy Risk Assessment Monitoring System (PRAMS), and the Behavioral Risk Factor Surveillance System (BRFSS). These surveys provide information on the health status and behaviors of the population. For many studies, however, the only way to obtain the needed information is to collect the required data in a study specifically designed to investigate a particular question. The design of such studies is discussed later. Global positioning system and geographic information system technology can be used to examine health issues such as access to prenatal care, mapping the distribution of health exposures or outcomes, linking data with geo-coded addresses of individuals to sources of potentially toxic exposures (McLafferty and Grady, 2005).

RATE ADJUSTMENT

Rates, which are essential in epidemiological studies, can be misleading when compared across different populations. For example, the risk for death increases considerably after 40 years of age, so a higher crude death rate is expected in a population of older people in contrast to a population of younger people (Gordis, 2013; Koepsell and Weiss, 2003;

Rothman, 2012). Comparing the overall mortality rate in an area with a large population of older adults with the rate in a younger population would be misleading. Methods that adjust for differences in populations can be used to compare death rates. Age adjustment is based on the assumption that a population's overall mortality rate is a function of the age distribution of the population and the age-specific mortality rates.

Age adjustment can be performed by direct or indirect methods. Both methods require a *standard population,* which can be an external population, such as the US population for a given year, a combined population of the groups under study, or some other standard chosen for relevance or convenience.

HOW TO Assess Health Problems in a Community

1. Examine local epidemiologic data (e.g., incidence, morbidity, mortality rates) to identify major health problems.
2. Examine local health services data to identify major causes of hospitalizations and emergency department visits. Consult with key community leaders (e.g., political, religious, business, educational, health, cultural) about their perceptions of identified community health problems.
3. Mobilize community groups to elicit discussions and identify perceived health priorities within the community (e.g., focus groups, neighborhood or community-wide forums).
4. Analyze community environmental health hazards and pollutants (e.g., water, sewage, air, toxic waste).
5. Examine indicators of community knowledge and practices of preventive health behaviors (e.g., use of infant car seats, safe playgrounds, lighted streets, seat-belt use, designated driver programs).
6. Identify cultural priorities and beliefs about health among different social, cultural, racial, or national origin groups.
7. Assess community members' interpretation of and degree of trust in federal, state, and local assistance programs.
8. Engage community members in conducting surveys to assess specific health problems.

A direct adjusted rate applies the age-specific death rates from the study population to the age distribution of the standard population. The result is the (hypothetical) death rate of the study population if it had the same age distribution as the standard population.

The indirect method, as the name suggests, is more complicated. The age-specific death rates of the standard population applied to the study population's age distribution result in an index rate that is used with the crude rates of both the study and standard populations to produce the final indirect adjusted rate, which is also hypothetical. The indirect method may be required when the age-specific death rates for the study population are unknown or unstable (e.g., based on relatively small numbers).

Often, instead of an indirect adjusted rate, a standardized mortality ratio (SMR) is calculated. This is the number of observed deaths in the study population divided by the number of deaths expected on the basis of the age-specific rates in the standard population and the age distribution of the study population (Gordis, 2013; Szklo and Nieto, 2012).

COMPARISON GROUPS

Comparison groups are often used in epidemiology. To decide if the rate of disease is the result of a suspected risk factor, the exposed group should be compared with a group of comparable unexposed persons. For example, you might investigate the effect of smoking during pregnancy on the rate of low-birth-weight infants by calculating the rate of low-birth-weight infants born to women who smoked during their pregnancy. However, the hypothesis that smoking during pregnancy is a risk factor for low birth weight is supported only when the low-birth-weight rate among smoking women is compared with the (lower) rate of low-birth-weight infants born to nonsmoking women.

Ideally you want to compare one group of people who all have a certain characteristic, exposure, or behavior with a group of people exactly like them except they all lack that characteristic, exposure, or behavior. In the absence of that ideal, you can either randomize people to exposure or treatment groups in experimental studies or select comparison groups that are comparable in observational studies. It is especially important in observational studies to control for confounding variables or factors.

DESCRIPTIVE EPIDEMIOLOGY

Descriptive epidemiology describes the distribution of disease, death, and other health outcomes in the population according to person, place, and time. This type of epidemiology provides a picture of how things are or have been and describes who, where, and when of disease patterns. In contrast, analytic epidemiology looks for the determinants of the patterns observed—the how and why. That is, epidemiological concepts and methods are used to identify what factors, characteristics, exposures, or behaviors might account for differences in the observed patterns of disease occurrence. Descriptive and analytic studies are observational. In these studies the investigator observes events as they are or have been and does not intervene to change anything or to introduce a new factor. Experimental or intervention studies, however, include interventions to test preventive or treatment measures, techniques, materials, policies, or drugs.

PERSON

Personal characteristics of interest in epidemiology include race, sex, age, education, occupation, income (and related socioeconomic status), and marital status. Age is the most important predictor of overall mortality. The mortality curve by age drops sharply during and after the first year of life to a low point in childhood, then begins to increase through adolescence and young adulthood, and after that increases sharply through middle and older ages (Gordis, 2013). Mortality and morbidity differ by sex. Of the 10 leading causes of death, as listed earlier in the chapter, males and females diverged in the ranking in unintentional injuries (3rd for males and 6th for females). Chronic lower respiratory disease ranked 4th for males and 3rd for females, and stroke ranked 5th for males and 4th for females. Diabetes ranked 6th for males and 7th for females, and Alzheimer's disease ranked 9th for males and 5th for females. For rheumatoid arthritis, the prevalence among women is greater than among men (Remington et al, 2010).

There are also mortality differences by age. Specifically, in 2013, the leading cause of death among people ages 1 to 44 years was unintentional injuries, whereas the leading cause for the population aged 45 to 64 years was cancer, and for the population aged 65 years and over, heart disease was the leading cause of death. For the younger age groups, external causes accounted for more deaths than other causes, whereas for the older age groups, chronic illnesses were more prevalent (Heron, 2016).

Data are collected by race and Hispanic origin. The race categories are white, black, American Indian or Alaska Native (AIAN), and Asian or Pacific Islander (API). In the 2013 collection of data, the four groups shared seven of the leading causes of death but had different relative disease burden. For example, heart disease ranked first among white, black, and AIAN persons but second among the API population.

The leading cause of infant death in 2013 was congenital malformations, and the second leading cause was disorders related to short gestation and low birth weight. There were differences in the leading cause of death in the neonatal period (under 28 days after birth), which was disorders related to short gestation and low birth weight, and in the postneonatal period, which was sudden infant death syndrome (Heron, 2016)

HOW TO Assess Health Problems in an Individual
1. Obtain a history of physical and mental health problems.
2. Ask the individual to identify major health problems. Always start interventions with what the individual views as important.
3. Obtain a family history of diseases. Identify a possible genetic link based on early age of onset of a disease or multiple family members with a disease.
4. Do a clinical examination, including laboratory work.
5. Evaluate health risk based on lifestyle. Include smoking status, dietary patterns of fiber and fat, exercise patterns, stress factors, and risk-taking behaviors.
6. Identify immediate and long-range safety concerns.
7. Assess the individual's cultural beliefs about health.
8. Assess social support.
9. Examine the knowledge and practice of preventive health care.
10. Provide appropriate age-based screening (e.g., cancer screening, hypertension screening).

PLACE

When looking at the distribution of a disease, examine geographic patterns. Does the rate of disease differ from place to place (e.g., with local environment)? If geography had no effect on disease occurrence, random geographic patterns might be seen, but that is often not the case. For example, at high altitudes, oxygen tension is lower, which might result in

smaller babies. Other diseases reflect distinctive geographic patterns. For example, Lyme disease is transmitted from animal reservoirs to humans by a tick vector. Disease is more likely to be found in areas in which there are animals carrying the disease, a large tick population for transmission to humans, and contact between the human population and the tick vectors (Heymann, 2014). Geographic variations can be caused by the following:
- Differences in the chemical, physical, or biological environment
- Differences in population densities, customary patterns of behavior and lifestyle, or other personal characteristics

Geographic variations might occur because of high concentrations of a religious, cultural, or ethnic group that practices certain health-related behaviors. The high rates of stroke found in the southeastern United States are likely to be the result of social and personal factors that have little to do with geographic features per se. Other neighborhood-level variables include the unemployment and crime rate, education levels, racial segregation, social cohesion, and access to important services (Bradman et al, 2005; Fuller et al, 2005; McLafferty and Grady, 2005).

TIME

Time is the third component of descriptive epidemiology. In relation to time, epidemiologists ask these questions: Is there an increase or decrease in the frequency of the disease over time? Are other temporal (and spatial) patterns evident? Temporal patterns could include secular trends, point epidemic, cyclical patterns and event-related clusters.

Secular Changes

Long-term patterns of morbidity or mortality rates (i.e., over years or decades) are called secular trends. Secular trends may reflect changes in social behavior or practices. For example, increased lung cancer mortality rates in recent years reflect a delayed effect of the increased smoking in prior years. Also, the decline in cervical cancer deaths is primarily the result of widespread screening with the Pap test (Remington et al, 2010).

Some secular trends may result from increased diagnostic ability or changes in survival (or case fatality) rather than in incidence. For example, case fatality from breast cancer has decreased in recent years, although the incidence of breast cancer has increased. Some, though not all, of the increased incidence is the result of improved diagnostic capability. These two trends result in a breast cancer mortality curve that is flatter than the incidence curve (Remington et al, 2010). Relying on mortality data alone does not accurately reflect the true situation. Secular trends also are affected by changes in case definition or revisions in the coding of a disease according to the International Classification of Diseases (ICD).

A point epidemic is a time-and-space–related pattern that is important in infectious disease investigations and as an indicator for toxic exposures. A point epidemic is most clearly seen when the frequency of cases is graphed against time. The sharp peak characteristic of such graphs indicates a concentration of cases over a short interval of time. The peak often indicates the population's response to a common source of infection or contamination to which they were all simultaneously exposed. Knowledge of the incubation or latency period (i.e., the time between exposure and development of signs and symptoms) for the specific disease entity can help determine the probable time of exposure. A common example of a point epidemic is an outbreak of gastrointestinal illness from a food-borne pathogen. Nurses who are alert to a sudden increase in the number of cases of a disease can chart the outbreak, determine the probable time of exposure, and, by careful investigation, isolate the probable source of the agent.

In addition to secular trends and point epidemics, there are also cyclical time patterns of disease. Seasonal fluctuation is a common type of cyclical variation in some infectious illnesses. Seasonal changes may be influenced by changes in the agent itself, changes in population densities or behaviors of animal reservoirs or vectors, or changes in human behaviors resulting in changing exposures (e.g., being outdoors in warmer weather and indoors in colder months). Also, calendar events may create artificial seasons, such as holidays and tax-filing deadlines, that are associated with patterns of stress-related illness. Patterns of accidents and injuries also may be seasonal, reflecting differing employment and recreational patterns. Some disease cycles, such as influenza, have patterns of smaller epidemics every few years, depending on strain, with major pandemics occurring at longer intervals (Heymann, 2014). Public health workers need to pay attention to cyclical patterns so that they are prepared to meet possible increased demands for service.

A third type of temporal pattern is nonsimultaneous, event-related clusters. These are patterns in which time is not measured from fixed dates on the calendar but from the point of some exposure, event, or experience presumably held in common by affected persons, though not occurring at the same time. An example of this pattern would be vaccine reactions during an immunization program. Clearly, if vaccinations are being given on a regular basis, nonspecific symptoms, such as fever, headaches, or rashes, might be seen fairly consistently over time, making identification of a cluster related to the vaccinations difficult. If, however, the occurrence of symptoms is plotted against the amount of time since vaccination, the number of vaccine reactions is likely to peak at some period after the immunization.

❓ CHECK YOUR PRACTICE

The Dean of the School of Nursing held an open house on August 26 to welcome new and returning nursing students. Approximately 50 nursing students and professors attended. Light appetizers and cider were served. On the morning of August 28, two nursing students reported to the student health clinic with nausea and vomiting. Later that day, three other students reported to the clinic with headache, nausea, and vomiting. Two of the five students reported that their symptoms began the evening of August 27, and the other three reported symptom onset the morning of August 28. Two nursing professors called in sick with nausea and diarrhea on August 28. Both attended the dean's open house and a reception earlier in the week.

Check Your Practice:
The student health nurse notified the nurse epidemiologist at the local health department that she has seen five nursing students with gastrointestinal symptoms. She reports their names, dates of birth, and dates and times of onset of symptoms.

1. The nurse epidemiologist at the health department develops a line list to organize the data. The line list includes the information reported by the student health nurse. What is the term used to describe the type of epidemiology associated with time, place, and person?
   A. Descriptive
   B. Analytic
   C. Scientific
   D. Environmental
2. The nurse epidemiologist notes that the infections are clustered in time, place, and person. She interviews all of the ill nursing students and learns that all of them attended the open house at the dean's home. What should the nurse do next?
   A. Close the nursing school
   B. Arrange to collect stool specimens
   C. Contact the dean
   D. Quarantine all of the open house attendees

3. The nurse epidemiologist notifies the student health nurse that all of the stool specimens were positive for norovirus. Based on the incubation period for norovirus (12–48 hours) and the dates of onset of symptoms, the nurse epidemiologist suspects the students were exposed to the virus at or around the same time. She hypothesizes that the nurses contracted norovirus from a contaminated item consumed at the open house event. She makes arrangements to meet with the dean to discuss the situation and gather additional information. What information would be useful to the nurse epidemiologist?
   A. A list of items served at the event
   B. A list of persons who prepared and served the refreshments
   C. A list of students, faculty, and staff who attended the event
   D. A list of faculty and student absences
   E. All of the above
4. The nurse epidemiologist decides to interview everyone (ill and well) who attended the open house. This type of study is called a:
   A. Case-control study
   B. Cohort study
   C. Longitudinal study
   D. Case study
5. Based on the data analysis, the nurse epidemiologist determined that the fresh vegetable tray is associated with illness. She also learned that two of the food handlers were not feeling well during the event. What measures should she take at this point to control the outbreak?
   A. Try to obtain stool specimens from the catering staff
   B. Educate catering and serving staff about safe food preparation
   C. Encourage food service staff not to prepare or serve food when they are ill with gastrointestinal symptoms
   D. Call the Better Business Bureau

Case prepared by Mary Beth White-Comstock, MSN, RN, CIC.

ANALYTIC EPIDEMIOLOGY

Descriptive epidemiology deals with the *distribution* of health outcomes. The goal of analytic epidemiology is to discover the *determinants* of outcomes—the how and the why. Analytic epidemiology deals with the factors that influence the observed patterns of health and disease and increase or decrease the risk for adverse outcomes. This section discusses analytic study designs and the related measures of association derived from them. Table 9.3 summarizes the advantages and disadvantages of each design.

COHORT STUDIES

The cohort study is the standard for observational epidemiological studies. It comes closest to the idea of a natural experiment

(Rothman, 2012). The term *cohort* is used in epidemiology to describe a group of persons who are born at about the same time. In analytic studies, cohort refers to a group of persons generally sharing some characteristic of interest. They are enrolled in a study and followed over time to observe some health outcome (Porta, 2008). Because of this ability to observe the development of new cases of disease, cohort study designs allow for calculation of incidence rates and therefore estimates of risk for disease. Cohort studies may be prospective or retrospective (Gordis, 2013; Rothman, 2012).

PROSPECTIVE COHORT STUDIES

In a prospective cohort study (also called a *longitudinal* or *follow-up study*), subjects who do not have the Outcome under investigation are classified on the basis of the exposure of

TABLE 9.3 Comparison of Major Epidemiologic Study Designs

Study Design	Advantages	Disadvantages
Ecologic	Quick, easy, inexpensive first study Uses readily available existing data May prompt further investigation or suggest other or new hypotheses May provide information about contextual factors not accounted for by individual characteristics	Ecologic fallacy: The associations observed may not hold true for individuals Problems in interpreting temporal sequence (cause and effect) More difficult to control for confounding and "mixed" models (ecologic and individual data); more complex statistically
Cross-sectional (correlational)	Gives general description of the scope of problem; provides prevalence estimates Often based on population (or community) sample, not just who sought care Useful in health service evaluation and planning Data obtained at once; less expense and quicker than cohort because of no follow-up Baseline for prospective study or to identify cases and controls for case-control study	No calculation of risk; prevalence, not incidence Temporal sequence unclear Not good for rare disease or rare exposure unless there is a large sample size or stratified sampling Selective survival can be a major source of selection bias; surviving subjects may differ from those who are not included (e.g., death, institutionalization) Selective recall or lack of past exposure information can create bias
Case-control (retrospective, case comparison)	Less expensive than cohort; smaller sample required Quicker than cohort; no follow-up Can investigate more than one exposure Best design for rare diseases If well designed, it can be an important tool for etiologic investigation Best suited to a disease with a relatively clear onset (timing of onset can be established so that incident cases can be included)	Greater susceptibility than cohort studies to various types of bias (selective survival, recall bias, selection bias in choice of both cases and controls) Information on other risk factors may not be available, resulting in confounding Antecedent-consequence (temporal sequence) not as certain as in cohort Not well suited to rare exposures Gives only an indirect estimate of risk Generally limited to a single outcome because of sampling effect on disease status
Prospective cohort (concurrent cohort, longitudinal, follow-up)	Best estimate of disease incidence Best estimate of risk Fewer problems with selective survival and selective recall Temporal sequence more clearly established Broader range of options for exposure assessment	Expensive in terms of time and money More difficult organizationally Not good for rare diseases Attrition of participants can bias the estimate Latency period may be very long; may miss cases May be difficult to examine several exposures
Retrospective cohort (nonconcurrent cohort)	Combines advantages of both prospective cohort and case-control Shorter time (even if follow-up into the future) than prospective cohort Less expensive than prospective cohort because it relies on existing data Temporal sequence may be clearer than case-control	Shares some disadvantages with both prospective cohort and case-control Subject to attrition (loss to follow-up) Relies on existing records that may result in misclassification of both exposure and outcome May have to rely on a surrogate measure of exposure (e.g., job title) and vital records information on cause of death

interest at the beginning of the follow-up period. The subjects are then followed for some period of time to determine the occurrence of disease in each group. The question is, "Do persons with the factor (or exposure) of interest develop (or avoid) the outcome more frequently than those without the factor (or exposure)?"

For example, a cohort of subjects could be recruited who would be classified as physically active ("exposed") or sedentary ("not exposed"). If you had adequate information you could quantify the amount of the "exposure." You could then follow these subjects over time to determine the development of CHD. This study design avoids the problem of selective survival seen in other designs. The cohort study also has the advantage of allowing estimation of the risk for acquiring disease for those who are exposed compared with those who are unexposed (or less exposed). This ratio of cumulative incidence rates is called the *relative risk.*

Suppose 1000 physically active and 1000 sedentary middle-aged men and women were enrolled in a prospective cohort study. All were free of CHD at enrollment. Over a 5-year follow-up period, regular examinations detect CHD in 120 of the sedentary men and women and in 48 of the active men and women. Assuming no other deaths or losses to follow-up, the data could be presented as shown in Fig. 9.2.

The incidence of CHD in the active group is $(a/[a + b]) = 48/1000$, and the incidence of CHD in the sedentary group is $(c/[c + d]) = 120/1000$. The relative risk is:

$$(48/1000) \div (120/1000) = 0.4.$$

Because physical activity is protective for CHD, the relative risk is less than 1. In this example over a 5-year period, the risk for CHD in persons who are physically active compared with the risk among sedentary persons was 0.4. In the cohort study design, subjects are enrolled before disease onset, and this allows the researcher to study more than one outcome, calculate incidence rates and estimate risk, and establish the temporal sequence of exposure and outcome with greater clarity and certainty. The researcher may need a large sample to ensure that enough cases are observed to provide statistical power to detect meaningful differences between groups and may have to wait a long time for some diseases to develop.

Retrospective Cohort Studies

Retrospective cohort studies combine some of the advantages and disadvantages of case-control studies and prospective cohort studies. These studies rely on existing records, such as employment, insurance, or hospital records, to define a cohort that is classified as having been exposed or unexposed at some time in the past. The cohort is followed over time using the records to determine if the outcome occurred. Retrospective cohort (also called *historical cohort*) studies may be conducted entirely using past records or may include current assessment or additional follow-up time after study initiation. This approach saves time; however, its accuracy relies on existing historical records.

CASE-CONTROL STUDIES

In the case-control study, subjects are enrolled *because* they are known to have the outcome of interest (these are the cases) or they are known *not* to have the outcome of interest (these are the controls). Case-control status is verified using a clear case definition and some previously determined method or protocol (e.g., by an examination, laboratory test, or medical chart review). Information is then collected on the exposures or characteristics of interest, frequently from existing sources, subject interview, or questionnaire (Rothman, 2012; Szklo and Nieto, 2012). The question in a case-control study is "Do persons with the outcome of interest (cases) have the exposure characteristic (or a history of the exposure) more frequently than those without the outcome (controls)?"

Because of the method of subject selection in case-control studies, neither incidence nor prevalence can be calculated directly. In a case-control study, an odds ratio tells us how much more (or less) likely the exposure is to be found among cases than among controls. The odds of exposure among cases (*a* and *c* in the table that follows) are compared with the odds of exposure among controls (*b* and *d*). The ratio of these two odds provides us with an estimate of the relative risk.

Suppose a research group wanted to study risk factors for suicide attempts among adolescents. To do so they would enroll 100 adolescents who had attempted suicide, and select 200 adolescents from the same community with no history of a suicide attempt. The research group's goal is to determine if the adolescents had a history of substance abuse (SA). Through a questionnaire and use of medical records they learned that 68 of the 100 adolescents who had attempted suicide had a history of substance abuse. They also found that 36 of the 200 adolescents with no suicide attempt had a history of substance abuse. The information could be presented as follows:

History	Suicide Attempt	No Attempt
History of substance abuse	68	36
	(a)	(b)
No history of substance abuse	32	164
	(c)	(d)

The odds of a history of substance abuse among suicide attempters are *a/c* or 68/32, whereas the odds of substance abuse

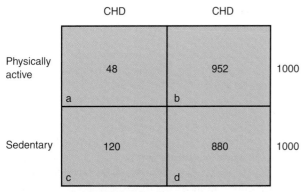

	CHD	CHD	
Physically active	48 a	952 b	1000
Sedentary	120 c	880 d	1000

FIG. 9.2 Cohort study.

among controls are *b/d* or 36/164. The odds ratio (equivalent to *ad/bc*) is the following:

$$\frac{68 \times 164}{36 \times 32} = 9.68$$

This would be interpreted to mean that adolescents who attempted suicide are almost 10 times more likely to have a history of substance abuse than are adolescents who have not attempted suicide. Note that an odds ratio of 1 is indicative of no association (i.e., the odds of exposure are similar for cases and controls). An odds ratio less than 1 suggests a protective association, that is, cases are less likely to have been exposed than controls. Because case-control studies know the number of cases involved, they do not require a large sample or take a long follow-up time. They may have biases. *Bias* is a systematic deviation from the truth. Because these studies begin with existing diseases, differential survival can produce biased results. The use of recently diagnosed (or "incident") cases may reduce this bias. Because exposure information is obtained from subject recall or past records, there may be errors in exposure assessment or misclassification.

CROSS-SECTIONAL STUDIES

The cross-sectional study provides a snapshot, or cross section, of a population or group (Gordis, 2013). Information is collected on current health status, personal characteristics, and potential risk factors or exposures all at once. In the cross-sectional study there is a simultaneous collection of information necessary for the classification of exposure. Historical information can also be collected (e.g., past diet, history of radiation exposures).

One way cross-sectional studies evaluate the association of a factor with a health problem is to compare the prevalence of the disease in those with the factor (or exposure) with the prevalence of the disease in the unexposed. The ratio of the two prevalence rates is an indication of the association between the factor and the outcome. If the prevalence of CHD in smokers were twice as high as the prevalence among nonsmokers, the prevalence ratio would be 2. If a factor is unrelated to the prevalence of a disease, the prevalence ratio will be close to 1. A value less than 1 may suggest a protective association. For example, the prevalence of CHD is lower among physically active people than among sedentary persons. Thus the prevalence ratio for the association between physical activity and CHD should be less than 1. Use caution in interpreting prevalence ratios because the prevalence measure is affected by cure, survival, and migration and does not estimate the risk for *getting* the disease.

Cross-sectional studies are subject to bias resulting from selective survival. That is, persons with existing cases who have survived to be in the study may be different from those diagnosed at about the same time who died and are unavailable for inclusion. Suppose physical activity not only reduced the risk for heart disease but also improved survival among those with heart disease. Sedentary persons with heart disease would then have higher fatality rates than physically active persons who developed heart disease. Higher rates of physical activity might be observed in a group of heart disease survivors than in a general population

without heart disease. This might occur because of the survival advantage and also because of the participation of the survivors in cardiac rehabilitation programs. It might, however, erroneously appear that physical activity was a risk factor for heart disease.

ECOLOGICAL STUDIES

An ecological study is a study that is a bridge between descriptive and analytic epidemiology. The descriptive component looks at variations in disease rates by person, place, or time. The analytic component tries to determine if there is a relation of disease rates to variations in rates for possible risk (or protective) factors or characteristics. The identifying characteristic of ecological studies is that only aggregate data, such as population rates, are used, rather than data on individuals' exposures, characteristics, and outcomes. Examples include the following:

1. Examination of information on per capita cigarette consumption in relation to lung cancer mortality rates in several countries, several groups of people, or the same population at different times
2. Comparisons of rates of breastfeeding and of breast cancer
3. Average dietary fat content and rates of CHD
4. Unemployment rates and level of psychiatric disorder
Ecological studies often use existing, readily available rates and are therefore quick and inexpensive to conduct. They are subject, however, to ecologic fallacy (i.e., associations observed at the group level may not hold true for the individuals who make up the groups, or associations that actually exist may be masked in the grouped data). This can occur when other factors operate in these populations for which the ecological correlations do not account. For that reason, ecological studies may suggest possible answers, but they require confirmation in studies that use individual data (Gordis, 2013; Koepsell and Weiss, 2003).

EXPERIMENTAL STUDIES

The study designs discussed so far are called *observational studies* because the investigator observes the association between exposures and outcomes as they exist but does not intervene to alter the presence or level of any exposure or behavior. In contrast, in experimental or intervention studies, the investigator initiates a treatment or intervention to influence the risk for or course of disease. These studies test whether interventions can prevent disease or improve health. Both observational and experimental studies generally use comparison (or control) groups. In experimental studies, persons can be randomly assigned to a particular group; an intervention (i.e., a treatment or exposure) is applied, and the effects of the intervention are measured. The two types of intervention studies are clinical trials and community trials.

CLINICAL TRIALS

The goal of a clinical trial is generally to evaluate the effectiveness of an intervention, such as a medical treatment for disease, a new drug or existing drug used in a new or a different way, a surgical technique, or other treatment. In clinical trials, subjects should be randomly assigned to groups. In randomization, treatments are assigned to patients (subjects) so that all possible treatment assignments have a predetermined probability, but neither subject nor investigator determines the actual assignment of any participant. Randomization avoids the bias that may result if subjects choose to be in one group or the other or if the investigator or clinician chooses subjects for each group.

Masking or "blinding" treatment assignments is a second aspect of treatment allocation. Generally it is best to use a double-blinded study in which neither subject nor investigator knows who is getting which treatment. Clinical trials usually are the best way to show causality because of the objective way in which subjects are assigned and the greater control over other factors that could influence outcome. Like cohort studies, they are prospective and provide the clearest evidence of correct temporal sequence.

They do tend to be conducted in a contrived (versus natural) situation, under controlled conditions, and with patient populations. That means that treatment may not be as effective when applied under more realistic clinical or community conditions in a more diverse patient population. There are also more ethical considerations involved in experimental studies than in observational studies. For example, is it fair to withhold a treatment, if the treatment truly appears to have the potential to alleviate a disease, to evaluate this treatment systematically using both an experimental and a control group? Finally, clinical trials are expensive in terms of time, personnel, facilities, and, in some cases, supplies.

COMMUNITY TRIALS

Community trials are similar to clinical trials in that an investigator determines what the exposure or intervention will be. However, community trials often deal with health promotion and disease prevention rather than treatment of existing disease. The intervention is usually undertaken on a large scale, and the unit of treatment is a community, region, or group rather than individuals. Although a pharmaceutical product such as fluoridation of water or mass immunizations may be involved in a community trial, these trials often involve educational, programmatic, or policy interventions. Examples of community interventions would be measuring the rates of diabetes or cardiovascular disease in a community in which the availability of exercise programs and facilities was increased or in which a much larger supply of healthful fresh foods was made available.

Although community trials provide the best means of testing whether changes in knowledge or behavior, policy, programs, or other mass interventions are effective, they do present some problems. For many interventions, it may take years for the effectiveness to be evident, for example, the effect of changing the availability of exercise and healthful food on the rates of either diabetes or heart disease. While the study is being carried out over time, other factors can influence the outcome either positively (i.e., making the intervention look more effective than it really is) or negatively (i.e., making the intervention look less effective than it really is). Comparable community populations without similar interventions for comparative analysis are

often difficult to find. Even when comparable comparison communities are available—especially when the intervention is improved knowledge or changed behavior—it is difficult and unethical to prevent the control communities from making use of generally available information, effectively making them less different from the intervention communities. Finally, because community trials are often undertaken on a large scale and over long periods, they can be expensive, require a large staff, have complicated logistics, and need extensive communication about the study.

CAUSALITY

STATISTICAL ASSOCIATIONS

Sample size, strength of association, and variance of measures can all affect statistical significance. For example, to determine if eating habits affect the onset of hypertension, a statistical association between the factor (diet) and the health outcome (hypertension) would need to be established. If the probability of disease seems unaffected by the presence or level of the factor, no association is apparent. If, on the other hand, the probability of disease does vary according to whether the factor is present, there is a statistical association. The earlier discussion of null values is pertinent at this point. When an observed measure of association (e.g., a risk ratio) does not differ from the null value, there is no evidence of an association between the factor and the outcome being studied. To say a result is statistically significant means that the observed result is unlikely to be due to chance. Sample size affects statistical significance.

BIAS

A statistically significant result may also be observed because of bias, a systematic error as a result of the study design, the way it is conducted, or a confounding factor. For example, if there were a gumball machine with colors randomly mixed and three red ones in a row came out, that would be due to chance. If, however, the person loading the gumball machine had poured in a bag of red ones first, then green ones, then yellow ones, it would not be surprising to get three red ones in a row because of the way the machine was loaded. In epidemiological studies, results are sometimes biased because of the way the study was "loaded" (i.e., the way the study was designed or the way subjects were selected, information was collected, and subjects were classified). Although the types of bias are numerous, there are three general categories of bias (Rothman, 2012). Bias can be attributed to the following:

1. **Selection or the way subjects enter a study:** Selection bias has to do with selection procedures and the population from which subjects are drawn, and it may involve self-selection factors. *Example:* Are teenagers who agree to complete a questionnaire on alcohol, tobacco, and other drug use representative of the total teenage population?
2. **Misclassification of subjects once they are in the study:** This is information, or classification (or misclassification), bias. It is related to how information is collected, including

the information that subjects supply or how subjects are classified.

3. **Confounding or bias resulting from the relationship between the outcome and study factor and some third factor not accounted for**. *Example:* There is a well-known association between maternal smoking during pregnancy and low-birth-weight babies. There is also an association between alcohol consumption and smoking that is not due to chance, nor is it causal (i.e., drinking alcohol does not cause a person to smoke, nor does smoking cause a person to drink alcohol). If we were to investigate the association between alcohol consumption and low birth weight, smoking would be a confounder because it is related to both alcohol consumption and low birth weight. Failure to account for smoking in the analysis would bias the observed association between alcohol use and low birth weight. In practice, we can often identify potentially confounding variables and adjust for them in the analysis.

ASSESSING FOR CAUSALITY

The existence of a statistical association does not necessarily mean that a causal relationship exists or that causality is present. As just discussed, the observed association may be a random event (due to chance) or may be the result of bias from confounding or from some aspect of the study design or execution. Statistical associations, although necessary to an argument for causal inference, are not adequate proof. Some epidemiologists refer to guidelines, a term originally established to evaluate the link between an infectious agent and a disease but revised and elaborated to apply also to other outcomes. Although various lists of guidelines have been proposed, the seven guidelines listed in Box 9.3 are often used (Gordis, 2013; Koepsell and Weiss, 2003).

APPLICATIONS OF EPIDEMIOLOGY IN NURSING

Nurses need to know and be able to use epidemiology. Nurses regularly collect, report, analyze, interpret, and communicate epidemiological data in many of the areas in which they work. Nurses involved in the care of persons with communicable diseases use epidemiology daily as they identify, report, treat, and provide follow-up on cases and contacts of TB, gonorrhea, and gastroenteritis. School nurses also function as epidemiologists, collecting data on the incidence and prevalence of accidents, injuries, and illnesses in the school population. They are also key players in the detection and control of local epidemics, such as outbreaks of lice. As described earlier in this chapter, nurses across practice settings are actively involved in activities related to primary, secondary, and tertiary prevention (see the discussion of levels of prevention and the Levels of Prevention box).

Some nursing jobs are specifically based in epidemiological practice. These include nurse epidemiologists and environmental risk communicators employed by local health departments, as well as hospital infection control nurses. Nurses are key members of local fetal and infant mortality review boards,

---

BOX 9.3 Guidelines for Causal Inference

1. **Strength of association:** A strong association between a potential risk factor and an outcome supports a causal hypothesis (i.e., a relative risk of 7 provides stronger evidence of a causal association than a relative risk of 1.5).
2. **Consistency of findings:** Repeated findings of an association with different study designs and in different populations strengthen a causal inference.
3. **Biological plausibility:** Demonstration of a physiological mechanism by which the risk factor acts to cause disease enhances the causal hypothesis. Conversely, an association that does not initially seem biologically defensible may later be discovered to be so.
4. **Demonstration of correct temporal sequence:** For a risk factor to cause an outcome, it must precede the onset of the outcome.
5. **Dose-response relationship:** The risk for developing an outcome should increase with increasing exposure (either in duration or quantity) to the risk factor of interest. For example, studies have shown that the more a woman smokes during pregnancy, the greater is the risk for delivering a low-birth-weight infant.
6. **Specificity of the association:** The presence of a one-to-one relationship between an agent and a disease (i.e., the idea that a disease is caused by only one agent and that agent results in only one disease lends support to a causal hypothesis, but its absence does not rule out causality). This criterion grows out of the infectious disease model in which it is more often though not always satisfied and is less applicable in chronic diseases.
7. **Experimental evidence:** Experimental designs provide the strongest epidemiologic evidence for causal associations, but they are not feasible or ethical to conduct for many risk factor–disease associations.

LEVELS OF PREVENTION
Related to Cardiovascular Disease

Primary Prevention
Discuss a low-fat diet and the need for regular physical exercise with clients.

Secondary Prevention
Implement blood pressure and cholesterol screening; give a treadmill stress test.

Tertiary Prevention
Provide cardiac rehabilitation, medication, and surgery.

---

which examine cases of newborn deaths for identifiable risk factors and quality of care measures. Members of these review boards may include public health and maternal and child nurses, as well as representatives from hospital labor and delivery and neonatal intensive care units. Nurses play a key role in disaster preparedness in their communities, and this work includes knowledge of epidemiology.

Nursing documentation on patient charts and records is an important source of data for epidemiological reviews. Patient demographics and health histories are often collected or verified by nurses. As nurses collect and document patient information, they might not be thinking about the epidemiological connection. However, the reliability and validity of such data can be key factors in the quality of future epidemiological studies.

QSEN FOCUS ON QUALITY AND SAFETY EDUCATION FOR NURSES

Targeted Competency: Informatics—Use information and technology to communicate, manage knowledge, mitigate error, and support decision making.

Important aspects of informatics include:

- **Knowledge:** Identify essential information that must be available in a common database to support client care.
- **Skills:** Use information management tools to monitor outcomes of care processes.
- **Attitudes:** Value nurses' involvement in design, selection, implementation and evaluation of information technologies to support client care.

Informatics Question
Determine If a Health Problem Exists in the Community
Nurses are involved in the surveillance and monitoring of health phenomena. Planning for resources and personnel often requires quantifying the level

of a problem in the community. For example, to know how different districts compare in the rates of infants with very low birth weight, you would calculate the prevalence of infants with very low birth weight in each district:

1. Determine the number of live births in each district from birth certificate data obtained from the vital records division of the health department.
2. Use the birth-weight information from the birth certificate data to determine the number of infants born weighing less than 1500 g in each district.
3. Calculate the prevalence of births of infants with very low birth weights by district as the number of infants weighing less than 1500 g at birth divided by the total number of live births.
4. If the number of births of infants with very low birth weights in each district is small, use several years of data to obtain a more stable estimate.

Prepared by Gail Armstrong, PhD, DNP, ACNS-BC, CNE, Associate Professor, University of Colorado College of Nursing.

PRACTICE APPLICATION

You are a nurse at a local health department where Rob Jones, a 46-year-old African American, comes for a routine blood pressure check. He mentions that his father recently died of prostate cancer and that he is worried about himself. Further assessment reveals that his father was diagnosed with prostate cancer when he was 52 years old and that Mr. Jones's uncle, who is 56, was recently diagnosed with prostate cancer. You know from Mr. Jones's health history that he smokes a pack of cigarettes per day and eats fried food frequently.

Which action would be your best choice?

A. Give Mr. Jones a digital rectal examination and prostate-specific antigen (PSA) test immediately to screen for prostate cancer.

B. Do not discuss or provide prostate cancer screening with him, because he is younger than 50 years.

C. Advise Mr. Jones to be tested immediately for the prostate cancer gene, because of his family history.

D. Inform him of the risks and benefits of prostate cancer testing and of his increased personal risk for prostate cancer because of his family history, smoking, and dietary habits. Involve him in the decision-making process about prostate cancer screening.

Answers can be found on the Evolve website.

REMEMBER THIS!

- Epidemiology is the study of the distribution and determinants of health-related events in human populations and the application of this knowledge to improving the health of communities.
- Epidemiology is a multidisciplinary science that recognizes the complex interrelationships of factors that influence disease and health at both the individual and the community level; it provides the basic tools for the study of health and disease in communities.
- Epidemiological methods are used to describe health and disease and to investigate the factors that promote health or influence the risk for, or distribution of, disease. This knowledge can be useful in planning and evaluating programs, policies, and services and in clinical decision making.
- Basic epidemiological concepts include the interrelationships among the agent, host, and environment (the epidemiologic triangle); the interactions of factors, exposures, and characteristics in a causal web affecting the risk for disease; and the levels of prevention corresponding to stages in the natural history of disease.

- Primary prevention involves interventions to reduce the incidence of disease by promoting health and preventing disease processes from developing.
- Secondary prevention includes programs (e.g., screening) designed to detect disease in the early stages, before signs and symptoms are clinically evident, to intervene with early diagnosis and treatment.
- Tertiary prevention provides treatments and other interventions directed toward persons with clinically apparent disease, with the aim of lessening the course of the disease, reducing disability, or rehabilitating the client.
- Epidemiological methods are also used in the planning and design of screening (secondary prevention) and community health intervention (primary prevention) strategies and in the evaluation of their effectiveness.
- Basic epidemiological methods include the use of existing data sources to study health outcomes and related factors and the use of comparison groups to assess the association between exposures or characteristics and health outcomes.

- Epidemiologists use rates and proportions to quantify levels of morbidity and mortality.
- Prevalence proportions provide a picture of the level of existing cases in a population at a given time.
- Incidence rates and proportions measure the rate of new case development in a population and provide an estimate of the risk for disease.
- Descriptive epidemiological studies provide information on the distribution of disease and health states according to personal characteristics, geographic region, and time. This knowledge enables practitioners to target programs and allocate resources more effectively and provides a basis for further study.
- Analytic epidemiological studies investigate associations between exposures or characteristics and health or disease outcomes, with the goal of understanding the etiology of disease. Analytic studies provide the foundation for understanding disease causality and for developing effective intervention strategies aimed at primary, secondary, and tertiary prevention.

ⓔ EVOLVE WEBSITE

http://evolve.elsevier.com/Stanhope/foundations
- Case Study, with Questions and Answers
- NCLEX® Review Questions
- Practice Application Answers

REFERENCES

American Nurses Association: *Essential nursing competencies and curricula guidelines for genetics and genomics*, Silver Spring, MD, 2006, ANA.

Bradman A, Chevier J, Tager I, et al: Association of housing disrepair indicators with cockroach and rodent infestations in a cohort of pregnant Latina women and their children, Environ Health Perspect 113:1795–1801, 2005.

Cohen IB: Florence Nightingale, *Sci Am* 250:128–137, 1984.

Council on Linkages between Academic and Public Health Practice: *Core competencies for public health professionals*, Washington DC, 2010, Public Health Foundation/Health Resources and Services Administration.

Fuller CM, Borrell LN, Latkin CA, et al: Effects of race, neighborhood, and social network on age at initiation of injection drug use, *Am J Public Health* 95:689–695, 2005.

Gordis L: *Epidemiology*, ed 5, Philadelphia, 2013, Saunders.

Heron M: Deaths: leading causes for 2013, *Natl Vital Stat Rep* 65(2):1–14, Hyattsville, MD, 2016, National Center for Health Statistics.

Heymann DL, editor: *Control of communicable diseases manual*, ed 20, Washington, DC, 2014, American Public Health Association.

Institute of Medicine: *The future of the public's health in the 21st century*, Washington, DC, 2002, National Academies Press. Retrieved May 2012 from http://www.iom.edu/Reports.

Koepsell TD, Weiss NS: *Epidemiologic methods: studying the occurrence of illness*, New York, 2003, Oxford University Press.

Macintyre S, Ellaway A: Ecological approaches: rediscovering the role of the physical and social environment. In Berkman LF, Kawachi I, editors: *Social epidemiology*, New York, 2000, Oxford University Press, pp 332–348.

McKeown RE, Learner RM: Ethics in public health practice. In Coughlin S, Beauchamp T, Weed T, editors: *Ethics and epidemiology*, ed 2, New York, 2009, Oxford University Press, pp 147–181.

McLafferty S, Grady S: Immigration and geographic access to prenatal clinics in Brooklyn, NY: a geographic information systems analysis, *Am J Public Health* 95:638–640, 2005.

Merrill RM, Timmreck TC: *Introduction to epidemiology*, ed 4, Sudbury, Mass, 2006, Jones & Bartlett.

Murphy SL, Xu JQ, Kochanek KD: Deaths: preliminary data for 2010, *Natl Vital Stat Rep* 60; 2012 for actual 2010 data.

Palmer IS: *Florence Nightingale and the first organized delivery of nursing services*, Washington, DC, 1983, American Association of Colleges of Nursing.

Porta M: *A dictionary of epidemiology*, ed 5, New York, 2008, Oxford University Press.

Remington PL, Brownson RC, Wegman MV: *Chronic disease epidemiology and control*, ed 3, Washington DC, 2010, American Public Health Association.

Rothman KJ: *Epidemiology: an introduction*, ed 2, New York, 2012, Oxford University Press.

Siu AL: Screening for high blood pressure in adults: US Preventive Services Task Force recommendation statement, *Annals of Internal Medicine* 163(10):778–786, 2015.

Snow J: On the mode of communication of cholera. In *Snow on cholera*, New York, 1855, The Commonwealth Fund.

Swider SM, Krothe J, Reyes D, Cravetz M: The Quad Council practice competencies for public health nursing, *Public Health Nursing* 30(6):519–536, 2013.

Szklo M, Nieto FJ: *Epidemiology beyond the basics*, ed 3, Boston, 2012, Jones & Bartlett.

US Department of Health and Human Services: *Healthy People 2020*, Washington, DC, 2010, US Government Printing Office.

Wiehe SE, Rosenman MC, Aalsma MC, Scanlon ML, Fortenberry JD: Epidemiology of sexually transmitted infections among offenders following arrest or incarceration, *American Journal of Public Health* 105(12):26–33, 2015.

Xu JQ, Murphy SL, Kochanek KD, Bastian BA: Deaths: Final data for 2013, *National Vital Statistics Reports* 64(2):1–119, Hyattsville MD, 2016, National Center for Health Statistics.

Evidence-Based Practice

Marcia Stanhope

OBJECTIVES

After reading this chapter, the student should be able to:

1. Define evidence-based practice.
2. Understand the history of evidence-based practice in health care.
3. Assess the relationship between evidence-based practice and the practice of nursing in the community.
4. Provide examples of evidence-based practice in the community.
5. Identify barriers to evidence-based practice.
6. Apply resources for evidence-based practice.

CHAPTER OUTLINE

Definition of Evidence-Based Practice
History of Evidence-Based Practice
Types of Evidence
Factors Leading to Change or Barriers to Evidence-Based Practice
Steps in the Evidence-Based Practice Process
Approaches to Finding Evidence
Approaches to Evaluating Evidence
Approaches to Implementing Evidence-Based Practice

Current Perspectives
   Cost versus Quality
   Individual Differences
   Appropriate Evidence-Based Practice Methods for Community-Oriented Nursing Practice
Healthy People 2020 Objectives
Example of Application of Evidence-Based Practice to Public Health Nursing

KEY TERMS

evidence-based medicine, 171
evidence-based nursing, 171
evidence-based practice, 171
evidence-based public health, 171
grading the strength of evidence, 176
integrative review, 174
meta-analysis, 174
narrative review, 174
randomized controlled trial (RCT), 172
research utilization, 171
systematic review, 174

Emphasis on evidence-based practice (EBP) is a recent development in health care delivery in the United States. It is a relevant approach to providing the highest quality of health care in all settings, which will result in improved health outcomes. EBP is important for all professionals who work in social and health care environments, regardless of the client or the setting with which professionals are dealing, including public health nurses who work with populations. Emphasis on EBP has resulted from increased expectations of consumers, changes in health care economics, increased expectations of accountability, advancements in technology, the knowledge explosion fueled by the Internet, and the growing number of lawsuits occurring when there is injury or harm as a result of practice decisions that are not based on the best available evidence (Makic et al, 2014). Nurses at all levels have an opportunity to improve the practice of nursing and client outcomes. The Institute of Medicine (IOM) has set a goal that by 2020, the best available evidence will be used to make 90% of all health care decisions, yet most nurses continue to be inconsistent in implementing EBP. An even greater concern in public health is that the field is lagging behind in developing evidence-based guidelines for the community setting. It is important to recognize that regardless of the level of education, undergraduate or graduate, nurses can be involved in the development, implementation, and evaluation of the effects of EBP (Florin et al, 2012; Gerrish and Cooke, 2013; Mattila et al, 2013; Merrill et al, 2013; Sprayberry, 2014).

The authors acknowledge the contribution of Sharon E. Lock to the content of this chapter.

DEFINITION OF EVIDENCE-BASED PRACTICE

The definition of evidence-based medicine by Sackett et al (1996) became the industry standard. Sackett et al (2000) defined evidence-based medicine as "the conscientious, explicit, and judicious use of current best evidence in making decisions about the care of individual clients" (p 71). Adapting the definition by Sackett et al (1996), Rychetnik et al (2003) defined evidence-based public health as "a public health endeavor in which there is an informed, explicit, and judicious use of evidence that has been derived from any of a variety of science and social science research and evaluation methods" (p 538). Brownson et al (2009) recently expanded the definition of evidence-based public health to include "making decisions on the basis of the best available evidence, using data and information systems, applying program planning frameworks, engaging the community in decision making, conducting evaluations, and disseminating what has been learned" (p 175).

In a position statement on evidence-based practice, the Honor Society of Nursing, Sigma Theta Tau International, defined evidence-based nursing as "an integration of the best evidence available, nursing expertise, and the values and preferences of the individuals, families, and communities who are served" (Honor Society of Nursing, Sigma Theta Tau International, 2005). The definition continues to be broadened in scope and now includes a life-long problem-solving approach to clinical practice, integrating both external and internal evidence to answer clinical questions and to achieve desired client outcomes (Melnyk and Fineout-Overholt, 2015). *External evidence* includes research and other evidence, whereas *internal evidence* includes the nurse's clinical experiences and the client's preferences.

Applied to nursing, evidence-based practice includes the best available evidence from a variety of sources, including research studies, evidence from nursing experience and expertise, and evidence from community leaders. Culturally and financially appropriate interventions need to be identified when working with communities. The use of evidence to determine the appropriate use of interventions that are culturally sensitive and cost-effective is a must.

HISTORY OF EVIDENCE-BASED PRACTICE

During the mid- to late 1970s there was growing consensus among nursing leaders that scientific knowledge should be used as a basis for nursing practice. During that time, the Division of Nursing in the U.S. Public Health Service began funding research utilization projects. Research utilization has been defined as "the process of transforming research knowledge into practice" (Stetler, 2001, p 272) and "the use of research to guide clinical practice" (Estabrooks et al, 2004, p 293).

Three projects funded by the Division of Nursing received the most attention and were the most influential in shaping nursing's view of using research to guide practice:

- The Nursing Child Assessment Satellite Training Project (NCAST) (Barnard and Hoehn, 1978; King et al, 1981)
- The Western Interstate Commission for Higher Education (WICHE) Regional Program for Nursing Research Development (WICHEN) (Krueger, 1977; Krueger et al, 1978; Lindeman and Krueger, 1977)
- The Conduct and Utilization of Research in Nursing Project (CURN) (Horsley et al, 1978; Horsley et al, 1983)

Using very different approaches and methods, each project tested interventions to facilitate research use in practice.

EVIDENCE-BASED PRACTICE

The second leading cause of cancer deaths among cancers that affect both men and women is colorectal cancer (CRC). However, CRC screening tests are underused, especially among racial/ethnic minority groups, persons without insurance, those with lower educational attainment, and those with lower household income levels. The Centers for Disease Control and Prevention's (CDC) Colorectal Cancer Control Program (CRCCP) has supported state health departments and tribal organizations in implementing evidence-based interventions to increase the use of CRC screening tests among their populations. CRCCP program funds were primarily used to implement evidence-based interventions or strategies recommended in *The Guide to Community Preventive Service (Community Guide)*. These strategies included: (1) client reminders, (2) high quality small media, (3) reduction of structural barriers, (4) provider reminder and recall systems, and (5) provider assessment and feedback. Joseph et al (2016) report on two successful evidence-based interventions to address disparities: The Alaska Native Tribal Health Consortium (ANTHC) and Washington State's Breast, Cervical, and Colon Health Program (BCCHP).

ANTHC is a statewide, tribal, nonprofit health services organization owned and managed by Alaska Native populations. To increase CRC screening, ANTHC facilitated implementation of provider and patient reminders and patient navigators, who provided one-on-one patient education, small media distribution, and reduction of structural barriers (e.g., assisting with transportation). After implementing the program, the statewide CRC screening rate increased by eight percent (from 50.9% in 2009 to 58.4% in 2012). Some regions reported increases as high as 43% (from 24.4% in 2010 to 67.6% in 2012).

BCCHP has contracts with six regional contractors to administer program services across Washington state. BCCHP identified patient care coordinators in each clinic who coordinated staff training on CRC screening and integrated client and provider reminder systems. After implementing the program, the CRC screening rate increased by 24% (from 24% in 2011 to 48% in 2014) among the seven participating clinics, with all clinics showing improvements.

Nurse Use

Nurses can be active in establishing evidence-based interventions in the community to meet a health care need and reduce health disparities. Using multicomponent interventions in a single clinical site or facility can support more organized screening programs and potentially result in greater increases in screening rates than relying on a single strategy. The focus on developing projects to meet needs and improve health care outcomes must be based on the evidence that shows these partnerships are needed to solve the health care need and improve health care outcomes.

From Joseph DA, Redwood D, DeGroff A, Butler EL: Use of evidence-based interventions to address disparities in colorectal cancer screening, *MMWR, 65*(1): 21-28, 2016.

Although nursing continued to focus on research utilization projects, medicine also began to call for physicians to increase their use of scientific evidence to make clinical decisions. In the late 1970s, David Sackett, a medical doctor and clinical epidemiologist at McMaster University, published a series of articles in the *Canadian Medical Association Journal* describing how to read research articles in clinical journals. The term *critical appraisal* was used to describe the process of evaluating the validity and applicability of research studies (Guyatt and Rennie, 2002). Later, Sackett proposed the phrase "bringing critical appraisal to the bedside" to describe the application of evidence from medical literature to client care. This concept was used to train resident physicians at McMaster University and evolved into a "philosophy of medical practice based on knowledge and understanding of the medical literature supporting each clinical decision" (Guyatt and Rennie, 2002, p xiv).

With Gordon Guyatt as Residency Director of Internal Medicine at McMaster, the decision was made to change the program to focus on "this new brand of medicine" that Guyatt eventually called *evidence-based medicine* (Guyatt and Rennie, 2002, p xiv). Guyatt and Rennie described the goal of evidence-based medicine as being "aware of the evidence on which one's practice is based, the soundness of the evidence, and the strength of inference the evidence permits" (2002, p xiv).

In 1992 the Evidence-Based Medicine Working Group published an article in the *Journal of the American Medical Association* expanding the concept of evidence-based medicine and calling it a "paradigm shift." A paradigm shift simply means a change from old ways of knowing to new ways of knowing and practicing. Ways of knowing in nursing have included the following:

* The empirical knowledge, or the science of nursing
* The aesthetic knowledge, or the art of nursing
* Personal knowledge, or interpersonal relationships and caring
* Ethical knowledge, or moral and ethical codes of conduct usually established by professional organizations (Bradshaw, 2010)

Nursing practice has often focused less on science and more on the other four ways of knowing described here.

According to the Working Group (Evidence-Based Medicine Working Group, 1992), the old paradigm viewed unsystematic clinical observations as a valid way for "building and maintaining" knowledge for clinical decision making (p 2421). In addition, principles of pathophysiology were seen as a "sufficient guide for clinical practice" (p 2421). Training, common sense, and clinical experience were considered sufficient for evaluating clinical data and developing guidelines for clinical practice. The Working Group cited developments in research over the past 30 years as providing the foundation for the paradigm shift and a "new philosophy of medical practice" (p 2421).

The new paradigm, evidence-based medicine, acknowledges clinical experience as a crucial, but not sufficient, part of clinical decision making. Systematic and unbiased recording of clinical observations in the form of research will increase confidence in the knowledge gained from clinical experience. Principles of pathophysiology are seen as necessary but not sufficient knowledge for making clinical decisions. The Working Group also stressed that physicians need to be able to critically appraise the research literature to appropriately apply research findings in practice. Knowledge gained from authoritative figures also was not sufficient for practice in the new paradigm (Evidence-Based Medicine Working Group, 1992).

In the years since the Working Group began, *evidence-based practice* has been proposed as a term that integrates all health professions. The underlying principle is that high-quality care is based on evidence rather than on tradition or intuition (Hoffmann, Bennett, Del Mar, 2013).

The current nursing literature on evidence-based practice is primarily associated with applications in the acute and primary care settings, and little is reported about its use in community settings. However, the basic principles of evidence-based practice can be applied at the individual level or at the community level. Although definitions of EBP vary widely in the literature, the common thread across disciplines is the application of the best available evidence to improve practice (Makic et al, 2014; Leufer and Cleary-Holdforth, 2009).

? CHECK YOUR PRACTICE

As a student at the health department, you have been asked to look for evidence that would support a community level intervention to improve outcomes related to diabetes self-management in the population. What would you do?

TYPES OF EVIDENCE

No matter which definition is supported, what counts as evidence has been the issue most hotly debated. A hierarchy of evidence, ranked in order of decreasing importance and use, has been accepted by many health professionals. The double-blind, randomized controlled trial (RCT) generally ranks as the highest level of evidence, followed by:

* Other RCTs
* Nonrandomized clinical trials
* Quasi-experimental studies
* Prospective cohort studies
* Case-control reports
* Qualitative studies
* Expert opinion (Russell-Babin, 2009)

Some nurses would argue that this hierarchy ignores evidence gained from clinical experience. However, the definition of evidence-based nursing presented earlier indicates that clinical expertise as evidence, when used with other types of evidence, is used to make clinical decisions. Also in the hierarchy of evidence, expert opinion can be gained from the following:

* Non–research-based published articles
* Professional guidelines
* National guidelines

- Organizational opinions
- Panels of experts
- The nurse's clinical expertise

Because it is difficult to find or perform RCTs in the community, other types of evidence have been highlighted as the best evidence in public health literature on which to base evidence-based public health practice:

- Scientific literature found in systematic reviews
- Scientific literature used or quoted in one or more journal articles
- Public health surveillance data
- Program evaluations
- Qualitative data obtained from community members and other stakeholders
- Media and marketing data, such as the results of a media campaign to reduce smoking, word of mouth, and personal or professional experience (Brownson, Fielding, Maylahn, 2013; Jacobs et al, 2012)

FACTORS LEADING TO CHANGE OR BARRIERS TO EVIDENCE-BASED PRACTICE

EBP represents a cultural change in practice. It provides an environment to improve both nursing practice and client outcomes. Nursing is known for providing care based on the following:

- Environmental and client assessments
- Critical observations
- Development of questions or hypotheses to be explored
- Collection of data from the environment through community or organizational assessments
- Client history
- Physical assessment
- Review of past health records
- Analyzing data to develop plans of care for the individual client, family, group, or community
- Drawing conclusions on which to base care for the purpose of improving client outcomes (Vanhook, 2009)

However, several factors have been identified in the literature that support implementation of EBP or that will need to be overcome for nursing and other disciplines to successfully implement EBP. These factors include the following:

- Knowledge of research and current evidence
- Ability to interpret the meaning of the evidence
- Individual professional's characteristics, such as a willingness to change, or personal viewpoints about the quality and credibility of evidence
- Commitment of the time needed to implement EBP and to engage in education and directed practice
- The hierarchy of the practice environment and the level of support of managers and the ability to engage in autonomous practice
- The philosophy of the practice environment and the willingness to embrace EBP
- The resources available to engage in EBP, such as amount of work, proper equipment, computer-based EBP programs, and information systems

- The practice characteristics, such as leadership and colleague attitudes
- Links to outside supports, for example, teaching facilities such as a teaching health department or a university
- Political constraints and the lack of relevant and timely public health practice research (Brownson, Fielding, Maylahn, 2013; Gerrish, Cooke, 2013; Layde et al, 2012; Lovelace et al, 2015; Rychetnik et al, 2012)

Although a community agency may subscribe to the use of EBP in theory, actual implementation may be affected by the realities of the practice setting. Community-focused nursing agencies may lack the resources needed for its implementation in the clinical setting, such as time, funding, computer resources, and knowledge. Nurses may be reluctant to accept findings and feel threatened when long-established practices are questioned. Cost also can be a barrier if the clinical decision or change will require more funds than the agency has available. Compliance can be a barrier if the client will not follow the recommended intervention. Public health departments are moving toward EBP and are seeking accreditation through the national public health accreditation board. The accreditation process began in 2012.

STEPS IN THE EVIDENCE-BASED PRACTICE PROCESS

EBP is a philosophy of practice that respects client values. Melnyk and Fineout-Overholt (2015) have described a seven-step EBP process (Box 10.1). Yes, the first step is step zero. This process was initially described as a five-step process by others (Craig and Smyth, 2007; Dawes et al, 2004; Dicenso et al, 2005). The unique features of the model by Melnyk et al is the emphasis on the spirit of inquiry and the sharing of the results of the process.

Step zero involves a curiosity about the interventions that are being applied. Do they work, or is there a better approach? In public health nursing, for example, are there better parenting outcomes if the parents attend classes at the health department?

BOX 10.1 Seven Steps in the Evidence-Based Practice Process

Evidence-based practice (EBP) is a philosophy of practice that respects client values. Melnyk et al (2015) have described the following seven-step EBP process:

0. Cultivating a spirit of inquiry
1. Asking compelling, clinical questions
2. Searching for the best evidence
3. Critically appraising the evidence
4. Integrating the evidence with clinical expertise and client preferences and values
5. Evaluating the outcomes of the practice decisions or changes based on evidence
6. Disseminating EBP results

From Melnyk BM, Fineout-Overholt E: *Evidence-based practice in nursing and healthcare: a guide to best practice*, ed 3, Philadelphia, 2015, Wolters Kluwer Health.

Or are home visits to new mothers and babies more effective for achieving a healthy baby? Step one requires asking questions in a "PICOT" format. Although Melnyk et al developed a specific process for the PICOT, the process was first described by Sackett et al (1996), who discussed the following:

- The need to define the *(P)opulation* of interest
- The *(I)ntervention* or practice strategy in question
- The population or intervention to be used for *(C)omparison*
- The *(O)utcome* desired
- The *(T)ime frame*

Step two involves searching for the best evidence to answer the question. This step involves searching the literature. In the case of the earlier example, a literature search would focus on a search of key terms such as *public health nursing, parenting of new babies, parenting classes,* and *home visits.*

Step three requires a critical appraisal of the evidence found in step two. To appraise the literature found, Melnyk et al suggest asking three questions about each of the articles found in the literature search: (1) the validity, (2) the importance, and (3) whether the results of the article will help you as a nurse provide quality care for your clients.

Step four is the step in which the evidence found is integrated with clinical expertise and client values. Institutional standards and practice guidelines, as well as cost of care and support of the health care environment to implement the findings, are all factors considered in this step.

Step five requires an evaluation of the outcomes of practice decisions and changes that were based on the answers to the first four steps. The goal in evaluation is a positive change in quality of care and health care outcomes. In the example of group parenting classes versus home visits to new mothers and babies, current literature suggests improved quality and health care outcomes with home visits (Doggett, 2013).

Step six is disseminating outcomes of the results to others, to colleagues, to the employing agency's administration, to faculty and other students, and through a poster or podium presentation of the student nurse organizations or professional organizations. Professional organizations often sponsor student presentations for undergraduates and graduate students. Sharing of information is most important because it prevents each individual nurse from trying to find the best answer to the same question answered by someone else and gives us the basis for asking new questions. Sharing makes practice more efficient and improves quality and health care outcomes.

In a busy community practice setting, it is often difficult for nurses to access evidence-based resources. Using evidence-based clinical practice guidelines is one way for nurses to provide evidence-based nursing care in an efficient manner. Clinical practice guidelines are usually developed by a group of experts in the field who have reviewed the evidence and made recommendations based on the best available evidence. The recommendations are usually graded according to the quality and quantity of the evidence. The Public Health Practice Reference is an example of practice guidelines developed for use by population-centered nurses.

APPROACHES TO FINDING EVIDENCE

Returning to the previous example, the clinical question has been stated, and the population has been defined as new mothers and babies. Two interventions will be compared. The outcome is stated as healthy babies, and the time frame may be 6 months, 1 year, or another time at which the outcomes of the interventions will be evaluated.

Four approaches are described that allow the nurse to read research and nonresearch evidence in a condensed format. The first, a systematic review, is "a method of identifying, appraising, and synthesizing research evidence. The aim is to evaluate and interpret all available research that is relevant to a particular research question" (Grove, Gray, and Burns, 2015, p. 513). A systematic review is usually done by more than one person and describes the methods used to search for the evidence and evaluate the evidence. Systematic reviews can be accessed from most databases, such as Medline and the Cumulative Index to Nursing and Allied Health (CINAHL). The Cochrane Library is an electronic database that contains regularly updated evidence-based health care databases maintained by the Cochrane Collaboration, a not-for-profit organization (http://www.cochrane.org). The Cochrane Library is composed of three main branches: systematic reviews, trials register, and methodology database. The Cochrane Library publishes systematic reviews on a wide variety of topics. Systematic reviews differ from traditional literature review publications in that systematic reviews require more rigor and contain less opinion of the author. Systematic reviews for public health can be found in the Guide to Community Preventive Services (2007, 2010), the Cochrane Public Health Group, the Center for Reviews and Dissemination, and the Campbell Collaboration (Box 10.2).

The second approach, meta-analysis, is "a specific method of statistical synthesis used in some systematic reviews, where the results from several studies are quantitatively combined and summarized" (Rychetnik et al, 2003, p 542). A well-designed systematic review or meta-analysis can provide stronger evidence than a single randomized controlled trial.

The integrative review is a form of a systematic review that does not have the summary statistics found in the meta-analysis because of the limitations of the studies that are reviewed (e.g., small sample size of the population). A narrative review is a review done on published papers that support the reviewer's particular point of view or opinion and is used to provide a general discussion of the topic reviewed. This review does not often include an explicit or systematic review process.

Undergraduate students often perform narrative reviews. However, it is important to learn the process for systematic reviews, especially the use of the results of systematic reviews. Reading systematic reviews that have been completed is helpful in answering the question related to the EBP process.

What counts as evidence also has been argued in the public health literature (Victora and Habicht, 2004). RCTs, which are the highest level of evidence used to make clinical decisions, are appropriate for evaluating many interventions in

BOX 10.2 Resources for Implementing Evidence-Based Practice

The following resources can assist nurses in developing evidence-based practice (EBP) in nursing:

1. The Evidence-Based Practice for Public Health Project (http://library. umassmed.edu/ebpph/) at the University of Massachusetts Medical School Library has developed a website for EBP in public health. Many bibliographic databases, such as Medline, do not list all the journals of interest to public health workers. The project provides access to numerous databases of interest concerning public health. From the project's website, nurses can access free public health online journals and databases.

2. The Agency for Healthcare Quality and Research (AHRQ) (http://www.ahrq. gov) developed clinical guidelines based on the best available evidence for several clinical topics, such as pain management. The guidelines are accessible via the agency's website and serve as a resource to nurses involved in individual client care.

3. The National Guideline Clearinghouse (http://www.guideline.gov/), an initiative of the AHRQ, is an online resource for evidence-based clinical practice guidelines. The AHRQ also supports Evidence-Based Practice Centers, which write evidence reports on various topics.

4. PubMed (http://www.pubmed.gov/) is a bibliographic database developed and maintained by the National Library of Medicine. Bibliographic information from Medline is covered in PubMed and includes references for nursing, medicine, dentistry, the health care system, and preclinical sciences. Full texts of referenced articles are often included. Searches can be limited to type of evidence (e.g., diagnosis, therapy) and systematic reviews.

5. The Cochrane Database of Systematic Reviews (http://www.cochrane.org) is a collection of more than 1000 systematic reviews of effects in health care internationally. These reviews are accessible at a cost via the website. Nurses may also have free access from a medical library.

6. The *Evidence-Based Nursing Journal* is published quarterly. The purpose of the journal is to select articles reporting studies and reviews from health-related literature that warrant immediate attention by nurses attempting to keep pace with advances in their profession. Using predefined criteria, the best quantitative and qualitative original articles are abstracted in a structured format, commented on by clinical experts, and shared in a timely fashion. The research questions, methods, results, and evidence-based conclusions are reported. The website for the journal is http://www.evidencebasednursing.com.

7. The Honor Society of Nursing, Sigma Theta Tau International (http://www. nursingsociety.org/), sponsors the online peer-reviewed journal *Worldviews on Evidence-Based Nursing*, which publishes systematic reviews and research articles on best evidence that supports nursing practice globally. The journal is available by subscription.

8. The Task Force on Community Preventive Services (http://www.the communityguide.org) is an independent, nonfederal task force appointed by the director of the Centers for Disease Control and Prevention (CDC). Information about the task force may be found at the website. The task force is charged with determining the topics to be addressed by the CDC's *Community Guide* and the most appropriate means to assess evidence regarding population-based interventions. The task force reviews and assesses the quality of available evidence on the effects of essential community preventive services. The multidisciplinary task force determines the scope of the *Community Guide* that will be used by health departments and agencies to determine best practices for preventive health in populations.

9. The U.S. Preventive Services Task Force (USPSTF) (http://www.ahrq.gov/ clinic/uspstfix.htm) is an independent panel of private-sector experts in prevention and primary care. The USPSTF conducts rigorous, impartial assessments of the scientific evidence for the effectiveness of a broad range of clinical preventive services, including screening, counseling, and preventive medications. Its recommendations are considered the gold standard for clinical preventive services. The mission of the USPSTF is to evaluate the benefits of individual services based on age, gender, and risk factors for disease; make recommendations about which preventive services should be incorporated routinely into primary medical care and for which populations; and identify a research agenda for clinical preventive care. Recommendations of the USPSTF are published as the *Guide to Clinical Preventive Services*. The guide is available online.

10. The Centers for Disease Control and Prevention (CDC) (http://www.CDC. gov) publishes guidelines on immunizations and sexually transmitted diseases. Guidelines are developed by experts in the field appointed by the U.S. Department of Health and Human Services and the CDC.

11. The Cochrane Public Health Group (PHRG) (http://www.ph.cochrane.org/), formerly the Cochrane Health Promotion and Public Health Field, aims to work with contributors to produce and publish Cochrane reviews of the effects of population-level public health interventions. The PHRG undertakes systematic reviews of the effects of public health interventions to improve health and other outcomes at the population level, not those targeted at individuals. Thus it covers interventions seeking to address macroenvironmental and distal social environmental factors that influence health. In line with the underlying principles of public health, these reviews seek to have a significant focus on equity and aim to build the evidence to address the social determinants of health.

12. The Center for Reviews and Dissemination (CRD) (http://www.york.ac.uk/ inst/crd/index.htm) is part of the National Institute for Health Research and is a department of the University of York. The CRD, which was established in 1994, is one of the largest groups in the world engaged exclusively in evidence synthesis in the health field. The CRD undertakes systematic reviews evaluating the research evidence on health and public health questions of national and international importance.

13. The Campbell Collaboration (http://www.campbellcollaboration.org/), named after Donald Campbell, was founded on the principle that systematic reviews on the effects of interventions will inform and help improve policy and services. The collaboration strives to make the best social science research available and accessible. Campbell reviews provide high-quality evidence of what works to meet the needs of service providers, policymakers, educators and their students, professional researchers, and the general public. Areas of interest include crime, justice, education, and social welfare.

Data from Titler MG, Kleiber C, Steelman VJ, et al: The Iowa model of evidence-based practice to promote quality care, *Crit Care Nurs Clin North Am* 13:497-509, 2001.

medicine but are often inappropriate for evaluating public health interventions. For example, an RCT can be designed ethically to test a new medication for diabetes, but not for a smoking cessation intervention. In a smoking cessation intervention, subjects could not be assigned randomly to smoking or nonsmoking groups because a smoking cessation intervention is not appropriate for someone who does not smoke. In this situation, a case-control study would be most appropriate. Today there are many community-based clinical trials assisting in finding answers to the questions of which population level intervention has the best outcomes. (Visit the CDC website to review these trials.)

HOW TO Develop an Evidence-Based Protocol

Evidence-based protocols are a recognized approach to providing quality client care. Such protocols enhance the abilities of providers and can reduce health care errors. The following are steps to developing a protocol:

- Identify the problem.
- Identify stakeholders.
- Form a team of others to help develop the protocol.
- Develop an action plan with project goals and a timeline.
- Review the available evidence.
- Examine current practice and identify gaps as well as best practices.
- Develop the protocol focusing on gaps.
- Initiate the approval process with the setting.
- Evaluate current practices and modify as needed.
- Educate others who will use the protocol.
- Implement the protocol.
- Evaluate protocol for safety, effectiveness, and adherence.

From McEuen JA, Gardner KP, Barnachea DF, et al: An evidence-based protocol for managing hypoglycemia, *Am J Nurs* 110:40-45, 2010.

APPROACHES TO EVALUATING EVIDENCE

One approach used in evaluating evidence is grading the strength of evidence. When evidence is graded, the evidence is assigned a "grade" based on the number and type of well-designed studies and the presence of similar findings in all of the studies. Grading evidence has been debated so strongly that in 2002 the Agency for Healthcare Research and Quality (AHRQ) commissioned a study to describe existing systems used to evaluate the usefulness of studies and strength of evidence. The report reviewed 40 systems and identified three domains for evaluating systems for the grading of evidence quality, quantity, and consistency:

- The *quality* of a study refers to the extent to which bias is minimized.
- *Quantity* refers to the number of studies, the magnitude of the effect, and the sample size.
- *Consistency* refers to studies that have similar findings, using similar and different study designs. (Melnyk and Fineout-Overholt, 2015)

An example of grading the strength of evidence is the process the U.S. Preventive Services Task Force used in developing the *Guide to Clinical Preventive Services* (2016a).

As indicated, many frameworks exist for evaluating the strength and usefulness of the evidence found in the literature and other sources, such as professional standards. A popular framework was developed by the AHRQ. Fineout-Overholt et al (2010) have also developed an approach for evaluating evidence. Although these approaches vary in the factors they evaluate, the best approach to choose is one that evaluates not only the strength but also the usefulness of the evidence. Table 10.1 provides an example of an approach for evaluating evidence.

The strength of the literature is measured by the type of evidence it represents. For example, the RCT is the evidence that has the greatest strength on which to make a clinical decision. In contrast, opinion articles, descriptive studies, and professional reports of expert committees have less strength. The usefulness of the evidence is measured by whether the evidence is valid, whether it is important, and whether it can be used to assist in making practice decisions or changes in the community environment and with the population of interest to improve outcomes (Facchiano, Snyder, 2012). The best RCT conducted in a hospital setting, using an intervention to prevent falls, may not be applicable in a community setting. Therefore, although it may be a strong study with outcomes that improve health, it may not have the usefulness for applicability in the community because of the setting in which it was conducted.

TABLE 10.1   Typology for Classifying Interventions by Level of Scientific Evidence

Type/Category	Strength/How Established	Considerations for the Level of Scientific Evidence—Quality	Quantity/Consistency Data Source Examples
Evidence-based I	Peer review via systematic or narrative review	Based on study design and execution External validity Potential side benefits or harms Costs and cost-effectiveness	*Community Guide* Cochrane reviews Narrative reviews based on published literature
Effective II	Peer review	Based on study design and execution External validity Potential side benefits or harms Costs and cost-effectiveness	Articles in the scientific literature Research-tested intervention programs Technical reports with peer review
Promising III	Written program evaluation without formal peer review	Summative evidence of effectiveness Formative evaluation data Theory-consistent, plausible, potentially high-reach, low-cost, replicable	State or federal government reports (without peer review) Conference presentations
Emerging IV	Ongoing work, practice-based summaries, or evaluation works in progress	Formative evaluation data Theory-consistent, plausible, potentially high-reaching, low-cost, replicable Face validity	Evaluability assessments Pilot studies National Institutes of Health Research Portfolio Online Reporting Tools (RePORT) database Projects funded by health foundations

From Brownson RC, Fielding JE, Maylahn CM: Evidence-based public health: a fundamental concept for public health practice, *Annu Rev Public Health* 30:175-201, 2009.

Shaughnessy et al (1994) proposed criteria for evaluating the usefulness of evidence, calling the process *patient-oriented evidence that matters* (POEM). In general, the reader should ask the following questions: "What are the results? (Are they important?) Are the results valid? How can the results be applied to client care?" (p 489). Application of POEM can be found at http://www.essentialevidenceplus.com. Brownson et al (2013) proposed that the following questions be asked for EBP (plus suggested application examples):

- What is the size of the public health problem? What is the need for improved health outcomes for new mothers and babies in our community?
- Can interventions be found in the literature to address the problem (e.g., home visits or parenting classes)?
- Is the intervention useful in this community, with this population, or with populations at risk (e.g., the low income or uninsured)?
- Is the intervention the best one or are there other ways to address the problem considering cost and potential health outcomes for the population? (Assess cost and health outcomes of both of the interventions before choosing, including the nurses available to make home visits or who have the skills to teach the parenting class.)

Several variables are considered important in determining the quality of evidence used to make clinical decisions (Polit and Beck, 2014):

- **Sample selection:** Sample selection should be as unbiased as possible. For example, a sample is randomly selected when each subject has an equal chance of being selected from the population of interest. Random selection offers the least bias of any type of sample selection. Other types of sample selection, such as convenience sampling, contain researcher or evaluator bias.
- **Randomization:** When testing an intervention, randomly assign participants to either the intervention or control group. This type of assignment is less biased than if participants are allowed to choose the group they want to join.
- **Blinding:** The researcher or evaluator should not know which participants are in the experimental (treatment) group or which are in the control group. The researcher or evaluator is "blinded" as to who is receiving the treatment and who is not receiving the treatment.
- **Sample size:** The sample size should be large enough to show an effect of the intervention. In general, the larger the sample size, the better.
- **Description of intervention:** The intervention should be described in detail and explicitly enough that another person could duplicate the study if desired.
- **Outcomes:** The outcomes should be measured accurately.
- **Length of follow-up:** Depending on the intervention, the participants should be followed for a long enough period to determine whether the intervention continued to work or if the results were just by chance.
- **Attrition:** Few subjects should have dropped out of the study.

- **Confounding variables:** Variables that could affect the outcome should be accounted for by either statistical methods or study measurements.
- **Statistical analysis:** Statistical analysis should be appropriate to determine the desired outcome.

APPROACHES TO IMPLEMENTING EVIDENCE-BASED PRACTICE

The first step toward implementing EBP in nursing is recognizing the current status of one's own practice and believing that care based on the best evidence will lead to improved client outcomes (Melnyk et al, 2015). EBP is a relatively new concept, and thus, many practicing nurses are not familiar with the application of EBP and may lack computer and Internet skills necessary to implement EBP. Also, implementation will be successful only when nurses practice in an environment that supports evidence-based care. Public health nurses consider EBP as a process to improve practice and outcomes and use the evidence to influence policies that will improve the health of communities.

CURRENT PERSPECTIVES
COST VERSUS QUALITY

Much of the pressure to use EBP comes from third-party payers and is a response to the need to contain costs and reduce legal liability. Nurses must question whether the current agenda to contain health care costs creates pressure to focus on those research results that favor cost saving at the expense of quality outcomes for clients. Outcomes include client and community satisfaction and the safety of care. Costs can be weighed against outcomes when EBP is used to show the best practices available to reduce possible harm to clients (Makic et al, 2014; Melnyk et al, 2014).

LEVELS OF PREVENTION
Using Evidence-Based Practice

According to evidence collected and averaged by the Task Force on Community Preventive Services, the following are interventions supported by the literature at each level of prevention:

Primary Prevention
Extended and extensive mass media campaigns reduce youth initiation of tobacco use.

Secondary Prevention
Client reminders and recalls via mail, telephone, e-mail, or a combination of these strategies are effective in increasing compliance with screening activities such as those for colorectal and breast cancer.

Tertiary Prevention
Diabetes self-management education in community gathering places improves glycemic control.

From Task Force on Community Prevention Services: All findings of the Community Preventive Services Task Force. In: *The Community Guide: The guide to community preventive services*, Atlanta, GA, 2016b, Centers for Disease Control and Prevention. Retrieved July 2016 from http://www.thecommunityguide.org/about/conclusionreport.html.

INDIVIDUAL DIFFERENCES

EBP cannot be applied as a universal remedy without attention to client differences. When EBP is applied at the community level, the best evidence may point to a solution that is not sensitive to cultural issues and distinctions and thus may not be acceptable to the community. Ethical practice in communities requires attention to community differences.

APPROPRIATE EVIDENCE-BASED PRACTICE METHODS FOR COMMUNITY-ORIENTED NURSING PRACTICE

Gaining various perspectives in a specific community is important for nurses using EBP. Nursing has a legitimate role to play in interprofessional community-focused practice and can contribute to its evidence base. Nurses are obliged to ensure that the evidence applied to practice is acceptable to the community. Establishing an EBP culture depends on the use of both qualitative and quantitative research approaches or the best evidence available at the time. For example, a quantitative research study of a community health center could provide information about patterns of client use, the cost of various services, and the use of different health care providers. However, when quantitative research is combined with qualitative research, the nurse can gain an understanding of why clients use or do not use the services and can help the health center be both clinically effective and cost-effective. Evidence from multiple research methods has the potential to enrich the application of evidence and improve nursing practice (Stevens, 2013). The Quality and Safety

Education for Nurses (QSEN) box gives an example of how to use evidence for making a change in a community's health.

The rising cost of health care will demand a more critical look at benefits and costs of EBP. Finding resources to implement EBP will continue to be a challenge requiring creative strategies. An emphasis on quality care, equal distribution of health care resources, and cost control will continue. Implementing EBP can assist nurses in addressing these issues in the clinical setting. However, EBP can save money by providing the best care possible.

As nurses implement EBP in an environment focused on cost savings, the potential for governments, managed care organizations, or other health care agencies to endorse reimbursement of health care options solely on the basis of cost, without allowing for individual variation or considering environmental issues, will continue to be a concern. Nurses must use caution in adopting EBP in a prescriptive manner in different community environments. One aspect of the Patient Protection and Affordable Health Care Act of 2010 (ACA; PL 111-148) addresses the development of task forces on preventive services and community preventive services to develop, update, and disseminate EBP recommendations of the use of community preventive services. In addition, grant programs to support EBP delivery in the community are addressed in the ACA.

Although the Internet is one source of evidence data (see Box 10.2), there may be a lack of quality indicators to evaluate the myriad websites claiming to contain evidence-based information. It is essential to evaluate the quantity of the information on the website, whether it comes from a reputable agency or scholar,

---

QSEN FOCUS ON QUALITY AND SAFETY EDUCATION FOR NURSES

Targeted Competency: Evidence-Based Practice—Integrate best current evidence with clinical expertise and client and family preferences and values for delivery of optimal interventions.
Important aspects of EBP include:

- **Knowledge:** Describe EBP to include the components of research evidence, clinical expertise, and client and family values.
- **Skills:** Locate evidence reports related to clinical practice topics and guidelines.
- **Attitudes:** Value the need for continuous improvement in clinical practice based on new knowledge.

Evidence-Based Practice Question:

As a nurse in the community, you are working within a Native American community that has a high prevalence of diabetes. As you visit with clients in their homes, you notice that many have a standardized "Diabetes Care" handout they received from the same primary care clinic. Your clients comment that the nutritional recommendations are unrealistic in the context of their regular diet. You decide to initiate a focus group with clients who attend the diabetes clinic at the health department to customize diabetic nutritional guidelines for this community.

1. Go to The National Guideline Clearinghouse website at http://www.guideline.gov. This website is an initiative of the Agency for Healthcare Research and Quality and is a reservoir for evidence-based clinical guidelines.
2. On the home page, type "diabetes" in the search box.
3. The second result is: Guideline Synthesis: Nutritional Management of Diabetes Mellitus.

4. Review the various areas of the guidelines: Medical Nutritional Therapy, Carbohydrates, Protein, Fiber, Sucralose, Alcohol Consumption, Dietary Fat and Cholesterol, Micronutrients, Nutritional Interventions for Preventing and Managing Complications, and Physical Activity and Weight Management.
5. What baseline data might you gather from your focus-group participants to be best informed in how to tailor the evidence-based recommendations for this community?
6. What might be effective strategies in writing up the community-specific guidelines and distributing them that might enhance their adoption?

Answer:
- Understanding the common elements of this community's diet is a good place to start. What carbohydrates, proteins, and sources of sugar, dietary fat, and cholesterol are commonly consumed?
- How does the common diet compare to the National Clearinghouse Guidelines? Are there healthy sources of carbohydrates and healthy fats that are part of the diet that can be emphasized?
- What are common alcohol consumption patterns in the community? Would educational efforts regarding the deleterious effects of alcohol on diabetes be helpful?
- Writing up community-based guidelines with assistance from leaders in the community would be a helpful strategy. You could include healthy recipes from community leaders in your guidelines. Your community-based guidelines might be distributed at a community celebration or gathering by members of the community who helped develop them.

Prepared by Gail Armstrong, DNP, ACNS-BC, CNE, Associate Professor, University of Colorado Denver College of Nursing.

APPLYING CONTENT TO PRACTICE

This chapter emphasizes that it is important for nurses to acknowledge and understand evidence-based practice. They can participate by using it or they can add to the research base for the public's health through active programs of research or reviewing the best available evidence by reading published systematic reviews. Nurses can demonstrate leadership in supporting evidence-based practice (EBP) by becoming change agents, fostering a cultural change in the practice environment, and assisting nurses who do not know how to use EBP to make a difference in practice.

For example, nurses who have recently graduated are knowledgeable about the use of evidence in practice. The new nurses can assist nurses who have been out of school for a while to find sources of evidence on which to base their practice, such as referring them to the *Guide to Community Preventive Services*. Using evidence in practice will demonstrate its value, but implementation can be difficult because of the sheer volume of evidence and increasing population needs. Sharing knowledge and engaging in teamwork can help overcome these barriers.

Nurses have an important role to play in developing and using clinical guidelines for community practices. Use of a community development model and engaging in community partnerships will ensure that the community's perspective is included (see Chapter 12).

Nurses active in EBP can devote attention to understanding how best to incorporate the guidelines into practice, demonstrating practice excellence. EBP offers the opportunity for shared decision making because it can help nurses focus their thinking, observe process outcomes, and thus improve care for clients by communicating with leaders and other nurses what they have observed. Participation in EBP offers continuing professional growth (Griffin and Titler, 2015).

and whether the source of the website has a financial interest in the acceptance of the evidence presented. (Refer to Chapter 11 on health education, which discusses the Internet as a source of data and how to evaluate its usefulness and reliability.)

HEALTHY PEOPLE 2020 OBJECTIVES

Healthy People 2020 objectives offer a systematic approach to health improvement. See the *Healthy People 2020* box for the most recent objectives to improving clients' understanding of EBP and how they can contribute to health care decisions.

❤ *HEALTHY PEOPLE 2020*

Information access is important to ensure clients and communities have the correct information to make evidence-based health care decisions. The *Healthy People 2020* objectives related to providing resources are as follows:

- **HC/HIT-6.3:** Increase the proportion of persons who use electronic personal health management tools.
- **HC/HIT-4:** Increase the proportion of patients whose doctor recommends personalized health information resources to help them manage their health.
- **HC/HIT-12:** Increase the proportion of crisis and emergency risk messages, intended to protect the public's health, that demonstrate the use of best practices.
- **HC/HIT-11:** Increase the proportion of meaningful users of health information technology.
- **HC/HIT-13:** Increase the social marketing in health promotion and disease prevention.

EXAMPLE OF APPLICATION OF EVIDENCE-BASED PRACTICE TO PUBLIC HEALTH NURSING

This example describes the Intervention Wheel, a population-based practice model for public health nursing. The model consists of three levels of practice at the community, systems, and individual and family levels. It also consists of 17 public health interventions for improving population health (Minnesota Department of Public Health, 2003). (See Appendix C.4.) The model was originally developed using a qualitative grounded theory process but did not include a systematic review of evidence to support the interventions or their application to practice. Initially, the model was developed from an extensive analysis of the actual work of 200 practicing public health nurses working in a variety of settings. The 17 interventions grew out of this analysis, as did the three levels of practice. The authors indicated that the original intent was to provide a description of the scope and breadth of public health nursing practice. Because of the positive response to the Intervention Wheel, the decision was made to complete a systematic review of the evidence supporting the use of the Intervention Wheel. The goal was to examine the evidence underlying the interventions and the levels of practice. The systematic review involved answering six questions, a comprehensive search of the literature, a survey of 51 bachelor of science in nursing (BSN) programs in five states, and a critique (by five graduate students) of the 665 pieces of evidence found in the literature review for rigor (strength and usefulness). After limiting the final review to 221 sources of evidence, each source was independently rated by at least two members of a 42-member panel of practicing public health nurses and educators. The 42-member panel met to reach consensus on the outcomes of the reviews. The outcomes were field-tested with 150 practicing nurses, then critiqued by a national panel of 20 experts. The Intervention Wheel is the result of this systematic review and critique (Keller et al, 2004). Although this critique may appear overwhelming, the undergraduate or graduate student may be involved in such a systematic critique as one of many participants contributing to the outcome of such a review. Table 10.2 applies some of the interventions to the core functions of public health.

CASE STUDY

Developing an Evidence-Based Health Promotion Program

Jamie Lee is the occupational health nurse at the T-shirt factory in town. Recently the health clinic at the T-shirt factory had budget cuts, resulting in the reduction of services and personnel. The once full-time clinic is now open only 3 days a week, and Ms. Lee no longer has support staff to help her with her paperwork responsibilities.

From her interactions with the workers, Ms. Lee has observed several risky health behaviors (e.g., unhealthy diets, smoking) among them. Although she is very busy in the clinic, Ms. Lee would like to develop a health promotion program to address these risky health behaviors, but she is not sure where to start.

TABLE 10.2   Core Public Health Functions and Related Evidence-Based Nursing Interventions

Core Functions	Related Nursing Interventions
Assessment	Diagnose and investigate health problems and hazards in the community
	Mobilize community partnerships to identify and solve health problems
	Link people to needed health services
	Use evidence-based practice for new insights and innovative solutions to health problems
Policy development	Inform, educate, and empower communities about health issues
	Develop policies and plans using evidence-based practice that supports individual and community health efforts
Assurance	Monitor health status to identify community health problems
	Enforce laws and regulations that protect health and ensure safety
	Ensure the provision of health care that is otherwise unavailable
	Ensure a competent public health and personal health care workforce
	Use evidence-based practice to evaluate effectiveness, accessibility, and quality of personal and population-based services

From U.S. Department of Health and Human Services: *Healthy People 2020: roadmap to improving all Americans' health,* Washington, DC, 2010, U.S. Government Printing Office..

PRACTICE APPLICATION

A nurse who is the director of a part-time, nurse-managed clinic is in the process of analyzing how best to expand services to operate as a full-time clinic in the most cost-effective and clinically effective manner. The director gathers evidence from the literature on nurse-managed clinics in other rural settings to evaluate the cost and clinical effectiveness of various models. The nurse also considers evidence from the following sources in the decision-making process: client satisfaction research data, knowledge of clinic staff, expert opinion of community advisory board members, evidence from community partners, and data on service needs in the state. Having examined the evidence, the nurse decides that incremental (step-by-step) growth toward full-time status is warranted. Evidence of needs in the community and analysis of statistical data indicate that the addition of services for children is a priority and a pediatric nurse practitioner is hired as a first step while planning for full-time status continues.

Evaluation of the evidence gathered demonstrates which of the following?
A. Effectiveness of the intervention in communities
B. Application of the data to populations and communities
C. Existence of positive or negative health outcomes
D. Economic consequences of the intervention
E. Barriers to implementation of the interventions in communities

Explain how this example applies principles of evidence-based practice.
Answers can be found on the Evolve website.

REMEMBER THIS!

* Evidence-based practice was developed in other countries before its use in the United States.
* Application of evidence-based practice in relation to clinical decision making in population-centered nursing concentrates on interventions and strategies geared to communities and populations rather than to individuals.

* The goals, as evidenced through *Healthy People 2020,* are to increase the quality and years of healthy life and to eliminate health disparities in populations (U.S. Department of Health and Human Services, 2010).

EVOLVE WEBSITE

http://evolve.elsevier.com/Stanhope/foundations
* Case Study, with Questions and Answers
* NCLEX® Review Questions
* Practice Application Answers

REFERENCES

Barnard K, Hoehn R: *Nursing child assessment satellite training: final report,* Hyattsville, Md, 1978, Department of Health, Education & Welfare, Division of Nursing.
Bradshaw WG: Importance of nursing leadership in advancing evidence-based nursing practice, *Neonatal Netw* 29:117–122, 2010.

Brownson RC, Fielding JE, Maylahn CM: Evidence-based public health: a fundamental concept for public health practice, *Annu Rev Public Health* 30:175–202, 2009.
Brownson RC, Fielding JE, Maylahn CM: Evidence-based decision making to improve public health practice, *Front Public Health Serv Syst Res* 2(2), 2013. doi:10.13023/FPHSSR.0202.02.
Carper BA: Fundamental patterns of knowing in nursing, *ANS* 1:13–24, 1978.
Craig JV, Smyth RL: *The evidence-based practice manual for nurses,* ed 2, Edinburgh, 2007, Churchill Livingstone.
Dawes M, Davies P, Gray A, et al: *Evidence-based practice: a primer for health care professionals,* ed 2, London, 2004, Churchill Livingstone.
Dicenso A, Guyatt G, Ciliska D, editors: *Evidence-based nursing: a guide to clinical practice,* St Louis, 2005, Mosby.

Doggett L: New research strengthens home visiting field, *Zero to Three* 33:5–9, 2013.

Estabrooks CA, Winther C, Derksen L: Mapping the field: a biliometric analysis of the research utilization literature in nursing, *Nurs Res* 53:293–303, 2004.

Evidence-Based Medicine Working Group: Evidence-based medicine: a new approach to teaching the practice of medicine, *JAMA* 268:2420–2425, 1992.

Facchiano L, Snyder CH: Evidence-based practice for the busy nurse practitioner: part 3: critical appraisal process, *J Am Acad Nurse Pract* 24:704–715, 2012.

Fineout-Overholt E, Melnyk B, Stillwell SB, et al: Critical appraisal of the evidence. I. An introduction to gathering, evaluating, and recording the evidence, *Am J Nurs* 110:47–52, 2010.

Florin J, Ehrenberg A, Wallin L, et al: Educational support for research utilization and capability beliefs regarding evidence-based practice skills—a national survey of senior nursing students, *J Adv Nurs* 68:888–897, 2012.

Gerrish K, Cooke J: Factors influencing evidence-based practice among community nurses, *JCN* 27:98–101, 2013.

Griffin E, Titler MG: Using evidence through collaboration to promote excellence in nursing practice. In Schmidt NA, Brown JM, editors: *Evidence-based practice for nurses: appraisal and application of research*, ed 3, Burlington, Mass, 2015, Jones & Bartlett Learning.

Grove SK, Gray JR, Burns N: *Understanding nursing research: building an evidence-based practice*, ed 6, St Louis, 2015, Elsevier Saunders.

Guyatt G, Rennie D, editors: *Users' guides to the medical literature: a manual for evidence-based clinical practice*, Chicago, Ill, 2002, American Medical Association.

Hoffmann T, Bennett S, Del Mar C: Introduction to evidence-based practice. In Hoffmann T, Bennett S, Del Mar C, editors: *Evidence-based practice across health professions*, ed 2, New York, 2013, Elsevier.

Honor Society of Nursing, Sigma Theta Tau International: *Position statement on evidence-based nursing*, Indianapolis, Ind, 2005, Sigma Theta Tau International. Retrieved July 2016 from http://www.nursingsociety.org.

Horsley JA, Crane J, Bingle JD: Research utilization as an organizational process, *J Nurs Admin* 8:4–6, 1978.

Horsley JA, Crane J, Crabtree MK, et al: Using research to improve nursing practice: a guide, San Francisco, 1983, Grune & Stratton.

Jacobs JA, Jones E, Gabella BA, et al: Tools for implementing an evidence-based approach in public health practice, *Prev Chronic Dis* 9:110324, 2012.

Joseph DA, Redwood D, DeGroff A, Butler EL: Use of evidence-based interventions to address disparities in colorectal cancer screening, *MMWR* 65:21–28, 2016.

King D, Barnard KE, Hoehn R: Disseminating the results of nursing research, *Nurs Outlook* 29:164–169, 1981.

Keller L, Strohschein S, Lia-Hoagbert B, Schaffer MA: Population-based public health interventions: practice-based and evidence-supported. I, *Public Health Nurs* 21:453–468, 2004.

Krueger JC: Utilizing clinical nursing research findings in practice: a structured approach, *Commun Nurs Res* 9:381–394, 1977.

Krueger JC, Nelson AH, Wolanin MO: *Nursing research: development, collaboration and utilization*, Germantown, Md, 1978, Aspen.

Layde PM, Christiansen AL, Peterson DJ, et al: A model to translate evidence-based interventions into community practice, *Am J Public Health* 102:617–624, 2012.

Lindeman CA, Krueger JC: Increasing the quality, quantity, and use of nursing research, *Nurs Outlook* 25:450–454, 1977.

Lovelace KA, Aronson RE, Rulison K, et al: Laying the groundwork for evidence-based public health: why some local health departments use more evidence-based decision-making practices than others, *Am J Public Health* 105:S189–S197, 2015.

Makic MBF, Rauen C, Watson R, et al: Examining the evidence to guide practice—challenging practice habits, *Crit Care Nurse* 34:28–30, 32–46, 2014.

Mattila L, Rekola L, Koponen L, et al: Journal club intervention in promoting evidence-based nursing—perceptions of nursing students, *Nurse Educ Pract* 13:423–428, 2013.

McEuen JA, Gardner KP, Barnachea DF, et al: An evidence-based protocol for managing hypoglycemia, *Am J Nurs* 110:40–45, 2010.

Melynk BM, Gallagher-Ford L, Long LE, Fineout-Overholt E: The establishment of evidence-based practice competencies for practicing registered nurses in real-world clinical settings: proficiencies to improve healthcare quality, reliability, patient outcomes, and costs, *Worldviews Evid Based Nurs* 11:5–15, 2014.

Melnyk BM, Fineout-Overholt E: *Evidence-based practice in nursing and healthcare: a guide to best practice*, ed 3, Philadelphia, 2015, Wolters Kluwer Health.

Merrill KC, Macintosh J, Mandleco B, et al: Overview—innovative methods to create a spirit of inquiry in undergraduate nursing students, *Commun Nurs Res* 46:184, 2013.

Minnesota Department of Health: *Public health interventions: applications for public health nursing practice*, St Paul, Minn, 2003, MDH.

Parkhurst JO, Abeysinghe S: What constitutes "good" evidence for public health and social policy-making? From hierarchies to appropriateness, *Soc Epistemol* 2016. doi:10.1080/02691728.2016.1172365.

Polit DF, Beck CT: *Essentials of nursing research: Appraising evidence for nursing practice*, ed 8, Philadelphia, 2014, Wolters Kluwer Health.

Rychetnik L, Hawe P, Waters E, et al: A glossary for evidence-based public health, *J Epidemiol Comm Health* 58:538–545, 2003.

Rychetnik L, Bauman A, Laws R, et al: Translating research for evidence-based public health: key concepts and future directions, *J Epidemiol Community Health* 66:1187–1192, 2012.

Sackett DL, Rosenberg WMC, Gray J, et al: Evidence-based medicine: what it is and what it isn't, *Br Med J* 312:71–72, 1996.

Shaughnessy AF, Slawson DC, Bennett JA: Becoming an information master: a guidebook to the medical information jungles, *J Fam Pract* 39:489–499, 1994.

Sprayberry LD: Transformation of America's healthcare system—implications for professional direct-care nurses, *Medsurg Nurs* 23:61–66, 2014.

Stetler CB: Updating the Stetler model of research utilization to facilitate evidence-based practice, *Nurs Outlook* 49:272–279, 2001.

Stevens KR: The impact of evidence-based practice in nursing and the next big ideas, *Online J Issues Nurs* 18:4, 2013.

Task Force on Community Prevention Services: All findings of the Community Preventive Services Task Force. In: *The Community Guide: The guide to community preventive services*, Atlanta, Ga, 2016b, Centers for Disease Control and Prevention. Retrieved July 2016 from http://www.thecommunityguide.org/about/conclusionreport.html.

U.S. Department of Health and Human Services: *Healthy People 2020: a roadmap for health*, Washington, DC, 2010, U.S. Government Printing Office.

Using Health Education and Groups in the Community

Jeanette Lancaster

OBJECTIVES

After reading this chapter, the student should be able to:

1. Discuss ways that people learn.
2. Identify the steps and principles that guide health education.
3. Describe the importance of literacy, especially health literacy, in health promotion and health education.
4. Describe factors that influence group functioning and how members of groups learn about health behaviors.
5. Describe how nurses can work with groups to promote the health of individuals and communities.
6. Explain strategies that nurses can use to provide effective health education.

CHAPTER OUTLINE

Healthy People 2020 Objectives for Health Education
Education and Learning
   The Nature of Learning
The Educational Process
   Identify Educational Needs
   Establish Educational Goals and Objectives
   Select Appropriate Educational Methods
   Skills of the Effective Educator
   Motivational Interviewing
   Developing Effective Health Education Programs
   Educational Issues and Barriers to Learning
   Population Considerations Based on Age and Cultural
     and Ethnic Backgrounds

   Educator-Related Barriers
   Learner-Related Barriers
   Use of Technology in Health Education
   Evaluation of the Educational Process
   Evaluation of Health and Behavioral Changes
Groups: A Tool in Health Education
   Group: Definitions and Concepts
   Choosing Groups for Health Change
   Beginning Interactions and Dealing with Conflict
   Evaluation of Group Progress

KEY TERMS

ACTS, 189
affective domain, 184
andragogy, 190
cognitive domain, 184
cohesion, 196
conflict, 199
democratic leadership, 198
education, 184
established groups, 199
evaluation, 194
formal group, 196
group, 195
group culture, 197
group purpose, 196

Health Belief Model (HBM), 193
health literacy, 192
informal group, 196
leadership, 197
learning, 184
long-term evaluation, 195
maintenance functions, 196
maintenance norms, 197
motivational interviewing, 188
National Assessment of Adult Literacy
  (NAAL), 192
norms, 197
patriarchal leadership, 198
pedagogy, 190

Precaution Adoption Process Model
  (PAPM), 193
process evaluation, 194
psychomotor domain, 184
reality norms, 197
role structures, 197
selected membership group, 199
short-term evaluation, 195
task function, 196
task norm, 197
teach-back, 189
Transtheoretical Model (TTM), 193

One of the best ways to manage health care costs is to help people stay healthier. Nurses are ideal health care practitioners to lead in health promotion through health education because (1) they educate clients across all three levels of prevention: primary, secondary, and tertiary; and (2) they work with individuals, families, groups, and communities. The goal is to help clients attain optimal health, prevent health problems, identify and treat health problems early, and minimize disability. Education allows individuals to make knowledgeable health-related decisions, assume personal responsibility for their health, and cope effectively with alterations in their health and lifestyles. Often the goal in health promotion and health education is helping clients change their behaviors; a key part of public health nursing practice is to teach people to promote health, prevent illness, and manage chronic illness.

This chapter discusses ways to develop individual, group, and community health promotion programs. Specific content in the chapter includes information about how people learn, the sequence of actions that a nurse follows when developing an educational program, using skills, such as motivational interviewing in health promotion, selected models of health promotion, and the important topic of literacy, especially health literacy. The role of groups in health promotion is also presented. Many of the objectives of *Healthy People 2020* address the importance of health promotion, and selected objectives are cited in this chapter.

HEALTHY PEOPLE 2020 OBJECTIVES FOR HEALTH EDUCATION

As mentioned in chapters throughout the text, *Healthy People 2020* lists national health needs and outlines goals and objectives designed to improve health. The *Healthy People 2020* educational objectives emphasize the importance of educating various populations (based on age and ethnicity) about health promotion activities in the priority areas of unintentional injury, violence, suicide, tobacco use and addiction, alcohol or other drug use, unintended pregnancy, human immunodeficiency virus (HIV) and acquired immunodeficiency syndrome (AIDS), sexually transmitted diseases (STDs), unhealthy dietary patterns, and inadequate physical activity (US Department of Health and Human Services [USDHHS], 2010).

In designing, implementing, and evaluating health education activities, it is important to learn about the primary health problems in the community, as well as education principles related to both learning and teaching. The goal of an educational program is to teach what people think they want to learn and in ways that facilitate their learning. In public health it is important for learners to participate in identifying their learning needs. Then education programs are designed to meet the health need or problem in that population. Generally these programs involve educating individual members of the population about health promotion, illness prevention, and treatment. For example, in a community in which childhood and adolescent asthma is a problem, a community-based asthma education and training program can be developed. If childhood obesity is a major health concern, a program to educate children in their schools and their parents or caregivers about healthy eating, cooking, and exercise may be useful.

To develop a community-based educational program for education about asthma or childhood obesity, the nurse would need to follow a set of steps. The steps are listed here and discussed in detail throughout the chapter. Typical steps to follow in developing a health education program include (1) *identify* a population-specific learning need for the community health client; (2) *select* one or more learning theories to use in the education program; (3) *consider* which educational principles are most likely to increase learning and choose those that are most appropriate and feasible; (4) *examine* educational issues, such as population-specific or cultural concerns, identify barriers to learning, such as limited literacy or limited or lack of health literacy, and choose the most appropriate teaching and learning strategies based on the age, gender, cultural background, education, and learning needs of the learners; (5) *design and implement* the educational program using carefully chosen strategies; (6) *evaluate* the effects of the educational program. The steps used in educational programs parallel those of the nursing process—assessment, planning, implementation, and evaluation.

♥ HEALTHY PEOPLE 2020

Selected examples related to health education are as follows:
- **ECBP-2:** Increase the proportion of elementary, middle, and senior high schools that provide comprehensive school health education to prevent health problems in the following areas: unintentional injury, violence, suicide, tobacco use and addiction, alcohol or other drug use, unintended pregnancy, HIV/AIDS and sexually transmitted infections (STIs), unhealthy dietary patterns, and inadequate physical activity.
- **ECBP-3:** Increase the proportion of college and university students who receive information from their institution on each of the priority health-risk behavior areas listed previously.
- **ECBP-8:** Increase the proportion of worksites that offer a comprehensive employee health promotion program to their employees.
- **ECBP-11:** Increase the proportion of local health departments that have established culturally appropriate and linguistically competent community health promotion and disease prevention programs.

HEALTH EDUCATION AND INFLUENCE OF GENOMICS

As has been discussed in many chapters of this text, there is a correlation among weight, health, and exercise. It has recently been determined that even if obesity is in your genes, regular exercise can help keep pounds from accruing to you. Researchers at the University of North Carolina at Chapel Hill found that people who carried the FTO gene variant that increases the risk of obesity could reduce the effects of their DNA by about one third by engaging in regular exercise. One thing that the study shows is that people do not have to be victims to their genes. They have choices. With this gene variant, regular exercise can interrupt to some extent the effects on weight. Overall the research team found that exercise weakened the gene variant's effects by about 30 percent.

Source: Graff M, Scott RA. Justice AE, et al: Genome-wide physical activity interactions in adiposity-A meta-analysis of 200,452 adults, PLOS, Genetics on Line, April 27, 2017.

EDUCATION AND LEARNING

Education is an activity designed to help people change their knowledge, attitudes, and skills about a specific topic. Knowledge is the least difficult area to change, followed by attitudes, and then the most difficult is behavior. Nurses provide people with health information so they can improve their decision-making abilities and thereby decide if they will change their behavior. Education emphasizes the provider of knowledge and skills. In contrast, learning emphasizes the recipient of knowledge and skills and the person(s) in whom a change is expected to occur. Remember that learning involves change, and change is difficult for many people.

People learn in a variety of ways. Many people learn best through active involvement in their learning, in contrast to learners who are like sponges and prefer to simply soak up the information that is presented. Learners accept information based on many factors, including what they already know, what they believe, the culture in which they have been raised, their generational experiences related to learning, and how well they can understand and relate to the information that they receive. What people hear is filtered through their past experiences; the social groups to which they belong; assumptions, values, level of attention, and knowledge; and the esteem in which they hold the person communicating the information. Effective health education is a competency that is included in many documents that describe the role of public health professionals, including nurses. The Applying Content to Practice box illustrates the relationship between health education and selected standards, expectations, and competencies in public health.

A variety of educational principles can be used to guide the selection of health information for individuals, families, communities, and populations. Three of the most useful categories of educational principles are those associated with the nature of learning, the educational process, and the skills of effective educators.

THE NATURE OF LEARNING

One way to think about the nature of learning is to examine the cognitive (thinking), affective (feeling), and psychomotor (acting)

> ## APPLYING CONTENT TO PRACTICE
>
> Just as objectives in *Healthy People 2020* (USDHHS, 2010) recommend that health education and promotion be used to provide public health care, so do other key documents, such as the American Nurses Association's *Scope & Standards of Practice: Public Health Nursing*. Standard 5b, labeled Health Education and Health Promotion, says that the "public health nurse employs multiple strategies to promote health, prevent disease, and ensure a safe environment for populations" (American Nurses Association [ANA], 2007, p 23). Similarly, the *Core Competences for Public Health Professionals* of the Council on Linkages between Academia and Public Health Practice (2010) lists six competencies related to communication skills; five of them relate directly to this chapter. These competencies, which are discussed and illustrated throughout the chapter, are as follows:
> 1. Assesses the health literacy of populations served
> 2. Communicates in writing and orally, in person, and through electronic means, with linguistic and cultural proficiency
> 3. Solicits input from individuals and organizations
> 4. Uses a variety of approaches to disseminate public health information
> 5. Applies communication strategies in interactions with individuals and groups

domains of learning. Each domain has specific behavioral components that form a hierarchy of steps, or levels. Each level builds on the previous one. Understanding these three learning domains is crucial in providing effective health education (Bloom et al, 1956). First, consider assumptions about how adults learn. Specifically, adults are motivated to learn when (1) they think they need to know something, (2) the new information is compatible with their prior life experiences, (3) they value the person(s) providing the information, and (4) they believe they can make any necessary changes that are implied by the new information (Knowles et al, 2015).

Cognitive Domain

The cognitive domain includes memory, recognition, understanding, reasoning, application, and problem solving and is divided into a hierarchical classification of behaviors. Learners master each level of cognition in order of difficulty and move up the learning hierarchy (Bloom et al, 1956). Start by assessing the cognitive abilities of the learners. This is especially important when learners have a limited level of literacy either of the language used in the instruction or of the content presented. A later section will discuss literacy in general and health literacy in particular. Teaching above or below a person's level of understanding can lead to frustration and discouragement. The components of the cognitive domain are as follows (Bloom et al, 1956):
1. **Knowledge:** Requires recall of information
2. **Comprehension:** Combines recall with understanding
3. **Application:** New information is taken in and used in a different way
4. **Analysis:** Breaks communication down into parts to understand both the parts and their relationships to one another
5. **Synthesis:** Builds on the first four levels by assembling them into a new whole
6. **Evaluation:** Learners judge the value of what has been learned

Affective Domain

The affective domain includes changes in attitudes and the development of values. For affective learning to take place, nurses consider and attempt to influence what learners feel, think, and value. Because the attitudes and values of nurses may differ from those of their clients, it is important to listen carefully to detect clues to feelings that learners have that may influence learning. It is difficult to change deeply rooted attitudes, beliefs, interests, and values. To make such changes, people need support and encouragement from those around them. Affective learning, like cognitive learning, consists of the following series of steps:
1. **Knowledge:** Receives the information
2. **Comprehension:** Responds to the information received
3. **Application:** Values the information
4. **Analysis:** Makes sense of the information
5. **Synthesis:** Organizes the information
6. **Evaluation:** Adopts behaviors consistent with new values

Psychomotor Domain

The psychomotor domain includes the performance of skills that require some degree of neuromuscular coordination and emphasizes motor skills (Bloom et al, 1956). Clients are taught a variety of psychomotor skills, including bathing infants, changing dressings, giving injections, measuring blood glucose levels, taking blood pressures, and walking with crutches, as well as many skills related to health promotion exercises.

When you are teaching a skill, first show clients how to do the skill. You can show the client using pictures, a model, or a device or via a live demonstration, video, CD, or the Internet. There are many helpful teaching materials available on YouTube. Next, allow clients to practice, which is a repeat demonstration or teach-back approach to validate that what was being taught was learned. Also, if the teaching is being done in a class, participants may learn by observing one another master a task. Psychomotor learning depends on learners meeting the following three conditions (Bloom et al, 1956; Dembo, 1994):

- The learner must have the *necessary ability,* including both cognitive and psychomotor ability. For example, you may find that a person with Alzheimer's disease can follow only one-step instructions. Thus you need to tailor your education plan to that person.
- The learner must have a *sensory image* of how to carry out the skill. For example, when teaching a group of women how to cook heart-healthy meals, ask the women to describe their kitchen and how they would actually go about the shopping and cooking process.
- The learner must have *opportunities to practice* the new skills. Provide practice sessions during the program to help the client adapt the skill to the home or work environment where the skill will be performed.

CASE STUDY

Teaching About Diabetes

To apply the three learning domains, consider this clinical situation: In the community being served, the nurse identifies a large number of women who are newly diagnosed as having diabetes. The goals of the nurse would include: (1) learning what the women know about their health condition; (2) providing basic information about diabetes and self-care (cognitive domain); and (3) teaching them how to correctly inject insulin and to determine the amount of insulin each would need at a given time (psychomotor domain). It is important to demonstrate insulin injection and ask each woman to do a repeat demonstration to verify that she has the necessary ability and dexterity to self-inject insulin. During the teaching session, the nurse learns that the women have a limited understanding of the possible long-term complications of diabetes. Teaching at this level will include the affective domain in that the women may be denying the seriousness of their illness. They may think that a disease that causes limited pain and discomfort in its early stages cannot lead to many complications if not properly managed. In this case the nurse would be guided by six principles of effective education. First, the nurse would convey the information clearly, using words that the women understand. A place for the teaching would be chosen that is private and comfortable, and the nurse would organize her teaching approach to fit the needs of the learner. In diabetes education, it is important not only to give information but to demonstrate and then ask the learners to practice in the class what they are learning. Evaluation of the effectiveness of the session(s) can be accomplished by asking the learners what they have learned and by watching and listening to them as they discuss and practice their new learning.

Application to other clinical examples: How would you apply the three domains of learning to developing an educational session for a group of women who have young children in the home and need to be better informed about safety practices in terms of water, stoves, poisons, medicines, tools, and so forth?

To summarize, when assessing a client's ability to learn a skill, be sure to evaluate intellectual, emotional, and physical ability and then teach at the level of the learner's ability. Some clients do not have the intellectual ability to learn the steps that

QSEN FOCUS ON QUALITY AND SAFETY EDUCATION FOR NURSES

Targeted Competency: Client-Centered Care—Key aspects of client-centered care include the following:

- **Knowledge:** Integrate understanding of multiple dimensions of client-centered care: information, communication, and education.
- **Skills:** Communicate client values, preferences, and expressed needs to other members of the health care team.
- **Attitudes:** Respect and encourage individual expression of client values, preferences, and expressed needs.

Client-centered care question:
Providing health information in a way that is not understandable or useful to the recipient is a poor form of client-centered communication. If you were teaching a group of four women about wound care after surgery, what steps would you take to ensure that the message the women received was the message that you intended to send?

Answer: Generally you would begin by providing the needed information by describing each step; you might include an easy-to-understand handout in the language the four women understand, or you might give them a CD to take home that has the information on it. Next, you would demonstrate how to clean the wound. Then you would ask each woman to repeat the cleaning process that you just demonstrated. Finally, you would ask each woman if she has the facilities and supplies to clean the wound at home; then you would ask each woman if she had any questions or concerns that you might answer. What else would you do?

Data from Cronenwett L, Sherwood G, Barnsteiner J, et al: Quality and safety education for nurses, *Nurs Outlook* 55:122-131 2007.

make up a complex procedure. Others may have cultural beliefs that conflict with healthy behaviors. Another person may be tremulous and have poor eyesight, making him incapable of learning insulin self-injection.

THE EDUCATIONAL PROCESS

The educational process builds on an understanding of education, learning, and how people learn. The five steps of the educational process are discussed next.

IDENTIFY EDUCATIONAL NEEDS

To learn about clients' health education needs, begin by conducting a systematic and thorough needs assessment. Assessment steps are listed in Box 11.1. Once needs are identified, prioritize them beginning with the most critical educational needs.

Factors that can influence a person's learning needs and ability to learn include the learner's demographic, physical, geographic, economic, psychological, social, and spiritual characteristics.

BOX 11.1 Steps of a Needs Assessment

1. Identify what the client wants to know. (Consider *Healthy People 2020* educational objectives.)
2. Collect data systematically to obtain information about learning needs, readiness to learn, and barriers to learning.
3. Analyze assessment data that have been collected and identify cognitive, affective, and psychomotor learning needs.
4. Think about what will increase the client's ability and motivation to learn.
5. Assist the client to prioritize learning needs.

Also consider the learner's knowledge, skills, and motivation to learn, as well as resources available to support and possibly prevent learning. Resources include printed, audio or visual materials, equipment, agencies, and other individuals. Barriers for the presenter include lack of time, skill, confidence, money, space, energy, and organizational support.

ESTABLISH EDUCATIONAL GOALS AND OBJECTIVES

After you identify the learner's needs, develop the goals and objectives for the educational program. Goals are broad, long-term expected outcomes, such as, "Each child in the third-grade class will participate in 30 minutes of daily physical exercise, 4 days per week for 2 months." Program goals should deal directly with the clients' overall learning needs. The learning need of the third graders is to know the importance of exercise and fitness to their health.

Objectives are specific, short-term criteria that are met as steps toward achieving the long-term goal, such as, "Within 2 weeks, each child will be able to demonstrate at least two exercises they have learned." Objectives are written statements of an intended outcome or expected change in behavior and should define the minimum degree of knowledge or ability needed by a client. Objectives must be stated clearly and defined in measurable terms, and they typically imply an action (Knowles et al, 2015).

SELECT APPROPRIATE EDUCATIONAL METHODS

Choose educational methods that will facilitate the efficient and successful accomplishment of program goals and objectives. The methods also should be appropriately matched to the strengths and needs of both the client and the presenter. Choose the simplest, clearest, and most succinct manner of presentation and avoid complex program designs. Try to vary the methods to hold the attention of the learners and to meet the needs of different learners. Some people learn best by being actively involved in the program (Fig. 11.1), such as by

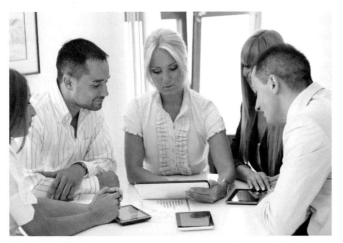

FIG. 11.1 The instructional methods need to meet the learning needs of the learners. (© 2012 Photos.com, a division of Getty Images. All rights reserved. Image 150854734.)

> **BOX 11.2   How to Effectively Teach Clients**
>
> Use the TEACH mnemonic:
>
> **T**une in. Listen before you start teaching. The client's needs should direct the content.
>
> **E**dit information. Teach necessary information first. Be specific.
>
> **A**ct on each teaching moment. Teach whenever possible. Develop a good relationship.
>
> **C**larify often. Make sure your assumptions are correct. Seek feedback.
>
> **H**onor the client as a partner. Build on the client's experience. Share responsibility with the client.

Modified from Hansen M, Fisher J: Patient-centered teaching from theory to practice, *Am J Nurs* 98:56-60, 1998.

---

brainstorming, role playing, simulation, games, group participation, demonstrations, and field trips. Others learn by a more solitary approach, such as watching a video, listening to a guest speaker, case studies, reading printed materials, or reflecting on how they might apply the content to their health situation.

Educators also need to be able to deliver presentations, lead group discussions, organize role-plays, provide feedback to learners, share case studies, use media and materials, and, where indicated, administer examinations. Consider the content to include, how to organize and sequence the information, what your rate of delivery will be, whether you need to include repetition, how much practice time should be included, how you will evaluate the effectiveness of the teaching, and ways that you can provide reinforcement and rewards (Box 11.2).

When choosing educational methods, consider age, gender, culture, developmental disabilities or special learning needs, educational level, knowledge of the subject, and size of the group. For example, clients with a visual impairment need more verbal description than those with no sight impairment. Persons who have hearing impairments or language limitations need more visual material and speakers or translators who can use sign language or speak their native language. Also, when the learners have limitations in attention and concentration, educators can use creative methods and tools to keep them focused. For example, you might include frequent breaks; provide simple surroundings with few or no distractions; use small-group interactions to keep learners involved and interested; and use hands-on equipment, such as mannequins, models, interactive games, and other materials and devices the learner can physically manipulate. Involve the learner appropriately, actively, and creatively in learning. Interactive educational programs often are more effective than noninteractive ones. Interactive strategies include discussion, small group work, games, and role-playing, whereas noninteractive strategies are lectures, videos, or demonstrations. Box 11.3 details descriptions of learning formats.

The goal of nurses who use *Healthy People 2020* as a guide in educating clients is to foster healthy communities, mainly through primary and secondary prevention.

BOX 11.3 Examples of Learning Formats

Presentation: This method can be used when the group is large and you want to be consistent in the message that is delivered to all participants. Remember, people tend to have a short attention span. So what can you do to keep them engaged? You might ask them to spend some time talking with one another in small groups and then have the group respond to questions or ask attendees to write answers to questions and invite several to share their answers. The presentation can take many forms, ranging from a health seminar to a town hall meeting.

Demonstration: This technique is often used to show attendees how to perform a task. For example, insulin injection demonstration, heart-healthy food preparation, and breastfeeding may be demonstrated.

Small informal group: Because learners often learn as much from one another as from the instructor, small groups can be valuable. This is especially true when the content lends itself to members sharing their own experiences. For example, in working with women in a shelter for abused women, participants may be able to share with one another actions they took to remove themselves safely from the violent environment. They might also be able to jointly plan how each might move to the stage of independent living outside the shelter.

Health fair: See the How To box on ways to plan, implement, and evaluate a health fair. For example, you might offer a health fair in a senior center and have displays, such as posters; videos; live demonstrations; handouts on such topics as reducing fat in selected recipes (including samples) and age-appropriate exercises for flexibility; as well as screenings for elevated blood pressure, glucose, or cholesterol or for osteoporosis and vision.

Nonnative language sessions: You could adapt the health fair approach for a Hispanic group by holding the session in Spanish and providing all of the materials in Spanish. Then ask Spanish-speaking nurses to staff each of the stations for health learning.

LEVELS OF PREVENTION

Primary Prevention

Education at health fairs regarding immunizations for children, older adults, and people with chronic illnesses.

Secondary Prevention

Education at health fairs regarding early diagnosis and treatment of diabetes and hypercholesterolemia, along with providing health screenings, with the goal of shortening disease duration and severity.

Tertiary Prevention

Education in rehabilitation centers or adult daycare centers to help individuals who have had a stroke maximize their functioning.

locations and can be either inside or outside (Fig. 11.2). The How To box lists guidelines to assist nurses who chair, co-chair, or serve on a planning committee for a health fair.

HOW TO Plan, Implement, and Evaluate a Health Fair

1. Form a planning committee with 2–12 people who represent the groups who will be part of the health fair (i.e., health professionals, representatives from health agencies, schools, churches, employers, the media, and the target audience).
2. Identify the target group. Develop a theme.
3. Establish goals, expected outcomes, and screening activities consistent with the needs and wishes of the target group. Your primary goal might be to improve the health of a specific population, such as workers at one plant or children in one school. You might have secondary goals, such as for the workers to reduce health care costs and for the children to reduce absenteeism.
4. Develop a timeline and schedule.
5. Choose a site and consider the site logistics. Do this about 1 year ahead. Think about the size of the site you will need and the traffic flow from one booth or demonstration to another, whether parking is available and free or low cost, and whether there are toilets and places to get food and drinks. If the site is inside, consider adequate exits; the possible risks to children, the elderly, or handicapped people; and other safety and security issues. You may need to create a map both for how to get to the fair and another one to help attendees get from one table, exhibit, or screening station to another. Be sure to include on the map the location of amenities like toilets and food vendors.
6. Plan for the needed supplies, such as tables, chairs, electronic equipment, and accessories such as extension cords, office supplies, sign-in sheets (and what information should be included), release forms for screenings, name tags, bags for attendees to gather the educational information, and evaluation forms. Set your budget. Obtain supplies in advance.
7. Recruit and manage exhibitors. Do this about 4 months ahead. Develop a list of possible exhibitors and sponsors and contact them via letter, fax, e-mail, telephone, or in person. Follow up with a confirmation letter (or fax) that outlines the details of the health fair.
8. Publicize the health fair. The planning committee will have many good ideas about how to publicize in the specific community. Examples might be fliers, posters, memos, brochures, e-mail blasts, local print, radio, or television.
9. On the day of the fair, greet attendees.
10. Evaluate the health fair by having exhibitors, participants, and volunteers fill out a form. You will need a specific form for each of these groups.
11. Stay after the event concludes to thank the committee and volunteers.
12. After the event, analyze the evaluations and develop a list of lessons learned. Include any recommendations for the next health fair. Pay bills. Send thank-you notes to the committee, volunteers, sponsors, and others who made the health fair a success.

Data from Rice CS, Pollard JM: *Health fair planning guide*, AgriLIFE EXTENSION, ed 2, College Station, Tex, 2011, Texas A&M System. Retrieved February 2016 from http://fcs.tamu.edu/health/hfpg/Health-Fair-Planning-Guide-with-Appendix.pdf. And Centers for Disease Control and Prevention, How to Plan a Health Fair, 2013. Retrieved February 2016 from www.cdc.gov/women/events/fair/index.htm.

The Centers for Disease Control and Prevention (CDC) offers excellent tips for planning health events. For example, these include (1) how to plan a health fair, (2) how to plan a health seminar, (3) how to plan a town hall meeting on a health issue, (4) how to plan a wellness walk, and (5) how to plan a health fair site (CDC, 2013). Health fairs are a popular way to provide primary and secondary health education. The objectives of holding health fairs are to increase awareness by providing health screenings, activities, information and educational materials, and demonstrations. A health fair can target a specific population or focus on a specific health issue, as well as target a range of groups and cover a variety of health education and health promotion topics. The fair can be held in many

SKILLS OF THE EFFECTIVE EDUCATOR

The educator needs to understand the basic sequence of instruction. The following steps are useful in planning an educational program. Begin by (1) *gaining the attention* of the learners and helping them understand that the information being presented is important and beneficial to them; then

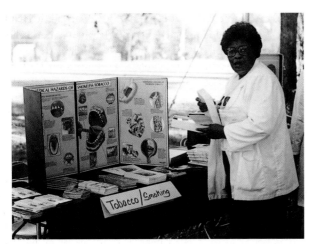

FIG. 11.2 A nurse conducts a health fair. (From Harkreader H, Hogan MA, Thobaben M: *Fundamentals of nursing,* ed 3, Philadelphia, 2007, Saunders.)

(2) *tell the learners the objectives of the instruction;* (3) *ask* learners to recall previous knowledge related to the topic of interest so they link new knowledge with previous knowledge; (4) *present the essential material* in a clear, organized, and simple manner and in a way consistent with the learners' strengths, needs, and limitations; (5) *help learners apply* the information to their lives and situations; (6) *encourage learners to demonstrate* what they have learned, which will help you correct any errors and improve skills; and (7) *provide feedback* to help learners improve their knowledge and skills. By using these steps, nurses may help clients maximize learning experiences. If steps of this process are omitted, superficial and fragmented learning may occur.

MOTIVATIONAL INTERVIEWING

Before developing a health education program or plan, do a careful assessment of the specific need. The health education goal is to engage the clients in wanting to learn ways in which they can change their behavior. Pay attention to the words you use, avoid medical jargon, and use simple language. Motivational interviewing (MI) is an evidence-based intervention used in clinical areas in which the goal is change in client behavior (Clancy and Taylor, 2016). It is a collaborative partnership between the teacher and the learner designed to help people make their own choices. This tool is useful in health education. MI can help clients resolve their ambivalence about change and uses the techniques of elaboration, affirmation, reflection, and summary to engage people in talking about change (Miller and Rose, 2009). MI combines warmth, respect, and empathy with a technique of focused listening to persuade the client to want to change. MI is generally used in conjunction with other communication techniques. MI has four essential steps: engaging, which includes person-centered, empathic listening; guiding, which includes a particular identified target for change; evoking of the client's own motivations for change; and planning. Using open-ended questions, reflections, and an understanding of the client's values, the clinician can form a partnership with the client. The nurse facilitates

rather than dictates in order to help the client state ideas and plans (Minkin et al, 2014; Treasure, 2004).

MI was initially designed to treat problem drinkers and is often used with individuals rather than groups. However, the principles can be applied to health education. For example, if a public health nurse determines that she has four women in a community group she leads who are overweight, eat high-calorie foods, and indicate they don't exercise, how could the nurse use MI? First, the nurse needs to form a partnership with each of the women, in which she and the clients can communicate easily and in which each woman trusts the nurse. The nurse draws each woman out and learns what, if anything, each wishes to change. The nurse also learns about each one's motivation to change and ability to do so.

> ### ❓ CHECK YOUR PRACTICE
>
> Consider the client, Anna, and examine her motivation to change her eating and activity patterns. Anna says that her family will only eat fried foods, so to get her husband and children to eat a meal, she fries their meats and vegetables. The family does eat fresh fruit and drink milk. Anna says that she gets exercise by walking to the bus stop en route to work and cleaning her home. She has not considered other forms of regular exercise. If you want to use MI with Anna and incorporate these principles, how would you design your nursing plan? The principles are as follows:
>
> 1. Expressing empathy by trying to see the world through Anna's eyes
> 2. Building on Anna's strengths and helping her believe that she has the ability to make a change (self-efficacy)
> 3. Rolling with resistance when Anna is ambivalent about her ability to change
> 4. Developing discrepancy by helping Anna recognize that her current actions conflict with her expressed goals of eating healthy foods and exercising regularly

Do you agree that you could incorporate into your strategy the counseling skills that are part of MI—open-ended questions, affirmations, reflections, and summaries (OARS)? These communication skills are useful in any nurse–client interaction. Open-ended questions refer to those that are not easily answered with yes or no or a short answer. These questions invite elaboration and more thinking about what is being asked. In helping Anna prepare healthier meals, ask her to describe the dinner she cooked the previous night. Affirmations are designed to recognize client strengths; they must be genuine and correct. Once Anna begins to explore the idea of preparing more nutritious food, you would affirm her progress and encourage her to continue working toward that goal. Reflections or reflective listening is possibly the most critical skill in that it conveys empathy because you are listening carefully. You can then guide Anna toward dealing with her ambivalence about change by examining the positive and negative aspects of the present situation. Using reflective listening, if Anna expresses concern or difficulty in her goal of preparing different meals, you can focus on her concern and possible ambivalence about sticking to the plan for change. What are other strategies you could use?

MI uses the term *change talk* to refer to statements by clients that they are motivated and willing to make a change. An easy-to-use mnemonic is "DARN-CAT," which refers to the following:

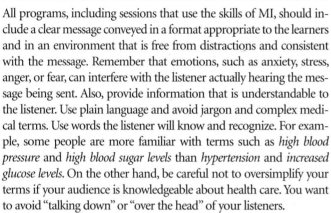

Preparatory Change Talk	**Implementing Change Talk**
Desire (I want to change)	**C**ommitment (I will make changes)
Ability (I can change)	**A**ctivation (I am ready, prepared, willing to change)
Reason (It's important to change)	
Need (I should change)	**T**aking steps (I am taking actions to change)

Apply the DARN-CAT to the goal you and Anna have for her to learn ways to prepare more nutritious meals. Although MI is a set of skills that requires training to use completely, nurses can incorporate some of the MI techniques into their communication with clients.

DEVELOPING EFFECTIVE HEALTH EDUCATION PROGRAMS

All programs, including sessions that use the skills of MI, should include a clear message conveyed in a format appropriate to the learners and in an environment that is free from distractions and consistent with the message. Remember that emotions, such as anxiety, stress, anger, or fear, can interfere with the listener actually hearing the message being sent. Also, provide information that is understandable to the listener. Use plain language and avoid jargon and complex medical terms. Use words the listener will know and recognize. For example, some people are more familiar with terms such as *high blood pressure* and *high blood sugar levels* than *hypertension* and *increased glucose levels*. On the other hand, be careful not to oversimplify your terms if your audience is knowledgeable about health care. You want to avoid "talking down" or "over the head" of your listeners.

Using plain language is more than a good idea. On October 3, 2010, President Obama signed the Plain Writing Act of 2010. Although this law requires that federal agencies use "clear government communication that the public can understand and use," this law can be transferred to health education programs. See *Plain Language.gov.* The CDC has developed guidelines for "plain language" communication your audience understands the first time. See the How To box on plain language in health education.

HOW TO Use Plain Language in Health Education
1. Organize the audience.
   - Know your audience and purpose before you begin.
   - Put the most important message first.
   - Present other information in order of importance to the audience.
   - Break text into logical chunks, and use headings.
2. Choose words carefully.
   - Write in the active voice.
   - Choose words and numbers the audience knows; do not use jargon or technical or slang words.
   - Keep words, sentences, and paragraphs short.
   - Include "you" and other pronouns.
   - Use upper- and lowercase words.
   - Use examples.
3. Make information easy to find.
   - Use headings and text boxes.
   - Delete unnecessary words sentences and paragraphs.
   - Create lists and tables. (CDC, n.d.)

The Quad Council Practice Competences for Public Health Nursing in Domain 3 list competences related to communication skills. They begin with assessing the health literacy of the individuals, families, groups, and communities being served. They emphasize the importance of effective written, oral, and electronic communication, as well as communication delivered in a culturally responsive and relevant fashion (Swider et al, 2013).

The type of learning format you select will depend on the learners. If they are young, you will want an interactive format, and many of your options will include the use of technology. You could use a game, such as developing a bingo game with food groups to teach about healthy eating. The old adage "A picture is worth a thousand words" still holds true. People tend to remember what they see or hear; a lively format rather than a passive one encourages learning. Most people have a short attention span, so you need to make your point quickly and directly. It may help to provide take-home written materials or a CD for further reminders and follow-up of what is taught. People often learn better when they are actively engaged in the learning; thus small-group discussion, role-playing, use of a computer-based program, and question-and-answer sessions may reinforce learning.

A patient education tool that is being increasingly used and has been briefly mentioned in the chapter is "teach-back." Teach-back is a health literacy tool that allows nurses to immediately assess what the individual, family, or group has learned by having the person or group immediately say or demonstrate what they learned during the session. It is considered to be a "show me" approach whereby the nurse can clarify immediately any misunderstandings (Caplin and Saunders, 2015). Nurses can also use ACTS (assess, collaborate, train, and survey) with clients and client groups. Assess the client's main concern (can be a person, family or community group); then assess learning needs and baseline level of knowledge, how they prefer to learn, their core values, and potential influential language, cultural, social or physical influences. Next compare the assessed needs with the resources available. The next step is to use Teach 3 or teach-back strategies. Teach 3 means that you teach the audience three or fewer key actions, pieces of information, or skills. Attendees then restate or demonstrate what was taught. Just as with teach-back, any misunderstandings can be immediately corrected. The key point in the two teaching strategies is to teach a small amount at any one time, and then immediately have the attendees provide feedback on what they heard or saw (French, 2015).

Fig. 11.3 shows a community group being educated, and Box 11.4 lists ways to design clear educational programs.

EDUCATIONAL ISSUES AND BARRIERS TO LEARNING

There are three important educational issues to consider when you are planning educational programs. First, different populations of learners require different teaching strategies. Second, be prepared to overcome barriers to learning. And third, consider the appropriateness of using technology in the programs.

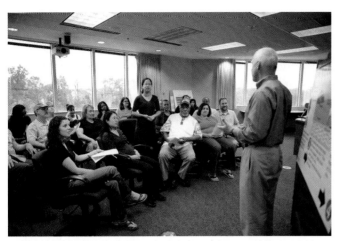

FIG. 11.3 A nurse educates a community group about environmental health issues and gathers their concerns. (From Centers for Disease Control and Prevention, 2009, courtesy Dawn Arlotta.)

BOX 11.4 Designing Clear Educational Programs

1. Develop the content for your message.
2. Identify the most appropriate format and location for your program, taking into account your budget, location, and other available resources and constraints. See Box 11.3 for examples of formats.
3. Organize the learning experience to suit the audience; consider how to engage the learners in the process.
4. Plan how you will deliver the material using the following points:
   - Limit the number of points you wish to cover to the most important ones.
   - Begin with a strong opening and close with a strong ending; people remember most what is said first and last.
   - Fit your use of language to the learners; use an active voice and emphasize the positive. For example, "Many people are able to lose weight by reducing their intake by 500 calories a day and exercising 45 minutes at least four times a week."
   - Use examples, stories, and other vivid messages. Limit statistics and complex terminology.
   - Refer to trustworthy sources. In general, government, educational, or professional association sources are peer reviewed by professionals and are dependable. The Centers for Disease Control and Prevention, National Cancer Institute, American Association of Public Health, and the American Academy of Pediatrics are four examples of organizations whose sites offer useful information.
   - Use aids to highlight your message. For example, you might have posters, handouts, or CDs to give to attendees. You might also incorporate a clip from a website, such as http://www.YouTube.com, to emphasize your point.
5. Do not forget to plan the evaluation when you are initially planning the program.

POPULATION CONSIDERATIONS BASED ON AGE AND CULTURAL AND ETHNIC BACKGROUNDS

Nurses are a trusted source of health education in the community; nurses continue to be rated via the Gallup Poll as the highest professional group in terms of honesty and ethics.

Nurses have held the number one position every year except one since they were added to the list in 1999. In 2001 firefighters were ranked number one (Saad, 2015). The increase in populations of varying cultural and ethnic backgrounds and the aging of Baby Boomers require that community health education cross age and cultural boundaries. In terms of age, children, adults, and older adults have different learning needs and respond to different educational strategies. In each age group, learners also vary in their cognitive ability, personality, and prior knowledge. Some people learn better with more direct instruction, supervision, and encouragement than do other people. As discussed in Chapter 5 culture can be "defined by group membership, such as racial, ethnic, linguistic or geographical groups, or as a collection of beliefs, values, customs, ways of thinking, communicating, and behaving" (CDC, 2015). Nurses need to tailor their education to the cultural group(s) they are teaching. The Quad Council Practice Competences for Public Health Nursing in Domain 4 discuss Cultural Competency Skills. They say that the public health nurse uses the social and ecological determinants of health to work effectively with diverse individuals, families, and groups and to develop culturally responsive interventions with communities and populations (Swider et al, 2013, p 530).

Learning strategies for children and individuals with little knowledge about a health-related topic are characterized as *pedagogy.* In the pedagogical model of learning, the teacher makes decisions about what will be learned and how and when it will be learned. This form of learning is teacher directed. Learning strategies for adults, older adults, and individuals with some health-related knowledge about a topic are called *andragogy.* In the andragogical model, learners influence what they need and want to learn. Andragogy is a more transactional way of learning than the pedagogical model. Each model has useful elements (Knowles et al, 2005). For example, when learners are dependent and entering a totally new content area, they may require more pedagogical experiences. Consider both the age of the learner population and their learning needs as you choose the pedagogical or andragogical principles for the program. In educational programs for children, provide information that matches the developmental abilities of the group. Nurses can use the following age-specific strategies to tailor educational programs for children.

- **With younger children, use more concrete examples and word choices.** You might tell 3-year-olds to brush their teeth two times per day; for 10-year-olds, you can explain to them the benefits of brushing their teeth and the risks in not brushing and talk about issues such as the care of the teeth with braces.
- **Using objects or devices, as opposed to discussion of ideas, will increase attention.** When teaching a group of children with asthma how to use inhalers, hand out inhalers to each one so he or she can practice proper technique with the inhalers rather than just giving them a handout with instructions or demonstrating how to use an inhaler while they watch you.
- **Incorporating repetitive health behaviors into games will help children retain knowledge and acquire skills.** Learning

to cook healthier food is often more effectively learned if the teacher demonstrates the new way of cooking, allows the participants to taste the food, discusses what changes would need to be made to prepare healthier food, and then has the participants each prepare one dish in the demonstration menu.

The average person, both adults and children, washes his or her hands too hastily to remove germs. The actual physical activity of washing hands is more beneficial in germ control than the soap used.

Check your practice: Assume that you are trying to teach a group of 5-year-olds how to effectively wash their hands before meals. You know that an activity often helps young children learn. So you:

- Ask each child to wash his or her hands while completely singing a favorite song.
- The song "Twinkle, Twinkle Little Star" takes about the exact amount of time to sing as is recommended for effective hand washing.
- Other songs can be used when they are appropriate to the season, such as "Jingle Bells."
- By singing a song as a group or one child at a time, learning the appropriate length to wash hands can be fun and easy to accomplish.

Children especially are able to learn health promotion behaviors when learning is fun and is appropriate to what they know and can actually do.

It is also important to consider characteristics of learners that depend on the generation to which they belong. People born after 1980 are considered the *net generation* because they have always had digital media and access to the Internet, use mobile devices to access and process information, and are "always on and connected to their devices." They typically prefer to work in groups or teams, are active learners who seek innovation, want an immediate response to their questions, and are able to multitask. These learners prefer "augmented reality," such as simulations and virtual reality, and they want to construct information on their own, which is consistent with their desire for independence. They do enjoy being mentored by older generations. *Generation X* members were born between 1960 and 1980, and they tend to be self-directed, like to work in teams, and may need to develop skills because they are not as likely to be as tech savvy as the net generation. Members of this group can tolerate delayed gratification, they want clear information with practical value, and they are able to have fun and engage in games and activities when appropriate. The *Boomers,* who were born between 1940 and 1960, are accustomed to being dependent on the teacher, want to be in charge of their own learning, respond positively to feedback, and want to do a good job. They prefer a caring environment and want to connect learning to the mission of the agency. They also want to be connected with other people. Clearly, these three generations have different characteristics, and the teacher is often a member of a generation different from that of the learner(s).

In thinking about culture, it is important to know that by 2050 approximately 50% of the US population will consist of ethnic minorities, such as Asians, African Americans, Hispanic Americans, Native Americans, and Pacific Islanders. Culture influences family structure and interactions, as well as views about health and illness. These demographic changes present new challenges to nurse educators. Nurses need to understand the health belief systems of the ethnic populations being served and be familiar with populations who are prone to develop certain health problems. When presenting seminars or providing written, audio, or visual information, make sure that the information is provided in a culturally competent manner.

For example, in a rural farming area, there might be a large population of Mexican migrant crop workers. Knowing that this Spanish-speaking group is more likely to have tuberculosis than other segments of the community, nurses may visit the migrant worker camp to present information on tuberculosis, such as prevention, symptom identification, early diagnosis, and treatment. An interpreter may accompany the nurses and provide oral content in Spanish. Written handouts can be in Spanish and designed to be read and understood on the level at which the group comprehends.

Barriers to learning fall into two broad categories: one concerning the educator and the other concerning the learner.

EDUCATOR-RELATED BARRIERS

Some common educator-related barriers to learning, together with strategies to minimize them, are as follows (Knowles et al, 2005):

- **Fear of public speaking.** Be well prepared, use icebreakers, recognize and acknowledge the fear, and practice in front of a mirror or video camera or with a friend.
- **Lack of credibility with respect to a certain topic.** Increase your confidence by carefully preparing for the talk so that you think you have included useful information and you understand the information. Avoid apologizing for lack of expertise and instead convey the attitude of an expert by briefly sharing your personal and professional background.
- **Limited professional experiences related to a health topic.** You may want to describe personal experiences (brief ones), share experiences of others, or use analogies, illustrations, or examples from movies, current news, or famous people. Be certain the examples fit the audience.
- **Inability to deal with difficult people who need to learn health-related information.** One strategy that may help with handling difficult learners is to confront the problem learner directly. Other strategies include using humor, using small groups to foster the participation of timid people, and asking disruptive people to give others a chance to speak, or, if this does not work, asking them to leave.
- **Lack of knowledge about how to gain participation.** You can foster participation by asking open-ended questions, inviting participation, and planning small-group activities in which a person responds based on the group rather than presenting individual information.
- **Lack of experience in timing a presentation so that it is neither too long nor too short.** Strategies to help determine

whether the length of the presentation is appropriate include planning well, practicing the presentation, and trying to speak during the practice at the same pace that you will speak to the group.

- **Uncertainty about how to adjust instruction.** You can more easily adjust instruction when you know the participants' needs, request feedback, and redesign the presentation during breaks based on what you have learned about the participants.
- **Discomfort when learners ask questions.** Try to anticipate questions, concisely paraphrase questions to be sure that you correctly understood the question, and recognize that it is appropriate to admit that you do not know the answer to a question.
- **Desire to obtain feedback from learners.** Solicit informal feedback during the program and at the end with program evaluation.
- **Concern about whether media, materials, and facilities will function properly.** Test the equipment before the program to make sure it runs and also that you know how to use it. Have back-up plans for how to get help if you have a problem.
- **Difficulty with openings and closings.** Strategies to foster successful openings and closings include developing several examples of openings and closings, memorizing the opening and closing, concisely summarizing information, and thanking participants for attending.
- **Overdependence on notes.** You may wish to use note cards or visual aids as prompts, and practicing in advance is a proved way to increase skill at presenting.

LEARNER-RELATED BARRIERS

Two of the most important learner-related barriers are low literacy and lack of motivation to learn information and make needed behavioral changes. Nurses often deal with individuals and populations who are illiterate or who have *low literacy levels.* These individuals may be embarrassed to admit this deficit to health care providers and educators and may try to appear to understand when they really do not. Specifically, they may not ask questions to clarify information even when they do not understand it. As society becomes more multicultural, the problem of low literacy can increase because of limited use of the primary language and limited education. It is essential to assess the literacy, especially health literacy of the learners. The next paragraphs discuss the significance of this problem and the need for nurses to address health literacy.

The National Assessment of Adult Literacy (NAAL) is the largest literacy assessment study done in the United States. This assessment was first conducted in 1992. At that time, of the five levels in the assessment, 50% of American adults were in the top two levels and 50% were in the bottom three levels of literacy. The minimal standard needed to function in the workplace is level 3 proficiency. In 2003 the tool measured literacy in four levels: *below basic, basic, intermediate,* and *proficient.* The literacy scales used in 2003 were prose literacy, document literacy,

and quantitative literacy. Prose examples include searching, comprehending, and using information from editorials, news stories, brochures, and instructional materials. Document literacy refers to searching, comprehending, and using information from documents such as job applications, payroll forms, transportation schedules, maps, tables, and drug and food labels. Quantitative literacy is the ability to identify and perform computations such as balancing a checkbook, completing an order form, or determining the interest on a loan from an advertisement. The 2003 test is more than just a survey and actually asks the test takers to perform tasks to demonstrate their literacy level (Kutner et al, 2006). The 2003 NAAL included information about health literacy, which is an important topic for nurses. The 2003 NAAL used the Institute of Medicine's definition of health literacy: "The degree to which individuals have the capacity to obtain, process, and understand basic health information and services needed to make appropriate health decisions" (Ratzan and Parker, 2000). Kutner et al (2006) found that the majority of participants had an intermediate (53%) literacy level, 12% were proficient, 22% were basic, and 14% had below basic levels of literacy. The assessment was given to over 19,000 adults in households or prisons. Interestingly, women had a higher literacy level than men; white and Asian/Pacific Islander adults had higher scores than African American, Hispanic, American Indian/Alaska Native, and multiracial adults; and adults 65 years of age or older and persons living below the poverty line had a lower average literacy level than others surveyed. The Health Resources and Services Administration (HRSA) added medically underserved people to the list of individuals who were more likely to have low health literacy (HRSA, n.d.). In addition, the *National Action Plan to Improve Health Literacy* (USDHHS, Office of Disease Prevention and Health Promotion, 2010) adds recent refugees and immigrants to the list of people who may have low health literacy including nonnative English speakers.

Of every five Americans, one reads below the fifth-grade level, and one of every three lacks the literacy ability needed to understand health care providers (Roberts, 2004). Typically, individuals read three to five grade levels below the last year of school completed. It has been found that most health instructions continue to be written at the 10th-grade reading level, which is too difficult for almost half of the adult readers in the United States (Health Literacy Innovations, 2010). Several tests are used to evaluate literacy levels, including the Fry-Based Electronic Readability Formula, Flesch Reading Ease Score, Precise SMOG, and Gunning-Fog (Health Literacy Innovations, 2010). Examine one of them and apply it to a paper you have written to learn at what level you typically write.

Individuals with limited literacy may be unable to understand instructions on prescription bottles, seek preventive care, understand the relationship between risky behavior and health, manage chronic health conditions, interpret health appointment cards, fill out health insurance forms, and read and understand self-care or hospital discharge instructions. Also, individuals may have weak literacy and numeracy skills in their native language, and even translated materials may be difficult for them to understand because not all languages have words that directly translate into English (CDC, 2015). The following may happen when someone has health illiteracy. The person may:

- Have limited vocabulary and general knowledge and not ask for clarification
- Focus on details and deal in literal or concrete concepts versus abstract concepts
- Select responses on a survey or questionnaire without necessarily understanding them
- Be unable to understand math (which is important in calculating medications)

Health illiteracy is expensive when people cannot understand their health care treatment or follow directions correctly. This inability can lead to increased numbers of emergency room visits, hospitalizations and health care complications resulting from those hospitalizations, poorer health care outcomes, and decreased life expectancy (Kleinbeck, 2005).

Some people are not motivated to learn. Although adults respond to some external motivators, the most powerful motivators are internal. People are motivated to learn if they value and feel they will benefit from the outcome of the learning, if they think they can follow through on what is being taught, and if it will improve their situation in life or increase their self-esteem (Ota et al, 2006).

A variety of health promotion models can be used to structure health education and health promotion plans. One model, the Health Belief Model (HBM) is an individual-level model that can be used to plan programs if you think the motivation of learners might be a concern. Specifically, the HBM was one of the first theories of health behavior. It began in an interesting way that is still applicable to the behavior of people today. In the 1950s the US Public Health Service sent mobile radiography units to communities to provide free chest radiographs as a way to screen for tuberculosis. The radiography examinations were free, convenient, and painless, yet people did not take advantage of the service. A group of social psychologists were asked to try to explain the failure to use this screening—specifically, to determine what would motivate people to seek health care.

The HBM includes six components that attempt to answer the question of what motivates an individual to do something. These components are (1) perceived susceptibility ("Will something happen to me?"), (2) perceived severity ("If something does happen to me, will it be a big problem?"), (3) perceived benefits ("If I do what is suggested, will it really help me?"), (4) perceived barriers ("Assuming I do what is suggested, will there be barriers that will be unpleasant, costly, and so forth?"), (5) cues to action ("What might motivate me to actually do something?"), and (6) self-efficacy ("Can I really do this?"). This model has been applauded and criticized. It does offer guidance in planning health education programs in that it reminds nurses to think carefully about what motivates people to change. To understand motivation, it is important to learn: (1) how people involved feel about the health problem, (2) whether

they think the problem is serious, (3) whether they think that action on their part will make a difference, and (4) whether they think they can both manage the barriers and actually perform the action (Edberg, 2015)

Consider the following example of how the HBM might be applied to a person in the community who has recently been diagnosed with diabetes. The person, June, is 25 years old and was diagnosed 2 months ago with diabetes mellitus. She has found it hard to follow the recommendations of the public health nurse she saw in the community clinic. When the nurse asked June what seemed to be getting in her way of complying, June said that she wondered what might happen to her if she did not follow the advice the nurse had given her about diet, exercise, and taking her insulin. June questioned whether something would really happen to her and, if that was the case, would it really be a problem? Her ambivalence about making this change led her to wonder: If she took her medication, ate a diabetic diet, exercised, and took her insulin correctly, would it really reduce the seriousness of her disease? She also questioned whether she could afford the food and insulin and had the time to cook appropriately and exercise regularly. June was afraid that insulin self-injection might be painful. If the nurse used motivational interviewing to help June develop and commit to a health change plan, what steps would the nurse take? June said that when she saw her friend Sue, who is also a diabetic patient, she noticed that Sue was careful about what she ate, talked about her regular exercise program, and looked better than she had in the past. How would the nurse use the information that June reported about her friend Sue?

A second set of models is presented. The selection of these three models—the HBM, the Transtheoretical Model (TTM), and Precaution Adoption Process Model (PAPM)—does not imply that they are the best or only models. They are, however, useful models in health promotion. The TTM and the PAPM are discussed together because they both deal with change that occurs in stages and over time. The TTM has the following six stages:

1. Precontemplation, in which the person does not plan to change; this may be because the person does not know there is a problem or does not want to do anything about it (Edberg, 2015). For example, the person may not know that it is not good to cook food in lard.
2. Contemplation, in which the person begins thinking about making a change in the future and examines the pros and cons of doing so. The person might have gone to a class in which he learned that it is better to cook food in canola oil rather than in lard and is beginning to wonder if his food would taste as good if he made that change.
3. Preparation, in which the person intends to do something. In the cooking example, the person might put canola oil on the shopping list.
4. Action, by which the person actually buys the canola oil and cooks a chicken with it instead of the lard.
5. Maintenance, when the person decides that he can get used to eating chicken cooked in oil and begins preparing his food in that way on a regular basis.

6. The person terminates the change process because he is able to continue the new, more health-conscious way of cooking.

Although the terms used are slightly different, the intent of the PAPM is much like that of the TTM. The stages are (1) unaware of the issue, (2) unengaged by the issue, (3) deciding about acting, (4) deciding not to act, (5) deciding to act, (6) acting, and (7) maintenance. You can apply the earlier cooking example to these stages, as well.

USE OF TECHNOLOGY IN HEALTH EDUCATION

Many kinds of technologies, such as computer games and programs, videos, CDs, and Internet resources, can increase learning. These technologies may enable the learner to control the pace of instruction, offer flexibility in the time and location of learning, present an appealing form of education, and provide immediate feedback. You may want to use a variety of technological applications in your teaching. It is also important to be aware that people increasingly are using the Internet as a source of health information. The Pew Research Center's unit studying society and Internet usage has since 2000 conducted 97 national studies. Highlights from 15 years of study found the following:

- Age: For young adults, especially those with higher levels of education and those in more affluent households, Internet use is at full saturation levels. Although older adults have lagged behind young people, about 85% of senior citizens use the Internet.
- Class differences: People with college educations are more likely to use the Internet than those without a high school diploma. The usage gap among different classes has shrunk over the past 15 years.
- Racial and ethnic differences: At present, 78% of blacks, 81% of Hispanics, 85% of whites, and 97% of English-speaking Asian Americans are Internet users.
- Community differences: Although people who live in rural areas are less likely to be online, at present, 78% of rural residents are Internet users (Perrin and Duggan, 2015).

Why do people use the Internet? A major benefit is its convenience: It is available 24 hours per day, 7 days per week, and there is no need to drive there, take public transportation, or find a parking place. Is the Internet a good source of health information? The answer depends on the site you use to find your information.

Educating people through the Internet has been shown to be more effective in fostering treatment adherence than in-person counseling, telephone counseling, or self-directed learning (Dauz et al, 2004). Clients may ask nurses to provide them with information about ways to evaluate the quality and reliability of this information. The following list provides some criteria for assessing the quality of Internet health information (VanBiervliet and Edwards-Schafer, 2004):

- **Authorship:** Are the credentials and affiliations of authors and contributors listed?
- **Caveats:** Does the site clarify whether its function is to provide information or to market products?

EVIDENCE-BASED PRACTICE

The use of technology as a way to provide health education and intervene in the progress of a chronic illness, hypertension, was presented in a case study. The authors used TXT2DASH, which is an mHealth program designed to improve self-management and increase nutritional self-efficacy in patients who sought care at free health care clinics and who had hypertension. In this program the patients were sent weekly educational text messages on the Dietary Approaches to Stop Hypertension (DASH) diet. This diet has been shown to reduce and control blood pressure. Messages were sent 3 days a week for 4 weeks; each week a different food category was discussed. Three health care clinics providing free care participated in the project, and 13 patients completed the final data collection and demonstrated dietary behavior improvements, especially in the areas of drinking soda and using fats and oils.

Nurse Use

It is important in any health education program to consider the readability and user-friendliness of the program. The cost of the program to the participants or to the clinic must be considered. If a text messaging program is used, it is important to determine whether there is any support to the patients to enable them to have cellular devices.

Welsh, P: Strategies in development of an mHealth technology for low socioeconomic groups in free healthcare clinics, *CIN: Computers, Informatics, Nursing*, 34(1): 3-5, January 2016.

- **Content:** Is the information accurate and complete, and is an appropriate disclaimer provided?
- **Credibility:** Does the site include the source, currency, relevance, and editorial review process for the information?
- **Currency:** Are dates listed for when the content was posted and updated?
- **Design:** Is the site accessible, capable of internal searches, easy to navigate, and logically organized?
- **Disclosure:** Is the user informed about the purpose of the site and about any profiling or collection of information associated with using the site?
- **Interactivity:** Does the site include feedback mechanisms and opportunities for users to exchange information?
- **Links:** Have the links been evaluated according to back-linkages, content, and selection?

The Evidence-Based Practice Box describes mHealth technology for use in a free clinic.

EVALUATION OF THE EDUCATIONAL PROCESS

Evaluation is important in both the educational process and the nursing process. Evaluation is a systematic and logical way to make decisions to improve the educational program. You will need to evaluate the educator, the process, and the product. Feedback to the *educator* provides the educator an opportunity to modify the teaching process and better meet the learner's needs. The educator may receive written feedback from learners, such as with an evaluation sheet. The educator also may ask for verbal feedback, as well as get nonverbal feedback by using return demonstrations to see what learners have mastered and by observing facial expressions when feedback is being given (Bastable, 2008). Process evaluation examines the dynamic components of the educational program. It follows and assesses the movements and management of information transfer and attempts to make sure that the objectives are being met. Process evaluation is necessary *throughout* the educational program to determine whether goals and objectives are being met and the time required for their accomplishment. Ongoing evaluation also allows the teacher to correct misinformation, misinterpretation, or confusion and to periodically reconsider the goals and objectives of the program.

The *educational product,* an outcome of the educational process, is measured both qualitatively and quantitatively (Bastable, 2008). For example, a qualitative assessment should answer the question, "How well does the learner appear to understand the content?" A quantitative assessment should answer the question, "How much of the content does the learner retain?" Thus the quality of the product is measured by improvement and increase, or the lack thereof, in the learner's knowledge, skills, and abilities related to the content of the educational program. Selected outcomes for the population of interest need to be identified when the educational program is designed so you can measure the program's effectiveness.

EVALUATION OF HEALTH AND BEHAVIORAL CHANGES

Various approaches, methods, and tools can be used to evaluate health and behavioral changes. These include questionnaires, rating scales, surveys, checklists, skills demonstrations, testing, subjective client feedback, and direct observation of improvements in client mastery of materials (Bastable, 2008). Qualitative or quantitative strategies may be used to measure changes in knowledge, skills, abilities, attitudes, behavior, health status, and quality of life. Choose the method of evaluation based on the situation. For example, when evaluating a person's ability to perform a psychomotor skill such as changing a dressing, it is best to watch the person perform the skill.

Also evaluate both short-term and long-term effects of the health teaching. A short-term evaluation of whether a client can perform a return demonstration of breast self-examination requires minimal energy, expense, or time and shows skill mastery within a matter of minutes. If the short-term objective is not met, the nurse determines why and identifies possible solutions so that successful learning can occur. If the short-term objective is met, the nurse then focuses on long-term evaluation designed to assess the lasting effects of the education program.

Long-term follow-up with clients is challenging, and it focuses on following and assessing the status of an individual, family, community, or population over time to determine whether specific goals and objectives were met. Often, for nurse educators, the goal of long-term evaluation is to analyze the effectiveness of the education program for the entire community, not the health status of a specific client. Nurses track the achievement of community objectives over time but not that of the individual community members. Thus in a changing population, long-term evaluation of the results of an education program is still possible. The percentage of objectives and goals met by sampling the target population gives valid statistics for program assessment, even though the population of individuals may have experienced a complete turnover.

For example, a nurse notes that according to annual health department data, 60% of the pregnant women in the nurse's catchment area received some prenatal care. Wanting to increase this percentage to 100%, the nurse tries an educational intervention in which radio and television stations make public service announcements about the importance and availability of prenatal services.

After 1 year, the nurse discovers that 80% of all pregnant women now receive prenatal care. The nurse continues to use public service announcements the following year because good results are evident. However, the long-term goal of the education program to influence the behavior of 100% of the pregnant women in the community has not yet been met. Therefore the nurse enlists volunteers to put informational posters in shopping malls, grocery stores, public transportation stops, laundries, and public transportation vehicles. In the second year after implementing the revised educational program, again using the statistics from the health department, the nurse finds that 95% of all pregnant women in the target area now receive prenatal care. The nurse can thus evaluate and modify a community educational program over time to increase the rate, range, and consistency of progress made toward meeting the long-term goals of the project.

It may be hard to keep track of the clients to complete the evaluation; some will move, and others will lose interest and fail to keep appointments or return calls, text messages, or e-mails.

A considerable amount of health education is carried out in the community in groups rather than provided to one person at a time. For this reason, the following section discusses how groups can be used as a tool for health education and the promotion of health.

GROUPS: A TOOL IN HEALTH EDUCATION

Nurses often provide health education to groups. Members of the group may support either beneficial or poor health practices. For example, a young person may be part of a group that abuses substances. Another youth might be part of a group that runs marathons. The health-oriented goals of each of these two groups are different. A group is an effective and powerful medium to initiate and implement changes for individuals, families, organizations, and the community. Groups form for various reasons. They may form for a clearly stated purpose or goal, or they may form naturally as shared values, interests, activities, or personal characteristics attract individuals to each other.

Community groups represent the collective interests, needs, and values of individuals; they provide a link between the individual and the larger social system. Throughout life, group membership influences thoughts, choices, behaviors, and values as people socialize and interact. Through groups, people may express personal views and relate them to the views of others.

Groups serve as communication networks and can help organize various aspects of communities.

Community groups may be informal or formal. Formal groups have a defined membership and a specific purpose. They may or may not have an official place in the community's organization. In informal groups, the ties among members are multiple, and the purposes are unwritten yet understood by members. These groups often form spontaneously when participants have a common interest or need. You can find out about what formal and informal groups exist in a community by reading the local newspaper or local Internet sites, listening to public service information on the radio or television, and asking residents about the groups to which they belong. Nurses can help form new groups or create linkages among existing groups.

Group support often helps people make needed changes for health that they are unable to accomplish on their own or with the help of just one individual. For example, groups may support physical activity and fitness, sound nutrition, conquering smoking or drug abuse, getting out of abusive relationships, and safe sexual practices. One of the core competencies for public health professionals is to "use group processes to advance community involvement" (Council on Linkages, 2010, p 10).

GROUP: DEFINITIONS AND CONCEPTS

A group is a collection of interacting individuals who have common purposes. To some extent, each member influences and is in turn influenced by every other member. Groups form for a variety of reasons. Families, an example of a community group, share kinship bonds, living space, and economic resources. There are many group purposes, such as teaching the members and providing psychological support and socialization.

Groups also form in response to community needs, problems, or opportunities. For example, community residents may form a neighborhood association to protect their health and welfare. Community groups occur spontaneously because of mutual attraction between individuals and to meet personal needs such as those for socialization and recreation. Health-promoting groups may form when people meet in community and health care settings and discover common challenges to their physical and emotional well-being.

Groups need to identify a clear purpose so they can establish criteria for member selection and determine an action plan. A clear statement of purpose proved valuable in forming a new group in one city's housing development. The local department of social services had received numerous reports of child abuse and neglect. Routine home visits for well-child care documented high stress between parents and their offspring, and some parents asked the nurse to teach them about child discipline. The nurse proposed that a parent group address this community need, and she chose this purpose for the group: *dealing with kids for child and parent satisfaction.* The purpose indicated both the process (to help parents deal with children)

and the desired outcome (satisfaction for parents and children). Having a group purpose stated enabled parents to decide if they wanted to join.

Cohesion is the attraction among individual members and between each member and the group. Individuals in a highly cohesive group identify themselves as a unit, work toward common goals, endure frustration for the sake of the group, and defend the group against outside criticism. Attraction increases when members feel accepted and liked by others, see similar qualities in one another, share similar attitudes and values, and work together to meet group goals. The following member traits can increase group cohesion and productivity: (1) attraction to a set of compatible personal and group goals, (2) attraction to members of the group, and (3) a good mix among members of problem-solving, leading, and following skills.

Groups have both task and maintenance functions. A task function is anything a member does that deliberately contributes to the group's purpose. Members with task-directed abilities become more attractive to the group. These traits include strong problem-solving skills, access to material resources, and skills in directing. Maintenance functions help members affirm, accept, and support one another, resolve conflicts, and create social and environmental comfort. Groups need members with both task and maintenance functions. In contrast, some member traits can decrease cohesion and productivity, such as (1) conflicts between personal and group goals, aversion to some members of the group, and not understanding the behaviors and attributes of one another; (2) lack of interest in group goals and activities; (3) poor problem-solving and communication abilities; and (4) lack of both leadership and supporter skills and disagreement about types of leadership. Usually, the more alike group members are, the stronger is a group's attraction. Differences tend to decrease attractiveness and may lead to competition and jealousy among members. At the same time, personal differences can increase group cohesion if they support complementary functioning or provide contrasting viewpoints necessary for decision-making. Cohesive factors are complex, and many factors influence member attraction to each other and to the group's goal. High group cohesion positively affects productivity and member satisfaction. The following example illustrates factors that influence group cohesion.

A nurse initiated a group for clients who had been treated for burns. Ten residents from the same town had been discharged after a month in the local burn unit. The stated purpose of the group was to teach coping skills to assist members in the transition from hospital to home. Each person had been treated for extensive burns in an intensive care treatment center; each had relied heavily on health care workers for physical, social, and emotional rehabilitation; and each had faced the challenge of resuming work and family roles. Individuals shared some similar experiences and hopes for the future but varied in the amount of trauma and stress experienced. They also differed widely in psychological readiness for return to ordinary daily routines. One woman in the group was able to return quickly to her job as a cashier in a large supermarket. The strength of her determination to overcome public reaction to her scars, coupled with an ability to "use the right words" and an empathy for others, distinguished her from others in the group. These differences proved attractive to other members, inspiring them to work toward a return to their own roles in life. These members saw her differences as attainable.

This group's cohesion was provided by the members' attraction to the common purpose of returning to successful life patterns and managing relationships with others. Members also thought that interaction with others with similar burn experiences could help them reach that goal. This example shows that certain member experiences, such as crises or traumas, may help individuals identify with each other and increase member attraction.

Being different from the general population and similar to the other group members is, for some, a compelling force for membership in the group. Other members may be repelled by the group because they do not want to be identified by an aversive characteristic such as disfigurement. Empathy for another's pain, learned only through mutual experience, may provide each individual with a required perspective for problem solving or affirming another's view. This nurse helped members use common experiences and learn from their differences. The group was effective.

Member attraction to the group also depends on the nature of the group. Factors include the group programs, size, type of organization, and position in the community. Attraction to the group is increased when individuals understand the goals and see group activities as effective. Cohesive groups tend to be more productive and able to accomplish their goals; cohesion can be increased as members better understand the experiences of others and identify common ideas and reactions to various issues. Nurses facilitate this process by pointing out similarities, contrasting supportive differences, or helping members redefine differences in ways that make those dissimilarities compatible.

Norms are standards that guide, control, and regulate individuals and communities. Group norms set the standards for group members' behaviors, attitudes, and perceptions. Group norms suggest what a group believes is important, what it finds acceptable or objectionable, or what it perceives as of no consequence. The task norm is the commitment to return to the central goals of the group. The strength of the task norm determines the group's ability to adhere to its work.

Maintenance norms create group pressures to affirm members and maintain their comfort. Maintenance behaviors include identifying the social and psychological tensions of members and taking steps to support those members at high-stress times. For example, maintenance norms often refer to things such as scheduling meetings at convenient times and in an accessible and comfortable space with parking as well as seating, refreshments, and toilets.

Groups also have reality norms, whereby members reinforce or challenge and correct their ideas of what is real.

Groups can examine the life situations facing members and help make sense of them. As individuals gather information, attempt to understand that information, make decisions, and consider the facts and their implications, they can take responsible action, not only in relation to themselves and their group but also for the community. Group (task, maintenance, and reality) norms combine to form a group culture. Reality norms influence each member to see relevant situations in the same way the other members see them. For example, suppose a group of individuals with diabetes defines an uncontrolled diet as harmful; members may try to influence one another to maintain diet control. The nurse can provide accurate information about diet and the disease process while continually conveying an assurance that health through diet control is attainable and desirable.

Group members with similar backgrounds may have a limited scope of knowledge. For example, women members of a spouse abuse group may think that men are exploitative and harmful based on their childhood and marriage experiences. Such a stereotypical view of men could be reinforced by similar perceptions in other members; this might lead to continuing anger, fear of interactions with men, and a hostile or helpless approach to family affairs. Nurses or group members who have known men in loving, helpful, and collaborative ways can describe these perceptions of men and offer positive examples. Nurses bring an important perspective to groups in which similar backgrounds limit the understanding and interpretation of personal concerns.

Groups have role structures that define the expected ways in which members behave toward one another. The role that each person assumes serves a purpose in the group. Roles might be as leader, follower, task specialist, maintenance specialist, evaluator, peacemaker, and gatekeeper. Box 11.5 includes descriptions of each of these group roles. Because leadership is an especially complex role, it will be discussed in greater detail.

Leadership is a complex concept. It consists of behaviors that guide or direct members and determine and influence group action. Positive leadership defines or negotiates the

---

BOX 11.5 Examples of Group Role Behavior

There are many examples; this is a representative list of the types of roles members may use.

Follower: Seeks and accepts the authority or direction of others
Gatekeeper: Controls outsiders' access to the group
Leader: Guides and directs group activity
Maintenance specialist: Provides physical and psychological support for group members, thereby holding the group together
Peacemaker: Attempts to reconcile conflict between members or takes action in response to influences that disrupt the group process and threaten its existence
Task specialist: Focuses or directs movement toward the main work of the group

group's purpose, selects and helps implement tasks that accomplish the purpose, maintains an environment that affirms and supports members, and balances efforts between task and maintenance. An effective leader pays attention to communications and interactions among the members, including spoken words and body language. This information provides continuous feedback about the members and the group process. By paying close attention to communications and interactions, members detect changing group needs and can take responsibility and pride in their own involvement. One or more members may lead the group, or leadership may be shared by one or more members. Generally, shared leadership increases productivity, cohesion, and satisfying interactions among members.

After initiating or establishing a group, nurses may facilitate leadership within and among members, frequently relinquishing central control and encouraging members to determine the ultimate leadership pattern for their group. In some settings and circumstances, a single authority is necessary (e.g., when members have limited skills or time or are uncomfortable with shared responsibility for leading). A leadership style that shares leading functions with other group members is effective when there are many alternatives and when issues of values and ethics are involved in the group's action. Leadership can be described as patriarchal, paternal, or democratic. Each of these styles has a particular effect on members' interaction, satisfaction, and productivity. Groups may reflect one or a combination of styles.

A patriarchal or paternal style is seen when one person has the final authority for group direction and movement. A person using patriarchal leadership may control members through rewards and threats, often keeping them in the dark about the goals and rationale behind prescribed actions. Patriarchal and paternal styles of leadership are authoritarian; they can be used in a disaster team, in which immediate task accomplishment is the goal. Group morale and cohesiveness are typically low under sustained authoritarian styles of leadership, and members may not learn how to function independently. Also, issues of authority and control may disrupt productivity if the group members challenge the power of the leader. Democratic leadership is cooperative and promotes and supports member involvement in all aspects of decision making and planning. Members influence each other as they explore goals, plan steps toward the goals, implement those steps, and evaluate progress.

CHOOSING GROUPS FOR HEALTH CHANGE

Nurses choose the type of group to use after considering the overall needs of the community and its people, including client contacts, expressed concerns of community spokespersons, health statistics for the area, available health resources, and the community's general well-being. These data point to the community's strengths and critical needs.

The nurse can identify goals for the community and for various groups through media reports and from community informants and colleagues. Community members should be involved in setting the goals and in planning the interventions. Alliances or coalitions unite diverse interest groups who share a common interest in perceived threats to community health to both analyze the community and develop the plan for change. Nurses and other professionals are active in groups formed to address community issues.

Nurses may work with existing groups or form new groups. Deciding whether to work in established groups or to begin new ones is based on client needs, the purpose of existing groups, and the membership ties in existing groups. The advantages to using established groups for individual health change are that membership ties already exist, the existing structure can be used, and it is not necessary to find new members because compatible individuals already form a working group. Established groups usually have operating methods that have proved successful; an approach for a new goal is built on this history. Members are aware of each other's strengths, limitations, and preferred styles of interaction and may be comfortable working together, and they may be able to influence one another. If you choose to work with an established group, be sure to determine whether the new focus is compatible with the existing group purposes. Fig. 11.4 shows a breakout session during a community forum.

Nurses can use existing community groups as a source of information to conduct a community assessment. Many community groups, such as health-planning groups, better business clubs, women's action groups, school boards, and neighborhood councils, are excellent resources for information because part of their purpose is to determine and respond to community needs. In addition, they are already established as part of the community structure. When a group representing one community sector is selected for community health intervention, the total community structure is studied. Groups reflect existing community values, strengths, and norms.

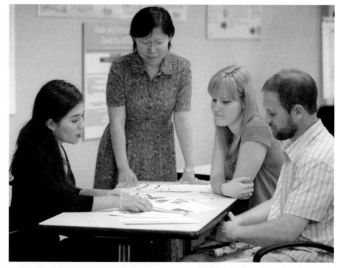

FIG. 11.4 Breakout session in a community forum on environmental health concerns. (From Centers for Disease Control and Prevention, 2009, courtesy Dawn Arlotta.)

How might nurses help established groups work toward community goals? The same interventions recommended for groups formed for individual health change can be used for groups focused on community health. Such interventions include the following:

- Building cohesion through clarifying goals and individual attraction to groups
- Building member commitment and participation
- Keeping the group focused on the goal
- Maintaining members through recognition and encouragement
- Maintaining member self-esteem during conflict and confrontation
- Analyzing forces affecting movement toward the goal
- Evaluating progress

When nurses enter established groups, they need to assess the leadership, communications, and normative structures. This facilitates group planning, problem solving, intervention, and evaluation. The steps for community health changes parallel those of decision making and problem solving in other methodologies.

CASE EXAMPLE

Nurse working with an established group to intervene in a community problem: A nurse was asked to meet with a neighborhood council to help them study and "do something about" the number of homeless living on the streets. Residents knew the nurse from a local clinic and from his consulting work at a shelter for the homeless in an adjacent community. When the council invited him, they stated that "our intent is to be part of the solution rather than part of the problem." The nurse agreed to meet, and he learned that the neighborhood council had addressed concerns of the neighborhood for 20 years—protecting zoning guidelines, setting up a recreational program for teens, organizing an after-school program for latchkey children, and generally representing the homeowners of the area. The neighborhood was composed of low-income families who took great pride in their homes. After meeting with the council and listening to their description of the situation, the nurse agreed to help, and he joined the council.

As the first step in addressing the problem, the council conducted a comprehensive problem analysis on the homeless situation. All known causes and outcomes of homeless persons on the street were identified, and the relationships between each factor and the problem were documented from literature and from the local history. The nurse brought expertise in health planning and knowledge of the homeless and their health risks. He suggested negotiation between the council and the local coalition for the homeless, recognizing that planning would be most relevant if homeless individuals participated. The council was cohesive and committed to the purpose, had developed working operations, and did not need help with group process. They made adjustments in their usual group operation to use the knowledge and health-planning skills of the nurse. Interventions for the homeless included establishing temporary shelters at homes on a rotating basis, providing daily meals through the city council or churches, and joining the area coalition for the homeless.

This example shows how an established, competent group addressed a new goal successfully by building on existing strengths in partnership with the nurse. Community groups, because of their interactive roles, are logical and natural vehicles for people who work together for community health change. As the decision-making and problem-solving capabilities of community groups are strengthened, the groups become more able representatives for the whole community. Nurses improve the community's health by working with groups toward that goal.

When it is neither desirable nor possible to use existing groups, the nurse can initiate a selected membership group. Choose members who have common health needs or concerns. For instance, individuals with diabetes can meet to discuss diet management and physical care and to share problem-solving remedies; community residents can meet for social support and rehabilitation after treatment for mental illness; or isolated older adults can meet to socialize, eat nutritious meals, and exercise. Consider members' attributes when composing a new group. Members are attracted to others from similar backgrounds, with similar experiences, and with common interests and abilities.

The size of the group influences effectiveness; generally, 8 to 12 is a good number for group work focused on individual health changes. Groups of up to 25 members may be effective when their focus is on community needs. Large groups often divide and assign tasks to the smaller subgroups, with the original large groups meeting less frequently for reporting and evaluation. Setting member criteria can facilitate recruitment and selection of the most appropriate members for any group. The criteria usually suggest a mixture of member traits, allowing for balance for the processes of decision making and growth.

BEGINNING INTERACTIONS AND DEALING WITH CONFLICT

Work on the stated purpose begins as soon as the group forms. It is important to help members interact with a degree of satisfaction. This requires close attention to maintenance tasks of attending, eliciting information, clarifying, and recognizing contributions of members. Begin by talking about what brought each member to the group. Encourage each person to participate; recognize and support them as they take on leadership functions. The new group begins to take shape in the early sessions as members try out familiar roles and test their individual abilities. The core competency skills for communication recommended by the Public Health Foundation (Council on Linkages, 2010) are useful to nurses who work with groups in the community. Box 11.6 lists these competencies. Subsequent steps are then planned not only according to the nurse's skill and preference but also according to the group composition and the skills brought by members

Conflict normally occurs in all human relations. However, people generally see conflict as the opposite of harmony and try to guard against it. This is an unfortunate view because the

BOX 11.6   Core Competencies for Communication Skills of Educators

Communication Skills
- Communicates effectively both in writing and orally, including via e-mail.
- Solicits input from individuals and organizations.
- Advocates for public health programs and resources.
- Leads and participates in groups to address specific issues.
- Uses the media, various technologies, and community networks to convey information.
- Effectively presents accurate demographic, statistical, programmatic, and scientific information for professional and lay audiences.

Attitudes
- Listens to others in an unbiased manner.
- Respects points of view of others.
- Promotes the expression of diverse opinions and perspectives.

tensions of difference and potential conflict actually help groups work toward their purposes. It is important to understand common causes of conflict and conflict management and resolution approaches. Conflict signals that antagonistic points of view must be considered and that one must reexamine beliefs and assumptions underlying relationships. Some people are concerned about security, control of self and others, respect between parties, and access to limited resources. In groups, members may express frustrations about trust, closeness and separation, and dependence and independence. These themes of interpersonal conflict operate to some extent in all interactions and are not unique to groups. Conflict can be overwhelming, especially when members think that expressing

controversy is unacceptable or unremitting or when it is suppressed over time and builds up to an explosive stage. A group that repeatedly avoids expressing conflict becomes fragile, unable to adapt, and helpless to face challenges. Conflict may be destructive if contentious parties fail to respect the rights and beliefs of others.

Approaches for conflict-acknowledging and problem solving that respect others and represent self-concerns are first learned in families and other small groups. These lessons teach people that conflict is natural and can support growth and change. Other people learn to avoid conflict or disregard others in the promotion of self. Teams that embrace a united desire for harmony and avoid conflict may hinder collaboration and personal growth (Gerow, 2001).

EVALUATION OF GROUP PROGRESS

It is important to evaluate individual and group progress toward meeting health goals. Early in the planning, specify the action steps that should be taken to meet the goals. These small steps may be responses to learning objectives (listed as action steps designed to support facilitative forces and deal with resistive forces), or they may reflect the group's problem-solving plan. The action steps and the indicators of achievement are discussed and written in a group record. Build recognition of accomplishments into the evaluation system. Recognition may include concrete rewards, such as special foods and drinks, or it may be the personal expression of joy and member-to-member approval. Celebration of group accomplishments marks progress, rewards members, and motivates each person to continue.

PRACTICE APPLICATION

Kristi, a bachelor of science in nursing student, is having her community health practicum at a local health department. The health department has gotten many calls from people wanting information about the H3N2 virus. For Kristi's community health intervention project, she decides to do a community educative piece on this topic.

What is her best course of action?

A. Develop a poster presentation to have on display at the health department.

B. Assemble an educative pamphlet to mail to anyone calling with questions.
C. Work with the health department staff to develop a community forum–style presentation and information brochures on this virus.
D. Develop an in-service program for health department staff on the potential spread of the virus and ways to prevent its spread.

Answers can be found on the Evolve website.

REMEMBER THIS!

- Health education is essential in nursing because the promotion, maintenance, and restoration of health rely on clients' understanding of health care topics.
- Nurse educators identify learning needs, consider how people learn, examine educational issues, design and implement educational programs, and evaluate the effects of the educational program on learning and behavior.
- Nurses often use the *Healthy People 2020* educational objectives as a guide to identifying community-based learning needs.
- Education and learning are different. Education is the establishment and arrangement of events to facilitate learning.

- Learning is the process of gaining knowledge and expertise and results in behavioral changes.
- Three domains of learning are cognitive, affective, and psychomotor. Depending on the needs of the learner, one or more of these domains may be important for the nurse educator to consider as learning programs are developed.
- Nine principles associated with community health education are gaining attention, informing the learner of the objectives of instruction, stimulating recall of prior learning, presenting the stimulus, providing learning guidance, eliciting

performance, providing feedback, assessing performance, and enhancing retention and transfer of knowledge.

- Often, theory can guide the development of health education programs. Two useful ones are the Health Belief Model and the Transtheoretical Model, which are discussed in connection with the Precaution Adoption Process Model.
- Principles that guide the effective educator include message, format, environment, experience, participation, and evaluation.
- Educational issues include population considerations, barriers to learning, and technological issues.
- Two important learner-related barriers are low literacy level, especially health literacy, and lack of motivation to learn information and make the needed changes.
- The five phases of the educational process are identifying educational needs, establishing educational goals and objectives, selecting appropriate educational methods, implementing the educational plan, and evaluating the educational process and product.
- Evaluation of the product includes the measurement of short-term and long-term goals and objectives related to improving health and promoting behavioral changes.
- Working with groups is an important skill for nurses. Groups are an effective and powerful vehicle for initiating and implementing healthful changes.
- A group is a collection of interacting individuals with a common purpose. Each member influences and is influenced by other group members to varying degrees.

- Group cohesion is enhanced by commonly shared characteristics among members and diminished by differences among members.
- Cohesion is the measure of attraction between members and the group. Cohesion or the lack of it affects the group's function.
- Norms are standards that guide and regulate individuals and communities. These norms are unwritten and often unspoken and serve to ensure group movement to a goal, to maintain the group, and to influence group members' perceptions and interpretations of reality.
- Some diversity of member backgrounds is usually a positive influence on a group.
- Leadership is an important and complex group concept. Leadership is described as patriarchal, paternal, or democratic.
- Group structure emerges from various member influences, including members' understanding and support of the group purpose.
- Conflicts in groups may develop from competition for roles or member disagreement about the roles ascribed to them.
- Health behavior is greatly influenced by the groups to which people belong and for which they value membership.
- An understanding of group concepts provides a basis for identifying community groups and their goals, characteristics, and norms. Nurses use their understanding of group principles to work with community groups toward needed health changes.

EVOLVE WEBSITE

http://evolve.elsevier.com/Stanhope/foundations
- Case Study, with Questions and Answers
- NCLEX® Review Questions
- Practice Application Answers

REFERENCES

American Nurses Association: *Scope & standards of practice: public health nursing*, Silver Springs, Md, 2007, ANA.
Bastable SB: *Nurse as educator*, ed 3, Boston, 2008, Jones and Bartlett.
Bloom BS, Englehart MO, Furst EJ, et al: *Taxonomy of educational objectives: the classification of educational goals—handbook. I. cognitive domain*, White Plains, NY, 1956, Longman.
Caplin M, Saunders T: Utilizing teach-back to reinforce patient education: A step-by-step approach, *Orthopaedic Nursing* 34(6):365–368, 2015.
Centers for Disease Control and Prevention: *How to plan a health fair*, Atlanta, 2013, CDC. Retrieved January 2016 from http://www.cdc.gov/women/fair/index.htm.
Centers for Disease Control and Prevention: *Tools for cross-cultural communication and language access can help organizations address health literacy and improve communication effectiveness*, Atlanta, 2015, Centers for Disease Control and Prevention. Retrieved January 2016 from http://www.cdc.gov/healthliteracy/culture.html.
Centers for Disease Control and Prevention: *Health literacy*, Atlanta, n.d. Retrieved January 2016 from http://www.cdc.gov/healthliteracy/pdf/checklist.pdf.
Clancy R, Taylor A: Engaging clinicians in motivational interviewing: Comparing online with face-to-face post-training consolidation,

International journal of mental health nursing 25(1):51–61, February 2016.
Council on Linkages between Academia and Public Health Practice: *Core competencies for public health professionals*, Washington, DC, 2010, Public Health Foundation. Retrieved February 2016 from http://www.phf.org.
Cronenwett L, Sherwood G, Barnsteiner J, et al: Quality and safety education for nurses, *Nurs Outlook* 55:122–131, 2007.
Dauz E, Moore J, Smith CE, et al: Installing computers in older adults' homes and teaching them to access a patient education web site: a systematic approach, *Comput Inform Nurs* 22:266–272, 2004.
Dembo MH: *Applying educational psychology*, ed 5, White Plains, NY, 1994, Longman.
Edberg M: *Essentials of health behavior: Social and behavioral theory in public health*, ed 2, Burlington, MA, 2015, Jones and Bartlett.
French KS: Transforming nursing care though health literacy ACTS, *Nurs Clin N Am* 50:87–98 2015.
Gerow SJ: Teachers in school-based teams: contesting isolation in schools. In Sockett HT, DeMulder EK, DePage PC, et al, editors: *Transforming teacher education: lessons in professional development*, Westport, Conn, 2001, Bergin & Garvey.
Hansen M, Fisher J: Patient-centered teaching from theory to practice, *Am J Nurs* 98:56–60. 1998.
Health Literacy Innovations: Focus on readability and readability indices, *Health Literacy Innovations Newslett* 1:1–9, 2010.
Health Resources and Services Administration: *Health literacy*, n.d. Retrieved February 2016 from http://www.hrsa.gov/publichealth/healthliteracy/.
Kleinbeck C: Reaching positive diabetes outcomes for patients with low literacy, *Home Healthcare Nurse* 23:16–22, 2005.

Knowles MS, Holton EF III, Swanson RA: *The adult learner: the definitive classic in adult education and human resource development*, ed 8, New York, 2015, Routledge.

Kutner M, Greenberg E, Jin Y, Paulsen C: *The health literacy of America's adults: results from the 2003 National Assessment of Adult Literacy*. NCES 2006-483, Washington, DC, 2006, US Department of Education, Center for Education. Retrieved March 2010 from http://www.edpubs.org.

Miller WR, Rose GS: Toward a theory of motivational interviewing, *Am Psychol* 64:527–537, 2009.

Minkin A, Snider-Meyer J, Olson D, Gresser S, Smith H, Kier FJ: Effectiveness of a motivational interviewing intervention on medication compliance, *Home Healthcare Nurse* 32(8):490–496, 2014.

Ota C, DiCarlo C, Burts D, et al: Training and the needs of adult learners, *J Extension* 44(6):2006. Retrieved from http://www.joe.org/joe/2006december/tt5.shtml.

Perrin A, Duggan M: *American's internet access: 2000-2015*, Philadelphia, June 2015, Pew Research Center.

Ratzan SC, Parker RM: Introduction. In Selden CR, Zorn M, Ratzan SC, et al, editors: *National Library of Medicine current bibliographies in medicine: health literacy, NLM Pub No. CBM 2000-1*, Bethesda, MD, 2000, National Institutes of Health, US Department of Health and Human Services.

Rice CS, Pollard JM: *Health fair planning guide, AgriLIFE EXTENSION*, ed 2, College Station, TX, 2011, Texas A&M System. Retrieved February 2016 from http://fcs.tamu.edu/health/hfpg/Health-Fair-Planning-Guide-with-Appendix.pdf.

Roberts K: Simplify, simplify: tackling health literacy by addressing reading literacy, *Am J Nurs* 104:118–119, 2004.

Saad L: *American's faith in honesty, ethics of police rebounds*, December 21, 2015, Gallup. Retrieved February 2016 Source: Gallup http://www.gallup.com/poll/187874/americans-faith-honesty-ethics-police-rebounds.aspx.

Swider SM, Krothe J, Reyes D, Cravertz M: The quad council practice competencies for public health nursing, *Public health nursing* 30(6):519–536, 2013.

Treasure J: *Motivational interviewing* (vol 10), Bedfordshire, UK, 2004, Advances in psychiatric treatment. Retrieved February 2016 from http://apt.rcpsych.org/.

US Department of Health and Human Services: *Healthy People 2020*, Washington, DC, 2010, DHHS. Retrieved February 2016 from http://www.healthypeople.gov/2020/default.aspx.

US Department of Health and Human Services, Office of Disease Prevention and Health Promotion: *National action plan to improve health literacy*, Washington, DC, 2010, Author.

VanBiervliet A, Edwards-Schafer P: Consumer health information on the web: trends, issues, and strategies, *Dermatol Nurs* 16:519–523, 2004.

Welsh P: Strategies in development of an mHealth technology for low socioeconomic groups in free healthcare clinics, *CIN: Computers, Informatics, Nursing* 34(1):3–5, January 2016.

CHAPTER 12

Community Assessment and Evaluation

Mary Gibson, Esther Thatcher, George F. Shuster

OBJECTIVES

After reading this chapter, the student should be able to:

1. Decide whether nursing practice is community oriented.
2. Understand selected concepts basic to community-oriented nursing practice: community, community client, community health, and partnership for health.
3. Compare the nursing process to community-oriented nursing practice.
4. Decide which methods of assessment, intervention, and evaluation are most appropriate in selected situations.
5. Develop a community-oriented nursing care plan.

CHAPTER OUTLINE

What Is a Community?
Community as Client
  The Community as Client and Partner in Nursing
    Practice
Goals and Means of Community-Oriented Practice
  Community Health
  Healthy People 2020
  Community Partnerships
  Strategies to Improve Community Health

Community-Focused Nursing Process: An Overview
  of the Process from Assessment to Evaluation
  Assessing Community Health
  Assessment Issues
  Identifying Community Problems
  Planning for Community Health
  Implementation in the Community
  Evaluating the Intervention for Community Health
Personal Safety in Community Practice

KEY TERMS

aggregate, 205
change agent, 216
change partner, 216
community, 205
community assessment, 204
community competence, 208
community health, 208
community health problems, 212
community health strengths, 212
community-oriented practice, 207
community partnership, 209
confidentiality, 214

database, 214
data collection, 211
data gathering, 212
data generation, 212
evaluation, 217
goals, 215
implementation, 216
informant interviews, 212
interdependent, 205
intervention activities, 216
objectives, 215
participant observation, 212

partnership, 209
population-centered practice,
  206
problem analysis, 215
problem prioritizing, 215
secondary analysis, 213
setting for practice, 205
surveys, 213
target of practice, 205
windshield survey, 211

In the past, nurses have viewed the community as a client and as a partner in improving the health status of its citizens. Since the days of Florence Nightingale and Lillian Wald, nurses have looked at what is going on in the communities and environments in which they found their clients. Florence Nightingale defined her community as war-torn Crimea and discovered that the lack of fresh air, sanitation, and hygiene was contributing to the illnesses of the soldiers. Lillian Wald found that the neighborhoods around the Henry Street Settlement were impoverished, with poor housing conditions and sanitation, improper nutrition, and crowding contributing to the problems of new mothers and children. Both women became political activists, worked with the leaders in their communities, and even solicited help from their respective governments to help change the conditions for the individuals and families in their communities.

Although in the past nurses have sometimes viewed the community as a client, many community-oriented nurses have come to consider the community their most important client and, more recently, their partner (Anderson and McFarlane, 2015; Caldwell et al, 2015). This chapter clarifies community concepts and provides a guideline for nursing practice with the community client. The core functions of public health nursing (PHN) include assessment, policy development, and assurance. A public and private group partnership, the Council on Linkages between Academia and Public Health Practice (2014), defined competencies for the core functions of public health practice (see Chapter 1 for more details). In the area of assessment, 11 competencies for the nurse and other health providers working in the community are listed (Box 12.1).

The nursing process from assessment through evaluation is used to promote community health. This process begins with community assessment, one of the core functions, which involves getting to know the community. It is a logical, systematic approach to identifying community needs, clarifying problems, and identifying community strengths and resources. This chapter provides the nurse with the knowledge necessary to develop the community assessment core competencies. Nurses in community health are interested in these concepts because they want to know how the community's health affects their individual, family, and group clients.

WHAT IS A COMMUNITY?

The concept of *community* varies widely. The World Health Organization (WHO) includes this definition:

> *A group of people, often living in a defined geographical area, who may share a common culture, values and norms, and are arranged in a social structure according to relationships which the community has developed over a period of time. Members of a community gain their personal and social identity by sharing common beliefs, values and norms which have been developed by the community in the past and may be modified in the future.*

This definition is similar to the one used by the Public Health Accreditation Board (2013, p. 8)

> *"Community is a group of people who have common characteristics; communities can be defined by location, race, ethnicity, age, occupation, interest in particular problems or outcomes, or other similar common bonds. Ideally, there would be available assets and resources, as well as collective discussion, decision-making, and action.*

(WHO, 2004, p 16)

The most frequently used single definition of community is "community of place" or geographic boundaries. With agency interactions (e.g., among schools, social services, and governmental agencies) extending the ability to solve problems, nurses working in communities quickly learn that society consists of many different kinds of communities. Neighborhood and face-to-face communities are two examples. Some other types of communities are listed in Box 12.2.

Other communities, such as communities of special interest or resource communities, are spread out across widely scattered geographic areas. They are brought together by long-term or short-term common concerns and interests. An example of another type of community is a community of problem ecology, which is created when environmental problems affect a widespread area. For instance, a problem such as water pollution can bring people together from areas that would not normally share a common interest. Nurses also may work in partnership with

---

BOX 12.1 Core Competencies for Public Health Professionals

Public health professionals should be able to do the following:
- Define a problem.
- Determine appropriate uses and limitations of both quantitative and qualitative data.
- Select and define variables relevant to the defined public health problems.
- Identify relevant and appropriate data and information sources.
- Evaluate the integrity and comparability of data, and identify gaps in data sources.
- Apply ethical principles to the collection, maintenance, use, and dissemination of data and information.
- Partner with communities to attach meaning to collected quantitative and qualitative data.
- Make relevant inferences from quantitative and qualitative data.
- Obtain and interpret information regarding risks and benefits to the community.
- Apply data collection processes, information technology applications, and computer systems storage and retrieval strategies.
- Recognize how the data illuminate ethical, political, scientific, economic, and overall public health issues

From Council on Linkages between Academia and Public Health Practice: *Core competencies for public health professionals*, Washington, DC, 2014, The Council. Retrieved July 2016 from phf.org/corecompetencies.

BOX 12.2 Types of Communities

- Face-to-face community
- Neighborhood community
- Community of identifiable need
- Community of problem ecology
- Community of concern
- Community of special interest
- Community of viability
- Community of action capability
- Community of political jurisdiction
- Resource community
- Community of solution

From Blum HL: *Planning for health*, New York, 1974, Human Sciences Press.

political communities, such as school districts, townships, or counties. Because the nature of each type of community varies, nurses planning interventions with communities must take into account the characteristics of that specific community. Each community is unique, and its defining characteristics will affect the nature of the partnership.

In most definitions, the concept of community includes three dimensions—*people, place,* and *function*—as follows:
1. The *people* are the community residents.
2. *Place* refers both to geographic and time dimensions.
3. *Function* refers to the aims and activities of the community.

Nurses in community health practice regularly need to examine how the personal, geographic, and functional dimensions of community shape their nursing practice with individuals, families, and groups. They can use both a conceptual definition and a set of indicators for the concept of *community* in their practice.

In this chapter, the following conceptual definition is used: community is a locality-based entity composed of systems of formal organizations reflecting society's institutions, informal groups, and aggregates. As defined in Chapter 1, an aggregate is a collection of individuals who have in common one or more personal or environmental characteristics. The components of community are interdependent, and their function is to meet a wide variety of collective needs. This definition of community includes personal, geographic, and functional dimensions and recognizes interaction among the systems within a community. Indicators of the dimensions of this definition are listed in Table 12.1.

The next section describes the community as client and partner of the nurse. The community is first the setting for practice for the nurse practicing health promotion and disease prevention interventions with individuals, families, and groups. Second, the community is the target of practice for the public health nurse whose practice is focused on the broader community rather than on individuals.

HOW TO Identify Community Systems

The following is a list of system categories found within a community:
1. Politics and government
2. Safety and transportation
3. Education
4. Physical environment
5. Recreation
6. Economics
7. Communication
8. Health and social services
9. Religion and beliefs

TABLE 12.1 Concepts of Community Specified

Dimensions	Measures	Examples of Data Sources
Place	Geopolitical boundaries	Maps
	Local or folk name for area	Local newspaper
	Size in square miles, acres, blocks, or census tracts	Census data
	Transportation avenues, such as rivers, highways, railroads, and sidewalks	Chamber of commerce, city, county, or township government
	History	Library archives and local histories
	Physical environment, such as land use patterns and condition of housing	Local housing office
People or person	Population: number and density	Census data
	Demographic structure of population, such as age, sex, socioeconomic factors, and racial distributions; rural and urban character, and dependency ratio	Census data
	Informal groups, such as block clubs, service clubs, and friendship networks	Churches, senior centers
		Civic groups
		Local newspaper
	Formal groups such as schools, churches, businesses, industries, governmental bodies, unions, and health and welfare agencies	Telephone directory
		United Way
		Social service agencies
		Chamber of commerce
		Local or state officials
	Linking structures (intercommunity and intracommunity contacts among organizations)	Tourist bureau
		Chamber of commerce
Function	Production, distribution, and consumption of goods and services	State departments
		Business and labor
		Local library
	Socialization of new members	Social and local research reports
	Maintenance of social control	Police station
	Adaptation to ongoing and expected change	Social and local research reports
	Provision of mutual aid	United Way
		Welfare agencies
		Churches and religious organizations

COMMUNITY AS CLIENT

Nurses who have a community orientation are often considered unique because of their target of practice. The idea of health-related care being provided within the community is not new. At the turn of the century, most persons stayed at home during illnesses. As a result, the practice environment for nurses was the home rather than the hospital.

As the range of community nursing services expanded, many different kinds of agencies were started and their services often overlapped. For instance, both privately established voluntary agencies and official local health agencies worked to control tuberculosis. The nurses employed by these agencies were called *community health nurses, public health nurses,* or *visiting nurses.* Nurses practiced in clients' homes, not in the hospital.

Early PHN textbooks in the 1940s included lengthy descriptions of the home environment and tools for assessing the extent to which that environment promoted the health of family members. Health education about the domestic environment was often a major part of home nursing care.

By the 1950s, schools, prisons, industries, and neighborhood health centers, as well as homes, had all become areas of practice for nurses in the community. Many of the new nurses in the community did not consider the environments in which they practiced. Although their practices took place within the community, they focused on the individual client or family seeking care. The care provided was not population centered; rather, it was oriented toward the individual or family who lived in the community, and this is now called community-*based* nursing practice. This commitment to direct, hands-on, clinical nursing care delivered to individuals or families in community settings remains a more popular approach to nursing practice than recognizing the whole community as the target of nursing practice. This remains true today. However, the American Public Health Association: Public Health Nursing Section (APHA: PHN, 2013) statement indicates that "Public health nursing activities comprise the domains depicted by the Public Health Intervention Wheel (see Appendix C.4) and the 10 Essential Public Health Services (see Chapter 1). These activities include community collaboration, health teaching, and policy development, in response to priorities derived from ongoing, comprehensive population-focused assessment. Public health nurses are members and leaders of interprofessional teams in diverse settings and in many different types of agencies and organizations, including all levels of government, community-based and other nongovernmental service organizations, foundations, policy think tanks, academic institutions, and other research settings. Increasing numbers of public health nurses work in global health in an effort to promote global responsibility and connectivity. Public health nurses that work with individuals and families do so within the context of a population focus—applying a systems perspective to factors that impact health." When the *location of practice* is the community and the *focus of practice* is the individual or family, the client remains the individual or family, and the nurse is practicing in the community as the setting; this is an example of community-based nursing practice.

The community is the client only when the nursing focus is on the collective or common good of the population instead of on individual health. Population-centered practice seeks healthful change for the whole community's benefit (Nash et al, 2016). Although the nurse may work with individuals, families or other interacting groups, aggregates, institutions, communities, or within a population, the resulting changes are intended to affect the whole community. For example, an occupational health nurse's target might be preventing illness and injury for the individual worker. This would result in maintaining or promoting the health of an entire company workforce. Because of this focus, the nurse would help an individual disabled worker become independent in activities of daily living. The nurse would also become involved with promoting vocational rehabilitation services in the community and seek reasonable employment policies for all disabled workers through the community government.

THE COMMUNITY AS CLIENT AND PARTNER IN NURSING PRACTICE

Population-focused health care is experiencing a rebirth, and the community as client is important to nursing practice for several reasons. When focusing on the community as client, direct clinical care can be a part of population-focused community health practice (Sidorov and Romney, 2016). For example, sometimes direct nursing care is provided to individuals and family members because their health needs are common community-related problems. Changes in their health will affect the health of their communities (Lathrop and Hodnicki, 2014).

In such cases, decisions are made at the individual level because the individual's health is related to the health of the population as a whole and because the individual has an effect on the community's health. Improved health of the community remains the overall goal of nursing intervention. Interventions to stop spouse abuse and elder abuse are two examples of nursing interventions done primarily because of the effects of abuse on society and therefore on the population as a whole. Also, the treatment of a client for tuberculosis reduces the risk to other community members. This care reduces the risk for an epidemic in the community.

The community client also highlights the complexity of the change process. Change for the benefit of the community client often must occur at several levels, ranging from the individual to society as a whole. For example, health problems caused by lifestyle, such as smoking, overeating, and speeding, cannot be solved simply by asking individuals to choose health-promoting habits. Society must also provide healthy choices. Most individuals cannot change their habits alone; they require the support of family members, friends, community health care systems, and relevant social policies. Individuals who have lifestyle health problems are often blamed for their illness because of their choices (e.g., to smoke). In his classic work, Ryan (1976) points out that the "victim" cannot always be blamed and expected to correct the problem without changes also being made at the same time in the helping professions and in public policy. Some communities have no-smoking areas in restaurants to prevent secondhand smoke from harming others. This is an example of a community-level policy to change behavior.

Commitment to the health of the community client requires a process of change at each of these levels. One nursing role emphasizes individual and direct personal care skills, another nursing role focuses on the family as the unit of service, and a third focuses on the community as a unit of service. Collaborative practice models involving the community and nurses in joint decision making and specific nursing roles are required (Green, 2015; Pilon et al, 2015). Korazim-Kőrösy et al (2014 note that nurses must remember that collaboration means shared roles and a cooperative effort in which participants want to work together. These participants must see themselves as part of a group effort and share in the process, beginning with planning and including decision making. This means sharing not only the power but also the responsibility for the outcomes of the intervention.

Viewing the community as client and thus as the target of service means embracing two key concepts: (1) community health and (2) partnership for community health. These two concepts form not only the goal (community health) but also the means of population-centered practice (partnership).

GOALS AND MEANS OF COMMUNITY-ORIENTED PRACTICE

In community-oriented practice, the nurse and community seek healthful change together (Mpofu, 2015). Their common goal of community health involves an ongoing series of health-promoting changes rather than a fixed state. The most effective means of completing healthy changes in the community is through this same partnership.

COMMUNITY HEALTH

Like the concept of community, *community health* has three common characteristics or dimensions: status, structure, and process. Each dimension reflects a unique aspect of community health (Cottrell, 1976).

Status

Community health in terms of status or outcome is the most well-known and accepted approach; it involves biological, emotional, and social parts. The *biological* (or physical) part of community health is often measured by traditional morbidity and mortality rates, life expectancy indices, and risk factor profiles. *Morbidity and Mortality Weekly Report* (Consensus set of health status indicators, 1991) published the work of a consensus committee involving representatives from a number of community health-related organizations. This committee identified by consensus 18 community health status indicators, presented in Box 12.3. More recently, the Centers for Disease Control and Prevention (CDC), in partnership with some public health organizations, has relaunched the Community Health Status Indicators (CHSI) project to provide an overview of key health indicators for local communities, such as those identified by the *Morbidity and Mortality Weekly Report* (Consensus set of health status indicators, 1991). Health status indicator data on thousands of communities can be found at http://wwwn.cdc.gov/CommunityHealth/.

The *emotional component* of health status can be measured by consumer satisfaction and mental health indexes. Crime rates and functional levels reflect the *social part* of community health. Other status measures, such as worker absenteeism and infant mortality rates, reflect the effects of all three parts.

BOX 12.3 Consensus Set of Indicators* for Assessing Community Health Status

Indicators of Health Status Outcome
1. Race-specific and ethnicity-specific infant mortality, as measured by the rate (per 1000 live births) of deaths among infants less than 1 year of age

Death Rates (per 100,000 Population)† for:
2. Motor vehicle crashes
3. Work-related injury
4. Suicide
5. Lung cancer
6. Breast cancer
7. Cardiovascular disease
8. Homicide
9. All causes

Reported Incidence (per 100,000 Population) of:
10. Acquired immunodeficiency syndrome (AIDS)
11. Measles
12. Tuberculosis
13. Primary and secondary syphilis

Indicators of Risk Factors
14. Incidence of low birth weight, as measured by percentage of total number of live-born infants weighing less than 2500 g at birth
15. Births to adolescents (females 10–17 years of age) as a percentage of total live births
16. Prenatal care, as measured by percentage of mothers delivering live infants who did not receive prenatal care during the first trimester
17. Childhood poverty, as measured by the proportion of children younger than 15 years of age living in families at or below the poverty level
18. Proportion of persons living in counties exceeding US Environmental Protection Agency standards for air quality during the previous year

From Consensus set of health status indicators for the general assessment of community health status: United States, *MMWR Morb Mortal Wkly Rep* 40:449-451, 1991 (updated August 2001).
*Position or number of the indicator does not imply priority.
†Age adjusted to the 1940 standard population.

Structure

Community health, when viewed from the structure of the community, is usually defined in terms of *services* and *resources*. Measures of community health services and resources include service use patterns, treatment data from various health agencies, and provider-to-client ratios. These data provide information, such as the number of available hospital beds or the number of emergency room visits to a particular hospital. The problems that can be found when structure measures are used are serious. For example, problems related to access to care and quality of care are well known through stories reported in local newspapers. Less well known, but of equal concern, is the false thought that simply *providing* health care improves health. Such problems require cautious use of health services and resources as measures of community health.

A structural viewpoint also defines the characteristics of the community structure itself. Characteristics of the community structure are commonly identified as social measures, or correlates, of health. Measures of community structure include demographics, such as socioeconomic and racial distributions, age, and educational level. Their relationships to health status have been thoroughly documented. For example, studies have repeatedly shown that health status decreases with age and improves with higher socioeconomic levels (Agency for Healthcare Research and Quality, 2015).

Process

The view of community health as the process of effective community functioning or problem solving is well established. However, it is especially appropriate to nursing because it directs the study of community health to promote effective community action for health promotion.

Community competence, defined originally in a classic work by Cottrell (1976), provides a basic understanding of the process dimension of community health. Community competence is a process whereby the parts of a community—organizations, groups, and aggregates—"are able to collaborate effectively in identifying the problems and needs of the community; can achieve a working consensus on goals and priorities; can agree on ways and means to implement the agreed-on goals; and can collaborate effectively in the required actions" (Cottrell, 1976, p 197).

Ruderman (2000) further expanded on Cottrell's definition by indicating that community competence indicates the capacity of a community to implement change by assessing the need or the demand for change. Once change is indicated, then the community must define and make available the resources for the change to occur.

The term community health, as used in this chapter, is the meeting of collective needs by identifying problems and managing interactions within the community itself and between the community and the larger society. This definition emphasizes the process dimension but also includes the dimensions of status and structure. Measures for all three dimensions are listed in Table 12.2.

The use of status, structure, and process dimensions to define community health, as shown in Table 12.2, is an effort to develop a broad definition of community health, involving indicators that often are not included when discussions focus only on individual and family risk factors as the basis for community health.

Consideration of health risks guides us to think upstream—to identify risks that could be prevented to make and keep people healthy. Most community-oriented and population-oriented approaches to health are grounded in the notion that the earlier in the causal process (or the more upstream) interventions occur, the greater the likelihood of improved health. Frequently, prevention or upstream action requires community-wide intervention

TABLE 12.2 Concept of Community Health Specified

Dimensions	Measures	Examples of Data Sources
Status	Vital statistics (live births, neonatal deaths, infant deaths, maternal deaths)	Census data
		State health department annual vital statistics
	Incidence and prevalence of leading causes of mortality and morbidity	Census data
		State health department
	Health risk profiles of selected aggregates	Local health department
		Support groups
		Local nonprofit organizations
	Functional ability levels	Census data
		US Department of Labor
Structure	Health facilities such as hospitals, nursing homes, industrial and school health services, health departments, voluntary health associations, categorical grant programs, and prepaid health plans	Local chamber of commerce
		United Way
	Health-related planning groups	Local newspapers
		Local magazines
		Local government
	Health manpower, such as physicians, dentists, nurses, environmental sanitarians, social workers	Telephone directory
		State and local labor statistics
		Professional licensing boards
	Health resource use patterns, such as bed occupancy days and client and provider visits	Medicare and Medicaid databases (federal and state government)
		Annual reports from hospitals, health maintenance organizations (HMOs), nonprofit agencies
Process	Commitment to community health	Local government
		Real estate agencies (e.g., turnover and vacancy rates)
	Awareness of self and others and clarity of situational definitions	Local history
		Neighborhood help organizations
	Effective communication	Local/neighborhood newspapers and radio programs
		Local government
	Conflict containment and accommodation	Social services department
	Participation	Existence of and participation in local organizations
	Management of relationships with society	Windshield survey—observation of interactions
	Machinery for facilitating participant interaction and decision making	Notices for community organizations and meetings in public places (e.g., supermarkets, newspapers, radio)

directed toward social, economic, and environmental conditions that correlate with low health status (Braveman and Gottlieb, 2014).

HEALTHY PEOPLE 2020

One important guideline available for nurses working to improve the health of the community is *Healthy People 2020,* a 2010 publication from the US Department of Health and Human Services (USDHHS). It offers a vision of the future for public health and specific objectives to help attain that vision. The *Healthy People 2020* vision recognizes the need to work collectively, in community partnerships, to bring about the changes that will be necessary to fulfill this vision. *Healthy People 2020* provides the foundation for a national health promotion and disease prevention strategy built on four goals:

1. Attain high-quality, longer lives free of preventable disease, disability, injury, and premature death.
2. Achieve health equity, eliminate disparities, and improve the health of all groups.
3. Create social and physical environments that promote good health for all.
4. Promote quality of life, healthy development, and healthy behaviors across all life stages.

In Section IV of the Advisory Committee Findings and Recommendations for the Role and Function of *Healthy People 2020,* there is a direct discussion about the relationship between individuals and their communities. It states,

> The Advisory Committee believes Healthy People 2020 can best be described as a national health agenda that communicates a vision and a strategy for the nation. Healthy People 2020 should provide overarching, national-level goals. On a practical level, it is a road map showing where we want to go as a nation and how we are going to get there.

COMMUNITY PARTNERSHIPS

The executive summary written by the advisory committee for *Healthy People 2020* identifies a model for action that will require community partnership as key to meeting program goals. **Community partnership** is necessary because when there is community partnership, lay community members have a vested interest in the success of efforts to improve the health of their community. Lay community members who are recognized as community leaders also possess credibility and skills that health professionals often lack. Therefore successful strategies for improving the community's health must include community partnership as the basic means, or key, for improvement (Adams and Canclini, 2008). Community partnership is a basic focus of such population-centered approaches as Mobilizing for Action through Planning and Partnerships (MAPP) (National Association of Community and City Health Officials [NACCHO], 2016).

Most changes must aim at improving community health through active partnerships between community residents and health workers from a variety of disciplines. Unfortunately, community residents are often viewed only as sources of information and receivers of interventions. This form of partnership is called *passive participation.* Passive participation is the opposite of the partnership approach in which all are involved in assessing, planning, and implementing needed community changes (Korazim-Kőrösy et al, 2014).

The community member–professional partnership approach specifically emphasizes active participation. Power is shared among lay and professional persons throughout the assessment, planning, implementation, and evaluation processes. **Partnership** means the active participation and involvement of the community or its representatives in bringing about healthful change (O'Donnell, 2009). For example, breast cancer is an issue for rural Native American women, and an active community partnership involving the Native American women helped develop and ensure an effective, ongoing program (Espey et al, 2014).

Partnership, as defined here, is a concept that is as essential for nurses to know and use as are the concepts of community, community as client, and community health. Experienced nurses know that partnership is important because health is not a static reality. Rather, it is continuously generated through new and increasingly effective means of community member–professional collaboration. However, such changes also require other active professional service providers, such as school teachers, public safety officers, and agricultural extension agents. Partnership in identifying problems and setting goals is especially important because it brings commitment from all persons involved, which is essential to successful change (Archer, Cary, and Malone, 2014).

A growing body of literature supports the significance and effectiveness of partnership in improving community health. Studies document the use of partnership models for a wide range of outcomes such as improving access to quality, low-cost snacks in after-school programs, reducing vehicle idling near public schools, improving breast and cervical cancer screening, and increasing flu vaccination rates of homeless populations (Beets et al, 2014; Eghbalnia et al, 2013; Espey et al, 2014; Metcalfe and Sexton, 2014). The roles of these partners in health have included listening sympathetically, offering advice, making referrals, and starting programs among a wide range of communities. These include working with vulnerable populations, such as American Indian and Alaska Native women, Hispanic/Latino men who have sex with men (MSM), and rural Hispanic migrant farm workers (Espey et al, 2014; Rhodes et al, 2015; Sánchez et al, 2012). They include partnerships with older adults in retirement communities, as well as smaller, more rural communities (Pinto, Waldemore, and Rosen, 2015; Perry et al, 2015). There are also examples of community partnerships for at-risk students at the grade school or middle school level, for building community capacity for advocating for policy change, and for disaster planning (Cheezum et al, 2013; Duff and Poole, 2016; Santibañez et al, 2015). Upvall and Leffers (2014) advocate using partnership models in global health nursing, provided certain ethical challenges and issues are addressed such as power imbalances between those receiving assistance and those providing it. In international health, partnership models generally are viewed as empowering people, through their lay leaders, to control their own health destinies and lives. In the United States, partnership models have often involved informal community leaders, organizations such as churches, and communities.

Partnerships involving nurses working with community organizations offer one of the most effective means for interventions because they actively involve the community and build on existing community strengths. Nurses working with community groups and organizations fulfill many different roles. These roles include media advocacy, political action, "grass roots health communication and social marketing," and outreach facilitation to get more community members involved, for example, in a school health fair. Regardless of what roles nurses fulfill as their contribution to the partnership, they must remember to "start where the people are" (Minkler, 2012).

 HEALTHY PEOPLE 2020

Community Consortium and Partners

Healthy People provides science-based, 10-year national objectives for improving the health of all Americans. For three decades, *Healthy People* has established benchmarks and monitored progress over time in order to do the following:

Encourage collaborations across sectors.

Guide individuals toward making informed health decisions.

Measure the impact of prevention activities.

For the implementation of *Healthy People 2020,* the development of a consortium is occurring. The consortium is a diverse, motivated group of agencies and organizations committed to achieving *Healthy People 2020* goals and objectives. Any agency or organization that supports *Healthy People 2020* is a welcome partner. Examples of partners include the following:

Health care providers

State and local public health professionals

Educators

Community members

Businesses

Environmental health professionals

Housing professionals

From USDHHS: *Healthy People 2020: a roadmap for health,* Washington, DC, 2010, US Government Printing Office.

EVIDENCE-BASED PRACTICE

The landmark Institute of Medicine 1988 report, *The Future of Public Health,* recommended all public health agencies to regularly and systematically collect and analyze information on the health of the community. Theoretically, such data would provide a logical order for public health practice decision-making and actions; however, implementation barriers, such as low capacity, lack of funds and infrastructure, and constrained resources, are well documented. Researchers Rabarison, Timsina, and Mays (2015) conducted a study investigating the connection between assessment and planning and its impact on decision making related to program activities. Rabarison et al (2015) analyzed the likelihood of chronic disease prevention activities delivery if the local health agencies (LHAs) implemented a community health assessment and improvement plan in their communities. The researchers linked data from the 2010 National Association of County and City Health Officials profile of LHAs and the 2010 County Health Rankings to create a statistically matched sample of implementation LHAs (those with a community health assessment and improvement plan) and comparison LHAs (those without an assessment and plan). Results indicated that implementation LHAs were twice as likely to deliver population-based chronic disease prevention programs than the comparison LHAs.

Nurse Use

Routine implementation of a community health assessment and improvement plan leads to improved public health decision-making and actions. The nurse may be involved in all steps of the assessment, from data collection to data analysis to planning and implementing interventions to strengthen the community.

STRATEGIES TO IMPROVE COMMUNITY HEALTH

Healthy People 2020 has stimulated joint efforts to develop strategies for achieving its goals. These efforts have involved such organizations as the CDC, the American Public Health Association (APHA), the Association of State and Territorial Health Officials (ASTHO), and the NACCHO. The results of these efforts are publications and guidelines that provide detailed strategies for achieving the objectives in the Assessment Protocol for Excellence in Public Health (APEXPH), the Planned Approach to Community Health (PATCH), and, more recently, MAPP. Each of these approaches offers step-by-step guidelines for community planning and interventions (see Chapter 16). Most recently, the CDC's Healthy Communities Program has developed the Community Health Assessment and Group Evaluation (CHANGE) Tool, which is designed to help assess for community change and establishing community priorities. It is available for free at http://www.cdc.gov/nccdphp/dch/programs/healthycommunitiesprogram/tools/change.htm.

In addition to these approaches, there have been efforts to apply the evidence-based practice approach to community-level interventions. The *Community Guide* provides recommendations for population-based interventions to promote health and to prevent disease, injury, disability, and premature death, and it is appropriate for use by communities and health care systems. The initial *Community Guide* was a result of the work of the Task Force on Community Preventive Services (2016a), which has been updated and continues to systematically review published scientific studies, weigh the evidence, and determine the effectiveness of interventions in a particular area. For instance, in regard to physical activity promotion, the Task Force recommends community-wide campaigns, individually adapted health behavior change programs, school-based physical education, social support interventions in community contexts, and creating or improving access to places for physical activity combined with informational outreach (Task Force on Community Prevention Services, 2016b). The work of this Task Force is ongoing, and updates as well as publications on a wide range of public health areas can be found at http://www.thecommunityguide.org/index.html.

The National Center for Chronic Disease Prevention and Health Promotion website (2017) includes links to CDC-supported public health programs that have been found to be effective. Links to guides and kits for the programs also can be found. Examples include the following:

- Well-Integrated Screening and Evaluation for Women Across the Nation—WISEWOMAN (lifestyle intervention programs addressing cardiovascular and other chronic disease risk factors)
- Kids in Parks (activity)
- Trailnets Healthy, Active, and Vibrant communities (activity)
- Eat Well Play Hard in child care settings (healthy eating and activity)

Several different population-centered health promotion approaches have been noted here. Regardless of what approach is taken, specific strategies to improve community health often depend on whether the status, structure, or process dimension of community health is being emphasized. If the emphasis is on the status dimension, the best strategy is usually at the level of primary or secondary prevention because the objective is either to prevent a disease or to treat it in its early stages. Immunization programs are an example of a nursing intervention at the primary prevention level.

Nursing intervention strategies focused on the structural dimension are directed to either health services or demographic characteristics. Interventions aimed at altering health services might include program planning. Interventions aimed at affecting demographic characteristics might include community development.

When the emphasis is on the process dimension, the best strategy is usually health promotion, which is also a primary prevention strategy. For example, if family-life education is lacking in a community because of ineffective communication among families, children, school board members, religious leaders, and health professionals, the most effective strategy may be to open discussion among these groups and help community members develop education programs.

COMMUNITY-FOCUSED NURSING PROCESS: AN OVERVIEW OF THE PROCESS FROM ASSESSMENT TO EVALUATION

Most nurses are familiar with the nursing process as it applies to individually focused nursing care. Using it to promote community health makes this same nursing process community focused (Anderson and McFarlane, 2011). The phases of the nursing process that directly involve the community client as partner begin at the start of the contract or partnership and include assessment, diagnosis, planning, implementation, and evaluation.

ASSESSING COMMUNITY HEALTH

Community assessment is one of three core functions of PHN and is the process of critically thinking about the community. This involves getting to know and understand the community as client. Nurses start an assessment by clearly defining their client in terms of the three dimensions of place, people, and function presented in Table 12.1. Before data are collected in the assessment phase, the nurse must be able to answer questions such as the following:

- What are the geographic boundaries of this community?
- Which people are members of this community?
- What characteristics do they have in common?

For example, homebound older adults in a particular city are a community of special interest individuals with shared needs, who are defined by their age and homebound status. Once the nurse is clear about the boundaries of the community as client,

the community assessment phase can be continued. (See QSEN box below).

The assessment helps the nurse in community health to understand individual, family, and group problems and to know what community strengths and resources are available to help the nurse solve the client's problems. The community assessment phase involves a logical, systematic approach to the initial phase of the nursing process. Community assessment helps in the following ways:

- To identify community needs
- To clarify problems
- To identify strengths and resources

There are different types of community assessment. Community assessments can be short and simple or long and complex. One example of a short and simple community assessment is the windshield survey, which is discussed on page 213. Comprehensive community assessment is the necessary initial phase of the nursing process in community health with the community client as partner.

Assessing community health requires the following three steps:

1. Gathering relevant existing data and generating missing data
2. Developing a composite database
3. Interpreting the composite database to identify community problems and strengths

Data Collection and Interpretation

The primary goal of data collection is to get usable information about the community and its health. The systematic collection of data about community health requires the following:

- Gathering or compiling existing data
- Generating missing data
- Interpreting data
- Identifying community health problems and community abilities

Gathering. Data gathering is the process of obtaining existing, readily available data. The following data usually describe the demography of a community:

- Age of the residents
- Gender distribution of the residents
- Socioeconomic characteristics
- Racial distributions
- Vital statistics, including selected mortality and morbidity data
- Community institutions, including health care organizations and the services they provide
- Health personnel characteristics

Often these data have been collected by others via structured interviews, questionnaires, or surveys and are available in published reports at the library or local public health department. These data give the nurse a snapshot of how the clients receiving services fit into the community.

Data Generation. Data generation is the process of developing data that do not already exist, through interaction with community members, individuals, families, or groups. This type of information is more difficult to obtain and is generally not statistical. Data that often must be generated include the following:

- Information about a community's knowledge and beliefs
- Values and sentiments
- Goals and perceived needs
- Norms
- Problem-solving processes
- Power
- Leadership
- Influence structures

These data are more likely to be collected by interviews and observation.

Composite Database Analysis. Combining the gathered and generated data creates a composite database. Data analysis seeks to make sense of the data, as follows:

1. First, data are analyzed and synthesized, and themes are noted.
2. Community health problems, or needs for action, and community health strengths, or abilities, are determined.
3. The resources available to meet the needs are identified.
4. Problems are indicated by differences between the nurse's and community's goals for community health.
5. Strengths, on the other hand, are suggested by similarities between the nurse's and community's concepts of community health and available data.
6. Finally, the resources available to meet the needs are identified.

Data-Collection Methods

Several methods to collect data are needed. Methods that encourage the nurse to consider the community's perception of its health problems and abilities are as important as methods structured to identify knowledge that the nurse considers essential.

Five useful methods of collecting data are as follows:

1. Informant interviews
2. Participant observation
3. Windshield surveys
4. Secondary analysis of existing data
5. Surveys

These methods can be grouped into the following two distinct but complementary categories:

1. Methods that rely on what is directly observed by the data collector
2. Methods that rely on what is reported to the data collector

Collection of Direct Data. *Informant interviews, participant observation,* and *windshield surveys* are three methods of directly collecting data. All three methods require the following:

- Sensitivity
- Openness
- Curiosity
- The ability to listen, taste, touch, and smell
- The ability to see life as it is lived in a community

Informant interviews, which consist of directed talks with selected members of a community about community members or groups and events, are basic to effective data collection. Talking to key informants is a critical part of the community assessment. Key informants are not always people who have a formal title or position; they often have an informal role within the community. Examples of informal key informants are a member of a minority group who is listened to by other members of the group, a church deacon, and a parent who is active and vocal about the school health curriculum.

Also basic is participant observation, the deliberate sharing, if conditions permit, in the life of a community. For example, if the nurse lives in the community, activities such as participating in clinical organizations and church life and reading the newspaper give the nurse "observations" of the community's life. Informant interviews and participant observation are good ways to generate information about community beliefs, norms, values, power and influence structures, and problem-solving processes. Such data can seldom be reported in numbers, so they are not often collected. Even worse, conclusions that are based on intuition and are unchecked are sometimes used to replace this type of data. Conclusions from direct data collection methods should be confirmed by those people providing the information.

CASE STUDY

Community-Based Health Service Needs of an Aging Population

Alan Thompson is a nurse in community health and a member of a committee assigned to assess the health care needs of the aging "Baby Boomers" in Duxbury County. Mr. Thompson and his committee are aware that as the Baby Boomer population ages, health care professionals need to prepare for a rapid increase in the number of people older than 65 years. The committee's purpose is to make suggestions to the health department and county officials about how to prepare for the influx in health services that will be needed for these older adults.

Currently, 25% of the population in Duxbury County is older than 65 years. However, in 25 years this percentage is expected to increase to more than 50%. Currently, five primary care providers are in the county, with service waiting lists ranging from 1 to 3 weeks; only one of these providers specializes in geriatric care. One 54-bed long-term nursing care facility is located in the northern region of the large county. Because of rural roads, there is no public transit system. However, residents may call a hospital shuttle program if they need transportation to a physician's appointment.

Informant interviews with social workers and religious leaders can provide data that describe a community that has well-defined clusters of persons with similar problems, such as persons of low income, persons with concerns about adolescent pregnancy, and persons with worries about the health of babies. These data could be difficult to acquire without personal interviews.

Windshield surveys are the motorized equivalent of simple observation. They involve the collection of data that will help define the community, the trends, stability, and changes that will affect the health of the community (The University of Kansas, 2016).

While driving a car or riding public transportation, the nurse can observe many dimensions of a community's life and environment through the windshield, such as the following:

- Common characteristics of people on the street
- Neighborhood gathering places
- The rhythm of community life
- Housing quality
- Geographic boundaries

Windshield surveys can be used by themselves for short and simple assessments. An example of a windshield survey is found in Table 12.3.

Collection of Reported Data. Secondary analysis and surveys are two methods of collecting reported data. In secondary analysis, the nurse uses previously gathered data, such as minutes from community meetings. This type of analysis is extremely valuable because it saves time and effort. Many sources of data are readily available and useful for secondary analysis, including the following:

- Public documents
- Health surveys
- Minutes from meetings
- Statistical data
- Health records

HOW TO Identify a Key Informant for Interviews

The following individuals may be key informants:

- County health department nurses or church leaders
- Many community members whom nurses know and who can identify other key informants
- President of the parent–teacher organization
- Mayor or other local politicians
- The mother who organized the local chapter of Mothers Against Drunk Driving (informal leader)

TABLE 12.3 Windshield Survey Guidelines

Each community has its own characteristics. These characteristics, along with demographic data, provide valuable information in understanding the population that lives within the community and the health status, strengths and limitations, risks, and vulnerabilities unique to the "population of interest." Once you have defined a "community of interest" to assess, a *windshield survey* is the equivalent of a community head-to-toe assessment. The best way to conduct a windshield survey is to have a designated driver and at least one other passenger to scan the outline and take notes. Having one pair of eyes on the road, you can benefit from having several other individuals noticing the unique characteristics of the community and a shared experience provides additional insight. As you analyze your findings, it may be necessary to make a second tour to fill in any blanks. Many of us take these characteristics for granted, but they provide a rich context for understanding communities and populations and have significant impact on the health status of the community in general. You will report your findings in practicum conference and use relevant findings in your Community Problem Analysis paper, so collect your findings and analysis in a useful format.

Elements	Description
Boundaries	What defines the boundary? Roads, water, railroads? Does the area have a name? A nickname?
Housing and zoning	What is the age of the houses? What kind of materials in the construction? Describe the housing, including space between houses, general appearance and condition, and presence of central heating, air conditioning, and modern plumbing.
Open space	Describe the amount, condition, use of open space. Is the space used? Safe? Attractive?
Commons	Where do people in the neighborhood congregate? Who congregates there and at what hours during the day?
Transportation	How do people get from one place to another? Is public transportation available? If so, what kind and how effective? How timely? Personal autos? Bikes, etc.?
Social service centers	Do you see evidence of recreation centers, parks, social services, offices of doctors and dentists, pharmacies?
Stores	Where do residents shop? How do they get to the shops? Do they have groceries or sources of fresh produce? Is this a "food desert"?
Street people and animals	Who do you see on the streets during the day? Besides the people, do you see animals? Are they loose or contained?
Condition of the area	Is the area well kept or is there evidence of trash or abandoned cars or houses? What kind of information is provided on the signs in the area?
Race and ethnicity	What is the race of the people you see? What do you see about indices of ethnicity? Places of worship, food stores, restaurants? Are signs in English or other languages? (If the latter, which ones?)
Religion	What indications do you see about the types of religion residents practice?
Health indicators	Do you see evidence of clinics, hospitals, mental illness, substance abuse?
Politics	What indicators do you see about politics? Posters, headquarters?
Media	Do you see indicators of what people read? If they watch television? Listen to the radio?
Business and industry	What type of business climate exists? Manufacturers? Light or heavy industry? Large employers? Small business owners? Retail? Hospitality industry? Military installation? Do people have to seek employment elsewhere?

Adapted from Mizrahi TM: School of Social Work, Virginia Commonwealth University, Richmond, VA, September 1992; Stanhope MS, Knollmueller RN: *Public and community health nurse's consultant: a health promotion guide*, St. Louis, 1997, Mosby.

Surveys report data from a sample of persons. They are equally useful, but they take more time and effort than observational methods and secondary analyses because they require time-consuming and costly data collection (see discussion of how to identify a key informant for interviews). Thus the nurse does not often use the survey method. However, surveys are necessary for identifying certain community problems. For example, a lack of accessible personal health services cannot be documented readily and accurately in any other way.

Community Reconnaissance

Community reconnaissance, that is, surfing the Web, requires a computer and access to the Web instead of the automobile commonly used in windshield surveys noted in the previous section. However, both windshield surveys and community reconnaissance require superb detective skills.

What can you learn about a community by surfing the Web? Many counties and municipalities have their own websites. Many are represented in statewide and national databases. You can often find the address of a website (URL) for a community by using the county format noted in the Bernalillo County, New Mexico, example (http://bernalillo.nmgenweb.us/) and substituting the name of the county and state in which a particular community is located, or by browsing several websites identified by a search engine.

Local and state sites are, for example, very revealing of community economics and civic engagement. These sites typically advertise their communities to potential residents and businesses. They seldom disclose data about community issues, however, although they may include links to community newspapers and radio and television stations that will report issues. Small communities, however, may lack resources to develop their own websites.

An assessment guide is a useful tool for a community reconnaissance (see the assessment checklist on page 218 as an example). A guide structures Web browsing and allows the community assessor (you!) to recognize the strengths and limitations of Web data. Demographic data and vital statistics about the populations living in the community and data about the eight community systems delineated by Anderson and McFarlane (2010) are one possible guide, although many students have found it helpful to add a ninth system to their assessment guide, called *Religion and Faith*.

ASSESSMENT ISSUES

Gaining entry or acceptance into the community is perhaps the biggest challenge in assessment. The nurse is usually an outsider and often represents an established health care system that is neither known nor trusted by community members who may therefore react with indifference or even active hostility to the nurse. In addition, nurses may feel insecure about their skills as a community worker and the community may refuse to acknowledge its need for those skills. Because the nurse's success depends largely on the way he or she is viewed, entry into the community is critical. Often the nurse can gain entry by:

- Taking part in community events
- Looking and listening with interest
- Visiting people in formal leadership positions
- Employing an assessment guide
- Using a peer group for support
- Keeping appointments
- Clarifying community members' perceptions of health needs
- Respecting an individual's right to choose whether he or she will work with the nurse

Maintaining confidentiality is important. Nurses must be very careful to protect the identity of community members who provide sensitive or controversial data. In some cases the nurse may consider withholding data; in other situations the nurse may be legally required to disclose data. For example, nurses are required by law to report child abuse.

IDENTIFYING COMMUNITY PROBLEMS

The windshield assessment activities and the creation of a composite database, will result in a list of community strengths and health problems. Each problem needs to be identified and stated clearly. The health risk to the community is stated, the person(s) affected is named, and the community factors that led to the problem are defined. This process is an important first step to planning. In the planning phase, priorities are established, and interventions are identified.

Each community has its own unique characteristics. Some of these characteristics are strengths on which the nurse can build, but others contribute to the problem identified.

Frequently, multiple community health problems will be identified during the assessment phase. When multiple problems exist, priorities for resolving the problems must be set based on the following (McKenzie and Pinger, 2014):

- Which problems are important to the community?
- Which segments of the population are most affected?
- What are the benefits to the community?
- What happens to the community or the population if the problem is or is not resolved?
- How much does it cost to implement solutions, in terms of money and resources, to improve the problem and to save lives?
- How do politics, community values, and community priorities affect efforts to solve the problem?
- What does the community expect to happen?

PLANNING FOR COMMUNITY HEALTH

The planning phase includes the following:

- Analyzing the community health problems identified in the community nursing diagnoses
- Establishing priorities among them
- Establishing goals and objectives
- Identifying intervention activities that will accomplish the objectives

Problem Analysis

During analysis, the nurse seeks to clarify the nature of the problems. The nurse identifies the following:

- The origins and effects of the problem
- The points at which intervention might be undertaken
- The parties who have an interest in the problem and its solution
Analysis often requires identifying the following:
- The direct and indirect factors that contribute to the problem
- The outcomes of the problem
- Relationships among the problems (i.e., whether one problem causes or is affected by other problems)
- Factors that contribute to the problem

This is important because the nurse can anticipate that several of the same factors that contribute to a problem and affect the outcomes of a problem also cause many other problems.

Problem analysis should be undertaken for each identified problem. It often requires organizing a special group composed of the nurse and the following:

- Persons whose areas of expertise relate to the problem
- Individuals whose organizations are capable of intervening
- Representatives of the community experiencing the problem—the client

Together they can identify the factors contributing to the problem and explain the relationships between each factor and the problem.

Problem Priorities

Infant malnutrition represents only one of several community health problems identified by the community assessment. In reality, several community health problems may be identified. They may include lack of clinics, poor housing conditions, a mortality rate from cardiovascular disease that is higher than the national norm, and—as expressed by many residents—a desire to quit smoking.

Each problem identified as part of the assessment process must be put through a ranking process to determine its importance. This is known as problem prioritizing.

Problem Priority Criteria. Answers to the following questions have been helpful in ranking identified problems:

- How aware is the community of the problem?
- Is the community motivated to resolve or better manage the problem?
- Is the nurse able to influence problem resolution?
- Are there available experts to solve the problem?
- How severe are the outcomes if the problem is unresolved?
- How quickly can the problem be solved?

The members of the partnership answer questions related to their ability to influence or change the situation, and the nurse and the community agree on the ability to resolve the problem. One example of the difference between the perceptions of the nurse and community members is smoking in public buildings; the community nurse might identify smoking as a public health problem, but community members might view smoking as an issue of individual choice and personal freedom. For example, recently a midsize community, through the local government and the health department, passed a regulation to forbid smoking in all public places, including restaurants and bars. The outcry from the community residents has been loud. Residents believe their individual rights and freedoms have been taken away by government regulations. It does not matter to the residents that lung cancer rates are high.

This process is repeated separately for each identified problem, and all of the problems are compared. Priorities among the identified problems are established.

Establishing Goals and Objectives

Once high-priority problems are identified, relevant goals and objectives are developed. Goals are generally broad statements of desired outcomes. Objectives are the precise statements indicating the means of achieving desired outcomes.

The objectives must be *precise, behaviorally stated,* and *measurable* and can be solved in a series of steps implemented over time rather than all at once.

As noted, establishing these goals and objectives involves collaboration between the nurse and representatives of the community groups affected by both the problem and the proposed intervention. This often requires a great deal of negotiation among everyone taking part in the planning process. One important advantage offered by the continuous active involvement of people affected by the outcomes is that they have a vested interest in those outcomes and therefore are supportive of and committed to the success of the intervention. Once goals and objectives are chosen, intervention activities to accomplish the objectives can be identified.

Identifying Intervention Activities

Intervention activities, the means by which objectives are met, are as follows:
- The strategies used to meet the objectives
- The ways change will be effected
- The ways the problem cycle will be broken

Because alternative intervention activities do exist, they must be identified and evaluated. Clearly it is more valuable in the long term to educate others in how to assess the community problems and interventions to solve them. It is also necessary to analyze the change process necessary to complete the objectives.

IMPLEMENTATION IN THE COMMUNITY

Implementation, the fourth phase of the nursing process, involves the work and activities aimed at achieving the goals and objectives. Implementation efforts may be made by the person or group who established the goals and objectives, or they may be shared with or even delegated to others.

Factors Influencing Implementation

Implementation is shaped by the following:
- The nurse's chosen roles
- The type of health problem selected as the focus for intervention
- The community's readiness to take part in problem solving
- Characteristics of the social change process

The nurse taking part in community-oriented intervention has knowledge and skills that the other interveners do not have; the question is how the nurse uses the position, knowledge, and skills.

Nurse's Role. Nurses can act as content experts, helping communities select and attain task-related goals. In the example of infant malnutrition, the nurse can use epidemiological skills to determine the incidence and prevalence of malnutrition. The nurse can serve as a process expert by increasing the community's ability to document the problem rather than by providing help only as an expert in the area.

Content-focused roles often are considered change agent roles, whereas process roles are called change partner roles. Change agent roles stress gathering and analyzing facts and implementing programs, whereas change partner roles include those of enabler-catalyst, teacher of problem-solving skills, and activist advocate.

The Problem and the Nurse's Role. The role the nurse chooses depends on the following:
- The nature of the health problem
- The community's decision-making ability
- Professional and personal choices
- Some health problems clearly require certain intervention roles, as follows:
  - If a community lacks democratic problem-solving abilities, the nurse may select teacher, facilitator, and advocate roles. Problem-solving skills must be explained, and the nurse becomes a role model.
  - A problem with determining the health status of the community, on the other hand, usually requires fact-gatherer and analyst roles.
  - Some problems require multiple roles. Managing conflict among the involved health care providers, a common problem, demands process skills.
  - Collecting and interpreting the data necessary to document a problem require both interpersonal and analytical skills.
  - The community's history of taking part in decision making is a critical factor. In a community skilled in identifying and successfully managing its problems, the nurse may best serve as technical expert or advisor.

Different roles may be required if the community lacks problem-solving skills or has a history of unsuccessful change efforts. The nurse may have to focus on developing problem-solving capabilities or on making one successful change so that the community becomes empowered to take on the job of promoting change on its own behalf.

Social Change Process and the Nurse's Role. The nurse's role also depends on the social change process. Not all communities are open to change. The ability to change is often related to the extent to which a community focuses on traditional norms. The more traditional the community, the less likely it is to change. The ability to change is often directly related to the following (Rogers, 2003):
- High socioeconomic status
- A perceived need for change
- The presence of liberal, scientific, and democratic values
- A high level of social participation by community residents

For example, people living in a community might go to an immunization clinic rather than to a private physician if the clinic is nearby and less expensive and if the physician is not always available when needed.

Changes also are easier to accept in the following situations (Rogers, 2003):
- The change is shared in ways that fit in with the community's norms, values, and customs.
- Information is spread by the best communication mode (e.g., mass media for early adopters [people open to change] and face to face for late adopters [people who have more difficulty with change]).
- Other communities support the change efforts.
- Opinion leaders are identified and used.
- Communication about the change is clear and straightforward.

EVALUATING THE INTERVENTION FOR COMMUNITY HEALTH

Simply defined, evaluation is the appraisal of the effects of some organized activity or program. An example of evaluation is provided in the Evidence-Based Practice box on page 210. Evaluation may involve the design and conduct of evaluation research, or it may involve the more elementary process of assessing progress by contrasting the objectives and the results (Fink, 2013). This section deals with the basic approach of contrasting objectives and results.

Evaluation begins in the planning phase, when goals and measurable objectives are established and goal-attaining activities are identified. After implementing the intervention, only the accomplishment of objectives and the effects of intervention activities have to be assessed. Nursing progress notes direct the nurse to perform such appraisals concurrently with implementation. In assessing the data recorded there, the nurse is requested to evaluate whether the objectives were met and whether the intervention activities used were effective. Such an evaluation process is oriented to community health because the intervention goals and objectives come from the nurse's and the community's ideas about health.

Fig. 12.1 presents a summary of the complete nursing process with a community client.

Role of Outcomes in the Evaluation Phase

The measurement of outcomes is a particularly important part of the evaluation process. This is one reason for placing emphasis on measurable objectives. Cashman et al (2008) emphasize outcomes questions about appropriate and effective interventions, such as the following:
- Was the appropriate intervention done ineffectively or effectively?

- Were the objectives sensitive enough to measure change?
- Was an inappropriate intervention used?
- Has the health problem been resolved or the risk reduced?

Emphasizing epidemiology and the correct use of rates and numbers are means of evaluating intervention outcomes among defined communities. Often data collected over time also can provide important outcomes information about health trends within the community. As indicated, epidemiological data and trends do not provide the only measure of success, but they do provide important information about the intervention. Nurses need to consider the collection of this type of outcomes data for use as part of the evaluation phase. Outcomes can be measured by looking at changes from before and after the intervention to solve the problems. Changes in the following can be used to see the outcomes of the interventions (Fink, 2013):
- Demographics
- Socioeconomic factors
- Environmental factors
- Individual and community health status
- Use of health services

PERSONAL SAFETY IN COMMUNITY PRACTICE

Effective nursing practice starts with personal safety, and this remains important throughout the process. An awareness of the community and common sense are the two best guidelines for judgment. For example, common sense suggests not leaving anything valuable on a car seat or leaving the car unlocked. Similar guidelines apply to the use of public transportation. Calling ahead to schedule meetings will help prevent delays or confusion, and it gives the nurse an opportunity to lay the groundwork for the meeting. If there is no telephone or access

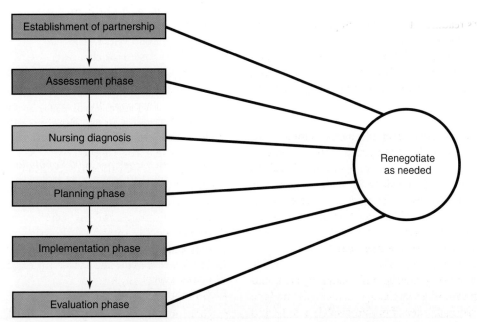

FIG. 12.1 Flowchart illustrating the nursing process with the community as client.

to a neighbor's telephone, plan to establish a time for any future meetings during the initial visit. Regardless of whether there has been telephone contact, there are rare situations when a meeting is postponed because the nurse arrives at a location where people are unexpectedly loitering by the entrance and the nurse has concerns about personal safety.

For nurses who are either just beginning their careers in community health or who are just starting a new position, the following three clear sources of information will help answer any questions about personal safety:

1. **Other nurses, social workers, or health care providers who are familiar with the dynamics of a given community.** They can provide valuable insights into when to visit, how to get there, and what to expect because they function in the community themselves.

2. **Community members.** The best sources of information about the community are the community members themselves, and one benefit of developing an active partnership with community members is their willingness to share their insight about day-to-day community life.

3. **The nurse's own observations.** Knowledge gained during the data collection phase of the process should provide a solid basis for an awareness of day-to-day community activity. Nurses with experience practicing in the community generally agree that if they feel uncomfortable in a situation, they should trust their feelings and leave.

CHECKLIST FOR A COMMUNITY ASSESSMENT

Asset Development
- ☐ Land
- ☐ Libraries
- ☐ Parks
- ☐ Police stations
- ☐ Fire stations

Community Organizations
- ☐ Crime Watch
- ☐ Neighborhood Watch
- ☐ Women's clubs
- ☐ Optimist
- ☐ Kiwanis
- ☐ Lions
- ☐ Businesses
- ☐ Schools
- ☐ Colleges

Government Assistance
- ☐ Number of families receiving Aid to Families with Dependent Children
- ☐ Number of persons receiving public assistance
- ☐ Number of persons receiving Medicaid
- ☐ Number of persons receiving food stamps

Health Risk Variables
Population Variables
- ☐ Population
- ☐ Total population density
- ☐ Population age groups (0–4 yr, 5–17 yr, 18–64 yr, ≥65 yr)

Ethnicity
- ☐ Percentage White
- ☐ Percentage African American
- ☐ Percentage Hispanic

Socioeconomic Data
- ☐ Percentage of persons below the federal poverty guideline
- ☐ Total number of households
- ☐ Estimated per capita income
- ☐ Estimated average household income
- ☐ Percentage of households with incomes less than $15,000

- ☐ Unemployment rate
- ☐ Occupational status
- ☐ Value of housing
- ☐ Educational level

Birth and Birth-Related Information
- ☐ Fertility rate
- ☐ Percentage of teen births
- ☐ Percentage of low birth weight
- ☐ Percentage of infant mortality

Age-Adjusted Death Rates
- ☐ Accident
- ☐ Cancer
- ☐ Cirrhosis
- ☐ Diabetes
- ☐ Heart disease
- ☐ Human immunodeficiency virus
- ☐ Homicide
- ☐ Pneumonia and flu
- ☐ Respiratory
- ☐ Stroke
- ☐ Suicides

Access to Primary Care
- ☐ Primary care physicians per population (family practice, general practice, pediatrics, internal medicine, and obstetrics and gynecology)
- ☐ Primary care providers per population (nurse-midwives, nurse practitioners, and physician assistants)

Inpatient Discharges per 1000 Population
- ☐ Discharges per 1000 population for each service area or the county as a whole excluding newborns
- ☐ Discharges per 1000 population for each service area or the county as a whole for the top five discharges

Survey Data
- ☐ Top five health concerns
- ☐ Insurance status
- ☐ Access to care

From Pickens S, Boumbulian P, Tietz M: Community assessment: strengths, assets & management, *Inside Prevent Care* 1(6), 1995.

PRACTICE APPLICATION

Lily, a nurse in a small city, became aware of the increased incidence of respiratory diseases through contact with families in the community and the local chapter of the American Lung Association. During family visits, Lily noted that many of the parents were smokers. Because most of the families Lily visited had small children, she became concerned about the effects of secondhand smoke on the health of the infants and children among her family caseload.

Further assessment of this community indicated that the community recognized several problems, including school safety and the risk for water pollution, in addition to the smoking problem that Lily had identified during her family visits. Talks with community members revealed that they wanted each of these identified problems "fixed," although these same community members also remained uncertain as to how to begin.

In deciding which of the three identified problems to address first, which criterion would be most important for Lily to consider?

A. The amount of money available
B. The level of community motivation to "fix" one of the three identified problems
C. The number of people in the community who expressed a concern about one of the three identified problems
D. How much control she would have in the process

Answers can be found on the Evolve website.

REMEMBER THIS!

- A community is defined as a locality-based entity composed of systems of formal organizations reflecting societal institutions, informal groups, and aggregates that are interdependent and whose function or expressed intent is to meet a wide variety of collective needs.
- A community practice setting is an insufficient reason for saying that practice is oriented toward the community client. When the location of the practice is in the community but the focus of the practice is the individual or family, the nursing client remains the individual or family, not the whole community.
- Community-oriented practice is targeted to the community, the population group in which healthful change is sought.
- *Community health,* as used in this chapter, is defined as the meeting of collective needs through identifying problems and managing interactions within the community itself and between the community and the larger society.
- Most changes aimed at improving community health involve, of necessity, partnerships among community residents and health workers from a variety of disciplines.
- Assessing community health requires gathering existing data, generating missing data, and interpreting the database.
- Five methods of collecting data useful to the nurse are informant interviews, participant observation, secondary analysis of existing data, surveys, and windshield surveys.

- Gaining entry or acceptance into the community is perhaps the greatest challenge in assessment.
- The nurse is usually an outsider and often represents an established health care system that is neither known nor trusted by community members, who may react with indifference or even active hostility.
- The planning phase includes analyzing and establishing priorities among community health problems already identified, establishing goals and objectives, and identifying intervention activities that will accomplish the objectives.
- Once high-priority problems are identified, broad relevant goals and objectives are developed.
- The goal, generally a broad statement of desired outcome, and objectives, the precise statements of the desired outcome, are carefully selected.
- Intervention activities, the means by which objectives are met, are the strategies that clarify what must be done to achieve the objectives, the ways change will be effected, and the way the problem will be interpreted.
- Implementation, the third phase of the nursing process, is transforming a plan for improved community health into the achievement of goals and objectives.
- Simply defined, evaluation is the appraisal of the effects of some organized activity or program.

ⓔ EVOLVE WEBSITE

http://evolve.elsevier.com/Stanhope/foundations
- Case Study, with Questions and Answers
- NCLEX® Review Questions
- Practice Application Answers

REFERENCES

Agency for Healthcare Research and Quality: *2014 National Healthcare Quality and Disparities Report,* Rockville, Md, 2015. AHRQ. Retrieved August 2016 from http://www.ahrq.gov/sites/default/files/wysiwyg/research/findings/nhqrdr/nhqdr14/2014nhqdr.pdf.

American Public Health Association: *Public Health Nursing Section: Public Health Nursing Section,* Washington, DC, 2009, APHA.

Anderson ET, McFarlane J: *Community as partner: theory and practice in nursing,* ed 7, Philadelphia, 2015, Wolters Kluwer.

Archer R, Cary AH, Malone B: The academic health department: the case for building partnerships to enhance the health of the public, *Public Health Nurs* 31:193–195, 2014.

Beets MW, Tilley F, Turner-McGrievy G, et al: Community partnership to address snack quality and cost in after-school programs, *J Sch Health* 84:543–548, 2014.

Blum HL: *Planning for health,* New York, 1974, Human Sciences Press.

Braveman P, Gottlieb L: The social determinants of health: it's time to consider the causes of the causes, *Public Health Rep* 129:19–31, 2014.

Caldwell WB, Reyes AG, Rowe Z, et al: Community partner perspectives on benefits, challenges, facilitating factors, and lessons learned from community-based participatory research partnerships in Detroit, *Prog Community Health Partnersh* 9:299–311, 2015.

Cheezum RR, Coombe CM, Israel BA, et al: Building community capacity to advocate for policy change: an outcome evaluation of the Neighborhoods Working in Partnership Project in Detroit, *J Comm Pract* 21:228–247, 2013.

Consensus set of health status indicators for the general assessment of community health status: United States, *MMWR Morb Mortal Wkly Rep* 40:449–451, 1991 (updated August 2001).

Cottrell LS: The competent community. In Kaplan BH, Wilson RN, Leighton AH, editors: *Further explorations in social psychiatry*, New York, 1976, Basic Books.

Council on Linkages between Academia and Public Health Practice: *Core competencies for public health professionals*, Washington, DC, 2014, The Council. Retrieved July 2016 from http://phf.org/corecompetencies.

Duff CL, Poole CR: School nurses coordinating care through a community/school health partnership, *NASN Sch Nurse*, 2016. doi:1942602S16639379.

Eghbalnia C, Sharkey K, Garland-Porter D, et al: A community-based participatory research partnership to reduce vehicle idling near public schools, *J Environ Health* 75:14–19, 2013.

Espey D, Flagg T, Henderson JA, et al: Strengthening breast and cervical cancer control through partnerships: American Indian and Alaska Native Women and the National Breast and Cervical Cancer Early Detection Program, *Cancer* 120:2557–2565, 2014.

Fink AG: *Evidence-based public health practice*, Los Angeles, CA, 2013, Sage Publications.

Green R: Community collaboration in caring for students with diabetes: a case study, *J Comm Health Nurs* 32:151–160, 2015.

Korazim Kőrösy Y, Mizrahi T, Bayne-Smith M, Carcia ML: Professional determinants in community collaborations: interdisciplinary comparative perspectives on roles and experiences among six disciplines, *J Comm Pract* 22:229–255, 2014.

Lathrop B, Hodnicki DR: The Affordable Care Act: primary care and the doctor of nursing practice nurse, *Online J Issues Nurs* 19:7, 2014.

McKenzie JF, Pinger RR: *An introduction to community health*, ed 8, Boston, 2014, Jones & Bartlett.

Metcalfe SE, Sexton EH: An academic-community partnership to address the flu vaccination rates of the homeless, *Public Health Nurs* 31:175–182, 2014.

Minkler M, Vasquez VB, Tajik M, et al: Promoting environmental justice through community-based participatory research: the role of community and partnership capacity, *Health Educ Behav* 35:119–137, 2008.

Minkler M: *Community organizing and community building for health and welfare*, New Brunswick, NJ, 2012, Rutgers University Press.

Mpofu E: *Community-oriented health services: practices across disciplines*, New York, 2015, Springer.

Nash DB, Fabius RJ, Skoufalos A, et al, editors: *Population health: creating a culture of wellness*, ed 2, Philadelphia, 2016, Jones & Bartlett.

National Association of Community and City Health Officials (NACCHO): *Mobilizing for action through planning and partnerships (MAPP)*, Washington, DC, 2016, NACCHO. Retrieved July 2016 from http://www.naccho.org/programs/public-health-infrastructure/mapp.

National Center for Chronic Disease Prevention and Health Promotion: National Center for Chronic Disease and Health Promotion: chronic disease prevention, Washington, DC, 2017, The Center. Retrieved March 2017 from http://www.cdc.gov/nccdphp/.

Pickens S, Boumbulian P, Tietz M: Community assessment: strengths, assets & management, *Inside Prevent Care* 1(6), 1995.

Pilon BA, Ketel C, Davidson H, et al: Evidence-guided integration of interprofessional collaborative practice into nurse managed health centers, *J Prof Nurs* 31:340–350, 2015.

Pinto BM, Waldemore M, Rosen R: A community-based partnership to promote exercise among cancer survivors: lessons learned, *Int J Behav Med* 22:328–335, 2015.

Perry TE, Wintermute T, Carney B, et al: Senior housing at a crossroads: a case study of a university/community partnership in Detroit, Michigan, *Traumatology* 21:244–250, 2015.

Rhodes SD, Alonzo J, Mann L, et al: Enhancement of locally developed HIV prevention intervention for Hispanic/Latino MSM: a partnership of community-based organizations, a university, and the Centers for Disease Control and Prevention, *AIDS Educ Prev* 27:312–332, 2015.

Rogers E: *Diffusion of innovations*, ed 5, New York, 2003, Free Press.

Ruderman M, editor: *Resources guide to concepts and methods for community-based and collaborative problem solving*, Johns Hopkins University, Baltimore, Md, 2000, Women's and Children's Health Policy Center.

Ryan W: *Blaming the victim*, New York, 1976, Vintage Books.

Sánchez J, Silvia-Suarez G, Serna CA, et al: The Latino migrant worker HIV prevention program: building a community partnership through a community health worker training program, *Fam Community Health* 35:139–146, 2012.

Santibañez S, Siegel V, O'Sullivan M, et al: Health communications and community mobilization during an Ebola response: partnerships with community and faith-based organizations, *Public Health Rep* 130:128–133, 2015.

Sidorov J, Romney M: The spectrum of care. In Nash DB, Fabius RJ, Skoufalos A, et al, editors: *Population health: creating a culture of wellness*, ed 2, Philadelphia, 2016, Jones & Bartlett.

Task Force on Community Prevention Services: Systematic Review Methods, *The Community Guide: The guide to community preventive services*, Atlanta, GA, 2016a, Centers for Disease Control and Prevention. Retrieved July 2016 from http://www.thecommunityguide.org/about/methods.html.

Task Force on Community Prevention Services: All findings of the Community Preventive Services Task Force. In: *The Community Guide: The guide to community preventive services*, Atlanta, Ga, 2016b, Centers for Disease Control and Prevention. Retrieved July 2016 from http://www.thecommunityguide.org/about/conclusionreport.html.

University of Kansas: *The community toolbox*, Retrieved August 14, 2016, from http://ctb.ku.edu.

Upvall M, Leffers J: *Global health nursing: building and sustaining partnerships*, New York, 2014, Springer.

U.S. Department of Health and Human Services: *Healthy People 2020: a roadmap for health*, Washington, DC, 2010, U.S. Government Printing Office. Retrieved January 2011 from http://www.healthypeople.gov/2020/default.aspx.

World Health Organization: *Centre for health development: ageing and health technical report: a glossary of terms for community health care and services for older persons*, vol 5, Kobe, Japan, 2004, WHO.

CHAPTER 13

Case Management

Ann H. Cary

OBJECTIVES

After reading this chapter, the student should be able to:

1. Define continuity of care, care management, case management, care coordination, transitional care, integrated care, social determinants of health, and advocacy.
2. Describe the scope of practice, roles, and functions of a case manager.
3. Identify the relationship between advocacy and case management.
4. Compare and contrast the nursing process with the process of case management and advocacy.
5. Identify methods to manage conflict, as well as the process of achieving collaboration.
6. Define and explain the legal and ethical issues confronting case managers.

CHAPTER OUTLINE

Concepts of Case Management
    Definitions of Case Management
    Healthy People 2020 and the Case Management Process
    Case Management and the Nursing Process
    Characteristics and Roles
    Knowledge and Skill Requirements
    Tools of Case Managers
Community Models of Case Management

Essential Skills for Case Managers
    Advocacy
    Conflict Management
    Collaboration
Issues in Case Management
    Legal Issues
    Ethical Issues

KEY TERMS

accountable care organizations, 222
advocacy, 222
affirming, 230
aggregate, 222
assertiveness, 232
autonomy, 227
beneficence, 233
care management, 222
CareMaps, 227
case management, 222
case manager, 222
case management plans, 227
collaboration, 229
conflict management, 229
constituency, 229
cooperation, 232
coordinating, 222
critical paths, 223
dashboard indicators, 222
demand management, 222
disease management, 222
informing, 230
information exchange process, 230
justice, 233
liability, 232
life care plan, 228
mediator, 229
negotiating, 231
nonmaleficence, 233
population management, 222
population manager, 222
problem-purpose-expansion method, 231
problem solving, 230
promoter, 229
risk sharing, 227
social mandate, 222
supporting, 222
telehealth, 223
timelines, 233
use management, 223
veracity, 233

Since the Patient Protection and Affordable Care Act (ACA) was initiated in 2010, the health care industry continues to reevaluate systems that attempt to integrate financing, management, quality, and service delivery models. Challenges abound for clients and providers as they attempt to coordinate care, transition clients among providers and systems, access and share information and documentation about clients and communities, and navigate the complexity of integrated care to optimize quality and access while managing costs. The new models of health care financing provide incentives to value care outcomes over the volume of care provided. Delivery of care is now organized through a network of providers, such as negotiated contracts with hospitals and other levels of care, physicians, nurse practitioners, pharmacies, ancillary health services, and outpatient centers.

Managing the health of populations served by the integrated systems is essential (Newman et al, 2014). These include accountable care organizations (ACOs). Nurse case managers and nurse care managers will play a pivotal role in innovative systems of delivery (Institute of Medicine [IOM], 2011). Population management includes the following:

- Wellness and health promotion
- Illness prevention
- Acute and subacute care
- Chronic disease
- Rehabilitation
- End-of-life care
- Care coordination
- Community engagement

Case managers are at the core of population health strategies to improve community outcomes (Noonan, 2014). Population health management can maintain and improve the physical and psychosocial status of clients through cost-effective and customized solutions, such as coordinating and transitioning of care to reduce gaps and costs; supporting evidence-based practices; selecting quality care that is culturally competent; and providing disease management and self-management educational programming (Case Management Society of America [CMSA], 2016; Noonan, 2014). Examples include planning and health delivery strategies for adolescents in a school system or the chronic disease management of elderly individuals in a rural community (Huber, 2010; McKesson Corporation, 2014). Like the earlier concept described by the American Hospital Association (AHA, 2016), the ACA endorses the use of integrated systems to attain the following objectives:

- Emphasis on population health management across the continuum, rather than on episodes of illness for an individual
- Management shifting from inpatient care as the point of management to primary care providers as points of entry
- Care management services and programs providing access and accountability for the continuum of health
- Successful outcomes measured by systems performance and pay for performance for providers to meet the needs of populations

The contemporary focus of integrated health systems defines the nature of the client as a population in addition to that as an individual. In these systems, population management involves the following activities:

- Assessing the needs of the client population through health histories (and, in the future, genograms), claims, use-of-service patterns, and risk factors; and communicating through information systems to ascertain patterns, trends, and responses to health programming in a population
- Creating benefits and network designs to address these needs
- Selecting dashboard indicators to measure performance
- Prioritizing actions to produce a desired outcome with available resources

- Selecting evidence-based programs related to wellness, prevention, health promotion, and demand management; patient/client engagement; and educating the population about them
- Instituting evidence-based care management processes that assure transitional and coordinated care across the health continuum for a population aggregate
- Deploying case managers within a variety of delivery and insurance systems to clients and providers
- Evaluating provider patterns of performance and client dashboard indicators for impact

Establishing a relationship between financing, managing, delivering, and coordinating services is critical to reach the goal of population health management—that is, achieving health outcomes at the population level. The *Healthy People 2020* goals are a social mandate for health care. In the second decade of the twenty-first century, case management will be an essential intervention to positively influence the leading health indicators, chronic disease outcomes, and focus areas of *Healthy People 2020.*

Establishing evidence-based strategies for all functions is critical to the success of case management for individuals and populations. Using the current best evidence blended with clinical expertise is a critical skill of the case manager (American Nurses Association [ANA], 2013; Lamb, 2013; CMSA, 2016). In their practice, nurse case managers have the following core values:

- Increasing the span of healthy life
- Reducing disparities in health among Americans
- Promoting access to care and to preventive services

Many of the interventions nurses use with clients and health care systems will further the *Healthy People 2020* objectives. These include case management interventions to minimize fragmented care and promote quality transitions of care; incorporate standardized practice tools and adherence guidelines; improve safety of care; and use interprofessional teams to deliver services.

In the intervention wheel model for public health nursing practice, the nursing actions of case management, collaboration, and advocacy comprise 3 of 17 evidence-based interventions for individuals, families, and populations served by public health nurses (Keller et al, 2004; see Appendix C.4). These three concepts and practice arenas for public health nurses are more fully described in this chapter. Case management incorporates many of the *Quad Council Competencies for Public Health Nursing* (Quad Council, 2011; see Appendix C.3) because it involves individual and family care as well as community resources, population health, interprofessional teams, and policy implementation.

CONCEPTS OF CASE MANAGEMENT

Case management is a strategy that is used in an overarching process called care management. Care management is an enduring process in which a population manager establishes systems and monitors the health status, resources, and outcomes for an aggregate—a targeted segment of the population or a group. Care management strategies were initially developed by health maintenance organizations (HMOs) in the late

BOX 13.1 Additional Definitions of Case Management Strategies

- **Use management** attempts to redirect care and monitors the appropriate use of provider care and treatment services for both acute and community and ambulatory services (Leonard and Miller, 2012).
- **Critical paths** are tools that name activities that can be used in a timely sequence to achieve the desired outcomes for care. The outcomes are measurable, and the critical path tools strive to reduce differences in client care.
- **Disease management** activities target chronic and costly disease conditions that require long-term care interventions (e.g., diabetes). These strategies address the entire cycle of a disease process, typically incorporating primary, secondary, and tertiary care interventions and self-care activities (Huber, 2015).
- **Demand management** seeks to control use by providing clients with correct information to empower them to make healthy choices, use healthy and health-seeking behaviors to improve their health status, and make fewer demands on the health care system (Pawson et al, 2016).

1970s to manage the care of different populations while promoting quality of care and ensuring appropriate use and costs. Care management strategies include use management, critical paths, disease management, demand management, and case management (Box 13.1).

The population manager is the architect for the target group's health in the care management delivery process. The building blocks used by the manager include the following (Mullahy, 2017):

- Risk analysis
- Data mapping
- Data monitoring for health processes, indicators, and unexpected illnesses
- Epidemiological investigation of unexpected illnesses
- Multidisciplinary development of action plans and programs
- Identifying case management triggers or events that promote earlier referrals of high-risk clients when prevention can have dramatic results

Case management, in contrast to care management, involves activities implemented with individual clients in the system. The case manager builds on the basic functions of the traditional role and adapts new competencies for managing the transition from one part of the system to another or to home.

Definitions of Case Management

A historical focus on collaboration is seen in the Commission for Case Manager Certification definition:

A collaborative process that assesses, plans, implements, coordinates, monitors and evaluates the options and services required to meet the client's health and human services needs. It is characterized by advocacy, communication, and resource management and promotes quality and cost-effective interventions and outcomes

(Mullahy, 2017, p. 33).

Case management is defined in public health nursing as the ability to "optimize self-care capabilities of individuals and families and the capacity of systems and communities to coordinate and provide services" (Minnesota Department of Health, 2003, p 93). Case management is viewed as only one competency, or skill, that nurses need to have to provide quality care. Case management is identified as one of 17 interventions in the scope of practice of nursing in the community (Minnesota Department of Health, 2003). The following knowledge and skills are required to achieve this competency (Mullahy, 2017):

- Knowledge of community resources and financing methods
- Written and oral communication and documentation skills
- Negotiation and conflict-resolution skills
- Critical thinking processes to identify and prioritize problems from the view of the provider and client
- Application of evidence-based practices and outcome measures

Case management practice is complex because of the coordinating activities of multiple providers, payers, and settings throughout a client's continuum of care. Care by multiple providers (the client, family, significant others, community organizations) must be assessed, planned, implemented, adjusted, and based on mutually agreed-upon goals. The nurse employed and located in one setting will be influencing the selection and monitoring of care provided in other settings by formal and informal care providers. With the use of electronic care delivery through telehealth activities, case management activities are now delivered via telephone, e-mail, fax, and video visits in a client's residence. They may also be delivered to a global network of clients located in different countries.

Although the activities in case management may differ among providers and clients, the goals are as follows (Mullahy, 2017):

- To promote quality services provided to clients
- To reduce institutional care while maintaining quality processes and satisfactory outcomes
- To manage resource use through protocols, evidence-based decision making, guideline use, and disease management programs
- To control expenses by managing care processes and outcomes (Mullahy, 2017)

A particularly challenging problem is the fragmenting of services, which can result in overuse, underuse, gaps in care, and miscommunication. This may ultimately result in costly client outcomes. Case management in rural settings is more complex because of the following:

- Fewer organized community-based systems
- Geographic distance to delivery
- Population density
- Finances
- Pace and lifestyle
- Values
- Social organization differences from the urban setting

The Effectiveness of a Registered Nurse Case Manager

This retrospective case-control study sought to assess the effectiveness of a registered nurse case manager's (RNCM's) certified diabetes educator (CDE) quality improvement case management program. The RNCMs provided chronic care interventions, particularly for high-risk diabetes populations with glycosylated hemoglobin (A1C) of 9% or higher. The RNCMs used protocols to titrate medications and assess patients for medication adherence, diabetes knowledge, and barriers to care. Researchers Watts and Sood (2016) reviewed computerized patient records over a period of 10 years for patients seen at 11 different community outpatient clinics. Results indicated that a large portion of high-risk patients with a baseline A1C of 9% or higher were seen by the RNCM. Patients who were seen by an RNCM had a statistically significant reduction in A1C after 14 to 26 months of intervention (t-test, $p < 0.001$). The RNCMs clinical intervention demonstrated a significant A1C reduction of approximately 2%.

Nurse Use

Nursing case management can improve health outcomes for high-risk diabetes populations. This finding may have additional implications for health care policy makers for planning interventions with respect to long-term management of diabetes mellitus.

From Watts SA, Sood A: Diabetes nurse case management: improving glucose control: 10 years of quality improvement follow-up data. *Appl Nurs Res* 29:202–205, 2016.

Healthy People 2020 and the Case Management Process

Nurse case managers in their practices have as core values the goals of *Healthy People 2020*. Many of the interventions that nurses use with clients, as well as the design of the health care system and the number of covered lives in those systems, promote further progress in meeting the objectives of *Healthy People 2020*. Case management strategies offer opportunities for nurses to help meet the objectives for specific population targets listed in *Healthy People 2020* (U.S. Department of Health and Human Services, 2010).

The target populations include those who do not have access to health care and those whose lifestyle or health conditions may limit the quality and length of healthy life; variables include ethnicity/race, low income, limited education, gender or sexual orientation, those living in the inner city or rural areas, those without health insurance, and the disabled or those experiencing chronic disease.

This chapter guides the reader through the nature and process of case management for individual and family clients. Case management has had a rich tradition in public health nursing and is frequently found in hospitals, transitional and long-term care, home and hospice care, and health insurance companies. Case management in public health nursing and in the community dates back to Lillian Wald and the Henry Street Settlement (Christopher et al, 2016). Nursing has maintained the leadership among health care providers in coordinating resources to achieve health care outcomes based on quality, access, and cost. As health care delivery moves to chronic disease management services, with an emphasis on pursuing the most efficient use of services to manage client outcomes, case management emerges to play a strong role.

Case Management and the Nursing Process

Case management activities with individual clients and families will reveal the larger picture of health services and health status of the community. Through a nurse's case management activities, general community weaknesses in quality and quantity of health services often are discovered. For example, the management of a severely disabled child by a nurse case manager may uncover the absence of respite services or parenting support and education resources in a community. The components of the nursing process are used when implementing the functions of a case manager with clients. The spectrum of case management consists of four activities: assessment, planning, facilitating, care coordination, evaluation, and advocacy (CMSA, 2016).

While managing the disability and injury claims at an industry, the nurse may discover that referrals for home health visits and physical therapy are generally underused by the acute care providers in the community. Community assessment, policy development, and assurance activities that frame core functions of public health actions are often the logical next steps for a nurse's practice. When observing lack of care or services at the individual and family intervention levels, the nurse can, through case management, intervene at the community level to make changes (Table 13.1). The case management process involving client and nurse is depicted in Fig. 13.1.

Characteristics and Roles

Case management can be labor intensive, time-consuming, and costly. Because of the rapid growth in the nature of complexity in clients' problems, the intensity and duration of activities required to support the case management function may soon exceed the demands that the direct caregiver can meet. Managers and clinicians in community health are exploring methods to make case management more efficient, including the use of providers who can perform to the limit of their licenses, auxiliary case management providers/services, and evidence-based practices.

 HEALTHY PEOPLE 2020

Objectives Achieved Using Case Management Strategies

Case management strategies offer opportunities for nurses to help meet the following *Healthy People 2020* objectives for target populations:

- **ECBP-14 and 14.1:** Increase the inclusion of clinical prevention and population content in undergraduate nursing, including counseling training for health promotion and disease prevention
- **SA-9:** Increase the portion of persons who are referred for follow-up for substance abuse problems

From U.S. Department of Health and Human Services: *Healthy People 2020: a roadmap for health,* Washington, DC, 2010, U.S. Government Printing Office.

TABLE 13.1 The Nursing Process and Case Management

Nursing Process	Case Management Process	Activities
Assessment	Case finding Identification of incentives for the target population Screening and intake Determination of eligibility Assessment	Develop networks with the target population Disseminate written materials Seek referrals Apply screening tools according to program goals and objectives Use written and onsite screens Apply comprehensive assessment methods (i.e., physical, social, emotional, cognitive, economic, self-care capacity) Obtaining consent for services if appropriate
Diagnosis	Identification of the problem or opportunity	Hold interprofessional, family, and client conferences Determine conclusions on the basis of assessment Use an interprofessional team
Planning for outcomes	Problem prioritizing Planning to address care needs Identification of resource match	Validate and prioritize problems with all participants Develop goals, activities, time frames, and options Gain the client's consent to implement Have the client choose options
Implementation	Advocating of clients' interests Frequent monitoring to assess alignment with goals and changing nature of client needs	Contact providers Negotiate services and price Adjust as implementation is needed Document processes and monitor progress
Evaluation	Measure attainment of activities and goals of service delivery plan Continued monitoring of clients during service Reassessment Bringing closure to care when client needs are achieved or change Discharge appropriately	Ensure quality of transitional communication and coordinate of service delivery Monitor for changes in client or service status Examine outcomes against goals Examine needs against service Examine costs Examine the satisfaction of client, providers, and the case manager Examine best practices and outcomes for this client

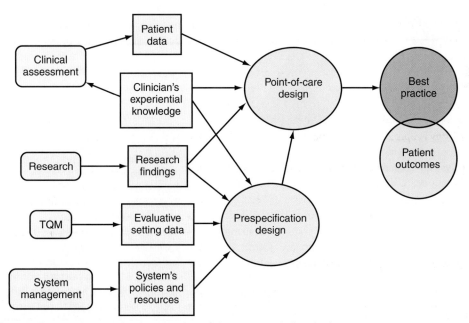

FIG. 13.1 Factors that require the attention of the nurse and client in the case management process.

In 1998, Cary described the roles that case managers assume in the practice setting. These roles are clearly affirmed today in the work of Leonard and Miller (2012) and by the Case Management Society of America (CMSA, 2016) (Box 13.2). The roles demanded of the nurse as case manager are vividly influenced by the forces at work in the employing agency.

Fig. 13.2 presents the continuum of care case management model.

Knowledge and Skill Requirements

Adopting the case management role for a nurse does not happen automatically with an agency position. Knowledge and

---

BOX 13.2 Case Manager Roles

- **Broker:** Acts as an agent for provider services that are needed by clients to stay within coverage according to the budget and cost limits of a health care plan
- **Consultant:** Case manager who works with providers, suppliers, the community, and other case managers to provide case management expertise in programmatic and individual applications
- **Coordinator:** Arranges, regulates, and coordinates needed health care services for clients at all necessary points of services
- **Educator:** Educates the client, family, and providers about the case management process, delivery system, community health resources, and benefit coverage so that informed decisions can be made by all parties
- **Facilitator:** Supports all parties in work toward mutual goals
- **Liaison:** Provides a formal communication link among all parties concerning the plan of care management
- **Mentor:** Case manager who counsels and guides the development of the practice of new case managers
- **Monitor and reporter:** Provides information to parties on the status of members and situations affecting patient safety, care quality, and patient outcome and on factors that alter costs and liability

- **Negotiator:** Negotiates the plan of care, services, and payment arrangements with providers; uses effective collaboration and team strategies
- **Client advocate:** Acts as an advocate, provides information, and supports benefit changes that assist member, family, primary care provider, and capitated systems
- **Researcher:** Case manager who uses and applies evidence-based practices for programmatic and individual interventions with clients and communities, participates in the protection of clients in research studies, and initiates and collaborates in research programs and studies
- **Standardization monitor:** Formulates and monitors specific public health nursing and disease management protocols that guide the type and timing of care to comply with predicted treatment outcomes for the specific client and conditions; attempts to reduce variation in resource use; targets deviations from standards so adjustments can occur in a timely manner. These protocols are usually found in agency policy books or in public health reference guides within governmental agencies
- **Systems allocator:** Distributes limited health care resources according to a plan or rationale

---

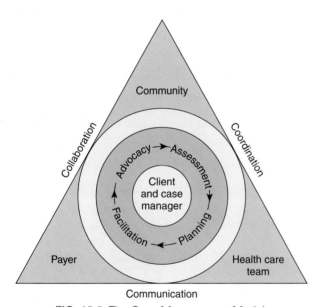

FIG. 13.2 The Case Management Model.

BOX 13.3 Knowledge Domains for Case Management

- Standards of practice for case management
- Evidence-based practice guidelines for specific health and disease conditions and communities
- Knowledge of the health care financial environment and the financial dimension of client
- Clinical knowledge, skill, and maturity to direct quality timing and sequencing of care activities
- Care resources for clients within institutions and communities: Facilitating the development of new resources and systems to meet clients' needs
- Transition planning for ideal timing and sequencing of care
- Management skills: communication, delegation, persuasion, use of power, consultation, problem solving, conflict management, confrontation, negotiation, management of change, marketing, group development, accountability, authority, advocacy, ethical decision making, and profit management
- Teaching, counseling, and education skills
- Program evaluation and research
- Performance improvement techniques
- Peer and team consultation, collaboration, and evaluation
- Requirements of eligibility and benefit parameters by third-party payers
- Legal and ethical issues
- Information management systems: clinical and administrative
- Health care legislation/policy
- Technical information skills, interoperable information systems, dashboard monitoring, data management and analysis, predictive modeling software, facile use of electronic health records (EHRs)
- Outcomes management and applied research

---

skills that are developed and refined are essential to success. Knowledge domains useful for nurses in systems desiring to implement quality case management roles are found in Box 13.3 (Cary, 1998; Tahan et al, 2015; Treiger, 2013). If a nurse seeks a case manager position, some of the skills and knowledge areas will need to be developed through academic and continuing education programs, literature reviews, orientation, and mentoring experiences.

Tools of Case Managers

The six "rights" of case management are right care, right time, right provider, right setting, and right price/value, and right outcomes. How does the nurse judge the effectiveness of case management? Three tools are useful for case management practice: case management plans, disease management, and life care

planning tools. An underlying principle for use of each of these tools is the need to use robust evidence as the basis for the selection of activities.

Telehealth is a contemporary intervention approach used by case managers. It is an organized health care delivery approach to triage and provides advice, counseling, and referral for a client's health problem using phones or computers with cameras. The client is usually in the home, and the nurse is at an office, health care facility, or phone bank location. Software is being refined for use in documentation, decision making, dashboard tools, predictive modeling, workflow, electronic medical records, patient engagement strategies, and social media remote monitoring as described earlier (Carneal and Pock, 2014; Stricker, 2014; Treiger, 2013).

Case management plans have evolved through various terms and methods (e.g., critical paths, critical pathways, Care-Maps, multidisciplinary action plans, nursing care plans). Today the activities that involve developing individual plans for clients are usually referred to as case management plans, Care-Maps, or integrated clinical pathways. Regardless of the title given, standards of client care, standards of nursing practice, and clinical guidelines using evidence-based practices for case management serve as core foundations of case management plans. Likewise, in interprofessional action plans, core professional standards of each discipline guide the development of the standard process.

Adaptation of the case management care plan to each client's characteristics is a crucial skill for standardizing the process and outcome of care. It links multiple provider interventions to client responses and offers reasonable predictions to clients about health outcomes. Institutions report that sharing case management plans with clients empowers the clients to assume responsibility for monitoring and adhering to the plan of care. Self-responsibility by clients incorporates autonomy and self-determination as the core of case management. For the nurse employed to function as a case manager, ample opportunity exists to develop, test, and revise case management plan prototypes for a target population experiencing acute and chronic health problems.

Disease management is an organized program of coordinated health care interventions and communications for populations with conditions in which client self-care efforts are critical (CMSA, 2016). This approach focuses on the natural progression of a disease. Disease management programs may contain many of the following components (Hisashige, 2012):

- Selection of high-risk patients, with a focus on a singular disease state (diabetes, asthma, congestive heart failure [CHF])
- Financial and risk sharing arrangements between payers and providers
- Programs for monitoring the use of clinical paths and evidence-based guidelines to assess outcomes and costs
- Protocols for clinical and administrative processes as well as cost allocations
- Services to educate clients and promote self-management skills
- Enhanced quality through evidence-based decision support and other registry technologies
- Support for provider–client relationships and plans of care
- Evaluation of clinical, humanistic, and economic outcomes to address the goal of improving overall health

The philosophy of disease management gives the clients the tools needed to better manage their lives (CMSA, 2016;

Newman et al, 2014). Clients with chronic diseases benefit from a disease management approach. The goals are to interrupt continued development of a disease and prevent future disease and complications through secondary and tertiary prevention interventions. Promotion of wellness is necessary for success. For specific client populations that consume a disproportionate share of resources, disease management programs allocate the correct resources in an efficacious manner (Berkowitz, 2016). Disease management programs also reduce emergency department visits and result in fewer inpatient days, greater client satisfaction, and reduced school absences (Caloyeras et al, 2014). As the science of disease management evolves to predict direct relationships between outcomes and protocols of care, case managers will be able to ensure cost-effective, optimal clinical care across the continuum—a goal of care management for populations. In fact, disease management is viewed as a top strategy by employers. For case managers, disease management strategies, which are part of the care management programs, shift the client interventions from specific, episodic care to holistic care functions that are proactive and population based (American Hospital Association, 2016). The Joint Commission (TJC) certifies and the American Accreditation HealthCare Commission accredits disease management organizations and programs on the basis of their respective standards (visit http://www.jointcommission.org and http://www.urac.org). This may influence the choice of programs a case manager selects to use with clients. The Focus on Quality and Safety Education for Nurses (QSEN) box emphasizes the importance of the interprofessional team in the community. It is important that the nurse understands roles and relationships and overlap in services to become more efficient in providing quality and safe care.

QSEN FOCUS ON QUALITY AND SAFETY EDUCATION FOR NURSES

Targeted Competency: Teamwork and Collaboration—Function effectively within nursing and interprofessional teams, fostering open communication, mutual respect, and shared decision making to achieve quality client interventions and outcomes.

Important aspects of teamwork and collaboration include the following:
- **Knowledge:** Describe scopes of practice and roles of health care team members
- **Skills:** Clarify roles and accountabilities under conditions of potential overlap in team member functioning
- **Attitudes:** Value the perspectives and expertise of all health team members

Teamwork and Collaboration Question:
Observe a typical workday of a community health or public health nurse, noting the types of activities that are done in coordination and case management and the amount of time spent in these areas. Interview several staff members to determine whether they perceive that the amount of their time spent in case management is changing. To what degree are the staff members involved in care management activities? Ask about common colleagues with whom case managers collaborate. Besides primary care physicians, which health care team members are often involved in managing clients' care across time and across settings? What skills are needed by the case management nurse to best facilitate these interdisciplinary teams?

Prepared by Gail Armstrong, DNP, ACNS-BC, CNE, Associate Professor, University of Colorado Denver College of Nursing.

The life care plan is another tool used in case management. It assesses the current and future needs of a client for catastrophic or chronic disease over the life span. The life care plan is a customized, medically based document that provides assessment of all present and future needs (i.e., medical, financial, psychological, vocational, spiritual, physical, and social), including services, equipment, supplies, and living arrangements for a client (Leonard and Miller, 2012). These plans may be used by either a plaintiff or defense lawyer to analyze damages. They are also used to set financial rewards, which can be used to pay for care in the future and create a lifetime care plan. Life care plans are typically used for clients experiencing catastrophic illness or adverse events resulting from professional malpractice. Another group of life care planning beneficiaries involves those who have sustained injury when younger and whose care requirements have changed as a result of aging (Day et al, 2015; Rutherford-Owen and Marini, 2012). A systematic process is used, and interprofessional input is required. The first phase of the plan is crafted to include a thorough assessment of the client, financial and billing agreements, an information release signed by the client, and a targeted date for report completion. Development of the plan is the second phase. Case management plans are based on several factors: social situation, leisure activities, educational and employment status, medical history, physical abilities, current status, and assistance required for completing the activities of daily living.

The plan includes projected costs and resources needed for the frequency and duration of treatments, equipment, and supplies. It also includes plans for future evaluations. The life care plan seeks to portray the needs of a client that are consistent with the changes in a client's life over the predicted life span, taking into account the injury or diagnosis (Apuna-Grummer and Howland, 2013).

All of these tools and programs, in coordination, constitute population health management strategies to educate clients and promote self-management, provide nurse coaching support, promote safe care transitions, improve care management and coordination, and enhance quality (Kizer, 2015).

COMMUNITY MODELS OF CASE MANAGEMENT

Liberty Mutual Insurance Company has used case management principles for more than 30 years in workers' compensation cases and has expanded services for employees whose conditions were noted to be chronic or catastrophic. Box 13.4 lists examples of case-managed conditions. Case managers coordinate all

BOX 13.4   Examples Of Case-Managed Conditions

- Acquired immunodeficiency syndrome
- Amputations
- Brain trauma
- Cerebrovascular accident
- Chronic diseases and disabilities (e.g., asthma, diabetes, mental illness, behavioral health)
- High-risk neonates
- High usage of services
- Multiple fractures
- Psychiatric conditions
- Severe burns
- Spinal cord injury
- Substance abuse
- Terminal illness
- Transplantation
- Ventilator dependency
- Work-related injuries

providers, clients, and services to reduce excessive expenses caused by lack of coordination, failure to use quality alternatives, duplication, and fragmentation. Some states through their Medicaid programs are developing disease management programs for high-cost chronic diseases, such as asthma and diabetes, among their populations.

The Agency for Healthcare Research and Quality (AHRQ) (2016) profiled the Elder Services of Merrimack Valley (ESMV), an Area Agency on Aging in Northeastern Massachusetts, as a service delivery innovation that included nursing case management. ESMV followed recently discharged Medicare patients in their homes and monitored them via telephone to identify and address declines in health status that increase the risk for readmission. Patients received an in-home visit 48 hours after hospital discharge and a weekly phone call. The nurse case manager collaborated with the family's assigned health coach. The nurse care manager facilitated the provision of needed services, such as primary care, specialty care, a change to the medication regimen, a home visit from a nurse, and/or an emergency department visit. The program reported a significant reduction in hospital readmissions among at-risk Medicare patients, which also generated a substantial cost savings for the hospitals and health care system.

Important guidance in developing a community-based case management program can be found in the United States. Case management is a key component of federally financed and many state-financed health delivery options. The experiences of states over the past two decades provide testimony to the importance of case management for populations at risk. For older clients, state-derived case management provides objective advice and assistance with care needs. It also provides access to multidisciplinary providers and services. For payers (i.e., federal, state, clients), case management serves as a way to ensure that funds are allocated appropriately to those in greatest need. Case management serves a policy assurance and accountability function for communities.

Within the states, the types of agencies designated to conduct case management are often district offices of state government, area agencies on aging, county social services departments, and private contractors. States maintain the oversight responsibilities for case management agencies to do the following:

1. Ensure they are complying with program standards, contracts, reporting, and fiscal controls
2. Identify emerging problems and issues to be resolved by additional state policies
3. Provide onsite technical assistance and consulting to improve performance. States' payment methods for case management include daily and monthly rates, hourly and quarterly rates, capped rates for services, and capped aggregate rates to cover both case management and provider costs (Mullahy, 2017).

ESSENTIAL SKILLS FOR CASE MANAGERS

Three specific skills essential to the role performance of the case manager are discussed: advocacy, conflict management, and collaboration.

Advocacy

Case managers report that they are first and foremost client advocates (CMSA, 2016; Sminkey and LeDoux, 2016; Tahan et al, 2015). The definition of nursing includes advocacy: "Nursing is the protection, promotion and optimization of health and abilities, prevention of illness and injury, alleviation of suffering through the diagnosis and treatment of human response, and advocacy in the care of individuals, families, communities and populations" (ANA, 2010, p 6). For nurses, advocacy involves various activities, ranging from exploring self-awareness to lobbying for health policy. Advocacy is essential for practice with clients and their families, communities, organizations, and colleagues on an interprofessional team. The functions of advocacy require scientific knowledge, expert communication, facilitating skills, and problem-solving and affirming techniques. As the Code of Ethics for Nurses (ANA, 2015) states, "Nurses consider the needs and respect the values of each person in every professional relationship and setting" (p 1). This means the nurse has the obligation to move beyond his or her own personal feelings of agreement or disagreement to respond compassionately. However, this goal is a contemporary one; the perspective regarding the advocacy function has shifted through time. The nurse advocate has been described in earlier writings as one who acted on behalf of or interceded for the client (Nelson, 1988). An example of the nurse interacting on behalf of the client is the nurse who calls for a well-child appointment for a mother visiting the family planning clinic when the mother is capable of making an appointment on her own. The contemporary goal of advocacy would direct the nurse to move clients toward making the call themselves.

The change over time in the advocacy role to that of mediator by the nurse advocate is described as a response to social change, reimbursers, and providers in the health care system. Mediation is an activity in which a third party attempts to provide assistance to those who may be experiencing a conflict in obtaining what they desire. The goal of the nurse advocate as mediator is to help parties understand each other on many levels so that agreement on an action is possible. In the example of a nurse as case manager for an HMO, mediation activities between an older client and the payer (i.e., the HMO) could accomplish the following results: the client may understand the options for community-based skilled nursing care, and the payer may understand the client's desires for a less restrictive environment for care, such as the home. Although the case manager as mediator does not decide the plan of action (in contrast to the role of arbitrator), he or she facilitates the decision-making process between the parties so that the desired care can be reimbursed within the range of options available to the client.

In today's practice, the nurse advocate makes the client's rights the priority. The goal of promoter for the client's autonomy and self-determination may result in a high degree of client independence in decision making. For example, when a group of young pregnant women is the collective "client" (i.e., the aggregate), the nurse advocate's role may be to inform the group of the benefits and consequences of breastfeeding their infants. However, if the new mothers decide on formula feeding, the nurse advocate should support the group and continue to provide parenting, infant, and well-child services.

A different perspective of the nurse advocate as promoter holds that the nurse's role as advocate may demand a variety of functions that are influenced by the client's physical, psychological, social, and environmental abilities. The nurse adapts the advocacy function to the client's dynamic capabilities as the client follows a path to a healthy status. Examples of advocacy in such cases might include promoting a client group's access to onsite physical fitness programs in the occupational setting or supporting parents' and students' concerns about the high fat content of vending machine food in the school system.

Process of Advocacy

The goal of advocacy is to promote self-determination in a constituency or client group. It is often critical in promoting a client's self-determination. Table 13.2 compares the nursing

TABLE 13.2 Nursing Process and Advocacy Process

Nursing Process	Advocacy Process
Assessment/diagnosis	Exchange information
	Gather data
	Illuminate values
Planning/outcomes	Generate alternatives and consequences
	Prioritize actions
Implementation	Make decisions
	Support the client
	Assure
	Reassure
Evaluation	Affirm
	Evaluate
	Reformulate

process with the advocacy process. The client may be an individual, family, peer, group, or community. The classic process of advocacy has been defined by Kohnke (1982), Mallik and Rafferty (2000), Smith (2004), and Choi (2015) to include informing, supporting, and affirming. All three activities are more complex than they may initially seem, and they require self-reflection by the nurse as well as skill development. It is often easier for the nurse to inform, support, and affirm another person's decision when it is consistent with the nurse's values. When clients make decisions within their value systems that are different from the nurse's values, the advocate may feel conflict about contributing to the process of informing, supporting, and affirming those decisions. Promoting self-determination in others demands that the nurse have a philosophy of free choice once the information necessary for decision making has been discussed.

Informing. Knowledge is essential but not sufficient to the outcome of decision making. The interpreting of knowledge is affected by the client's values and the meaning the client assigns to the knowledge. Informing clients about the nature of their choices, the content of those choices, and the consequences to the client is not a one-way activity. More active participation of clients in conversations with providers has been linked to better treatment compliance and health outcomes (Hibbard and Greene, 2013). Although the exchange may be initiated at the factual level, it will likely proceed to include the opinions of both parties—the client and the nurse (see the How To box on information exchange.

HOW TO Use the Information Exchange

Guidelines for exchanging information in the advocacy process include the nurse's responsibility to do the following:
1. Assess the client's present understanding of the situation.
2. Provide correct information.
3. Communicate with the client's literacy level in mind, making the information as understandable as possible.
4. Use a variety of media and sources to increase the client's comprehension.
5. Discuss other factors that affect the decision, such as financial, legal, and ethical issues.
6. Discuss the possible consequences of a decision.

Supporting. Upholding a client's right to make a choice and to act on the choice involves supporting. People who become aware of clients' decisions fall into three general groups: supporters, dissenters, and obstructers. Supporters approve and support the actions of the clients. *Dissenters* do not approve of and do not support the actions of the clients. *Obstructers* cause difficulties as clients try to implement their decisions. There is the need for the nurse advocate to assure clients that they have the right and responsibility to make decisions and reassure them that they do not have to change their decisions.

Affirming. Affirming is based on an advocate's belief that a client's decision is consistent with the client's values and goals. The advocate validates that the client's behavior is purposeful and consistent with the choice that was made. The advocate

expresses a dedication to the client's wishes; as a result, purposeful exchange of new information may occur so that the client's choice remains viable.

The importance of affirming activities cannot be emphasized strongly enough. It is not the advocate's role in the decision-making process to tell the client which option is "correct" or "right"; instead, the advocate's role involves the following:

- Providing the opportunity for information exchange, thus giving clients the tools that can empower them in making the best decision from their perspective.
- Enabling the client to make an "informed decision." This is a powerful tool for building self-confidence. It gives the client the responsibility for selecting the options and experiencing the success and consequences of the options based on current data.
- Empowering clients in their decision making when they can recognize events that are beyond their control and can link events that occur by chance with predictable events to make decisions they want.

Nurses can promote client decision making in the following ways:

- Using the information exchange process
- Promoting the use of the nursing process
- Including written techniques (i.e., contracts, lists)
- Using reflection and prioritizing decisions
- Using role playing to "try on" and determine the "fit" of different options and consequences for the client
- Helping clients recognize the progression of activities they experience as they build their "informed decision-making base"
- Empowering clients with skills that can strengthen their autonomy and confidence in the future

Advocacy is a complex process that maintains a delicate balance between "doing for" and "promoting autonomy." The process is influenced by the client's physical, emotional, and social abilities. The goal of advocacy is to promote the maximum degree of client self-determination possible for the client given the client's current and potential status; for most clients, this goal can be realized.

Skill Development

Skills needed by nurse advocates are not unique to their profession. Nursing demands scientific, technical, relationship, and problem-solving knowledge and skills. Advocacy applies nursing skills of communication and competency to promote client self-determination.

Knowledge of nursing and other disciplines, as well as of human behavior, is essential for the advocacy role in establishing authority, promoting authenticity, and developing skills. The capacity to be assertive for personal rights and the rights of others is essential.

Systematic Problem Solving

The nursing process—assessment, diagnosis, goal identification, planning, implementation, and evaluation—constitutes an example of a method of problem solving that can be used in the advocacy role. Advocates can be particularly helpful with clients in illuminating values and generating alternatives as described in the following sections.

Illuminating values. People's values affect their behavior, feelings, and goals. The advocate seeks to understand a client's values. The role of the advocate is to assist clients in discovering their values, which can be particularly demanding in the information exchange and affirming process. One way to help clients state their values is through a process called *clarification*. A simple way to do this is to ask questions such as the following:

• What are 10 things you enjoy doing?
• What are the most important things to you in life (e.g., family, money, happiness, health, comfort, pleasure, recognition)?
• How do you spend a typical day?

Generating alternatives. Clients and advocates may feel limited in their options if they generate solutions before completely analyzing the problems, needs, desires, and consequences. Several techniques can be used to generate alternatives, including brainstorming and a technique known as the problem-purpose-expansion method (Box 13.5).

Impact of Advocacy

Advocacy empowers clients to participate in problem-solving processes and decisions about health care. Clients try to understand changing opportunities in the health care system for access, use, and achieving continuity of care. Nurse advocates promote client self-determination and management of behavior as it relates to health and the adherence to therapeutic regimens. Clients are part of larger systems: the family, the work environment, and the community. Each system interacts with the client to shape the available options through resources, needs, and desires. Each system also has both confirming and conflicting goals and processes that need to be understood for client self-determination to be successful. For example, the practice of advocacy among minority groups may involve the ability to focus attention on the magnitude of problems caused by diseases affecting minority clients. Whether the client is an individual, family, group, or community, the advocacy function can promote the interest of self-determination that characterizes progressive societies.

Advocacy is not without opposition. Clients and advocates may find barriers to services, vendors, providers, and resources. A community may experience a shortage in nursing home beds, a childcare facility may experience staffing shortages, a family may not have the financial resources to keep a child at home, or a client may find that the school system cannot fund a full-time nurse for its clinic. The reality of scarce resources creates a difficult barrier for advocates. However, events such as these often stimulate a community's self-determination and lead to innovative actions to correct gaps in service (see the Levels of Prevention box).

Conflict Management

Case managers help clients manage conflicting needs and scarce resources. Mutual benefit with limited loss for everyone is a goal of conflict management. Techniques for managing conflict include the following:

• Using a range of active communication skills directed toward learning all parties' needs and desires
• Detecting areas of agreement and disagreement
• Determining abilities to collaborate
• Assisting in discovering alternatives and valuable activities for reaching a goal.

Negotiating is a strategic process used to move conflicting parties toward an outcome. Parties must see the possibility of achieving an agreement and the costs involved in not achieving an agreement. Preparations must be made as to time, place, and ground rules concerning participants, procedures, and confidentiality. In a conflict situation, parties engage in behaviors that reflect the dimensions of assertiveness and cooperation.

BOX 13.5 Techniques of Generating Alternatives for Problem Solving

Brainstorming
1. The nurse, client, professionals, or significant others generate as many alternatives as possible, without critical evaluation.
2. They examine the list for the critical elements the client seeks to preserve (e.g., environmental preferences, degree of control).
3. They analyze the list for consequences, the probability of chance events occurring, and the effect of the alternatives on self and others.

Problem-Purpose-Expansion Method
1. Restate the problem.
2. Expand the problem statement so different solutions can be generated. For example, if the purpose of the problem statement is to convince the insurance company to approve a longer hospital stay, the nurse and client have narrowed their options. If the purpose of the problem statement is to make the client's convalescence as beneficial and safe as possible, several solutions and options are available, as follows:
   • Obtaining skilled nursing facility placement
   • Obtaining home health skilled services
   • Arranging physician home visits
   • Paying for custodial care
   • Paying for private skilled care
   • Obtaining informal caregiving

 LEVELS OF PREVENTION
Related to Case Management

Primary Prevention
Use the information exchange process to increase the client's understanding of how to use the health care system and the health promotion strategies that will maintain health.

Secondary Prevention
Use case finding to identify existing health problems in your caseload and the population served by your agency. Timely, holistic assessments and interventions can slow disease trajectories and promote healing and health.

Tertiary Prevention
Monitor the use of prescription medications and adherence to treatment to reduce risk for illness complications. Use models such as the *CSMA Case Management Adherence Guidelines* at (http://www.cmsa.org) to prevent subsequent consequences of issues in medication compliance as part of the treatment plan. Institutionalize this model in your agency.

BOX 13.6 Categories Of Behaviors Used in Conflict Management

- **Competing:** An individual pursues personal concerns at another's expense.
- **Accommodating:** An individual neglects personal concerns to satisfy the concerns of another.
- **Avoiding:** An individual pursues neither personal concerns nor another's concerns.
- **Collaborating:** An individual attempts to work with others toward solutions that satisfy the work of both parties.
- **Compromising:** An individual attempts to find a mutually acceptable solution that partially satisfies both parties.

Modified from Thomas KW, Kilmann RH: *Thomas-Kilmann conflict mode instrument,* New York, 1974, Xicom. *History and Validity of the Thomas-Kilmann Conflict Mode Instrument (TKI).* Mountain View, CA, CPP, Inc. Retrieved January 2015 from: https://www.cpp.com/products/tki/tki_info.aspx.

Assertiveness is the ability to present one's own needs. **Cooperation** is the ability to understand and meet the needs of others. Behaviors seen in conflict management are described in Box 13.6. The Thomas-Kilmann categories of behaviors noted in this box, although written some time ago, outline a variety of behaviors that can be valuable in a given situation.

Clearly, flexibility in conflict management behavior can encourage an outcome that meets the client's goals. Helping parties navigate the process of reaching a goal requires effective personal relations, knowledge of the situation and alternatives, and a commitment to the process.

Collaboration

In case management, the activities of many disciplines (e.g., social workers, nurses, physicians, insurers, physical therapists) are needed for success. Clients, the family, significant others, payers, and community organizations contribute to achieving the goal. Collaboration is achieved through a developmental process. It occurs in a sequence, yet it is reciprocal between those involved.

The goal of communication in the collaborative development process is to promote respect for, understanding of, and the accuracy of all team members' points of view. Although communication is an essential component in collaboration, it is not sufficient to result in or maintain collaboration. Although the collaboration model recognizes the contributions inherent in joint decision making, one member of the team should be held accountable to the system and to the client. This team member should be responsible for monitoring the entire process.

Teamwork and collaboration clearly demand knowledge and skills about the following:
- Clients
- Health status
- Resources
- Treatments
- Community providers
- Clients' and families' complex needs
- Intrapersonal, interpersonal, medical, nursing, and social dimensions
- Team member and leadership skills

CASE STUDY

Defining Deficiencies through Case Management Activities

Through a nurse's case management activities, general community deficiencies in quality and quantity of health services are often discovered. When observing lack of care or services at the individual and family intervention levels, the nurse can, through case management, intervene at the community level to make changes.

George Stone is a nurse in community health practice working as a case manager for the pediatric asthmatic population. He is studying the use of service patterns among children with asthma. Mr. Stone would like to see if the services offered for asthmatic children are being used and, if not, the reasons they are underused.

Mr. Stone learns that many families without insurance are not using the free inhalers and spacers that the local Lion's Lodge provides to children without insurance. In fact, the families do not know this service exists. Mr. Stone makes it a priority to educate these families about this service so that they can save money and still receive the necessary medication for their children. Through school nurses, Mr. Stone identifies the current asthmatic students in the area who are eligible for free inhalers and spacers. Flyers are sent to their homes advertising the Lion's Lodge service. Mr. Stone also visits the physicians in the area who specialize in asthma. He educates the physicians and their staff about who is eligible for the free inhalers and spacers and how to get the service for their current and new clients. One year later, Mr. Stone collects new usage data and compares them with his original findings. He finds a 50% increase in families receiving inhalers and spacers from the Lion's Lodge.

It is unlikely that any single professional has the expertise required in all of these. It is likely, however, that the synergy produced by all involved can result in successful outcomes.

ISSUES IN CASE MANAGEMENT

Legal Issues

Liability concerns of case managers exist when the following three conditions are met:
1. The provider had a duty to provide reasonable care.
2. A breach occurred through an act or omission to act.
3. The act or omission caused injury or damage to the client.

Case managers must strive to reduce risks, practice wisely within acceptable standards, and limit legal defense costs through professional insurance coverage (Box 13.7).

Legal citings related to case management and managed care include the following:
- Negligent referrals
- Provider liability
- Payer liability
- Breach of contract
- Bad faith

As in any scope of nursing practice, proactive risk-management strategies can lower the provider's exposure to legal liability (Box 13.8). When courts find that cost considerations affect decisions related to medical care, all parties to the decision, such as the nurse, the agency, and all other health care providers, will be liable for any resulting damages.

Ethical Issues

Case managers as nursing professionals are guided in ethical practice by the *Code of Ethics for Nursing* (ANA, 2015) and the

BOX 13.7   Five General Areas Of Risk For Case Managers

1. Liability for managing care (Leonard and Miller, 2012; Sminkey and LeDoux, 2016)
   - Inappropriate design or implementation of the case management system
   - Failure to obtain all pertinent records on which case management actions are based
   - Failure to have cases evaluated by appropriately experienced and credentialed clinicians
   - Failure to confer directly with the treating provider at the onset of and throughout the client's care
   - Substituting a case manager's clinical judgment for that of the medical provider
   - Requiring the client or provider to accept case management recommendations instead of any other treatment
   - Harassment of clinicians, clients, and family in seeking information and setting unreasonable deadlines for decisions or information
   - Claiming orally or in writing that the case management treatment plan is better than the provider's plan
   - Restricting access to otherwise necessary or appropriate care because of cost
   - Referring clients to treatment furnished by providers who are associated with the case management agency without proper disclosure
   - Connecting case managers' compensation to reduced use and access
2. Negligent referrals (Leonard and Miller, 2012; Sminkey and LeDoux, 2016)
   - Referral to a practitioner known to be incompetent
   - Substituting inadequate treatment for an adequate but more costly option
   - Curtailing treatment inappropriately when curtailment caused the injury
   - Referral to a facility or practitioner inappropriate for the client's needs
   - Referral to another facility that lacks care requirements
3. Experimental treatment and technology (Sminkey and LeDoux, 2016)
   - Failure to apply the contractual definition of "experimental" treatment found in the client's insurance policy
   - Failure to review sources of information referenced in the client's insurance policy (e.g., Food and Drug Administration determination, published medical literature)
   - Failure to review the client's complete medical record
   - Failure to make a timely determination of benefits in light of timelines of treatment
   - Failure to communicate to the insured client or participant how coverage was determined
   - Improper financial considerations determining the coverage
4. Confidentiality (Leonard and Miller, 2012)
   - Failure to deny access to sensitive information awarded special protection by state law
   - Failure to protect access allowances to computerized medical records
   - Failure to adhere to regulations, such as the Health Insurance Portability and Accountability Act of 1996 (HIPAA) and the Americans with Disabilities Act
5. Fraud and abuse (Leonard and Miller, 2012)
   - Making false statements on claims or causing incorrect claims to be filed
   - Falsifying the adherence to conditions of participation of Medicare and Medicaid
   - Submitting claims for excessive, unnecessary, or poor-quality services
   - Engaging in payment, bribes, kickbacks, or rebates in exchange for referral
   - Coding intervention requirements improperly

BOX 13.8   Elements That Reduce Risk Exposure

1. Clear documentation of the extent of participation in decision making and the reasons for decisions
2. Records demonstrating accurate and complete information on interactions and outcomes
3. Use of reasonable care in selecting referral sources, which may include verification of the provider licensure
4. Written agreements when arrangements are made to modify benefits other than those in the contract
5. Good communication with clients
6. Informing clients of their rights of appeal

Code of Professional Conduct for Case Managers (Commission for Case Manager Certification [CCMC], 2015), by performance indicators for ethics in the *Standards of Practice for Case Management* (CMSA, 2016), and by the contract expressed in the *Nursing's Social Policy Statement*:

Nursing is the protection, promotion, and optimization of health and abilities, prevention of illness and injury, alleviation of suffering through the diagnosis and treatment of human response, and advocacy in the care of individuals, families, communities and populations

(ANA, 2010, p 2)

This contractual philosophy of nursing practice is ideally suited to preserving the principles of autonomy, beneficence, and justice in the case management processes. Leonard and Miller

(2012) and Sminkey and LeDoux (2016) describe how case managers may confront dilemmas in each of these areas, as follows:

- Case management may hamper a client's autonomy of individual right to choose a provider if a particular provider is not approved by the case management system. If a new provider must be found who can be approved for coverage, continuity of care may be disrupted.
- Beneficence, or doing good, can be impaired when excessive attention to containing costs supersedes or impairs the nurse's duty to improve health or relieve suffering.
- Justice, as an ethical principle for case managers, considers equal distribution of health care with reasonable quality. Tiers of quality and expertise among provider groups can be created when quality providers refuse to accept reimbursement allowances from the managed system, leaving less-experienced or lower-quality providers as the caregiver of choice for clients being managed.
- Nonmaleficence is "doing no harm." When case managers incorporate outcomes measures, evidence-based practice, and monitoring progress in their plans of care, this principle is addressed.
- Veracity, or truth telling, is absolutely necessary to the practice of advocacy and building a trusting relationship with a client. Clients particularly complain that in the changing health care system, payers do not seem to be able to provide comprehensive yet inexpensive options for care.

Maintaining familiarity with ethical issues published in the case management literature can offer specific assistance for practicing case managers.

⟫ APPLYING CONTENT TO PRACTICE

The clinical practice skill of advocacy is an inherent concept in the practice of case management. Of the 16 interventions by public health nurses described in the Wheel of Intervention model, both advocacy and case management are described in accordance with best practices and operational definitions of 3 of the 16 interventions. Advocacy can be applied at the community, systems, individual, or family level. In fact, when a public health nurse advocates for clients at any of these levels, the source of conflict and collaboration will likely come from competing values, that is, those of the client and any of the other levels of population values. For example:

- A client may want access to unlimited treatment, but financial values may pose a source of conflict as the system attempts to justify the comparative effectiveness or costs.

- Family members may pose conflicting values for the nature of care they wish a family member to receive, even as the client refuses care.
- Communities can divert budget allotments to needs that are in competition for other population services such as community policing, health care access, and environmental services.

The nurse as advocate must listen carefully to his or her client in order to truly represent the interest of the client and encourage "win-win" processes and outcomes for the client. Advocacy occurs in all three of the core functions of public health: assessment, policy development, and assurance.

▮ CLINICAL APPLICATION

During her visit to the regularly scheduled blood pressure clinic in a local apartment cluster, Mrs. Barnes, a 45-year-old woman, complained of feeling dizzy and forgetful. She could not remember which of her six medications she had taken during the past few days. Her blood pressure readings on reclining, sitting, and standing revealed extreme elevations. The nurse and Mrs. Barnes discussed the danger of her present status and the need to seek medical attention. Mrs. Barnes called her physician from her apartment and agreed to be transported to the emergency department.

While in the emergency department, Mrs. Barnes manifested the progressive signs and symptoms of a cerebrovascular accident (CVA, stroke). During hospitalization, she lost her capacity for expressive language and demonstrated hemiparesis and loss of bladder control. Her cognitive function became intermittently confused, and she was slow to recognize her physician and neighbors who came to visit. The utilization management nurse contacted the case manager from the health department to screen and

assess for the continuum of care needs as early as possible because Mrs. Barnes lived alone and family members resided out of town.

It became apparent that family caregiving in the community could be only intermittent because members lived too far away. Mrs. Barnes had residual functional and cognitive deficits that would demand longer-term care.

As the case manager contracted by the plan, place the following actions in the sequence needed to construct a case management plan:
A. Discuss with the family their schedule of availability to offer care in the client's home.
B. Call the client and introduce yourself as a prelude to working with her.
C. Obtain information on the scope of services covered by the benefit plan for your client.
D. Arrange a skilled nursing facility site visit for the patient and family.
Answers can be found on the Evolve website.

▮ REMEMBER THIS!

- An important role of the nurse in community health is that of client advocate.
- The goal of advocacy is to promote the client's self-determination.
- When performing in the advocacy role, conflicts may emerge regarding the full disclosure of information, territoriality, accountability to multiple parties, legal challenges to client's decisions, and competition for scarce resources.
- The functions of advocacy and allocation can pose dilemmas in practice.
- Skills important in fulfilling the role of client advocate include the helping relationship, assertiveness, and problem solving.
- Problem solving is a systematic approach that includes understanding the values of each party and generating alternative solutions.
- Brainstorming and the problem-purpose-expansion method are two techniques to enhance the effectiveness of problem-solving skills.
- During conflict, negotiations can move conflicting parties toward an outcome.
- Care management is a strategic program to maintain the health of a population enrolled in a health care delivery system.

- Continuity of care is a goal of community health nursing practice. It requires making linkages with services to improve the client's health status.
- As the structure of the health care system moves toward delivering more services in the community, the achievement of continuity of care will present a greater challenge.
- Case management is typically an interdisciplinary process in which the client is the focus of the plan.
- Documenting case management activities and outcomes is essential to nursing practice in the community.
- Case management is a systematic process of assessment, planning, service coordination, referral, monitoring, and evaluation that meets the multiple service needs of clients.
- Nurses in community health have advocacy and case management functions within their scope of practice.
- Nurses functioning as advocates and case managers need to be aware of the ethical and legal issues confronting their practice.
- Standardization of care for predictable outcomes can be achieved through critical paths, disease management protocols, and multidisciplinary action plans.
- Telehealth application provides new alternatives within resource delivery options but must be customized for clients.

EVOLVE WEBSITE

http://evolve.elsevier.com/Stanhope/foundations
- Case Study, with Questions and Answers
- NCLEX® Review Questions
- Practice Application Answers

REFERENCES

Agency for Healthcare Research and Quality: *Health Care Innovations Exchange: Community-based health coaches and care coordinators reduce readmissions using information technology to identify and support at-risk Medicare patients after discharge*, Rockville, Md, 2016. AHRQ. Retrieved July 2016 from http://www.innovations.ahrq.gov.

American Hospital Association: *Guide to the health care field*, Chicago, 2016, AHA.

American Nurses Association (ANA): *Framework for Measuring Nurses' Contributions to Care Coordination,* Silver Spring, MD, 2013, ANA.

American Nurses Association: *Code of ethics for nursing, with interpretive statements*, Silver Spring, Md, 2015, ANA.

American Nurses Association: *Nursing's social policy statement*, ed 3, Silver Spring, Md, 2010, Nursing Books.

Apuna-Grummer D, Howland WA: *A core curriculum for nurse life care planning*, Bloomington, IN, 2013, American Association of Nurse Life Care Planners.

Berkowitz AL: Managing acute stroke in low-resource settings, *Bulletin of the World Health Organization*, 94:554–556, 2016.

Caloyeras JP, Hangsheng L, Exum E, Broderick M, Mattke S: Managing manifest diseases, but not health risks, saved PepsiCo money over seven years, *Health Aff* 33:124–131, 2014.

Carneal G, Pock R: Six year of study reveals the impact of IT on the practice of case management, *CMSA Today* 2:16–17, 2014.

Cary AH: Advocacy or allocation, *Nurs Connect* 11:1, 1998.

Case Management Society of America: *Standards of practice for case management*, Little Rock, Ark, 2016, CMSA.

Choi PP: Patient advocacy: the role of the nurse, *Nurs Stand* 29: 52–58, 2015.

Christopher MA, Hawkey R, Jared MC: Lillian D. Wald: pioneer of public health. In Forrester DA, editor: *Nursing's greatest leaders: a history of activism*, New York, NY, 2016, Springer.

Commission for Case Manager Certification: *Code of professional conduct for case managers with standards, rules, procedures, and penalties*, Mt. Laurel, NJ, 2015, CCMC.

Day SM, Reynolds RJ, Kush SJ: The relationship of life expectancy to the development and valuation of life care plans, *NeuroRehabilitation* 36:253–266, 2015.

Hibbard JH, Greene J: What the evidence shows about patient activation: better health outcomes and care experiences; fewer data on costs, *Health Aff* 32:207–214, 2013.

Hisashige A: The effectiveness and efficiency of disease management programs for patients with chronic diseases, *Glob J Health Sci* 5:27–48, 2012.

Huber DL: *Leadership & nursing care management*, ed 5, St Louis, MO, 2014, Elsevier Saunders.

Institute of Medicine (IOM): *The Future of Nursing: Leading Change, Advancing Health,* Washington, DC, 2011, National Academies Press.

Keller LO, et al: Population-based public health interventions: innovations in practice, teaching and management, part II, *Public Health Nurs* 21:469–487, 2004.

Kizer KW: Clinical integration: a cornerstone for population health management, *J Health Manag* 60:165–168, 2015.

Kohnke MF: *Advocacy risk and reality*, St Louis, 1982, Mosby.

Lamb G: *Care Coordination: The Game Changer*, Silver Spring, MD, 2013, Nursesbooks.org.

Leonard M, Miller E: *Nursing case management: review and resource manual*, ed 4, Silver Spring, MD, 2012, American Nurses Credentialing Center.

Mallik M, Rafferty AM: Diffusion of the concept of advocacy, *J Adv Nurs* 32:399–404, 2000.

McKesson Corporation: *How Care Management Evolves with Population Management—A White Paper.* 2014. Retrieved January 2015 from http://www.healthleadersmedia.com/content/SPR-300965/How-Care-Management-Evolves-with-Population-Management.

Minnesota Department of Health: *Public health interventions: applications for public health nursing practice*, St. Paul, Minn, 2003, Minnesota Department of Health.

Mullahy CM: *The case manager's handbook*, ed 6, Burlington, MA, 2017, Jones & Bartlett Learning.

Nelson ML: Advocacy in nursing, *Nurs Outlook* 36:136–141, 1988.

Newman MB, Kowlsen T, Beckworth V: An integrated approach: the impact of health care reform from a managed care perspective, *CMSA Today* 1:20–23, 2014.

Noonan P: The case manager's role in population health, *CSMA Today* 3:16–17, 2014.

Pawson R, Greenhalgh J, Brennan C: Demand management for planned care: a realist synthesis, *Health Services and Delivery Research* 4:1–21, 2016.

Quad Council: *Quad Council Competencies for Public Health Nursing.* 2011. Retrieved January 2015 from http://www. achne.org/files/Quad%20Council/ QuadCouncilCompetenciesforPublicHealthNurses.pdf.

Rutherford-Owen T, Marini I: Life care planimplementation among adults with spinal cord injuries, *J Life Care Planning* 10:5–20, 2012.

Sminkey PV, LeDoux J: Case management ethics: high professional standards for health care's interconnected worlds, *Prof Case Manag* 21:193–198, 2016.

Smith AP: Patient advocacy: roles for nurses and leaders, *Nurs Econ* March-April, 2004. Retrieved January 2011 from http://findarticles.com/p/articles/mi_m0FSW/is_2_22/ai_n17206874/?tag=rbxcra.2.a.44.

Stricker P: Data analytics: a critical tool, *CMSA Today* 4:20–23, 2014.

Tahan H, Watson A, Sminkey PV: What case managers should know about their roles and functions: a national study from the Commission for Case Manager Certification, *Prof Case Manag* 20:271–296, 2015.

Thomas KW, Kilmann RH: *Thomas-Kilmann conflict mode instrument*, New York, 1974, X.com. History and Validity of the Thomas-Kilmann Conflict Mode Instrument (TKI). Mountain View, CA, CPP, Inc. Retrieved January 2015 from https:// www.cpp.com/products/tki/tki_info.aspx.

Treiger TM: Case management today and its evolution into the future, *CMSA Today* 7:16–20, 2013.

U.S. Department of Health and Human Services: *Healthy People 2020: a roadmap for health*, Washington, DC, 2010, U.S. Government Printing Office.

Watts SA, Sood A: Diabetes nurse case management: improving glucose control: 10 years of quality improvement follow-up data, *Appl Nurs Res* 29:202–205, 2016.

14 | CHAPTER

Disaster Management

Sharon A. R. Stanley, Sharon L. Farra, Susan B. Hassmiller

OBJECTIVES

After reading this chapter, the student should be able to:

1. Discuss types of disasters, including natural and human-made.
2. Evaluate the effects of disasters on people and their communities.
3. Describe the disaster management phases of prevent, preparedness, response, and recovery, and explain the nurse's role in each phase.
4. Describe the steps to take to initiate and maintain a disaster clinic.
5. Identify how community groups and other organizations such as the American Red Cross can work together to prepare for, respond to, and recover from disasters.

CHAPTER OUTLINE

Disasters
   Healthy People 2020 Objectives
The Disaster Management Cycle and the Nursing Role
   Prevention (Mitigation)

Preparedness
Response
Recovery
Future of Disaster Management

KEY TERMS

chemical, biological, radiological, nuclear, and explosive (CBRNE) disasters, 241
community emergency response team (CERT), 241
delayed stress reactions, 250
disaster, 236
disaster medical assistance teams (DMATs), 241
Emergency Support Function 8: Public Health and Medical (ESF), 238

Homeland Security Act of 2002, 238
human-made disasters, 236
Medical Reserve Corps (MRC), 241
mitigation, 239
National Health Security Strategy (NHSS), 243
National Preparedness Guidelines (NPG), 238
National Preparedness Goal, 238
National Response Framework (NRF), 238
natural disasters, 237

Pandemic and All-Hazards Preparedness Reauthorization Act (PAHPRA), 238
preparedness, 240
Presidential Policy Directive 8: National Preparedness, 238
prevention, 239
rapid needs assessment, 239
recovery, 250
response, 244
triage, 239

Around the world, people are experiencing unprecedented disasters from natural causes such as hurricanes, earthquakes, and tsunamis that can lead to nuclear power plant meltdowns, human-made disasters (e.g., oil spills), and acts of terrorism. Disasters occur suddenly and unexpectedly, and they often cannot be prevented. However, communities can be helped to prepare for, respond to, and recover from disaster. This chapter describes management techniques to be used in the prevention, preparedness, response, and recovery phases of disaster. The nursing role is discussed for each phase.

DISASTERS

A disaster is any **natural** or human-made incident that causes disruption, destruction, or devastation requiring external assistance. Disasters can affect a single family or a small group, as in a house fire, or they can kill thousands and have economic losses in the millions, as with floods, earthquakes, tornadoes, hurricanes, and bioterrorism. Disasters are expensive in terms of lives affected and property lost or damaged. Although natural events such as earthquakes or hurricanes often trigger disasters, predictable and preventable human-made factors can

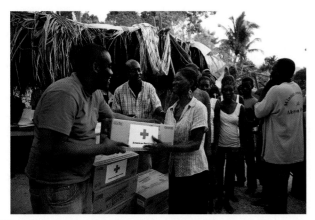

FIG. 14.1 One week after the earthquake struck and tsunami surged through northeastern Japan, a Japanese Red Cross volunteer surveys the damage to Otsuchi in Iwate Prefecture. (Courtesy of the American Red Cross Disaster Online Newsroom, Washington, DC. Retrieved January 2015 from http://newroom.redcross.org).

increase the effect of the disaster. Each year hurricanes in the United States batter the coasts and inland areas. A 9.0 magnitude earthquake struck Northeastern Japan on March 11, 2011. The earthquake was quickly followed by a tsunami (Fig. 14.1). These dual natural disasters caused an estimated death toll of 20,000, but there was a third, human-made component to complete the incident triad: a nuclear reactor crisis. An independent parliamentary investigation later found the Fukushima nuclear disaster to be the result of a mix of several human-made factors (Inajima et al, 2012). Box 14.1 lists examples of natural and human-made disasters.

Unfortunately, developing countries experience a disproportionate burden from natural disasters. These countries are usually poor and have limited resources for dealing with the effects of the disaster. To add to the misery, the governments of some countries thwart the efforts of international aid workers to bring relief to their people, as seen in recent years in Syria. Disasters have political aspects in addition to the enormous losses to the people. For example, some countries will not accept aid from nations they do not consider their allies or supporters.

The urbanization and overcrowding of cities have increased the danger of natural disasters because communities have been built in areas that are vulnerable to disaster, such as in known tornado zones or near rivers or flood plains. Increases in population and developing for habitation of areas vulnerable to natural disasters have led to major increases in insurance payouts in the United States in every decade. Projections suggest that by 2050, at least 46% of the world's population will live in areas vulnerable to natural floods, earthquakes, and severe storms.

In recent years, we have learned more about what is called a "complex humanitarian emergency (CHE). These emergencies result from a "humanitarian crisis in a country, region or society where there is total or considerable breakdown of authority resulting from internal or external conflict and which requires an international response that goes beyond the mandate or capacity of any single and/or ongoing UN country programme" (Downes, 2015, p. 12). Downes developed a course at Emory University in Atlanta, Georgia, to teach health care students to learn how to respond when a CHE occurred. She used the example of the Ebola outbreak in West Africa in 2015. She noted that the countries most affected by the Ebola virus were those with a long history of political instability and weak health systems. The students in the course learned not only about the complexity of health care in an emergency setting, but they also learned how central the nursing role was to dealing with the emergency.

Overcrowding and urban development have also increased human-made disasters. The stress caused by overcrowding has caused civil unrest and riots. In some parts of the world, modern wars waged over land rights and space have markedly

---

BOX 14.1 Types of Disasters

Natural	Human-Made
• Hurricanes	• Conventional warfare
• Tornadoes	• Nonconventional warfare (e.g., nuclear, chemical)
• Hailstorms	• Transportation accidents
• Cyclones	• Structural collapse
• Blizzards	• Explosions and bombings
• Droughts	• Fires
• Floods	• Hazardous materials incident
• Mudslides	• Pollution
• Avalanches	• Civil unrest (e.g., riots)
• Earthquakes	• Terrorism (e.g., chemical, biological, radiological, nuclear, explosives)
• Volcanic eruptions	• Cyberattacks
• Communicable disease epidemics	• Airplane crashes
• Lightning-induced forest fires	• Radiological incidents
• Tsunamis	• Nuclear power plant incidents
• Thunderstorms and lightning	• Critical infrastructure failures
• Extreme heat and cold	• Water supply contamination

From U.S. Department of Health and Human Services: Healthy People 2020: a roadmap to improve all Americans' health, Washington, DC, 2010, USDHHS.

increased the risk for injury and death from disaster. In the United States and other countries, school violence, a human-made disaster, has increased in intensity and magnitude. Disaster recovery efforts are expensive, and the costs are growing because of the number of people involved and the amount of technology that must be restored. People in industrialized countries are becoming less self-sufficient because they rely heavily on technology and social and economic systems within their community. People who live on the brink of disaster every day, physically, emotionally, or economically, are among the first to be affected when disaster strikes.

Although the number of disasters worldwide continues to grow, the number of lives lost has decreased. The increase in the number of lives saved may be due to better disaster forecasting and early warning systems that help people better prepare for the impending disaster. Disaster disproportionably strikes at-risk individuals, whether their day-to-day risk is physical, emotional, or economic. Disasters in less developed communities can also destroy decades of progress in a matter of hours, in a manner that rarely happens in more developed countries. The poor, elderly, ethnic minorities, people with disabilities, and women and children in developing communities are excessively affected and least able to rebound (World Health Organization, 2012). Economic losses from disasters such as tsunamis, cyclones, earthquakes and flooding now reach an annual average of US $250 to $300 billion. Also, the mortality and economic loss associated with risk in low- and middle-income countries are increasing. Unfortunately, by 2050, the percentages of population areas more vulnerable to disasters will increase. Eighty percent of the world's population will live in developing countries, with 46% living in tornado and earthquake zones, near rivers, and on coastlines (UNISDR, 2015; Dilley et al, 2005).

Although natural disasters cannot be prevented, much can be done to prevent further increases in accidents, death, and destruction after impact. A concise, realistic, and well-rehearsed disaster plan is essential. Open, clear, and ongoing communication among involved workers and organizations is critical. Also, many of the human-made disasters listed in Box 14.1 can be prevented (e.g., major transportation accidents and fires resulting from substance abuse).

The U.S. Department of Homeland Security (DHS) was created through the Homeland Security Act of 2002 (DHS, 2008a), consolidating more than 20 separate agencies. Presidential Policy Directive 8: National Preparedness (PPD-8) was signed and released by President Barack Obama on March 30, 2011. PPD-8 replaced Homeland Security Presidential Directive 8 from the Bush era, and guides how the nation, from the federal level to private citizens, can "prevent, protect against, mitigate the effects of, respond to, and recover from those threats that pose the greatest risk to the security of the Nation" (DHS, 2011). The National Preparedness Guidelines (NPG) (DHS, 2015) and the National Response Plan (NRP), which provide a national doctrine for preparedness that includes the National Response Framework [NRF]), was promulgated in January 2008. The second edition of the National Response Framework, updated in 2013, provides context for how the whole community works together and how response

efforts relate to other parts of national preparedness (DHS, 2013). Each of the five frameworks covers one mission area: Prevention, Protection, Mitigation, Response, or Recovery. In that framework, there are also 15 emergency support functions. Emergency Support Function 8: Public Health and Medical provides coordinated federal assistance to supplement state, local, and tribal resources in response to public health and medical care needs (Federal Emergency Management Agency [FEMA], 2016).

The National Preparedness Goal was first released in September 2011, and the second edition in 2015 maintains the goal of "A secure and resilient nation with the capabilities required across the whole community to prevent, protect against, mitigate, respond to, and recover from the threats and hazards that pose the greatest risk" (FEMA, 2015, p. 1). The five mission areas in the goal are the same five frameworks in the National Response Framework.

Homeland Security Presidential Directive 5 (HSPD 5) directed the Secretary of Homeland Security to develop and administer the National Incident Management System (NIMS), a unified, all-discipline, and all-hazards approach to domestic incident management (FEMA, 2017). The NIMS was established to provide a common language and structure to help those involved in disaster response to communicate together more effectively and efficiently.

Two national preparedness documents specifically guide disaster health preparedness, response, and recovery: HSPD 21: Public Health and Medical Preparedness and the National Health Security Strategy (NHSS). HSPD 21 established a national strategy that enables a level of public health and medical preparedness sufficient to address a range of possible disasters. It does so through four critical components of public health and medical preparedness: (1) biosurveillance, (2) countermeasure distribution, (3) mass casualty care, and (4) community resilience. The NHSS focuses on the national goals for protecting people's health in the case of disaster in any setting. The U.S. system for homeland security includes public health preparedness and response as a core part of its national strategies. Every aspect of disaster management involves public health nursing. The NHSS was directed by the 2006 Pandemic and All-Hazards Preparedness Act (PAHPA). The goal of this act is to improve the nation's ability to detect, prepare for, and respond to a variety of public health emergencies. The PAHPA was reenacted in 2013 and is now called the Pandemic and All-Hazards Preparedness Reauthorization Act (PAHPRA). The PAHPRA funds public health and hospital preparedness programs, medical countermeasures under the BioShield Project, and enhances the authority of the Food and Drug Administration (FDA) (USDHHS, 2017).

Healthy People 2020 Objectives

Because disasters affect the health of people in many ways, they have an effect on almost every *Healthy People 2020* objective. Disasters clearly affect the objectives that relate to unintentional injuries, occupational safety and health, environmental health, and food and drug safety. Disasters affect many of the objectives in the areas of Access to Health Services and Public Health

Infrastructure (USDHHS, 2010). In the past few years, with the many incidents and scares related to possible bioterrorism, people have become even more aware of the importance of disaster preparedness and how the things they take for granted such as safe food, water, and housing can be threatened. Public health professionals study the effect that disasters have on population health and develop new prevention strategies. Other organizations, such as the American Red Cross (ARC), work with communities in the preparedness, response, and recovery phases of a disaster. The Healthy People 2020 box provides examples of objectives related to disaster mitigation.

THE DISASTER MANAGEMENT CYCLE AND THE NURSING ROLE

Disaster management includes four stages: prevention (including mitigation and protection), preparedness, response, and recovery. Fig. 14.2 shows the disaster management cycle. Nurses have skills that enable them to work in all aspects of disasters, such as assessment, priority setting, collaboration, health education, disease screening, and mass clinic expertise. Nurses also have the ability to provide essential public health services, make referrals, serve as a liaison among organizations and health care and social service providers, and provide psychological first aid, triage, and rapid needs assessment.

Prevention (Mitigation and Protection)

All-hazards mitigation (prevention) is an emergency management term for reducing risks to people and property from natural hazards before they occur. Prevention can include structural measures, such as protecting buildings and infrastructure from the forces of wind and water, and nonstructural measures, such as land development restrictions. Prevention

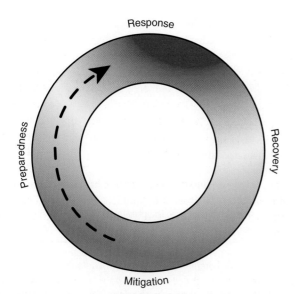

FIG. 14.2 Disaster management cycle. (From Ontario Agency for Health Protection and Promotion [Public Health Ontario]. Public health emergency preparedness: an IMS-based workshop. Base scenario, Toronto, ON: Queen's Printer for Ontario, 2015 July (p. 7).

also includes human-made hazards and the ability to deter potential terrorists, detect terrorists before they strike, and take action to eliminate the threat (DHS, 2007). Prevention activities may include heightened inspections; improved surveillance and security operations; public health and agricultural surveillance and testing; immunizations, isolation, or quarantine; and halting chemical, biological, radiological, nuclear, and explosive (CBRNE) threats (DHS, 2007). The nurse should be familiar with the region's local cache of pharmaceuticals and how the Strategic National Stockpile (SNS) will be distributed. Nurses are involved in many aspects of prevention, including the following:

- **Awareness and education:** Holding or attending community meetings on disaster preparedness, including informing the community about the many educational resources available to them. One resource is an in-depth citizen guide for preparing for a disaster called "Are you ready?" The guide is available at http://www.fema.gov.
- **Organizing and participating** in mass prophylaxis and vaccination campaigns to prevent, treat, or contain disease.
- **Advocacy** identifying environmental hazards, serving on the public health team for mitigation work, supporting actions and efforts for effective building codes and proper land use.

Because disasters are both natural and human-made, nurses need to assess for and report environmental health hazards, including unsafe equipment and faulty structures. They must be aware of high-risk targets and current vulnerabilities and what can be done to eliminate or mitigate the vulnerability. Targets may include military and civilian government facilities, health care facilities, international airports and other transportation systems, large cities, and high-profile landmarks. Terrorists might also target large public gatherings, water and food supplies, banking and finance, information technology, postal and shipping services, utilities, and corporate centers (DHS, 2007).

Preparedness
Personal Preparedness

Nurses who are disaster victims themselves and must provide care to others will experience considerable stress. Conflicts between family and work-related duties are inevitable. For example, a nurse who is also the mother of a young child will not be able to participate fully, if at all, in disaster relief efforts until she has made arrangements for her child. Advance personal and family preparation can help ease some of the conflicts that arise and allow nurses to attend to client needs sooner. In addition, the nurse assisting in disaster relief efforts must be as healthy as possible, both physically and mentally, to serve clients, families, and other disaster victims.

Disasters require nurses to respond quickly. Public health nurses need to have their own personal plans in place before a disaster. Preparedness is multifaceted. The family of each nurse must also be included and informed about the disaster plan. One way a nurse can ensure that his or her family is protected is by providing them with the skills and knowledge to help them cope with a disaster. Long-term benefits will come by involving children or adolescents in activities such as writing preparedness or response plans, rehearsing the plan, preparing disaster kits, becoming familiar with their school emergency plan and where families should reunite in the event of an emergency, finding out where the evacuation shelters are located and identifying the evacuation routes, and learning about the range of potential hazards in their vicinity. Natural and human-made hazards, including terrorism, should be discussed. Vulnerable types of infrastructure such as dams, chemical plants, bridges, and transportation should be pointed out. Discussion offers children and adolescents an opportunity to express their feelings. The ability to control as much as they can during each phase of a disaster provides them with the ability to bounce back (Figure 14.3). The How To box is an excellent guide for developing and putting together the supplies needed for a disaster plan.

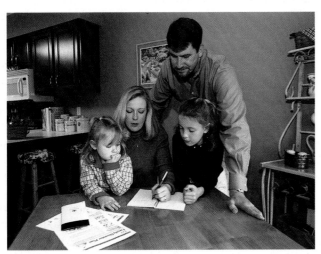

FIG. 14.3 Personal preparedness. Public health nurses need to develop their own disaster plan as a part of their community disaster activities. (Courtesy of the Wichita Falls Health District, Wichita Falls, TX. Retrieved January 2015 from http://tx-wichitafalls2. civicplus.com/index.aspx?NID=1301).

HOW TO Be Red Cross Ready
1. Get a Kit
   Consider the following when assembling or restocking your kit to ensure that you and your family are prepared for any disaster:
   - Store at least 3 days of food, water, and supplies in your family's easy-to-carry preparedness kit. Keep extra supplies on hand at home in case you cannot leave the affected area.
   - Keep your kit where it is easily accessible.
   - Remember to check your kit every 6 months and replace expired or outdated items.
2. Make a Plan
   When preparing for a disaster, always:
   - Talk with your family.
   - Plan.
   - Learn how and when to turn off utilities and how to use life-saving tools such as fire extinguishers.
   - Tell everyone where emergency information and supplies are stored. Provide copies of the family's preparedness plan to each member of the family. Always ensure that information is up to date and practice evacuations, following the routes outlined in your plan. Don't forget to identify alternative routes.
   - Include pets in your evacuation plans.
3. Get Informed
   There are three key parts to becoming informed:
   - Get Info: Learn the ways you would get information during a disaster or an emergency.
   - Know Your Region: Learn about the disasters that may occur in your area.
   - Action Steps: Learn first aid from your local ARC chapter.

Emergency Supplies That Nurses Should Have Ready
- Identification badge and driver's license
- Proof of licensure and certification (e.g., RN, CPR/AED, First Aid)
- Pocket-size reference books (e.g., nursing protocols and intervention standards)

Blood Pressure Cuff (Adult and Child) and Stethoscope
- Gloves, mask, and other personal protective equipment (PPE) for general care
- First aid kit with mouth-to-mouth cardiopulmonary resuscitation (CPR) barrier
- Radio with batteries and cell phone charger
- Cash, credit card
- Important papers and contact information in hard copy
- Sun protection
- Sturdy shoes with socks
- Medical identification of allergies, blood type
- Medications for self
- Weather-appropriate clothing to include rain gear
- Toiletries
- Watch, cell phone, PDA with preentered emergency numbers
- Flashlight, extra batteries
- Record-keeping materials, including pencil/pen
- Map of area

(Courtesy of the American Red Cross. Retrieved January 2016 from http://www.redcross.org/flash/brr/english-html/default.asp).

In addition to the items in the How To box, include these items:
- A change of clothing and protective footwear per person and one blanket or sleeping bag per person.
- A manual can opener

- A first-aid kit that includes 1 week's supply of your family's prescription medications and over-the-counter medications you take. Make a list of your medications and dosages, allergies, and physician names.
- Candles and matches.
- Sanitation supplies, including toilet paper, soap, feminine hygiene items, and plastic garbage bags.
- Special items for infants, older adults, or disabled family members.
- An extra pair of eyeglasses.
- Pet supplies if you have animals.
- Documents: Identification, passport, birth certificate, insurance policies, family contact information, local maps with marked evacuation routes, some money.
- Gather emergency supplies, and store them in a sturdy, easy-to-carry container. Keep important documents in a waterproof container.

Nurses should consider several contingencies for children and seniors with a plan to seek help from neighbors in the event of being called to a disaster. Many special-needs shelters encourage preregistration for physically or mentally challenged people. Because most shelters do not allow pets other than "pocket" pets, other arrangements will need to be made, such as going to a special pet shelter or placing the pet in a bathroom with sufficient food and water. A note should be placed on the front door for emergency personnel as to where the pet might be found. Currently, many local emergency management offices are considering incorporating pets into the local disaster plans. Useful sites for information about being prepared are as follows:

Prepare for emergencies now: Information for people with disabilities. https://www.fema.gov/media-library/assets/documents/90360.

Professional Preparedness

One of the essentials for baccalaureate prepared nurses is to be informed about disaster preparedness. Public health nurses need to be aware of and understand the disaster plans at the workplace and in the community. These nurses take time to read and understand workplace and community disaster plans and participate in disaster drills and community mock disasters. Adequately prepared nurses can serve as leaders and enable others to have a smoother recovery phase.

Disaster management in the community is about population health, and the three core public health functions are used just as in day-to-day operations. You would rely on assessment, policy development, and assurance in disaster work. Although disaster work is not highly technological, there is increasing information provided in a wireless format. Fieldwork, including shelter management, requires that nurses be creative and willing to improvise in delivering care. All workers should be certified in first aid and CPR. In addition, the ARC provides a comprehensive program of disaster training for health professionals, to enable them to provide assistance within their own communities and to other affected communities and countries. The courses teach nurses how to adapt their existing nursing skills to a disaster setting and to the scope of ARC

disaster nursing. Note that the knowledge the nurse will need for chemical, biological, radiological, nuclear, and explosive (CBRNE) disasters and those involving weapons of mass destruction (WMD) requires a base of specialized information. Box 14.2 describes competencies for all public health workers in the event of a disaster.

Nurses who want to know more about disaster management and be more actively involved can become involved in several community organizations. The National Disaster Medical System (NDMS) enables nurses to work on specialized teams such as the Disaster Medical Assistance Team (DMAT). In a presidentially declared disaster, including overseas war, the U.S. Public Health Service can activate disaster medical assistance teams (DMATs) to an area to supplement local and state medical care needs. DMATs can also be activated by the Assistant Secretary for Health if requested to do so by a state health officer. Teams of specially trained civilian physicians, nurses, and other health care personnel can be sent to a disaster site within hours of activation. DMATs can provide triage and continuing medical care to victims until they can be evacuated to a national network of hospitals prearranged by the NDMS (DHS, 2015). Because of the nature of this country's disasters since the initiation of DMATs, these teams have been used primarily to staff community health outpatient clinics in the affected areas. The Medical Reserve Corps (MRC) and the Community Emergency Response Team (CERT) provide opportunities for nurses to support emergency preparedness and response in their local jurisdictions. The ARC offers training in disaster health services and disaster mental health for both response in local jurisdictions and national deployment opportunities. After participation in disaster training, nurses can take the following steps: join a local disaster action team, act as a liaison with local hospitals, determine health-services support for shelter

---

BOX 14.3   Websites Providing Education and Training Opportunities

Public Health Workforce Development Centers
- Centers for Disease Control and Prevention: https://www.slu.edu/public-health-social-justice/training/center_heartlandphp
- Heartland Centers for Public Health and Community Capacity Development: http://www.heartlandcenters.slu.edu/
- National Public Health Training Centers Network, HRSA: http://bhpr.hrsa.gov/grants/publichealth/trainingcenters/index.html
- Northwest Center for Public Health Practice: http://www.nwcphp.org/training

Government and Other Nurse-Specific Courses
- American Red Cross Disaster Health and Sheltering Course for Nursing Students: http://www.drc-group.com/library/exercise/osc/OSC-DHS-FactSheet.pdf
- Emergency Management Institute: http://training.fema.gov/
- Federal Emergency Management Agency (FEMA) Training: http://www.fema.gov/prepared/train.shtm
- National Nurse Emergency Preparedness Initiative: http://www.nnepi.org/

Public Health Organizations
- American Public Health Association (APHA): http://www.apha.org
- Association of Public Health Nurses (APHN): http://www.phnurse.org/
- Association of Schools and Programs of Public Health (ASPPH): http://www.aspph.org/
- National Association of County and City Health Offices (NACCHO): http://www.naccho.org
- Public Health Foundation (PHF): http://www.phf.org

---

sites, plan on a multidisciplinary team for optimal client service delivery, address the logistics of health and medical supplies, and teach disaster nursing in the community. A list of education and training opportunities is shown in Box 14.3.

The importance of being adequately trained and properly associated with an official response organization to serve in a disaster cannot be overstated. In a disaster, many untrained and ill-equipped individuals rush in to help. Spontaneous volunteer overload creates added burden on an already tense situation to include role conflict, anger, frustration, and help-lessness. Box 14.4 provides a list of volunteer opportunities in disaster work.

BOX 14.4   Volunteer Opportunities in Disaster Work

American Red Cross (ARC): http://www.redcross.org
Buddhist Compassion Relief (Tzu Chi): http://www.tzuchi.org/
Certified Emergency Response Team (CERT): https://www.citizencorps.gov/cert/
Citizen Corps: http://ready.gov/citizen-corps
Disaster Medical Assistance Team (DMAT): http://www.phe.gov/preparedness/responders/ndms/teams/Pages.dmat.aspx
Medical Reserve Corps (MRC): mrc.hhs.gov
National Voluntary Organizations Active in Disaster (NVOAD): http://www.nvoad.org
The Salvation Army: http://www.salvationarmyusa.org

Community Preparedness

The level of community preparedness for a disaster is only as good as the people and organizations in the community make it. Some communities stay prepared for a possible disaster by having a written disaster plan and participating in yearly disaster drills. Other communities are less prepared and depend on luck and the fact that they are unlikely to experience a disaster. Some organizations within the community may be more prepared than others. For example, most health care facilities have written disaster plans and require employees to perform annual mock drills, but many businesses lack these requirements. In recent years, hospitals and health departments in cities with nursing, medical, and other health professional schools have included their faculty in the disaster planning work so that if a disaster occurs, faculty and students can easily be mobilized to assist.

Presidential Policy Directive (PPD)-8 emphasizes that true preparedness is a *whole* community event. PPD-8 urges the strengthening of our nation's security and resilience through an integrated set of guidance, programs, and processes to implement the national preparedness goal, described earlier in this chapter (DHS, 2011).

This planning and implementation require a coordinated response that involves many stakeholders, including first and foremost the general public. Community preparedness also involves all levels of government, public health agencies, hospitals, first responders, emergency management, health care providers within the community, schools and universities, the private sector, and business and nongovernmental organizations (NGOs) such as the ARC. Mutual aid agreements and prior planning help to bridge perceived and actual barriers; establish relationships before the incident at the local, regional, state, and national levels; and ensure seamless service. Sometimes barriers involve regulatory authority and jurisdictional boundaries; sometimes the barriers involve organizational control versus the common good.

Emergency management is responsible for developing and coordinating emergency response plans within their defined area, whether local, state, federal, or tribal. The Federal Emergency Management Agency (FEMA) coordinates comprehensive, all-hazard planning at the national level, assuring a menu of exercises and plan templates to address plausible incidents in any given community. Emergency management personnel at the state and local levels work closely with their communities and response partners, providing opportunities to train, exercise, evaluate, and update disaster plans. Stronger predisaster partnerships, which include all stakeholders, produce a more coordinated response.

Disaster planning involves simplicity and realism with backup contingencies because (1) the disaster will never be an "exact fit" for the plan, and (2) all plans must be implementation ready, no matter who is present to start them (DHS, 2015). The following Quality and Safety Education for Nurses box describes safety guidelines for the nurse's family.

Finally, the community must have an adequate warning system and a backup evacuation plan to remove those individuals from areas of danger who hesitate to leave. Some people refuse

QSEN FOCUS ON QUALITY AND SAFETY EDUCATION FOR NURSES

Targeted Competency: Safety—Minimize risk for harm to clients and providers through both system effectiveness and individual performance. Selected knowledge, skills, and attitudes are cited here to develop a disaster safety plan:

- Knowledge: Examine human factors and other basic safety design principles, as well as commonly used unsafe practices (such as workarounds and dangerous abbreviations). Specific steps might be:
  1. Learn how you can get information during the disaster or emergency.
     - Determine what types of disasters are most likely to happen.
     - Learn about warning signals in your community.
     - Ask about postdisaster pet care (shelters usually will not accept pets).
     - Review the disaster plans at your workplace, school, and other places where your family spends time.
     - Determine how to help older adult or disabled family members or neighbors.
     - WHAT should you do?
- Skills: Demonstrate effective use of strategies to reduce risk for harm to self or others.
  1. Create a disaster plan:
     - Talk with your family and create two places to meet, including outside your home and outside your neighborhood. Give each member of the family a copy of the plan.
     - Discuss the types of disasters that are most likely to happen, and review what to do in each case and make a plan.
     - Choose an out-of-state friend to be your family contact; this person will verify the location of each family member. After a disaster, it may be easier to call long distance than to make local calls.
     - Review evacuation plans, including care of pets. Have alternative routes for evacuation.
  1. Complete this checklist:
     - Post emergency phone numbers next to telephones.
     - Teach everyone how and when to call 9-1-1.

- Determine when and how to turn off water, gas, and electricity at the main switches.
- Check adequacy of insurance coverage for yourself and your home.
- Locate and review the use of fire extinguishers.
- Install and maintain smoke detectors.
- Conduct a home hazard hunt, and fix potential hazards.
- Stock emergency supplies, and assemble a disaster supplies kit.
- Acquire first aid and cardiopulmonary resuscitation (CPR) certification.
- Locate all escape routes from your home. Find two ways out of each room.
- Find safe spots in your home for each type of disaster.
  2. Practice and maintain your plan:
     - Review the plan every 6 months.
     - Conduct fire and emergency evacuation drills.
     - Replace stored water every 3 months and stored food every 6 months.
     - Test and recharge fire extinguishers according to manufacturer's instructions.
     - Test your smoke detectors monthly, and change the batteries at least once a year.
  3. What more should you do?
     - Attitudes: Appreciate the cognitive and physical limits of human performance.
     - Monitor your personal reactions to the disaster, and seek assistance if the stress of the losses and the potential work to reestablish a new normal seem overwhelming. Monitor also the reactions of your colleagues and the clients you serve, and provide or refer to others anyone who needs stress-management intervention.

Safety Question: To prepare more effectively for the event of a future disaster, list the steps that you would take to ensure the safety of your family, including any pets you may have.

---

to leave their homes because they are afraid their possessions will be lost or destroyed by the disaster or from looting after the disaster. Law enforcement personnel or others in authority may have to speak directly to these reluctant residents to convince them to leave their homes and go to safer quarters. Also, some people mistakenly believe that experience with a particular type of disaster is enough preparation for the next one. People must be convinced that predisaster warnings are official, serious, and personally important before they are motivated to take action.

The National Health Security Strategy

The purpose of the National Health Security Strategy (NHSS), which was developed in 2009 with a goal to do a revision every 4 years, is to reconnect public health and medical preparedness, response, and recovery strategies to ensure the nation's resilience in the face of health threats or incidents with potentially negative health consequences. Outcomes of the NHSS include community strengthening, integration of response and recovery systems, and seamless coordination among all levels of the public health and medical system (USDHHS, 2017). Community resilience has become a central theme in disaster planning. The NHSS is built on the premise that healthy individuals, families, and communities with access to health care and knowledge become some of our nation's strongest assets in

disaster incidents. Healthier communities have better bounce-back ability.

Disaster and mass casualty exercises. Although practice will not ensure a perfect response to disaster, disaster and mass casualty drills and exercises are extremely valuable components of preparedness. After the exercise, the lessons learned through after-action reports are used to update disaster plans and subsequent operations. Exercise categories include discussion-based simulations, or "tabletops," and operations-based events, such as drills and functional and full-scale exercises (FEMA, 2016). Operations-based events involve escalating scope and scale testing of the disaster preparedness and response network using a specific plan.

National Level Exercise 2009 (NLE09) was the first major exercise conducted by the U.S. government that focused exclusively on terrorism prevention and protection, as opposed to incident response and recovery. NLE09 was designated a Tier I National Level Exercise. These exercises started out as the Top Officials exercise series [TOPOFF]) but now incorporate the whole community, with an understanding that the practice must reach all levels of the public, private, and government sectors to be effective.

The National Exercise Program (NEP) serves to test and validate core capabilities. Participation in exercises, simulations, or other activities, including real world incidents, helps organizations

CASE STUDY

Use of the Mock Attack Strategy to Prepare for Potential Disasters

The Saber city disaster preparedness (DP) team wanted to coordinate a mock terrorist attack to study the effectiveness of its disaster management plan. The goal of the mock attack was to promote confidence, develop skills, coordinate activities, and coordinate participants of the disaster management team. The DP team planned a commonly seen terrorist attack: a bus carrying important politicians would explode outside the federal courthouse in downtown Saber. All participating organizations (including the health department, hospital, police department, and fire department) were notified of the date the mock attack would be held. Volunteers were found to play the victims on the scene.

After months of planning, the day of the mock attack came. The members of the DP team watched how well the organizations worked together during the events of the mock attack. At noon, reports of an exploded bus in front of the courthouse came across police scanners: "Several people are dead and many more injured." Emergency medical response teams and hazardous material response crews were called to the scene to care for the injured and attend to the potential hazardous exposure. Police officers quickly cleared the area of people and established a barrier around the scene. Firefighters put out the fire on the burning bus.

From the mock attack, the DP team learned that the city of Saber was prepared for a terrorist attack. Communication among organizations flowed smoothly, and the disaster management team was skillful in controlling the situation. Participants in the mock attack stated they were happy to have the practice and felt more confident in their ability to provide care in the case of a major disaster.

---

validate their capabilities and identify shortfalls, pulling in their partners and stakeholders including citizen participation (FEMA, 2014). An annual Capstone Exercise, formerly titled the National Level Exercise (NLE), is conducted every 2 years as the final component of each NEP progressive exercise cycle. The Capstone Exercise for 2014 examined the nation's collective ability to coordinate and conduct risk assessments and implement National Frameworks and associated plans to deliver core capabilities (FEMA, 2014).

The Homeland Security Exercise and Evaluation Program (HSEEP) was developed to help states and local jurisdictions improve overall preparedness with all natural and human-made disasters. It provides a standardized methodology and terminology for exercise design, development, conduct, evaluation, and improvement planning and assists communities to create exercises that will make a positive difference before a real incident (FEMA, 2016). HSEEP is the national standard for all exercises.

Whether conducted as drills, tabletops, functional scenarios, or full-scale scenarios, and whether the scope is local or national, nurses and other health care providers must be included as a part of the exercise's planning, response, and after-action activities. Nurses, as client and community advocates, are essential players in the exercise and preparedness arena.

Response

The first level of disaster response occurs at the local level with the mobilization of responders such as the fire department, law enforcement, public health, and emergency services. If the disaster stretches local resources, the county or city emergency management agency will coordinate activities through an emergency operations center. Generally, local responders within a county sign a regional or statewide mutual aid agreement to allow the sharing of needed personnel, equipment, services, and supplies.

The initial scope of disaster assessment is usually measured in dollars, health risk and injury, and/or lives lost. The more destruction and lives at risk, the greater is the degree of attention and resources provided at the local, regional, and state levels. When state resources and capabilities are overwhelmed, governors may request federal assistance under a presidential disaster or emergency declaration. If the event is considered an incident of national significance (a potential or high-impact disaster), appropriate response personnel and resources are provided.

National Response Framework

Once a federal emergency has been declared, the National Response Framework (NRF) may take effect, depending on the specific needs arising from the disaster. The NRF was released by the USDHS in January 2008 as a successor to the National Response Plan. The NRF focuses on response and short-term recovery and is seemingly less cumbersome to use than the NRP. This framework "helps define the roles, responsibilities, and relationships critical to effective emergency planning, preparedness, and response to any emergency or disaster" (DHS, 2013). The online component, the NRF Resource Center (http://www.fema.gov/emergency/nrf/), contains supplemental materials, including annexes, partner guides, and other supporting documents and learning resources. This information is dynamic and is designed to change with lessons learned from real-world events. The framework involves the entire community and is scalable, flexible, and adaptable to the given situation. It is a living document that is revised every 18 months in response to evolving conditions and real-world applications (DHS, 2013).

This framework should be used by government executives, private sector business, nongovernmental leaders, and emergency management practitioners. It is built on these five principles: engaged partnerships; tiered response; scalable, flexible, and adaptable operational capabilities; unity of effort through unified command; and readiness to act.

The NRF includes Emergency Support Functions (ESFs). The 15 ESFs provide a mechanism to bundle federal resources and capabilities to support the nation. Functions include transportation, communications, public works and engineering, firefighting, information and planning, mass care, emergency assistance, temporary housing and human services, logistics, public health and medical services, search and rescue, oil and hazardous materials, agriculture and natural resources, energy, public safety and security, long-term community recovery, and external affairs/standard operating procedures (FEMA, 2014b) and energy. Each ESF includes a coordinator function, and both primary and support agencies that work together to coordinate and deliver the full breadth of federal capabilities. The ESFs provide the structure for coordinating federal interagency support for a federal response to an incident.

ESF 8 (described previously) is Public Health and Medical Services. It provides guidance for medical and mental health personnel, medical equipment and supplies, assessment of the status of the public health infrastructure, and monitoring for potential disease outbreaks. The ESF 8 primary agency is the USDHHS; supporting agencies include the USDHS, the ARC, the Department of Defense, and the Department of Veterans Affairs.

The NDMS is part of ESF 8 and includes the DMATs. These teams of specially trained civilian physicians, nurses, and other health care personnel can be sent to a disaster site within hours of activation (FEMA, 2017).

National Incident Management System

The National Incident Management System (NIMS) is the national platform for disaster response, and it includes universal protocols and language. The NIMS identifies concepts and principles that answer how to manage emergencies from preparedness to recovery regardless of their cause, size, location, or complexity. "NIMS provides a consistent, nationwide approach and vocabulary for multiple agencies or jurisdictions to work together to build, sustain and deliver the core capabilities needed to achieve a secure and resilient nation" (FEMA, 2017, p. 1).

No matter what type of nursing practice or which agency a nurse chooses, he or she will come into direct contact with NIMS, which includes the Incident Command System (ICS). The NIMS includes varying levels of education and training, with many organizations requiring a base level of familiarization to comply with federal funding requirements. A well-developed training program promotes nationwide NIMS implementation. The training program also grows the number of adequately trained and qualified emergency management/response personnel.

🔲 CHECK YOUR PRACTICE

Nurses working as members of a disaster assessment team need to provide accurate information to others in the National Incident Management System (NIMS) environment. A part of that communication involves the rapid and on-going needs assessment. Accurate information helps in providing the most appropriate and needed resources. In a time of crisis or great uncertainty, there is a crucial need for accurate and timely information. Health care personnel are the best sources of essential health information, especially technical information. The NIMS approach uses public affairs spokespersons for formal communication. The Public Information Officer (PIO) is a person with the authority and responsibility to communicate information to the public. Nurses are considered highly trustworthy, and they are often asked by members of the media for an interview. If the nurse is asked for an interview, what is the best first approach?

1. Set up a time for the interview later in the day after you prepare your notes.
2. Refer the media to the PIO representing the agency.
3. Politely say that you are extremely busy dealing with victims of the disaster and you do not have time for an interview.

Furthermore, terrorists are capable of spreading fear by sending explosives or chemical and biological agents through the mail. The nurse should also observe for and report any psychological or sociological health hazards such as overcrowding, extreme disrespect, and anger in vulnerable populations that could lead to unrest and violence.

Response to Bioterrorism

Biological or chemical terrorist attacks require a very different response. An unannounced dissemination of a biological agent may easily go unnoticed, and the victims may have left the area of exposure long before the act of terrorism is recognized. The first signs that a biological agent has been released may not be apparent for days or weeks, when the victims become ill and seek a health evaluation. In this case the health care professionals, including nurses, are considered the "first on the scene." The five components of a comprehensive public health response to outbreaks of illness are (1) detecting the outbreak; (2) determining the cause; (3) identifying factors that place people at risk; (4) implementing measures to control the outbreak; and (5) informing the medical and public communities about treatments, health consequences, and preventive measures (Rotz et al, 2000).

People who experience or witness a terrorist attack may experience a stress response as well as one or more of the following symptoms (International Council of Nurses, 2009): (1) repeated thoughts about the attack; (2) immense fear of everything, which may prevent them from even leaving their homes; (3) survivor guilt or questioning why they lived and others did not; (4) a sense of great loss; and (5) hesitation to express feelings.

Although many of the nursing actions for dealing with terrorism are similar to those in any other disaster, the following list summarizes key actions. The International Council of Nurses Fact Sheet on terrorism and bioterrorism provides useful details on each of the following actions:

- Help people cope with the aftermath of terrorism
- Allay public concerns and fears of bioterrorism
- Identify the feelings that you and others may be experiencing
- Assist victims to think positively and to move to the future
- Prepare nursing personnel to be effective in a crisis or emergency situation

Identifying the chemical or biological agent is the first priority. Rapid identification is vital to protect health care workers and any others affected. Results of a biological release are hard to recognize because many biological agent symptoms mimic influenza or other viral syndromes. Pathogens such as bacteria, viruses, and toxins can be used to create biological weapons. Although an aerosol release may be a likely vehicle for dissemination, certain biological agents could also be released through the water and food supply. Only about a dozen pathogens pose a major threat, even though there are thousands of pathogens, some highly contagious. Quarantine of those exposed to contagious agents may be considered in some instances. A few vaccines have been developed to combat bacterial pathogens. The Centers for Disease Control and Prevention (CDC) provides an excellent source of biological agent information to include the latest agent fact sheets for health practitioners (CDC, 2014a.). Important information provided includes the methods of transmission and communicability period. Through the Pandemic and All-Hazards Preparedness Reauthorization Act (PAHPRA), several biodefense programs exist to help public health professionals mount a proactive response to these events (USHHS, 2017):

- BioWatch is an early warning system for biothreats that uses an environmental sensor system to test the air for biological agents in several major metropolitan areas.

- BioSense is a data-sharing program to facilitate surveillance of unusual patterns or clusters of diseases in the United States. It shares data with local and state health departments and is a part of the BioWatch system.
- Project BioShield is a program to develop and produce new drugs and vaccines as countermeasures against potential bioweapons and deadly pathogens.
- Cities Readiness Initiative is a program to aid cities in increasing their capacity to deliver medicines and medical supplies during a large-scale public health emergency such as a bioterrorism attack or a nuclear accident.
- Strategic National Stockpile (SNS) is a CDC-managed program with the capacity to provide large quantities of medicine and medical supplies to protect the American public in a public health emergency to include bioterrorism. The SNS is deployed through a combination of state level request and the public health system.

Some of the most common lessons from exercises as well as live incidents involve communication. In an effort to keep the public health community informed, the CDC developed the Public Health Information Network (PHIN). The PHIN provides for the electronic exchange of information among governmental agencies. It focuses on six components that help ensure information access and sharing: early event detection, outbreak management, connecting laboratory systems, countermeasure and response administration, partner communications and alerting, and cross-functional components, and is critical to information exchange (CDC, 2014b).

How Disasters Affect Communities

The pain and suffering of people who lose their possessions, are injured, or lose loved ones are immeasurable. When disaster hits, people in a community will be affected physically and emotionally, depending on the type, cause, and location of the disaster; its magnitude and extent of damage; the duration; and the amount of prewarning provided.

The first goal of any disaster response is to reestablish sanitary barriers as quickly as possible (Veenema, 2012). Water, food, waste removal, vector control, shelter, and safety are basic needs. Difficult weather conditions such as extreme heat or cold can hamper efforts, especially if electricity is affected. Continuous monitoring of the environment proactively addresses potential hazards. Disease prevention is an ongoing goal, especially if there is an interruption in the public health infrastructure. Infectious disease outbreaks occur in the recovery phase of disasters, and occasionally disaster workers introduce new organisms into the area.

The psychological effects of September 11, 2001, were different from those of more contained, single-event disasters. The attack was totally unexpected and of great magnitude, with much uncertainty and fear about what might happen next. Not knowing when or if a subsequent attack will occur may prevent individuals from moving beyond their fear and anger (ARC, 2002).

Also, Hurricane Katrina, which started as a natural disaster, had its consequences compounded by a human-made disaster caused by flooding from levee failure. Later followed by Hurricane Rita, Hurricane Katrina affected the Gulf Coast and the nation in ways that will be felt for generations to come. It is the costliest U.S. disaster ever, with economic estimates of more than $125 billion (National Oceanic and Atmospheric Administration, 2017). The hurricane, floods, and more than 1800 confirmed deaths created traumatic stress that rose to unbearable levels in New Orleans, resulting in a tense and sometimes violent aftermath (Reagan, 2005). New Orleans was typically described as a war zone in the weeks after the disaster, as was the Gulfport-Biloxi coastline in Mississippi, where 90% of the buildings were demolished. Hundreds of thousands of people lost access to their homes and their jobs as a result of Hurricane Katrina, and the rebuilding has been slow and costly.

Stress reactions in individuals. A traumatic event can cause moderate to severe stress reactions. Individuals react to the same disaster in different ways depending on their age, cultural background, health status, social support structure, and general ability to adapt to crisis. Symptoms that may require assistance are listed in Box 14.5.

BOX 14.5   Tips for Survivors of a Disaster or Other Traumatic Event: Managing Stress*

You may feel emotionally:
- Anxious, fearful, or sad
- Extreme sense of urgency or panic
- Angry, especially if the event involved violence
- Guilty, even when you had no control over the traumatic event
- Heroic, like you can do anything
- Like you have too much energy or no energy
- Disconnected, not caring about anything or anyone
- Numb, unable to feel either joy or sadness

You may have physical reactions such as:
- Stomachaches and diarrhea
- Headaches or other physical pains for no obvious reason
- Eating too much or too little
- Sweating or having chills
- Having tremors or muscle twitches\being jumpy or easily startled

Behavior reactions may include:
- Trouble remembering things, thinking, making decisions, or concentrating

- Feeling confused or numb
- Worrying excessively
- Trouble talking about what happened and listening to others
- Trouble sleeping
- Increase or decrease in energy or activity levels
- Feeling sad or crying often
- Using alcohol, tobacco, illegal drugs, or prescription medicines to reduce distress
- Having outbursts of anger, or feeling irritated and blaming others or to forget
- Having difficulty helping others and accepting help or making decisions when around people
- Being reluctant to abandon property

Children
- Regressive behaviors (e.g., bedwetting, thumb sucking, crying, clinging to parents)
- Fantasies that disaster never occurred
- Nightmares
- School-related problems, including inability to concentrate and refusal to go back to school

*The tips in Box 14.5 are not an entire list. For further details, see Substance Abuse and Mental Health Services Administration. *Tips for survivors of a disaster or other traumatic event: Managing stress, 2013.* Retrieved from http://www.disasterdistress.samhsa.gov.

People who are affected by a disaster often have an exacerbation of an existing chronic disease. For example, the emotional stress of the disaster may make it difficult for people with diabetes to control their blood glucose levels. Grief results in harmful effects on the immune system. It reduces the function of cells that protect against viral infections and tumors. Hormones produced by the body's flight-or-fight mechanism also play a role in mediating the effects of grief.

Older adults' reactions to disaster depend a great deal on their physical health, strength, mobility, independence, and income. They can react deeply to the loss of personal possessions because of the sentimental value attached to the items and their irreplaceable value. Their need for relocation depends on the extent of damage to their home or their compromised health. They may try to conceal the seriousness of their health conditions or losses if they fear loss of independence. Box 14.6 lists other populations at higher risk for serious disruption after a disaster. Many of them are the same populations who are also at risk for adverse health effects before a disaster.

The effect of disasters on young children can be especially disruptive (National Institute of Mental Health [NIMH], 2015) (Fig. 14.4). Regressive behaviors such as thumb sucking, bedwetting, crying, and clinging to parents can occur. Children tend to reexperience images of the traumatic event or have recurring thoughts or sensations, or they may intentionally avoid reminders, thoughts, and feelings related to disaster events. Children may have arousal or heightened sensitivity to sights, sounds, or smells and may experience exaggerated responses or difficulty with usual activities. Children not immediately affected by a disaster also can experience effects from it. The constant bombardment of disaster stories on television can cause fear in children. They may believe that the event could happen to them or their family, believe someone will be injured or killed, or think they will be left alone. It is best to turn off the television news and engage in activities with family, friends, and neighbors. The parents' reaction to a disaster greatly influences children (NIMH, 2015).

One special population that may be overlooked is children in childcare facilities. Children are cared for in many different

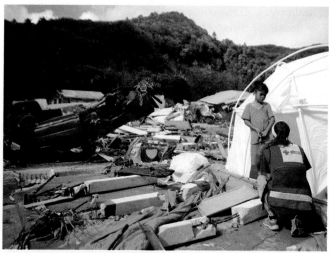

FIG. 14.4 The effects of disaster on children can be especially disruptive. In 2013, 1 week after Typhoon Haiyan made landfall, residents of Tanauan, the Philippines, struggle to cope amid the devastation. Every house in the city of 50,000 was badly damaged or destroyed. The effects of a disaster on young children can be especially disruptive. (Courtesy of the American Red Cross Photo Library. Photo by Patrick Fuller/International Federation of Red Cross and Red Crescent Societies, Geneva, Switzerland. Retrieved January 2015 from: http://media.redcross.org/sites/.)

locations, ranging from freestanding buildings to provider homes. They tend to have little, if any, security against a disaster, and people come in and go out of the facility all day. Also, if a disaster occurs, a plan must be in place for how the children can be reunited with their parents. Because of their small size, they may have to be helped to leave the facility. In addition, they are more vulnerable to chemical and biological agents because of their immature physiological and psychological development, and they have less fluid reserve than adults so are more susceptible to dehydration. With all populations, review individual strategies, including available specific resources, in the event of an emergency. The following actions are recommended regarding childcare emergency supplies (Gaines and Leary, 2004):

- Put together a family readiness kit and disaster supply kit (see the American Academy of Pediatrics at http://www.aap.org).
- Gather the supplies recommended by the ARC (http://www.redcross.org).
- Store things such as first-aid supplies, emergency blankets, medications, ice packs, and nonperishable food in backpacks or rolling containers.
- Put copies of each child's medical information, parent contact information, and local emergency telephone numbers in a portable container.
- Take with you the attendance list of children and some comfort items such as games, toys, blankets, crayons, and paper.

Public health nurses should help those in the affected community talk about their feelings, including anger, sorrow, guilt, and perceived blame for the disaster or the outcomes of the disaster. Community members should be encouraged to engage

---

BOX 14.6   Populations at Greatest Risk for Disruption After Disaster

- Disabled
- Older adults
- Visually or hearing impaired
- Health care providers and first responders
- Women
- Pregnancy
- Children
- Diabetes
- American Indians
- Latino Communities

From National Institutes of Health, National Library of Medicine: Special populations: emergency and disaster preparedness, Washington, DC, 2014, NIH. Retrieved January 2016 from http://sis.nlm.nih.gov/outreach/specialpopulationsanddisasters.html.

in healthy eating, exercise, rest, daily routine maintenance, limited demanding responsibilities, and time with family and friends.

Stress reactions in the community. Communities reflect the individuals and families living in them, both during and after a disaster incident. Four community phases are commonly recognized: (1) heroic, (2) honeymoon, (3) disillusionment, and (4) reconstruction. The first two phases—the heroic and honeymoon phases—are most often associated with response efforts. The latter two phases—disillusionment and reconstruction—are most often linked with recovery. For purposes of continuity, all phases will be discussed in this response section.

During the heroic phase, there is overwhelming need for people to do whatever they can to help others survive the disaster. First responders, who include health and medical personnel, will work hours on end with no thought of their own personal or health needs. They may fight needed sleep and refuse rest breaks in their drive to save others. Moreover, imported responders may be unfamiliar with the terrain and inherent dangers. Those with oversight responsibilities may need to order helpers to take necessary breaks and attend to their health needs. Exhausted, overworked responders present a danger to themselves and the community served.

In the honeymoon phase, survivors may be rejoicing that their lives and the lives of loved ones have been spared. Survivors will gather to share experiences and stories. The repeated telling to others creates bonds among the survivors. A sense of thankfulness over having survived the disaster is inherent in their stories.

The disillusionment phase occurs after time elapses and people begin to notice that additional help and reinforcement may not be immediately forthcoming. A sense of despair results, and exhaustion starts to take its toll on volunteers, rescuers, and medical personnel. The community begins to realize that a return to the previous normal is unlikely and that they must make major changes and adjustments. Nurses need to consider the psychosocial impact and the consequent emotional, cognitive, and spiritual implications. Public health nurses should identify groups and population segments particularly at risk for burnout and exhaustion, to include responders and volunteers involved in rescue efforts. They may need breaks and reminders for nourishment. In addition, those in shock and those consumed by grief related to loss of loved ones will need compassionate care, with possible referrals to mental health counseling resources.

The last phase—reconstruction—is the longest. Homes, schools, churches, and other community elements need to be rebuilt and reestablished. The goal is to return to a new state of normalcy. Because the scope of human need may still be extensive, the nurse will continue to function as a member of the interprofessional team to provide and ensure provision of the best possible coordinated care to the population.

Role of the Nurse in Disaster Response

The nurse's role during a disaster depends largely on the nurse's experience, professional role in a community disaster plan,

specialty training, and special interest. Flexibility is essential because the only certainty is that there will be continuing changes (Stanley et al, 2008). Nurses serve in many roles in the community. They advocate for a safe environment. They also know that disasters are both natural and human-made, so they assess for and report environmental health hazards. For example, the nurse should be aware of and report unsafe equipment, faulty structures, and the beginning of disease epidemics such as measles or influenza. The public health nurse brings leadership, policy, planning, and practice expertise to disaster preparedness and response (Association of Public Health Nurses [APHN], 2014).

Assessment is a major nursing role during a disaster. In completing an assessment, use the skills of interview, observation, individual physical examinations, health and illness screening, surveys (i.e., sample and special health), and records (i.e., census, school, vital statistics, disease reporting). The traditional model of community assessment presents the foundation for the rapid community assessment process. The acute needs of populations in disaster turn the community assessment into rapid appraisal of a sector or region's population, social systems, and geophysical features. Elements of a rapid needs assessment include determining the magnitude of the incident, defining the specific health needs of the affected population, establishing priorities and objectives for action, identifying existing and potential public health problems, evaluating the capacity of the local response, including resources and logistics, and determining the external resource needs for priority actions (Stanley et al, 2008). Also, assessments in sudden-impact disasters, such as tornadoes and earthquakes, are more concerned with ongoing hazards, injuries and deaths, shelter requirements, and clean water. Triage should begin immediately and is the process of separating casualties and allocating treatment on the basis of the individuals' potentials for survival. Highest priority is given to individuals with life-threatening injuries, but also those who have a high probability of survival once they are stabilized (Veenema, 2012). Second priority is given to victims with injuries that have systemic complications that are not yet life threatening and could wait 45 to 60 minutes for treatment. Last priority is given to those victims with local injuries without immediate complications and who can wait several hours for medical attention.

Assessments in gradual-onset disasters, such as famines, are most concerned with mortality rates, nutritional status, immunization status, and environmental health.

Nurses also should understand what the available community resources will be after a disaster strikes, and, most important, how the community will work together. A community-wide disaster plan serves as a roadmap for what "should" occur before, during, and after the response and the role of each participant in the plan. As shown in Box 14.4, there are a variety of community organizations in which nurses can become involved to assist in a disaster.

There may be times when the nurse is the first to arrive on the scene of a disaster. If so, the more usual skills of community assessment, case finding and referring, prevention, health education, surveillance, and working with aggregates will be put aside temporarily so that the nurse can deal with life-threatening problems. Once rescue workers arrive on the scene, plans for triage should begin immediately.

Nurses can help initiate or update the agency's disaster plan, provide educational programs and materials regarding disasters specific to the area, and organize disaster drills. Nurses also can provide an updated record of vulnerable populations within the community. When calamity strikes, disaster workers must know what kinds of populations they are attempting to assist. For example, if a tornado strikes a retirement village, the needs are quite different from those seen after the tornado hits a church filled with families or a center for the physically challenged. In addition to knowing where special populations exist, the nurse can educate groups about what effect the disaster might have on them. Nurses should review individual strategies, including available specific resources, in the event of an emergency.

Lack of or inaccurate information regarding the scope of the disaster and its initial effects contributes to the misuse of resources. Often, too many volunteers who lack official sponsorship convene at the site of disaster and are disappointed when their help cannot be used. Similarly, well-meaning people may send clothes and food to disaster sites that lack storage and distribution abilities. Contributions that add to the stress of coping with the disaster can be a burden. Local and regional emergency management and public health resources need to be readjusted as assessment reports continue to come in. Establishing a priority of needs that benefit the largest aggregate of affected individuals with the most correctable problems is consistent with the basic tenets of triage.

Ongoing assessments or surveillance reports are just as important as initial assessments. Surveillance reports indicate the continuing status of the affected population and the effectiveness of ongoing relief efforts. They continue to inform relief managers of needed resources. Nurses involved in ongoing surveillance can use the methods listed in the "How To" box to gather information. Surveillance continues into the recovery phase of a disaster.

HOW TO Gather Disaster Information

1. Interview
2. Observation
3. Individual physical examinations
4. Health and illness screening
5. Surveys (sample and special health)
6. Records (census, school, vital statistics, disease reporting)

From Landesman L: *Public health management of disasters: the practice guide*, Washington, DC, 2001, American Public Health Association.

Shelter Management

Shelters are generally the responsibility of the local ARC chapter, although in massive disasters the military may set up "tent cities" or bring in trailers for the masses who need temporary shelter. Nurses, because of their comfort with delivering aggregate health promotion, disease prevention, and emotional support, make ideal shelter managers and team members. Each person who comes to the shelter is assessed to determine what type of facility is most appropriate. Although initially physical health needs are the priority, especially among older adults and the chronically ill, many of the predominant problems in shelters revolve around stress. The shock of the disaster itself, the loss of personal possessions, the fear of the unknown, living in proximity to total strangers, and even boredom can cause stress.

Nurses working in shelters, in addition to providing assessments, also provide referrals and meet health care needs such as helping clients get prescription glasses, medications, first aid, and appropriate diet adjustments; keeping client records; ensuring emergency communications; and providing a safe environment (ARC, 2013). The ARC provides training for shelter support and use of appropriate protocols and partners with other agencies such as the MRC and local public health agencies to ensure adequate health care to those in shelters. Nurses can use common-sense approaches to help shelter residents. These measures include listening to victims tell and retell their disaster story and current situation; encouraging residents to share their feelings with one another if it seems appropriate to do so; helping residents make decisions; delegating tasks (e.g., reading, crafts, playing games with children) to teenagers and others to help combat boredom; providing the basic necessities (i.e., food, clothing, rest); attempting to recover or get needed items (e.g., prescription glasses, medication); providing basic compassion and dignity (e.g., privacy when appropriate and if possible); and referring to a mental health counselor or other source of help.

Nurses need to be aware of the surrounding medical facilities and services provided in their area, including special needs shelters. Individuals who are medically dependent and not acutely ill but have varied physical, cognitive, and psychological conditions should be directed to a special needs shelter. The federal government provides assistance to special needs shelters

---

EVIDENCE-BASED PRACTICE

Veenema and Thornton (2015) reviewed the disasters at Chernobyl, Three Mile Island, and the Fukushima Daiichi nuclear power plant to develop the information that would be useful to inform nurses in preparedness efforts. In reviewing these historic power plant disasters, they found that nurses played a significant role in the response and recovery phases of the disasters. Nurses screened individuals for exposure to radiation, decontaminated victims, provided clinical care to those experiencing radiation syndrome symptoms, and provided mental health counseling and emotional support to both individuals and communities. Their review reinforced the belief that nurses can only provide quality care to others when they are safe. Some of the specific care that nurses and other health care personnel provide include triage, screening, treatment including decontamination, transporting, and referring.

Nurse Use:

It is important for nurses and public health preparedness workers to learn the key expectations if they are to be called to provide care during a radiological disaster. They will need to understand the basic effects of high-level radiation exposure, how they should intervene, and, equally important, how to protect themselves from exposure.

Veenema TG, Thornton CP: Understanding nursing's role in health systems response to large-scale radiological disasters. *J Radiol Nurs* 34:63–72, 2015.

through one of the emergency support functions (ESF 8) of the National Response Plan, which provides assessment of public health and medical needs, health surveillance, supplies, and medical care personnel, such as teams from the National Disaster Medical System (DHS, 2015).

Special needs shelters reduce the surge demands on hospitals and long-term care facilities that often occur during disasters. Although helpful in reducing surge, too many referrals can create tension among the special needs shelters, the regular shelters, and the health care facilities as roles and responsibilities become blurred and overall resources and personnel are limited. Careful preplanning for a community's special needs populations is essential.

International Relief Efforts

Disasters occur throughout the world, and people suffer from natural disasters and human-made disasters. Civil strife leads to war, famine, and communicable disease outbreaks. Sometimes disaster or relief workers are sent to these international disasters at the request of the affected country's government. At other times, workers are not welcomed but instead may go with the support of the United Nations. When workers are not welcomed, their lives may be in danger, even though they go as peacekeeping agents of the Federation of the Red Cross and Red Crescent societies and the International Committee of the Red Cross or as health representatives from the World Health Organization. International disaster or relief workers generally have intensive training and preparation before embarking on a mission.

Psychological Stress of Disaster Workers

Disaster relief work can be rewarding because it provides an opportunity to have a profound and positive impact on the lives of those who may be experiencing their greatest time of need. However, the work is also challenging and stressful. During an assignment, responders may be exposed to chaotic environments, long hours, rapidly changing information and directives, long wait times before getting to work, noisy environments, and living quarters that are less than ideal. According to the National Institute of Occupational Health and Safety (NIOSH, 2013), responders may not recognize the need for self-care, and to monitor their own emotional and physical health. As recovery efforts span time frames of weeks to months, there is increasing risk for adverse effects to responders.

No one who experiences a disaster either personally or in a professional capacity is untouched by it. Nurses who work with survivors of disasters may be at risk for stress reactions. Self-care is as important as the care that is provided to community members. Symptoms that may signal a need for stress management assistance include: being reluctant or refusing to leave the scene until the work is finished; denying needed rest and recovery time; feeling overriding stress and fatigue; engaging in unnecessary risk-taking activities; having difficulty communicating thoughts, remembering instructions, making decisions, or concentrating; engaging in unnecessary arguments; having a limited attention span; and refusing to follow orders (ARC, 2013). Physical symptoms such as tremors, headaches, nausea,

and colds or flulike symptoms can also occur. Suppressing feelings of guilt, powerlessness, anger, and other signs of stress will eventually lead to symptoms such as irritability, fatigue, headaches, and distortions of bodily functions. It is normal to experience stress, but it must be dealt with. The worst thing anyone can do is to deny that it exists.

The nurse should understand that everyone reacts differently after a disaster assignment. Most reactions are considered normal and are temporary, resolving in days to a few weeks. For some workers, disasters bring forth strong thoughts and emotions, both positive and negative. Other workers may experience mild reactions or hardly any reaction at all. There are some common strategies that will help individuals returning from the incident: rest and recovery time, focusing on accomplishments, using calming strategies such as relaxation techniques or working on hobbies, and concentrating on self-care to include healthy food and drink, exercise, and sleep, take time to debrief (ARC, 2013). **Delayed stress reactions,** or those that occur once the disaster is over, include exhaustion and an inability to adjust to the slower pace of work or home (Bryce, 2001).

Workers may be disappointed if family members and friends do not seem as interested in what they have been through and if coming back home, in general, does not live up to expectations. Also, they may feel frustration and conflict if their needs seem inconsistent with those of their family and co-workers or if they have left the disaster site thinking that so much more could have been done (Bryce, 2001). Issues or problems that once seemed pressing may now seem trivial. Anger may emerge as others present problems that seem trivial in contrast to those faced by the victims who were left behind. Disaster workers may fantasize about returning to the disaster site if they think their actions are appreciated more there than at home or the office. Mood swings are common and serve to resolve conflicting feelings. Feelings or actions that persist or that the worker perceives are interfering with daily life should be dealt with by a trained mental health professional.

Recovery

Recovery is about returning to the new normal with the goal of reaching a level of organization that is as near the level before the disaster as is possible. This is often the hardest part of the disaster. During the recovery period, all involved agencies pull together to restore the institutions and properly rebuild. For example, the government takes the lead in rebuilding efforts, whereas the business community tries to provide economic support. Many religious organizations help with rebuilding efforts as well. The Internal Revenue Service educates victims as to how to write off losses, and the Housing and Urban Development Department provides grants for temporary housing. The CDC provides continuing surveillance and epidemiological services. Voluntary agencies continue to assess individual and community needs and meet those needs as they are able. When housing is destroyed, groups such as Habitat for Humanity play a valuable role in the rebuilding. The best time to start thinking about the lessons learned from a recent disaster is during the recovery phase of the disaster cycle.

Role of the Nurse in Disaster Recovery

The role of the nurse in the recovery phase of a disaster is as varied as in the prevention, preparedness, and response phases, and the three levels of prevention are used (see the Levels of Prevention box). Flexibility is essential in the recovery operation. Community cleanup efforts can cause many physical and psychological problems. For example, the physical stress of moving heavy objects can cause back injury, severe fatigue, and even death from heart attacks. Nurses also must continue to teach proper hygiene and make sure immunization records are current given the threat of disease.

The reality of the recovery effort is that the rapid needs assessment continues into an ongoing community needs assessment. To determine effective interventions to ensure the best possible outcomes, it is essential to have ongoing accurate data about the population. Some conditions are manifest only after time elapses. A major advantage of the recovery community assessment efforts is that they can be more in-depth, with greater confidence in the results. Some examples of community data points in the recovery phase include the following: ongoing illness and injuries related to the disaster; diseases related to disruption of environmental or health services; health facility infrastructure in terms of adequate personnel, beds, medical and pharmaceutical supplies; and environmental health assessment to include water quantity and quality, sanitation, shelter, solid waste disposal, and vector populations.

Disruption of the public health infrastructure, including water and food supply, the sanitation system, the vector control program, and access to primary and mental health care, can lead to increased disease and community dysfunction. Nurses will engage in ongoing community assessments during the recovery phase. It is important to be alert for environmental health hazards during the recovery phase of a disaster. During home visits, nurses may uncover situations such as a faulty housing structure or lack of water or electricity. Objects that have been blown into the yard by a tornado or that floated in from a flood may be dangerous and must be removed. Also, the nurse should assess the dangers of live or dead animals and rodents that are harmful to a person's health. An example of this would be finding poisonous snakes in and around homes once the waters from a flood start to recede. Case finding and referral are critical during the recovery phase and may continue for a long time.

Other examples of community data points to watch for during the recovery phase include ongoing illnesses and injuries related to the disaster, disease and acute respiratory infections related to disruption of environmental health services, health facility infrastructure in terms of adequate personnel, beds, and medical and pharmaceutical supplies (Landesman, 2006).

The hurricanes in the United States over the past several years changed how the health care system prepares for, responds to, and recovers from a disaster. People have learned how critical it is for communities to have a well-organized plan and for key players to know their roles and be flexible and collaborative. The value of an electronic medical record became more apparent in recent years when hospitals, clinics, and health departments lost records during a disaster and when people were relocated for substantial periods of time without access to their medications or their medical records (Cary, 2008).

It is important to have a realistic perspective related to how long recovery may take. It will take months or years to return to a semblance of normal, and this new normal may be different from the predisaster state. Also, postdisaster cleanup may lead to unintentional injuries, including those resulting from falls, contact with live wires, accidents while cutting items, heart attacks from overexertion and stress, and auto accidents caused by road conditions and absent traffic signals. Nurses need to educate the community about the hazards described earlier, as well as hazards related to carbon monoxide poisoning from using lanterns, gas ranges, or generators or from burning charcoal to heat an enclosed area.

Nurses play a key role in helping survivors by providing psychological support. Acute and chronic illness may become worse after a disaster. The psychological stress of loss, cleanup, or moving can lead to feelings of hopelessness, depression, and grief in the disillusionment phase. Referrals to mental health professionals should continue throughout the recovery phase and as long as the need exists. The role of the nurse in case finding and referral remains critical during this phase. In the end, it is the concept of community resilience that will lead the community to its new normal. The public health nurse is the community and client advocate who ensures that resilience is supported in partnership with the population.

FUTURE OF DISASTER MANAGEMENT

In the last several years, the terrorist events of September 11, 2001, Hurricane Katrina, the H1N1 pandemic, the Haiti earthquake of 2010, the earthquake and tsunami in Japan, and the civil war in Syria continued to underscore the need for nursing involvement at every step of the disaster management cycle. To fully participate in this mission, nurses must continue to plan and train in an all-hazards environment, regardless of their specialty practice. Public health nurses are especially critical members of the multidisciplinary disaster health team given their population-based focus and specialty knowledge in epidemiology and community assessment. Although sophisticated technology and surveillance will continue to advance in response to both human-made and **natural disasters**, the nature

LEVELS OF PREVENTION

Related to Disaster Prevention Management

Primary Prevention
Participate in developing a disaster management plan for the community.

Secondary Prevention
Assess disaster victims and triage for care.

Tertiary Prevention
Participate in home visits to uncover dangers that may cause additional injury to victims or cause other problems (e.g., house fires from faulty wiring).

of disasters will retain the element of unpredictability. That unpredictability and the medical and public health surge requirements in disaster makes prevention and preparedness activities on the part of individuals and communities even more important. Disaster information changes rapidly because of the learning that occurs during and after each incident, producing progressive best practices. Staying current in disaster training requires the public health nurse's commitment in community planning activities, exercise participation, and actual disaster work.

 APPLYING CONTENT TO PRACTICE

Throughout this chapter, how nurses work in disaster management is applied to standards of public health nursing and the core competencies of health professionals in disaster work. Other applicable areas include discussion about the continuous processes of assessment, planning, implementation, evaluation, collaboration, and cooperation. The role of the nurse in disaster management relates to both standards of nursing and public health practice. Specifically, the nurse must first assess, then plan, implement, and evaluate while simultaneously working with a variety of other concerned and involved agencies and individuals.

CLINICAL APPLICATION

Paula Miller, a nurse in a medium-sized public health department in Lincoln, Nebraska, was called to serve on her first national disaster assignment. Her disaster skills were tested when a level 1 hurricane hit Miami and its surrounding areas. Ms. Miller left Lincoln to help manage a shelter in an elementary school cafeteria in Homestead, Florida, near Miami.

The devastation that she saw en route to the school had a negative effect on her. Assigned to help with client intake, she patiently listened to the disaster victims, referred many of her most distraught clients to the mental health counselor, and set priorities for other needs as they arose. For example, she found that many of her clients had left their medications behind and needed therapy. Other needs included diapers and formula for infants, prescription eyeglasses, and clothing. By identifying their needs, Ms. Miller helped ensure that the master "needs list" was complete.

As the days went on, the stress level in the shelter grew. The crowded living conditions and lack of privacy took its toll on the residents. Around the tenth day of her assignment, Ms. Miller began to experience pounding headaches and had difficulty concentrating. She thought she would be fine, but the mental health counselor said that she was experiencing a stress reaction.

Which of the following actions would probably be the most useful for this nurse to take?
A. Share her feelings with the onsite mental health counselor on a regular basis.
B. Call home to share her feelings with family members.
C. Meet the needs of her clients to the best of her ability, and accept the fact that stress is a part of the job.

Answers can be found on the Evolve website.

REMEMBER THIS!

- The number of disasters, both human-made and natural, continues to increase, as does the number of people affected by them.
- The cost to recover from a disaster has risen sharply because of the amount of technology that must be restored.
- Professional preparedness involves an awareness and understanding of the disaster plan at work and in the community.
- Nurses are increasingly getting involved in disaster planning, response, and recovery through their local health department or local government.
- Disaster health and disaster mental health training from an official agency such as the ARC can prepare nurses for the many opportunities that await them in disaster prevention, preparedness, response, and recovery.
- Being knowledgeable about community resources available to vulnerable populations before a disaster incident ensures a more coordinated response and recovery.
- Helping clients maintain a safe environment and advocating for environmental safety measures in the community are key roles for the nurse during all phases of disaster management.
- People in a community react differently to a disaster depending on the type, cause, and location of the disaster; its magnitude and extent of damage; its duration; and the amount of warning that was provided.

- People react differently to disasters depending on factors such as their age, cultural background, health status, social support structure, and general adaptability to crisis.
- The stress of nurses is compounded if they are both victims and caregivers in a disaster.
- Disaster shelter nurses are exposed to a variety of physical and emotional complaints, including stress. Stress may be instigated by the shock of the disaster, the loss of personal possessions, the fear of the unknown, living in proximity to strangers, and boredom.
- The degree of worker stress during disasters depends on the nature of the disaster, the worker's role in the disaster, individual stamina, noise level, adequacy of workspace, potential for physical danger, stimulus overload, and, especially, being exposed to death and trauma.
- Symptoms of worker stress during disasters include minor tremors, nausea, decreased concentration, difficulty thinking and remembering, irritability, fatigue, and other somatic disorders.
- A key attribute in aiding disaster victims is flexibility.
- The stage of disaster known as recovery occurs as all involved agencies pull together to restore the economic and civic life of the community.

WHAT WOULD YOU DO?

1. If you thought a hurricane might affect your community, what steps would you take to adequately prepare for the possible disaster? What steps would you take to ensure safety and preparedness for your family and for the clients for whom you care? Whose help would you enlist? To whom would you go for advice? Talk with two classmates, and compare your answers; then prepare an action plan.
2. Assume your community has the potential to be hit by a tornado. List the groups who would be most vulnerable.

What steps could you take in advance to reduce their vulnerability? What community resources are available?
3. If you and your classmates saw a tornado moving across the street in a small town as you drove to your clinical site, what steps would you take to determine whether people were injured? What would you do first? Who else would you involve? Discuss your replies with a classmate and come up with a consolidated plan.
4. Describe the role of the nurse in the preparedness, response, and recovery stages of disaster. Does all of this make sense to you?

EVOLVE WEBSITE

http://evolve.elsevier.com/Stanhope/foundations
• Case Study, with Questions and Answers
• NCLEX® Review Questions
• Practice Application Answers

REFERENCES

American Red Cross: *Disaster mental health services: an overview,* ARC Pub no. 3077-2A, Washington, DC, 2002, ARC.

American Red Cross: *Disaster health services guidance,* Washington, DC, 2013, Disaster Health Services.

Association of Public Health Nurses: *The Role of the Public Health Nurse in Disaster Preparedness Response, and Recovery: A position paper,* 2014. Retrieved from http://www.achne.org/.

Bryce CP: *Stress management in disasters,* Washington, DC, 2001, Pan American Health Organization.

Cary S: Caring for patients on kidney dialysis in a disaster, *Am J Nurs* 108:26–32, 2008.

Centers for Disease Control and Prevention: *Public Health Information Network (PHIN),* 2014b. Retrieved February 2016 from http://www.cdc.gov/phin/.

Department of Homeland Security: *National disaster medical system: DMAT,* Washington, DC, 2015, USDHS. Retrieved February 2016 from http://www.phe.gov.

Department of Homeland Security: *Target capabilities list, version 2.0,* Washington, DC, 2007, USDHS. Retrieved January 2015 from http://www.fema.gov/pdf/government/training/tcl.pdf.

Department of Homeland Security: *Homeland Security Act of 2002: Title 1—Department of Homeland Security,* Washington, DC, 2002a, USDHS.

Department of Homeland Security: *Homeland security presidential directives,* Washington, DC, 2008a, updated March 2011. USDHS. Retrieved January 2015 from http://www.dhs.gov/presidential-policy-directive-8-national-preparedness.

Department of Homeland Security: *National Preparedness Guidelines,* 2015. Retrieved February 2016 from http://www.dhs.gov/national-preparedness-guidelines.

Department of Homeland Security: *National Response Framework (NRF),* 2013. Retrieved February 2016 from http://www.fema.gov/national-response-framework.

Dilley M, Chen RS, Deichmann U, et al: *Natural Disaster Hotspots: A Global Risk Analysis (Disaster Risk Management Series No. 5),* Washington, DC, 2005, World Bank.

Downes E: Nursing and complex humanitarian emergencies: Ebola is more than a disease, *Nurs Outlook* 63:12–15, 2015.

Federal Emergency Management Agency: *Emergency Support Function#8-Public Health and Medical Services Annex,* 2016. Retrieved July 28, 2017 from http://www.fema.gov/media-library/ESF_8_Public_Health_Medical_20160705_508.pdf.

Federal Emergency Management Agency: *Homeland Security Exercise and Evaluation Program (HSEEP),* Washington, DC, June 2016. Retrieved July 27, 2017 from http://www.fema/gov/hseep.

Federal Emergency Management Agency: *National Incident Management System (NIMS),* 2017. Retrieved July 27, 2017 from http://www.fema.gov/national-incident-management-system.

Federal Emergency Management Agency: *National Preparedness Report,* 2013d. Retrieved February 2016 from http://www.fema.gov/media-library/assets/documetns/32509.

Federal Emergency Management Agency: *National Exercise Program (NEP)-Capstone Exercise 2014,* 2014a. Retrieved January 2015 from http://www.fema.gov.national-exercise-program-nep-capston-exercise-2014.

Federal Emergency Management Agency: *Disaster Declarations for 2013,* 2014b. Retrieved January 2015 from https://www.fema.gov/disasters.

Federal Emergency Management Agency: *National Preparedness Goal, Second Edition-What's New,* 2015. Retrieved February 2016 from http:www.fema.gov/national-preparedness-goal.

Gaines SK, Leary J: Public health emergency preparedness in the setting of child care, *Fam Commun Health* 27:263–268, 2004.

Inajima T, Adelman J, Okada Y: *Fukushima disaster was manmade, investigation finds,* Bloomberg Businessweek, July 5, 2012. Retrieved January 2015 from http://www.bloomberg.com/news/2012-07-05/fukushima-nuclear-disaster-was-man-made-investigation-rules.html.

Landesman L: *Public health management of disasters: the practice guide,* Washington, DC, 2001, American Public Health Association.

National Institute of Occupational Health and Safety: *Traumatic Incident stress,* 2013. Retrieved February 2016 from http://www.cdc.gov/niosh/topics/traumaticincident/.

National Oceanic and Atmospheric Administration: *Hurricanes in history,* Washington DC, 2007. Retrieved July 28, 2017 from http://www.nhc.noaaa.gov/outreach/history/n.d.

National Institute of Mental Health: *Helping children and adolescents cope with violence and disasters: What parents can do,* 2015. Retrieved July 28, 2017 from http://www/nimh.nih.gov/health/publications/helping-children-and-adolescents-cope-with-violence-and-disasters-parents/index.shtml.

Reagan M, editor: *CNN reports: Katrina state of emergency*, Kansas City, Mo, 2005, Andrews McMeel.

Rotz LD, Koo D, O'Carroll PW, et al: Bioterrorism preparedness: planning for the future, *J Public Health Manag Pract* 6:45, 2000.

Substance Abuse and Mental Health Services Administration: *Tips for survivors of a disaster or other traumatic event: Managing stress*, 2013. Retrieved from http://www.disasterdistress.samhsa.gov.

Stanley S, Polivka B, Gordon D, et al: The ExploreSurge trail guide and hiking workshop: discipline specific education for public health nurses, *Public Health Nurs* 25:166–175, 2008.

United Nations Office for Disaster Risk Reduction: *Making development sustainable: The future of disaster risk management. Global Assessment Report on Disaster Risk Reduction*, Geneva, Switzerland, 2015, UNISDR.

U.S. Department of Health and Human Services: *Healthy People 2020: a roadmap to improve America's health*, Washington, DC, 2010,

U.S. Government Printing Office. Retrieved June 2012 from http://www.healthypeople.gov.

U.S. Department of Health and Human Services: *National Health Security Strategy of the United States of America*, 2017. Retrieved July 27, 2017 from http://www.phe.gov/nhss.

U.S. Department of Health and Human Services: *Public Health Emergency Pandemic and All-Hazards Preparedness Reauthorization Act of 2013*, 2017. Retrieved July 27, 2017 from https://www.phe.gov/Preparedness/legal/pahpra/Pages/pahpra.aspx.

Veenema TG: *Disaster Nursing and emergency preparedness for chemical, biological, and radiological terrorism and other hazards*, New York, 2012, Springer Publishing.

Veenema TG, Thornton CP: Understanding nursing's role in health systems response to large-scale radiologic disasters, *Radiol Nurs* 34(2):63–72, 2015.

Vinter S, Lieberman DA, Levi J: Public health preparedness in a reforming health care system, *Harv Law Policy Rev* 4:339–360, 2010.

CHAPTER 15

Surveillance and Outbreak Investigation

Marcia Stanhope

OBJECTIVES

After reading this chapter, the student should be able to:

1. Define public health surveillance.
2. List types of surveillance systems.
3. Identify steps in planning, analyzing, interviewing, and evaluating surveillance.
4. Recognize sources of data used when investigating a disease or condition outbreak.
5. Describe the role of the nurse in surveillance and outbreak investigation.
6. Relate the nurse's role in investigation to the national core competencies for public health nurses.

CHAPTER OUTLINE

Disease Surveillance/Public Health Surveillance
  Definitions and Importance
  Uses of Public Health Surveillance
  Purposes of Surveillance
  Collaboration Among Partners
  Nurse Competencies
  Data Sources for Surveillance
National Notifiable Diseases
  State Notifiable Diseases
  Types of Surveillance Systems

  Passive System
  Active System
  Sentinel System
  Special Systems
The Investigation
  Investigation Objectives
  Patterns of Occurrence
  When to Investigate
Interventions and Protection

KEY TERMS

biological terrorism, 256
chemical terrorism, 256
common source outbreak, 261
disease surveillance, 255
endemic, 261
epidemic, 261
event, 256
holoendemic, 261

hyperendemic, 261
intermittent or continuous
  source, 261
mixed outbreak, 261
National Notifiable Disease
  Surveillance System
  (NNDSS), 258
outbreak, 261

outbreak detection, 261
pandemic, 261
point source outbreak, 261
propagated outbreak, 261
sentinel, 260
sporadic, 261
syndromic surveillance
  systems, 260

Disease surveillance has been a part of public health protection since the 1200s during the investigations of the bubonic plague in Europe. The Constitution of the United States provides for "police powers" necessary to preserve health safety as well as other events (see Chapter 7). These powers include public health surveillance. State and local "police powers" also provide for surveillance activities. Health departments usually have the legal authority to investigate unusual clusters of illness as well (Shannon, 2015).

DISEASE SURVEILLANCE/PUBLIC HEALTH SURVEILLANCE

DEFINITIONS AND IMPORTANCE

Disease surveillance is "the ongoing systematic collection, analysis, interpretation and dissemination of specific health data for use in public health" (Lee et al, 2010; McNabb et al, 2016; Centers for Disease Control and Prevention [CDC], 2015a). Surveillance provides a means for nurses to monitor

---

BOX 15.1   Features of Surveillance

- Is organized and planned
- Is the principal means by which a population's health status is assessed
- Involves ongoing collection of specific data
- Involves analyzing data on a regular basis
- Requires sharing the results with others
- Requires broad and repeated contact with the public about personal health issues
- Motivates public health action as a result of data analyses to:
  - Reduce morbidity
  - Reduce mortality
  - Improve health

---

disease trends to reduce morbidity and mortality and improve health (McNabb et al, (2016) also use the term **public health surveillance** as "the systematic collection of health information for the purpose of monitoring, preventing, or controlling the spread of disease in a population (p. 13)." The Centers for Disease Control and Prevention indicates that public health surveillance is the foundation of public health practice (2015a).

Surveillance is a critical role function for nurses practicing in the community. It is important because it generates knowledge of a disease or event outbreak patterns (including timing, geographic distribution, and susceptible populations).

Although surveillance was initially devoted to monitoring and reducing the spread of infectious diseases, it is now used to monitor and reduce chronic diseases and injuries, as well as "environmental and occupational exposures" (McNabb et al, 2016) and personal health behaviors. Surveillance systems help nurses and other professionals monitor emerging infections and bioterrorist outbreaks (McNabb et al, 2016) and personal health behaviors. Bioterrorism is one example of an event creating a critical public health concern that involves environmental exposures that must be monitored. This event also requires serious planning to be able to respond quickly and effectively. Biological terrorism is "the deliberate release of viruses, bacteria, or other germs (agents) used to cause illness or death in people, animals, or plants" www.emergency.cdc.gov/bioterrorism/overview.asp (CDC, 2012a). Chemical terrorism is the intentional release of hazardous chemicals into the environment for the purpose of harming or killing (U.S. Department of Homeland Security, n.d.). In the event of a bioterrorist attack, imagine how difficult it would be to control the spread of biological agents such as botulism or anthrax or chemical agents such as sarin or ricin if no data were available about these agents, their resulting diseases or symptoms, and their usual incidence (new cases) patterns in the community. (See Box 15.1 for a summary of the features of surveillance.)

USES OF PUBLIC HEALTH SURVEILLANCE

Public health surveillance can be used to facilitate the following (CDC, 2014):

- Estimate the magnitude of a problem (disease or event)
- Determine the geographic distribution of an illness or symptoms

- Portray the natural history of a disease
- Detect epidemics and define a problem
- Generate hypotheses and stimulate research
- Evaluate control measures
- Monitor changes in infectious agents
- Detect changes in health practices
- Facilitate planning

PURPOSES OF SURVEILLANCE

Surveillance helps public health departments identify trends and unusual disease patterns, set priorities for using scarce resources, and develop and evaluate programs for commonly occurring and universally occurring diseases or events (Box 15.2).

Surveillance activities can be related to the core functions of public health—assessment, policy development, and assurance. Disease surveillance helps establish baseline (endemic) rates of disease occurrence and patterns of spread. Surveillance makes it possible to initiate a rapid response to an outbreak of a disease or event that can cause a health problem. Surveillance data are assessed and analyzed, and interpretations of these data analyses are used to develop policies that better protect the public from problems such as emerging infections, bioterrorist biological and chemical threats, and injuries from problems such as motor vehicle accidents. Surveillance makes it possible to have ongoing monitoring in place to ensure that disease and event patterns improve rather than deteriorate. It can also make it possible to study whether the clinical protocols and public health policies that are in place can be enhanced based on current science so that disease rates actually decline.

Surveillance data are very helpful in determining whether a program is effective. Such data make it possible to determine whether public health interventions are effective in reducing the spread of disease or the incidence of injuries.

COLLABORATION AMONG PARTNERS

A quality surveillance system requires collaboration among various agencies and individuals: federal agencies, state and local public health agencies, hospitals, health care providers, medical examiners, veterinarians, agriculture, pharmaceutical agencies, emergency management, and law enforcement agencies, as well as 9-1-1 systems, ambulance services, urgent care

---

BOX 15.2   Purposes of Surveillance

- Assess public health status
- Define public health priorities
- Plan public health programs
- Evaluate interventions and programs
- Stimulate research

From Centers for Disease Control and Prevention (CDC): Introduction to public health. In: *Public Health 101 Series,* Atlanta, GA, 2014, U.S. Department of Health and Human Services, CDC. Available at: http://www.cdc.gov/publichealth101/surveillance.html.

and emergency departments, poison control centers, nurse hotlines, schools, and industry. Such collaboration promotes the development of a comprehensive plan and a directory of emergency responses and contacts for effective communication and information sharing. The type of information to be shared includes the following:

- How to use algorithms to identify which events should be investigated (i.e., using a precise step-by-step plan outlining a procedure that in a finite number of steps helps identify the appropriate event)
- How to investigate
- Whom to contact
- How and to whom information is to be disseminated
- Who is responsible for appropriate action

Nurses are often in the forefront of responses to be made in the surveillance process whether working in a small rural agency or a large urban agency; within the health department, school, or urgent care center; or on the telephone performing triage services during a disaster. It is the nurse who sees the event first (Association of Public Health Nurses, 2014; Veenema, 2013).

NURSE COMPETENCIES

The national core competencies for public health nurses were developed from the work of the Council on Linkages Between Academia and Public Health Practice (2014) and by the Quad Council of Public Health Nursing Organizations (2011). These competencies are divided into eight practice domains: analytic assessment skills, policy development/program planning skills, communication skills, cultural competency skills, community dimensions of practice skills, public health sciences skills, financial planning and management skills, and leadership and systems thinking skills.

To be a participant in surveillance and investigation activities, the staff nurse must have the following knowledge related to the core competencies:

1. Analytic assessment skills
   - Defining the problem
   - Determining a cause
   - Identifying relevant data and information sources
   - Partnering with others to give meaning to the data collected
   - Identifying risks
2. Communication
   - Providing effective oral and written reports
   - Soliciting input from others and effectively presenting accurate demographic, statistical, and scientific information to other professionals and the community at large
3. Community dimensions of practice
   - Establishing and maintaining links during the investigation
   - Collaborating with partners
   - Developing, implementing, and evaluating an assessment to define the problem

4. Basic public health science skills
   - Identifying individual and organizational responsibilities
   - Identifying and retrieving current relevant scientific evidence
5. Leadership and systems thinking
   - Identifying internal and external issues that have an effect on the investigation
   - Promoting team and organizational efforts
   - Contributing to developing, implementing, and monitoring of the investigation

Whereas the staff nurse participates in these activities, the advanced practice public health nurse should be proficient in applying these competencies.

The Minnesota Model of Public Health Interventions: Applications for Public Health Nursing Practice (Center for Public Health Nursing, 2001, pp 15, 16) suggests that surveillance is one of the interventions related to nursing practice in public health. The model provides seven basic steps of surveillance for nurses to follow:

1. Consider whether surveillance as an intervention is appropriate for the situation.
2. Organize the knowledge of the problem, its natural course of history, and its aftermath.
3. Establish clear criteria for what constitutes a case.
4. Collect sufficient data from multiple valid sources.
5. Analyze the data.
6. Interpret and disseminate the data to decision makers.
7. Evaluate the impact of the surveillance system.

DATA SOURCES FOR SURVEILLANCE

Clinicians, health care agencies, and laboratories report cases to state health departments. Data also come from death certificates and administrative data such as discharge reports and billing records (McNabb et al, 2016). The following are select sources of mortality and morbidity data:

1. Mortality data are often the only source of health-related data available for small geographic areas. Examples include the following:
   - Vital statistics reports (e.g., death certificates, medical examiner reports, birth certificates)
2. Morbidity data include the following:
   - Notifiable disease reports
   - Laboratory reports
   - Hospital discharge reports
   - Billing data
   - Outpatient health care data
   - Specialized disease registries
   - Injury surveillance systems
   - Environmental surveys
   - Sentinel surveillance systems

A good example of a process in place to collect morbidity data is the National Program of Cancer Registries. This program provides for monitoring of the types of cancers found in a state and the locations of the cancer risks and health problems in the state.

HEALTHY PEOPLE 2020

Surveillance Objectives

- **EH-5:** Reduce waterborne disease outbreaks arising from water intended for drinking among persons served by community water systems.
- **FS-2:** Reduce infections associated with foodborne outbreaks from pathogens commonly transmitted through food.
- **GH-1:** Reduce the number of cases of malaria reported in the United States.
- **IID-16:** (Developmental) Increase the scientific knowledge on vaccine safety and adverse events.
- **PHI-2:** Increase the proportion of tribal, state, and local public health agencies that incorporate core competencies for public health professionals into the job.
- **PHI-7:** Increase the proportion of population-based *Healthy People 2020* objectives for which national data are available for all population groups identified for the objective.

From U.S. Department of Health and Human Services: *Healthy People 2020: a roadmap to improve all Americans' health,* Washington, DC, 2010, U.S. Government Printing Office.

Each of the data sources has the potential for underreporting or incomplete reporting. However, if there is consistency in the use of surveillance methods, the data collected will show trends in events or disease patterns that may indicate a change needed in a program or a needed prevention intervention to reduce morbidity or mortality (CDC, 2014).

Mortality data assist in identifying differences in health status among groups, populations, occupations, and communities; monitoring preventable deaths; and examining cause and effect factors in diseases. Vital statistics can be used to plan programs and monitor programs to meet *Healthy People 2020* goals.

The sentinel surveillance system provides for the monitoring of key health events when information is not otherwise available or for calculating or estimating disease morbidity in vulnerable populations (McNabb et al, 2016).

NATIONAL NOTIFIABLE DISEASES

Box 15.3 shows the national notifiable infectious diseases. Reporting of disease data by health care providers, laboratories, and public health workers to state and local health departments is essential if trends are to be accurately monitored.

The data provide the basis for detecting disease outbreaks, for identifying person characteristics, and for calculating incidence, geographic distribution, and temporal trends. They are used to initiate prevention programs, evaluate established prevention and control practices, suggest new intervention strategies, identify areas for research, document the need for disease control funds, and help answer questions from the community. (https://wwwn.cdc.gov/nndss/conditions/notifiable/2016/)

(CDC, 2016a)

The CDC and the Council of State and Territorial Epidemiologists have a policy that requires state health departments to report certain diseases to the CDC National Notifiable Disease

---

BOX 15.3 Infectious Diseases Designated as Notifiable at the National Level: United States, 2016

- Anthrax
- Arboviral neuroinvasive and nonneuroinvasive diseases
- California serogroup virus disease
- Chikungunya virus disease
- Eastern equine encephalitis virus disease
- Powassan virus disease
- St. Louis encephalitis virus disease
- West Nile virus disease
- Western equine encephalitis virus disease
- Babesiosis
- Botulism
- Botulism, foodborne
- Botulism, infant
- Botulism, other
- Botulism, wound
- Brucellosis
- Campylobacteriosis
- Cancer
- Carbon monoxide poisoning
- Chancroid
- *Chlamydia trachomatis* infection
- Cholera
- Coccidioidomycosis/ Valley fever
- Congenital syphilis
- Cryptosporidiosis
- Cyclosporiasis
- Dengue virus infections
- Dengue

- Dengue-like illness
- Severe dengue
- Diphtheria
- Ehrlichiosis/anaplasmosis
- *Anaplasma phagocytophilum* infection
- *Ehrlichia chaffeensis* infection
- *Ehrlichia ewingii* infection
- Undetermined human ehrlickiosis/Anaplasmosis
- Foodborne disease outbreak
- Giardiasis
- Gonorrhea
- *Haemophilus influenzae,* invasive disease
- Hansen's disease/leprosy
- Hantavirus infection, non-Hantavirus pulmonary syndrom
- Hantavirus pulmonary syndrome (HPS)
- Hemolytic uremic syndrome, post-diarrheal (HUS)
- Hepatitis A, acute
- Hepatitis B, acute
- Hepatitis B, chronic
- Hepatitis B virus, perinatal infection
- Hepatitic C, acute
- Hepatitis C, past or present
- HIV infection (AIDS has been reclassified as HIV stage III) (AIDS/HIV)
- Influenza-associated pediatric mortality
- Invasive pneumococcal disease (IPD)/*Streptococcus pneumoniae,* Invasive disease
- Lead, elevated blood levels
- Lead, elevated blood levels, adult (≥16 years)
- Lead, elevated blood levels, children (<16 years)

BOX 15.3 Infectious Diseases Designated as Notifiable at the National Level: United States, 2016—cont'd

- Legionellosis/ Legionnaire's disease or Pontiac fever
- Leptosriosis
- Listeriosis
- Lyme disease
- Malaria
- Measles/ Rubeola
- Meningococcal disease
- Mumps
- Novel influenza A virus infections
- Pertussis/ Whooping cough
- Pesticide-related illness and injury, acute
- Plague
- Poliomyelitis, paralytic
- Poliovirus infection, nonparalytic
- Psittacosis/ ornithosis
- Q fever
- Acute
- Chronic
- Rabies, animal
- Rabies, human
- Rubella/ German measles
- Rubella, congenital syndrome (CRS)
- Salmonellosis
- Severe acute respiratory syndrome–associated coronavirus disease (SARS)
- Shiga toxin-producing *Escherichia coli* (STEC)
- Shigellosis
- Silicosis
- Smallpox/ Variola
- Spotted fever rickettsiosis
- Streptococcal toxic shock syndrome (STSS)

- Syphilis
- Early latent
- Late latent
- Late with clinical manifestations (including late benign syphilis and cardiovascular syphilis)
- Primary
- Secondary
- Stillbirth
- Tetanus/*c. tetani*
- Toxic shock syndrome (other than streptococcal) (TSS)
- Trichinellosis/ trichinosis
- Tuberculosis (TB)
- Tularemia
- Typhoid fever
- Vancomycin-intermediate *Staphylococcus aureus* (VISA)
- Vancomycin-resistant *Staphylococcus aureus* (VRSA)
- Varicella/ Chickenpox
- Varicella deaths
- Vibriosis
- Viral hemorrhagic fevers (VHF)
- Crimean-Congo hemorrhagic fever virus
- Ebola virus
- Lassa virus
- Lujo virus
- Marburg virus
- New World arenaviruses (Gunarito, Machupo, Junin, and Sabia viruses)
- Waterborne disease outbreak
- Yellow fever
- Zika virus disease
- Zika virus, congenital infection

Modified from Centers for Disease Control and Prevention: *Nationally notifiable infectious diseases: United States,* Atlanta, 2016, CDC. Retrieved July 2016 from https://wwwn.cdc.gov/nndss/conditions/notifiable/2016/.

Surveillance System (NNDSS). The data for nationally notifiable diseases from 50 states, the US territories, New York City, and the District of Columbia are published weekly in the Morbidity and Mortality Weekly Report (MMWR). Data collection about these diseases and revision of statistics are ongoing. Annual updated final reports are published in the *CDC Summary of Notifiable Diseases: United States* (CDC, 2016a).

STATE NOTIFIABLE DISEASES

Requirements for reporting diseases are mandated by law or regulation. Although each state differs in the list of reportable diseases, the usefulness of the data depends on "uniformity, simplicity, and timeliness." Because state requirements differ, not all nationally notifiable diseases are legally mandated for reporting in a state. For legally reportable diseases, states compile disease incidence data (new cases) and transmit the data electronically, weekly, to the CDC through the National Electronic Disease Surveillance System (NEDSS) (CDC, 2015b) (https://wwwn.cdc.gov/nndss/nedss.html). To determine which of the national notifiable diseases are

QSEN FOCUS ON QUALITY AND SAFETY EDUCATION FOR NURSES

Targeted Competency: Safety—Minimizes risk for harm to clients and providers through both system effectiveness and individual performance.
- **Knowledge:** Discuss potential and actual impact of national client safety resources, initiatives, and regulations.
- **Skill:** Use national resources for own development and to focus attention on safety in the community.
- **Attitude:** Value relationships between national safety campaigns and implementation in locales, times and settings.

Safety Question

The Quad Council competency for communication skills indicates that the public health nurse uses a variety of methods to disseminate public health information to populations within a community and provides a presentation of targeted health information to multiple audiences at a local level: groups, professionals, and agency peers.

How would the nurse use the national sentinel surveillance system to identify health conditions and risks in the community? What types of data sources in this system would the nurse collect? After careful analysis of the data sources, what would the nurse include in a presentation to multiple audiences?

reportable in your state, go to your state health department website.

TYPES OF SURVEILLANCE SYSTEMS

Informatics is essential to the mission of protecting the public's health. Surveillance systems are designed to assist public health professionals in the early detection of disease and event outbreaks to intervene and reduce the potential for morbidity or mortality or to improve the public's health status (CDC, 2014). Surveillance systems in use today are defined as passive, active, sentinel, and special.

PASSIVE SYSTEM

In the passive system, case reports are sent to local health departments by health care providers (i.e., physicians, nurses) or laboratory reports of disease occurrence are sent to the local health department. The case reports are summarized and forwarded to the state health department, national government, or organizations responsible for monitoring the problem, such as the CDC or an international organization such as the World Health Organization.

ACTIVE SYSTEM

In the active system, the nurse, as an employee of the health department, may begin a search for cases through contact with local health care providers and agencies. In this system, the nurse names the disease or the event and gathers data about existing cases to try to determine the magnitude of the problem (how widespread it is).

SENTINEL SYSTEM

In the sentinel system, trends in commonly occurring diseases or key health indicators are monitored (*Healthy People 2020*). A disease or an event may be the sentinel, or a population may be the sentinel. In this system a sample of health providers or agencies is asked to report the problem. The system is useful because it helps monitor trends in commonly occurring diseases and events.

SPECIAL SYSTEMS

Special systems are developed for collecting particular types of data; these may be a combination of active, passive, or sentinel systems. As a result of bioterrorism, newer systems called syndromic surveillance systems are being developed to monitor illness syndromes or events. This approach requires the use of automated data systems to report continued (real time) or daily (near real time) disease outbreaks (CDC, 2016b) (Box 15.4).

The CDC's Syndromic Surveillance website discusses the impact of increasing electronic health record systems: "Public health syndromic surveillance using inpatient and ambulatory clinical care electronic health record (EHR) data is a relatively new practice. As eligible health professionals and hospitals adopt, implement, and upgrade their EHR systems

through the Centers for Medicare and Medicaid services EHR Incentive programs (Meaningful Use programs), there is an opportunity for public health agencies (PHAs) to routinely receive health data from settings other than emergency departments and urgent care centers. Given the number of factors and complex relationships that affect EHR data quality, a collaborative approach that includes public health, healthcare, and EHR technology developers is the best way to determine how EHR data can be meaningfully used for surveillance." (http://www.cdc.gov/ehrmeaningfuluse/syndromic.html

Although all of the systems are important, the public health nurse is most likely to use the active or passive systems. A passive system may use the state reportable disease system to complete a community assessment or Mobilizing for Action through

EVIDENCE-BASED PRACTICE

Cancer Screening Interventions for Surveillance

An analysis was conducted to identify uses of spatial analysis in cancer screening interventions. Researchers used a spatial analysis tool called *cluster detection* to identify geographic areas with populations at high risk for colorectal cancer. Specifically, the investigators used the free cluster detection software application SaTScan to map the at-risk population. The researchers sought to identify which spatial analysis method was most successful in identifying at-risk populations. Various methods were used to detect areas in Florida where the population was at high risk. Although no single method emerged as being able to detect all significant clusters, all methods did detect one area as high risk. This area could be seen as a priority area to implement a screening intervention to improve early identification of disease and early treatment.

Nurse Use

Cluster detection is a surveillance tool that public health nurses can use to determine geographic priority areas for health promotion and disease prevention interventions. Being able to focus on a specific area would enable the nurse to use public health resources in an efficient manner and provide outreach to the populations at highest risk for disease.

From Sherman RL, Henry KA, Tannenbaum SL, et al: Applying spatial analysis tools in public health: an example using SaTScan to detect geographic targets for colorectal cancer screening interventions. *Prev Chronic Dis* 11:130264, 2014. DOI: http://dx.doi.org/10.5888/pcd11.130264. Sherman RL, Henry KA, Tannenbaum SL, et al: Applying spatial analysis tools in public health: an example using SaTScan to detect geographic targets for colorectal cancer screening interventions. *Prev Chronic Dis* 11:130264, 2014. DOI: http://dx.doi.org/10.5888/pcd11.130264

Planning and Partnerships (MAPP) (see Chapters 12 and 16). The active system is used when several school children become ill after eating lunch in the school cafeteria or at the local hot dog stand, to investigate the possibility of food poisoning, or to follow up with the contacts of a client newly diagnosed with tuberculosis or a sexually transmitted disease (STD) at the local homeless shelter (CDC, 2014).

THE INVESTIGATION

INVESTIGATION OBJECTIVES

Any unusual increase in disease incidence (new cases) or an unusual event in the community should be investigated. The system used for investigation depends on the intensity of the event, the severity of the disease, the number of people or communities affected, the potential for harm to the community or the spread of disease, and the effectiveness of available interventions (CDC, 2012b). The objectives of an investigation are as follows:

- To control and prevent disease or death
- To identify factors that contribute to the outbreak of the disease and the occurrence of the event
- To implement measures to prevent occurrences

Defining the Magnitude of a Problem or an Event

The following definitions provide a way to describe the level of occurrence of a disease or an event for purposes of communicating the magnitude of the problem. A disease or an event found to be present (occurring) in a population is defined as endemic if there is a persistent (usual) presence with a low to moderate number of cases of the disease or event. The endemic levels of a disease or an event in a population provide the baseline for establishing a public health problem. For example, foodborne botulism is endemic to Alaska. The baseline must be known to determine the existence of a change or increase in the number of cases from the baseline. If a problem is considered hyperendemic, there is a persistently (usually) high number of cases. An example is the high cholera incidence rate among Asians and Pacific Islanders. Sporadic problems are those with an irregular pattern with occasional cases found at irregular intervals. Epidemic means that the occurrence of a disease within an area is clearly in excess of expected levels (endemic) for a given time period. This is often called the outbreak. Pandemic refers to the epidemic spread of the problem over several countries or continents (e.g., severe acute respiratory syndrome [SARS] outbreak). Holoendemic in a population implies a highly prevalent problem that is commonly acquired early in life. The prevalence of this problem decreases as age increases (Nmadu et al, 2015). Outbreak detection, or identifying an increase in the frequency of disease above the usual occurrence of the disease, is the function of the investigator (CDC, 2015c).

Patterns of Occurrence

Patterns of occurrence can be identified when investigating a disease or event. These patterns are used to define the boundaries of a problem to help investigate possible causes or sources of the problem. A common source outbreak refers to a group exposed to a common noxious influence such as the release of noxious gases (e.g., ricin in the Japanese subway system several years ago and more recently in a water system in the United States) (Merrill, 2017). In a point source outbreak, all persons exposed become ill at the same time, during one incubation period. A mixed outbreak is "when a victim of a common source epidemic has person-to-person contact with others and spreads the disease, further propagating the health problem" (Merrill, 2017, p. 316), as in the spreading of influenza. Intermittent or continuous source cases may be exposed over a period of days or weeks, as in the recent food poisonings at a restaurant chain throughout the United States as a result of the restaurant's purchase of contaminated green onions. A propagated outbreak does not have a common source and spreads gradually from person to person over more than one incubation period, such as the spread of tuberculosis from one person to another.

Causal Factors From the Epidemiological Triangle

Factors that must be considered as causes of an outbreak are categorized as agents, hosts, and environmental factors (see Chapter 9). The belief is that these factors may interact to cause the outbreak and therefore the potential interactions must be examined. Box 15.5 presents definitions used to classify agents in an attack. Box 15.6 lists the types of agent factors that may be present. The host factors associated with cases may be age, sex, race, socioeconomic status, genetics, and lifestyle choices (e.g., cigarette smoking, sexual practices, contraception, eating habits).

BOX 15.5 Classification of Agents

Infectivity: Refers to the capacity of an agent to enter a susceptible host and produce infection or disease
Pathogenicity: Measures the proportion of infected people who develop the disease
Virulence: Refers to the proportion of people with clinical disease who become severely ill or die

---

BOX 15.6 Types of Agent Factors

1. Biological
   - Bacteria (e.g., tuberculosis, salmonellosis, streptococcal infections)
   - Viruses (e.g., hepatitis A, herpes)
   - Fungi (e.g., tinea capitis, blastomycosis)
   - Parasites (e.g., protozoa-causing malaria, giardiasis; helminths [roundworms, pinworms]; arthropods [mosquitoes, ticks, flies, mites])
2. Physical
   - Heat
   - Trauma
3. Chemical
   - Pollutants
   - Medications/drugs
4. Nutrients
   - Absence
   - Excess
5. Psychological
   - Stress
   - Isolation
   - Social support

WHAT WOULD YOU DO

You have joined the community emergency response team to investigate a suspected disease outbreak in the area. How would you determine the existence of an unusual outbreak?

The environmental factors that may be related to a case are physical (e.g., weather, temperature, humidity, physical surroundings) or biological (e.g., insects that transmit the agent). Some of the socioeconomic factors that might affect the development of a disease or an event are behavior (e.g., terrorist behaviors), personality, cultural characteristics of the group, crowding, sanitation, and the availability of health services.

WHEN TO INVESTIGATE

An unusual increase in disease incidence should be investigated. The amount of effort that goes into an investigation depends on the severity or magnitude of the problem, the numbers in the population who are affected, the potential for spreading the disease, and the availability and effectiveness of intervention measures to resolve the problems. Most of the outbreaks of diseases (or increased incidence rates) occur naturally or are predictable compared with the consistent patterns of previous outbreaks of a disease such as influenza, tuberculosis, or common infectious diseases. When a disease or an event outbreak occurs as a result of the purposeful introduction of an agent into the population, then the predictable patterns may not exist. Sobel and Watson (2009) provide clues to be used when trying to determine the existence of bioterrorism. These clues are simplified and appear in Box 15.7.

BOX 15.7   Epidemiological Clues that may Signal a Covert Bioterrorism Attack

- Large numbers of ill persons with a similar disease or syndrome
- Large numbers of unexplained disease, syndrome, or deaths
- Unusual illness in a population
- Higher morbidity and mortality than expected with a common disease or syndrome
- Failure of a common disease to respond to usual therapy
- Single case of the disease caused by an uncommon agent
- Multiple unusual or unexplained disease entities coexisting in the same person without any other explanation
- Disease with an unusual geographic or seasonal distribution
- Multiple atypical presentations of disease agents
- Similar genetic type among agents isolated from temporally or spatially distinct sources
- Unusual, atypical, genetically engineered, or antiquated strain of agent
- Endemic disease with an unexplained increase in incidence
- Simultaneous clusters of similar illness in noncontiguous areas, domestic or foreign
- Atypical aerosol, food, or water transmission
- Ill people presenting at about the same time
- Deaths or illness among animals that precedes or accompanies illness or death in humans
- No illness in people not exposed to common ventilation systems, but illness among those people in proximity to the systems

The How To box provides a brief guide to conducting the investigation.

HOW TO   Conduct an Investigation

- Confirm the existence of an outbreak.
- Verify the diagnosis and/or define a case.
- Estimate the number of cases.
- Orient the data collected to person, place, and time.
- Develop and evaluate a hypothesis.
- Institute control measures and communicate findings.

From the Centers for Disease Control and Prevention (CDC): Steps to Investigation Retrieved January 2015 from http://www.cdc.gov.

 LEVELS OF PREVENTION

For Surveillance Activities

Primary Prevention
Develop an approach for mass immunizations of citizens to prevent the occurrence of H1N1 (H1N2 or H3N3) in the community.

Secondary Prevention
Investigate an outbreak of flulike illness in a local school.

Tertiary Prevention
Provide health care and treatment for those infected by H1N1 or the new strains of the virus.

INTERVENTIONS AND PROTECTION

Remember that disease and event surveillance systems exist to help improve the health of the public through the systematic and ongoing collection, distribution, and use of health-related data. A nurse can contribute to such systems and best use the data collected through such systems to help manage endemic health problems and those that are emerging, such as evolving infectious diseases and bioterrorist (human-made) health problems. The functions of surveillance and investigation include detecting cases, estimating the impact of disease or injury, showing the natural history of a health condition, determining the distribution and spread of illness, generating hypotheses, evaluating prevention and control measures, and facilitating planning (McNabb et al, 2016). Response to bioterrorism or to a large-scale infectious disease outbreak may require the use of emergency public health measures such as quarantine, isolation, closing public places, seizing property, mandatory vaccination, travel restrictions, and disposal of the deceased. Suggestions for protecting health care providers from exposure include the use of standard precautions when coming into contact with broken skin or body fluids, the use of disposable nonsterile gowns and gloves followed by adequate hand washing after removal, and the use of a face shield (CDC, 2016c).

> ▶ **APPLYING CONTENT TO PRACTICE**

Remember that disease and event surveillance systems exist to help improve the health of the public through the systematic and ongoing collection, distribution, and use of health-related data. A nurse can contribute to such systems and best use the data collected through such systems to help manage endemic health problems and those that are emerging, such as evolving infectious diseases and bioterrorist (human-made) health problems. The functions of surveillance and investigation include detecting cases, estimating the impact of disease or injury, showing the natural history of a health condition, determining the distribution and spread of illness, generating hypotheses, evaluating prevention and control measures, and facilitating planning (McNabb et al, 2016). Response to bioterrorism or to a large-scale infectious disease outbreak may require the use of emergency public health measures such as quarantine, isolation, closing public places, seizing property, mandatory vaccination, travel restrictions, and disposal of the deceased. Suggestions for protecting health care providers from exposure include the use of standard precautions when coming

in contact with broken skin or body fluids, the use of disposable nonsterile gowns and gloves followed by adequate hand washing after removal, and the use of a face shield (CDC, 2016c). This chapter focuses on the importance of using informatics to identify, monitor, and intervene in unusual occurrences and events to protect the public and to keep communities safe. Informatics the use of information and technology to communicate, manage knowledge, mitigate error, and support decision making. The knowledge requirement for the public health nurse and student is to explain why information and technology skills are essential for safety. The skill to be developed is the seeking of education about how information is managed in the setting before providing an intervention. This chapter applies this by looking at trends of occurrences and events before investigating the situation and deciding on an intervention. It is also important to be able to use the databases and the tools of investigation to ensure safe processes of care. The attitude of engaging in continuous learning and the development of new technology skills is essential.

PRACTICE APPLICATION

As a clinical project the health department asked the public health nursing class at the university to develop a community service message to air on local radio about the potential of a pandemic flu.

What does the message need to contain to help the community prepare?
Answers can be found on the Evolve website.

REMEMBER THIS!

- Disease surveillance has been a part of public health protection since the 1200s during the investigations of the bubonic plague in Europe.
- Surveillance provides a means for nurses to monitor disease trends to reduce morbidity and mortality and to improve health.
- Surveillance is a critical role function for nurses practicing in the community.
- Surveillance is important because it generates knowledge of a disease or event outbreak patterns.
- Surveillance focuses on the collection of process and outcome data.
- Although surveillance was initially devoted to monitoring and reducing the spread of infectious diseases, it is now used to monitor and reduce chronic diseases and injuries, as well as environmental and occupational exposures.
- Surveillance activities can be related to the core functions of public health assessment, policy development, and assurance.
- A quality surveillance system requires collaboration among agencies and individuals.
- The Minnesota Model of Public Health Interventions: Applications for Public Health Nursing Practice (Center for Public Health Nursing, Office of Public Health Practice, 2001) suggests that surveillance is one of the interventions related to public health nursing practice.
- Clinicians, health care agencies, and laboratories report cases to state health departments. Data also come from death certificates and administrative data such as discharge reports and billing records.
- Each of the data sources has the potential for underreporting or incomplete reporting. However, if there is consistency in

the use of surveillance methods, the data collected will show trends in events or disease patterns that may indicate a change needed in a program or a needed prevention intervention to reduce morbidity or mortality.
- The sentinel surveillance system provides for the monitoring of key health events when information is not otherwise available or for calculating or estimating disease morbidity in vulnerable populations.
- Reporting of disease data by health care providers, laboratories, and public health workers to state and local health departments is essential if trends are to be accurately monitored.
- Requirements for reporting diseases are mandated by law or regulation.
- Surveillance systems in use today are defined as passive, active, sentinel, and special.
- Any unusual increase in disease incidence (i.e., new cases) or an unusual event in the community should be investigated.
- Patterns of occurrence can be identified when investigating a disease or event. These patterns are used to define the boundaries of a problem to help investigate possible causes or sources of the problem.
- Factors that must be considered as causes of outbreak are categorized as agents, hosts, and environmental factors.
- An unusual increase in disease incidence should be investigated.
- Functions of surveillance and investigation include detecting cases, estimating the impact of disease or injury, showing the natural history of a health condition, determining the distribution and spread of illness, generating hypotheses, evaluating prevention and control measures, and facilitating planning.

EVOLVE WEBSITE

http://evolve.elsevier.com/Stanhope/foundations
- NCLEX® Review Questions
- Practice Application Answers

REFERENCES

Association of Public Health Nurses: *The role of the public health nurse in disaster preparedness, response, and recovery: a position paper*, APHN Public Health Preparedness Committee, 2014, Columbus, Ohio.

Centers for Disease Control and Prevention: *Steps to investigation*, 2014. Retrieved January 2015 from http://www.cdc.gov.

Centers for Disease Control and Prevention: Introduction to public health. *In: Public Health 101 Series*, Atlanta, Ga, 2014, U.S. Department of Health and Human Services, CDC. Retrieved from http://www.cdc.gov/publichealth101/surveillance.html.

Centers for Disease Control and Prevention: *Surveillance Resource Center*, 2015a. Retrieved July 2016 from http://www.cdc.gov/surveillancepractice/.

Centers for Disease Control and Prevention: *National Notifiable Disease Surveillance System (NNDSS)*, 2015b. Retrieved July 2015 from https://www.cdc.gov/nndss/nedss.html.

Centers for Disease Control and Prevention: *Outbreak response and prevention branch, Division of Foodborne, Waterborne, and Environmental Diseases (DFWED)*, 2015c. Retrieved July 2015 from http://www.cdc.gov/ncezid/dfwed/orpb/index.html.

Centers for Disease Control and Prevention: *Nationally notifiable infectious diseases: United States*, 2016a, CDC. Retrieved July 2016 from https://www.cdc.gov/nndss/conditions/notifiable/2016/.

Centers for Disease Control and Prevention: *Syndromic surveillance (SS)*, 2016b. Retrieved July 2016 from http://www.cdc.gov/ehrmeaningfuluse/syndromic.html.

Centers for Disease Control and Prevention: *Preparation & planning*, 2016c, Emergency Preparedness and Response. Retrieved July 2016 from https://emergency.cdc.gov/planning/.

Council on Linkages between Academia and Public Health Practice: *Core competencies for public health professionals*, Washington, DC, 2014, The Council. Retrieved July 2016 from http://www.phf.org/resourcestools/pages/core_public_health_competencies.aspx.

Lee LM, Michael L, Teutsch SM, Thacker SB: *Principles and practice of public health surveillance*, ed 3, New York, 2010, Oxford University Press.

McNabb SJN, Conde JM, Ferland L, et al, editors: *Transforming public health surveillance: proactive measures for prevention, detection, and response*, Amman, Jordan, 2016, Elsevier.

Merrill RM: *Introduction to epidemiology*, ed 7, Burlington, Mass, 2017, Jones & Bartlett.

Nmadu PM, Peter E, Alexander P, et al: The prevalence of malaria in children between the ages 2–15 visiting Gwarinpa General Hospital Life-Camp, Abuja, Nigeria, *J Health Sci* 5:47–51, 2015.

Pryor ER: Early recognition and detection of biological events. In Veenema TG, editor: *Disaster nursing and emergency preparedness for chemical, biological, and radiological terrorism and other hazards*, ed 3, New York, 2013, Springer.

Public Health Nursing Section: *Public health interventions: applications for public health nursing practice*, St Paul, Minn, 2001, Minnesota Department of Health. Retrieved from http://www.health.state.mn.us/divs/opi/cd/phn/docs/0301wheel_manual.pdf.

Quad Council of Public Health Nurse Organizations: *Quad Council PHN Competencies*, Grand Rapids, Mich, 2011, The Council. Retrieved July 2016 from http://www.quadcouncilphn.org/documents-3/competencies/.

Shannon K: *Suspicious biological outbreaks: benefits of conducting joint law enforcement and public health investigations*, October 15, 2015, National Association of County & City Health Officials, Preparedness Brief. Retrieved July 2016 from http://nacchopreparedness.org/suspicious-biological-outbreaks-benefits-of-conducting-joint-law-enforcement-and-public-health-investigations/.

Sherman RL, Henry KA, Tannenbaum SL, et al: Applying spatial analysis tools in public health: an example using SaTScan to detect geographic targets for colorectal cancer screening interventions, *Prev Chronic Dis* 11:130264, 2014.

U.S. Department of Health and Human Services: *Healthy People 2020: a roadmap for health*, Washington, DC, 2010, U.S. Government Printing Office.

U.S. Department of Homeland Security: *Chemical Threats*, n.d. Retrieved July 2016 from https://www.ready.gov/chemical-threats.

Veenema TG: *Disaster nursing and emergency preparedness for chemical, biological, and radiolocal terrorism and other hazards*, ed 3, New York, 2013, Springer.

CHAPTER 16

Program Management

Marcia Stanhope

OBJECTIVES

After reading this chapter, the student should be able to:

1. Compare the program management process with the nursing process.
2. Describe the application of the program planning process in the community.
3. Identify the benefits of program planning and evaluation.
4. Apply the components of a program evaluation method in practice.
5. Describe the types of program evaluation measures.
6. Name the sources and techniques of program evaluation.

CHAPTER OUTLINE

Definitions and Goals
Benefits of Program Planning
Planning Process
    Basic Program Planning
    Program-Planning Models for Public
      Health

Program Evaluation
    Benefits of Program Evaluation
    Evaluation Process
    Formulation of Objectives
    Sources of Program Evaluation
    Aspects of Program Evaluation

KEY TERMS

case registers, 271
community indexes, 271
epidemiological data, 272
evaluation, 266
evaluation of processes, 273
evaluation of program
    effectiveness, 274

formative evaluation, 273
health program planning, 266
needs assessment, 266
outcome, 272
planning process, 266
program, 266
program evaluation, 270

strategic planning, 266
summative evaluation, 273

Program management consists of assessing, planning, implementing, and evaluating a program. This chapter focuses primarily on planning and evaluation. Although presented in separate discussions, these factors are related and dependent processes that work together to bring about a successful program. This chapter does not deal with implementing programs because the majority of the chapters in this book focus on implementation.

The program management process is like the nursing process. One is applied to a program, and the other is applied to clients. The process of program management, like the nursing process, consists of a rational decision-making system designed to help nurses determine the following:

- When to make a decision to develop a program
- Where they want to be at the end of the program
- How to decide what to do to have a successful program
- How to develop a plan to go from where they are to where they want to be
- How to know that they are getting there
- What to measure to know whether what they are doing is appropriate

Today there is a greater need for the nurse to be accountable for nursing actions and client outcomes. Prospective payment systems, pay for performance, health care reform, and integrated care delivery models have changed the focus of nursing. Planning for nursing services is necessary today if the nurse is to survive in the field of health care delivery.

The authors acknowledge and thank Doris Glick for contributions to previous editions of this text.

This chapter examines how nurses can *act* instead of *react* by planning programs that can be evaluated for their effectiveness. These programs may be single health promotion programs for a client group, an ongoing program to provide health care services to a client group, or a program designed to address a population problem at the community level.

DEFINITIONS AND GOALS

Community health planning is population focused, and it positions the well-being of the public above private interests (American Planning Association, 2015). A program is an organized approach to meet the assessed needs of individuals, families, groups, or communities by reducing or eliminating one or more health problems. The following are examples of specific programs in nursing in the community:

- Immunization programs
- Health risk screening programs for industrial workers
- Family planning programs
- The following are more broadly based group and community programs:
- Community school health programs
- Home health programs
- Occupational health and safety programs
- Environmental health programs
- Community programs directed at specific illnesses through special interest groups (e.g., American Heart Association, American Cancer Society, March of Dimes)

The planning process is defined as the selecting and carrying out of a series of actions to achieve stated goals (Issel, 2014). The goal of planning is to ensure that health care services are acceptable, equal, efficient, and effective. Evaluation is defined as the methods used to determine whether a service is needed and likely to be used, whether it is conducted as planned, and whether it actually helps people in need (Royse, Thyer, and Padgett, 2016). The two levels of evaluation are defined in Box 16.1.

BENEFITS OF PROGRAM PLANNING

Systematic planning for meeting client needs does the following:
- Benefits clients, nurses, employing agencies, and the community
- Focuses attention on what the organization and health provider are attempting to do for clients

- Assists in identifying the resources and activities that are needed to meet the objectives of client services
- Reduces role ambiguity (uncertainty) by giving responsibility to specific providers to meet program objectives
- Reduces uncertainty within the program environment
- Increases the abilities of the provider and the agency to cope with the external environment
- Helps the provider and the agency anticipate events
- Allows for quality decision making and better control over the actual program results

Today this type of planning is referred to as strategic planning, and it involves the successful matching of client needs with specific provider strengths and competencies and agency resources. Everyone involved with the program can anticipate the following:
- What will be needed to implement the program
- What will occur during implementation
- What the program outcomes will be

PLANNING PROCESS

Program planning is required by federal, state, and local governments; by charitable organizations; and by the employing agency. Planning programs and planning for the evaluation of programs are two very important activities, whether the program being planned is a national health insurance program such as Medicare, a state health care program such as early childhood developmental screening programs, a local program such as vision screening for elementary school children, or a health education program on diet and exercise for a group of obese clients. Regardless of the type of program, the planning process is the same.

BASIC PROGRAM PLANNING

Definition of Problem and Need

The initial and most critical step in health program planning is defining the problem and assessing client need. The target population, or client, to be served by any program must be identified and involved in designing the program to be developed. Program planners must verify that a current health problem exists and is being ignored or is being unsuccessfully treated in a client group. Needs assessment is defined as a systematic appraisal of type, depth, and scope of problems as perceived by clients, health providers, or both (Box 16.2).

BOX 16.1   Two Levels of Evaluation

- **Formative evaluation:** Evaluation for the purpose of assessing whether objectives are met or planned activities are completed. This type of evaluation begins with an assessment of the need for a program and is ongoing as the program is implemented.
- **Summative evaluation:** Evaluation to assess program outcomes or as a follow-up of the results of the program activities and usually occurs when a program is completed or at a specific point in time (e.g., at the end of 1 year or 5 years).

BOX 16.2   Stages Used in Assessing Client Need

- **Preactive:** Projecting a future need.
- **Reactive:** Defining the problem based on past needs identified by the client or the agency.
- **Inactive:** Defining the problem based on the existing health status of the population to be served.
- **Interactive:** Describing the problem using past and present data to project future population needs.

Needs assessment includes the steps in section A1 of the How To box on this page. The client may be identified as a community or group, as families, or as individuals. The client should be defined by biological and psychosocial characteristics, by geographic location, and by the problems to be addressed. For example, in a community with a large number of preschool children who require immunizations to enter school, the client population may be described as all children between 4 and 6 years of age residing in Central County who have not had up-to-date immunizations. This example identifies the client, specifies the need, and states the population size and where they are located.

A health education program may be necessary to alert the population to the existing need. In the example of the need for immunization of preschool children, public service announcements on television and radio and in newspapers may be used to alert parents to laws requiring immunizations, to the continuing problems with communicable diseases, and to the outcomes of successful immunizing programs, such as vaccination programs that have been successful in eliminating smallpox worldwide. A good example of the use of media occurred during an outbreak of rubella in Los Angeles. Local and national television was used to bring attention to the problem, to encourage parents to have children immunized, and to encourage other communities to launch campaigns to prevent additional outbreaks. More recent campaigns relate to the epidemic of pertussis in the United States, the Ebola outbreak, and the Zika virus scares within the United States.

EVIDENCE-BASED PRACTICE

The Meharry Community Networks Program (CNP) conducted a needs assessment to examine demographic and lifestyle factors that influenced decisions and obstacles to being screening for breast cancer among low-income African Americans in three urban areas in Tennessee. A 123-item survey was administered to women aged 40 years and older (n = 355) from the CNP community database inquiring about demographic characteristics, health care access and utilization, and screening practices for various cancers. Marital status and having health insurance were significant predictors of breast cancer screening (p < 0.05). Lack of transportation and lack of enough information about screenings were significantly associated as barriers to screening (p < 0.05). Additional obstacles included trouble remembering to schedule.

Three themes emerged: (1) cultural health perceptions, (2) perceived barriers to screenings, difficulties finding childcare or care for elders, not knowing where to go for screenings, not having health insurance, the cost of screening, pain and discomfort of screening, and fear of getting a positive cancer diagnosis. Future programing for improving screening should include educational interventions aimed at improving breast cancer knowledge and screening rates and needs to incorporate information about obstacles and predictors to screening.

Nurse Use

A community needs assessment helps the nurse to identify gaps in health care and to identify the strengths and weaknesses of a community. Such information is vital in planning effective strategies for assisting underserved populations in obtaining necessary health care services.

Data from Patel K, et al: Factors influencing breast cancer screening in low-income African Americans in Tennessee, *J Community Health*, 39(5): 943-950, 2014.

HOW TO   Develop a Program Plan

A. Describe the problem.
B. Formulate the plan.
1. Assess population need.
   - Who is the program population?
   - What is the need to be met?
   - How large is the client population to be served?
   - Where are they located?
   - Are there other programs addressing the same need? (Describe)
   - Why is the need not being met?
2. Establish program boundaries.
   - Who will be included in the program?
   - Who will not be included? Why?
   - What is the program goal?
3. Assess program feasibility.
   - Who agrees that the program is needed (i.e., stakeholders: administrators, providers, clients, funders)?
   - Who does not agree?
4. Assess resources (general).
   - What personnel are needed? What personnel are available?
   - What facilities are needed? What facilities are available?
   - What equipment is needed? What equipment is available?
   - Is funding available to support the project? Is additional funding needed?
   - Are resources being donated (e.g., space, printing, paper, medical supplies)?
     (1) Type
     (2) Amount
5. Determine tools used to assess need.
   - Census data
   - Key informants
   - Community forums
   - Existing program surveys
   - Surveys of the client population
   - Statistical indicators (e.g., demographic and morbidity/mortality data)
C. Conceptualize the problem.
1. List the potential solutions to the problem.
2. What are the risks of each solution?
3. What are the consequences?
4. What are the outcomes to be gained from the solutions?
5. Draw a decision tree to show the problem-solving process used.
D. Detail the plan.
1. What are the objectives for each solution to meet the program goal?
2. What activities will be done to conduct each of the alternative solutions listed under C1 and based on objectives?
3. What are the differences in the resources needed for each of the alternative solutions?
4. Which of the alternative solutions would be chosen if the resources described under B4 were the only resources available?
5. Who would be responsible or accountable for implementing the plan?
E. Evaluate the plan.
1. Which of the alternative solutions is most acceptable to:
   - The client population
   - The agency administrator
   - You
   - The community
2. Which of the alternative solutions appears to have the most benefits to the following:
   - The client population

Continued

- The agency administrator
- You
- The community
3. Based on costs, which alternative solution would be chosen by:
   - The client population
   - The agency administrator
   - You
   - The community
F. Implement the program plan.
   1. On the basis of data collected, which of the solutions has been chosen?
   2. Why should the agency administrator approve your request? Give your rationale.
   3. Will additional funding be sought?
   4. When can the program begin? Give date.

When determining the size and distribution of a client population for a program, more is involved than counting the number of persons in the community who may be eligible for the program. It involves determining the number of persons with the problem who are not being served by existing programs and the number of eligible persons who have and have not taken advantage of existing services. For example, consider again the community need for a preschool immunization program. In planning the program, the size of the population of preschool children in the county may be obtained from census data or state vital statistics. The nurse then must determine the number of children unserved and the number of children who have not used services for which they are eligible. Today there are many opportunities to locate the unserved children through early start programs for preschool children.

The client population to be served by the program is established by defining the size and distribution of the client population. Setting these factors as boundaries will stipulate who is included in and who is excluded from the health program. If the fictional immunization program were designed to serve only preschool children of low-income families, all other preschool children would be excluded.

What people think about the need for a program might differ among health providers, agency administrators, policymakers, and potential clients. These groups are considered the stakeholders in the program. Collecting data on the opinions and attitudes of all persons, whether directly or indirectly involved with the program, is necessary to determine whether the program is feasible, if there is a need to redefine the problems, or if a new program should be developed or an existing program expanded or modified. If a new or changed program is to be successful, it must not only be *available* but also be *accessible* and *acceptable* to the people who will use it.

Before implementing a health program, *available resources* must be identified. Program resources include personnel, facilities, equipment, and financing. If any one of the four categories of resources is unavailable, the program is likely to be inadequate to meet the needs of the client population.

Various *needs assessment* tools exist to assist the nurse in the needs assessment process. The major tools used for needs assessment, summarized in Table 16.1, are census data, key informants, community forums, surveys of existing community agencies with similar programs, surveys of residents of the community to be served (client population), and statistical indicators (Wambeam, 2014).

TABLE 16.1　Summary of Needs Assessment Tools

Name	Definition	Advantages	Disadvantages
Community forum	Community, group, organization, open meeting	Low cost Learn perspectives of large number of persons	Limited data Limited expression of views Discourages the less powerful Becomes an arena to discuss political issues
Focus groups	Open discussion with small representative groups	Low cost Clients participate in identification of need Initiates community support for the program	Time consuming Allows focus on irrelevant or political issues
Key informant	Identify, select, and question knowledgeable leaders	Provides picture of services needed	Bias of leaders Community characteristics may be incorrectly perceived by informants
Indicators approach	Existing data used to determine the problem	Excellent data on problems and characteristics of client groups	Growth and change in population may make data outdated
Survey of existing agencies	Estimates of client populations via services used at similar community agencies	Easy method to estimate the size of the client group Know the extent of services offered in existing programs	All cases of need may not be reported Exaggeration of services may occur
Surveys	Measurement of total or sample client population by interview or questionnaire	Direct and accurate data on the client population and their problems	Expensive Technically demanding Need many interviews or observations Interviews may be biased

| Solution | Alternatives | Uncertain risks | Consequences |

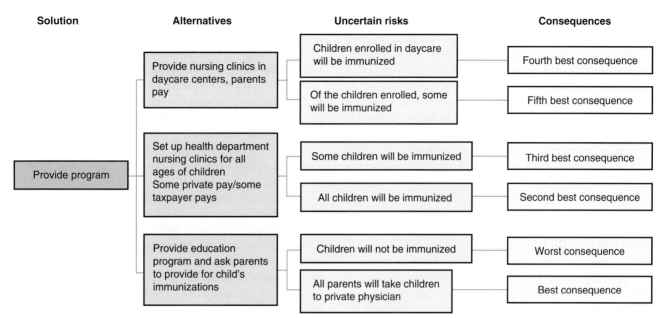

FIG. 16.1 A preschool immunization program for low-income children: using a decision tree to rank solutions to the problem.

Name the Problem. The need and demand for a program are determined by working with the client. This stage of planning creates options for solving the problem and considers several solutions. Each option for program solution is examined for its uncertainties (risks) and consequences, leading to a set of outcomes.

Considering alternative solutions to the problem, some will have more risks or uncertainties than others, as follows:

- The nurse must decide between the solution that involves more risk and the solution that is free from risk.
- A "do nothing" decision is always the decision with the least risk to the provider.
- When choosing a solution, the nurse looks at whether the desired outcome can be achieved.
- After careful consideration, the nurse rethinks the solutions.
- Information collected with the tool is used to develop these alternative solutions.
- Decision trees are useful graphic aids that will provide a picture of the solutions and the consequences and risks of each solution.

Decision trees are useful graphic aids that give a picture of the solutions and the risks of each solution. Such a picture graph of the process of identifying a solution helps clients and administrators rank the consequences of a decision. Fig. 16.1 shows the process of using a decision tree.

In the immunization example, the best consequence would be for families to provide for immunizations. The value of this action to the parents, the odds that immunizations will be given if a formal clinic is not available, the cost to the parents versus the taxpayer, and the cost to the community must be considered. Costs to the community include a possible increased incidence of communicable disease or mortality and an increased need for more expensive services to treat the diseases if children

are not immunized. If the parents provide the immunizations, costs to the taxpayer and to the community are low.

Identify Objectives and Activities for Alternatives

In this phase the nurse who is the provider, with client input, considers the possibilities of solving a problem using one of the solutions identified. The provider details (or is specific about) the costs, resources, and program activities needed to choose one of the solutions. For each of the three proposed alternatives in Fig. 16.1, the program planner must list activities that would need to be implemented to use each of the alternatives.

To illustrate, consider again the immunization scenario. Using the proposed solution of encouraging the parents to provide the immunizations (the best consequence), examples of activities include developing a script for a health education program and implementing a television program to encourage parents to take children to the physician. If the second, third, or fourth best consequence was chosen, offering a clinic 8 hours per day at the health department and providing a mobile clinic to each day care center for 4 hours each day to provide the immunizations would be possible activities.

For each alternative the nurse lists the resources needed to implement each activity. In the example, personnel could include nurses, volunteers, and clerks; supplies might include handouts, Band-Aids, medications, records, and consent forms; equipment might include syringes, needles, stethoscopes, and blood pressure cuffs; and facilities might include a television studio for a media blitz on the education program and a room with examination tables, chairs, and emergency carts. The costs of each solution must be considered by listing the costs of personnel, supplies, equipment, and facilities for each solution. As indicated, clients should review each solution for acceptance.

Evaluate Problem Solutions

In the evaluation phase of the plan, each alternative is weighed to judge the costs, benefits, and acceptance of the idea to the client, community, and nurse. The information outlined in section C in the How To box on page 273, would be used to rank the solutions for choice by client and nurse based on cost, benefit, and acceptance. The solution that will provide the desired outcomes must be considered. Looking at available information through literature reviews or interviews might suggest whether each of the options had been tried in another place or by someone else. The results from other sources would be helpful in deciding whether a chosen solution would be useful.

Choose the Solution

Clients, nurses, and administrators select the best solution. Providing reasons why a particular solution was chosen will help the nurse obtain the approval of the administration for the plan. Involving clients and administrators throughout the planning process helps promote acceptance of the plan. On approval, the plan is implemented.

PROGRAM PLANNING MODELS FOR PUBLIC HEALTH

Program planning began as a public health effort to address health problems (Issel, 2014). The first plans were related to environmental planning for city, water, and sewer services (Rosen, 1958). Population-based program planning began with the need for mass immunizations, such as the program to administer the first polio vaccine. The following are the three models of program planning used in public health today (Box 16.3):

1. **PATCH:** Planning Approach to Community Health
2. **APEXPH:** Assessment Protocol for Excellence in Public Health
3. **MAPP:** Mobilizing for Action through Planning and Partnership

The PATCH Model of program planning was developed using Green's PRECEDE model of health education (Sharma, 2017). The PATCH Model does the following (Issel, 2014):

- Considers health education a process that helps people be more in control of their health
- Provides ways for people to be in control of their health
- Incorporates clients viewed as essential to planning success through the following:
  - Community participation
  - Use of data to develop a comprehensive health promotion strategy
  - Evaluation for improvement
  - Setting long-term goals on increasing community capacity

APEXPH addresses the three core competencies of public health: assessment, assurance, and policy development. This model provides a framework to assess the organization and management of health departments and to work with communities in assessing the health status of the community (Issel, 2014).

MAPP is the newer approach and is a strategic planning model that helps community health workers be facilitators as communities establish priorities in their public health issues and identify resources to address the issues (Issel, 2014).

PROGRAM EVALUATION

BENEFITS OF PROGRAM EVALUATION

The major benefit of program evaluation is that it shows whether the program is meeting its purpose. It should answer the following questions:

- Are the needs for which the program was designed being met?
- Are the problems it was designed to solve being solved?

Quality assurance audits are prime examples of formative program evaluation in health care delivery (see Chapter 17). Evaluation data are used to justify continuing programs in community health. Program records—including client evaluations,

---

BOX 16.3 **Elements of Three Programming Planning Models**		
PATCH (Planning Approach to Community Health)	**APEXPH (Assessment Protocol for Excellence in Public Health)**	**MAPP (Mobilizing for Action Through Planning and Partnership)**
1. Mobilize the community to act	1. Assess internal organizational capacity	1. Mobilize community members and organizations
2. Collect data	2. Assess priorities for health problems	2. Generate shared visions and common values
3. Choose health priorities	3. Set priorities for health problems	3. Develop a framework for long-range planning
4. Develop a comprehensive intervention plan	4. Implement the plan	4. Conduct needs assessments in four areas:
5. Evaluate the process		Community strengths
		Local public health system
		Community health status
		Forces of change
		5. Implement plan

From Issel LM: *Health program planning and evaluation: a practical, systematic approach for community health*, Burlington, MA, 2014, Jones & Bartlett Learning.
Websites: PATCH: http://www.cdc.orghttp://www.NACHO.org; APEXPH/MAPP:
PATCH, Planning Approach to Community Health; *APEXPH*, Assessment Protocol for Excellence in Public Health; *MAPP*, Mobilizing for Action through Planning and Partnership.

CASE STUDY

Using Evidence to Develop an Occupational Health Program for Factory Workers

Jean Carpenter is the occupational nurse at the regional car factory. She noticed that many of the workers exhibit poor health habits, such as smoking and eating high-fat foods. Through talking with workers who visited the clinic, Ms. Carpenter learned that many of them wanted to take better care of themselves but believed they could not because of the long hours they worked and the high stress of their jobs. She decided to determine whether poor health habits were a problem for everyone working in the factory or if they were common only to those who visited the nursing clinic.

Ms. Carpenter sent surveys to all 2000 employees at the factory and received responses from 40% of the employees. From the surveys, she learned that 30% of the workers worked 10 to 12 hours per day each week, 40% smoked a half to two packs of cigarettes per day, and the most recent meal of 85% did not include any fruits or vegetables.

Ms. Carpenter went to the president of the car factory, shared this information with him, and discussed how poor health could decrease productivity. The president supported her suggestion to implement a health promotion program for the factory employees and offered to provide any space and office materials she needed for the program. Ms. Carpenter is now faced with developing a program plan so she can apply for grant money to fund any other supplies or personnel needed.

CDC FRAMEWORK	ROSSI ET AL FRAMEWORK
Engage stakeholders	Goal setting
Describe the program	Determining goal measurement
Focus the evaluation design	Identifying goal-attaining activities
Gather credible evidence	Making the activities operational
Justify conclusions	Measuring the goal effect
Ensure use and share lessons learned	Evaluating the program

FIG. 16.2 Using elements of the evaluation process.

community indexes, and case registers—serve as the major source of information for program evaluation. Surveys, interviews, observations, and diagnostic tests are ways to assess consumer and client responses to health programs. Planning for the evaluation process is an important part of program planning. When the planning process begins, program evaluation begins with the needs assessment (formative evaluation).

CHECK YOUR PRACTICE

You are having your public health nursing clinical rotation at the local health department. The health department is currently working on a framework for evaluating the Healthy Start Program for preschool children offered by the health department. You were asked to develop an evaluation process for conducting this evaluation. What would you suggest as the process to be used?

EVALUATION PROCESS

A framework for evaluation in public health has been developed by the Centers for Disease Control and Prevention (CDC) to guide understanding about program evaluation and facilitate integration of evaluation in the public health system. Royse et al (2016) further expand this approach. This framework defines program evaluation as a systematic way to improve and to account for public health actions by using methods that are useful, feasible, ethical, and accurate. Six interdependent steps are identified that must be part of an evaluation process (CDC, 2016) (Fig. 16.2):

1. **Engage stakeholders:** This includes those who are involved in planning, funding, and implementing the program; those who are affected by the program; and the intended users of its services.
2. **Describe the program:** The program description should address the need for the program and should include the

mission and goals. This sets the standard for judging the results of the evaluation.

3. **Focus the evaluation design:** Describe the purpose for the evaluation, the users who will receive the report, how it will be used, the questions and methods to be used, and any necessary agreements.
4. **Gather credible evidence:** Specify the indicators that will be used, sources of the data, quality of the data, quantity of information to be gathered, and the logistics of the data gathering phase. Data gathered should provide credible evidence and convey a well-rounded view of the program.
5. **Justify conclusions:** The conclusions of the evaluation should be validated by linking them to the evidence gathered and then appraising them against the values or standards set by the stakeholders. Approaches for analyzing, synthesizing, and interpreting the evidence should be agreed on before data collection begins, to ensure that all needed information will be available.
6. **Ensure use and share lessons learned:** Use and dissemination of findings require deliberate effort so that the lessons learned can be used in making decisions about the program.

It should be noted that the steps are very similar to the steps in the planning process.

FORMULATION OF OBJECTIVES

The *objectives* identified in the planning process set the stage for conducting the program and provide the method for evaluating the activities of the program. The following discussion helps in the development of clear, concise objectives.

Specifying Objectives (Goals)

If the objectives are too general, program evaluation becomes impossible. The objectives must be specific and stated so that anyone reading them could conduct the program without further instruction. To be truly effective, the program plan should begin with a general program goal and move on to specific objectives that will help meet the program goal. Useful program objectives include the following:

- A statement of the specific behaviors
- Accomplishments
- Success criteria, or expected result, for the program

Each program objective requires the following:
- A strong, action-oriented verb to specify the behavior
- A statement of a single purpose
- A statement of a single result (an outcome)
- A time frame for achieving the expected result

In this continuing example about childhood immunizations, a program objective that meets these criteria may be as follows: to decrease (action verb) the incidence of early childhood disease in Center County (outcome) by providing immunization clinics in all schools (purpose) between August and December of 2015 (time frame).

As objectives are developed, an operational indicator for each objective should be considered so that the evaluator knows when and if the objective has been met. For instance, an operational indicator for the previous objective would be a 10% to 25% decrease in the incidence rates of the most frequently occurring childhood vaccine–preventable illnesses in Center County. Such indicators provide a target for persons involved with program implementation. A review of *Healthy People 2020* objectives will give the reader examples of objectives that include all the elements just listed.

Levels of Program Objectives

It is customary for objectives to be stated in levels from general to specific. The first level consists of general and broad objectives that are sometimes called *goals.* Their purpose is to focus on the major reason for the program.

For example, a general program goal may be to reduce the incidence of low-birth-weight babies in Center County by 2020 by improving access to prenatal care. Several specific objectives are required to meet a general program goal. A specific objective for this program may be to open (action verb) a prenatal clinic in each health department within the county by January 2020 (time frame) to serve the population within each census tract of the county (purpose) to improve pregnancy outcomes (result).

As objectives are developed, an operational indicator for each objective should be considered so that the evaluator knows when and if the objective has been met. For instance, an operational indicator for the earlier objective would be a 10% to 25% increase in the use of prenatal care by women in Center County. Such indicators provide a target for persons involved with program implementation. A review of *Healthy People 2020* objectives will give the reader examples of objectives that include all the elements just listed.

Specific program activities are then planned to meet each specific objective, and resources, such as number of nurses, equipment, supplies, and location, are planned for each of the objectives. It is

assumed that as each specific objective is met, the general program objective will also be achieved. Remember that several specific objectives are required to meet a general program objective or goal.

SOURCES OF PROGRAM EVALUATION

Major sources of information for program evaluation are program clients, program records, and community indexes. The program participants, or clients of the service, have a unique and valuable role in program evaluation. Whether the clients for whom the program was designed accept the services will determine to a large extent whether the program achieves its goal. Thus their reactions, feelings, and judgments about the program are important to the evaluation.

To assess the response of participants in a program, the evaluator may use the following:
- Written survey in the form of a questionnaire
- Attitude scale
- Interviews
- Observations

Attitude scales are probably used most often and are usually phrased in terms of whether the program met its objectives. The client satisfaction survey is an example of an attitude scale often used in the health care delivery system to evaluate the program objectives.

The second major source of information for program evaluation is *program records,* especially clinical records. Clinical records provide information about the care given to the client and the results of that care. Whether a program goal has been met can be determined by summarizing the data from a group of records. For example, if one overall goal is to reduce the incidence of low-birth-weight babies through prenatal care, records would be reviewed to obtain the number of mothers who received prenatal care and the number of low-birth-weight babies born to them.

A third major source of evaluation is epidemiological data. Mortality and morbidity data measuring health and illness indicators are probably cited more frequently than any other single index for program evaluation. Incidence and prevalence are valuable indexes used to measure program effectiveness and impact, and these data are readily available on the Internet. (See Chapter 9 for a further discussion of rates and ratios.)

An example of a national program based on a needs assessment of the US population is the national health objectives program *Healthy People 2020* (US Department of Health and Human Services [USDHHS], 2010). *Healthy People* documents have been published every 10 years since 1980. The data gathered from each 10-year period have been used to evaluate the population needs met and the assessment of needs for the next *Healthy People* document.

The Healthy Communities Program (USDHHS, 2010) suggests activities to evaluate national health objectives related to communities. The example shown in the *Healthy People 2020* box on this page highlights injury and violence prevention. This box shows that objectives include an action verb, a result, an operational indicator, and a time frame for implementing the objective (10 years, begun in 2010).

The Levels of Prevention box provides examples of applying levels of prevention to program planning and evaluation.

❤ *HEALTHY PEOPLE 2020*

Example of a Measurable National Health Objective

In the *Healthy People* focus area of immunization and infectious diseases, one objective is:

IID-1.10 Reduce (action verb) cases of varicella (purpose) from 586,000 (operational indicator) to 100,000 persons (outcome) aged 17 years of age and under (target) between 2008-2020 (time frame).

From U.S. Department of Health and Human Services: *Healthy People 2020: a roadmap for health,* Washington, DC, 2010, U.S. Government Printing Office.

ASPECTS OF PROGRAM EVALUATION

The aspects of program evaluation include the following (Longest Jr, 2015):
- **Relevance:** The need for the program
- **Adequacy:** The program addresses the extent of the need
- **Progress:** Tracking of program activities to meet the program objectives
- **Efficiency:** Relationship between the program outcomes and the resources spent
- **Effectiveness:** The ability to meet the program objectives and the results of program efforts
- **Impact:** Long-term changes in the client population
- **Sustainability:** Enough resources (usually money) to continue the program

The How To box suggests questions that may be asked about program evaluation using this process.

Relevance

Evaluation of *relevance* is an important component of the initial planning phase. As money, providers, facilities, and supplies for delivering health care services are more closely monitored, the needs assessment done by the nurse will determine whether the program is needed.

Adequacy

Evaluation of adequacy looks at the extent to which the program addresses the entire problem defined in the needs assessment. The magnitude of the problem is determined by vital statistics, incidence, prevalence, and expert opinion.

Progress

The monitoring of program activities—such as hours of services, number of providers used, number of referrals made, and amount of money spent to meet the program objectives—provides an evaluation of the *progress* of the program. This type of evaluation is an example of formative evaluation or evaluation of processes, which occurs on an ongoing basis while the program exists. *Progress evaluation* occurs primarily while implementing the program. The nurse who completes a daily or weekly log of clinical activities (e.g., number of clients seen in the clinic or visited at home, number of phone contacts, number of referrals made, number of community health-promotion activities) is contributing to progress evaluation of the nursing service.

Efficiency

If the reason for the evaluation is to examine the *efficiency* of a program, it may occur on an ongoing basis as a formative evaluation or at the end of the program as a summative evaluation that looks at the end result of the program. The evaluator may be able to determine whether the program provides better benefits at a lower cost than a similar program or whether the benefits to the clients or number of clients served justify the costs of the program.

HOW TO   Do a Program Evaluation

To do a program evaluation, first choose the type of evaluation you wish to do. Second, identify the goal and objectives for evaluation. Third, decide who will be involved in the evaluation. Fourth, answer the questions related to the type of evaluation as follows:

A. Program relevance: Needs assessment (formative)
   1. Use answers to all questions listed in section B of "How to Develop a Program Plan" on page 268.
   2. On the basis of the needs assessment, was the program necessary?
B. Adequacy
   1. Is the program large enough to make a positive difference in the problem/need?
   2. Are the boundaries of the services defined so that the problem or need can be addressed for the target population?
C. Program progress (formative)
   1. Monitor activities (circle which this reflects: daily, weekly, monthly, annually)
      - Name the activities provided.
      - How many hours of service were provided?
      - How many clients have been served?
      - How many providers are there?
      - What types of clients have been served?
      - What types of providers were needed?
      - Where have services been offered (e.g., home, clinic, organization)?
      - How many referrals have been made to community sources?
      - Which sources have been used to provide support services?
   2. Budget
      - How much money has been spent to carry out the activities?
      - Will more or less money be needed to conduct activities as outlined?
      - Will changes to objectives and activities be needed to keep the program going?
      - What changes do you recommend and why?
D. Program efficiency (formative and summative)
   1. Costs
      - How do costs of the program compare with those of a similar program to meet the same goal?
      - How do the activities outlined in section C1 compare with the activities in a similar program?
      - Although this program costs more/less than expected, is it needed? Why?
   2. Productivity (may use national or state averages for comparison)
      - How many clients does each type of staff see per day (e.g., registered nurses, clinical nurse specialists, nurse practitioners)?
      - How does this compare with similar programs?
      - Although the productivity level of this program is low/high, is the program needed? Why?

Continued

3. Benefits
  - What are the benefits of the program to the clients served?
  - What are the benefits to the community?
  - Are the benefits important enough to continue the program? Why? (Look at cost, productivity, and outcomes of care.)
E. Program effectiveness (summative)
  1. Satisfaction
     - Is the client satisfied with the program as designed?
     - Are the providers satisfied with the program outcomes?
     - Is the community satisfied with the program outcomes?
  2. Goals
     - Did the program meet its stated goal?
     - Are the client needs being met?
     - Was the problem solved for which the program was designed?
F. Impact (summative)
  1. Long-term changes in health status (1 year or more)
     - Have there been changes in the community's health?
     - What are the changes seen (e.g., in morbidity or mortality rates, teen pregnancy rates, pregnancy outcomes)?
     - Have there been changes in individuals' health status?
     - What are the changes seen?
     - Has the initial problem been solved or has it returned?
     - Is new or revised programming needed? Why?
     - Should the program be discontinued? Why?
G. Sustainability
  1. Was the program funded as a demonstration or by an external agency?
  2. Can money and resources be found to continue the program after the initial funding is gone?
Depending on the answers to the questions, the program can be found to be successful or not.

Developed by Marcia Stanhope using the framework in Veney J, Kaluzny A: *Evaluation and decision making for health service programs,* Englewood Cliffs, NJ, 2008, Prentice Hall.

Effectiveness and Impact

An evaluation of program effectiveness may help the nurse evaluator determine both client and provider satisfaction with the program activities, as well as whether the program met its stated objectives. However, if the evaluation of *impact* is the goal, long-term effects such as changes in morbidity and mortality must be investigated. Both effectiveness and impact evaluations are usually summative evaluation functions primarily performed as end-of-program activities.

Sustainability

A program can be continued if there are resources for the program. Ongoing evaluation of sustainability is important! As an example, in past research, the combination of prenatal care programs delivered by nurses and the Special Supplemental Nutrition Program for Women, Infants, and Children (WIC) produces better pregnancy and postnatal outcomes for mothers and babies

than does traditional medical care. Looking at the program evaluation process in the How to box above and given this example, how would you determine whether this program could be sustained?

QSEN FOCUS ON QUALITY AND SAFETY EDUCATION FOR NURSES

Targeted Competency-Quality Improvement —Uses data to monitor outcomes of care processes and uses improvement methods to design and test changes to continually improve quality and safety of health care systems.
- **Knowledge:** Describe approaches for changing processes of care
- **Skill:** Identify gaps between local and best practice
- **Attitude:** Value measurement and its role in good client care

QI Question

The PHN Quad Council has identified a beginning PNH competency as policy development and program planning skills. The beginning PHN participates in developing organizational plans to implement programs and policies and participates in evaluating programs as a team member. How could the new PHN best contribute to program management? What type of activity might the PHN participate in to determine gaps in existing programs?

▶ **APPLYING CONTENT TO PRACTICE**

Program planning skills and knowledge are essential for public health nurses. In *Public Health Nursing: Scope and Standards of Practice* (ANA, 2013), the first standard is that of assessment. This addresses the issue of conducting needs assessments and having the ability to collect multiple sources of data, analyze population characteristics, problem solve, and set priorities based on the data collected. Standard 2 speaks to using the assessment data to diagnosis health problems with input from the client population. Standards 3 through 5 address the nurses' roles in identifying health status outcomes, planning and implementing processes to address the health problem, and directing strategies to meet the outcomes. Standard 6 discusses the nurses' role in evaluation including participating in process and outcome evaluation by monitoring activities in programs.

The four professional organizations dedicated to public health nursing—The Association of State and Territorial Directors of Nursing (now APHN), The Association of Community Health Nursing Educators, The Public Health Nursing section of the APHA, and the School Health Nurses Association—have banded together to form an organization called the Quad Council Coalition. This council, which at one time included the ANA, developed a document identifying the domains of practice for public health nurses. One of the domains is Policy Development and Program Planning Skills. The competencies the nurse needs for this domain of practice related to program management are:
- Manages public health programs consistent with public health laws and regulations.
- Develops a plan to implement policy and programs.
- Develops mechanisms to monitor and evaluate programs for their effectiveness and quality (Quad Council, 2011).

New baccalaureate nurses will want to be knowledgeable and be able to participate in program management; graduate nurses will want to be able to direct programs.

▌ PRACTICE APPLICATION

The following is a real-life example of the application of the program management process by an undergraduate nursing student. This activity resulted in the development and implementation of a nurse-managed clinic for the homeless.

This example shows how students and providers can make a difference in health care delivery. It also shows that no mystery surrounds the program management process.

Eva was listening to the radio one Sunday afternoon and heard an announcement about the opening of a soup kitchen within the community for the growing homeless population. She was beginning her nursing course in community health and wanted to find a creative clinical experience that would benefit her as well as others. The announcement gave her an idea. Although it mentioned food, clothing, shelter, and social services, nothing was said about health care.

Eva was interested in finding a way to provide nursing and health care services at the soup kitchen. Which of the following should she do?

A. Talk with key leaders to determine their interest in her idea.

B. Review the literature to find out the magnitude of the problem.
C. Survey the community to find out if others are providing services.
D. Discuss the idea with members of the homeless population.
E. Consider potential solutions to the health care problems.
F. Consider where she would get the resources to open a clinic.
G. Talk with church leaders and nurse faculty members to seek acceptance for her idea.

Answers can be found on the Evolve website.

REMEMBER THIS!

- Planning and evaluation are essential elements of program management and vital to the survival of the nursing discipline in health care delivery.
- A program is an organized approach to meet the assessed needs of individuals, families, groups, or communities by reducing or eliminating one or more health problems.
- Planning is defined as selecting and carrying out a series of actions to achieve a stated goal.
- Evaluation is defined as the methods used to determine whether a service is needed and will be used, whether a program to meet that need is carried out as planned, and whether the service actually helps the people it is intended to help.
- To develop quality programs, planning should include four essential elements: problem diagnosis and assessment of need, identification of problem solutions, analysis and comparison of alternative methods, and selection of the best plan and planning methods.
- The initial and most critical step in planning and evaluating a health program is assessment of need.
- Some of the major tools used in needs assessment are census data, community forums, surveys of existing community agencies, surveys of community residents, and statistical indicators.
- The major benefit of program evaluation is the determination of whether a program is fulfilling its stated goals.

- Quality assurance programs are prime examples of program evaluation.
- Plans for implementing and evaluating programs should be developed at the same time.
- Program records and community indexes serve as major sources of information for program evaluation.
- Planning programs and planning for their evaluation are two of the most important ways in which nurses can ensure successful program implementation.
- The program management process, like the nursing process, is a rational decision-making process.
- Program planning helps nurses and agencies focus attention on services that clients need.
- Planning helps everyone involved understand their role in providing services to clients.
- The assessment of needs process provides an evaluation of the relevance that a new service may have to clients.
- A decision tree is a useful tool to choose the best alternative for solving a problem.
- Setting goals and writing objectives to meet the goals are necessary to evaluate program outcomes.
- *Healthy People 2020* is an example of a national program based on needs assessment that has stated goals and objectives on which the program can be evaluated.

ⓔ EVOLVE WEBSITE

http://evolve.elsevier.com/Stanhope/foundations
- Case Study, with Questions and Answers
- NCLEX® Review Questions
- Practice Application Answers

REFERENCES

American Planning Association: *Annual report*, 2015. Retrieved August 2016 from https://www.planning.org/annualreport/.

Centers for Disease Control and Prevention: *A framework for program evaluation*, 2016. Retrieved August 2016 from http://www.cdc.gov/eval/framework/.

Issel LM: *Health program planning and evaluation: a practical, systematic approach for community health*, Burlington, Mass, 2014, Jones & Bartlett.

Longest, Jr BB: *Health program management: from development through evaluation*, ed 2, San Francisco, 2015, Jossey-Bass.

Patel K, Kanu M, Liu J, et al: Factors influencing breast cancer screening in low-income African Americans in Tennessee, *J Community Health* 39:943–950, 2014.

Rosen G: *A history of public health*, Baltimore, Md, 1958, Johns Hopkins University.

Royse D, Thyer BA, Padgett DK: *Program evaluation: an introduction to an evidence-based approach*, ed 6, Boston, Mass, 2016, Cengage Learning.

Sharma S: *Theoretical foundations of health education and health promotion*, ed 3, Burlington, Mass, 2017, Jones & Bartlett.

U.S. Department of Health and Human Services: *Healthy People 2020: a roadmap for health*, Washington, DC, 2010, U.S. Government Printing Office.

Veney J, Kaluzny A: *Evaluation and decision making for health service programs*, Englewood Cliffs, NJ, 2008, Prentice Hall.

Wambeam RA: *The community needs assessment workbook*, Chicago, Ill, 2014, Lyceum Books.

Managing Quality and Safety

Marcia Stanhope

OBJECTIVES

After reading this chapter, the student should be able to:

1. Describe differences in total quality management/continuous quality improvement (TQM/CQI).
2. Explain the role of quality assurance/quality improvement (QA/QI) in CQI.
3. Understand the historical development of the quality process in nursing.
4. Describe the changes developing in managing quality and safety within managed care.
5. Evaluate approaches and techniques for implementing CQI and the method of documentation.
6. Plan a model QA/QI program.
7. Identify the purposes for the types of records kept by public health agencies.

CHAPTER OUTLINE

Historical Developments
Quality and Nursing Practice
Definitions and Goals
 What Is Quality?
 How Does Quality Assurance Relate to Total Quality Management?
Approaches to Quality Improvement
 General Approaches
 Specific Approaches
 Total Quality Management and Continuous Quality Improvement

Model Continuous Quality Improvement Program
 Structure
 Process
 Outcome
 Evaluation, Interpretation, and Action
Documentation
 Records
 Community Health Agency Records
 Healthy People 2020 and Quality Health Care

KEY TERMS

accountability, 280
accreditation, 280
audit process, 284
certification, 281
charter, 281
concurrent audit, 284
continuous quality improvement (CQI), 277
credentialing, 280
customer, 282

licensure, 280
malpractice lawsuits, 284
managed care, 278
managed care organizations, 277
outcome, 285
process, 285
quality, 276
quality assurance, 276
quality improvement organization, 278

recognition, 281
retrospective audit, 284
risk management, 285
sentinel method, 286
structure, 285
total quality management (TQM), 277
tracer method, 285
utilization review, 284

Although the concept of quality assurance has been a part of the health care arena for many years, it is only in the past few years that a major movement to improve health care quality has begun in the United States. The Institute of Medicine (IOM, 2001), not confident in the ability of the current health care system to deliver the quality of care expected, set forth a series of recommendations to transform current systems to meet Americans' expectations. Very little is known about the quality of care in this country for the following two reasons:

1. A variety of definitions of quality are used.
2. It is difficult to obtain comparable data from all providers and health care agencies.

In a changing health care market, the demand for quality has become a rallying point for health care consumers. All consumers, including private citizens, insurance companies, industry, and the federal government, are concerned about achieving the highest-quality outcomes at the lowest possible cost (Knickman, 2015). In addition to the demand for higher quality and lower cost, the public wants health care to be delivered with greater access and wants health care that is accountable, efficient, and effective.

Moreover, consumers want information about quality. Information is empowering to the consumer. With the expanded use of the Internet, access to information on the quality of health care is readily available on topics ranging from talking to consumers about quality health care (e.g., https://talkingquality.ahrq.gov/) to clinical practice guidelines that promise to improve care for all (e.g., http://www.guideline.gov). Total quality management (TQM) is a management philosophy that includes a focus on client, continuous quality improvement (CQI), and teamwork (Ross, 2014). Although relatively new in health care, TQM/CQI has been tried and proven in industry.

Both consumers and providers have a vested interest in the quality of the health care system, as follows (Claxton et al, 2015):
1. Improving safety of care saves lives
2. Costs reduction by using effective interventions
3. Increases in client confidence in health care delivery regardless of setting

In health care, a direct link exists between doing a good job and individual and professional survival. Health care providers pride themselves on individual achievement and responsibility for good client outcomes (Kovner and Knickman, 2015). Health care organizations are natural extensions of health care providers and thus can demonstrate their responsibility for optimal outcomes through a rigorous quality improvement process. The application of quality improvement strategies in the following five areas of performance could affect both the process and outcomes of health care (US Department of Health and Human Services [USDHHS], 2015):
1. Transform health care
2. Strengthen the nation's health and human services infrastructure and workforce
3. Advance the health, safety, and well-being of the American people
4. Advance scientific knowledge and innovation
5. Increase the efficiency, transparency, and accountability of HHS programs

In the 1990s the United States entered a new era of population-centered, community-controlled delivery of care in which managed care organizations (MCOs) played an integral role. MCOs are agencies such as health maintenance organizations (HMOs) and preferred provider organizations (PPOs) designed to monitor and deliver health care services within a specific budget. Currently, providers, clients, payers, and policymakers all have input into the quality measurement process. The Health Plan Employer Data and Information Set (HEDIS), a data collection arm of the National Committee for Quality Assurance (NCQA), provides performance information, or report cards, for 90% of America's health plans. In 2012, 538 health insurance plans, including HMOs (now called managed care organizations) and PPOs (now called quality improvement organizations), reported audited HEDIS data to show the level of quality performance (NCQA, 2013). In the Affordable Care Act (KHN, 2014), accountable care organizations (ACOs) are being promoted. The ACO may involve a network of physicians for the clients.

Although introduced in the 1990s, report cards for public health agencies are currently being used to measure quality health care in communities. The term community health report card refers to different types of reports, community health profiles, needs assessments, scorecards, quality-of-life indicators, health status reports referred to as community health status indicators (e.g., http://:www.cdc.gov/community health), and progress reports. All of these reports are critical components of community-based approaches to improving the health and quality of life of communities.

Community health report cards can be a useful tool in efforts to help identify areas in which change is needed, to set priorities for action, and to track changes in population health over time. The Centers for Disease Control and Prevention (CDC) has an interactive website referred to as the Community Health Status Indicators (CHSI) so that states and communities can download data collected through the report card process for comparison of progress within the state and across the United States. The report card may be used to track leading causes of morbidity and mortality in a community, looking at trends over time to see if public health interventions have improved health care outcomes. The card also may be used to assess a specific chronic disease, such as diabetes, to determine the health status of the community for this particular disease (CDC, 2015a). The report card may be used as an internal measure of public health program outcomes and CQI measures within the agency (CDC, 2015a).

In 2017, HEDIS measures of care included several that address public health issues, including breast and cervical cancer screening, childhood immunization status, comprehensive diabetes care, flu shots for adults, lead screening in children, physical activity in older adults, and prenatal and postpartum care, to name a few (NCQA, 2017).

As a part of a movement to provide quality health care in communities, health departments are examining their place in promoting this quality (Public Health Foundation, 2015). Lesneski et al (2013) state that public health and CQI are connected because of the use of systems approaches that public health takes in identifying problems and developing interventions. Aspects of planning, implementing, and evaluating by TQM fall under each of the core public health functions of assessment, assurance, and policy development. However, it is with the assurance core function, related to ensuring available access to the health care services essential to sustain and improve the health of the population, that TQM programs must be undertaken. Public health cannot ensure services that improve health if those services lack quality. Public health will want to maintain quality in its workforce and continually evaluate the effectiveness of its services whether the service is delivered to the individual, the community, or the population.

Nurses in community practice are in a perfect position to implement strategies to improve community-oriented health care through the following (Swider et al, 2013; Quad Council of Public Health Nursing Organizations, 2011):

- Community assessments
- Identifying high-risk individuals
- Targeting interventions, case management
- Managing illnesses across a continuum of care

These strategies have long been used by nurses. They are gaining attention because they are cost-effective; healthy consumers obviously use fewer health care resources than do sick people. Thus everyone—consumers, providers, and those who pay the health care bills—benefits if people stay healthy. The growth of the managed care industry has changed the face of health care in the United States, both in how health care is delivered and how it is received by consumers. Consumers are forming partnerships in their communities to counteract the power of MCOs by holding them accountable for the quality of health outcomes in relation to costs. Partnerships are using data-based community assessments to improve health and ensure that communities receive quality services and the establishing of quality indicators for ACOs (KHN, 2014; Howrey et al, 2015). Consumers are no longer willing to have care just given to them. Instead, they want to be partners in making decisions on their care.

The competencies for public health leadership developed by the Council on Linkages (2001, updated 2010 and 2014) are crucial to ensure the quality and performance of the public health workforce (Rowitz, 2014). (See Appendix C.3 for a list of the competencies.) Records are maintained on all health care system clients to provide complete information about the client and indicate the quality of care being given to the client within the system. Records are a necessary part of a CQI process, as are the tools and methods for evaluating quality.

HISTORICAL DEVELOPMENTS

Improving the quality of care has been a part of nursing since the days of Florence Nightingale. In 1860 Nightingale called for the development of a uniform method to collect and present hospital statistics to improve hospital treatment. Nightingale was a pioneer in setting standards for nursing care. The movement to establish nursing schools in the United States came in the late 1800s from a desire to set standards that would upgrade nursing care. In the early 1900s, efforts were begun to set similar standards for all nursing schools. From 1912 to 1930, interest in quality nursing education led to the development of nursing organizations involved in accrediting nursing programs. Licensure has been a major issue in nursing since 1892. By 1923 all states had permissive or mandatory laws directing nursing practice.

After World War II the attention of the emerging nursing profession focused on establishing a scientific method of practice. The nursing process was the chosen method and included evaluation of how nursing activities helped clients (Maibusch, 1984). Quality assurance (QA) and quality improvement (QI) were the evaluative steps in the nursing process.

The 1950s brought the development of QA measurement tools. One of the first tools was Phaneuf's nursing audit method (1965), which has been used extensively in population-centered nursing practice.

In 1966 the American Nurses Association (ANA) created the Divisions on Practice. As a result, in 1972 the Congress for Nursing Practice was charged with developing standards to institute QA programs. The Standards for Community Health Nursing Practice were distributed to ANA Community Health Nursing Division members in 1973, 1986, 1999, and 2005, with updates in 2007. In 2013 the scope and standards were again revised to strengthen the focus on the population as client and on evidence-based practice.

In 1972 the Joint Commission on Accreditation of Hospitals (JCAH) clearly stated the responsibilities of nursing in its description of standards for nursing services. The JCAH called on the nursing industry to clearly plan, document, and evaluate nursing care provided. In the mid-1980s the JCAH became the Joint Commission on Accreditation of Healthcare Organizations (JCAHO) and began developing quality control standards for hospital and home health nursing. JCAHO is now known simply as The Joint Commission (TJC) and presently incorporates CQI principles in its standards.

Also in 1972 the Social Security Act (PL 92-603) was amended to establish the Professional Standards Review Organization (PSRO) and to mandate the process for the review of the delivery of health care to clients of Medicare, Medicaid, and maternal and child health programs. The PSRO program later became the Professional Review Organization (PRO) under the 1983 Social Security Amendments. The purpose of the PRO was to monitor the implementation of the prospective reimbursement system for Medicare clients (the diagnosis-related groups [DRGs]). Although PSROs were intended for physicians, PROs have made QI a primary issue for all health care professionals. The PRO has now been renamed the Quality Improvement Organization and is mandated to improve the quality and efficiency of Medicare-funded services (Centers for Medicare and Medicaid Services [CMS], 2014).

In response to increasing charges of malpractice claims, the government passed the National Health Quality Improvement Act of 1986. Although it was not funded until 1989, its two major goals were to (1) encourage consumers to become informed about their practitioner's practice record and (2) create a national clearinghouse of information on provider malpractice records. The emphasis of this act continued to be on the structure of care rather than the process or outcomes of care (National Association for Healthcare Quality, 1993; Oster and Braaten, 2016).

QUALITY AND NURSING PRACTICE

Efforts to strengthen nursing practice in the community have been carried out by several nursing organizations, including the ANA, the Public Health Nursing Section of the American Public Health Association (APHA), the Association of State and Territorial Directors of Nursing (ASTDN), and the Association of Community Health Nursing Educators (ACHNE). These organizations are now called the *Quad Council for Public Health Nursing.* The quality of nursing education is a major concern of the ACHNE, which was established in 1978. In 1993, 2000, 2003, 2007, and 2009 five reports published by this organization identified the curriculum content required to prepare nurses for practice in the community (ACHNE, 1993, 2000a, 2000b, 2003, 2007, 2009). In 2005 and again in 2007 the Quad Council organizations reviewed scopes and standards of population-focused (public health) and community-based nursing practice and developed new standards to guide the profession in obtaining the best health outcomes for the populations they served. These Scopes and Standards of Public Health Nursing Practice were updated and published again in 2013 (ANA, 2013). QA/QI programs remain the enforcers of standards of care for many agencies that have not elected to engage in a program of CQI. These activities are called *assurance activities* because they make certain that those policies and procedures are followed so that appropriate quality services are delivered.

The Council on Linkages Between Academia and Public Health Practice (the Council) is a coalition of representatives from 17 national public health organizations. Since 1992 the Council has worked to further academic and practice collaboration to ensure a well-trained, competent workforce and a strong, evidence-based public health infrastructure. The Council is funded by the Centers for Disease Control and Prevention and staffed by the Public Health Foundation. The most recent core competencies were updated in 2014. These competencies are used in QA/QI as performance measurements of providers to ensure quality of services (Council on Linkages, 2014). In 2003 and using the work of the Council on Linkages, the Quad Council of Public Health Nursing developed a set of core competencies for public health nurses. This was updated in 2009 and 2011 and can be used as a performance measure for public health nursing practice (Quad Council, 2011).

DEFINITIONS AND GOALS

WHAT IS QUALITY?

Quality is a hard term to define. To some extent, quality has to be defined in relation to the product and service under consideration. Also, quality is often determined differently by the provider than by the person receiving the product or service. Quality is defined by the client as the improvement in health status. The Institute of Medicine, now known as the Health and Medicine Division (HMD) of the National Academies of Science, definition of quality is "the degree to which health services for individuals and populations increase the likelihood of desired health outcomes and are consistent with current professional knowledge" (IOM 2001, p. 1000, 2011). The Agency for Healthcare Research and Quality (AHRQ, 2016) defines quality health care as doing the right thing, for the right client, and having the best possible results. Quality in public health is defined as "the degree to which policies, programs, services, and research for the population increase desired health outcomes and conditions in which the population can be healthy" (IOM, 2013, p 3).

However, a definition of quality rests largely on the perception of the client, the provider, the care manager, the purchaser,

the payer, or the public health official. Whereas the physician views quality in a more technical sense, the client may look at the personal outcome; the manager, purchaser, or payer may consider the cost-effectiveness; and the public health official will look at the appropriate use of health care resources to improve population health (USDHHS, 2015).

According to AHRQ (2016), problems with the quality of health care were divided into five groups: variations in services, overuse of service, underuse of service, misuse of service, and disparities in quality. Variation in service refers to the lack of standards of practice continuity. This variation is often seen among regional, state, and local health care services and stems from lack of evolutionary health care practice and not keeping abreast of the constant changes taking place in health care (evidence-based practice) (AHRQ, 2016). Underuse of service refers to conservative treatment practices. As an example, adolescents ages 16 to 17 in nonmetropolitan areas were less likely to have received meningococcal conjugate vaccine than were adolescents in metropolitan areas (AHRQ, 2015). Overuse of service refers to the excessive ordering of unnecessary tests, surgeries, and treatments. This overuse drives up the cost of already expensive health care. Misuse of service refers to client safety issues and how disability and mortality can be reduced. With diligent care by health care providers, client injury and death can be avoided (National Quality Forum [NQF], 2016). Disparities in quality refer to racial, ethnic, and socioeconomic disparities in accessibility and affordability of health care (AHRQ, 2016).

The term *health services* applies to a wide range of health delivery institutions. Of particular interest to public health are the following:
- The question of access to appropriate and needed services
- A well-prepared workforce
- Improvement in the status of the population's health
- Client satisfaction and well-being
- The processes of client-provider interaction

HOW DOES QUALITY ASSURANCE RELATE TO TOTAL QUALITY MANAGEMENT?

Total quality management provides direction for managing a system of care, whereas continuous quality improvement using quality assurance and quality improvement focuses on the care a client receives within the system. TQM is a process-driven, customer-oriented management philosophy that includes leadership, teamwork, employee empowerment, individual responsibility, and continuous improvement of system processes to yield improved outcomes (Oakland, 2014). Under TQM, quality is defined as customer satisfaction. QA/QI is the promise or guarantee that certain standards of excellence are being met for the client in the delivery of care.

QI is defined as a structured approach to improving performance (IOM, 2013). QI in public health is the use of a deliberate and defined improvement process, such as plan-do-check-act (PDCA), which is focused on activities that are responsive to community needs and improving population health. It refers to a continuous and ongoing effort to achieve measurable improvements in the efficiency, effectiveness, performance, accountability, outcomes, and other indicators of quality in services or processes that achieve equity and improve the health of the community (IOM, 2013).

QA is concerned with the accountability of the provider and is only one tool in achieving the best client outcomes. Accountability means being responsible for care and answerable to the client (Sollecito and Johnson, 2013). Under QA/QI, quality may have a variety of definitions. According to the National Health and Medical Research Council (NHMRC, 2014), QA should consist of peer review leading to QI to improve health care delivery. Client standards of care and safety issues are the core of QA.

The goals of QA and QI are on a continuum of quality, and in public health they are (1) to continuously improve the timeliness, effectiveness, safety, and responsiveness of programs and (2) to optimize internal resources to improve the health of the community, which in this case is the client (IOM, 2013).

Under a continuous quality improvement (CQI) philosophy, QA and QI are but two of the many approaches used to ensure that the health care agency fulfills what the client thinks are the requirements for the service. QA focuses on finding what providers have done wrong in the past (e.g., deviations from a standard of care found through a chart audit). CQI operates at a higher level on the quality continuum but requires the commitment of more organization resources to move in a positive direction. CQI focuses on the sources of differences in the ongoing process of health care delivery and seeks to improve the process (Ross, 2014; Sollecito and Johnson, 2013).

The How To box lists differences between quality assurance and continuous quality improvement.

Traditional approaches to quality include the following:
- Focus on assessing or measuring performance
- Ensure that performance conforms to standards
- Take action to bring about change when care does not meet standards

CQI requires constant attention and should involve surveillance of all records while there is still the opportunity to intervene in both the client's care and the practitioner's actions. Comprehensive data analysis is necessary to detect process failure. Many agencies use some of the TQM/CQI concepts, such as client satisfaction questionnaires, but have not adopted the entire management philosophy. However, because QA/QI methods have traditionally been used and are still in use in many agencies, the QA/QI concepts will be covered.

HOW TO Differentiate between Quality Assurance and Continuous Quality Improvement

Quality Assurance	Continuous Quality Improvement
External determinants	Internal determinants
Detects errors	Determines requirements and deficiencies and expectations
Fixes blame and responsibility	Identifies process improvement opportunities
Postevent investigation	Prevention
Quality assurance department is responsible	All members in the organization are responsible
Inspires fear	Inspires hope

APPROACHES TO QUALITY IMPROVEMENT

Two basic approaches exist in quality improvement: general and specific. The general approach involves a large governing or official body's evaluation of a person's or an agency's ability to meet criteria or standards. Specific approaches to QI are methods used to manage a specific health care delivery system in an attempt to deliver care with outcomes that are acceptable to the consumer.

GENERAL APPROACHES

General approaches to protect the public by ensuring a level of competency among health care professionals are *credentialing, licensure, accreditation, certification, charter, recognition,* and *academic degrees.*

Credentialing is generally defined as the formal recognition of a person as a professional with technical competence or of an agency that has met minimum standards of performance. These mechanisms are used to evaluate the agency structure through which care is provided and the outcomes of care given by the provider. Credentialing can be mandatory or voluntary. Mandatory credentialing requires laws. State nurse practice acts are examples of mandatory credentialing. Voluntary credentialing is performed by an agency or an institution. The certification examinations offered by the ANA through the American Nurses Credentialing Center (ANCC) are examples of voluntary credentialing. Licensing, certification, and accreditation are examples of credentialing.

Licensure is one of the oldest general QA approaches in the United States and Canada. Individual licensure is a contract between the profession and the state whereby the profession is granted control over who can enter into and who exits from the profession. Licensure controls entry into a profession. Exit is generally punitive for some infraction. The licensing process requires that written regulations define the scope and limits of the professional's practice. Job descriptions based on these regulations set minimum and maximum limits on the functions and responsibilities of the practitioner. All 50 states have mandatory nurse licensure, and nurses take the same computerized examination in all 50 states to become licensed to practice nursing. A new approach to interstate practice requires a pact between states so that nurses can practice across state borders. Although reciprocity (which means nurses can have their license accepted through an application process if there is agreement among the states requiring application) exists among states for nursing licensure, interstate practice without approval is an issue for state boards of nursing (National Council of State Boards of Nursing, 2016).

Accreditation, a voluntary approach to QA, is used for institutions. The American Association of Colleges of Nursing (AACN) through the Commission on Collegiate Nursing Education accredit baccalaureate and higher degree nursing programs (Commission on Collegiate Nursing Education, 2016). The NLN accredits programs across the spectrum of diploma, associate degree, baccalaureate, and higher degree programs. In addition, state boards of nursing accredit basic nursing education programs so that their graduates are eligible for the licensing examination.

Although supposedly voluntary, accreditation is considered quasivoluntary because it is often linked to governmental regulations that encourage programs to participate in the accrediting process to be reimbursed for services. For example, only accredited public health and home health agencies are eligible for reimbursement for Medicare clients. During accreditation, programs do a thorough review of their strengths and limitations in response to a set of criteria they must address. The program is next reviewed by individuals who are familiar with similar programs; that is, the reviewers may work in comparable programs or agencies. Accreditation processes have evaluated an agency's physical structure, organizational structure, personnel qualifications, and the educational qualifications of its staff. However, beginning in 1990, more emphasis was placed on the evaluation of the outcomes of care and on the educational qualifications of the person providing the care.

Certification, another general and voluntary approach to quality, combines features of licensure and accreditation. Educational achievements, experience, and performance on an examination determine a person's qualifications for functioning in an identified specialty area, such as nursing in the community. The ANCC provides certification in several areas of nursing. Many other professional nursing specialty credentialing organizations also provide for individual certification.

Although usually a voluntary process, certification also can be a quasivoluntary process. For example, to function as a nurse practitioner in some states, the person must show proof of educational credentials and take an examination to be certified to practice within the boundaries of that state. Major concerns exist about certification as a quality assurance mechanism. Certification examinations measure competency using a written test; however, limited clinical performance has been measured. Although the nursing profession has recognized the certification process as a means of establishing minimal competence, professional organizations and nurses must communicate the importance of certified nurses to the public.

Charter, recognition, and academic degrees are other general approaches to quality assurance. Charter is the mechanism by which a state governmental agency grants corporate status to institutions with or without rights to award degrees (e.g., university-based nursing programs). Recognition is defined as a process by which one agency accepts the credentialing status of and the credentials conferred by another agency. An example is when state boards of nursing accept nurse practitioner credentials that are awarded by the ANCC or one of the specialty credentialing agencies. A recent approach to recognition is the Magnet Health Care Organization Recognition program, which emphasizes status given by the ANCC to organizational nursing services that, after an extensive review, are considered excellent. This program began with reorganization of excellent hospital nursing services and was extended to include all health care organizations who wished to apply for Magnet status for excellent nursing services. Studies indicate many positive benefits of magnet hospitals, including lower mortality rates and better

patient satisfaction (McHugh et al, 2013; Stimpfel et al, 2016). In 2016, 441 hospitals and health care organizations were awarded Magnet recognition (ANCC, 2016). Reapplication for Magnet status must occur every 4 years to ensure that Magnet organizations stay at the top of their game (ANCC, 2016). Academic degrees are titles awarded by degree-granting institutions to individuals who have completed a predetermined program of studies. Four academic degrees are awarded in nursing, with some variety at each degree level: Associate of Arts or Sciences; Bachelor of Science in Nursing; master's degrees, such as Master of Science in Nursing and Master of Nursing; and doctoral degrees, such as Doctor of Philosophy and Doctor of Nursing Practice.

SPECIFIC APPROACHES

Historically, QA programs conducted by health care agencies have measured or accessed the performance of individuals and conformed to standards set forth by accrediting agencies. TQM as a management philosophy uses CQI methods that incorporate many tools, including QA, to increase customer satisfaction with quality care (Table 17.1).

As previously indicated, the Agency for Healthcare Research and Quality (AHRQ, 2016) defines quality health care as doing the right thing, at the right time, in the right way, for the right people, and having the best possible results. To the IOM (2001, p 3), quality health care is care that is the following:

- Effective: Providing services based on scientific knowledge to all who could benefit and refraining from providing services to those not likely to benefit
- Safe: Avoiding injuries to clients from the care that is intended to help them
- Timely: Reducing waits and sometimes harmful delays for both those who receive and those who give care
- Client centered: Providing care that is respectful of and responsive to individual client preferences, needs, and values and ensuring that client values guide all clinical decisions
- Equitable: Providing care that does not vary in quality because of personal characteristics such as gender, ethnicity, geographic location, and socioeconomic status
- Efficient: Avoiding waste, including waste of equipment, supplies, ideas, and energy

TABLE 17.1   Traditional Management Model Compared With a Total Quality Management Model

Traditional Management Model	Total Quality Management Model
Legal or professional authority	Collective or managerial responsibility
Specialized accountability	Process accountability
Administrative authority	Participation
Meeting standards	Meeting process and performance expectations
Longer planning horizon	Shorter planning horizon
Quality assurance	Continuous improvement

TOTAL QUALITY MANAGEMENT AND CONTINUOUS QUALITY IMPROVEMENT

In health care, a major group of customers is clients. Health care agencies have only recently begun using TQM.

If an agency uses TQM, it must be focused on the customer (client), and everyone in the organization must be "committed to quality" (Rowitz, 2014). There are both internal and external customers. Internal customers are employees in other departments or work units, such as environmental health workers, statisticians, or physicians. External customers are those who pay for the service: regulators, accrediting bodies, clients, and families. The internal customer is often overlooked. Employees forget that their professional colleagues are often customers for their services. For example, nurses working in community settings are often customers of the agency's laboratories or data offices. It is easy to take coworkers for granted and forget that they deserve efficient, effective service just as do clients, families, and other service recipients. Several key determinants that can lead to customer satisfaction are listed in the How To box.

HOW TO Ensure Customer Satisfaction with Services Provided

Tangibles
- Facility attractiveness
- Employee appearance
- Characteristics of other customers

Reliability
- Dependability
- Consistency of service delivery

Responsiveness
- Employee willingness
- Promptness in service delivery

Competence
- Employee knowledge

Understanding the Customer
- Effort to learn customer needs
- Individualized attention

Access
- Distance to facility
- Waiting time
- Hours of operation

Courtesy
- Staff politeness and mannerisms

Communication
- Ability of employees to explain the material in an understandable way
- Openness to questions

Credibility
- Trustworthiness of staff

Security
- Physical safety
- Confidentiality

Customer satisfaction for both internal and external users of services can be assessed through the use of focus groups (of clients or employees), surveys (written or telephone), and response cards. Personnel policies that are motivating and provide continuous training and learning opportunities are important parts of a quality improvement program. In quality improvement, people are not blamed for failures in the system and therefore are supported in their efforts to look for problems and seek ways to improve system performance.

Guidelines provided by the 1991 APHA *Model Standards* linked standards to meeting the health goals for the nation in the year 2000 (Lesneski et al, 2013). *Healthy People 2000* and APHA (1991) *Model Standards* provided not only lists of priority health objectives for the nation and a way for public health to implement TQM/CQI but also the most current statistics and scientific knowledge about health promotion and disease prevention. *Healthy People in Healthy Communities* (USDHHS, 2001) provided the objectives with their stated targets, measurement tools, and reflected intended performance expectations.

Healthy People 2010 built on *Healthy People 2000* and contained modified and additional objectives for promoting health and preventing disease (USDHHS, 2000). An important part of the framework of *Healthy People 2010* was eliminating health disparities and ensuring access to quality health care for all. After extensive review of the *Healthy People 2010* objectives, new goals and objectives were developed for *Healthy People 2020*. Of the four goals for *Healthy People 2020* (USDHHS, 2010), although all of the goals speak to quality of life and health, goal two specifically addresses issues related to quality of health care delivery—achieve health equity, eliminate disparities, and improve the health of all groups.

In addition, the *Planned Approach to Community Health* (PATCH) (CDC, 1995 with update in 2010, 2015b); the Assessment Protocol for Excellence in Public Health (APEXPH), *APEXPH in Practice* (National Association of City and County Health Officials [NACCHO], 1995); and most recently the *Mobilizing for Action through Planning and Partnerships* (MAPP) process (NACCHO, 2016) provide methods of assessing community needs to see how well health departments are operating to meet existing standards (see Chapter 16).

As health care reform continues, especially with the implementation of the Patient Protection and Affordable Care Act, public health agencies face competition and are trying to reform themselves. A promising outcome of reform is private health care and public health coming together in a community-level effort to monitor performance and improve health.

Recognizing the many factors that cause health problems and the fragmenting that continues to exist in the health care system, this public-private collaborative framework supported by the *Healthy People* documents involves many stakeholders, including public health, in monitoring the health of entire communities. Performance monitoring is defined as "a continuing community-based process of selecting indicators that can be used to measure the process and outcomes of an intervention strategy for health improvement (making the results available to the community as a whole) to inform assessments of an effective intervention and the contributions of accountable agencies to this" (*Healthy People, Map It,* 2011; University of Kansas, 2016).

Home health care agencies have increasingly adopted QI programs because of the competition that exists. Congruent with the TQM philosophy, meeting customer expectations is essential for home health care agencies. Models for QA/QI in home health care have been developed to improve the quality of care in TQM/CQI frameworks, emphasizing processes, empowerment, collaboration, consumers, data and measurement, and standards and outcomes (Oakland, 2014). Data sets of clinical information, such as those developed through the Omaha System and the OASIS toolkit from the National Association of Home Care and Hospice (NAHC) (CMS, 2016; Martin and Kessler, 2017; NAHC, 2016; The Omaha System, 2016), are useful in measuring the quality of care. In 2003 the Home Health Care Quality Initiative (HHQI) was developed by the USDHHS to provide consumers with data on the quality of home health services. *Home Health Compare,* posted on the Medicare website, is a home health report card available to consumers nationwide (USDHHS, 2016).

Finally, in the area of standards and guidelines, USDHHS (2015) address five areas of performance that need improvement. One of these areas is consistently providing appropriate and effective care. This area is applicable to all health care practitioners, including nurses. Evidence-based practice guidelines are one way to deliver consistent, up-to-date care and improve outcomes for individuals, communities, and populations. Every year the American Cancer Society (ACS) provides a summary of current cancer screening guidelines for health care professionals and updates the guidelines at least every 5 years, or sooner if new evidence warrants an update (Smith et al, 2016). The use of guidelines helps gather data on the effectiveness and outcomes of nurse interventions (Matthew-Maich et al, 2013; Rohmer, 2016). The AHRQ, formerly the Agency for Healthcare Policy and Research (AHCPR), has played a major role in developing clinical practice guidelines.

Guidelines are protocols or statements of recommended practice developed by governmental and health care agencies and professional organizations; they are based on the distilling of scientific evidence and expert opinion that guide a clinician in decision making. Guidelines provide research-based evidence for interventions and promote improved health outcomes. Using research findings as guidelines or frames of reference can improve nurses' awareness of new or better ways to practice, allow for documentation of nurse interventions, and improve outcomes at all levels of public health nursing practice (Matthew-Maich et al, 2013; Rohmer, 2016). Keystones of evidence-based practice guidelines arise from client concerns, clinical experience, best practices, and clinical data and research (Boswell and Cannon, 2017). Clinical practice guidelines are systematically developed statements to assist practitioner and client decisions about appropriate health care for specific clinical circumstances. See the Evidenced-Based Practice box for an example.

EVIDENCE-BASED PRACTICE

This mixed-methods study sought to identify factors that support or hinder the development of a quality improvement culture in public health agencies. The researchers conducted case studies of ten agencies that participated in early quality improvement efforts. Agency staff who participated in National Association of County and City Health Officials (NACCHO)–sponsored quality improvement trainings were invited to complete a survey. Health directors and quality improvement teams from these agencies were also interviewed. The investigators found that agencies that were successful in creating a positive quality improvement culture had the following characteristics: had leadership support; had participated in national quality improvement initiatives; had a greater number of staff trained in quality improvement; had quality improvement teams that met regularly with decision-making authority; reported that accreditation was a major driver to quality improvement work; and had a history of evidence-based decision making and use of quality improvement to address emerging issues. The investigators reported that the role of accreditation preparation as a driving force in quality improvement appears to diminish as an agency develops a quality improvement culture. The researchers noted that common barriers to creating a quality improvement culture included lack of time and resources and relevance of quality improvement to daily work. However, they also reported that staff used quality improvement to overcome these barriers.

Nurse Use

Leadership and teamwork within an organization play a key role in creating a positive quality improvement environment. Community health nurses are in a prime position to be leaders in their organizations in developing a quality improvement environment.

Modified from Davis MV, Mahanna E, Joly B, et al: Creating quality improvement culture in public health agencies, *Am J Public Health,* 104(1): e98-e104, 2014.

CHECK YOUR PRACTICE

One approach useful for measuring quality of care to clients of an agency is the audit process. You have been asked to suggest a process for conducting an audit for the school health program at the health department. There are three approaches to audits. Which would you choose to audit this program and how would you do it?

Traditional Quality Assurance

Traditional QA programs can fit well with the CQI process. In most health care systems, the overall goal of specific QA approaches is to monitor the process and outcomes of client care. The goals of CQI are as follows:

1. To identify problems between the provider and client through QA methods
2. To intervene in problem cases
3. To provide feedback regarding interactions between the client and provider
4. To provide documentation of interactions between the client and provider

Specific approaches are often implemented voluntarily by agencies and provider groups interested in the quality of interactions in their setting. However, state and federal governments require mandatory programs within public health agencies. For example, periodic utilization review, peer reviews (audits), and other QA measures are required in public health agencies that receive funds from state taxes, Medicaid, Medicare, and other public funding sources. Examples of specific approaches to QA are agency staff review committees (peer review), utilization review committees, research studies, PRO (now QIO), monitoring, client satisfaction surveys, risk management, and malpractice lawsuits.

Staff Review Committees. Staff review committees are the most common specific approach to QA in the United States. Staff review (or peer review) committees are designed to monitor the client-specific aspects of certain levels of care. The audit is the major tool used to determine the quality of care.

The audit process consists of the following six steps:
1. Selecting a topic for study
2. Selecting explicit criteria for quality care
3. Reviewing records to determine whether the criteria are met
4. Having peer review of all cases that do not meet the criteria
5. Making specific recommendations to correct problems
6. Implementing follow-up to determine whether the problems have been solved

Two types of audits are used in nursing peer review: concurrent and retrospective. The concurrent audit is a process audit that evaluates the quality of ongoing care by examining the nursing process. Concurrent audit is used by Medicare and Medicaid to evaluate the care received by public health and home health clients. The audit data look at the group, population, or community served. The advantages of this method are as follows:
- Identification of problems at the time care is given
- Provision of a mechanism for identifying and meeting client needs during care
- Implementation of measures to fulfill professional responsibilities
- Provision of a mechanism for communicating on behalf of the client
The disadvantages of the concurrent audit are as follows:
- It is time consuming.
- It is more costly to implement than the retrospective audit.
- Because care is ongoing, it does not present the total picture of care that the client ultimately will receive.

The retrospective audit, or outcome audit, evaluates the quality of care through evaluation of the nursing process at the end of a program or as an audit of the long-term impact of a program within the health care system. The advantages of the retrospective audit are that it provides the following:
- Comparisons of actual practice to standards of care
- Analysis of actual practice findings
- A total picture of care given
- More accurate data for planning corrective action
Disadvantages of the retrospective audit are as follows:
- The focus of evaluation is directed away from ongoing care.
- Client problems (group, population, community) are identified after care is offered through the program; thus, corrective action can be used only to improve the care of future clients.

Currently, in public health, program record audits are done to determine the processes and outcomes of care, such as family planning audits, Special Supplemental Nutrition Program for Women, Infants, and Children (WIC) audits, breast and cervical cancer screening audits, billing coding (to audit costs), and registration audits. Programs regarding physical activity, nutrition, obesity, arthritis, smoking cessation, and others are all designed to address the major causes of morbidity and mortality locally, statewide, and nationwide. The audits assist in determining the progress being made in reducing morbidity and mortality.

Utilization Review. The purpose of utilization review is to ensure that care is needed and that the cost is appropriate. Utilization review is more likely used in HMOs and other MCOs, including Medicaid or Medicare state-level managed care programs. The three types of utilization review are as follows:
1. Prospective: An assessment of the necessity of care before giving service
2. Concurrent: A review of the necessity of services while care is being given
3. Retrospective: An analysis of the necessity of the services received by the client after the care has been given
Each of these reviews provides an assessment of the appropriateness of the cost of care. Prospectively, care can be denied and money saved. Concurrently, services can be cut if they are not found to be essential. Retrospectively, payment can be denied to the provider if the care was not necessary.

Utilization review began in the middle of the 20th century because of concerns for increasing health care costs. The first committees were developed by insurance companies and professional groups. Utilization review committees became mandatory under the 1965 Medicare law as a way to control hospital costs.

The utilization review process includes development of explicit criteria regarding the need for services and the length of service. Utilization review has been used primarily in hospitals to establish the need for client admission and to determine the length of the hospital stay. In community health and public health, especially home health care, utilization review establishes criteria for admission to agency service, the number of visits a client may receive, the eligibility for client services (e.g., a nursing aide or physical therapist), and discharge.

Utilization review has several advantages:
- It helps clients avoid unnecessary care.
- It may encourage the consideration of alternative care options, such as home health care, rather than hospital care.
- It can provide guidelines for staff and program development.
- It provides for agency accountability to the consumer.
The major disadvantage of utilization review is that not all clients fit the classic picture presented by the criteria used to determine approval or denial of care. For example, an older adult client was admitted to a home health care agency for management after hospital discharge. The client was paraplegic as a result of a cerebrovascular accident. After several weeks of

physical and speech therapy, the client showed little sign of progress. The utilization review committee considered the client's condition to be stable and did not recognize the continued need for management to prevent future complications; therefore, Medicare payment was denied.

Appeal mechanisms have been built into the utilization review process used by Medicare and Medicaid. The appeal allows providers and clients to present additional data that may help reverse the original decision to deny payment. This is a tedious process and is often difficult for clients to understand and manage.

Risk Management. Risk management committees often are a part of the CQI program of a community agency. Risk management seeks to reduce the agency's liability because of the grievances brought against them. The risk management committee reviews all risks to which an agency is exposed. It reviews client and personnel safety policies and procedures and determines whether personnel are following the rules. Examples of problems reviewed by a risk management committee in public health clinics include administering an incorrect vaccination dosage, pediatric client injury caused by a fall from an examining table, or injury to a nurse from a needlestick in the sexually transmitted diseases clinic at the health department or as a result of an accident while making a home visit. Incident reports are reviewed by the risk management committee for appropriate, accurate, and thorough documentation of any problem that occurs relating to clients or personnel. In addition, patterns are identified from looking at program data that may require changes in policy or staff development to correct the problem. As a part of risk management, grievance procedures are established for both clients and personnel.

Professional Review Organizations

The PSRO was established in 1972 in an amendment to the Social Security Act (PL 92-603) as a publicly mandated utilization and peer review program. This law provided that medical, hospital, and nursing home care under Medicare, Medicaid, and Title V maternal and child health programs would be reviewed for appropriateness and necessity and such care would be reimbursed accordingly. In 1983 Congress passed the Peer Review Improvement Act (PL 97-248), creating PROs. PROs, now called Quality Improvement Organizations (QIOs), replaced PSROs and are directed by the federal government to reduce hospital admissions for procedures that can be performed safely and effectively in an ambulatory surgical setting on an outpatient basis. The goal was to reduce inappropriate or unnecessary admissions or invasive procedures by specific practitioners or hospitals. Quality measures include the reduction of unnecessary admissions caused by previous substandard care, avoidable complications and deaths, and unnecessary surgery or invasive procedures (Sollecito & Johnson, 2013).

Institutions contract with PROs (QIOs) for quality reviews. PROs are local (usually state) organizations that establish criteria for care based on local patterns of practice. They can be for-profit or not-for-profit organizations. They have access to physicians or may include physicians in their membership.

PROs must define their operational objectives and are required to consult with nurses and other nonphysician health care providers when reviewing the activities of those professionals. PROs monitor access to care and cost of care. Professionals working under the regulation of PROs should develop accurate and complete documentation procedures to ensure compliance with the criteria of the PRO.

Debate has occurred over the limitations and benefits of the federally mandated quality review process. Limits include jeopardizing professional autonomy because decision making regarding care includes professionals, consumers, and government representatives. Another limitation of this process is the development of costly control mechanisms whereby client care activities may be determined by cost rather than by professional criteria and judgment. The benefit of the QIO system has been the development of standards and the peer review mechanisms to increase accountability for the care provided.

In 1985 PRO authority was expanded to include the review of services offered by HMOs (now called MCOs) and competitive medical plans. In addition, the Medicare Quality Assurance Act was passed to strengthen QA programs and to improve access to care after hospitalization. This act required hospitals receiving Medicare payments to provide to Medicare beneficiaries written forms of discharge planning supervised by registered nurses and social workers.

Evaluative Studies

Evaluative studies for quality health care increased during the 20th century. Studies demonstrate the effect of nursing and health care interventions on client populations. Three key models have been used to evaluate quality: Donabedian's structure-process-outcome model, the tracer method, and the sentinel method.

Donabedian's model (1981, 1985, 2003) introduced three major methods for evaluating quality care:

1. **Structure**: Evaluating the setting and instruments used to provide care; examples of structure are facilities, equipment, characteristics of the administrative organization, client mix, and the qualifications of health providers
2. **Process**: Evaluating activities as they relate to standards and expectations of health providers in the management of client care
3. **Outcome**: The net change or result that occurs as a result of health care

The three methods may be used separately to evaluate a part of care. However, to get an overall picture of the quality of care, they should be used together (Table 17.2).

The tracer method described by Kessner and Kalk (1973) is a measure of both process and outcome of care and is used today. This method is more effective in evaluating the health care of groups than of individual clients. It is also more effective in evaluating care delivered by an institution than care delivered by an individual provider. The following are essential characteristics for implementing the tracer method (The Joint Commission, 2016):

• A tracer, or a problem, that has a definite impact on the client's level of functioning

TABLE 17.2   Quality Assurance Measures

Structure	Process	Outcome
Internal Agency	*Peer Review Committees*	*Internal Agency Committees*
Self-study	Prospective audit	Evaluative studies
Review agency documents	Concurrent audit	Survey health status
	Retrospective audit	
External Agency	*Client*	*Client*
Regulatory audit	Satisfaction survey	Malpractice suits
	Utilization review	Satisfaction survey

- Well-defined and easily diagnosed characteristics
- Population prevalence high enough to permit adequate data collection
- A known variation resulting from use of effective health care
- Well-defined management techniques in prevention, diagnosis, treatment, or rehabilitation
- Understood (documented) effects of nonmedical factors on the tracer

Groups are selected for tracer outcome studies in nursing. The client groups would have the following:

1. A shared disease
2. A similar intervention
3. Similar needs
4. Be located in the same community
5. A similar lifestyle
6. Be at the same illness stage

The tracer method provides nurses with data to show the differences in outcomes as a result of nursing care standards.

The sentinel method of quality evaluation is based on epidemiological principles. This method is an outcome measure for examining specific instances of client care (Ross, 2014). Changes in the sentinel indicate potential problems for others. For example, increases in encephalitis in certain communities may result from increases in mosquito populations. Data may be collected at the health department through a state or local required disease reporting system. The health department would be notified, and an immediate mosquito control strategy would be put into place. Such an intervention would include, for example, nurses notifying the population to remove standing water around the outside of homes, such as animal water bowls, rain barrels, and gutter downspout water collection pools. Flyers may be sent home with schoolchildren or given to clients visiting the public health clinics, and media announcements may be used. In addition, the environmental office at the health department may inspect local swimming pools and also may implement a nighttime mosquito spraying program throughout the community.

The characteristics of the sentinel method are described in the How To box.

MODEL CONTINUOUS QUALITY IMPROVEMENT PROGRAM

The primary purpose of a QA/AI program is to ensure that the results of an organized activity are consistent with the expectations. All personnel affected by a QI program should be involved in its development and implementation. Although administration and management are responsible for the quality of services, the key to that quality is in the personnel who deliver the service—their knowledge, skills, and attitudes.

HOW TO Conduct a Sentinel Evaluation

- Identify cases of unnecessary disease, disability, and complications. Example: Tuberculosis (TB).
- Count the deaths from these causes.
- Examine the circumstances surrounding the unnecessary event (or sentinel) in detail.
- Review morbidity and mortality rates as an index for comparison; determine the critical increase in the untimely event, which may reflect changes in quality of care. Example: Compare the incidence and prevalence of TB cases before the increased population occurred.
- Explore health status indicators, such as changes in social, economic, political, and environmental factors, that may have an effect on health outcomes. Example: Overcrowding in the shelter in which migrant workers stay (environmental) and the inability to follow up on testing because of the transient nature of the population (social).

Fig. 17.1 shows a model that identifies the basic components of a QI program. QI programs answer the following questions about health care services and nursing care:

- What is being done now?
- Why is it being done?
- Is it being done well?
- Can it be done better?
- Should it be done at all?
- Are there improved ways to deliver the service?
- How much does it cost?
- Should certain activities be abandoned or replaced?

The PDCA model and Donabedian's framework for evaluating health care programs using the components of structure, process, and outcome can be used in developing a QI program. *Outcome* is the most important ingredient of a program because it is the key to the evaluating providers and agencies by accrediting bodies, by insurance companies, and by Medicare and Medicaid through QIOs, report cards, and other accrediting agencies.

STRUCTURE

The vision, values, philosophy, and objectives of an agency serve to define the structural standards of the agency. Evaluation of structure is a specific approach to looking at quality. In evaluating the structure of an organization, the evaluator determines whether the agency is adhering to the stated philosophy and objectives and to its vision and stated values. Is the agency providing services to populations across the life span? Are primary, secondary, or tertiary preventive services offered? Standards of structure are defined by the licensing or accrediting agency (e.g., the Community Health Accreditation Program [CHAP] standards for accrediting home health agencies).

Identifying values, the first step in a QA program, serves to define the beliefs of the agency about humanity, nursing, the

Structure

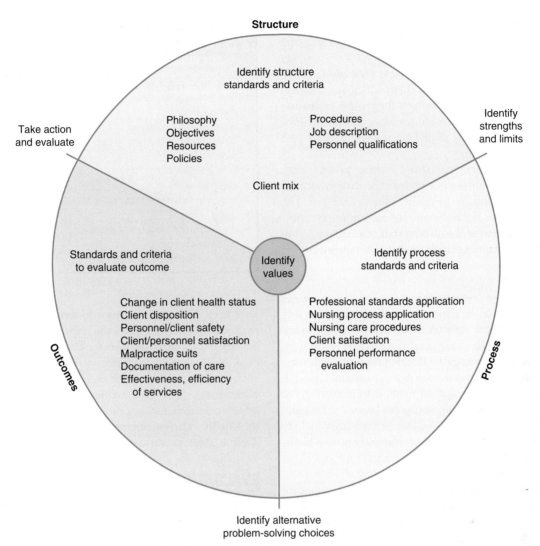

Identify structure
standards and criteria

Philosophy
Objectives
Resources
Policies

Procedures
Job description
Personnel qualifications

Take action
and evaluate

Identify
strengths
and limits

Client mix

Standards and criteria
to evaluate outcome

Identify
values

Identify process
standards and criteria

Change in client health status
Client disposition
Personnel/client safety
Client/personnel satisfaction
Malpractice suits
Documentation of care
Effectiveness, efficiency
  of services

Professional standards application
Nursing process application
Nursing care procedures
Client satisfaction
Personnel performance
  evaluation

Outcomes

Process

Identify alternative
problem-solving choices

FIG. 17.1 Model quality assurance programs.

community, and health. The beliefs of the community, the population to be served, and the providers of care are equally important to the agency, and all need to be considered to provide quality service.

Identifying standards and criteria for QA begins with writing the philosophy and objectives of the organization. The philosophy includes values identification or the beliefs of the agency about humanity, nursing, the community, and health. The beliefs of the community, the population to be served, and the providers of care are equally important to the agency beliefs, and all need to be considered. Program objectives define the intended results of nursing care, descriptions of client behaviors, or changes in health status to be demonstrated on discharge.

Once objectives are formulated, the resources needed to accomplish the objectives should be identified. The personnel, supplies and equipment, facilities, and financial resources that are needed should be described. Once resources are determined, policies, procedures, and job descriptions should be formed to serve as behavioral guides to the employees of the agency. These documents should reflect the essential nursing

and other health provider qualifications needed to implement the services of the agency.

Standards of structure are evaluated internally by a committee composed of administrative, management, and staff members for the purpose of doing a self-study. Standards of structure are also evaluated by a utilization review committee, often composed of an external advisory group with community representatives for all services offered through an agency, such as a nurse, a public health physician, an environmental engineer, a sanitation engineer, a health educator, a board member, and an administrator from a similar agency. The data from these committees identify the strengths and weaknesses of the agency structure.

PROCESS

The evaluation of process standards is a specific look at the quality of care being given by agency providers, such as nurses. Agencies use a variety of methods to determine criteria for evaluating provider activities: conceptual models; the standards of care of the provider's professional organization, such as the ANA's *Scope and Standards of Public Health Nursing Practice* (2013) (see Chapter 1); or the nursing process. The activities of the nurse are evaluated to see if they are the same as the nursing care procedures defined by the public health agency.

The primary approaches used for process evaluation include the peer review committee and the client (often community) satisfaction survey. The techniques used for process evaluation are direct observation, focus groups, questionnaires, interviews, written audits, and video or digital recordings of client and provider encounters.

Once data are collected to evaluate nursing process standards, the peer review committee reviews the data to identify strengths and weaknesses in the quality of care delivered. The peer review committee is usually an internal committee composed of representatives of the nursing staff who are trained to administer audit instruments and conduct client interviews.

OUTCOME

The evaluation of outcome standards, or the result of nursing care, is one of the more difficult tasks facing nursing today. Identifying changes in the client's health status that result from nursing care provides nursing data that demonstrate the contribution of nursing to the health care delivery system. Research studies using the tracer or sentinel method to identify client outcomes and client satisfaction surveys can be used to measure outcome standards. Measures of outcome standards include client data about the changes in the community in low-birth-weight babies as a result of improved prenatal care and client compliance with care through the WIC program.

From these data, strengths and weaknesses in nursing care delivery can be determined. The most common measurement methods are direct physical observations and interviews. Instruments have been developed to measure general health status indicators in home health. The Omaha Visiting Nurse Association problem classification system includes nursing diagnoses, protocols of care, and a problem rating scale to measure nursing care outcomes. In addition, the ANA has developed 10 areas for data collection of outcome criteria in community-based, non–acute care settings, including the following (Rowitz, 2014):

1. Pain management
2. Consistency of communication
3. Staff mix
4. Client satisfaction
5. Prevention of tobacco use
6. Prevention of cardiovascular disease
7. Caregiver activity
8. dentification of the primary caregiver
9. Activities of daily living
10. Psychosocial interactions

Nursing has been involved primarily in evaluating program outcomes to justify program expenses rather than in evaluating client outcomes.

Outcome evaluation assumes that health care has a positive effect on client status. The major problem with outcome evaluation is determining which nursing care activities are primarily responsible for causing changes in client status. Recently studies

BOX 17.1   Types of Problems Studied in a Quality Assurance Program

- Client death (population mortality)
- Client injury (population morbidity)
- Personnel and client safety
- Agency liability
- Increased costs
- Denied reimbursement by third-party payers (decreased program funding by government)
- Client complaints
- Inefficient service
- Staff noncompliance with standards of structure
- Lack of resources
- Unnecessary staff work and overtime
- Documenting of care
- Client health status (population health status)

have been conducted on nursing-sensitive indicators, such as readmission rates, that show the importance of nurse staffing in adverse client outcomes (Brooks-Carthon et al, 2016; Giuliano et al, 2016). In nursing, many uncontrolled factors in the field, such as environment and family relationships, have an effect on client status (Box 17.1). Often it is difficult to determine whether these factors are the cause of changes in client status or whether nursing interventions have the most effect. See Table 17.2 for a summary of QA measures.

EVALUATION, INTERPRETATION, AND ACTION

Interpreting the findings of a quality care evaluation is an important part of the process. It allows differences between the quality care standards of the agency and the actual practice of the nurse or other health providers to be identified. These patterns reflect the total agency's functioning over time and generate information for decisions to be made about the strengths and limitations of the agency. Regular intervals for evaluation should be established within the agency, and periodic reports should be written so that the combined results of structure, process, and outcome efforts can be analyzed and health care delivery patterns and problems identified. These reports should be used to establish an ongoing picture of changes that occur within an agency to justify nursing services.

Identification and choices of possible courses of action to correct the weaknesses within the agency should involve both the administration and the staff. The courses of action chosen should be based on their importance, cost, and timeliness. For example, if there is a nursing problem in the recording of client health education, the agency administration and staff may analyze the problem to see why it is occurring. Reasons for lack of recordkeeping given by the nurses include a lack of time to do paperwork properly, workloads that reduce the amount of time spent with clients, and lack of available resources for health education. If such reasons are given, it would not be appropriate for management to deal with the problem by providing a staff development program on the importance of doing and recording health education; it would be more important to assess how to provide the time and resources necessary for the nurses to offer health education to the clients. Economically, it may be more beneficial to provide personal data assistants or laptop computers and clerical assistance so that nurses can make notes at the point of implementation, thereby providing more client contact time, or it may be more beneficial economically to employ an additional nurse and reduce workloads.

Taking action is the final step in the QA/QI model. Once the alternative courses of action are chosen to correct problems, actions must be implemented for change to occur in the overall operation of the agency. Follow-up and evaluation of the actions taken must occur to improve quality of care. Although health provider evaluation will continue to be included in a QI effort, the focus of a CQI effort is the process and not the person. It is assumed that health care professionals and other employees want to do the best job possible for the client, and problems or differences in a process should not be automatically attributed to their behavior. Although frequent feedback should be given to all employees, the hallmark of QI is continuous learning. Staff development must be ongoing for all employees. (See the Levels of Prevention box.)

QSEN FOCUS ON QUALITY AND SAFETY EDUCATION FOR NURSES

Targeted Competency: Quality Improvement—Use data to monitor the outcomes of intervention processes, and use improvement methods to design and test changes to continuously improve the quality and safety of health care systems.

Important aspects of quality improvement include:

- **Knowledge:** Recognize that nursing and other health professions students are parts of systems and intervention processes that affect outcomes for clients and families.
- **Skills:** Identify gaps between local practices and best practice.
- **Attitudes:** Value own and others' contributions to outcomes in local community settings.

Quality Improvement Question:

You are working as a home care nurse and are discovering a trend of frequent readmissions to the hospital of many of your clients with heart failure. Using the quality assurance approach, consider the following questions:

- What is being done now?
- Why is it being done?
- Is it being done well?
- Can it be done better?
- Should it be done at all?
- Are there improved ways to deliver service?
- How much is it costing?
- Should certain activities be abandoned or replaced?

To which aspects of your clients' quality of life and care transitions will you apply these questions?

Answer: It would be helpful to look at a group of clients discharged from the hospital. Are they receiving adequate education and preparation to return home? You could also gather data about how clients are being managed by the community. How often are they following up with their primary care clinician? Are clients adequately educated to monitor their own fluid status, weight, and dietary restrictions? Are there community-based cardiovascular care programs that can help clients maintain optimum health and avoid exacerbations?

Prepared by Gail Armstrong, DNP, ACNS-BC, CNE, Associate Professor, University of Colorado Denver College of Nursing.

CASE STUDY

Nursing and Quality Assurance

Ms. Miller is a nurse and the quality assurance director at the Best Care Home Health Agency. Incident report data showed that in the past 3 months, the number of incidents in which a fall resulted in an injury doubled from 9 falls to 18 falls. Another nurse, Ms. Collins, would like to find out what the agency is currently doing to assess for risk for falls and if it could be done better.

First, Ms. Miller researched the risk factors for falls resulting in injury so that she would know what should be assessed to predict the potential risk for a fall. She found that a history of falls, use of an ambulatory aid, mental status, type of gait, medications, urinary alterations, improper footwear, diagnoses, alcohol abuse, age (older than 65 years), and gender (female) were risk factors for falls, especially falls resulting in an injury such as a fractured hip. Furthermore, in a literature review, Ms. Collins also found several fall assessment tools that were well documented for their effectiveness in predicting the risk for a fall and reducing the occurrences of a fall.

Because an incident report was written for each fall, Ms. Miller was able to backtrack through each client's file to evaluate the client's initial assessment. Looking at the initial assessment, Ms. Collins found that although several risk assessment tools were used for other items, such as the risk for depression, there was no risk assessment tool for falls. Ms. Collins recommended that the agency begin to use one of the fall risk assessment tools to improve assessment for this incident, with the goal of decreasing the incidence of injuries resulting from falls.

LEVELS OF PREVENTION

Related to Quality Management

Primary Prevention

The nurse participates in a parent education program to improve the immunization level of children in the local elementary school and develops a strategy for follow-up.

Secondary Prevention

Agency evaluation, using a retrospective audit of records of the immunization program, determines that the vaccine-preventable infectious disease rates have declined in the elementary school after the implementation of the parent education program.

Tertiary Prevention

A review of the public health report card indicated that community incidence of complications from vaccine-preventable diseases have declined over a 2-year period after the implementation of the parent education program.

DOCUMENTATION

Documentation is essential to the evaluation of quality care in any organization. The following text focuses on the kinds of documentation that normally occur in a community agency.

RECORDS

Records are an important part of the communication structure of the health care organization. Accurate and complete records are required by law and must be kept by all agencies, both governmental and nongovernmental. In most states, the state departments of health stipulate the kinds of records to be kept and their content requirements for community agencies.

Records provide complete information about the client (whether a family, group, population, or community), indicate the extent and quality of the services being given, resolve legal issues in malpractice suits, and provide information for education and research.

COMMUNITY HEALTH AGENCY RECORDS

Within the community or public health agency, many types of records are kept and used to predict population trends in a community, to identify health needs and problems, to prepare and justify budgets, and to make administrative decisions. The kinds of records the agency keeps can include reports of accidents, births, census, chronic disease, communicable disease, mortality, life expectancy, morbidity, child and spouse abuse, occupational illness and injury, and environmental health.

Agencies also keep records to maintain administrative contact and control of the organization. These records are clinical, provider service, and financial. The *clinical record* is the client health record. The *provider service records* include information about the numbers of clinic clients seen daily, the immunizations given, home visits made daily, transportation and mileage, the provider's time spent with the client, and the amount and kinds of supplies used. The service record is completed on a daily basis by each provider and is summarized monthly and annually to indicate trends in health care activities and costs relative to personnel time, transportation, maintenance, and supplies. The *financial records* include salaries, overhead, and transportation costs, and they serve as the basis for the cost accounting system (see Chapter 16). These records are basic to peer review and audit.

As an outgrowth of QA efforts in the health care system, comprehensive methods are being designed to document and measure client progress and client outcome from agency admission through discharge. An example of such a method is the client classification system developed by the Visiting Nurses Association of Omaha, Nebraska (Martin and Kessler, 2017; The Omaha System, 2016). This comprehensive method for evaluating client care has several components: a classification system for assessing and categorizing client problems, a database, a nursing problem list, and anticipated outcome criteria for the classified problem. Such schemes are viewed as having the potential to improve the delivery of nursing care, documentation of care, and the descriptions of client care. Briefly, the implementation of comprehensive documentation methods improve nursing assessment, planning, implementation, and evaluation of client care; it also allows for the organization of important client information for more effective and efficient nurse productivity and communication.

 HEALTHY PEOPLE 2020

Goal of Improving Access to Comprehensive, High-Quality Health Care and Examples of Objectives to Eliminate Health Disparities

Quality Health Care

Clinicians and public health officials have used Health Risks and Quality of Life (HRQoL) and well-being to measure the effects of chronic illness, treatments, and short-term and long-term disabilities. Although there are several existing measures of HRQoL and well-being, methodological development in this area is still ongoing. Over the decade, *Healthy People 2020* will evaluate the following measures for monitoring HRQoL and well-being in the United States:

- **Patient Reported Outcomes Measurement Information System (PROMIS) Global Health Measure:** Assesses global physical, mental, and social HRQoL through questions on self-rated health, physical HRQoL, mental HRQoL, fatigue, pain, emotional distress, social activities, and roles.
- **Well-Being Measures:** Assess the positive evaluations of people's daily lives—when they feel very healthy and satisfied or contented with life, the quality of their relationships, their positive emotions, resilience, and realization of their potential.
- **Participation Measures:** Reflect individuals' assessments of the impact of their health on their social participation within their current environment. Participation includes education, employment, civic, social, and leisure activities. The principle behind participation measures is that a person with a functional limitation—for example, vision loss, mobility difficulty, or intellectual disability—can live a long and productive life and enjoy a good quality of life.

From U.S. Department of Health and Human Services: *Healthy People 2020*, Washington, DC, 2010, U.S. Government Printing Office.

HEALTHY PEOPLE 2020 AND QUALITY HEALTH CARE

One of the goals of *Healthy People 2020* is to increase the quality and years of healthy life. This will be accomplished by helping individuals of all ages increase their life expectancy and improve their quality of life. According to *Healthy People 2020*, there are substantial differences in life expectancy among population groups within the nation. This is influenced by gender, race, and income. Quality of life reflects a sense of happiness and personal satisfaction. Health-related quality of life reflects a personal sense of physical and mental health and the ability to react to the physical and social environments. Basically, all the objectives are directed toward meeting this goal.

To assess the quality of the outcomes of the objectives related to individuals and communities, several objectives specifically address how the quality assessment will occur, as listed in the *Healthy People 2020* box.

▮ PRACTICE APPLICATION

Oscar, a nursing student, has been working in the migrant farmworker clinic and has noted that each practitioner uses a different educational method for teaching good nutrition practices to clients with newly diagnosed diabetes. The clinic has seen a substantial increase in the number of new clients with diabetes in the Hispanic farmworker population. Oscar knows that practice guidelines for teaching nutrition practices exist in his clinical facility and that charts have an area in which to note nutrition education information. He also knows that for nurses to be most effective and ensure quality client outcomes, research-based practice guidelines should be used by all nurses in the health department.

As part of his course, Oscar must prepare a teaching plan and conduct a class on a health care problem. He obtains permission from his instructor and the director of the clinic to conduct an in-service program. The purpose of Oscar's in-service program is to instruct the nursing staff in how to teach good nutrition practices to clients with newly diagnosed diabetes. He obtains and studies the guidelines about teaching good nutrition practices and researches the methodological background for the development of the guidelines. Oscar's native language is Spanish, so this will help him determine whether brochures regarding good nutrition for clients with newly diagnosed diabetes convey the appropriate message.

As part of his in-service program, Oscar maintains demographic records on attendees and conducts before-and-after tests of knowledge, adding questions about the present use of the guidelines. He plans to follow up with the nurses in 6 months with a further test and questions about use of the guidelines. The director will help him determine an outcome measure that can be used with the client population to show effective use of the guidelines.

1. What outcome measure would be useful in this project?
2. How will this help in the overall assessment of quality in the nursing service?

Answers can be found on the Evolve website.

REMEMBER THIS!

- The health care delivery system is the largest employing industry in the United States; society is demanding increased efficiency and effectiveness from the system.
- Quality control is the tool used to ensure effectiveness and efficiency.
- The managed care industry is changing the face of the American health care delivery system and thus how quality will be defined and measured.
- The objective and systematic evaluation of nursing care is a priority within the profession for several reasons, including the effects of cost on health care accessibility, consumer demands for better quality care, and the increasing involvement of nurses in public and health agency policy formulation.
- Total quality management/continuous quality improvement is a management philosophy used in health care. It is prevention oriented and process evaluation focused.
- The concept of quality includes customer satisfaction.
- Efforts are being made by the public and private sectors to form partnerships to monitor the performance of all players in health care delivery for the purpose of improving the health of communities.
- Quality assurance is the monitoring of the activities of care to determine the degree of excellence attained in the implementation of the activities.
- Quality assurance has been a concern of the profession since the 1860s, when Florence Nightingale called for a uniform format to gather and disseminate hospital statistics.

- Licensure has been a major issue in nursing since 1892.
- Two major categories of approaches exist in quality assurance and improvement today: general approaches and specific approaches.
- Accreditation is an approach to quality control used for institutions, whereas licensure is used primarily for individuals.
- Certification combines features of both licensing and accreditation.
- Three major models have been used to evaluate quality: Donabedian's structure-process-outcome model, the sentinel model, and the tracer model.
- The seven basic components of a quality assurance program are (1) identifying values; (2) identifying structure, process, and outcome standards and criteria; (3) selecting measurement techniques; (4) interpreting the strengths and weaknesses of the care given; (5) identifying alternative courses of action; (6) choosing specific courses of action; and (7) taking action.
- Records are an integral part of the communication structure of a health care organization. Accurate and complete records are required by law of all agencies, whether governmental or nongovernmental.
- Quality assurance and improvement mechanisms in health care delivery are the mechanisms for controlling the system and requesting accountability from individual providers within the system. Records help establish a total picture of the contribution of the agency to the client community.

ⓔ EVOLVE WEBSITE

http://evolve.elsevier.com/Stanhope/foundations
- Case Study, with Questions and Answers
- NCLEX® Review Questions
- Practice Application Answers

REFERENCES

Agency for Healthcare Research and Quality [AHRQ]: *2014 national healthcare quality and disparities report, AHRQ Pub. No. 15-0007,* Rockville, MD, 2015, USDHHS.

Agency for Healthcare Research and Quality [AHRQ]: *2015 national healthcare quality and disparities report and 5th anniversary update on the national quality strategy, AHRQ Pub. No. 16-0015,* Rockville, MD, 2016, AHRQ, National Quality Strategy.

American Nurses Association: *Public health nursing: scope and standards of practice,* Silver Spring, MD, 2013, ANA.

American Nurses Credentialing Center: *Magnet recognition program,* Silver Spring, MD, 2016, ANCC. Retrieved August 2016 from http://www.nursecredentialing.org/Magnet/Program Overview.

American Public Health Association: *Healthy communities 2000: model standards, guidelines for community attainment of the year 2000 national health objectives,* ed 3, Washington, DC, 1991, APHA.

Association of Community Health Nursing Educators: *Perspectives on doctoral education in community health nursing,* Lexington, KY, 1993, ACHNE.

Association of Community Health Nursing Educators: *Graduate education for advanced practice education in community/public health nursing*, Chapel Hill, NC, 2000a, ACHNE.

Association of Community Health Nursing Educators: *Essentials of baccalaureate nursing education for entry level community health nursing practice*, Chapel Hill, NC, 2000b, ACHNE.

Association of Community Health Nursing Educators: *Graduate education for advanced practice in community public health nursing*, New York, 2003, ACHNE.

Association of Community Health Nursing Educators: *Graduate education for advanced practice public health nursing: at the cross-roads*, Chapel Hill, NC, 2007, ACHNE.

Association of Community Health Nursing Educators: *Essentials of Baccalaureate Nursing Education for entry level community health nursing practice*, Chapel Hill, NC, 2009, ACHNE.

Boswell C, Cannon S: *Introduction to nursing research: incorporating evidence-based practice*, ed 4, Burlington, MA, 2017, Jones & Bartlett Learning.

Brooks-Carthon JM, Lasater KB, Rearden J, Holland S, Douglas S: Unmet nursing care linked to rehospitalizations among older black AMI patients: a cross-sectional study of US hospitals, *Medical Care* 54(5):457–465, 2016.

Centers for Disease Control and Prevention [CDC]: *Planned Approach to Community Health: guide for local coordinators*, Atlanta, GA, 1995, CDC, National Center for Chronic Disease Prevention and Health Promotion, and updated 2010.

Centers for Disease Control and Prevention [CDC]: *About CHSI 2015*, Atlanta, GA, 2015a, CDC. Retrieved August 2016 from http://wwwn.cdc.gov/CommunityHealth/info/AboutProject.

Centers for Disease Control and Prevention [CDC]: *Assessment & planning models, frameworks & tools*, Atlanta, GA, 2015b. Retrieved August 2016 from https://www.cdc.gov/stltpublichealth/cha/assessment.html.

Centers for Medicare and Medicaid Services [CMS]: *OASIS User Manuals*, 2016. Retrieved August 2016 from https://www.cms.gov/Medicare/Quality-Initiatives-Patient-Assessment-Instruments/HomeHealthQualityInits/HHQIOASISUserManual.html.

Centers for Medicare and Medicaid Services [CMS]: Quality Improvement Organizations 2014. Retrieved September 2016 at http://www.cms.gov.

Claxton G, Cox C, Gonzales S, Kamal R, Levitt L: *Measuring the quality of healthcare in the US, Kaiser Family Foundation Insight Brief*, 2015. Retrieved August 2016 from http://www.healthsystemtracker.org/insight/measuring-the-quality-of-healthcare-in-the-u-s/.

Commission on Collegiate Nursing Education: *CCNE Accreditation*, 2016. Retrieved August 2016 from http://www.aacn.nche.edu/ccne-accreditation.

Council on Linkages between Academia and Public Health Practice: *Core competencies for public health professionals*, Washington, DC, 2014, The Public Health Foundation.

Davis MV, Mahanna E, Joly B, et al: Creating quality improvement culture in public health agencies, *Am J Public Health* 104(1): e98–e104, 2014.

Donabedian A: *Explorations in quality assessment and monitoring* (vol 2), Ann Arbor, MI, 1981, Health Administration Press.

Donabedian A: *Explorations in quality assessment and monitoring* (vol 3), Ann Arbor, MI, 1985, Health Administration Press.

Donabedian A: *An introduction to quality assurance in health care*, New York, 2003, Oxford University Press.

Giuliano KK, Danesh V, Funk M: The relationship between nursing staffing and 30-day readmission for adults with heart failure, *J Nurs Adm* 46(1):25–29, 2016.

Healthy People 2020 MAP-IT: *Implementing Healthy People 2020 MAP-IT: a guide to using Healthy People 2020 in your community*, February 2011. Retrieved June 2011 from http://www.healthypeople2020.gov.

Howrey BT, Thompson BL, Borkan J, Kennedy LB, Hughes LS, Johnson BH, Likumahuwa S, Westfall JM, Davis A, deGruy F: Partnering with patients, families, and communities, *Fam Med* 47(8):604–611, 2015.

Institute of Medicine [IOM]: *Crossing the quality chasm*, Washington, DC, 2001, National Academy.

Institute of Medicine [IOM]: *Health matters*, Washington, DC, 2011, National Academy Press.

Institute of Medicine [IOM]: *Toward quality measures for population health and the leading health indicators*, Washington DC, 2013, The National Academies Press.

Kaiser Health News: *Accountable Care Organizations Explained.* 2014. Kaiser Family Foundation. Available at: www.khn.org

Kessner DM, Kalk CE: Assessing health quality: the case for tracers, *New Engl J Med* 288:189–194, 1973.

Knickman JR: Health care financing. In Knickman JR, Kovner AR, editors: *Jonas & Kovner's health care delivery in the United States*, ed 11, New York, 2015, Springer Publishing Company.

Kovner A, Knickman JR, editors: *Jonas and Kovner's health care delivery in the United States*, ed 11, New York, 2015, Springer Publishing Company.

Lesneski CD, Massie SE, Randolph GD: Continuous Quality improvement in U.S. public health organizations: moving beyond quality assurance. In Sollecito WA, Johnson JK, editors: *McLaughlin and Kaluzny's Continuous quality improvement in healthcare*, ed 4, Burlington, MA, 2013, Jones and Bartlett Learning.

Maibusch RM: Evolution of quality assurance for nursing in hospitals. In Schrolder PS, Maibusch RM, editors: *Nursing quality assurance*, Rockville, MD, 1984, Aspen.

Martin KS, Kessler PD: The Omaha System: improving the quality of practice and decision support. In Harris MD, editor: *The handbook of home health care administration*, ed 6, Burlington, MA, 2017, Jones and Bartlett Learning.

Matthew-Maich N, Ploeg J, Dobbins M, Jack S: Supporting the uptake of nursing guidelines: what you really need to know to move nursing guidelines into practice, *Worldviews on Evidence-Based Nursing* 10(2):104–115, 2013.

McHugh MD, Kelly LA, Smith HL, Vanak JM, Aiken LH: Lower mortality in magnet hospitals, *Med Care* 51(5):382–388, 2013.

National Association for Healthcare Quality: *Risk management: NAHQ guide to quality management*, Skokie, IL, 1993, NAHQ.

National Association of City and County Health Officials [NACCHO]: *APEXPH in practice*, Washington DC, 1995, NACCHO.

National Association of City and County Health Officials [NACCHO]: *Mobilizing for Action through Planning and Partnerships (MAPP)*, Washington DC, 2016, NACCHO. Retrieved August 2016 from http://naccho.org/programs/public-health-infrastructure/mapp.

National Association of Home Care and Hospice [NAHC]: *About NAHC*, 2016. Retrieved August 2016 from http://www.nahc.org/about/.

National Committee for Quality Assurance: *HEDIS: health plan for employee and data information set*, Washington, DC, 2017, NCQA.

National Committee for Quality Assurance: *National Health Care Quality Report*, Rockville, MD, 2013, AHRQ, USDHHS.

National Committee for Quality Assurance: *Measuring quality improvement health care report cards*, Rockville, MD, 2016, AHRQ, USDHHS.

National Committee for Quality Assurance: *HEDIS 2017 measures: summary table of measures, product lines and changes*, Washington,

DC, 2017, NCQA. Retrieved August 2016 from http://www.ncqa.org/hedis-quality-measurement/hedis-measures/hedis-2017.

National Council of State Boards of Nursing: *Nurse licensure compact*, Chicago, 2016, The Council. Retrieved August 2016 from https://www.ncsbn.org/nurse-licensure-compact.htm.

National Health and Medical Research Council: *Ethical considerations in quality assurance and evaluation activities*, Austrailian Government, Victoria Australia, 2014, NHMRC.

National Quality Forum: *Patient safety 2015*, Washington, DC, 2016, USDHHS.

Oakland JS: *Total quality management and operational excellence: text with cases*, ed 4, New York, 2014, Routledge.

Oster CA, Braaten JS: *High reliability organizations: a healthcare handbook for patient safety and quality*, Indianapolis, IN, 2016, Sigma Theta Tau International.

Phaneuf M: A nursing audit method, *Nurs Outlook* 5:42–45, 1965.

Public Health Foundation: *National public health performance standards*, Washington, DC, 2015, NACCHO, ASTHO.

Quad Council of Public Health Nursing Organizations: *Quad Council competencies for public health nurses*, Washington, DC, 2011, Public Health Foundation. Retrieved August 2016 from http://www.phf.org/resourcestools/Pages/Public_Health_Nursing_Competencies.aspx.

Rohmer F: *Public health and evidence-based healthcare*, New York, 2016, Callisto Reference.

Ross TK: *Health care quality management: tools and applications*, San Francisco, 2014, Jossey-Bass.

Rowitz L: *Public health leadership: putting principles into practice*, ed 3, Burlington, MA, 2014, Jones & Bartlett Learning.

Smith RA, Andrews K, Brooks D, DeSantis CE, Fedewa SA, Lortet-Tieulent J, Manassaram-Baptiste D, Brawley OW, Wender RC: Cancer screening in the United States, 2016: a review of current American Cancer Society guidelines and current issues in cancer screening, *CA Cancer J Clin* 66(2):96–114, 2016.

Sollecito WA, Johnson JK, editors: *McLaughlin and Kaluzny's continuous quality improvement in health care*, ed 4, Burlington, MA, 2013, Jones & Bartlett Learning.

Stimpfel AW, Sloane DM, McHugh MD, Aiken LH: Hospitals known for nursing excellence associated with better hospital experience for patients, *Health Services Research* 51(3):1120–1134, 2016.

Swider SM, Krothe J, Reyes D, Cravetz M: The Quad Council practice competencies for public health nursing, *Public Health Nursing* 30(6):519–536, 2013.

The Joint Commission: *Facts about the tracer methodology*, 2016. Retrieved August 2016 from https://www.jointcommission.org/facts_about_the_tracer_methodology/.

The Omaha System: *Omaha system overview*, 2016. Retrieved August 2016 from http://www.omahasystem.org/overview.html.

University of Kansas: *The community tool kit*, 2016. Retrieved September 2016 from edu.ku.edu.

US Department of Health and Human Services: *Healthy People 2010: understanding and improving health*, ed 2, Washington, DC, 2000, US Government Printing Office.

US Department of Health and Human Services: *Healthy people in healthy communities*, Washington, DC, 2001, US Government Printing Office.

US Department of Health and Human Services: *Healthy People 2020*, Washington, DC, 2010, US Government Printing Office.

US Department of Health and Human Services: *HHS action plan to reduce racial and ethnic health disparities implementation progress report*, Washington, DC, 2015, Office of the Assistant Secretary for Planning and Evaluation.

US Department of Health and Human Services: *Home health compare: Medicare*, Washington, DC, 2016, US Government Printing Office. Retrieved August 2016 from https://www.medicare.gov/home-healthcompare/search.html.

18 | CHAPTER

Family Development and Family Nursing Assessment

Joanna Rowe Kaakinen, Jackie F. Webb

OBJECTIVES

After reading this chapter, the student should be able to:

1. Explain the multiple ways public health nurses work with families and communities.
2. Identify challenges to working with families in the community.
3. Describe family function and structure.
4. Describe family demographic trends and demographic changes that affect the health of families.
5. Work with families using a strength-based approach to assess, develop, and evaluate family action plans.

CHAPTER OUTLINE

Family Nursing in the Community
Family Demographics
Definition of Family
Family Functions
Family Structure
Family Health
    Family Health, Nonhealth, and Resilience
Four Approaches to Family Nursing
Theories for Working with Families in the Community
    Family Systems Theory
    Family Developmental and Life Cycle Theory
    Bioecological Systems Theory

Working with Families for Healthy Outcomes
    Preencounter Data Collection
    Determining Where to Meet the Family
    Making an Appointment with the Family
    Planning for Personal Safety
    Interviewing the Family: Defining the Problem
    Designing Family Interventions
    Evaluation of the Plan
Family Nursing Assessment
    Friedman Family Assessment Model
Social and Family Policy Challenges
Healthy People 2020 and Family Implications

KEY TERMS

dysfunctional families, 297
family, 295
family demographics, 295
family functions, 295

family health, 297
family nursing, 294
family nursing assessment, 305
family nursing diagnosis, 303

family nursing theory, 299
family structure, 295
functional or balanced families, 297

Family nursing is practiced in all settings. The trend in the delivery of health care has been to move health care to community settings; thus, family nursing is pertinent to nurses in community health. Family nursing is a specialty area that has a strong theory base and is more than just "common sense" or viewing the family as the context for individual health care. Family nursing consists of nurses and families working together to ensure the success of the family and its members in adapting to responses to health and illness. The purpose of this chapter is to present a current overview of families and family nursing, theoretical frameworks, and strategies for assessing and intervening with families in the community.

FAMILY NURSING IN THE COMMUNITY

Health care decisions are made within the family, the basic social unit of society. Health care occurs in families, who are in the

The authors acknowledge and thank Linda K. Birenbaum for contributions to previous editions of this text.

larger community and society. Families are responsible for providing or managing the care of their members. In the current health care system, families are significant members of health care teams because they are the ever-present force over the lifetime of care. Families are more responsible than ever for assisting in the health care of ill family members.

Nurses are responsible for the following:

- Helping families promote their health
- Meeting family health needs
- Coping with health problems within the context of the existing family structure and community resources
- Collaborating with families to develop useful interventions

Nurses must be knowledgeable about family structures, functions, processes, and roles. In addition, nurses must be aware of and understand their own values and attitudes pertaining to their own families, as well as being open to different family structures and cultures.

FAMILY DEMOGRAPHICS

Family demographics is the study of the structure of families and households and of family-related events, such as marriage, divorce, and death that alter the structure through their number, timing, and sequencing.

An important use of family demography by nurses is to forecast stressors and developmental changes experienced by families and to identify possible solutions to family problems. It is important to note that the structure of families has changed over time. The rapid changes that occurred at the close of the twentieth century have implications for family relationships and the ability of families to meet the changing needs of their members.

DEFINITION OF FAMILY

The definition of family is critical to the practice of nursing. Family has traditionally been defined using the legal concepts of relationships such as genetic ties, adoption, guardianship, or marriage. Since the 1980s a broader definition of family has been used that moves beyond the traditional blood, marriage, and legal constrictions.

Family refers to two or more individuals who depend on one another for emotional, physical, and/or financial support. The members of the family are self-defined (Kaakinen and Hanson, 2015a). Nurses working with families should ask people whom they consider to be their family and then include those members in health care planning. The family may range from traditional nuclear and extended family to "postmodern" family structures such as single-parent families, stepfamilies, same-gender families, and families consisting of friends.

FAMILY FUNCTIONS

Historically, families have performed a variety of functions (Kaakinen and Hanson, 2015a). Five of these **family functions** are summarized in Box 18.1.

BOX 18.1   Historical Family Functions

Economic function: Family income is a substantial part of family economics, but it is also related to family consumerism, money management, housing decisions, insurance choices, retirement, and savings. Family economics affect and reflect the nation's economy.

Reproductive function: The survival of a society is linked to patterns and rates of reproduction. The family has been the traditional structure in which reproduction was organized. Today the reproductive function of family has become more separated from traditional family structure as more children are born outside of marriage and into nontraditional family structures.

Socialization function: A major expectation of families is that they are responsible for raising their children to fit into society and take their place in the adult world. In addition, families disseminate their culture, including religious faith and spirituality.

Affective function: Families provide boundaries and structure that give a sense of belonging and identity of who the family members are individually and to their family. The purpose of the affective function is to learn about intimate reciprocal caring relationships, dependency, and how to nurture future generations.

Health care function: It is in the family that one learns the concepts of health, health promotion, health maintenance, disease prevention, and illness management. Family members provide informal caregiving to ill family members and are primary sources of support.

Families who performed all of these functions were considered healthy and good. In contemporary times, the traditional functions of families have been modified and new functions have been added. For example, the financial function of families has changed so that family members do not need each other to stay financially healthy as much as they did in the past. Many married couples are electing not to have children. Families depend on agencies to provide safety, such as law enforcement, and other agencies, such as churches, synagogues, and other religious organizations, are involved in the passing on of religious faith. Education (socialization function) is relegated to the schools. Family names are no longer needed to confer status as in the past, when names were important in a community.

The functions that served families have evolved and changed over time. Some have become more important and others less so. The following new functions are more prominent in modern families:

- The relationship function has become important in contemporary families, thus emphasizing how people get along and their level of satisfaction.
- The health function has become more evident because it is the basis of a lifetime of physical and mental health or the lack thereof.

FAMILY STRUCTURE

Family structure refers to the characteristics and demographics (i.e., gender, age, number) of individual members who make up family units. More specifically, the structure of a family defines the roles and the positions of family members (Box 18.2).

Family structures have changed over time, and the speed of these changes is increasing. Social norms have become more tolerant of a range of choices in relation to managing one's life; thus, there is no longer a general consensus that the traditional nuclear family model is the only "right" model. No "typical family" model exists. As a consequence, the number of family and household types is growing. There is an increasing awareness that more variety exists within and among particular family structures. For example, a single-mother household may include an unmarried teenage mother with an infant (unplanned pregnancy), a divorced mother with one or more children, or a career-oriented woman in her late thirties who elects to have a baby and remain single.

An individual may participate in various family life experiences over a lifetime (Fig. 18.1).

The following are examples of family life experiences:
- Spending the early, formative years in the family of origin (mother, father, sibling)
- Experiencing some years in a single-parent family because of divorce or death
- Participating in a stepfamily relationship when the single parent who has custody remarries
- Participating in several additional family types as an adult, building on childhood experience

The following are examples of what an adult may experience:
- Cohabitating while completing a desired education
- Marrying and having a commuter-type marriage while developing a career
- Divorcing and becoming the custodial parent
- Eventually cohabitating with another partner
- Marrying another partner who also has children

As couples age, they will address issues of the aging family, and subsequently the woman may become an elderly single widow. Nurses work with families representing various structures and living arrangements.

Future prospects for families are numerous. New family structures that currently are experimental will emerge as everyday "natural" families (e.g., families in which the members are not related by blood or marriage or who are of the same gender but who provide the services, caring, love, intimacy, and interaction needed by all persons to experience a quality life).

BOX 18.2 Family and Household Structures

Married Family
- Traditional nuclear family
- Dual-career family
- Spouses reside in the same household
- Commuter marriage
- Husband or father is away from the family
- Stepfamily
- Stepmother family
- Stepfather family
- Adoptive family
- Foster family
- Voluntary childlessness

Single-Parent Family
- Never married
- Voluntary singlehood (with children, biological or adopted)
- Involuntary singlehood (with children)
- Formerly married
- Widowed (with children)
- Divorced (with children)
- Custodial parent
- Joint custody of children
- Binuclear family

Multiadult Household (With or Without Children)
- Cohabitating couple
- Commune
- Affiliated family
- Extended family
- New extended family
- Home-sharing individuals
- Same-sex partners

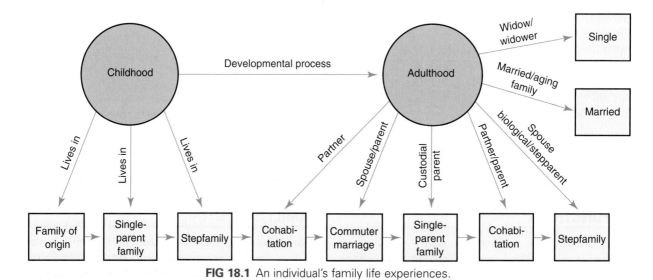

FIG 18.1 An individual's family life experiences.

FAMILY HEALTH

Despite the focus on family health in nursing, the meaning of family health lacks consensus and is not precise. The term family health is often used interchangeably with the concepts of family functioning, healthy families, or familial health. Kaakinen and Hanson (2015a) define family health as a dynamic changing relative state of well-being, which includes the biological, psychological, spiritual, sociological, and cultural factors of individual members and the whole family system.

This biopsychosocial/cultural/spiritual approach refers to individual members as well as the family unit as a whole. An individual's health affects the entire family's functioning, and in turn the family's functioning affects the health of individuals. Thus assessment of family health involves simultaneous assessment of individual family members and the family system as a whole.

Family Health, Nonhealth, and Resilience

Health professionals have tended to classify clients and their families into two groups: healthy families and nonhealthy families, or those in need of psychosocial evaluation and intervention. The term family health implies mental health rather than physical health. A popular term for nonhealthy families is dysfunctional families. Box 18.3 provides a description of healthy families. Terms related to healthy versus nonhealthy families have varied in the literature. Health professionals have tended to classify clients and their families into two groups: "good families," or functional families or balanced families, and "bad families," or families in need of psychosocial evaluation and intervention (Coyne et al, 2011). The term *family health* implies mental health rather than physical health. Recently the popular term for nonhealthy families is dysfunctional families—also called noncompliant, resistant, or unmotivated; these phrases denote families who are not functioning well with each other or the world. The label dysfunctional family does not allow for family change and intervention and needs to be dropped from the nursing language. Families are neither all good nor all bad; therefore nurses need to view family behavior on a continuum of need for intervention when the family comes in contact with the health care system. All families have both strengths and difficulties. All families have seeds of resilience. The Levels of Prevention box discusses ways to help families improve their nutrition.

Families with strengths, functional families, and resilient families are terms often used to refer to healthy families. Research has been conducted about healthy families, but it is clear that the issues examined all concern relational needs. This means that in healthy families the basic survival needs are met. The traits ascribed to healthy families are based on attachment and are affectionate in nature (Walsh, 2012a).

Studies have reported traits of healthy families as well as family stressors that are useful for nurses to include in their assessment (Criss et al, 2015; Price et al, 2017; Walsh, 2012b). Box 18.3 lists characteristics of families who are healthy and functioning well in society.

LEVELS OF PREVENTION

Levels of Prevention

Primary Prevention
- Educate parents about healthy nutritional choices for young children and the risks associated with obesity.
- Provide counseling and weight management for overweight children and teens.
- Help mothers who qualify for the Special Supplemental Nutrition Program for Women, Infants and Children (WIC) complete the extensive paperwork.

Secondary Prevention
- Screen teens for obesity with body mass index (BMI) greater than or equal to 30.
- Analyze children's height and weight growth as part of annual health assessments.

Tertiary Prevention
- Work with schools to improve the quality of food offered in school lunches.
- Help communities establish local farm-to-school networks, create school gardens, and ensure that more local foods are used in the school setting.

BOX 18.3   Characteristics of Healthy Families

1. The family tends to communicate well and listen to all members.
2. The family affirms and supports all of its members.
3. Teaching respect for others is valued by the family.
4. The family members have a sense of trust.
5. The family plays together, and humor is present.
6. All members interact with each other, and a balance in the interactions is noted among the members.
7. The family shares leisure time together.
8. The family has a shared sense of responsibility.
9. The family has traditions and rituals.
10. The family shares a religious core.
11. The privacy of members is honored by the family.
12. The family opens its boundaries to admit and seek help with problems.

From Kaakinen JR, Hanson SMH: Family health care nursing: An introduction. In Kaakinen JR, Coehlo DP, Steele R, et al, editors: *Family health nursing: theory, practice & research*, ed 5, Philadelphia, 2015a, FA Davis, pp 3–32.

FOUR APPROACHES TO FAMILY NURSING

Central to the practice of family nursing is conceptualizing and approaching the family from four perspectives (Kaakinen and Hanson, 2015a). All have legitimate implications for nursing assessment and intervention (Figs. 18.2 and 18.3). Which approach nurses use is determined by many factors, including the health care setting, family circumstances, and resources available to the nurse:

- **Family as a context or structure.** This has a traditional focus that places the individual first and the family second. The family as context serves as either a resource or a stressor to individual health and illness. A nurse using this focus might ask an individual client, "How has your diagnosis of type 1

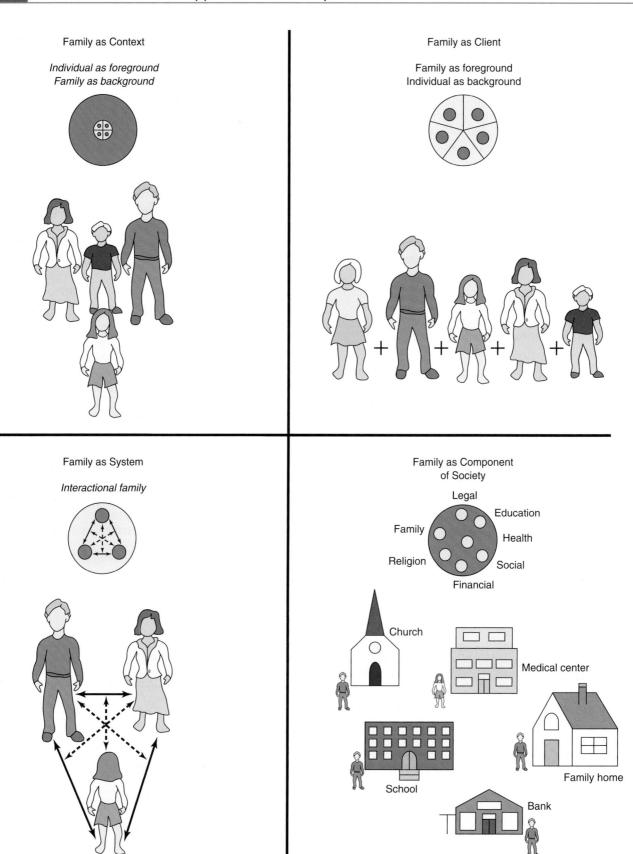

FIG. 18.2 Approaches to family nursing. (From Kaakinen JR, Hanson SMH: Family health care nursing: An introduction. In Kaakinen JR, Coehlo DP, Steele R, et al, editors: *Family health nursing: theory, practice & research,* ed 5, Philadelphia, 2015a, FA Davis, p. 11.)

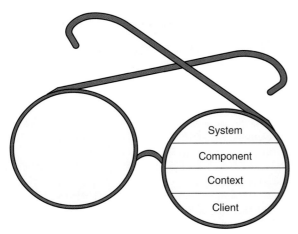

FIG. 18.3 Four views of the family. (From Kaakinen JR, Hanson SMH: Family health care nursing: An introduction. In Kaakinen JR, Coehlo DP, Steele R, et al, editors: *Family health nursing: theory, practice & research*, ed 5, Philadelphia, 2015a, FA Davis, p. 12.)

diabetes affected your family?" or "Will your need for medication at night be a problem for your family?"

- **Family as a client.** The family is first, and individuals are second. The family is seen as the *sum* of individual family members. The focus is concentrated on each individual as he or she affects the family as a whole. From this perspective, a nurse might say to a family member who has just become ill, "Tell me about what has been going on with your own health and how you perceive each family member responding to your mother's recent diagnosis of liver cancer."
- **Family as a system.** The focus is on the family as a client, and the family is viewed as an interacting system in which the whole is more than the sum of its parts. This approach simultaneously focuses on individual members and the family as a whole at the same time. The interactions among family members become the target for nursing interventions (e.g., the direct interactions between the parents, or the indirect interaction between the parents and the child). The systems approach to family always implies that when something happens to one family member, the other members of the family system are affected. Questions nurses ask when approaching a family as system are, "What has changed between you and your spouse since your child's head injury?" or "How do you feel about the fact that your son's long-term rehabilitation will affect the ways in which the members of your family are functioning and getting along with one another?"
- **Family as a component of society.** The family is seen as one of many institutions in society, along with health, education, religious, or financial institutions. The family is a basic or primary unit of society, as are all the other units, and they are all a part of the larger system of society. The family as a whole interacts with other institutions to receive, exchange, or give services and to communicate. Nurses have drawn many of their tenets from this perspective as they focus on the interface between families and community agencies.

THEORIES FOR WORKING WITH FAMILIES IN THE COMMUNITY

Family nursing theory is an evolving synthesis of the scholarship from three different traditions: family social science, family therapy, and nursing (Fig. 18.4). Of the three categories of theory, the family social science theories are the most well-developed and informative with respect to how families function, the environment-family interchange, interactions within the family, how the family changes over time, and the family's reaction to health and illness. Therefore, in this chapter, three family social science theories that blend well with public health nursing are reviewed. These social science theories are the **family systems theory, family developmental and life cycle theory**, and the **bioecological systems theory**.

Family Systems Theory

Families are social systems, and much can be learned from the systems approach. A system is composed of a set of organized, complex, interacting elements. Nurses use family systems theory to understand how a family is an organized whole as well as composed of individuals (Kaakinen and Hanson, 2015b). The purpose of the family system is to maintain stability through adaptation to internal and external stressors that are created by change (Kaakinen and Hanson, 2015b; White et al, 2015).

Family Developmental and Life Cycle Theory

Family developmental and life cycle theory provides a framework for understanding normal predicted stressors that families experience as they change and transition over time. In the original theory of family development, Duvall and Miller (1985) applied the principles of individual development to the family as a unit. The stages of family development are based on the age of the eldest child. Overall family tasks are identified that need to be accomplished for each stage of family development.

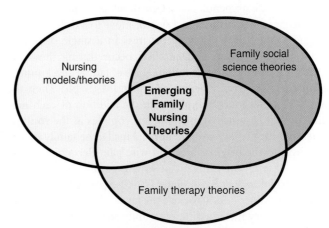

FIG. 18.4 Theory-based family nursing. (Modified from Kaakinen JR, Hanson SMH: Family health care nursing: An introduction. In Kaakinen JR, Coehlo DP, Steele R, et al, editors: *Family health nursing: theory, practice & research*, ed 5, Philadelphia, 2015, FA Davis, pp 3–32.)

TABLE 18.1   **Traditional Family Life Cycle Stages and Family Developmental Tasks**

Stages of Family Life Cycle	Family Developmental Tasks
Married couple	Establish relationship as a family unit, role development
	Determine family routines and rituals
Childbearing families with infants	Adjust to pregnancy and then birth of infant
	Learn new roles as mother and father
	Maintain couple time, intimacy, and relationship as a unit
Families with preschool children	Understand growth and development, including discipline
	Cope with energy depletion
	Arrange for individual time, family time, and couple time
Families with school-age children	Learn to open family boundaries as child increases amount of time spent with others outside of the family
	Manage time demands in supporting child's interest and needs outside of the home
	Establish rules, new disciplinary actions
	Maintain couple time
Families with adolescents	Adapt to changes in family communication, power structure, and decision making as teen increases autonomy
	Help teen develop as individual and family member
Families launching young adults	As young adult moves in and out of the home, allocate space, power, communication, roles
	Maintain couple time, intimacy, and relationship
Middle-aged parents	Refocus on couple time, intimacy, and relationship
	Maintain kinship ties
	Focus on retirement and the future
Aging parents	Adjust to retirement, death of spouse, and living alone
	Adjust to new roles (i.e., widow, single, grandparent)
	Adjust to new living situations, changes in health

BOX 18.4   **Examples of Assessment Questions Nurses Can Ask Based on the Family Developmental and Life Cycle Theory**

- How has time that the family spends together been affected?
- How has communication among and between the family members been altered?
- Has physical space in the home been changed to meet the needs of the evolving family?
- In what ways have the informal roles of the family been changed?
- What changes are being experienced in family meals, recreation, spirituality, or sleep habits?
- How are the family finances affected as the family members age?
- Who should be included in the family decision making?

Table 18.1 shows the stages of the family life cycle and some of the family developmental tasks. One developmental concept of this theory is that families as a system move to a different level of functioning, thus implying progress in a single direction. Family disequilibrium and conflicts occur during these expected transition periods from one stage of family development to another. The family begins as a married couple. Then the family becomes more complex with the addition of each new child until it becomes simpler and less complex as the younger generation begins to leave the home. Finally, the family comes full circle to the original husband-wife pair. Recognizing that families of today are different in structure, function, and processes, McGoldrick and colleagues (2015) expanded the work of Duvall and Miller (1985) to have the family developmental and life cycle theory include different family structures such as divorced families and blended families.

Family developmental and life cycle theory explains and predicts the changes that occur to families and family members over time. Achievement of family developmental tasks helps individual family members accomplish their tasks. This theory assists nurses in anticipating stressors families may experience based on the stage of the family life cycle and whether the family is experiencing these changes "on time" or "off time." Nurses can also use these predictable stressors to identify family strengths in adaptation to the changes. Box 18.4 provides examples of assessment questions for using this theory in conducting assessment of families.

Nursing intervention strategies that derive from the family developmental and life cycle theory help individuals and families understand the growth and development stages and to manage the normal transition periods between developmental periods (e.g., tasks of the school-age family member versus tasks of the adolescent family member) with the least amount of stress possible. Family nurses must recognize that in every family there are both individual and family developmental tasks that need to be accomplished for every stage of the individual or family life cycle that are unique to that particular family.

The major strength of this approach is that it provides a basis for forecasting normative stressors and issues that families will experience at any stage in the family life cycle. The major weakness of the model is that it was developed at a time when the traditional nuclear family was emphasized and that some theory development has been conducted on how family life cycles or stages are affected in divorced families, stepfamilies, and domestic-partner relationships (McGoldrick et al, 2015).

Bioecological Systems Theory

The bioecological systems theory was developed by Urie Bronfenbrenner (1972, 1979, 1997) to describe how environments and systems outside of the family influence the development of a child over time. Even though this theory was designed around how both nature and nurture shape the development of a child, the same underlying principles can be applied when the client is the family. This theory is very useful for community and public health nurses because it helps identify the stressors and potential resources that can affect family adaptation. Fig. 18.5 depicts the four systems in this theory at different levels of engagement that can affect family development and adaptation. The family as the client is at the center of the concentric circles. Each of the levels contains roles, norms, and rules that influence the current situation of the family.

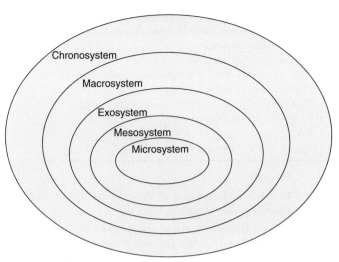

FIG. 18.5 Bioecological family systems model: Level of systems.

Microsystems are composed of the systems and individuals with which the family directly interacts on a daily basis. These systems vary for each family, but could include their home, neighborhood, place of work, school systems, extended family, health care system, community and public health system, or close friends.

Mesosystems are the systems with which the family interacts frequently but not on a daily basis. These systems vary based on the situation in which the community or public health nurse is working with a family. These systems might include a home health aide who comes to the home twice per week, a hospice nurse who comes to the home once per week, a social worker, church members who deliver food to the family, the transportation system, the school system, specialty physicians, a pharmacy, or extended family members.

Exosystems are external environments that have an indirect influence on the family. For example, some of these systems could be the economic system, local and state political systems, a religious system, the school board, community/health and welfare services, the Social Security office, or protective services.

Macrosystems are broad, overarching social, ideological, and cultural values, attitudes, and beliefs that indirectly influence the family. Examples include a Jewish religious ethic, a cultural value of autonomy in decision making, and ethnicity.

Chronosystems refer to time-related contexts in which changes that have occurred over time may influence any or all of the other levels and systems. Examples include the death of a young parent, a divorce and remarriage, war, and natural disasters.

One assumption of this model is that what happens outside the family is equally as important as what happens inside the family. The interaction between the family and the systems in which it interacts is bidirectional in that the outside systems affect the family, and the family affects these systems. The strength of this model is that it provides a holistic view of interactions between the family and society. In working with the family, a critical intervention strategy is drawing a family ecomap that shows the systems with which the family interacts, including the flow of energy from that system into the family or out of the family into the system. A family ecomap is a visual diagram of the family unit in relation to other units or subsystems in the community. It can serve to organize and present factual information and show the nature of relationships among family members, and between family members and the community. The weakness of this model is that it does not address how families cope or adapt to the interaction with these systems.

WORKING WITH FAMILIES FOR HEALTHY OUTCOMES

Nurses who work with families should transcend the traditional nursing approach as a service model and change their practice to a capacity-building model (Rusch et al, 2015). In a capacity-building model, nurses assume the family has the most knowledge about how their health issues affect the family, support family decision-making, empower the family to act, and facilitate actions for and with the family. The goal of family nursing is to focus care, interventions, and services to optimize the self-care capabilities of families and achieve the best possible outcomes.

Nurses work with all types of family structures in a variety of settings. Each family is unique in how it responds to the stressors that evolve when a family member experiences a health event. Community and public health nurses are in a unique position to help families by providing direct care, removing barriers to needed services, and improving the capacity of the family to take care of its members (Kaakinen and Tabacco, 2015).

Preencounter Data Collection

Nurses need to use excellent communication skills to help families prioritize the issues they are confronting, identify their needs, and develop a plan of action. Family members are experts in their own health. They know the family health history, their health status, and their health-related concerns (Pelletier and Stichler, 2013).

Determining Where to Meet the Family

Before contacting the family to arrange for the initial appointment, the nurse decides the best place to meet with the family, which might be in the home, clinic, or office. The decision may be determined by the type of agency with which the nurse works (e.g., home health is conducted in the home), or the mental health agency may choose to have the family meet in the neighborhood clinic office.

Advantages to meeting in the family home include the following:
- It enables the nurse to view the everyday family environment.
- Family members are likely to feel more relaxed and thereby demonstrate typical family interactions.
- It emphasizes that the problem is the responsibility of the whole family and not one family member.
- It may increase the probability of having more family members present.

The following are two important disadvantages of meeting in the family's home:
- The home may be the only sanctuary or safe place for the family or its members to be away from the scrutiny of others.
- Meeting with the family on their ground requires the nurse to be highly skilled in communication by setting limits and guiding the interaction.

Making an Appointment with the Family

Conducting the family appointment in the office or clinic allows easier access to other health care providers for consultation. An advantage of using the clinic may be that the family situation is so intense that a more formal, less personal setting may be necessary for the family to begin discussion of emotionally charged issues. A disadvantage of not seeing the everyday family environment is that it may reinforce a possible culture gap between the family and the nurse. See the How To box for information on making an appointment with the family.

HOW TO Make an Appointment with the Family

The assessment process starts immediately on referral. The following are suggestions that will make the process of arranging a meeting with the family easier:

1. Remember that the assessment is reciprocal and the family will be making judgments about you when you call to make the appointment.
2. Introduce yourself, and state the purpose for the contact.
3. Do not apologize for contacting the family. Be clear, direct, and specific about the need for an appointment.
4. Arrange a time that is convenient for the greatest possible number of family members.
5. If appropriate, ask if an interpreter will be needed during the meeting.
6. Confirm the place, time, date, and directions.

After the decision is made regarding where to meet the family, the nurse contacts the family. It is important to remember that the family gathers information about the nurse from this initial phone call to arrange a meeting, so the nurse should be confident and organized. After the introduction, the nurse concisely states the reason for requesting the family visit and encourages all family members to attend the meeting. Several possible times, including late afternoon or evening, for the appointment can be offered, which allows the family to select the most convenient time for all members to be present.

HOW TO Plan for the Assessment Process

Assessment of families requires an organized plan before you see the family. This planning includes the following:

1. Why are you seeing the family?
2. Are there any specific family concerns that have been identified by other sources?
3. Is an interpreter needed?
4. Who will be present during the interview?
5. Where will you see the family, and how will the space be arranged?
6. What are you going to be assessing?
7. How are you going to collect the data?
8. What services do you anticipate the family will need?
9. What are the insurance sources for the family?

Planning for Personal Safety

It is critical to plan for your own safety when you make a home visit. Learn about the neighborhood you will be visiting, anticipate the needs you may have, and determine whether it is safe

---

BOX 18.5 Home Visiting Safety Tips

- Leave a schedule at your office.
- Plan the visit during safe times of day.
- Dress appropriately, bringing little jewelry or money.
- Avoid secluded places if you are by yourself.
- Obtain an escort; take a co-worker or neighborhood volunteer.
- Sit between the client and the exit.
- If you feel unsafe, do not visit or leave immediately.
- Check in with your agency at the end of the day.

---

for you to make the home visit alone or if you need to arrange to have a security person with you during the visit. Always have your cell phone fully charged and readily available. In addition, as described in Box 18.5, the following strategies will help to ensure your own safety when you visit families in their homes (National Institute for Occupational Safety and Health, 2012).

Interviewing the Family: Defining the Problem

It is important to build a trusting family-nurse relationship. Working with families requires nurses to use therapeutic communication efficiently and skillfully by moving between informal conversation and skilled interviewing strategies. Prepare your family questions before your interview based on the best family theory given what is known about the family situation.

Although it seems commonplace, it is important for nurses to introduce themselves to the family and initiate conversation with each member present. Spending some initial time on informal conversation helps put the family at ease, allows them time to assess the person or nurse, and disperses some of the tension surrounding the visit (Wright and Leahey, 2013). Involving each family member in the conversation, including children, the elderly, or any disabled family member, demonstrates respect and caring and sends the message that the purpose of the visit is to help the whole family and not just the individual family member.

Shifting the conversation into a more formal interview can be accomplished by asking the family to share their story about the current situation. If the nurse focuses only on the medical aspect or illness story, much valuable information and the priority issue confronting the family may be missed in the data collection. The purpose of the interview is to gather information and help the family focus on their problem and determine solutions. The specific therapeutic questions given in Box 18.6 have been found to provide important family information (Leahey and Svavarsdottir, 2009, p 449).

BOX 18.6 Interview Questions for the Family Interview

- What is the greatest challenge facing your family now?
- On which family member do you think the illness has the most impact?
- Who is suffering the most?
- What has been most and least helpful to you in similar situations?
- If there is one question you could have answered now, what would it be?
- How can we best help you and your family?
- What are your needs and wishes for assistance now?

Encourage several members of the family to provide input into the discussion. One strategy is to ask the same question of several different family members. It is critical for the nurse to not take sides in the family discussion and to focus on guiding them in their decision making. In addition to the family story, the nurse will likely need to ask specific assessment questions about the family member who is in need of services.

Designing Family Interventions

Nurses will be challenged to help families identify the primary problem confronting them and to step aside and accept the family priority as they work in partnership with the family to keep their interventions simple, specific, timely, and realistic. It is essential that the family participate in determining the primary need and in designing interventions. As the nurse designs interventions for the family, it is important to consider the health literacy of the client. See Chapter 11 for a discussion of health literacy for individuals and families.

It is important to view the family with an open approach, because the central issue identified by the referral source may not be the actual problem the family is experiencing. See the following case study.

CHECK YOUR PRACTICE

The nurse works with the family to help them design realistic steps or a plan of action based on their ability to successfully adapt to the health issue given the strengths of the family. Working with the family, the following action plan approach helps focus the family on things they can immediately do to help address the problem:

1. We need the following type of help.
2. We need the following information.
3. We need the following supplies.

4. We need to involve or tell the following people.
5. We need to list five things in the order in which they need to happen to make our family action plan. Provide examples of these five things.

Using knowledge and evidence-based practice, you would guide the family in outlining ways to prevent a potential problem, minimize the problem, stabilize the problem, or help the family recognize it as a growing problem. What would be some steps that you would now take with the Raggs family?

CASE STUDY

A physician refers the Raggs family to the home health clinic for medication management. Sam, the 73-year-old husband, has had diabetes for 13 years and has developed type 1 diabetes mellitus. He is being discharged from the hospital. The potential area of concern that prompted the referral was the administration of insulin. After the initial meeting with the family, the primary problem the family uncovers is really not the administration of the medication, but managing his nutrition. The inference of the referral source was that the family knew how to manage the dietary aspects of diabetes because Sam has had a form of diabetes for 13 years.

If the primary family issue is not accurately identified, the family and the nurse will collect data, design interventions, and implement plans of care that do not meet the most pressing family needs. The importance of identifying the family issue of concern and accurately making the **family nursing diagnosis** is demonstrated by comparing the following two scenarios:

Scenario 1: The hypothesized central issue for the Raggs family was identified by the referral source: Is insulin being administered correctly? Based on this question from the referral source, the nurse asked only for information pertaining to this specific problem. The nurse asked questions that elicited information about the following:

1. Concerns of giving injections
2. Difficulty drawing up the accurate amount of insulin
3. The storage of insulin
   The nurse focused the interventions on:
1. The psychomotor skills of family members necessary to give the insulin injection
2. The correct amount of insulin to give according to blood glucose level
3. The correct storage and handling of the medication and the equipment. By not looking at the whole family, the care was based on the nurse's perception of the problem confronting the family.

Scenario 2: The central question asked by a nurse who knows how to integrate family theory into practice was, "What is the best way to ensure that the Raggs family understands how to manage the new diagnosis of type 1 diabetes mellitus?" By asking the family to share their story of the situation together, they determined that the primary issue was not medication administration but rather a

lack of family knowledge related to health care management of a family member who has been newly diagnosed with type 1 diabetes mellitus.

Asking broader-based questions uncovers the whole picture of the family dealing with this specific health concern and directs a more comprehensive holistic data-collection process. More evidence was collected in this case scenario because more options for possible interventions were considered concurrently. Areas of data collection based on the whole family story were as follows:

1. Administration of medication
2. Nutritional management
3. Blood glucose monitoring
4. Activity/exercise
5. Coping with a changed diagnosis
6. Knowledge of pathophysiology of diabetes

The following scenario shows how nurses work with families to determine their strengths, identify the problem, and design interventions.

Scenario 3: The home hospice nurse has been working with the Brush family for 3 weeks. The Brush family consists of Dylan (father), Myra (mother), William (10 years of age), Jessica (7 years of age), and Beatrice (maternal grandmother, 73 years of age).

Beatrice was diagnosed with terminal liver cancer 4 weeks ago. The Brush family—Beatrice, Dylan, Myra, William, and Jessica—agreed that Beatrice should live with them and be cared for until her death in their home. Beatrice has other children who live in the same city. The hospice nurse in collaboration with the Brush family identified that the primary problem is that Myra is experiencing role stress, strain, and overload in her new role as the family caregiver. Myra showed her role conflict by stating, "Sometimes I do not know who I am—daughter, nurse, mother, or wife." Myra took a family leave from her job to stay home to care for her mother. Some family members were surprised by her statement because they did not realize she was so overwhelmed. The family worked with the nurse to find ways to minimize Myra's role strain by spreading the caregiver role among the extended family members.

Continued

By understanding family systems theory, you know that what affects one family member affects all family members. One of the strengths this family has is the shared belief that caring for the dying grandmother in their home is the "right" ethical choice for them. The nurse brings knowledge and evidence into this situation because the nurse knows that the disruption to the family and their expected roles will be short term because the grandmother will probably not live for more than 4 months. However, experience with families also supports the nurse's knowledge that Myra's role conflict may likely increase when her caregiver role becomes more intense as her mother's health declines. A strength of this family is uncovered: it has a strong internal and external support system. The family determines that the extended family is willing to be involved in the care of Beatrice. The intervention is aimed at mobilizing resources to minimize Myra's role conflict. Using the simple action plan outlined previously, the family determined the following:

1. We need the following type of help:
   - Other family members will come every day to relieve Myra.
   - Every other weekend, one of Beatrice's other daughters (Sally or Peggy) will provide care through the night to relieve Myra.
   - Jobs in the family will be shared to relieve Myra. Dylan will do the shopping, William will clear the table and put dishes in the dishwasher, and Jessica will help fold the clothes and put them away. William and Jessica agreed to help by spending some time each evening with Beatrice, such as reading to her or watching TV with her.

2. We need the following information:
   - How to call the hospice nurse when Beatrice gets worse or when we need immediate help
   - A list of who to call when an emergency occurs
   - A list with names and numbers of Beatrice's health care team
3. We need the following supplies: None at this time
4. We need to involve or tell the following people: Sally and Peggy
5. To make our family action plan happen, we need to . . . (list five things in the order in which they need to happen):
   - Invite Sally and Peggy over for a family meeting and include the home hospice nurse.
   - Make a list of what weekends Sally and Peggy will help with Beatrice.
   - Make a calendar with whose turn it is to spend time with Beatrice every evening, which will relieve Myra of the care.

Based on the family story just described, as viewed through the frame of family systems theory, the following interventions were implemented:

1. Assisting the family in the role negotiation of tasks and who performs them
2. Educating family members so they can safely care for Beatrice now and when she enters the stage of active dying
3. Determining what additional resources the family needs. After a plan is put into place, it needs to be evaluated periodically.

Of all of these problems, the nurse worked with the family to help them identify that their major concern centered on nutritional management, which ultimately affects the administration of medication.

The major difference between the two scenarios presented here was the way in which the nurse framed questions while listening to the family story. In the first scenario, the nurse asked questions that allowed for consideration of only one aspect of family health. This type of step-by-step nurse-led linear problem-solving process is tedious and time-consuming, and will likely cause errors in the identification of the most pressing family concern. In the second scenario, the nurse asked questions that allowed for critical thinking about the family view of their challenges. The nurse gathered information from the referral source, conducted an assessment of the impact of the new diagnosis on the whole family, and collaboratively the nurse and family identified the critical family issue that had a more far-reaching effect on the health of the whole family.

Evaluation of the Plan

In evaluating the outcome, nurses use critical thinking to determine whether the plan is working. When the plan is not working, the nurse and the family work together to determine the barriers interfering with the plan or figure out if something changed in the family story. Family apathy and indecision are known to be barriers in family nursing (Friedman et al, 2003). Friedman and colleagues also identified the following nurse-related barriers that can affect achievement of the outcome:

1. Nurse-imposed ideas
2. Negative labeling
3. Overlooking family strengths
4. Neglecting cultural or gender implications

Family apathy may occur when there are value differences between the nurse and family; the family is overcome with a sense of hopelessness; the family views the problems as too overwhelming; or family members fear failure. Additional factors must be considered because family members may be indecisive for the following reasons:

- They cannot determine which course of action is better.
- They have an unexpressed fear or concern.
- They have a pattern of making decisions only when faced with a crisis.

An important part of the judgment step in working with families is the decision to terminate the relationship between the nurse and family. Termination is phasing out the nurse from family involvement. When termination is built into the interventions, the family benefits from a smooth transition process. The family is given credit for the outcomes of the interventions that they helped design. Strategies often used in the termination component are as follows:

- Decreasing contact with the nurse
- Extending invitations to the family for follow-up
- Making referrals when appropriate

The termination should include a summative evaluation meeting in which the nurse and family put a formal closure to their relationship.

When termination with a family occurs suddenly, it is important for the nurse to determine the forces bringing about the closure. The family may be initiating the termination prematurely, which requires a renegotiating process. The insurance or agency requirements may be placing a financial constraint on the amount of time the nurse can work with a family. Regardless of how termination comes about, it is important to recognize the transition from depending on the nurse on some level to having no dependence. Strategies that help with the termination are as follows:

- Increase time between the nurse's visits
- Develop a plan for the transition
- Make referrals to other resources
- Provide a written summary to the family

EVIDENCE-BASED PRACTICE

Reducing obesity in the United States is a *Healthy People 2020* objective. A study by the Centers for Disease Control and Prevention (2013) shows that there was a 43% drop in obesity rates among children 2 to 5 years of age over the last 10 years. Part of this decline is directly related to the change in the social policy of improvements in the food packages available to these parents through the Special Supplemental Nutrition Program for Women, Infants and Children (WIC). The improvements include adding healthy items like fruits and vegetables and whole-grain foods while reducing the amount of fruit juice and whole milk. This change, coupled with nutrition education for families with infants and young children, helped parents select healthier food choices and improved access to healthy foods for at-risk families.

Nurse Use

Nurses can advocate for social policies that improve the health of families and educate parents of young children to make healthy food choices. Public health nurses should be actively involved in helping to decrease childhood obesity. The Levels of Prevention box provides information on reducing childhood obesity.

From Centers for Disease Control and Prevention: *Vital signs: obesity among low income, preschool aged children—United States, 2008–2011*, 2013. Retrieved July 2016 from http://www.cdc.gov/mmwr/preview/mmwrhtml/mm6231a4.htm.

QSEN FOCUS ON QUALITY AND SAFETY EDUCATION FOR NURSES

Targeted Competency: Client-Centered Care—Recognize the client or designee as the source of control and full partner in providing compassionate and coordinated care based on respect for the client's preferences, values, and needs.

Important aspects of client-centered care include:

- **Knowledge:** Describe strategies to empower clients or families in all aspects of the health care process
- **Skills:** Assess the level of the client's decisional conflict, and provide access to resources
- **Attitudes:** Value active partnership with clients or designated surrogates in planning, implementing, and evaluating care

Client-Centered Care Question

Describe how a family assessment is different from an individual client assessment. Beyond immediate family members, who might be included in a client's "family"? Think about the difference between being an advocate for an individual (the client) and an advocate for a family. What different skills are needed?

Prepared by Gail Armstrong, PhD, DNP, ACNS-BC, CNE, Associate Professor, University of Colorado College of Nursing.

CASE STUDY

Assessing Family Resilience to Improve Family Interactions

Marty Belfair, a 55-year-old accountant, is the father of three children and has been married to his wife, Joanne, for the past 25 years. Mr. Belfair's children are Joshua (20 years of age), Mary (17 years of age), and Kyle (14 years of age). Mr. Belfair's mother, Delia, has lived in the Belfair household since her husband, Martin, passed away 4 years ago from lung cancer. A few months ago, Mr. Belfair was diagnosed with bladder cancer. After surgery and chemotherapy, the cancer still has not receded. The family physician estimates Mr. Belfair has only 5 months to live.

Alex Von Bremen is the hospice nurse working with the Belfair family. Mr. Von Bremen explains to the Belfairs that his goal is to work with the whole family in coping with Mr. Belfair's illness. Mr. Von Bremen asks each family member, "How do you feel Mr. Belfair's illness will affect the way in which the members of your family function and interact with one another?"

Joanne Belfair responds, "Right now we do not talk about Marty being sick. It is the elephant in the room. I am afraid that if Marty does not get better, the whole family will fall apart and never see each other."

Delia Belfair shared, "I do not know where I will live. We don't talk about it. I don't know if I'm welcome to stay if Marty's not here."

Mr. Belfair encourages his family: "I know my illness is hard to accept now, but we have been through tough times in the past and the family stayed together then. Remember when I lost my job? We all made sacrifices for the family and were a stronger family as a result." What other questions would you ask? What referrals would you recommend or initiate?

FAMILY NURSING ASSESSMENT

Family nursing assessment is the cornerstone for family nursing interventions. By using a systematic process, family problem areas are identified and family strengths are emphasized as the building blocks for interventions. Building the interventions with family-identified problems and strengths allows for equal family and provider commitment to the solutions and ensures more successful interventions. Some family assessment models that are available have been developed by nurses (Kaakinen and Hanson, 2015b). See the How To box for information on how to plan for the assessment process.

The Family Assessment Intervention Model and the Family Systems Stressor-Strength Inventory (FS3I) measure very specific dimensions of stressors and strengths in the family and give a microscopic view of family health. It is a more extensive and specific model that demands in-depth knowledge of family analysis and is useful for doing family research (Kaakinen and Hanson, 2015b).

One family assessment model and approach developed by a nurse is the Friedman Family Assessment Model and Short Form (Friedman et al, 2003). The Focus on Quality and Safety Education for Nurses (QSEN) box addresses the difference between family assessment and individual assessment.

Friedman Family Assessment Model

The Friedman Family Assessment Model (Friedman et al, 2003) draws heavily on the structure-function framework and on developmental and systems theory. The model takes a broad approach to family assessment, which views families as a subsystem of society. The family is viewed as an open social system. The family's structure (organization) and functions (activities and purposes) and the family's relationship to other social systems are the focus of this approach.

This assessment approach is important for family nurses because it enables them to assess the family system as a whole, as part of the whole of society, and as an interaction system. The general assumptions for this model are (1) the family is a social system with functional requirements; (2) the family is a small group possessing certain generic features common to all small groups; (3) the family as a social system accomplishes functions that serve the individual and society; and (4) individuals act in accordance with a set of internalized norms and values that are learned primarily in the family through socializations.

The guidelines for the Friedman Family Assessment Model consist of the following six broad categories of interview questions:

1. Identifying data
2. Developmental family stage and history
3. Environmental data
4. Family structure, including communication, power structures, role structures, and family values
5. Family functions, including affective, socialization, and health care
6. Family coping

Each category has several subcategories. There are both long and short forms of this assessment tool.

In summary, this approach was developed to provide guidelines for family nurses who are interviewing a family to gain an overall view of what is going on in the family. The questions are extensive, and it may not be possible to collect all the data at one visit. All the categories may not be pertinent for every family.

SOCIAL AND FAMILY POLICY CHALLENGES

Social and family policy challenges are part of the nurse's practice. As professionals, public health nurses are accountable for participating in the three core public health functions: assessment, policy development, and assurance.

Family policy refers to government actions that have a direct or indirect effect on families. The range of social policy decisions that affect families is vast, such as health care access and coverage, low-income housing, Social Security, welfare, food stamps, pension plans, affirmative action, and education. Although all government polices affect families in both negative and positive ways, the United States has little overall explicit family policy (Daiski et al, 2015). Most government policy indirectly affects families. The Family Medical Leave legislation passed in 1993 by the US Congress is an example of a type of family policy that has been positive for families. A family member may take a defined amount of leave for family events (e.g., births, deaths) without fear of losing his or her job. Despite its controversial introduction, The Patient Protection and Affordable Care Act of 2010 is a long-awaited example of family policy. Many programs that exist for families, such as Social Security and Temporary Assistance to Needy Families, are not available to all families. State assistance for families varies by state.

The challenges of social policy for families are numerous. Given the ongoing debate as to what constitutes a family, social policies may specify a definition that is not consistent with the family's own definition. Examples include same-sex partnerships and marriage, legal definition of parents, reproductive and fertility issues (e.g., a surrogate mother decides she wants to keep the baby), or issues involving care of older adults (e.g., a niece wants to institutionalize an older aunt with dementia because her children are not available). Besides how families define themselves, governments define health care services that affect families.

Teen pregnancy prevention is a monitored health status throughout the United States and a good example of the challenges of family health policy. In some states, any child who is sexually active may have access to reproductive health services. This is a family policy to which some families object, yet the sexually active teenager is protected by laws, both state and federal. The teenager who requests confidential services is protected by Title X and the Health Insurance Portability and Accountability Act (HIPPA) federal regulations, given the state law allowing access to services. Providers can encourage the teen to talk with his or her parents, but ultimately it is the teen's decision. Nurses need to know about these policies because they participate in carrying out family policy and have a responsibility to inform state policy regarding the services they provide.

Nurses participate in enforcing laws and regulations that affect the family, such as state immunization laws. Most states have some school immunization laws that exclude children from school who are not vaccinated. If the child does not have that particular set of immunizations and the parents do not want the child vaccinated, two sets of laws are in conflict—the immunization laws and the school attendance laws. The state could provide a mechanism for a waiver, or the child could be excluded from school, thus making home schooling the only option.

Health care insurance is a social and family policy issue. Ensuring that health services are available or providing those services is problematic for many states and county health departments. Medicare and Medicaid, enacted in 1965, provide some health care for the elderly and low-income families. Insuring the elderly has proved to be beneficial. Both living wills and durable power of attorney for health care, which are legal contracts that designate a person to make health care decisions when the individual is incapacitated, are increasingly being used by families. However, without these legal instruments, families are faced with making end-of-life decisions for their loved ones. Although Medicare and Medicaid provide health care to many, a significant population is still uninsured. For the uninsured, often the only access to health care is through the emergency department. Using the emergency department for primary care results in charity care that frequently gets relegated to the insured through higher premiums.

The H1N1 pandemic is an excellent example of mobilizing community partnerships to solve health problems. In one county health department, space for storing vaccines was insufficient in the county health clinics, so arrangements were made with the law enforcement departments to store vaccines in their secure evidence refrigerators. Other examples of partnering included collaboration with Health and Human Service departments and homeless programs to get at-risk populations and the homeless vaccinated. County health departments and pediatricians worked together to get family members who had infants younger than 6 months of age vaccinated, because these infants were too young to receive the H1N1 vaccine.

These are only a few examples of social and family policy in which nurses are involved. Population-focused nurses need to be involved in making policy that affects families at the local, state, and national levels. Using the core public health functions as a framework allows the population-focused nurse to view the broad spectrum of activities that improve the lives of communities, families, and the individuals within those families.

HEALTHY PEOPLE *2020* AND FAMILY IMPLICATIONS

Although *Healthy People 2020* emphasizes individual and community issues, some objectives relate specifically to families or homes, as shown in the *Healthy People 2020* box.

 HEALTHY PEOPLE 2020

New Objectives Specific to Families and Family Nursing

EMC-2: Increase the proportion of parents who use positive parenting, and communicate with their health care providers about positive parenting.

FP-13: Increase the proportion of adolescents who talk to a parent or guardian about reproductive health topics before they are 18 years old.

MHMD-11: Increase depression screening by primary care providers.

MICH-30: Increase the proportion of children, including those with a special need, who have a medical home.

NWS-4: (Developmental) Increase the proportion of Americans who have access to a food retail outlet that sells a variety of foods that are encouraged by the dietary guidelines for Americans.

FN-12: Increase the proportion of sexually active women who receive instruction on reproductive health before they are 18 years old.

From U.S. Department of Health and Human Services: Healthy People 2020, Washington, DC, 2010, U.S. Government Printing Office.
Note: The term *developmental* means the objective continues to be worked on to set targets, additional subobjectives, and timelines.

⟫ APPLYING CONTENT TO PRACTICE

This chapter describes how nurses and families work together to ensure the success of the family and its members in adapting to responses to health and illness. Family nursing is linked to several foundational public health nursing documents. The Quad Council's (2011) *Core Competencies for Public Health Nurses* clarifies that one of the assumptions of the document is that although PHNs engage in population-focused practice, they can and often do, apply public health concepts at the individual and family level. The Public Health Nurse Intervention Wheel identifies "Individuals/Families" as one of the three levels of public health practice (Public Health Nursing Section, 2001). Within that level, the focus of nursing practice is to change knowledge, attitudes, beliefs, practices, and behaviors of individuals, either alone or as part of a family, class, or group. The American

Nurses Association's (2013) *Public Health Nursing: Scope and Standards of Practice* lists the following competencies related to family nursing:

- The public health nurse incorporates individual and/or family care management to include broad community coordination of public health services (Standard 5A: Coordination of Care).
- The public health nurse describes how individual, family, group, and community-focused programs contribute to meeting the core public health foundations and the 10 essential public health services (Standard 8: Education).
- The public health nurse abides by the vision, the associated goals, and the plan to implement and measure progress of an individual, family, community, or population (Standard 12: Leadership).

▎ CLINICAL APPLICATION

The idealized family portrayed in the media during the twentieth century consists of a working father, a mother who stays home, and their children. Many families today compare their turbulent, hectic lives with those of the fictionalized past and find their situations wanting.

A. Did the idealized version of the traditional family ever really exist?

B. Some people believe that American families are in decline, whereas others believe that families are healthy. What do you think?

C. What seems to be happening with the definition of American families?

D. How does a definition of family influence our care and society's support of families?

Answers can be found on the Evolve website.

▎ REMEMBER THIS!

- Families are the context within which health care decisions are made. Nurses are responsible for assisting families in meeting health care needs.
- Family nursing is practiced in all settings.
- Family nursing is a specialty area that has a strong theoretical base and is more than just common sense.

- Family demographics is the study of structures of families and households, as well as events that alter the family, such as marriage, divorce, births, cohabitation, and dual careers.
- Demographic trends affecting the family include the age of individuals when they marry, an increase in interracial marriages with subsequent children, an increase in the number

of divorced individuals remarrying, an increase in dual-career marriages, an increase in the number of children from families in which marriage is disrupted, a large increase in the divorce rate, a dramatic increase in cohabitation, an increase in the number of children who spend time in a single-parent family, a delay of childbirth, an increase in the number of children born to women who are single or who have never married, and an increase in the number of children who live with grandparents.

- Traditionally, families have been defined as a nuclear family: mother, father, and young children. A variety of family definitions exist, such as a group of two or more, a unique social group, and two or more individuals joined together by emotional bonds.

- The five historical functions performed by families are economic survival, reproduction, protection, cultural heritage, socialization of young, and conferring status. Contemporary functions involve relationships and health.

- Family structure refers to the characteristics, gender, age, and number of the individual members who make up the family unit.

- Family health is difficult to define, but it includes the biological, psychological, sociological, cultural, and spiritual factors of the family system.

- The four approaches to viewing families are family as context, family as a client, family as a system, and family as a component of society.

- Nurses should ask clients whom they consider to be family and then include those members in the health care plan.

- The purpose of the initial family interview is based on the identified issue.

- It is important for the nurse to recognize that the family has the right to make its own health care decisions.

- The nurse, in working with families, must evaluate the family outcomes and response to the plan, not the success of the interventions.

- The Friedman Family Assessment Model takes a macroscopic approach to family assessment, which views the family as a subsystem of society.

- The future of the family, health care, and nursing is not an exact science. However, all areas are changing and many challenges are to be understood and overcome in this new century.

ⓔ EVOLVE WEBSITE

http://evolve.elsevier.com/Stanhope/foundations

- Case Study, with Questions and Answers
- NCLEX® Review Questions
- Practice Application Answers

REFERENCES

American Nurses Association: *Public health nursing: scope and standards of practice*, ed 2, Silver Spring, MD, 2013, ANA.

Bronfenbrenner U: *Influences on human development*, Hinsdale, Ill, 1972, Dryden Press.

Bronfenbrenner U: *The ecology of human development*, Cambridge, Mass, 1979, Harvard University Press.

Bronfrenbrenner U: Ecology of the family as a context for human development: research perspectives. In Paul JL, Churton M, Rosselli-Kostoryz H, et al: *Foundations of special education*, Pacific Grove, Calif, 1997, Brooks/Cole.

Centers for Disease Control and Prevention: *Vital signs: obesity among low income, preschool aged children—United States, 2008–2011*, 2013. Retrieved July 2016 from http://www.cdc.gov/mmwr/preview/mmwrhtml/mm6231a4.htm.

Coyne I, O'Neill C, Murphy M, et al: What does family-centered care mean to nurses and how do they think it could be enhanced in practice, *J Adv Nurs* 67:2561–2573, 2011.

Criss MM, Henry CS, Harrist AW, Larzelere RE: Interdisciplinary and innovative approaches to strengthening family and individual resilience: an introduction to the special issue, *Family Relations* 64:1–4, 2015.

Daiski I, Shillam CR, Casper LM, Florian SM: Family social policy and health disparities. In Kaakinen JR, Coehlo DP, Steele R, et al, editors: *Family health nursing: theory, practice & research*, ed 5, Philadelphia, 2015, FA Davis, pp 137–164.

Duvall EM, Miller BL: *Marriage and family development*, ed 6, New York, 1985, Harper & Row.

Friedman MM, Bowden VR, Jones EG: *Family nursing: research, theory and practice*, ed 5, Upper Saddle River, NJ, 2003, Prentice Hall.

Kaakinen JR, Coehlo DP, Steele R, et al (editors): *Family health nursing: theory, practice & research*, ed 5, Philadelphia, 2015a, FA Davis, pp. 3–32.

Kaakinen JR, Hanson SMH: Theoretical foundations for the nursing of families. In Kaakinen JR, Coehlo DP, Steele R, et al (editors): *Family health nursing: theory, practice & research*, ed 5, Philadelphia, 2015b, FA Davis, pp. 67–104.

Kaakinen JR, Tabacco A: Family nursing assessment and intervention. In Kaakinen JR, Coehlo DP, Steele R, et al (editors): *Family health nursing: theory, practice & research*, ed 5, Philadelphia, 2015, FA Davis, pp. 105–136.

Leahey M, Svavarsdottir EK: Implementing family nursing: how do we translate knowledge into clinical practice? *J Fam Nurs* 15:445–460, 2009.

Lietz CA: Family resilience in the context of high-risk situations. In Becvar SD, editor: *Handbook of family resilience*, New York, NY, 2013, Springer Science+Business Media, pp 153–172.

McGoldrick M, Preto NAG, Carter BA, editors: *The expanded family life cycle: individual, family and social perspectives*, ed 5, New York, 2015, Pearson.

National Institute for Occupational Safety and Health: *Home health workers: how to prevent violence on the job, U.S. Department of Health and Human Services, Centers for Disease Control and Prevention*, Publication No. 2012-118, February 2012. Retrieved from http://www.cdc.gov/niosh/docs/2012-118/pdfs/2012-118.pdf.

Pelletier LR, Stichler JF: Action brief: patient engagement and activation: a health reform imperative and improvement opportunity for nurses, *Nurs Outlook* 61:51–54, 2013.

Price CA, Bush KR, Price SJ, editors: *Families & change: coping with stressful events and transitions*, ed 5, Washington DC, 2017, Sage Publications.

Public Health Nursing Section: *Public Health Interventions: applications for public health nursing practice*, St. Paul, Minnesota, 2001, Minnesota Department of Health.

Quad Council of Public Health Nursing Organizations: *Quad Council core competencies for public health nurses*, Washington, DC, 2011, Public Health Foundation. Retrieved August 2016 from http://www.phf.org/resourcestools/Pages/Public_Health_Nursing_Competencies.aspx.

Rusch D, Frazier SL, Atkins M: Building capacity within community-based organizations: new directions for mental health promotion for Latino immigrant families in urban poverty, *Adm Policy Mental Health* 42:1–5, 2015.

U.S. Department of Health and Human Services: *Healthy People 2020*, Washington, DC, 2010, U.S. Government Printing Office.

Walsh F: The new normal: diversity and complexity in 21st century families. In Walsh F, editor: *Normal family processes: growing diversity and complexity*, ed 4, New York, 2012a, The Guilford Press, pp 3–27.

Walsh F: Family resilience: strengths forged through adversity. In Walsh F, editor: *Normal family processes: growing diversity and complexity*, ed 4, New York, 2012b, The Guilford Press, pp 399–427.

White JM, Klein DN, Martin TF: *Family theories: an introduction*, ed 4, Thousand Oaks, Calif, 2015, Sage Publications.

Wright LM, Leahey M: *Nurses and families: a guide to family assessment and intervention*, ed 6, Philadelphia, 2013, F.A. Davis.

Family Health Risks

Debra Gay Anderson, Hartley Feld, Mollie Aleshire, and Amanda Fallin

OBJECTIVES

After reading this chapter, the student should be able to:

1. Analyze the various approaches to defining and conceptualizing family health.
2. Determine the major risks to family health.
3. Understand the interrelationships among individual health, family health, and community health.
4. Explain the relevance of knowledge about family structures, roles, and functions for family and community-focused nursing.
5. Discuss the implications of policy and policy decisions, at all government levels, for families.
6. Explain the application of the nursing process (assessment, planning, implementation, evaluation) to reducing family health risks and promoting family health.

CHAPTER OUTLINE

Early Approaches to Family Health Risks
    Health of Families
    Health of the Nation
Concepts in Family Health Risk
    Family Health
    Health Risk
    Health Risk Appraisal
    Health Risk Reduction

    Family Crisis
Major Family Health Risks and Nursing Interventions
    Family Health Risk Appraisal
Nursing Approaches to Family Health Risk Reduction
    Home Visits
    Contracting with Families
    Empowering Families
Community Resources

KEY TERMS

behavioral risk, 313
biological risk, 315
contracting, 327
economic risk, 319
empowerment, 311
environmental risks, 313
family crisis, 314
family health, 311

genomics, 318
health risk appraisal, 313
health risk reduction, 313
health risks, 313
home visits, 323
in-home phase, 325
initiation phase, 323
life-event risks, 315

policy, 321
postvisit phase, 326
previsit phase, 324
risk, 312
social risks, 319
termination phase, 326
transitions, 315

Fineberg (2012, p 1020) says that a "successful health system has three attributes: healthy people meaning a population that attains the highest level of health possible, superior care . . . and fairness . . . ." The family is the building block for having healthy people, and many would say that there is much work to be done in the United States to have the highest level of health possible for the population. Today many families experience a fast pace of life and have economic problems they may never have expected; Also,

more families now have two rather than one adult in the workforce. This fast pace often interferes with families eating healthy, nutritious food, exercising to both maintain health and enjoy the company of one another, and actually having time to play together. A focus on the family is vital in promoting the health of individuals and the health of the community. The family of the 21st century faces challenges to maintaining their health different from those of their predecessors. Building support for families within society will lead to healthier families. It is important for nurses to be involved in community assessment, planning, development, and evaluation activities that emphasize family issues and ways to sustain families.

The authors acknowledge the contributions of Diane C. Hatton and Heather Ward to the content of this chapter.

A nation's family health care policy is a primary determinant of family health. Family policy means anything done by the government that directly or indirectly affects families. Family health policy and its relative effectiveness demonstrate a government's understanding of families and its role in promoting their health, with an important desired outcome being that families derive a sense of empowerment and are able to take responsibility for their own health (Chinn, 2012). Local, state, and federal government share the responsibility for family health programs. Each state, as well as each region within states, has programs and laws related to family services. Although the United States is an affluent and technologically advanced country, many disparities remain in health status between different populations of families (Agency for Healthcare Research and Quality [AHRQ], 2015). Factors contributing to the lack of effectiveness of the family health and services policies relate to the absence of a comprehensive, cohesive, and coordinated system for providing care. The United States could benefit from a cohesive family policy designed to improve the health and well-being of all families. Such a policy could help prevent future crises in vulnerable family populations, such as those in or on the verge of poverty or families overwhelmed with abuse and neglect, by providing a safety net to help families maintain their health in times of disaster, economic downturns, unemployment, health crises, and other situations. An effective family health policy might begin with developing an infrastructure of programs designed to provide access to primary and preventive health care. Nurses would be key builders of this process. Nurses who are educated in community assessment, planning, development, and evaluation activities that can help promote and maintain primary family health should be key builders in this process.

In establishing health objectives for the nation, an emphasis has been placed on both health promotion and risk reduction. Reducing the risks to segments of the population is a direct way to improve the health of the general population. Objectives have been identified related to specific health risks for families. The family is an important aggregate that affects the health of individuals, as well as a social unit whose health is basic to that of the community and the larger population. It is within the family that health values, health habits, and health risk perceptions are developed, organized, and carried out. Individuals' health behaviors are affected by and acted out within the family environment, the larger community, and society. Family health habits are developed in the same manner in the context of community norms and values and on the basis of availability and accessibility. For example, in a television commercial for an over-the-counter stimulant, a man is featured who is able to coach his child's basketball team, work at a rehabilitation center, and work as a borough inspector for the city, all while pursuing a college degree at night. The commercial credits the drug for providing the man with the energy needed to be successful in all of these areas. The message is clear: you can, and must, do it all, and taking drugs to succeed is a viable option. The health risks to individual and family health are affected by the societal norms—in this example, the norm is increasing productivity through drugs, and this is not a message that is conducive to good family health care.

To intervene effectively and appropriately with families to reduce their health risks and thereby promote their health, nurses need to understand not only family structure and functioning, but also family theory, nursing theory, and models of health risk (see Chapter 18). In addition, nurses need to look beyond the individual and the family in order to understand the complex environment in which the family exists. Increasing evidence of the effects of social, biological, economic, and life events on health requires a broader approach to addressing health risks for families. Nurses and the communities they serve have a vital interest in exploring new and appropriate options for structuring nursing interventions with families to decrease health risks and to promote health and well-being for all families. It is important for the nurse to focus on families who share similar health risks as a population. Working and planning interventions to reduce health risks in family populations provides a mechanism for shared communication and support among families as well as efficient and effective health care interventions that will not only make the families, but the community as a whole, healthier.

EARLY APPROACHES TO FAMILY HEALTH RISKS

HEALTH OF FAMILIES

Historically, studies of the family in health and illness focused on the following three major areas: (1) the effect of illness on families, (2) the role of the family in the cause of disease, and (3) the role of the family in its use of services. In his classic review of the family as an important unit, Litman (1974) described the important role that the family (as a primary unit of health care) plays in health and illness and emphasized that the relationships among health, health behavior, and family "is a highly dynamic one in which each may have a dramatic effect on the other" (p 495). Mauksch (1974) proposed the idea of distinguishing between family health and individual health. Pratt's (1976) examination of the role of the family in health and illness included the role of the family in promoting healthy behavior. Pratt proposed the *energized family* as being an ideal family type that was most effective in meeting health needs. The energized family is characterized as one that promotes freedom and change, is actively engaged with a variety of other groups and organizations, has flexible role relationships and an equal power structure, and exhibits a high degree of autonomy in family members. Doherty and McCubbin (1985) proposed a family health and illness cycle comprising six phases beginning with family health promotion and risk reduction and continuing through the family's vulnerability to illness, their illness response, their interaction with the health care system, and finally their ways of adapting to illness.

HEALTH OF THE NATION

Increased attention has been given to improving the health of everyone in the United States. As a result of major public health and scientific advances, the leading causes of morbidity and mortality have shifted from infectious diseases to chronic diseases, accidents, and violence, all of which have strong lifestyle and environmental components. A population-focused study in Alameda County, California (Belloc and Breslow, 1972) demonstrated relationships between the following seven lifestyle habits and decreased morbidity and mortality. These habits that were identified in 1972 remain beneficial today for health promotion. They include (1) sleeping 7 to 8 hours a day, (2) eating breakfast almost every day, (3) never or rarely eating between meals, (4) being at or near the recommended height-adjusted weight, (5) never smoking cigarettes, (6) never or rarely drinking alcohol, (7) regularly participating in physical activity.

Considerable evidence supports the belief that lifestyle and the environment interact with heredity to cause disease. In response to these findings and the limited effect of medical interventions on the growing numbers of injuries and chronic disease, the government launched a major effort to study the health status of the population. Part of this effort was a report by the Division of Health Promotion and Disease Prevention of the Institute of Medicine that examined how the physical, socioeconomic, and family environments related to decreasing risk and promoting health (Nightingale et al, 1978). The Surgeon General's Report on Health Promotion and Disease Prevention (Califano, 1979) described the risks to good health. Health objectives for the nation were established and then evaluated and restated for the years 2000, 2010, and 2020. See Chapter 2 for a description of the history of how the *Healthy People* document was developed.

The concept of risk, which refers to a factor predisposing or increasing the likelihood of ill health, is important in family health. It is important to pay attention to the environmental and behavioral factors that lead to ill health with or without the influence of heredity. Reducing health risks is a major step toward improving the health of the nation. Although the family is considered an important environment related to achieving important health objectives, limited attention has been given to (or research done on) family health risk and the role of society in promoting healthy families. The *Healthy People 2020* box shows objectives that relate to families.

CONCEPTS IN FAMILY HEALTH RISK

Pender's Health Promotion Model states that two factors motivate individuals to engage in positive health behaviors (Pender et al, 2015). One is a desire to promote one's own health using behaviors that can increase the well-being of the individual, family, community, and society and, in the process, be able to move toward not only individual self-actualization but also society actualization. The second factor is a desire to protect health, using those same behaviors in an effort to decrease the probability of ill health and provide active protection against illness and dysfunction in families (Pender et al, 2015). A person can reduce health risk by participating in health-protecting and health-promoting behavior. It is important to understand the following seven concepts: family health, family health risk, risk appraisal, risk reduction, life events, lifestyle, and family crisis. These concepts will be defined and discussed. It is important to remember that *health* can be defined in various ways and that individuals define health based on their own culture and value system. The concepts of life events and lifestyles are discussed throughout the other five concepts.

FAMILY HEALTH

Family theorists refer to healthy families but generally do not define family health. Based on the variety of perspectives of the family (see Chapter 18), definitions of healthy families can be seen within the guidelines of any one of the frameworks. For example, within the developmental framework, family health can be defined as having the abilities and resources to accomplish family developmental tasks. Thus the accomplishment of stage-specific tasks is one indicator of family health.

Because the family unit is a part of many societal systems, the systems perspective can explain many family health concepts and actions. Using the Neuman Systems Model (Neumann and Fawcett, 2011), family health is defined in terms of system stability as characterized by five interacting sets of factors: physiological, psychological, sociocultural, developmental, and spiritual. The client family is seen as a whole system with the five interacting factors. The Neuman Systems Model is a wellness-oriented model in which the nurse uses the strengths and resources of the family to maintain system stability while adjusting to stress reactions that may lead to health change and affect wellness.

In other words, this model focuses on family wellness in the face of change. Because change is inevitable in every family, the Neuman Systems Model proposes that families have a flexible external line of defense, a normal line of defense, and an internal line of resistance. When a life event is big enough to contract the flexible line of defense (a protective mechanism) and breaks through the normal line of defense, the family feels stress. The degree of wellness is determined by the amount of energy it takes for the system to become and remain stable. When more energy is available than is being used, the system remains stable. Examples of energy-building characteristics in this system are social support, resources, and prevention (or avoidance) of stressors. Nurses can use preventive health care to both reduce the possibility that a family encounters a stressor and help strengthen the family's flexible line of defense. The following clinical example illustrates the application of the Neuman Systems Model to one family's situation.

The Harris family consists of Ms. Harris (Gloria), 12-year-old Kevin, 8-year-old Leisha, and Ms. Harris's mother, 75-year-old Betty. Kevin was recently diagnosed with type 2 diabetes mellitus, and the family was referred by the endocrinology clinic to the local health department to work with the family in adjusting to the diagnosis.

The focus of the Neuman Systems Model would be to assess the family's ability to adapt to this stressful change (the diagnosis of type 2 diabetes mellitus) and then focus on their strengths to stabilize the family reaction. The answers to questions about the following *five interacting variables* would be an important component of the assessment:

1. **Physiological:** Is the Harris family physically able to deal with Kevin's illness?
   Is everyone else in the family currently healthy? Are there current health stressors?
2. **Psychological:** How well will the family be able to deal with the illness psychologically?
   Are their relationships stable and healthy? Are there any memories of other family members with diabetes?
3. **Sociocultural:** How will the sociocultural variable come into play in Kevin's illness?
   Does the family have social support? Are the treatment and diagnosis culturally sensitive? Can family members support each other?
4. **Developmental:** How will Kevin's development as a preadolescent be affected by diabetes? How will the family's development change? How will Kevin's diagnosis affect Leisha?
5. **Spiritual:** How will the family's spiritual beliefs be affected by the diagnosis? What effect will they have on Kevin's treatment and willingness to adhere to therapy?

HEALTH RISK

Several factors contribute to the development of healthy or unhealthy outcomes. Clearly, not everyone exposed to the same event will have the same outcome. The factors that determine or influence whether disease or other unhealthy results occur are called health risks. Health promotion and disease prevention efforts help control health risks, and these risks can be classified into general categories. *Healthy People 2020* (US Department of Health and Human Services [USDHHS], 2010) identified the major categories as being inherited biological risk, including age-related risks, social and physical environmental risks, behavioral risks, and health care risks. The rapid development of the effect of the Zika virus upon pregnant women is an example of an environmental risk that affects selected groups of people.

Although single risk factors can influence outcomes, the combined effect of several risks has greater influence. For example, a family history of cardiovascular disease is a single biological risk factor that is affected by smoking (a behavioral risk that is more likely to occur if other family members also smoke) and by diet and exercise. Society and family norms and behaviors affect the diet and exercise habits of their members. For example, people in the Northwest and West are more likely to eat heart-healthy diets and to exercise than are people who live in the Midwest and South; thus communities in the Northwest and West are often more supportive of exercise and bicycle paths and diets lower in fat than are communities in other parts of the United States. Therefore the health outcomes for the Northwest and West should be more positive because they support healthy diet and exercise. The combined effect of a family history, family behavioral risks, and society's influences is greater than each of the three individual risk factors (smoking, diet, and exercise).

HEALTH RISK APPRAISAL

Health risk appraisal refers to the process of assessing for the presence of specific factors in each of the categories that have been identified as being associated with an increased likelihood of an illness, such as cancer, or *an unhealthy event*, such as an automobile accident. Several techniques have been developed to accomplish health risk appraisal, including computer software programs and paper-and-pencil instruments. One technique is the Youth Risk Behavior Surveillance System instrument (YRBSS) of the Centers for Disease Control and Prevention (CDC, 2016). This system monitors priority health-risk behaviors and the prevalence of obesity and asthma among youth and young adults. The general approach is to determine whether a risk factor is present and to what degree. On the basis of scientific evidence, each factor is weighted, and a total score is derived. This appraisal method provides an individual score that can be examined as a whole within the family, thus appraising the health risks likely to be experienced by other members of the family.

HEALTH RISK REDUCTION

Health risk reduction is based on the assumption that decreasing the number or the magnitude of risks will decrease the probability of an undesired event occurring. For example, to decrease the likelihood of adolescent substance abuse, family behaviors such as parents not drinking, alcohol not available in the home, and family contracts related to alcohol and drug use

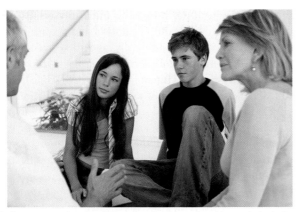

It is important for families to talk about health and their family health risk. (© 2012 Photos.com, a division of Getty Images. All rights reserved. Image #78631212.)

may be useful. Also, family discussions about the pros and cons of drinking and the potential adverse effects of excessive drinking or consuming other substances can influence risks. Health risks can be reduced through a variety of approaches, such as those just described. It is important to note the specific risk and the family's tolerance of it. Pender et al (2015) cite the following examples of different kinds of risks:

- Voluntarily assumed risks, such as overeating, are tolerated better than those imposed by others.
- Risks about which scientists debate and are uncertain are more feared than risks about which scientists agree, such as the causes of colon cancer.
- Risks of natural origin, such as hurricanes, are often considered less threatening than those created by humans.

Risk reduction is a complex process that requires knowledge of the specific risk and the family's perceptions of the nature of the risk. A public health approach to risk reduction would say that it is always more effective to prevent disease or health disruption than to treat, cure, or rehabilitate.

FAMILY CRISIS

A family crisis occurs when the family is not able to cope with an event and becomes disorganized or dysfunctional. Some life events can lead to stress and increase the risk for health disruptions. Examples include when a child leaves home to go to college or to work and live independently, divorce or death in the family, job loss or job change, or relocation. Price, Bush, and Price (2017) differentiate between family resources and family coping strategies. A family crisis exists when the demands of the situation exceed the resources of the family. When families experience a crisis or a crisis-producing event, they try to gather their resources to deal with the demands created by the situation. Examples of family resources are money and extended family members. Families cope by using known processes and behaviors to help them manage or adapt to the problem. Thus, if the primary wage earner has an unexpected illness, family resources might include financial assistance from relatives or emotional support. Family coping strategies, in

contrast, would include being able to ask a relative to loan them emergency funds or being able to talk with relatives about the worries they were experiencing.

It is important to note that the amount of support available to families in times of crisis from government and nongovernment agencies varies in different locales. In addition, the rules and conditions of support often differ and may inhibit families from seeking support, particularly if the conditions are demeaning.

MAJOR FAMILY HEALTH RISKS AND NURSING INTERVENTIONS

As mentioned previously, risks to a family's health typically come from these three major areas: biological and age-related risks, environmental risks, and behavioral risks. In most instances, a risk in one of these areas may not be enough to threaten family health, but a combination of risks from two or more categories could threaten health. For example, there may be a family history of cardiovascular disease, but often the health risk is increased by an unhealthy lifestyle. An understanding of each of these categories provides the basis for a comprehensive approach to family health risk assessment and intervention.

Healthy People 2020 targets areas in health promotion, health protection, preventive services, and surveillance and data systems to describe age-related objectives (USDHHS, 2010). Physical activity and fitness, nutrition, tobacco use, use of alcohol and other drugs, family planning, mental health and mental disorders, and violent and abusive behavior are included as potential factors to be addressed in the area of health promotion. Health protection activities include issues related to the prevention of unintentional injuries, occupational safety and health, environmental health, food and drug safety, and oral health. A variety of preventive services designed to reduce risks for illness have been identified for various health-related situations. These include maternal and infant health, heart disease and stroke, cancer, diabetes and other chronic disabling conditions such as human immunodeficiency virus (HIV) infection and other sexually transmitted diseases. These preventive services consist of immunization for infectious diseases and other clinical preventive services. The interrelationships among the various groups of risk are clear when the objectives for the nation are considered. Most of the national health objectives are based on risk factors of groups or populations in a variety of categories, such as age, gender, and health problems. However, it is important to recognize that some of these factors also relate to and have potential effects on the individuals' families, work, school, and communities.

FAMILY HEALTH RISK APPRAISAL

Assessment of family health risk requires many approaches. As in any assessment, the first and most important task is to get to know the family, their strengths, and their needs (see Chapter 18). This section focuses on appraisal of family health risks in the areas of biological and age-related risk, social and physical environmental

BOX 19.1 Definitions Related to Family Health

- **Determinants of health:** An individual's biological makeup influences health through interactions with social and physical environments, as well as behavior.
- **Behaviors:** These may be learned from other family members.
- **Social environment:** This includes the family; it is where culture, language, and personal and spiritual beliefs are learned.
- **Physical environment:** Hazards in the home may affect health negatively, and a clean and safe home has a positive influence on health.

TABLE 19.1 Family Life-Cycle Stages

STAGES	TASKS
Launching: single young adult leaves home	Coming to terms with the family of origin
	Development of intimate relationships with peers
	Establishment of self: career and finances
Marriage: joining of families	Formation of identity as a couple
	Inclusion of spouse in realignment of relationships with extended families
	Parenthood: making decisions
Families with young children	Integration of children into family unit
	Adjustment of tasks: childrearing, financial, and household
	Accommodation of new parenting and grandparenting roles
Families with adolescents	Development of increasing autonomy for adolescents
	Midlife reexamination of marital and career issues
	Initial shift toward concern for the older generation
Families as launching centers	Establishment of independent identities for parents and grown children
	Renegotiation of marital relationship
	Readjustment of relationships to include in-laws and grandchildren
	Dealing with disabilities and death of older generation
Aging families	Maintenance of couple and individual functioning while adapting to the aging process
	Support role of middle generation
	Support and autonomy of older generation
	Preparation for own death and dealing with the loss of spouse and/or siblings and other peers

Data from Wright LM, Leahey M: *Nurses and families: a guide to family assessment and intervention*, ed 2, Philadelphia, 1994, FA Davis.

risk, and behavioral risk. Box 19.1 includes several definitions related to family health.

Biological and Age-Related Risk

The family plays an important role in both the development and management of a disease or condition. Several illnesses are associated with either genetics or lifestyle patterns. These factors contribute to the biological risk for certain conditions. Patterns of cardiovascular disease, for example, often can be traced through several generations of a family. Such families are said to be at risk for cardiovascular disease. How or whether cardiovascular disease is found in a family is often influenced by the lifestyle of the family. Research findings support the positive effects of diet, exercise, and stress management on preventing or delaying cardiovascular disease. The development of hypertension can be managed by consuming a low-sodium diet, maintaining a normal weight, exercising regularly at the age-appropriate type and amount, and practicing effective stress management techniques, such as meditation.

Type 2 diabetes mellitus is another disease with a strong correlation with a family's genetic pattern; the family also plays a major role in the management of the condition. Family patterns of obesity increase individuals' risks for heart disease, hypertension, diabetes, some types of cancer, and gallbladder disease. It is often difficult to separate biological risks from individual lifestyle factors (USDHHS, 2010).

Transitions that occur when individuals or families move from one stage or condition to another are times of potential risk for families. Examples of these are age-related or life-event risks. See Table 19.1 for a list of family stages and the developmental tasks associated with each stage. Transitions present new situations and demands for families. These experiences often require families to change behaviors, schedules, and patterns of communication; make new decisions; reallocate family roles; learn new skills; and identify and learn to use new resources. The demands that transitions place on families have implications for the health of the family unit and individual family members and can be life-event risks. The nature of a transition event influences how prepared families are to deal with that particular transition. If the event is normative, or anticipated, families may be able to identify needed resources, make plans to cope with the change, learn new skills, and prepare for the event and its consequences. This kind of anticipatory preparation can increase the family's coping ability and

decrease stress and negative outcomes. However, when the event is nonnormative, or unexpected, families have little or no time to prepare, and the outcome can be increased stress, crisis, or even dysfunction.

Several normative events have been identified for families. The developmental model organizes these events into stages and identifies important transition points. It provides a useful framework for identifying normative events and preparing families to cope successfully with related demands. The developmental tasks associated with each stage identify the types of skills families need. The kinds of normative events families experience are usually related to the addition or loss of a family member, such as the birth or adoption of a child, death of a grandparent, a child moving out of the home to go to school or take a job, or the marriage of a child. Health-related responsibilities are associated with each of these tasks. For example, the birth or adoption of a child requires that families learn about human growth and development, parenting, immunizations, management of childhood illnesses, normal childhood nutrition, and safety issues. Adding a new person to the family also requires that members learn new ways to manage all of their roles and partner with one another to meet the changing needs of the family.

Nonnormative events present different kinds of issues for families. Unexpected events can be either positive or negative. A job promotion or inheriting a substantial sum of money may

CASE STUDY

The six members of the Mitchell family are Mr. Mitchell, Mrs. Mitchell, 18-year-old Annie, 15-year-old Michelle, 13-year-old Sean, and 7-year-old Bobby. Mr. Mitchell has been the pastor of Faith Baptist Church for the last 15 years. Mrs. Mitchell is a homemaker and primary caretaker for the children.

For the past year, Mrs. Mitchell has felt tired and "run down." At her annual physical, she describes her symptoms to her physician. After several tests, Mrs. Mitchell is diagnosed with stomach cancer. She starts to cry and says, "How will I tell my family?"

Mrs. Mitchell's primary physician refers the family to Trisha Farewell, a nurse in community health. Ms. Farewell calls the household and speaks with Mrs. Mitchell. Ms. Farewell tells Mrs. Mitchell that she was referred by the physician and she can help Mrs. Mitchell cope with the diagnosis. Mrs. Mitchell confides in Ms. Farewell that it has been 2 weeks since she received the diagnosis but she has yet to tell her husband and children. Mrs. Mitchell asks Ms. Farewell if she can help her tell her family and explain what it all means. Ms. Farewell makes an appointment to go to the Mitchell household and facilitate the family meeting. As seen in this case, the nurse often can help a family talk about a difficult subject and help the family examine ways in which they will cope with the difficulty.

be unexpected but is usually a positive event. However, for some families, a new job for one member may include more responsibility, stress, or travel, which could affect all members of the family. Likewise, inheriting money can change family dynamics in a variety of ways, including who decides how the money will be used. More often, nonnormative events are unpleasant, such as when a family member has a major illness, or when there is a divorce, a new marriage or partner living arrangement, the death of a child, or the family income substantially decreases because of loss of a job or other changes in the ways the family gets income.

Lorenz, Wickrama, and Conger (2004) supported a systems-oriented concept of family stress. They pointed out that families develop a series of processes to manage or transform inputs to the system (e.g., energy, time) to outputs (e.g., cohesion, growth, love), known as *rules of transformation*. Over time, families develop these patterns in enough quantity and variety to handle most changes and challenges. However, when families do not have an adequate variety of rules to allow them to respond to an event, the event becomes stressful. Rather than being able to deal with the situation, they fall into a pattern of trying to figure out what they need to do, and the usual tasks of the family are not adequately addressed. Rules that were implicit in the family are now reconsidered and redefined.

The family stress theory of Lorenz et al (2004) proposes three levels of stress:

- Level I is change in the more specific patterns of behavior and transforming processes, such as change in who does which household chores.
- Level II is change in processes at a higher level of abstraction, such as changes in what are considered as family chores.
- Level III is change in highly abstract processes, such as family values.

Coping strategies can be identified to address each level of stress that families go through in sequence, if necessary. Masarik and Conger (2017) completed a review of the Family Stress Model to understand how family stress influences children throughout their development in terms of physical, social-emotional, and cognitive domains. In their review they concluded that economic hardships and pressures increase child and adolescent maladjustment due to the distress of the parents.

CHECK YOUR PRACTICE

Assume that you are the nurse, Ms. Farewell. What would your questions be to Mrs. Mitchell?

How would you proceed to help her speak with her family about her serious diagnosis?

What steps, in what order, would you take to implement your nursing plan?

Biological Health Risk Assessment

One of the most effective techniques for assessing the patterns of health and illness in families is the genogram. Briefly, a genogram is a drawing that shows the family unit of immediate interest and includes several generations using a series of circles, squares, and connecting lines. Basic information about the family, relationships in the family, and patterns of health and illness can be obtained by completing the genogram with the family. (See Fig. 19.1.) Note that the symbols are depicted in this way: squares indicate males, circles indicate females, an X through either a square or a circle indicates a death, marriage is indicated by a solid horizontal line, and offspring and children are noted by a solid vertical line. A broken horizontal line indicates a divorce or separation. The dates of birth, marriage, death, and other important events can be indicated where appropriate. Major illnesses or conditions can be listed for each individual family member. Patterns can be quickly assessed and provide a guide for the health interviewer about health areas that need further exploration.

The genogram in Fig. 19.1 was completed for the fictional Graham family. Some of the interesting health patterns that can be seen from the genogram are the repetition of the following chronic health conditions: hypertension, type 2 diabetes mellitus, cancer, and hypercholesterolemia. Completing a genogram requires interviews with as many family members as possible. It is important to develop a family chronology, a timeline of family events over three generations, to extend the genogram for a better description of family patterns.

A more intensive and quantitative assessment of a family's biological risk can be achieved using a standard family risk assessment. Because such assessments involve other areas in addition to biological risk, one will be described later, after the description of the assessment of other types of risk.

As discussed earlier, both normative and nonnormative life events pose potential risks to the health of families. Even events that are generally viewed as being positive require changes and can place stress on a family. The normative event of the birth of a child, for example, requires considerable changes in family

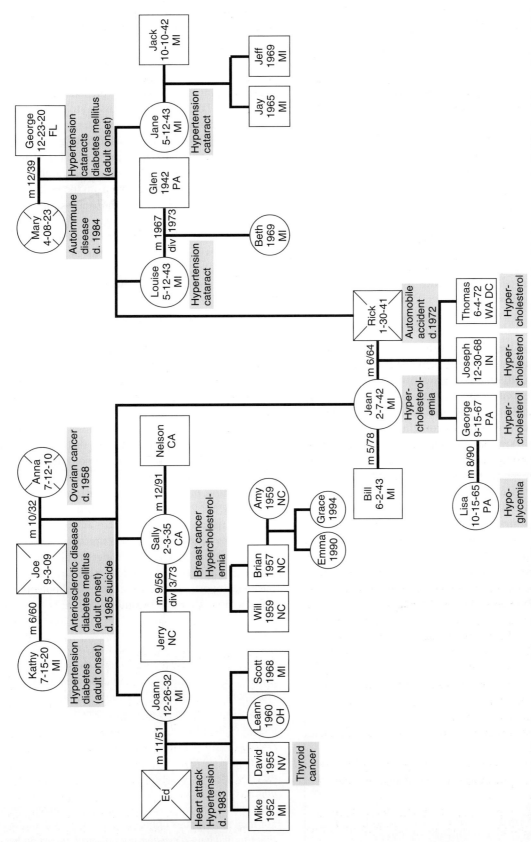

FIG. 19.1 Family genogram of the Graham family. (Developed by Carol Loveland-Cherry. In Stanhope M, Lancaster J: *Public health nursing*, ed 9, St Louis, 2016, Mosby.)

structures and roles. Furthermore, family functions are expanded from previous levels, requiring families to add new skills and establish additional resources. These changes in turn can result in strain and, if adequate resources are not available, stress. Therefore to adequately assess life risks, both normative and nonnormative events occurring in the family need to be considered. Community-level support groups can help families deal with a variety of stressful situations and crises (e.g., Families Anonymous, Bereaved Parents, Parents and Friends of Lesbian and Gay Persons, Single Parents) that arise from both life events and age-related events. Nurses can develop and moderate such groups.

Genetics and Family Health Risks

Much has been learned about how genetics and genomics affect health risks since the completion of the Human Genome Project (HGP) in 2003. As a result of this project, genetic research has expanded to genomics, which is the study of all of the genes in the human genome and their interactions with other genes, the individual's environment, and the influence of cultural and psychosocial factors (Tinley, 2016). The results of this vast project led to a new era in health care known as *genomic health care.* Genomic health care can give health care providers the tools they need to use a person's unique genomic information to design and prescribe the most effective treatment for each person and help clients and families understand some of their health risks that are influenced by their genetic makeup (Lea, 2016). The recently updated *Scope and Standards of Practice for Genetics/Genomics Nursing* provides guidelines and competencies for nurses working in this specialty area (American Nurses Association and the International Society of Nurses in Genetics, 2016). When nurses obtain a family history and learn about the illnesses and causes of the death of biologically related family members, they can then learn about shared genes, environmental factors, and lifestyle behaviors that can increase a person's risks for the same diseases that other family members experienced.

> **HOW TO** **Help Families Complete a Family Health History**
> 1. Inform the family that a family history is a written or graphic record of diseases or health conditions present in their family.
> 2. Encourage the family to develop a three-generation history of biological relatives, their age of diagnosis of a chronic disease, and the age and cause of death of any deceased family members.
> 3. Explain to the family that this type of history is a useful tool to help them know about their health risks and to prevent disease in themselves and their close relatives.
> 4. Tell the family that the health history is not a static document and that it should be updated regularly.
>   Suggest that the family consider using the Centers for Disease Control and Prevention online tool "My Family Health Portrait" to collect and organize their family health history. The tool is available free at https://familyhistory.hhs.gov in both English and Spanish. See also the Surgeon General's Family Health History Initiative which includes the My Family Health Portrait Tool: at http://www.hhs.gov/familyhistory/ or at the National Human Genome Research Institute site http://www.genome.gov/27527640. My Family Health Portrait has many tools and resources related to family health history.

Tests are now available to evaluate the risks for more than 1600 genetic disorders ranging from single-gene disorders, such as cystic fibrosis, to more complex disorders, such as diabetes (National Human Genome Research Institute, 2015). As will be discussed in a later section of the chapter, obtaining a family history is a useful place to begin when considering a genetic connection before the onset of testing.

DNA testing was first used in the late 1970s; today the indications for a DNA test have expanded to include predicting the development of genetic disorders, screening populations, confirming clinical diagnoses, prenatal testing, and DNA testing to develop and apply individualized medical treatment. The next few years will see an explosion in the number of DNA tests driven by information generated from the HGP. Improved technology will make DNA testing more accessible. These advances in genetics and genomics will necessitate that nurses continue to learn about this area of science to respond appropriately to the challenges of effectively using this new knowledge.

An example of this challenge is that of genetic testing for mutations associated with a hereditary cancer syndrome. The best way to identify whether there is a mutation in a family in which a hereditary cancer syndrome is suspected is to test the person who displays the most evidence of being a mutation carrier. This is usually a relative who has had a cancer that occurs typically as part of the hereditary cancer syndrome (e.g., breast, ovarian) that is suspected in the family.

The example just described could present difficulty because family members who have had cancer may not agree to being tested for genetic mutations. This refusal presents challenges to the person who desires information that might affect decision making and his or her health. An additional difficulty is that some individuals do not have an insurance carrier that reimburses for genetic testing, or they may have a high deductible in the insurance policy. Some people also think that testing will decrease the quality of their life and make them anxious about the future if they were to discover they have a mutation. Other people fear a positive test result may lead to feelings of guilt about passing along a disease to children and grandchildren. The following case illustrates the importance of genetic testing and potential concerns in regard to its relationship to family health risks.

Ms. Smith is a 42-year-old mother with three daughters, ages 16, 18, and 22. She has an extensive family history of ovarian cancer. Because of her family history, Ms. Smith is regularly screened per current treatment guidelines. Her mother, who was diagnosed with ovarian cancer at age 55, underwent genetic testing and was discovered to be a carrier of the BRCA-2 gene mutation predisposing to breast and ovarian cancer. Despite undergoing frequent screening, several of Ms. Smith's aunts have died of ovarian cancer at an early age, and her husband wants her to be tested for the BRCA-2 gene, and, if the test is positive, has encouraged her to undergo a prophylactic salpingo-oophorectomy. Ms. Smith fears that a positive genetic test may result in loss of insurance coverage. She is also concerned that this will have a negative psychological impact on her children.

Joan Akins is a public health nurse at the county health department serving the area where this family lives. Ms. Akins has recently conducted a cancer awareness campaign that included public health education on hereditary cancer syndromes. Ms. Smith contacts the nurse to seek advice on whether to undergo genetic testing. Ms. Akins actively listens to the client's concerns and provides general information about genetic testing and the implications of the test results for Ms. Smith and for her children. She also discusses the newly enacted Genetic Information Nondiscrimination Act legislation, which protects the public from genetic discrimination by employers and insurers. The nurse encourages Ms. Smith to talk with her gynecologist about her concerns and make an appointment for genetic counseling, providing names and contact information for local genetic counselors who specialize in cancer genetics.

As mentioned, genetic testing decisions are personal and complex and can be controversial, leading to conflict and confusion in families. It is important for nurses to respect individuals' and family members' decision-making processes. They must, at the same time, be well informed about genetic testing to provide accurate education to members of the public to support appropriate decision making.

Also, current methods of testing do not detect all of the mutations that can occur in some diseases, including hereditary cancer syndrome–related genes. If a mutation is detected during DNA testing, this would not confirm an absolute risk for cancer, but rather would indicate that a person is at increased risk to develop the cancers that are part of the particular hereditary cancer syndrome and may need high-risk management. Such a finding has implications for family members who might have inherited the same mutation, enabling them to undergo DNA testing specific to the identified mutation. Such focused testing is more accurate and cost-effective than testing for multiple potential mutations (National Human Genome Research Institute, 2015). In contrast, if DNA testing in a cancer-affected relative is negative, this does not indicate family members are not at risk. There might be a mutation in a hereditary cancer syndrome gene different from those tested. It is important to remember that many mutations associated with cancer susceptibility and familial syndromes have yet to be identified.

For these reasons, family history also must be considered. However, caution is needed in interpreting family history for several reasons: an inherited syndrome may not be evident for someone with a small family; not everyone is informed of their family's history of disease; the death of a family member may be unrelated to cancer, such as early accidental death; or members may have been adopted, and this may not be known to others in the family. Finally, because most cancers are not hereditary, family history should be accompanied by assessment of shared familial environments. Later in the chapter, gathering a family health history will be discussed further.

Environmental Risk

The importance of social risks to family health is gaining increased recognition. A family's health risk increases if they are living in high-crime neighborhoods, communities without adequate recreation or health resources, communities with major noise pollution or chemical pollution, or other high-stress environments. For example, consider the stress of a mother with children 6, 8, and 12 years of age who are unable to play outside their one-bedroom apartment because the area lacks parks or other green areas, the apartment is on a busy street, and the area has two aggressive youth gangs who are known to bully younger children.

Discrimination—whether racial, cultural, economic, or other—is also a social stress. The psychological burden resulting from discrimination is itself a stressor, and it adds to the effects of other stressors. The implication of these examples of risky social situations is that they contribute to the stressors experienced by the families. If adequate resources and coping processes are not available, breakdowns in health can occur.

The poor are at greater risk for health problems. Economic risk, which is related to social risk, is determined by the relationship between the financial resources of a family and the demands on those resources. Having adequate financial resources means that a family is able to purchase the necessary services and goods related to health. These include adequate housing, clothing, food, education, and health or illness care. The amount of money that a family has available is related to situational, cultural, and social factors. A family may have an income well above the poverty level, but because of a devastating illness of a family member, they may not be able to meet current financial demands. Likewise, families from ethnic populations or families with same-sex parents may experience discrimination in finding housing. Even if they find housing, they may not be welcome and may be harassed, resulting in increased stress.

Unfortunately, not all families have access to health care insurance. For families at the poverty level, programs such as Medicaid are available to pay for health and illness care. Families in the upper-income brackets usually have health insurance through an employer, or they can afford to either purchase health insurance or pay for health care out of pocket. An increasing number of middle-income families have major wage earners in jobs that do not have health benefits. These people often do not have enough income to purchase health care but earn too much money to qualify for public assistance programs. The implementation of the Affordable Care Act has had mixed results. Some insurers are removing themselves from the exchanges because they say the cost to them to cover people via this mechanism is too high. Insurance companies are continuing to merge, and this reduces the competition among insurers for consumers. As discussed in Chapters 21 and 23, the economic downturn in recent years has affected many families. Some of these families have lost their homes, jobs, automobiles, and health insurance. Other families have financial resources that allow them to maintain themselves but that limit the quality of their purchasing power for preventive health care or fresh, healthy, nutritious food. Families with limited resources may qualify for programs such as Medicaid; Special Supplemental Nutrition Program for Women, Infants, and Children (WIC); or Temporary Assistance to Needy Families (TANF). See Chapter 23 for more information on support for families with limited resources. The U.S. Department of Agriculture (USDA) published a report reviewing the history of WIC and current trends and issues of the program (Oliveira and Frazão, 2015). Some of the positive outcomes noted in the report were improved diets among children and higher utilization of preventative and curative health care services for primary care and dental care (Oliveira and

Frazao, 2015). Nurses play an important role in teaching families about the resources available to them and giving them clear directions about how and where to apply for needed services.

Environmental Risk Assessment

Assessment of environmental health risk is less defined and developed than are social risks. Information on relationships the family has with others, such as relatives and neighbors; their connections with other social units (e.g., church, school, work, clubs, organizations); and the flow of energy—positive or negative—can be assessed through the use of an ecomap.

An ecomap represents the family's interactions with other groups and organizations, accomplished by using a series of circles and lines. The family illustrated in Fig. 19.2 is represented

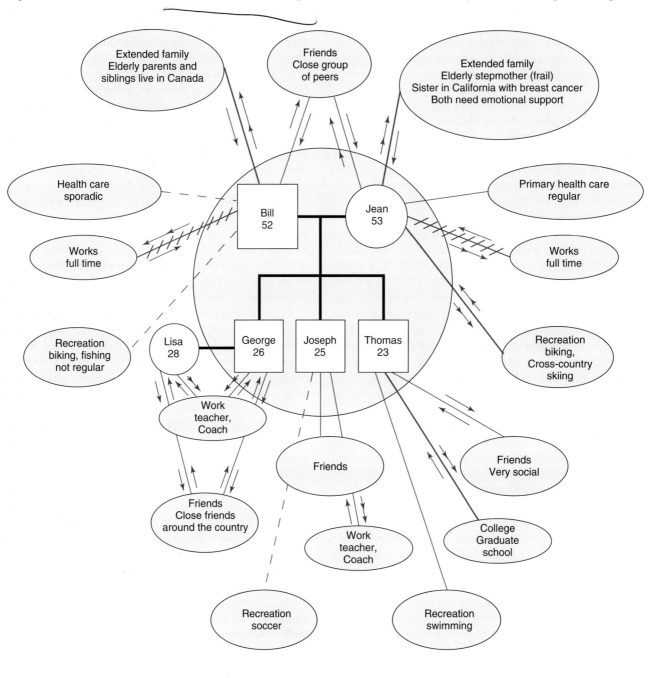

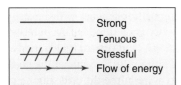

FIG. 19.2 Ecomap of the Graham family. (Developed by Carol Loveland-Cherry. In Stanhope M, Lancaster J: *Public health nursing,* ed 8, St. Louis, 2012, Mosby.)

by a *circle* in the middle of the page; other groups and organizations are indicated by other *circles*. *Lines*, representing the flow of energy, are drawn between the family circle and the circles representing other groups and organizations. An *arrowhead* at the end of each line indicates the direction of the flow of energy (into or out of the family), and the *darkness* of the line indicates the intensity of the energy.

The Graham family ecomap demonstrates that much of the family energy goes into work (also a source of stress for the parents). Major sources of energy for the Grahams are their immediate and extended families and friends.

In addition to the support network shown by the ecomap, other aspects of social risk include characteristics of the neighborhood and community in which the family lives. A nurse who has worked in the general geographic area may already have done a community assessment and have a working knowledge of the neighborhood and community. It is helpful for the nurse to obtain certain information from the family to understand how the family views the community. For example, information about the origins of the family is useful to understand other social resources and stressors. Information about how long the family has lived in their current location and the immigration patterns of the family and their ancestors helps the nurse understand some of the pressures they may experience.

Economic risk is a key predictor of health, as discussed in Chapter 22, which talks about rural and migrant health, and Chapter 23, which discusses poverty, homelessness, teen pregnancy, and mental illness. Families often consider financial information private, and both the nurse and the family may be uncomfortable when discussing finances. The nurse would only need to know the actual family income to help the family determine whether they are eligible for programs or benefits. It is helpful to know if the family's resources are adequate to meet their needs. It is important to remember that the family may have a standard of living different from that of the nurse, and they may be comfortable or at least accepting of their standard of living. Be careful to avoid imposing your financial values onto the family. In terms of health risk, be aware that the resources available to the family need to be used to obtain health and illness care; adequate shelter, clothing, and food; and access to recreation. As mentioned earlier, in an increasing number of families, the main wage earner is employed but receives no medical benefits, and the salary is insufficient for health promotion or illness-related care. This is a policy issue for which nurses can help draft legislation and provide testimony using stories of families in their caseloads.

Behavioral (Lifestyle) Risk

Personal health habits continue to contribute to the major causes of morbidity and mortality in the United States. The pattern of personal health habits and behavioral risk defines individual and family lifestyle risk. The family is the basic unit within which health behavior—including health values, health habits, and health risk perceptions—is developed, organized, and performed. Families maintain major responsibility for

determining what food is purchased and prepared, setting sleep patterns, planning family activities, setting and monitoring norms and expected behaviors about health and health risks, determining when a family member is ill, deciding when health care should be obtained, and carrying out treatment regimens.

Many family health risks can be reduced by careful attention to diet, exercise, and stress management. For example, most of the US population consumes an excessive amount of sodium. The daily guidelines call for less than 2300 mg overall and 1500 for specific populations. Consuming excessive sodium raises blood pressure, which is a major risk factor for heart disease and stroke. It has been found that 44% of sodium comes from 10 food categories: bread and rolls, cold cuts and cured meats, pizza, poultry, soups, sandwiches, cheese, pasta mixed dishes, meat mixed dishes, and savory snacks (CDC, 2012). It is important for nurses to counsel patients about checking food labels and choosing foods that are lower in sodium (CDC, 2012b). Also, although more people are exercising and not smoking, obesity continues to be a major health problem in the United States. For example, results from the 2013-2014 National Health and Nutrition Examination Survey (NHANES) indicated an estimated 32.7% of Americans over the age of 20 are overweight, 37.9% are obese, and 7.7% are obese (Fryar et al, 2016). About one in five adults 65 years of age and older (22.1%) has diabetes in contrast to 1 in 10 among people between the ages of 45 and 64 years (12.3%) (CDC, 2014). Obesity is related to diabetes, which demonstrates the association between health behaviors and health outcomes. General guidelines from the USDHHS and the US Department of Agriculture (USDA) include the following: eating a variety of foods, including fresh vegetables and fruits and grain products; maintaining a healthy weight; choosing a diet low in fat and cholesterol; limiting the use of sugars, salt, and sodium; and consuming alcohol only in moderation.

Regular physical exercise is effective in promoting and maintaining health and in preventing disease. Physical activity can help prevent obesity, diabetes, heart disease, cancer, osteoporosis, and depression (Reiner et al, 2013; van Uffelen, 2015). Benefits of regular physical activity include increased muscle strength, endurance, and flexibility; management of weight; prevention of colon cancer, stroke, and back injury; and prevention and management of coronary heart disease, hypertension, diabetes, osteoporosis, and depression (USDHHS, 2010). Families can structure time and activities for family members. It is helpful when the community in which they live promotes exercise by having accessible parks and walking or biking paths that help families select activities that provide moderate, regular physical exercise, rather than sedentary activities in the home setting. For example, adolescents from families who have close, supportive interactions, have clearly set and enforced rules, and have parents who are involved with their children are at decreased risk for alcohol use or misuse. These family patterns can be enhanced through family-focused intervention sessions in the home.

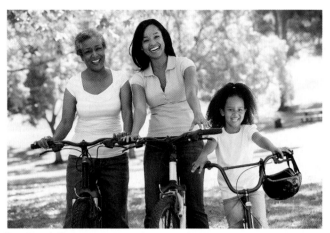

Families influence one another in using time to promote health. (© 2012 Photos.com, a division of Getty Images. All rights reserved. Image #95664337.)

Substance use and abuse are major contributors to morbidity and mortality in the United States. When caring for a family in which one or more members smoke, not only consider talking with them about smoking cessation but also provide education about the effects of secondhand smoke. As discussed in Chapter 24, passive or secondhand smoke has been associated with several types of cancer, heart disease, chronic obstructive pulmonary disease, low birth weight, premature births, and sudden infant death syndrome (USDHHS, 2010).

Similarly, drug use, including alcohol, is a major social and health problem that affects individuals, families, and communities. Drug use is associated with transmission of human immunodeficiency virus (HIV), fetal alcohol syndrome, liver disease, unwanted pregnancy, delinquency, school failure, violence, and crime (Maisto, Galizio, and Connors, 2015).

The literature consistently identifies the following family factors that decrease the risk for substance use in children:

- Family closeness
- Families doing activities together
- Behavior modeled in the family

Although violence and abusive behavior are not limited to families, the amount of intrafamilial violence is thought to be underestimated. It is difficult to collect data and obtain accurate statistics on family violence because the issue is so sensitive for families. Evidence supports the intergenerational nature of violence and abuse—that is, abusers were often abused as children. It is important for nurses to be watchful and observant for signs of neglect and abuse. This is not a topic that clients and families readily bring up in a visit. Often it is what is not said as much as what is said that will provide a clue to violent behavior in the family. Observe closely for nonverbal behavior and listen carefully to what families say when they describe their interactions with one another. Chapter 25, which discusses violence and human abuse, provides guidelines on signs to observe to identify violence and abusive behavior in families.

Behavioral (Lifestyle) Health Risk Assessment

Families are the major source of factors that can promote or inhibit positive lifestyles. They regulate time and energy and the boundaries of the system. Various tools exist for assessing individuals' lifestyle risks, but few are available for assessing family lifestyle patterns. Although assessment of individual lifestyles contributes to determining the lifestyle risk of a family, it is important to look at risks of the family as a unit. One approach is to identify family patterns for each of the lifestyle components included in *Healthy People 2020.* In the areas of health promotion, health protection, and preventive services, lifestyle can be assessed in several dimensions. From the literature on health behavior research, the critical dimensions include the following:

- Value placed on the behavior
- Knowledge of the behavior and its consequences
- Effect of the behavior on the family
- Effect of the behavior on the individual
- Barriers to performing the behavior
- Benefits of the behavior

It is important to assess the frequency, intensity, and regularity of specific behaviors. It is also important to evaluate the resources available to the family for implementing the behaviors. Physical activity as a family has many positive outcomes, including health benefits from the activity, the potential for quality time spent with one another, and the chance to be outside and active. You could assess physical activity in a family by looking at the value a family places on physical activity, the hours a family spends in exercise, the kinds of exercise the family does, the resources available for exercise, and the family's description and self-report of the activity.

NURSING APPROACHES TO FAMILY HEALTH RISK REDUCTION

HOME VISITS

Nurses work with families in a variety of settings, including clinics, schools, support groups, and offices. However, an important aspect of the nurse's role in reducing health risks and promoting the health of populations has been providing services to families in their homes.

Purpose

Home visits, in contrast to clinic visits, give a more detailed assessment of the family structure, the natural or home environment, and behavior in the home environment. Home visits also provide opportunities to identify both barriers and supports for reaching family health promotion goals. The nurse can work with the client directly to modify interventions to match resources. Visiting the family in their home may also contribute to the family's sense of control and active participation in meeting its health needs.

Home visiting provides a broad range of services to achieve a variety of health-related goals. Long-term effects of home visits are positive and can be cost effective for society in contrast to caring for individuals in hospitals or other inpatient sites. As a result, several states have reinstituted home visits for high-risk families. If the home visit is to be a valuable and effective intervention, careful and systematic planning must occur (Avellar et al, 2016; Robling et al, 2016). It is important to remember that a home visit is more than just taking care of people in a different setting. Instead, it is a useful intervention format.

Advantages and Disadvantages

The effectiveness of health promotion services in the home has been critically reexamined by agencies such as health departments and visiting nurses associations. Advantages include the convenience for clients, especially those with mobility issues or those who are unable or unwilling to travel; client control and comfort of the setting; the ability to individualize services; and a natural, relaxed environment for the discussion of concerns and needs. Costs, on the other hand, are a major disadvantage. The cost is high because of preparation for the previsit, travel time and expense to and from the home, the amount of time spent with one client, and postvisit follow-up. Many agencies have considered alternative modes of providing services to families, such as group education, counseling, or other interventions. The important issue is determining

TABLE 19.2   Phases and Activities of a Home Visit

Phase	Activity
I. Initiation	Clarify the source of referral for the visit
	Clarify the purpose for the home visit
	Share information on the reason and purpose of the home visit with the family
II. Previsit	Initiate contact with the family
	Establish a shared perception of purpose with the family
	Determine the family's willingness for a home visit
	Schedule the home visit
	Review the referral and/or family record
III. In-home	Introduce self and professional identity
	Interact socially to establish rapport
	Establish the nurse–client relationship
	Implement the nursing process
IV. Termination	Review the visit with the family
	Plan for future visits
V. Postvisit	Record the visit
	Plan for the next visit

Data from Whitley DM, Kelley SJ, Sipe TA: Grandmothers raising grandchildren: are they at increased risk of health problems? *Health Soc Work* 26:105-114, 2001.

which families would benefit the most and how home visits can most effectively be structured and scheduled. With increasing demands for home health care, the home visit is again becoming a prominent mode for delivery of nursing services.

Process

The components of a home visit are summarized in Table 19.2. The phases include the initiation phase, the previsit phase, the in-home phase, the termination phase, and the postvisit phase. Building a trusting relationship with the family client is the cornerstone of successful home visits. The following five skills are fundamental to effective home visits: observing, listening, questioning, probing, and prompting. The need for these skills is evident in all phases of the home visit process.

Initiation Phase. Usually, a home visit is initiated as the result of a referral from a health care or social agency. However, a family may request services, or the nurse may initiate the home visit as a result of case-finding activities. The initiation phase is the first contact between the nurse and the family. It provides the foundation for an effective therapeutic relationship. Subsequent home visits should be based on need and mutual agreement between the nurse and the family. Frequently, nurses are not sure of the reason for the visit. As a result, the visit may be compromised and come aimlessly or abruptly to a premature halt. The nurse must be clear about the purpose of the home visit, and this purpose or understanding must be shared with the family.

HOW TO   Prepare for the Home Visit: Initiation Phase

- First, if at all possible, nurses should contact the family by telephone before the home visit to introduce themselves, to identify the reason for the contact, and to schedule the home visit. A first telephone contact should be a maximum of 15 minutes. Nurses should give their name and professional identity—for example, "This is Karen Smith. I'm a nurse from the Fayette County Health Department."
- The family should be informed of how they came to the attention of the nurse—for example, as the result of a referral or a contact from observations or records in the school. If a referral was received, it is important and useful to learn if the family is aware of the referral.
- A brief summary of the nurse's knowledge about the family's situation will allow the family to clarify their needs. For example, the nurse might say, "I understand that your baby was discharged from the hospital yesterday and that you requested some assistance with learning more about how to care for your baby at home."
- A visit should be scheduled as soon as possible. Letting the family know agency hours available for visits, the approximate length of the visit, and the purpose of the visit is helpful to the family in determining when to set the visit. Although the length of the visit may vary, depending on circumstances, approximately 30 to 60 minutes is usual.
- If possible, the visit should be arranged when as many family members as possible will be available for the entire visit. It is important to tell clients about any fee for the visit and subsequent visits and possible methods for payment.
- The telephone call can terminate with a review by the nurse of the time, place, and purpose for the visit and a means for the family to contact the nurse in case they need to verify or change the time for the visit or to ask questions. If the family does not have a telephone, another method for setting up the visit can be used. A note can be dropped off at the family home or sent by mail informing the family of when and why the home visit will occur and providing a way for the family to contact the nurse if necessary.

Previsit Phase. The previsit phase has several components. For the most part, these are best accomplished in order, as presented in the How To box. Be aware that the family may refuse a home visit. Do not immediately interpret this as a personal rejection. Families may have a variety of reasons when they make decisions about when and which outsiders are allowed entry into their homes. The nurse needs to explore the reasons for the refusal. For example, there may be a misunderstanding about the reason for a visit, or there may be a lack of information about services, including payment for them. The contact for a visit may be terminated as requested (1) if the nurse determines that either the situation has been resolved or services have been obtained from another source and (2) if the family understands that services are available and how to contact the agency if desired. However, the nurse should leave open the possibility of future contact. In some instances the nurse will be mandated to persist in requesting a home visit because of legal obligations, such as follow-up of certain communicable diseases.

Before visiting a family, the nurse should review the referral or, if this is not the first visit, the family record. If time has lapsed between the contact and the visit, a brief telephone call to confirm the time often ensures that someone will be at home.

Personal safety is an issue that may arise either in approaching the family home or once the family has opened the door to the nurse. Nurses need to examine personal fears and objective threats to determine whether safety is indeed an issue. Certain precautions can be taken in known high-risk situations. Agencies may provide escorts for nurses or have them visit in pairs, readily identifiable uniforms may be required, or a sign-out process indicating the timing and location of home visits may be used routinely. Home visits are generally safe; however, as with all worksites, the possibility of violence exists. Therefore the nurse needs to use caution and exercise good judgment. If a reasonable question exists about the safety of making a visit, the nurse should not make the visit.

The nurse should be aware that families may think the nurse is checking up on them, that the nurse views them as being inadequate or dysfunctional, or that the nurse is impinging on their privacy. Nursing services, especially those from health departments, have been identified by the public as being "public services" for needy families or those with inadequate funds to pay for care. These potential areas of concern underlie the need for sensitivity on the part of the nurse, the need for clarity in information regarding the reason for the visits, and the need to establish collaborative, trusting relationships with the family.

Another factor that may affect the nature of the home visit is whether the visit is viewed as voluntary or required. A *voluntary* home visit (a visit requested by the client) is characterized by easier entry for the nurse, client-controlled interaction, a more informal tone, and a mutual discussion of the frequency of future visits. For example, a voluntary visit would be when a new mother requests that the nurse come to the home and assist her with effective breastfeeding for the infant. In contrast, the client may feel little need for *required* home visits (often legally mandated). When a visit is required, entry into the home may be more difficult than during a voluntary visit. The interaction is often more nurse controlled, and there may be a more formal, investigatory tone to the visit, with distorted nurse–client communication. There may not be any mutual discussion of the frequency of future visits. An example of a required visit might be when a family member has been diagnosed with tuberculosis and the nurse needs to verify that the client is taking medication regularly.

The changing nature of the American family can make it difficult to schedule visits during what have been traditional agency hours. The number of working single-parent or dual-income, two-parent families is increasing, which means that families have more demands on their time. Even if one parent is at home during the usual workday, the ideal is to visit when the entire family is present. This often is not possible because of conflict between agency hours and school or work schedules. It may be possible to schedule a visit at the beginning or end of a day to meet with working or school-age members. In some parts of the country, agencies are reconsidering traditional hours and Monday through Friday visits. These issues are important to assess and address during the previsit phase so that the nurse and the family will be better prepared for the visit.

Culture influences a person's interpretation of and response to health care (Shi and Singh, 2014). It is impossible, given the diversity of the United States and the diversity within cultural groups, to cover every group extensively. Instead, practitioners need to take the responsibility to learn about their client's culture as they prepare for visits with families or communities. See Chapter 5 for more information on cultural differences that influence the provision of health care.

In-home Phase. The actual visit to the home is the in-home phase and gives the nurse the opportunity to assess the family's home, lawn, neighborhood, and community resources, as well as the family interactions. When making the home visit, once at the home, the nurse provides personal and professional identification and tells the client where the agency is located. Next, a brief social period allows the client to assess the nurse and establish rapport. The next step is for the nurse to describe his or her role, responsibilities, and limitations. Another important component of this phase is to determine the client's expectations.

The major portion of the home visit involves establishing the relationship and implementing the nursing process. Assessment, intervention, and evaluation are ongoing. The reason for the visit then determines what will occur in the home visit. Schaffer, Keller, and Reckinger (2015) reported that the most frequent types of home visits involved health promotion, case management, directly observed therapy (DOT), contact investigation, families with newborns, abuse and neglect, parenting, prenatal child growth and development, postpartum, special needs child, and elevated blood lead levels. Keller et al (2004a, 2004b) recommend using the Intervention Wheel to guide nursing practice during home visits. The Intervention Wheel provides guidelines for the purpose of home visits. Some reasons for visits are listed in Box 19.2.

It is important that the nurse be realistic about what can be accomplished in a home visit. In some situations, one visit may

---

BOX 19.2   Reasons for the Home Visit

Nursing interventions may include some or all of the following 17 resources identified by the Minnesota Department of Health, Section of Public Health Nursing:

- Advocacy
- Case management
- Coalition building
- Collaboration
- Community organizing
- Consultation
- Counseling
- Delegated medical treatment and observations
- Disease and other health investigation
- Health teaching
- Outreach
- Policy development and enforcement
- Case finding
- Referral and follow-up
- Screening
- Social marketing
- Surveillance

From Keller LO, Strohschein S, Lia-Hoagberg B, et al: Population-based public health interventions: practice-based and evidence-supported. I. *Public Health Nurs* 21:453-468, 2004a.

be all that is possible or appropriate. In this instance the nurse needs to discuss with the family their needs and the resources available to meet them and determine whether further services are desired or indicated. If further services are indicated and the nurse's agency is not appropriate, the nurse can help the family identify other services available in the community and help initiate referrals. Although it is not unusual to have only one home visit with a family, often multiple visits are made. The frequency and intensity of home visits vary not only with the needs of the family but also with the eligibility of the family for services as defined by agency policies and priorities.

QSEN FOCUS ON QUALITY AND SAFETY EDUCATION FOR NURSES

Targeted Competency: Safety—Minimizes risk for harm to clients and providers through both system effectiveness and individual performance.
Important aspects of safety include:
- **Knowledge:** Examine human factors and other basic safety design principles as well as commonly used unsafe practices (e.g., workarounds and dangerous abbreviations)
- **Skills:** Use national client safety resources for own professional development and to focus attention on safety in care settings
- **Attitudes:** Value the contributions of standardization/reliability to safety

Safety Question: Assume that you are a home care nurse, planning a predischarge visit to the home of your client, Bill Jones. Mr. Jones is 78 years old and has recently suffered a left-sided cerebrovascular accident (CVA). This CVA affected his cognitive, motor, and sensory functioning. You know that individuals who suffer a left-sided stroke may experience memory deficits. Mr. Jones is experiencing moderate expressive aphasia and right-sided weakness, which make it difficult for him to carry out simple tasks of daily living.

Mr. Jones lives with his wife, Helen Jones, who is in good health. Their 45-year-old daughter lives an hour away, and visits monthly. The family is concerned about Mr. Jones's safety and asks for assistance in setting up safety systems in the home.

Specifically, the family has asked for aid in setting up a safe system for the complex medication regimen, adjusting the physical environment to minimize the risk for Mr. Jones falling, and a communication system to accommodate his aphasia. You are aware that Mr. Jones is concerned about maintaining his autonomy.

Use the phases and activities outlined in contracting (Table 19.3) in outlining how to address the concerns of the client and his family.

1. Which data will you collect to address the three requests of the family? What data will you collect from Mr. Jones?
2. What might be some mutually agreeable goals related to medications, the home environment, and a communication system?
3. How might you involve Mr. Jones in the development of a plan for these goals?
4. How might you guide his wife and daughter in exploring the division of responsibilities?
5. What processes might be effective in evaluation of goals and renegotiation?
6. How will you, Mr. Jones, and his family know when the time is right to terminate your contract with this family?

Answer:
1. As you begin contracting with this family, determine Mr. Jones's baseline functioning after the CVA. Review evaluation and plans of care by physical

Continued

cont**QSEN FOCUS ON QUALITY AND SAFETY EDUCATION FOR NURSES—cont'd**

and occupational therapy. How much can Mr. Jones contribute to his own care? What have been Mr. Jones's habits around his medications before the CVA? Did he use pill boxes? How many of these medication administration habits can be maintained with his new medication regimen? Having a physical therapist evaluate the home environment for fall risks would be helpful. Is the client able to write? If so, having a dry erase board handy throughout the home would be an effective means of communication. Otherwise, Mr. and Mrs. Jones will need to develop effective sign language so Mr. Jones can contribute to conversations.

2. Goals around medication administration management might be for Mr. Jones to initiate taking his own medications at the correct time each day, with assistance from his wife only when needed. This approach will allow him to maintain some autonomy, which he has stated is important to him.

   A goal around adjustment of the physical environment might be to have the home environment evaluated and the suggested alterations implemented within a week of Mr. Jones returning home. It would also be a helpful goal to monitor near falls so that Mr. and Mrs. Jones can continue to monitor the effectiveness of the environmental adjustments. Subtle

alterations may continue to be needed as they adjust to Mr. Jones's lack of balance.

   A goal around communications systems might be for you and the family to check in with Mr. Jones weekly to ensure that he thinks he has adequate opportunity to contribute to family communication and processes.

3. Use alternative communication strategies so Mr. Jones can actively participate in care decisions.

4. Depending on the degree of Mr. Jones's care, it would be easy for his wife to become overwhelmed. As the health care professional most in touch with the family dynamics on a regular basis, it is important to discuss how the daughter's visits can provide respite for Mrs. Jones. Are the monthly visits adequate? Does Mrs. Jones need more support when Mr. Jones first comes home? Are there responsibilities (e.g., refilling medication prescriptions) that the daughter can assume?

5. Facilitate regular communication among the family members about new routines and care rhythms.

6. At what point does the family feel independent and autonomous in their care of Mr. Jones? This point would be a good time to begin discussing termination of your contract with this family.

Prepared by Gail Armstrong, PhD, DNP, ACNS-BC, CNE, Associate Professor, University of Colorado Denver College of Nursing.

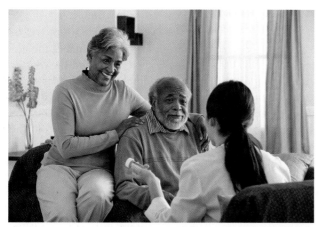

Home visits are important for families to help them effectively manage their health. (© 2012 Photos.com, a division of Getty Images. All rights reserved. Image #86497397.)

Families may or may not be able to control interruptions during the visit. Telephones ring, pets join in the visit, people come and go, and televisions are left on. The nurse can ask that, for a limited time, televisions be turned off or that other disruptive activities be limited. Families may be so used to the background noises and routine activities that they do not recognize them as being potentially disruptive.

Termination Phase. When the purpose of the visit has been accomplished, the nurse reviews with the family what has occurred and what has been accomplished. This is the major focus of the termination phase, and it provides a basis for planning further home visits.

- Ideally, termination of the visit and, ultimately, termination of service begin at the first contact with the establishment of a goal or purpose.

- If communication has been clear to this point, the family and nurse can now plan for future visits, specifically the next visit.
- Planning for future visits is part of setting goals and planning service.
- Contracting is a constructive approach to working with clients and is receiving increasing attention by health professionals.
- The purpose and components of contracting with clients are discussed in more detail later in the chapter.

Postvisit Phase. Even though the nurse has concluded the home visit and left the client's home, responsibility for the visit is not complete until the interaction has been recorded. A major task of the postvisit phase is documenting the visit and services provided. It is important to consider that agencies may organize their records by families. That is, the basic record may be a "family" folder with all members included. However, this often does not occur, although it is useful for the family history and background. More often, in agencies, each family member has a separate record, and other family members' records are cross-referenced. This is because the focus often shifts from the family to the individual. Consequently, nursing diagnoses, goals, and interventions are directed toward individual family members rather than the family unit. This approach has its shortcomings, and it is important for the nurse to recognize these limitations. It is important for the nurse to focus on the continuing assessment of the individual behaviors, responses, and work health status, and the impact on the family. Interventions at the family level may become necessary, such as educating all family members on hygiene and cleanliness or on the appropriate disposal of supplies of the client with tuberculosis in the home.

Record systems and formats vary from agency to agency. The nurse needs to become familiar with the particular system used in the agency. All systems should have a database, list a nursing diagnosis and problem list, specify a plan, including specific goals, actual actions and interventions, and evaluation. These are the basic elements needed for legal and clinical purposes. The format may consist of narratives; flow sheets; a problem-oriented medical record (POMR); a subjective, objective, assessment plan (SOAP); or a combination of formats. It is important that recording be current, dated, and signed.

The nurse should use theoretical frameworks appropriate to the family-centered nursing process. For example, a nursing diagnosis of *ineffective mothering skill* related to lack of knowledge of normal growth and development is an individual-focused nursing diagnosis. *Inability of a family to accomplish the stage-appropriate task of providing a safe environment for a pre-schooler* related to lack of knowledge and resources is a family-focused nursing diagnosis based on knowledge of the developmental approach to families. At times, it may be necessary to present information for a specific family member. However, the emphasis should be on the individual as a member of, and within the structure of, the family.

CONTRACTING WITH FAMILIES

Increasingly, health professionals look at working with clients in an interactive, collaborative style. This approach is consistent with a more knowledgeable public and the recent self-care movement in the United States. However, it may not be consistent with other cultures that look to health care providers for more direct guidance; therefore, it is important to determine the family's value system before assuming that contracting will work.

Contracting, which is making an agreement between two or more parties, involves a shift in responsibility and control toward a shared effort by the client and professional as opposed to an effort by the professional alone. The premise of contracting is family control. It is assumed that when the family has legitimate control, its ability to make healthful choices is increased. This active involvement of the client is reflected in several nursing models—for example, that of Orem (1995). Contracting is a strategy aimed at formally involving the family in the nursing process and jointly defining the roles of both the family members and the health professional.

Purposes

The nursing contract is a working agreement that is continuously renegotiable and may or may not be written. It may be either a contingency or a noncontingency contract. A *contingency contract* states a specific reward for the client after completion of the client's portion of the contract. In contrast, a *noncontingency contract* does not specify rewards. Instead the implied rewards are the positive consequences of reaching the goals specified in the contract.

For family health risk reduction, it is essential that the contract be made with all responsible and appropriate members of the family. Involving only one individual is not sufficient if the goal is family health risk reduction, which requires a total family system effort and change. Scheduling a visit with all family members present may require extra effort; if meeting with the entire family is not possible, each family member can review a contract, give input, and sign it. This allows active participation by all family members without the necessity of finding a time when everyone involved can be present.

Process of Contracting

Contracting is a learned skill on the part of both the nurse and the family. All persons involved need to know the purpose and process of contracting. The three general phases are *beginning*, *working*, and *termination*. The three phases can be further divided into eight sets of activities, as summarized in Table 19.3.

First collect and analyze the data. This activity involves both the family and the nurse. An important aspect of this step is obtaining the family's view of the situation and its needs and problems. The nurse can present his or her observations and validate them with the family and then obtain the family's view.

It is important that goals be mutually set and realistic. At times nurses and clients who are new to contracting may set overly ambitious goals. The nurse should recognize that there may be discrepancies between professional priorities and those of the client and decide if negotiating is required. The goals of contracting are not static because the process includes renegotiating when appropriate.

Throughout the process, the nurse and family continually learn and recognize what each can contribute to meeting the health needs of the family. By exploring resources both the nurse and the family learn about their own and one another's strengths, which requires a review of the nurse's skills and knowledge, the family support systems, and community resources.

Developing a plan to meet the goals involves specifying activities, prioritizing goals, and selecting a starting point. Next, the nurse and the family decide who will be responsible for which activities. Setting time limits involves deciding on a deadline for accomplishing (or evaluating progress toward accomplishing) a goal and the frequency of contacts. At the agreed-on time, the nurse and family together evaluate the progress in both process and outcome. The contract can be modified, renegotiated, or terminated on the basis of the evaluation.

TABLE 19.3 **Phases and Activities in Contracting**	
Phase	**Activity**
I. Beginning phase	Mutual data collection and exploration of needs and problems
	Mutual establishment of goals
	Mutual development of a plan
II. Working phase	Mutual division of responsibilities
	Mutual setting of time limits
	Mutual implementation of a plan
	Mutual evaluation and renegotiation
III. Termination	Mutual termination of a contract

Advantages and Disadvantages of Contracting

Contracting takes time and effort and may require the family and nurse to reorient their roles. Increased control on the part of the family also means increased responsibility. Some nurses may have difficulty relinquishing the role of the controlling expert professional. Contracts are not always successful, and contracting is neither appropriate nor possible in every case. Some clients do not want to have this kind of involvement; they prefer to defer to the "authority" of the professional. Clients who may not choose to contract include persons with minimal cognitive skills, those who are involved in an emergency situation, persons who are unwilling to be more active in their own care, and those who do not see control or authority for health concerns as being within their domain. Some of these clients may learn to contract; others never will be able to do so.

The nursing process does not necessarily provide an active role for the family as a client; the assumption that a need exists is based on professional judgment only, and it is also assumed that changes can and should be made within the family unit. Contracting is one alternative approach that depends on the value of input from both the nurse and family, the competency of the family, the family's ability to be responsible, and the dynamic nature of the process. Contracting not only allows for but also requires continual renegotiating. Although it may not be appropriate in all situations or with all families, contracting can provide direction and structure to health risk reduction and health promotion in families.

EMPOWERING FAMILIES

Approaches for helping individuals and families assume an active role in their health care should focus on empowerment rather than enabling or help-giving (Chinn, 2012). Help-giving interventions do not always have positive outcomes for clients. If families do not perceive a situation as a problem or need, offers of help may cause resentment. Help-giving also may have negative consequences if there is not a match between what is expected and what is offered. A nurse's failure to recognize a family's competencies and to define an active role for them can lead to the family's dependency and lack of growth. This can be frustrating for both the nurse and the family. For families to become active participants, they need to feel a sense of personal competence and a desire for and willingness to take action. Definitions of empowerment reflect the following three characteristics of the empowered family seeking help:

- Access and control over needed resources
- Decision-making and problem-solving abilities
- The ability to communicate and to obtain needed resources

The last characteristic refers to the fact that families may need to learn how to identify sources of help, how to contact agencies, how to ask critical questions, and how to negotiate with agencies to meet family needs. These characteristics often reflect a process by which people (i.e., individuals, families, organizations, communities) take control of their own lives. The outcomes of empowerment can be positive self-esteem, the ability to set and reach goals, a sense of control over life and

LEVELS OF PREVENTION
Strategies for Prevention Related to Families

Primary Prevention
Complete a family genogram and assess health risks with the family to contract for family health activities to prevent diseases from developing.

Secondary Prevention
Use a behavioral health risk survey to identify the factors leading to health problems, such as obesity in the family.

Tertiary Prevention
Develop a contract with the family to change nutritional patterns to reduce further complications from the specified health problem.

change processes, and a sense of hope for the future (Cleek et al, 2012; Collins and Rochfort, 2016).

The Levels of Prevention box shows prevention strategies applied to families.

Empowerment requires a viewpoint that often conflicts with the views of many helping professions, including nursing. Empowerment's underlying assumption is one of a partnership between the professional and the client as opposed to one in which the professional is dominant. Families are assumed to be either competent or capable of becoming competent. This implies that the professional is not an unchallenged authority who is in control. Empowerment promotes an environment that creates opportunities for competencies to be used. Finally, families need to determine that their actions result in behavior change. A nursing intervention that incorporates the principles of empowerment is directed toward the building of nurse–family partnerships and emphasizes health risk reduction and health promotion. The nurse's approach to the family should be positive and focused on competencies rather than on problems or deficits. The interventions need to be consistent with family cultural norms and the family's perception of the problem. Rather than making decisions for the family, the nurse supports the family in their decision making and bolsters their self-esteem by recognizing and using family strengths and support networks. Interventions that promote desired family behaviors increase family competency, decrease the need for outside help, and result in families seeing themselves as being actively responsible for bringing about desired changes. The goal of an empowering approach is to create a partnership between the nurse and the family characterized by cooperation and shared responsibility.

Vulnerable Populations: LGBTQ Families at Risk

Lesbian, gay, bisexual, transgendered, and queer/questioning (LGBTQ) families are another vulnerable group (the Q stands for someone questioning their sexual orientation). Q may also refer to "queer" as some LGBTs have reclaimed that term for political reasons) (Stanley, 2014). Over the past decade, there has been an explosion of visibility for this population. Debates and legal battles centering on LGBTQ rights have taken place nationally and in states all across the country. Notable examples include same-sex marriage, adoption, and antidiscrimination laws. In June 2015 the Supreme Court ruled that states cannot ban same-sex marriage, thus requiring all states to issue marriage licenses to same-sex couples (National Conference of State Legislatures [NCSL], 2015). Prior to this ruling, 37 states, the District of Columbia, and Guam allowed same-sex marriage (NCSL, 2015). Since the court's ruling, states have been divided by a backlash of new legislation considered anti-LGBTQ (Steinmetz, 2016).

As noted in the introduction to this chapter, nurses have an ethical obligation to provide culturally competent care to LGBTQ families. To begin, nurses should provide a safe environment for clients to discuss their sexual orientation. Some nurses may feel a degree of discomfort discussing sexual orientation with their clients. However, it is important to overcome this barrier to care for LGBTQ families.

Nurses should assess LGBTQ family dynamics. Just as there is great variation among heterosexual families, all LGBTQ families are not the same. In addition, same-sex couples have historically had special barriers within the health care system. For example, it may be difficult for LGBTQ couples to make medical decisions or visit their partners in the hospital. Also, there is great variation in LGBTQ adoption rights across the nation, thus there are similar barriers for same-sex households with children.

Nurses are in an optimal position to fulfill a vital role in helping LGBTQ families achieve equitable access to health care following the 2010 Presidential directive instructing hospitals that accept Medicaid and Medicare to allow adult clients to designate specific individuals who can visit them in the hospital. Nurses can assist with assessing the implementation of President Obama's directive. In addition, nurses can help to advocate for more policies designed to reduce barriers within the health care system for LGBTQ families.

Additionally, same-sex couples have historically had special barriers within the health care system. Some problems may stem from the lack of legal recognition for LGBTQ relationships in most areas of the country. Same-sex marriage laws vary widely from state to state. Certain states (e.g., Massachusetts) have legalized same-sex marriage, whereas others (e.g., Kentucky) have constitutional amendments defining marriage as a union between one man and one woman. Similarly, there is great variation in LGBTQ adoption rights across the nation (Gates et al, 2007).

These legal barriers present challenges for LGBTQ families in the health care system. For example, it may be difficult for LGBTQ couples living in states without same-sex marriage to make medical decisions or visit their partners in the hospital. There are similar barriers for same-sex–headed households with children. Consider the following case example.

Sarah and Maria have been in a long-term relationship for 10 years. Five years ago, the couple decided to have a baby. Sarah is the child's biological mother, but the couple has raised Mark together since he was born. The couple lives in a state that does not recognize same-sex adoption. Last year, the couple married. One day, Sarah and Mark were in a serious car accident. What are Maria's legal rights regarding making decisions or accessing medical information for Sarah? Is it different regarding her rights with Mark? As the nurse caring for Sarah and Mark, what support and/or advice can you offer Maria?

▶ APPLYING CONTENT TO PRACTICE

Vulnerable Populations: Teenage Parent Families at Risk

Although endless hours have been spent researching ways to help parents of teenagers, it is also important to remember the teenagers who are parents. This family structure faces multiple health-related and social challenges, the most prominent being affordable and accessible health care. A closely related challenge is the recruitment and development of mentors to help teen parents acquire this health care, as it is uncharted water for nearly all teenagers. The humiliation teens experience when visiting doctors and agencies is a pain analyzed and discussed incessantly, and yet little has been done for the teenage parents.

The most common issue raised by teenage parents is their uncertainty and low self-confidence in handling adult responsibilities other than actual parenting. There is a great need for more teenage-instructional literature on family health policy information and health care service accessibility written from the perspective of teenagers. Single teenage parents need to be able to understand welfare and how to apply, as well as how to find support communities. Teenage parents who decide not to be involved in a child's life must be able to understand child support, adoption, and legal visitation and involvement issues.

The rising numbers of teenagers giving birth must be met with stronger and more extensive plans for families led by teens. Education, vocational opportunity, and social acceptance are "luxuries" often missed by adolescent parents. While the last of these issues can only be solved by eventual cultural assimilation, schooling and careers should be made possible.

Although it is not advisable to simply hand out opportunities to teenagers with children, it is definitely necessary to offer assistance, not only so that they may have a second chance at a successful life, but for their children as well. It is recognized that the children of teenage parents often make the same mistakes as their parents, due to factors of poor living conditions, low socioeconomic status, and a rough childhood. Without adequate family care, there will be no end to the cycle of child parents. Today, many people are advocating for sex education and prevention, but it is also time *now* for postpregnancy programs, which accept that there is a child born to two teenagers; although they may have made a poor choice, these teenagers now have no choice but to accept parental responsibility and be shown the tools to do so.

Another type of family highlighted in this section is a more "traditional" family with a nonheterosexual member. After a family member comes out, families may need initial support to process the information. Nurses may be in a position to provide support during this time. Nurses also may refer families to community resources, such as Parents and Friends of Lesbians and Gays (http://www.pflag.org). Check within your local community for other appropriate resources.

In addition to providing support for the family unit as a whole, nurses may also be in a position to assess LGBTQ individuals. As in all family units, the health of individual members of a family affects the entire family unit. Sexual minorities face a higher risk for depression, anxiety, substance abuse, thoughts of suicide, and suicide. Addressing mental health issues in this population may help reduce the mental health disparities the LGBTQ population faces.

COMMUNITY RESOURCES

Families have varied and complex needs and problems. The nurse is often involved in mobilizing several resources to effectively and appropriately meet family health promotion needs. Although the specific resources vary from community to community, general types include state and national government resources, such as Medicare, Medicaid, TANF, WIC, Supplementary Security Income, food stamps, and the State Children's Health Insurance Program (SCHIP). These programs primarily provide support for basic needs (e.g., illness or health care, nutrition, funds for housing, clothing), and funds are based on meeting eligibility criteria.

In addition to government agencies providing health-related services to families, most communities have voluntary (nongovernment) programs. Local chapters of such organizations provide education, support services, and some direct services to individuals and families. Examples are the American Cancer Society, American Heart Association, American Lung Association, and Muscular Dystrophy Association. These agencies provide primary prevention and health promotion services, as well as screening programs and assistance after the disease or condition is diagnosed. Local social service agencies (e.g., Catholic Social Services) provide direct services such as counseling to families. Other voluntary organizations provide direct services (e.g., shelters for homeless or battered individuals, substance abuse counseling and treatment, Meals on Wheels, transportation, clothing, food, furniture).

Health resources in the community may be *proprietary*, *voluntary*, or *public*. In addition to private health care providers, nurses should be aware of voluntary and public clinics, screening programs, and health promotion programs. Identifying resources in a community requires time and effort. The telephone book and the Internet are good places to begin the search for local community resources. Also, community service organizations, such as the local chamber of commerce and health department, publish community resource listings. Brochures listing services are often available in clinics and health care providers' offices. Regardless of how the resource is identified, the nurse needs to be familiar with the types of services offered and any requirements or costs involved. If this information is not available, the nurse can contact the resource.

Locating and using these systems often requires skills and patience that many families lack. Nurses work with families to identify community resources, and, as client advocates, they help families learn to use resources. This may involve sharing information with families, rehearsing with families what questions to ask, preparing required materials, making the initial contact, and arranging transportation. The appropriateness and effectiveness of resources should be evaluated with families afterward. It is important to remember that navigating the maze of resources is often difficult for the nurse. If a family is in crisis or does not have a phone or a home base from which to call or receive return calls, this process is even more difficult, and their sense of helplessness may be increased. Therefore the nurse's assistance, while promoting the family's sense of empowerment, is a necessary and often complex undertaking.

Another resource and type of service that is growing in acceptance and availability is that of *telehomecare*. This type of care may be called *telehealth* or *telemedicine*. The goal is for clients to communicate with and transfer information to providers from their home. Telehomecare monitoring requires less time per client interaction, so it allows nurses to feasibly care for more clients per day. In addition, clients (including elderly individuals), as well as their caregivers, report few technological problems (Radhakrishnan et al, 2016). Telehomecare can be a particularly useful option in situations in which ongoing and frequent monitoring of a family member's condition is necessary; however, be aware that it is not a substitute for the in-home trust and relationship building and assessment of both family and community resources that can be accomplished only by an attentive and engaged nurse spending time with the family in their home environment. This kind of health care delivery is well suited to areas of the country where the distance from the client and the source of health care is either a large distance or might take a long time because of traffic patterns or when the client does not have transportation.

Policies have long had influence on family health care, and one national policy passed to strengthen and support the family is the Family Medical Leave Act (FMLA). On February 5, 1993, President Clinton signed the FMLA (PL 103-3). This act allows covered employees to take up to 12 weeks of leave each year for certain family and medical reasons (U.S. Department of Labor [USDOL], 2016). Many states have added more leave time and benefits for employees in their state (National Conference of State Legislatures, 2016). Under the FMLA, employees may take an unpaid leave of absence for many reasons: for their own serious illness; for the illness of their child, parent, or spouse; and for the birth or adoption of a child (PL 103-3). While on leave, employees still receive their medical benefits and are guaranteed that their position or one similar to it will be available to them on returning to work. The FMLA was needed to help Americans meet the needs of their families while maintaining employment. Women in particular were experiencing hardship in keeping a job while having a family. A relatively recent emerging family policy issue is paid leave for fathers. Internationally, paternity leave policies vary greatly from country to country. Family policy such as this reflects a growing recognition and valuing of the healthy family unit as a key factor and contributor to the health of not only individuals but our communities and society at large.

PRACTICE APPLICATION

The initial contact between a nursing service and a family provides limited information, and the situation that develops may be much more complex than anticipated. The following example, based on an actual case, illustrates the issues and approaches outlined in this chapter.

The Fayette County Health Department was notified that Amy Cress, age 16 years, had been referred by the school counselor at the local high school for prenatal supervision. Amy was 4 months pregnant, in apparently good health, in the 10th grade, and living at home with her mother, stepfather,

and younger sister. The family lived in a rural area outside of a small farming community. The father of the baby also lived in the community and continued to see Amy on a regular basis. The referral information provided the nurse with a beginning, but limited, assessment of the family situation.
A. What would you do first as the nurse assigned to this family?

B. How would you help this family learn to take responsibility for this situation?
C. After the initial contact, how would you extend the assessment to the entire family system?
D. Would you contract with this family? How? What would be the terms of the contract?
Answers can be found on the Evolve website.

REMEMBER THIS!

- The importance of the family as a major client system for nurses in reducing health risks and promoting the health of individuals and populations is well documented.
- The family is a basic unit within which health behavior, including health values, health habits, and health risk perceptions, is developed, organized, and performed.
- Knowledge of family structure and functioning is fundamental to implementing the nursing process with families in the community.
- Nurses need to go beyond the individual and family and to understand the complex environment in which the family functions to be effective in reducing family health risks. Categories of risk factors that are important to family health are biological, environmental (including economic factors), and behavioral risk.
- Several factors contribute to the experience of healthy or unhealthy outcomes. Not everyone exposed to the same event will have the same outcome. The factors that influence whether disease or other unhealthy results occur are called *health risks*. The accumulated risks are synergistic; their combined effect is more important than individual effects.

- An important aspect of nursing's role in reducing health risk and promoting the health of populations has been providing services to individual families in their homes.
- Home visits offer the opportunity to gain a more accurate assessment of the family structure and behavior in the natural environment. They also provide opportunities to observe the home environment and identify both barriers and supports to reducing health risks and increasingly look toward working with clients in an interactive, collaborative style.
- Contracting, which is making an agreement between two or more parties, involves a shift in responsibility and control from the professional alone to a shared effort by client and professional.
- Families have varied and complex needs and problems. The nurse often mobilizes several resources to effectively and appropriately meet family health needs.
- Nurses have an ethical obligation to provide culturally competent care to LGBTQ families and are in an optimal position to fulfill a vital role in helping LGBTQ families achieve equitable access to health care.

EVOLVE WEBSITE

http://evolve.elsevier.com/Stanhope/foundations
- Case Study, with Questions and Answers
- NCLEX® Review Questions
- Practice Application Answers

REFERENCES

Agency for Healthcare Research and Quality: *2014 National Healthcare Quality and Disparities Report*, Rockville, Md: 2015, AHRQ. AHRQ Pub. No. 15-0007.
American Nurses Association and the International Society of Nurses in Genetics: *Scope and standards of practice for genetics/genomics nursing*, ed 2, Silver Spring, Md, 2016, American Nurses Association.
Avellar S, Paulsell D, Sama-Miller E, et al: *Home visiting evidence of effectiveness review: executive summary*, OPRE Report #2015-85a, *Mathematica Policy Research*, 2016.
Belloc NB, Breslow L: Relationship of physical health in a general population survey, *Am J Epidemiol* 93:328–336, 1972.
Califano JA Jr: *Healthy people: the Surgeon General's report on health promotion and disease prevention*, Washington, DC, 1979, U.S. Government Printing Office.

Centers for Disease Control and Prevention: Vital signs: food categories contributing the most to sodium consumption: United States, 2007–2008, *Morb Mortal Wkly Rep* 61:92–98, 2012.
Centers for Disease Control and Prevention: *Summary Health Statistics: National Health Interview Survey, 2014*, Atlanta, Ga, 2014, CDC. Retrieved July 2015 from http://www.cdc.gov/nchs/nhis/shs/tables.htm.
Centers for Disease Control and Prevention: *Youth Risk Behavior Surveillance System (YRBSS)*, Atlanta, Ga, 2016, CDC. Retrieved July 2016 from http://www.cdc.gov/healthyyouth/data/yrbs/index.htm.
Chinn PL: *Peace and power: new directions for building community*, ed 8, Sudbury, Mass, 2012, Jones & Bartlett.
Cleek EN, Wofsy M, Boyd-Franklin N, et al: The family empowerment program: an interdisciplinary approach to working with multi-stressed urban families, *Fam Process* 51:207–217, 2012.
Collins C, Rochfort A: Promoting self-management and patient empowerment in primary care. In Capelli O, editor: *Primary care in practice—integration is needed, InTech*, 2016. Retrieved from http://www.intechopen.com/.
Doherty WJ, McCubbin HI: Family and health care: an emerging arena of theory, research and clinical intervention, *Family Relat* 34:5–11, 1985.
Fineberg HV: A successful and sustainable health system—how to get there from here, *N Engl J Med* 366:1020–1027, 2012.

Fryar CD, Carroll MD, Ogden CL: *Prevalence of overweight, obesity, and extreme obesity among adults ages 20 and over: United States, 1960–1962 through 2013–2014*, National Center for Health Statistics Health E-Stats, Division of Health and Nutrition Examination Survey, July 2016. Retrieved July 2016 from http://www.cdc.gov/nchs/data/hestat/obesity_adult_13_14/obesity_adult_13_14.pdf.

Gates GJ: *Same-sex couples and the gay, lesbian, and bisexual population: new estimates from the American Community Survey*, Los Angeles, Calif, 2007, The Charles R. Williams Institute on Sexual Orientation Law and Public Policy.

Keller LO, Strohschein S, Lia-Hoagberg B, et al: Population-based public health interventions: practice-based and evidence-supported. I, *Public Health Nurs* 21:453–468, 2004a.

Keller LO, Strohschein S, Schaffer MA, et al: Population-based public health interventions: innovations in practice, teaching, and management. II, *Public Health Nurs* 21:469–487, 2004b.

Lea DH: Genetics and genomics in professional nursing. In Friberg EE, Creasia JL, editors: *Conceptual foundations: the bridge to professional nursing practice*, ed 6, St Louis, 2016, Mosby, pp 292–304.

Litman TJ: The family as a basic unit in health and medical care: a social behavioral overview, *Soc Sci Med* 8:495–519, 1974.

Lorenz F, Wickrama KAS, Conger R, editors: *Family Research Consortium Summer Institute (1996); continuity and change in family relations: theory, methods, and empirical findings* (Advances in Family Research), Mahwah, NJ, 2004, Lawrence Erlbaum Associates.

Maisto SA, Galizio M, Connors GJ: *Drug use and abuse*, ed 7, Stanford CT, 2015, Cengage Learning.

Masarik AS, Conger RD: Stress and child development: A review of the Family Stress Model, *Curr Opin Psychol* 13:85–90, 2017.

Mauksch HO: A social science basis for conceptualizing family health, *Soc Sci Med* 8:521–528, 1974.

National Conference of State Legislatures: *Same-Sex marriage laws*, June 26, 2015. Retrieved July 2016 from http://www.ncsl.org/research/human-services/same-sex-marriage-laws.aspx.

National Conference of State Legislatures: *Employee Leave*, 2016. Retrieved July 2016 from http://www.ncsl.org/research/labor-and-employment/employee-leave.aspx.

National Human Genome Research Institute: *Frequently asked questions about genetic testing*, 2015, National Institutes of Health. Retrieved July 2016 from https://www.genome.gov/19516567/faq-about-genetic-testing/.

Neuman B, Fawcett J: *The Neuman Systems Model*, ed 5, Upper Saddle River, NJ, 2011, Pearson.

Nightingale EO, Cureton M, Kamar V, et al: *Perspectives on health promotion and disease prevention in the United States*, Washington, DC, 1978, Institute of Medicine, National Academy of Sciences.

Oliveira V, Frazão E: *The WIC Program: background, trends, and economic issues, 2015 edition*, EIB-134, U.S. Department of Agriculture, Economic Research Service, Washington, DC, January 2015.

Oneal GA, Eide P, Hamilton R, et al: Rural families' process of re-forming environmental health risk messages, *J Nurs Scholarsh* 47:354–362, 2015.

Orem DE: *Nursing: concepts of practice*, ed 5, St Louis, 1995, Mosby.

Pender NJ, Murdaugh CL, Parsons MA: *Health promotion in nursing practice*, ed 7, Boston, Mass, 2015, Pearson Education.

Pratt L: *Family structure and effective health behavior*, Boston, 1976, Houghton-Mifflin.

Price CA, Bush KR, Price SJ: *Families and change: coping with stressful events and transitions*, ed 5, Los Angeles, 2017, Sage.

Radhakrishnan K, Xie B, Berkley A, et al: Barriers and facilitators for sustainability of tele-homecare programs: a systematic review, *Health Res Educ Trust* 51:48–75, 2016.

Reiner M, Niermann C, Jekauc D, et al: Long-term health benefits of physical activity—a systematic review of longitudinal studies, *BMC Public Health* 13:813, 2013.

Robling M, Bekkers M, Butler CC, et al: Effectiveness of a nurse-led intensive home-visitation programme for first-time teenage mothers (Building Blocks): a pragmatic randomised controlled trial, *The Lancet* 387:146–155, 2016.

Schaffer MA, Keller LO, Reckinger D: Public health nursing interventions: visible or invisible, *Public Health Nurs* 12:711–720, 2015.

Shi L, Singh DA: *Delivering health care in America: a systems approach*, ed 6, Sudbury, Mass, 2014, Jones & Bartlett.

Stanley K: *LGBTQ pamphlet*, 2014, Texas Tech University, Student Counseling Center.

Steinmetz K: Why so many states are fighting over LGBT rights in 2016, *Time*, March 31, 2016. Retrieved July 2016 from http://time.com/4277247/north-carolina-georgia-lgbt-rights-religious-liberty-bills/.

Tinley ST: Introduction to basic genetics and genomics. In Seibert DC, Edwards QT, Maradiegue AH, et al, editors, *Genomic essentials for graduate level nurses*, Lancaster, Penn, 2016, DEStech Publications.

U.S. Department of Health and Human Services: *Healthy People 2020, a roadmap for health*, Washington, DC, 2010, U.S. Government Printing Office.

U.S. Department of Labor: *Employee rights under the Family and Medical Leave Act*, USDOL Wage and Hour Division, WH1420, 2016. Retrieved July 2016 from https://www.dol.gov/whd/regs/compliance/posters/fmlaen.pdf.

Van Uffelen J: Active and healthy ageing: the benefits of physical activity and exercise, *Sport Health* 33:36, 2015.

Worden A, Couloumbis A: *Pennsylvania governor won't appeal gay marriage ruling*, 2014. Retrieved September 2016 from http://www.governing.com/news/headlines/mct-corbett-wont-appeal-ruling.html.

Whitley DM, Kelley SJ, Sipe TA: Grandmothers raising grandchildren: are they at increased risk of health problems? *Health Soc Work* 26:105–114, 2001.

CHAPTER 20

Health Risks Across the Life Span

Judy L. Ponder, contributing editor, and Cynthia Rubenstein, Monty Gross,
Linda Hulton, Sharon Strang, Lynn Wasserbauer

OBJECTIVES

After reading this chapter, the student should be able to:

1. Discuss major health problems of children and adolescents.
2. Describe nursing measures to promote child and adolescent health within the community.
3. Discuss risk factors for adults, including those that are different for men and women.
4. Describe risk factors for older adults.
5. Discuss risk factors for persons in the community who have special health needs.
6. Explain nursing measures designed to reduce risks for adults in the community.

CHAPTER OUTLINE

Status of Children
Children's Health and Major Public Health Issues
  Obesity
  Injuries and Accidents
  Alterations of Behavior and Mental Health Problems
  Acute Illnesses
  Chronic Health Conditions
Target Areas for Prevention with Children
  Smoking
  Nutrition
  Immunizations
  Environmental Health Hazards
Health Policy, Legislation, and Ethics Related to Adult Health
  Ethical and Legal Issues and Legislation for Older Adults

Major Health Issues and Chronic Disease Management of Adults Across the Life Span
  Health Status Indicators
  Chronic Disease
  Women's Health Concerns
  Men's Health Concerns
Health Disparities Among Special Groups of Adults
  Adults of Color
  Incarcerated Adults
  Lesbian and Gay Adults
  Adults with Physical and Mental Disabilities
  Frail Elderly
Family Caregiving
Community-Based Models for Care of Adults
  Community Care Settings

KEY TERMS

advance directives, 343
anorexia nervosa, 347
bulimia, 347
caregiver burden, 343
child maltreatment, 339
chronic illness, 344
durable power of attorney, 343
health status indicators, 345

hormone replacement therapy (HRT), 348
immunization, 342
living will, 343
long-term care, 352
menopause, 348
neglect, 344
obesity, 334

overweight, 334
Patient Self-Determination Act, 343
prostate cancer, 349
sudden infant death syndrome, 340
testicular cancer, 349
unintentional injuries, 336

This chapter examines the health status of individuals across the life span and describes nursing interventions in the community for these groups. Emphasis is on the health status, leading causes of death and disease, and health risks of children and adolescents, adults, older adults, and selected at-risk populations. Consideration is also given to special needs populations in the community in terms of how to assess health risks. This chapter also discusses major public health problems of populations across the life span as identified in *Healthy People 2020* (US Department of Health and Human Services [USDHHS], 2010). Nurses who work in the community using a population-centered approach can have a significant influence on teaching individuals of all ages ways to increase their health promotion activities and reduce risk for disease and disability.

STATUS OF CHILDREN

To provide population-centered nursing care, it is important to understand the changing demographics of American children. The number of children determines the need for schools, health care, and other services. In 2014 there were 73.6 million children in the United States. This is 1.2 million more children than in 2000, and it is projected that by 2050 there will be 79.9 million children in the United States (DeNavas-Walt and Proctor, 2015). The racial composition of the children in the United States is changing, with fewer white non-Hispanic children and a growing number of Hispanic children. Also, family composition can affect the well-being of children. In 2014, 69% of children 0 to 17 years of age lived with two parents, 27.5% with one parent, and 4% with no parent. The number of children born to unmarried mothers increased by 14.5% between 1980 and 2014; the largest increase in births was in women between 25 to 29 years of age. The number of births to adolescent mothers has been decreasing, and between 1989 and 2014, the adolescent birth rate dropped 9.6% (Federal Interagency Forum on Child and Family Statistics [FIFCFS], 2016). Interestingly, the number of children whose parents are foreign-born increased from 15% in 1994 to 25% in 2015 (FIFCFS, 2016). Children of foreign-born parents often speak a language other than English in the home, and this may cause the children to have difficulty in school and could influence their ability to understand health care practices and instructions. Chapter 25 discusses violence in the community and includes abuse to children, which can affect a child's development, health, and overall well-being. Living in poverty affects many aspects of a child's well-being, including health. However, the 21% of children 0 to 17 years of age who lived in poverty in 2014 (15.5 million) was a decrease from 22% in 2010, and this number has even decreased slightly from the 16% in 2000 and 2001. The children most likely to live in poverty were those living in a family with a female head of household (46% in 2014). Poverty affects many aspects of well-being, including that of being able to purchase nutritious food (FIFCFS, 2016).

CHILDREN'S HEALTH AND MAJOR PUBLIC HEALTH ISSUES

The health and well-being of children have a significant impact on the future of any country. Effective health care includes getting immunizations and having regular dental and primary care visits that include health education. Children with health insurance, whether public or private, are more likely to have regular access to health care than are children without insurance. Access to quality health is one of the focus areas of *Healthy People 2020*. Both Medicaid and the State Children's Health Insurance Plan (SCHIP) are discussed in Chapter 7. They are federal and state plans to provide publicly funded health care to children. Because physical, cognitive, and emotional changes occur more rapidly during childhood and adolescence than any other time in the life span, access to regular health visits at key ages is important to monitor these changes. Recommendations for well-child care are found in Resource Tools 7A and 20A on the Evolve website. Nursing assessments include evaluation of growth, development, health status, quality of the parent–child relationship, and family support systems.

OBESITY

Obesity rates in American children have risen to epidemic levels over the past few decades. These increases are noted for all children aged 2 to 18 years regardless of gender or ethnicity. The Centers for Disease Control and Prevention (CDC) defines overweight as a body mass index (BMI) at or above the 85th percentile and lower than the 95th percentile, and obesity is defined as a BMI at or above the 95th percentile for children of the same age and sex when plotted on the CDC growth charts (Table 20.1) (CDC, 2015a). In 2011–2014, the prevalence of obesity was 9.4%% in children ages 2 to 5 years, 17.4% for children ages 6 to 11 years, and 20.6% for adolescents 12 to 19 years (National Center for Health Statistics (NCHS), 2016a).

Many factors contribute to the likelihood that a child will become overweight or obese. Factors include genetics, family eating and physical activity patterns, and time spent inactively viewing television, playing computer games, or using other electronic devices. The environment in which children live influences obesity. For example, if the area is heavily built up and does not allow space for parks, walking paths, or recreation sites, children have reduced areas to expend energy in games, sports, and play. At least 70% of overweight children will become overweight adults. Many children live in households that are unable to put adequate amounts of nutritious food on the table. In 2014 the percentage of children living in households that lacked consistent access to adequate food were substantially above the national average (FIFCFS, 2016).

TABLE 20.1 Classification of Body Mass Index (BMI) for Children Age 2 Years and Above	
Plotted Percentile for Age and Gender	**Weight Status Category**
<5th percentile	Underweight
5th to <85th percentile	Normal or healthy weight
85th to <95th percentile	Overweight
≥95th percentile	Obese

From Centers for Disease Control and Prevention: *About Child and Teen BMI*, Atlanta, GA, 2015a, CDC. Retrieved September 2016 from https://www.cdc.gov/healthyweight/assessing/bmi/childrens_bmi/about_childrens_bmi.html

The physiological consequences of childhood obesity are significant and have long-term effects. Specifically, an obese child has an increased disease risk for cardiovascular, metabolic, musculoskeletal, respiratory, and renal problems (May et al, 2012; Papandreou et al, 2012; Papoutsakis et al, 2013; Paulis et al, 2014; Morandi and Maffeis, 2013). These problems may be manifested as hypertension, respiratory problems, hyperlipidemia, bone and joint difficulties, hyperinsulinemia, and menstrual problems. Another critical consequence for children is the negative psychological and social impact of obesity with decreased self-esteem; higher incidence of depression, sadness, and anxiety; problems with social relationships; and higher reports of being the victim of bullying (Puhl et al, 2012; Ting et al, 2012).

Of particular concern is the rising association between childhood obesity and type 2 diabetes mellitus. Approximately 208,000 US children and adolescents have been diagnosed with type 2 diabetes (CDC, 2014). Although type 2 diabetes mellitus affects all ethnic groups, it occurs more often in nonwhite groups—in particular, African Americans, Latinos, Native Americans, Asian Americans, and Pacific Islanders (CDC, 2014; Temneanu et al, 2016). Screening for type 2 diabetes mellitus is recommended for children with a BMI from the 85th to the 95th percentile with two or more of the following risk factors:

- Family history of type 2 diabetes in a first- or second-degree relative
- Native American, African American, Latino, Asian American, or Pacific Islander descent
- Signs of insulin resistance or conditions associated with insulin resistance
- Maternal history of diabetes or gestational diabetes mellitus during the child's gestation (American Diabetes Association [ADA], 2016)

Excessive body fat at a young age is likely to persist into adulthood and is associated with physical and psychosocial comorbidities, as well as lower cognitive, school, and later life achievement (Martin et al, 2014).

High-fat diets and inactivity are the major contributors to obesity. The American diet in general tends to be high in fat, calories, and sugar, with generous serving sizes. School lunches and "fast-food" meals tend to be oversized and nutritionally poor. Vending machines with nonnutritious food choices can be found in schools. Colas and sugary fruit drinks add calories without nutritional value. Also, the increasing popularity among children of using technology and watching television contribute to a sedentary lifestyle, and schools do not consistently have physical education on a regular basis.

Genetics and genetic susceptibility are certainly contributing components, although the genetic composition of the population has been stable over time, thereby failing to account for a sudden rise in obesity in recent years (Garver et al, 2013). Within the literature, three modifiable risk factors for the development of childhood obesity have been identified. These risk factors are screen time (including television, computer/tablet,

phone, and video games), physical activity engagement, and dietary intake/eating behaviors (Hoelscher et al, 2013; Vollmer and Mobley, 2013; Fakhouri et al, 2013).

Interventions need to be based on goals of family lifestyle changes. The goal is to modify the way the family eats, exercises, and plans daily activities. Strategies for working with families for obesity prevention are discussed in Box 20.1. The goal of managing weight in children and adolescents is to normalize weight. This may involve slowing the rate of weight gain and allowing children to "grow" into their weight, improving dietary habits, increasing physical activity, improving self-esteem, and improving parent relationships. The "Let's Move!" campaign promoted by Michelle Obama is a comprehensive initiative to prevent childhood obesity. It has four primary

BOX 20.1 Family Recommendations for Obesity Prevention

- Breastfeeding is associated with a lower risk for developing childhood obesity.
- Parents' responsibilities include providing healthy meals and snacks for their children.
- Limit 100% fruit juices and avoid all other sugary beverages. These are empty calories and fill children up so they are not hungry at meals. Appropriate beverages are milk and water.
- For toddlers and preschoolers, it sometimes takes 10 to 15 tastes of a new food before learning to like that food. Be persistent!
- Parents should role model good eating behaviors—lots of fruits and vegetables, no sugary beverages, and little to no "junk food" or "fast food."
- Family meals are important for teaching manners, listening to hunger cues, and having quality family time together.
- Encourage children to help with food selection and preparation as appropriate to developmental skills. Allow them to select new foods to try in the produce section of the grocery store.
- Avoid using food as a punishment or reward. Do not expect your child to "clean the plate." These feeding techniques have been associated with increased risk for obesity.
- Turn off the television during meals and do not let your child eat in front of the television. Children do not listen to their cues of satiety when distracted.
- Cook meals at home. Broil, bake, stir-fry, or poach foods rather than frying.
- Modify family eating habits to include low-fat food choices. Serve calorically dense foods that incorporate the food guide pyramid: whole grains, fruits, vegetables, lean protein foods, and low-fat dairy products.
- Encourage family members to stop eating when they are satisfied. Encourage recognizing hunger and satiation cues.
- Schedule regular times for meals and snacks. Include breakfast and do not skip meals.
- Have low-calorie, nutritious snacks ready and available. Avoid having empty-calorie junk foods in the home. Plan for healthy snacks when eating "on the run"—granola, fruits, and nuts.
- Decrease salt, sugar, and fat. Increase complex carbohydrates—whole grains.
- Maintain regular activity (e.g., exercise, sports) and limit television viewing.
- Select family activities and vacations that include or focus on physical activity (hiking, bicycling, swimming).

TABLE 20.2   Daily Dietary Recommendations: Childhood and Adolescence

Food Group*	2–3 Years	4–8 Years	9–13 Years	14+ Years
Calorie level	1000–1400	1200–2000	1600–3200	1600–3200
Dairy	2 – 2.5 cups	2.5 cups	3 cups	3 cups
Try to select low-fat or fat-free sources of milk, cheese, yogurt.				
Protein	2–4 oz	3–5.5 oz	5–7 oz	5–7 oz
Mix up your protein foods to include seafood, beans and peas, unsalted nuts and seeds, soy products, eggs, and lean meats and poultry.				
Vegetables	1–1.5 cups	1.5–2.5 cups	2–4 cups	2–4 cups
Choose a variety of colorful fresh, frozen, and canned vegetables.				
Fruits	1–1.5 cups	1–2 cups	1.5–2.5 cups	1.5–2.5 cups
Focus on whole fruits that are fresh, canned, or dried.				
Grains	3–5 oz	4–6 oz	5–10 oz	5–10 oz
Find whole-grain foods (wheat, rice, oats, cornmeal, barley).				
Activity	Children 2–5 years old should play actively every day.			
	Children 6–18 years old should move at least 60 minutes every day.			
Limit	All age groups: Drink and eat less sodium, saturated fat, and added sugars.			

Modified from US Department of Agriculture, MyPlate Daily Checklist, 2016. Retrieved September 2016 from https://www.choosemyplate.gov/MyPlate-Daily-Checklist.
*Recommendations are per day for each group.

components: healthy schools, access to affordable and healthy food, raising children's physical activity levels, and helping parents make healthy choices. It offers easy-to-understand information on how to eat healthily, get active, and take action to prevent obesity on the website at http://www.letsmove.gov. See Table 20.2 for daily guidelines for food for children and adolescents.

Healthy People 2020 objectives include improving the nutritional status and physical activity patterns of the nation's youth. The American Academy of Pediatrics (AAP) recommends that each child and adolescent needs 60 minutes of moderate, aerobic physical activity per day (AAP, 2014). It is important for families to be active together because this promotes both physical exercise and family engagement. Schools can be a source of physical activity when they have regularly scheduled recess that promotes activity, as well as when they have forms of structured activity for the students.

INJURIES AND ACCIDENTS

Injuries and accidents are the most common causes of preventable disease, disability, and death among children. Unintentional injuries are any injuries sustained by accident, such as falls, fires, drowning, suffocation, poisoning, sports, or recreation or motor vehicle accidents. In the past, two dozen children have died each day from an unintentional injury in the United States (CDC, National Center for Injury Prevention and Control (NCIPC), 2012). Each year, approximately 8.7 million children and teens are treated in emergency departments for unintentional injuries, and over 9000 of those have resulted in death in 1 year (CDC, NCIPC, 2012). Most injuries are predictable and preventable. Because of their size, growth and development, inexperience, and natural curiosity, children and teens are especially at risk for injury. The key to

changing behaviors is teaching age-appropriate safety. The National Action Plan for Child Injury Prevention provides an overarching framework to guide those working to prevent injuries and promote the safety of children and adolescents (CDC, NCIPC, 2012).

The leading causes of unintentional injuries in children are motor vehicle accidents, suffocation, drowning, poisoning, fire, and falls (CDC, 2016a). Motor vehicle injuries are a leading cause of death among children in the United States (CDC, 2016a). During 2014 in the United States, 602 children ages 12 years and younger died as occupants in motor vehicle crashes, and more than 121,350 were injured (National Highway Traffic Safety Administration [NHTSA], 2016). However, many of these deaths can be prevented by buckling up all children in age- and size-appropriate car seats, booster seats, and seat belts. This reduces serious and fatal injuries by more than half (CDC, 2016b).

In addition to the deaths from injury, millions of children are injured and live with the consequences of the injury. The most vulnerable groups for an injury are males, children of lower socioeconomic status, members of American Indian and Alaska Native groups, and children younger than 1 year of age (CDC, NCIPC, 2012). In 2012, 18% of children aged 0 to 17 years visited the ER at least once. (Gindi and Jones, 2014). The most common reasons for children being seen in emergency departments are accidents related to falls, being struck by or against a person or object, overexertion, a motor vehicle crash, and being cut or pierced (Gindi and Jones, 2014).

Age-related development is an important issue in identifying risks to children. Table 20.3 lists the five leading causes and number of nonfatal unintentional injuries among children treated in emergency departments, by age group.

TABLE 20.3 Five Leading Causes and Number of Nonfatal Unintentional Injuries Among Children Treated in Emergency Departments, by Age Group: United States, 2013

Rank	Age <1	Ages 1–4	Ages 5–9	Ages 10–14	Ages 15–24
1	Unintentional fall 134,229	Unintentional fall 852,884	Unintentional fall 624,890	Unintentional struck by/against 561,690	Unintentional struck by/ against 905,659
2	Unintentional struck by/against 28,786	Unintentional struck by/against 336,917	Unintentional struck by/against 403,522	Unintentional fall 558,177	Unintentional fall 814,829
3	Unintentional other: bite/sting 12,186	Unintentional other: bite/sting 158,587	Unintentional cut/pierce 112,633	Unintentional overexertion 294,669	Unintentional overexertion 672,946
4	Unintentional foreign body 10,650	Unintentional foreign body 139,597	Unintentional other: bite/ sting 107,975	Unintentional cut/pierce 114,285	Unintentional motor vehicle— occupant 627,565
5	Unintentional other: specified 10,511	Unintentional cut/pierce 83,575	Unintentional overexertion 93,612	Unintentional pedal cyclist 84,732	Unintentional cut/pierce 431,691

From Centers for Disease Control and Prevention, Ten leading causes of death and injury, 2016a. Accessed through WISQARS Fatal Injury and Nonfatal Injury. Retrieved September 2016 from https://www.cdc.gov/injury/wisqars/leadingcauses.html.

QSEN FOCUS ON QUALITY AND SAFETY EDUCATION FOR NURSES

Targeted Competency: Client-Centered Care—Recognize the client or designee as the source of control and full partner in providing compassionate and coordinated care based on respect for the client's preferences, values, and needs.

Important aspects of client-centered care include the following:

* **Knowledge:** Describe strategies to assist clients and their families in all aspects of the health care process.
* **Skills:** Communicate client values, preferences, and expressed needs to other members of the health care team.
* **Attitudes:** Willingly support client-centered care for individuals and groups whose values differ from your values.

Client-Centered Care Question: You are making a home visit to the Jones family—Mr. and Mrs. Jones and their children, John (10 years), Sally (6 years), and Tommy (3 years). Mr. and Mrs. Jones are considered obese using the body weight index measures of the American Heart Association. John is considered overweight by this same measure, and you note that both Sally and Tommy are at the upper range for weight for their age. You observe during the visit that the family appears to eat a lot of processed food, including lunch meats, chips, and carbonated drinks with sugar. What steps would you take to help this family (1) understand the importance of maintaining an average weight, (2) learn about the different ways in which foods can be prepared, and (3) learn about the relationship among calorie consumption, physical activity, and weight?

Answer: First, you would need to assess their knowledge about weight management. Next, you would need to determine whether they have the skill to purchase and prepare lower-calorie, nutritious food and if they are capable of engaging in physical activities. You would also need to evaluate their attitude toward body size and image. Their willingness to change their behavior will be influenced by whether they view themselves as needing to change. If there is a willingness to make weight management behavior change, you can refer them to a nutrition expert for a consultation or to attend a class(es). You can find out how they spend their leisure time and what options they can identify that would include the entire family in a physical activity such as a walk, a game, or a trip to the park.

Developmental Considerations

Infants. Infants have the second highest injury rate of all groups of children; their small size contributes to some types of injury. The small airway may be easily occluded. The small body fits through places where the head may be entrapped. In motor vehicle crashes, small size is a great disadvantage and increases the risk for crushing or being propelled into surfaces.

The second half of infancy brings major accomplishments in gross motor activities. Rolling, sitting, pulling up, and walking bring safety concerns. Their developing motor skills remain immature, which limits their ability to escape from injury and places them at risk for drowning, suffocating, and burns (CDC, NCIPC, 2012).

Toddlers and Preschoolers. This population experiences a large number of nonfatal falls and being struck by or against an object. They are active and lack an understanding of cause and effect, and their increasing motor skills make supervision difficult (CDC, NCIPC, 2012). They are inquisitive and have relatively immature logic abilities.

School-Age Children. The school-age group has the lowest injury death rate. At this age, it is difficult to judge speed and distance, placing them at risk for pedestrian and bicycle accidents. Boys are twice as likely as girls to sustain a nonfatal bicycle injury, and the highest injury rate is at 10 to 14 years of age. Universal use of bicycle helmets would prevent most deaths. Peer pressure and lack of parental role modeling often inhibit the use of protective devices such as helmets and limb pads (CDC, NCIPC, 2012).

Adolescents. Motor vehicle–related injuries and violence are the leading causes of morbidity and mortality for adolescents.

Risk-taking becomes more conscious at this time, especially among boys. The injury death rates for boys are twice as high as those for girls. Adolescents are at the highest risk of any age group for motor vehicle deaths and fatal poisonings. Use of weapons and drug and alcohol abuse play an important role in injuries in this age group. Homicides are the third leading cause of death for US adolescents (Heron, 2016).

In a survey of adolescents, 24.7% reported being in a physical fight at least one time in the previous 12 months, and 7.1% reported missing school at least 1 day in the previous month because they felt unsafe at school or on their way to school (Kann et al, 2014). Suicide is the second leading cause of death among youths between the ages of 15 and 24 years (Heron, 2016). Poor social adjustment, psychiatric problems, and family disorganization increase the risk for suicide (FIFCFS, 2016).

For all ages, families should be given anticipatory guidance in the high-risk areas for each age group to promote safety and injury prevention. Nurses can use community centers, schools, workplaces, and health centers to provide teaching to families on how to prevent injuries in their children (Fig. 20.1).

Most states have enacted laws allowing health care providers to treat adolescents in certain situations without parental consent. These include emergency care, substance abuse, pregnancy, and birth control. All 50 states recognize the "mature minors doctrine." This allows youths 15 years of age and older to give informed medical consent if it is apparent that they are capable of understanding the risks and benefits and if the procedure is medically indicated.

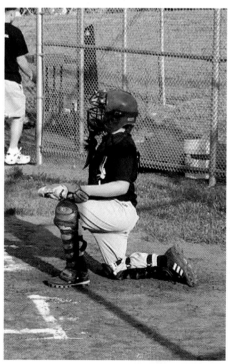

FIG. 20.1 Involvement in developmentally appropriate sports promotes physical activity and skills acquisition.

Injury Prevention

Nurses play a role in the prevention of accidents and injuries. Nurses can identify risk factors by assessing the characteristics of the child, family, and environment. Interventions include anticipatory guidance, environmental modification, and safety education. Education focuses on age-appropriate interventions based on knowledge of the leading causes of death and the leading risk factors. Topics to consider are listed in Box 20.2. Health care provider offices, schools, and daycare facilities provide opportunities to teach children, adolescents, and their families how to prevent injuries. Safety can be incorporated into required health education courses. There are *Healthy People 2020* objectives related to falls, fires and burns, road traffic injuries, drowning, bullying, date violence, and sexual violence among youth (USDHHS, 2010). Community-sponsored car seat and seat belt safety checks and safety fairs are another way to educate families, as are early home visitation programs to high-risk families. Injury prevention should be addressed at all health visits. Schools, day-care centers, and community groups often need guidance toward developing safe places for children to play.

The US Consumer Product Safety Commission has published guidelines for playground safety that cover structure, materials, surfaces, and maintenance of equipment (Box 20.3).

BOX 20.2   Injury Prevention Topics

- Car restraints, seat belts, air-bag safety
- Preventing fires, burns
- Preventing poisoning
- Preventing falls
- Preventing drowning, water safety
- Bicycle safety
- Safe driving practices
- Sports safety
- Pedestrian safety
- Gun safety
- Decreasing gang activities
- Preventing substance abuse

BOX 20.3   Guidelines for Playground Safety

- Playgrounds should be surrounded by a barrier to protect children from traffic.
- Activity centers should be distributed to avoid crowding in one area.
- Surfaces should be finished with substances that meet Consumer Product Safety Commission (CPSC) regulations for lead.
- Durable materials should be used.
- Sand, gravel, wood chips, and wood mulch (not CCA treated) are acceptable surfaces for limiting the shock of falls.
- Equipment should be inspected regularly for protrusions that could puncture skin or entangle clothes.
- Inspect equipment for openings and angles that allow for possible head entrapment.
- Multiple-occupancy swings, animal swings, rope swings, and trampolines are not recommended.

From US Consumer Product Safety Commission [USCPSC]: *Public playground safety handbook*, Bethesda, MD, 2010, USCPSC.

The developmental skills of specific ages are incorporated, as well as recommendations for physically challenged children. Nurses can use these guidelines to help the community establish standards for play areas.

Gun violence is another risk factor for children in that children may be curious and pick up guns without understanding the danger involved. Characteristics associated with gun violence include history of aggressive behaviors, poverty, school problems, substance abuse, and cultural acceptance of violent behavior. A significant number of accidental firearm injuries and deaths in children occur in the homes of friends and family members. Interventions must begin early and address each of these factors.

The *Healthy People 2020* objectives seek to reduce the number of high school students who carry weapons. Nurses can actively participate in efforts to reduce gun violence among young people in the following ways:

- Urge legislators to support gun control legislation.
- Collaborate with schools to develop programs to discourage violence among children.
- Encourage families to remove guns from their homes. If unable to do this, educate families to (1) store all firearms unloaded and uncocked in a securely locked container, with only the parents knowing where the container is located; (2) store the guns and ammunition in separate locked locations; (3) never leave a gun unattended when handling or cleaning it, even for a moment; it should be in the parent's view at all times.
- Initiate community programs focusing on gun storage and safety at school.
- Educate parents on communicating with the homeowners of the homes their children visit about gun access and safety.
- Children and adolescents learning to hunt in rural areas should take gun safety courses.
- Identify populations at risk for violence and target aggression or anger management.
- Discourage mixing alcohol or drugs with guns.

Child Maltreatment

According to the Administration for Children and Families (ACF, 2016), in 2014, there were an estimated 702,000 victims of abuse and neglect nationally, resulting in a rate of 9.4 victims per 1000 children in the population. Two factors contributed to the increase in the national estimate for 2014—an increase in the number of victims reported by states and a decrease in the child population. At the national level, the estimated number of victims increased less than 1% from 2010 to 2014. Also in 2014, it was nationally estimated that 1580 children died of abuse and neglect, which is a rate of 2.13 per 100,000 children in the national population.

Child maltreatment is defined as any act or series of acts of commission or omission by an adult that results in harm, potential for harm, or threat of harm to a child. Acts of commission (abuse) include physical abuse, sexual abuse, and psychological abuse; acts of omission (neglect) include failure to provide (physical neglect, emotional neglect, medical or dental neglect, educational neglect) and failure to supervise (inadequate supervision, exposure to violent environments) (ACF, 2016).

Child maltreatment occurs in all socioeconomic, racial, and ethnic groups. Yet African American, American Indian, and multiracial children experienced higher rates of victimization. Children under the age of 4 years and children with special needs are at highest risk. Children are most likely to be maltreated by their parents, and common parental characteristics include a poor understanding of child development and children's needs, history of abuse in the family of origin, substance abuse in the household, and nonbiological transient caregivers in the home (e.g., mother's boyfriend). Families at highest risk for maltreatment are those experiencing social isolation, family violence, parenting stress, and poor parent–child relationships (ACF, 2016).

ALTERATIONS OF BEHAVIOR AND MENTAL HEALTH PROBLEMS

Behavioral problems in children and adolescents are highly variable and may include eating disorders; attention problems, including attention deficit disorder with or without hyperactivity (ADD/ADHD); substance abuse; elimination problems; conduct disorders and delinquency; sleep disorders; anxiety disorders; autism spectrum disorder; depression; bipolar disorder; or school maladaptation (American Academy of Child and Adolescent Psychiatry [AACAP], 2015). The *Diagnostic and Statistical Manual of Mental Disorders*, 5th edition (American Psychiatric Association, 2013), is the most comprehensive and up to date source of information for practitioners who care for children with or suspected of having mental health issues. Early recognition and coordinated management of pediatric mental health issues are critical to the child's functioning in school, at home, and in the community.

Psychosocial stressors for children have increased over the years. There are many underlying causes for mental health problems in children, ranging from lead poisoning to exposure to violence in the home.

Many families do not understand the behaviors or symptoms they observe in their child. Embarrassment may prevent parents from seeking help. Nurses can promote community awareness about common mental health problems in children and identify resources for families. The use of the medical home to coordinate management of mental health problems is important to provide oversight of subspecialties, medications, and therapies.

A healthy self-concept is supported by positive interactions with others. Problem behaviors may provide negative feedback, which may generate low self-esteem. A child's coping mechanisms are influenced by the individual developmental level, temperament, previous stress experiences, role models, and support of parents and peers. Maladaptive coping mechanisms present as problem behaviors. Inappropriate behaviors may lead to further physical or developmental problems.

ACUTE ILLNESSES

Many of the acute health problems of children also affect adults and are discussed in detail in other chapters of this book. Many of the communicable diseases discussed in Chapter 26 affect children, and their transmission can be reduced by prevention strategies. For example, colds, influenza, and many other communicable diseases are transmitted by droplets or direct contact, so effective hand washing and covering one's nose and mouth when coughing or sneezing can reduce risk. Nurses can focus on preventive measures and promote high vaccination rates, good hand-washing hygiene, and early identification to prevent the spread of illness. See Box 20.4 for guidelines about teaching families good hand-washing techniques. If a child or adolescent is diagnosed with influenza, parents can be instructed to keep the child at home until symptoms have improved and fever has been gone for 24 hours. Nurses can help develop community-based policies in the event of a pandemic, and this may include plans for mass immunizations, specific flu clinics, and protocols for school closures.

One acute illness, sudden infant death syndrome (SIDS) is discussed here. SIDS is defined as the sudden death of an infant younger than 1 year of age, which remains unexplained after a thorough case investigation, including performance of a complete autopsy, examination of the death scene, and review of the clinical history (AAP, 2011). The peak age for SIDS deaths occurs between 2 and 3 months of age, although SIDS may occur up to 1 year of age. The specific independent risk factors for SIDS include (1) prone or side-lying sleep position; (2) sleeping on a soft surface; (3) maternal smoking during pregnancy; (4) overheating; (5) late or no prenatal care; (6) young maternal age; (7) preterm birth or low birth weight; or (8) male gender. The rate of SIDS in African American, American Indian, and Alaska Native infants is two to three times the national average. The incidence has decreased more than 50% since the "Back to Sleep" campaign was promoted in 1994. There is no test to identify infants who may die, making this a frustrating clinical problem. When an infant dies from SIDS, the family requires tremendous support. The nurse provides empathetic support and assists the family as they progress through the grief process and provides guidance for siblings and other family members. Referral to support groups may be helpful.

CHRONIC HEALTH CONDITIONS

Improved medical technology has increased the number of children surviving with chronic health problems. In addition, environmental factors are leading to an increase in certain chronic health conditions (Perrin et al, 2014). Examples of common chronic conditions in children are Down syndrome, spina bifida, cerebral palsy, asthma, ADHD, diabetes, congenital heart disease, cancer, hemophilia, bronchopulmonary dysplasia, and AIDS.

Despite the differences in the specific diagnoses, all of these families have complex needs and face similar problems. Several variables exist to assess for each child and family:

- What is the actual health status? Is the condition stable or life threatening?
- What is the degree of impairment to the child's ability to develop?
- What types of treatments and therapy are required and with what frequency?
- How often are health care visits and hospitalizations required?
- To what degree are the family routines disrupted?

The common issues nurses will want to evaluate for these families include the following:

- All children and adolescents with chronic health problems need routine health care. The same issues of pediatric health promotion and acute health care need to be addressed with this group. The use of the medical home, in which one provider or clinic has all of the child's records, is important for this population.
- Ongoing medical care specific to the health problem needs to be provided. Examples include monitoring for complications of the health problem, medications management, dietary adjustments, and coordination of therapies. Evaluation of the effectiveness of the treatment plan is critical.
- Because care is often provided by multiple specialists, it is important to coordinate the scheduling of visits, tests or procedures, and the treatment regimen.
- Skilled care procedures are often necessary, such as suctioning, positioning, medications, feeding techniques, breathing treatments, physical therapy, and use of appliances.
- Equipment needs are often complex and may include monitors, oxygen, ventilators, positioning or ambulation devices, infusion pumps, and suction machines.
- Educational needs are often complex. Communication among the family, the team of health care providers, school

---

BOX 20.4 Teaching Families About Hand Washing

Always wash your hands *before*:
- Preparing foods
- Eating
- Touching someone who is sick
- Inserting or removing contact lenses

Always wash your hands *after*:
- Preparing foods, particularly raw meats or poultry
- Using the toilet
- Changing a diaper
- Touching animals, animal toys, leashes, or animal waste
- Blowing your nose, coughing, or sneezing into your hands
- Touching someone who is sick

Or anytime you feel that your hands need washing!

How to wash your hands:
- Wet your hands with warm running water.
- Apply soap (liquid, bar, or powder).
- Lather your hands well.
- Rub your hands vigorously for at least 20 seconds (sing the "Happy Birthday" song)—scrub all surfaces, including between your fingers, under your nails, the backs of your hands, and your wrists.
- Rinse your hands well.
- Dry your hands with a clean towel, disposable towel, or air dryer.
- Use your towel to turn off the faucet if possible.

administrators, and teachers is essential to meet the child's health and educational needs.

- Safe transportation to health care services and school must be available. Several barriers may exist, including family resources, location, and the burden of supportive equipment.
- Financial resources may not be adequate to meet the needs.
- Behavioral issues include the effect of the condition on the child's behavior, as well as on other family members.

The ultimate goal is for children with chronic health conditions to achieve optimal health and functioning. Nurses can work to identify barriers for individual families and overall community barriers. Developing support groups, advocating for improved community access to resources, and educating those working with these children on their conditions and needs will promote the family's functioning.

Many children with chronic health conditions have physical limitations requiring adaptive devices and the use of wheelchairs. All children love to play, but most playgrounds are designed with equipment that is not friendly to children with physical disabilities. Should communities be required to adapt or build playgrounds with wheelchair access and swings for disabled children so that all children can enjoy outdoor play?

Asthma is a chronic disease that is on the rise. In 2014 an estimated 6.3 million children under the age of 18 were affected (NCHS, 2016b). Asthma is characterized by excessive lung sensitivity to various stimuli, including viral infection to allergies, irritating gases, and particles in the air. Secondhand smoke can worsen asthma, and asthma is the third leading cause of hospitalization in children under the age of 15 years. Asthma is a major cause of school absenteeism. Preschool children are increasingly among the newly diagnosed cases. Low-income and minority groups are more likely to be hospitalized for or to die of asthma. Population-focused strategies for asthma management include the following:

- Education programs for families of children and adolescents who have asthma
- Development of home and environmental assessment guides to identify triggers
- Education and outreach efforts in high-risk populations to aid in case finding (e.g., in areas with low income, high unemployment, and substandard housing, where there is exposure to secondhand smoke)
- Development of community clean air policies (e.g., no burning of leaves, use of smoke-free zones)
- Improved access to care for asthmatic patients (e.g., developing clinic services with consistent health care providers to decrease emergency department use)
- Assessment of schools and daycare centers for lack of asthma triggers

TARGET AREAS FOR PREVENTION WITH CHILDREN

In addition to the prevention of acute illnesses, selected areas, including smoking, nutrition, immunizations, and environmental health, will be discussed briefly. Many of these topics are discussed in depth in other chapters in the book.

EVIDENCE-BASED PRACTICE

The purpose of this descriptive research study was to investigate parental perception and childhood obesity. The report focused on the perception of weight status in relationship to actual obesity. Parents participated in a telephone survey to describe their child's weight status, as well as their own weight status. Participants answered questions such as, "What would you say best describes your own weight?" and "What would you say best describes (your child's) weight?" The body mass index (BMI) category options were as follows: underweight, healthy weight, overweight, or obese. Parents reported the weights as falling in one of the aforementioned categories, then height and weight were calculated for BMI score. The primary investigator would check parental perception of category with the BMI results for accuracy. The study participants consisted of a random sample of public school parents between 2009 and 2012. Study results revealed that more than 2 out of 5 parents misperceived the weight status of their children. Parents who misperceived their child's weight were nearly 12 times more likely to have an obese child.

Nurse Use

Nurses can play an important role in educating parents and children, as only 54.5% of children in this study had a healthy weight. It is imperative that nurses partner with nutritionists, social workers, teachers, and school health councils in assisting families to recognize an unhealthy weight. Practice implications that were learned from the study included that parental misperception of their child's weight was the strongest predictor of childhood obesity.

Data from McKee C, Long L, Southward L, Walker B, McCown J: The role of parental misperception of child's body weight in childhood obesity, *Journal of Pediatric Nursing, 31:* 196-203, 2016.

SMOKING

Smoking and the effects of tobacco affect both children and adults. Many times parents do not understand the effects of smoking on children. These effects are particularly harmful to children under age 5 years and those living in poverty. An added risk has been the introduction of electronic cigarettes. An initial study by Goniewicz et al (2013) found cancer-causing substances in all of the e-cigarette samples that were tested. Secondhand smoke continues to be harmful to young children. It is responsible for between 150,000 and 300,000 lower respiratory tract infections in infants and children under 18 months of age, which accounts for approximately 7500 and 15,000 hospitalizations each year (CDC, 2015b). Also, 430 SIDS deaths in the United States annually have been attributed to secondhand smoke exposure. It may also cause a buildup of fluid in the middle ear, which has resulted in 790,000 doctor's office visits per year, as well as more than 202,000 asthma flareups among children each year. More than 24 million children in the United States, or about 37%, have been exposed to secondhand smoke (American Lung Association [ALA], 2016). Parents may not understand or believe the effects of smoking on children. Children of smokers are more likely to smoke, and it is especially hard for adults to quit smoking if they began as a teen.

Interventions to discourage smoking focus on the parent, the child or adolescent, and public policy. Parents should be offered (1) educational programs dealing with the negative effects of smoking on children, (2) interventions to stop smoking,

(3) ways to create a smoke-free environment, and (4) behavior modification techniques. Antismoking programs directed toward children and teenagers are more successful if the focus is on short-term effects rather than on long-term effects. Developmentally, children and teenagers cannot visualize the future consequences of smoking. The immediate health risks and the cosmetic effects should be emphasized. Teaching should include how advertising puts pressure on people to smoke. Music, sports, and other activities, including stress-reducing techniques, should be encouraged.

NUTRITION

Maintaining child health relies on good nutrition and dietary habits. The first 6 years are the most important for developing sound lifetime eating habits. The quality of nutrition influences growth and development and prevention of disease. Atherosclerosis begins during childhood. Other diseases, such as obesity, diabetes, osteoporosis, and cancer, may also have early beginnings. Low-income and minority families are at increased risk for poor nutrition, but all groups show poor dietary habits. Many variables, including ethnicity, race, culture, and socioeconomic status, influence what a family eats. Also, children have some characteristics that affect their nutrition, such as being slow eaters, having picky food choices, allergies, acute or chronic health problems, and changes in growth patterns. It is important for nurses to help parents learn about the daily requirements of their children. A useful source of information is the website for the American Academy of Pediatrics (http://www.app.org), which has a section on childhood nutrition that offers sections such as childhood nutrition, healthy snacks, nutritional needs of young athletes, and vitamin supplements. Because nutritional needs for children vary at each developmental stage, it is important for nurses to understand the difference in what an infant needs versus what a toddler needs, as well as what an active 9-year-old needs versus what a 16-year-old male athlete needs. Nurses can guide families to improve their nutrition by providing information on good nutrition in individual or group sessions, conducting diet assessment, delivering educational activities that focus on the effects of fad foods and diets, giving attendees at educational sessions information about the daily food needs and suggesting healthy snacks, and assessing for risks for eating disorders.

IMMUNIZATIONS

Routine immunization of children has been successful in preventing some diseases. The challenge is making sure that children receive immunizations at the appropriate times and in their entirety. In recent years, more families are choosing not to vaccinate their children, and this has an effect on the community. Not all parents appreciate the seriousness of vaccine-preventable diseases because the prevalence is low in the world. They are confused by media misinformation about the consequences of vaccines, including autism. They have concerns about the data showing the safety of vaccines. They doubt the agencies making recommendations and the companies that manufacture

vaccines. It is important to understand their concerns and to educate them about vaccine safety.

The goal of immunization is to protect the individual by using immunizing agents to stimulate antibody formation. For some people, cost and convenience are critical issues in determining whether children are immunized. In many communities, successful programs combine low-cost or free immunizations provided at convenient times and locations. It is important to repeatedly urge parents to obtain immunizations for their children. Immunization recommendations rapidly change as new information and products are available. Two major organizations are responsible for guidelines: the AAP and the US Public Health Service's Advisory Committee on Immunization Practices (ACIP). Resource Tools 20C and 20D list current recommendations from the CDC. The main goal of the guidelines is to provide flexibility to ensure that the largest number of children will be immunized. All health care providers are urged to access immunization status at every encounter with children and to update immunizations whenever possible. See Resource Tools 20C, 20D, 20E, and 20F on the Evolve website for immunizing agents, contraindications, and side effects.

ENVIRONMENTAL HEALTH HAZARDS

The quality of the environment directly affects the health of children and adults. Growth, size, and behaviors place the pediatric population at greater risk for damage from toxins. Lead poisoning is the most common environmental health hazard. Pesticides and poor air quality also pose serious risks. Indoor air pollutants increased as houses were built "tightly" to conserve energy and as more chemicals were used in production. Growing tissues absorb toxins readily. Developing organ systems are more susceptible to damage. Smaller size means an increased concentration of toxins per pound of body weight. The fact that children are short exposes them to lower air spaces, where heavy chemicals tend to concentrate. Outdoor play, especially during summer months, increases the opportunity for exposure to air pollutants. When they are playing, children often run and breathe hard, which increases the volume of pollutants inhaled. Chewing and mouthing behaviors offer contact to toxins such as lead. Playing on the floor increases exposure to chemicals in rugs and flooring, and rolling in grass can expose children to pesticides. Playground materials may be treated with chemicals. Exposure risks for adolescents are similar to those for adults and are primarily through work, school, and hobbies.

Children at greatest risk are those with respiratory diseases and those from low-income families. Children with asthma and other respiratory problems are at risk from poor air quality and chemical irritants. The problems increase in urban and industrialized areas, where pollutant levels are high. Low-income populations are more likely to have substandard housing. Poor nutritional status increases the risk for complications. Screening and treatment may be delayed if access to health care is limited. Low-income neighborhoods are likely to be located closer to waste areas, and they often have higher levels of contaminants in the water source than the general population. It is critical to assess environmental health hazards during health care visits. Referral for treatment may be necessary, and counseling families on risk reduction is important. Bringing screening programs into neighborhoods at risk may facilitate early case finding and interventions. Lobbying efforts and education can effect public policy changes to make the environment healthier (AAP, 2012).

HEALTH POLICY, LEGISLATION, AND ETHICS RELATED TO ADULT HEALTH

Historically, men have dominated the medical and research professions because of cultural and societal norms. Early research typically was conducted on men, with mental health, reproduction, and the role of women as mothers being the exceptions (McKenzie et al, 2016). In the 1980s, recommendations were made by the US Public Health Services Task Force on Women's Health Issues to increase gender equity in biomedical research and the establishment of guidelines for including women in federally sponsored studies (Alexander et al, 2007). As discussed in other chapters in the book, especially Chapter 7, health policy is action taken by public and private agencies to promote health. It is a reflection of the values held in society and can greatly influence the health of the citizens overall. Legislation consists of laws that regulate health care and promote health. Nursing practice and the care provided is affected by policy and legislation. To be fully engaged in improving the health care from the bedside to the community level, nurses must understand how policy and legislation, along with other system factors such as social, cultural, and economic forces, can be incorporated into planning care for clients (Payne, 2015).

Five examples of federal legislation that have influenced the health of adults and their lives in communities include the Older Americans Act of 1965, the Americans with Disabilities Act of 1990, the Patient Self-Determination Act of 1990, the Family and Medical Leave Act of 1993, and the Personal Responsibility and Work Opportunity Reconciliation Act of 1996.

The Older Americans Act established the Administration on Aging (AOA) and state agencies to provide for the social service needs of older people. The mission of the AOA is to help older adults maintain dignity and live independently in their communities through a comprehensive and coordinated network across the United States (AOA, 2015). Considerable portions of AOA funds support state and community grants for social and nutritional service programs. Title III of the Older Americans Act authorizes funding for nonprofit area agencies on aging to coordinate social services that provide supportive and nutritional services, family caregiver support, and disease prevention and health promotion activities. The services are available to all people 60 years of age or older, specifically targeted to those with the greatest economic or social need.

The Americans with Disabilities Act was passed in 1990, providing protection against discrimination to millions of Americans with disabilities. This legislation requires government and businesses to provide disabled individuals with equal opportunities for jobs, education, access to transportation and public buildings, and other accommodations for both physical and mental limitations. The disabled as well as the nondisabled and businesses benefit from the changes.

The Patient Self-Determination Act of 1990 (PL 103-43) requires that providers receiving Medicare and Medicaid funds give clients written information regarding their legal options for treatment choices if they become incapacitated. A routine discussion of advance medical directives can help ease the difficult discussions faced by health care professionals, family, and clients. The nurse can assist an individual to complete a values history instrument. These instruments ask questions about specific wishes regarding different medical situations.

This clarifying process then leads to completion of advance directives to document these preferences in writing. The advance directives have two parts. The living will allows the client to express wishes regarding the use of medical treatments in the event of a terminal illness. A durable power of attorney is the legal way for the client to designate someone else to make health care decisions when he or she is unable to do so. A Do-Not-Resuscitate (DNR) order is a specific order from a physician not to use cardiopulmonary resuscitation. State laws vary widely regarding the implementing of these tools, so it is important to consult a knowledgeable source of information. It is also important to involve the family, especially the designated decision maker or agent, in these discussions so that everyone understands the client's choices (Marco et al, 2012).

Legislated rights of the elderly include individualized care; freedom from discrimination; privacy; freedom from neglect and abuse; control of one's own funds; ability to sue; freedom from physical and chemical restraint; involvement in decision making; the right to vote; access to community services; the right to raise grievances, obtain a will, and enter into contracts; the right to practice the religion of one's choice; and the right to dispose of one's own personal property.

The Family and Medical Leave Act, initially passed in 1993, provides job protection and continuous health benefits where applicable for eligible employees who need extended leave for their own illness or to care for a family member. Frequently, caregivers provide unpaid care for their family members, including aging parents, children, grandchildren, and partners. Often adults find themselves struggling to balance work and caring for a family member. More families find themselves in this struggle as more women enter the workforce and work full time. Caregivers' multiple roles and responsibilities are frequently coupled with financial strain, which can lead them to experience caregiver burden. In 2008 the Family and Medical Leave Act was amended to increase military family entitlements (Rogers et al, 2009).

In 1996, Congress passed the Personal Responsibility and Work Opportunity Reconciliation Act, commonly known as "welfare reform." This law targeted women who received public assistance and changed the previous Aid to Families with Dependent Children (AFDC) to Temporary Assistance for Needy

Families (TANF)—a work program that mandates that women heads of households find employment to retain their benefits. The Administration for Children and Families, within the USDHHS, is responsible for federal programs such as TANF that promote the economic and social well-being of families, children, individuals, and communities (ACF, 2016).

Nurses can advocate for and support health legislation and policy that support the physical, mental, and social well-being of adults. Advocacy can be accomplished in a variety of ways, such as lobbying, public speaking, participating in grassroots activities, and staying abreast of proposed legislation that influences the health of men and women, their families, and communities.

ETHICAL AND LEGAL ISSUES AND LEGISLATION FOR OLDER ADULTS

Ethical issues regarding the care and treatment of older adults arise regularly. As the population continues to age and technological advances continue to be developed, complex ethical and legal questions will increase. The most common of these issues involve decision making—assessment of the ability of the client to make decisions, the appropriate surrogate decision maker, disclosure of information to make informed decisions, level of care needed on the basis of function, and termination of treatment at the end of life. A routine discussion of advance medical directives can help ease the difficult discussions faced by health care professionals, family, and clients. The nurse can assist an individual to complete a values history instrument, which asks questions about specific wishes regarding different medical situations.

One often overlooked concern of elders is abuse. *Elder abuse* encompasses physical, psychological, financial, and social abuse or violation of an individual's rights. The National Center on Elder Abuse, within the AOA, notes that abuse encompasses physical, emotional, and sexual abuse, as well as exploitation, neglect, and abandonment. Abuse consists of the following:
- The willful infliction of physical pain or injury
- Debilitating mental anguish and fear
- Theft or mismanagement of money or resources
- Unreasonable confinement or the deprivation of services

Only one in six cases of elder abuse are reported, although nearly all states have enacted mandatory reporting laws and have services available to provide assistance (Robinson et al, 2016).

Neglect refers to a lack of services that are necessary for the physical and mental health of an individual by the individual or a caregiver. Older persons can make independent choices with which others may disagree. Their right to self-determination can be taken from them if they are declared incompetent. Exploitation is the illegal or improper use of a person or their resources for another's profit or advantage. During the assessment process, nurses need to be aware of conflicts between injuries and explanation of cause, dependency issues between client and caregiver, and substance abuse by the caregiver. Nearly all 50 states have enacted mandatory reporting laws and have instituted protective service programs. The local social services agency or area agency on aging can help with information on reporting requirements.

Many older persons have at least one chronic condition, and many have multiple conditions, putting them at risk for experiencing frailty while living in a community setting. The prevalence of frailty in the older population poses a major public health dilemma because the majority of this group will reside in a community setting, placing new demands on health care systems, family caregivers, and community resources. To improve the health of frail elderly, community-based nursing programs need to address racial/ethnic and socioeconomic disparities.

MAJOR HEALTH ISSUES AND CHRONIC DISEASE MANAGEMENT OF ADULTS ACROSS THE LIFE SPAN

Although there are some similarities in the health threats that adults and children share, some issues are unique to adults. As people live longer, they need to learn ways to promote health to maintain the best possible level of health, and when that is not possible, adults need to learn ways to effectively cope with chronic disease and in some cases disability. In chronic illness, cure is not expected, so nursing activities need to be more holistic, addressing function, wellness, and psychosocial issues. With chronic illness, the focus is on healing (i.e., a unique process resulting in a shift in the body/mind/spirit system) rather than curing (i.e., elimination of the signs and symptoms of disease). Eliopoulos (2013) lists the following goals for chronic care: (1) maintain or improve self-care capacity; (2) manage the disease effectively; (3) boost the body's healing abilities; (4) prevent complications; (5) delay deterioration and decline; (6) achieve the highest possible quality of life; and (7) die with comfort, peace, and dignity.

Chronic illness requires a shift in perspective in contrast to the rapid onset and focus on curing of an acute problem. The focus is on the development of self-management skills. The nurse partners with the client, paying attention to the client's self-concept and self-esteem, as well as to the resources needed to manage the disease outside the medical system. Goals for care are structured to help clients adjust their day-to-day choices to maintain the highest level of functional ability possible within the limits of their conditions. The motivation to make lifestyle changes necessary to cope with chronic illness stems from the fear of death; disability; pain; and negative effects on work, family, or activity.

According to the National Center for Chronic Disease Prevention and Health Promotion (NCCDPHP, 2016), the most common chronic diseases and conditions are heart disease, stroke, cancer, type 2 diabetes, obesity, and arthritis. They are not only the most common; they are also the most costly and preventable of all health problems. As of 2012, about half of all adults—117 million people—had one or more chronic health conditions; and one of four adults had two or more chronic health conditions (NCCDPHP, 2016). The most common effects of chronic conditions noted are intellectual impairment, including dementia (progressive intellectual impairment), depression (mood disorder), and delirium (acute confusion); immobility; instability; incontinence; and iatrogenic drug reactions. The average older adult in the community averages up to 20 different prescriptions filled each year. Hazards of this situation include drug interactions, side effects, and overmedication, which lead to chemically induced impairment.

HEALTH STATUS INDICATORS

Health status indicators are the quantitative or qualitative measures used to describe the level of well-being or illness present in a defined population or to describe related attributes or risk factors. They can be represented in the form of rates, such as mortality and morbidity, or proportions, such as percentages of a given population who receive immunizations (World Health Organization [WHO], 2016). Life expectancy is a measure that is often used to gauge the overall health of a population. Although the United States spends more money per capita on health than any other country, other developed countries have a longer life expectancy for both genders (NCHS, 2016a). In 2014 Hispanic females had the longest life expectancy in the United States (84.0 years), followed by white females (81.4), Hispanic males (79.2), black females (78.4), white males (76.5), and black males (72.5) (NCHS, 2016a).

When healthy years of life are increased, longer life spans are generally considered desirable. However, chronic diseases and other conditions associated with aging can increase functional limitations and affect quality of life. Also, being male or female leads to different socialization, expectations, and lifestyles that affect and interact with health in complex ways. Of particular concern is the high prevalence of adults with risk factors such as tobacco use, high cholesterol, obesity, and insufficient exercise habits, which are associated with chronic disease. Cholesterol levels have been dropping, in particular for older adults, because of a large increase in drug therapies (NCHS, 2016b). However, obesity rates remain high (NCHS, 2016b).

 HEALTHY PEOPLE 2020

Selected Objectives Relevant to Major Health Issues and Chronic Disease of Adults

- **AOCBC-10:** Reduce the proportion of adults with osteoporosis.
- **C-1:** Reduce the overall cancer death rate.
- **D-1:** Reduce the annual number of new cases of diagnosed diabetes in the population.
- **ECBP-9:** (Developmental) Increase the proportion of employees who participate in employer-sponsored health promotion activities.
- **HDS-2:** Reduce coronary heart disease deaths.
- **HRQOL/WB-1:** Increase the proportion of adults who self-report good or better health
- **MICH-11:** Increase abstinence from alcohol, cigarettes, and illicit drugs among pregnant women.
- **OA-1:** Increase the proportion of older adults who are up to date on a core set of clinical preventive services.
- **PAF-2:** Increase the proportion of adults that meet current federal physical activity guidelines for aerobic physical activity and for muscle strength training.

CHRONIC DISEASE

Cardiovascular Disease

A committee of the American Heart Association (AHA) in 2011 set a goal to improve the cardiovascular health of Americans by 29% by 2020. The committee developed definitions for "ideal," "intermediate," or "poor" cardiovascular health for adults and children based on seven CVD risk factors. More than one in three, or an estimated 81.1 million, American adults have one or more types of CVD. Heart disease is the leading cause of death in the United States (AHA, 2016; Xu et al, 2016).

The AHA has a new focus that emphasizes three things regarding cardiovascular health: CVD prevention and promotion of positive "cardiovascular health" (in addition to treatment), healthy behaviors and biomarker levels throughout the life span, and population-level cardiovascular health promotion, thus supporting the *Healthy People 2020* objectives that focus on CVD (AHA, 2016).

Hypertension

High blood pressure (HBP), or hypertension, is estimated to occur in one in three US adults, and because hypertension does not have symptoms, one-third of these people do not know they have the disease. HBP is a major risk factor for CVD, and stroke as uncontrolled hypertension leads to heart attack, stroke, kidney damage, and many other complications. Statistics showed that in 2011–2012, 82.3% of children and 42.2% of adults met these criteria (AHA, 2016). From 2009 to 2012, the age-adjusted prevalence of hypertension was 44.9% and 46.1% among non-Hispanic black men and women, respectively; 32.9% and 30.1% among non-Hispanic white men and women, respectively; and 29.6% and 29.9% among Hispanic men and women, respectively (AHA, 2016).

Lack of routine medical care influences blood pressure control and many other chronic health conditions. Routine physical activity has been found to prevent early death and chronic diseases, including coronary heart disease, stroke, type 2 diabetes mellitus, depression, and some types of cancer. The *2008 Physical Activity Guidelines for Americans* recommends that adults should engage in aerobic physical activity of moderate intensity, such as brisk walking for 150 minutes per week or vigorous exercise such as jogging for at least 75 minutes per week (USDHHS, 2008). Walking is desirable because many people are able to walk, and it can have a social as well as an aerobic effect when done with one or more other people.

CHECK YOUR PRACTICE

While at a health fair for your community, you screen a 40-year-old man for hypertension. His vital signs are as follows: BP 200/90, P 77, R 18.

The man tells you, "My dad and grandfather both had high blood pressure. Does that mean I have it too?"

What should you do?

Stroke

Approximately every 40 seconds, someone in the United States has a stroke. Projections show that by 2030, an additional 3.4 million people aged 18 years and older will have had a stroke, a 20.5% increase in prevalence from 2012. The highest increase (29%) is projected to be in Hispanic men (AHA, 2016). *Healthy People 2020* retained Objective 12-7 from *Healthy People 2010* to reduce stroke deaths to 48 per 100,000. Collaboration between health care institutions, community leaders, emergency medical services, and support groups within the community is needed for programs to be effective. Nurses can advocate for smoking cessation because the incidence of ischemic stroke is twice as high in smokers as in adults who do not smoke (AHA, 2016).

Diabetes

Diabetes is a serious public health challenge for the United States. According to the National Diabetes Statistics Report 2014, 29.1 million people, or 9.3% (1 out of every 11 people) of the US population, have diabetes (CDC, 2014). People with diabetes are at a higher risk for serious health complications, such as blindness, kidney failure, heart disease, stroke, and loss of toes, feet, or legs. Due to these health complications, medical costs are twice a high for people with diabetes as those without diabetes. In 2012 the estimated total costs, including direct and indirect costs, of diabetes in the United States was $245 billion, and the direct medical costs were $174 billion of this total amount (ADA, 2014). At least 18 of the goals of *Healthy People 2020* are related to diabetes. Diabetes is a public health problem. Primary prevention includes educating adults about nutrition and the risks of obesity, smoking, and physical inactivity. Community interventions addressing healthy eating, exercise, and weight reduction also can benefit adults at risk for diabetes. Secondary prevention includes screening for diabetes with finger-stick blood glucose tests or glucose tolerance tests. Screening is also accomplished by obtaining a thorough history and performing a detailed physical examination. Tertiary prevention targets activities aimed to reduce the complications of the disease. The following example discusses levels of prevention for CVD in women.

📋 LEVELS OF PREVENTION

Example of Cardiovascular Disease in Women

Primary Prevention
Collaborate with organizations such as the American Heart Association to design and implement interventions to reduce women's risk for cardiovascular disease.

Secondary Prevention
Establish screening clinics in community settings for measuring cholesterol and hypertension.

Tertiary Prevention
Develop a community-based exercise program for a group of women who have cardiovascular disease.

Mental Illness

Many adults and children are affected by a mental illness. According to the National Institute of Mental Health (NIMH) and the Substance Abuse and Mental Health Services Administration (SAMHSA), the 12-month prevalence rate for all psychological disorders, excluding developmental, childhood, and substance-related disorders, in US adults is 18.6% (NIMH, SAMSHA, 2013). Although the prevalence is high, people with a mental illness continue to be labeled, as negative attitudes toward mental illness continue today. Mental illness is prevalent across the globe, and despite advances in treatment, there is little evidence that prevalence rates are decreasing (Furber et al, 2015).

Key approaches to treating mental illness can include the use of effective behavioral therapies and medications (Clement et al, 2014). Community education programs can educate attendees and help dispel the stereotypes and fears often applied by society to individuals with mental illness. Local and mass media outlets can broadcast positive aspects of those living with mental disabilities and functioning as a productive part of society. Chapter 23 has more detailed information on mental illness in the community.

Cancer

Cancers of all types are a serious public health concern. Cancers (malignant neoplasms) are the second leading cause of death in the United States. In 2013 approximately 13,793,147 men and women alive in the United States had a history of cancer (Howlader et al, 2016). From 2009 to 2013 the median age of a cancer diagnosis was 65 years, with the highest percentage being 26.2% for people between the ages of 65 and 74 and the lowest being 1.0% for people under the age of 20 (Howlader et al, 2016). Approximately 1,685,210 new cases of cancer were expected to be diagnosed in 2016, and about 595,690 people were expected to die of cancer (Howlader et al, 2016). The survival rate for cancers is improving, although the rate varies depending on the type of cancer (American Cancer Society [ACS], 2016).

The ACS's 2016 Cancer Facts and Figures report based on data from the National Institutes of Health (NIH) estimated the overall costs of cancer in 2013 at $74.8 billion (ACS, 2016). Of this total, 44% was for hospital outpatient or office-based provider visits and 40% was for inpatient hospital stays (ACS, 2016). These costs could be reduced by removing barriers to care such as lack of health insurance and improving the health literacy of Americans.

Early screening and detection, promotion of healthy lifestyles, expansion of access to services, and improvement in cancer treatments will help reduce the burden of cancer and disparities. Men and women need to consistently use sun protection when outside and observe for signs of skin cancer. Colorectal cancer has been declining because of screening and risk factor reduction (ACS, 2016). Finding cancer lesions in a precancerous state, such as those found in skin, cervical, colorectal, and breast cancer, allows for treatment while in a highly treatable stage. Obesity, physical inactivity, smoking, heavy alcohol consumption, a diet high in red or processed meats, and insufficient intake of fruits and vegetables are risk factors for colorectal cancer. Reducing these risk factors will reduce the incidence of the disease.

Public health agencies, health care providers, and communities must work together to reduce the burden of cancer on society. The *Healthy People 2020* goal is to reduce the number of overall cancer cases, as well as the illness, disability, and death caused by cancer. Education on the hazards of tobacco use and secondhand smoke, eating a healthy diet, and limiting daily consumption of alcohol and exposure to ultraviolet rays are examples of topics for education programs that will reduce the burden of cancer on society.

Although sexually transmitted diseases (STDs) or sexually transmitted infections (STIs), human immunodeficiency virus (HIV), and acquired immunodeficiency syndrome (AIDS) will not be discussed in detail here because they are covered in depth in Chapter 27, it is important to note that these diseases affect a large number of adults, and each one is amenable to prevention. STDs refer to more than 25 infectious organisms transmitted primarily through sexual activity. STDs are caused by infectious organisms, such as viruses, bacteria, or parasites, typically passed through sexual contact. Other transmission modes include lice, mother-to-child transmission during pregnancy or breastfeeding, or contaminated needles used during drug use or surgery. Recently, with input from public health experts, the term *sexually transmitted infection* (STI) is used synonymously with STD, although there are distinctions that are discussed in Chapter 27 (American Sexual Health Association (ASHA, 2016). Opportunities to access treatment for STDs have improved due to the Affordable Care Act (ACA) expanding insurance coverage that includes consumer protection and prevention (Hoover et al, 2015).

Weight Control

Americans spend a great deal of time, energy, and money trying to control their weight. In 1998 the NIH began using the calculation of BMI to define overweight and obesity. BMI is the relationship between body weight and height. A BMI of 25 to 29.9 is defined as overweight, whereas a BMI of 30 and above is considered obese (CDC, 2015a).

Overweight and obesity are topics addressed numerous times in *Healthy People 2020* and have been discussed earlier in the chapter, especially regarding the association with diabetes. Almost 38% of adults in the United States are obese, with nearly 8% classified as extremely obese (BMI $\geq$40 kg/m2) (Flegal et al, 2016). The obesity rate is higher among women (40.4%) than in men (35 %), and women were nearly twice as likely to be extremely obese (Flegal et al, 2016). There are also significant racial and ethnic inequities, with higher obesity rates among blacks (48.4%) and Latinos (42.6%) compared with whites (36.4%) and Asian Americans (12.6%) (Flegal et al, 2016).

Obesity has many effects on health and is linked to major health problems. Nurses can provide education regarding obesity's risks to health. The educational offerings can be fashioned after a community health model using the levels of prevention to establish effective interventions for adults at risk for weight control issues. Although exercise levels have increased in the United States, a community prevention project aimed at increasing activity levels would help in prevention of obesity and the subsequent illnesses of diabetes and heart disease.

WOMEN'S HEALTH CONCERNS

Although there are more commonalities than differences between the health concerns of women and those of men, some notable differences are discussed here. For both sexes, prevention is important, and this includes screening, immunizations, and having a healthy lifestyle.

Eating Disorders

In addition to obesity, other eating disorders have increased among US women. Common eating disorders seen in women include anorexia nervosa and bulimia. Men may exhibit eating disorders, although these are more common in women. Anorexia nervosa is defined as a fear of gaining weight coupled with disturbances in perceptions of the body. Excessive weight loss is the most noticeable clue. Individuals with anorexia rarely complain of weight loss because they view themselves as normal or overweight. Many of these women also struggle with psychological problems, including depression, obsessive symptoms, and social phobias. Bulimia is characterized by a persistent concern with the shape of the body along with body weight, recurrent episodes of binge eating, a loss of control during these binges, and use of extreme methods to prevent weight gain, such as purging, strict dieting, fasting, use of laxatives or diuretics, or vigorous exercise (NIMH, 2014).

Through comprehensive physical and psychosocial assessments, as well as histories of dietary practice, nurses identify women with eating disorders and provide appropriate referrals. Weight control strategies include promoting healthy eating habits and regular physical activity. At a population level, nurses advocate against advertising that promotes exceptionally thin bodies for women. They also promote community-wide exercise and healthy eating programs.

Reproductive Health

Healthy People 2020 objectives address areas related to women's reproductive health. Nurses can advocate for policies that increase women's access to reproductive health services. They can also discuss contraception with women of childbearing age. Contraceptive counseling requires accurate knowledge of current contraceptive choices and a nonjudgmental approach. The goal of contraceptive counseling is to ensure that women have appropriate instruction to make informed choices about reproduction. The choice of contraceptive method depends on many factors, including the woman's health, frequency of sexual activity, number of partners, and plans to have future children. Except for abstinence, no method provides a 100% guarantee against unintended pregnancy or disease (CDC, 2016c).

Preconceptual counseling addresses risks before conception and includes education, assessment, diagnosis, and intervention. The purpose is to reduce and/or eliminate health risks for women and infants. One major health problem that could be significantly affected by preconceptual counseling is the problem of neural tube defects (birth defects of the brain and spinal cord), which can be prevented by the mother taking folic acid vitamins during pregnancy. Approximately 3000 babies annually are born with neural tube defects (March of Dimes, 2016). The goal of one *Healthy People 2020* objective is to increase the proportion of pregnancies begun with the recommended folic acid level and that women capable of or planning a pregnancy take 400 mcg of folic acid daily (USDHHS, 2010).

Another concern critical to preconception awareness is exposure to substances such as alcohol. A major preventable cause of birth defects, mental retardation, and neurodevelopmental disorders is fetal exposure to alcohol during pregnancy. Although fetal alcohol syndrome disorders (FASDs) are declining in the United States, they remain a preventable public health problem. The CDC and the AAP recommend no alcohol during pregnancy. Nurses can be involved in community interventions for women. They can conduct classes and participate in campaigns that print and broadcast advertisements informing women of childbearing age that drinking during pregnancy can cause birth defects. Nurses can serve as advocates not only to encourage their clients to use prenatal care services, but also to work toward establishing services that are accessible, affordable, and available to all pregnant women.

Gestational Diabetes

Gestational diabetes mellitus (GDM) is a condition characterized by carbohydrate intolerance that is first identified or develops during pregnancy. Women with GDM are at high risk for pregnancy and delivery complications, including infant macrosomia (extra-large baby), neonatal hypoglycemia, preeclampsia, and cesarean delivery (CDC, 2015c; DeSisto et al, 2014). The incidence of GDM is increasing in the United States, following the trend of the rise in obesity and type 2 diabetes prevalence (DeSisto et al, 2014). The prevalence of GDM increases with maternal age, number of children, and WIC use and decreases with higher education (DeSisto et al, 2014).

Menopause

During menopause the levels of the hormones estrogen and progesterone change in a woman's body. This change leads to the cessation of menstruation. The decline in these hormone levels can affect the vaginal and urinary tract, cardiovascular system, bone density, libido, sleep patterns, memory, and emotions (National Institute on Aging [NIA], 2012). Women's attitudes toward menopause vary greatly and are influenced by culture, age, support, and the recounted experiences of other women. For decades, however, the prevailing medical view of menopause was a state of deficiency that required hormone replacement to reduce heart disease and osteoporosis. A more positive outlook of menopause encourages women to view it as a transitional and natural stage in the life of a woman.

For decades, many US women used hormone replacement therapy (HRT), although HRT remained untested by rigorous scientific study. A clinical trial launched in 1991, the Women's Health Initiative, set out to test specific effects HRT had on women's health, especially its effect on heart disease and osteoporosis. Researchers concluded that HRT did not prevent heart disease and that to prevent heart disease women should avoid

smoking, reduce fat and cholesterol intake, limit salt and alcohol intake, maintain a healthy weight, and be physically active. The National Osteoporosis Foundation's (NOF's) Clinician's Guide to Prevention and Treatment provides a comprehensive overview of osteoporosis (NOF, 2014).

Breast Cancer

The ACS (2016) reports that breast cancer is the most frequently diagnosed cancer in women. In 2016 an estimated 246,660 US women were diagnosed with breast cancer, of whom an estimated 40,890 women will die (ACS, 2016). The breast cancer death rate in the United States has been steadily declining (ACS, 2016). Secondary prevention, which includes screening activities such as mammography and clinical breast examination, makes a difference in death rates. Early detection can promote a cure, whereas late detection typically ensures a poor prognosis (ACS, 2016).

Osteoporosis

Osteoporosis, or "*porous bone*," is a disease characterized by low bone mass and structural deterioration of bone tissue, leading to bone fragility and an increased risk for fractures of the hip, spine, and wrist (National Institute of Arthritis and Musculoskeletal and Skin Diseases [NIAMSD], 2014). Women are more likely than men to develop osteoporosis, and age increases the likelihood because of bones becoming thinner and weaker as people age. Small, thin-boned women are at greater risk, and Caucasian and Asian women are at highest risk.

Prevention includes diets rich in calcium and vitamin D and avoiding medications that cause bone loss. Always check with the pharmacist and read medication labels to determine which medications to avoid. Exercise also improves bone density, especially weight-bearing activities such as walking, running, stair climbing, and weight lifting. Limiting alcohol consumption and avoiding smoking are also important. Finally, several medications are approved for the prevention of osteoporosis in the United States (NIAMSD, 2014).

It is important to realize that the health status of one gender affects the health status of the other gender, the family, and society. When a man is ill and cannot work, the family and society are affected economically and work productivity is reduced (Giorgianni et al 2013). The family can suffer from lack of income. If the man dies, the widow generally experiences the loss of companionship and assumes the responsibilities of the lost spouse. Resources to promote and sustain health outcomes of both genders must be balanced for the overall health of the community. However, although a vital aspect of community health, men's health is often overlooked and barriers exist that prevent men from reaching their full health potential (Giorgianni et al, 2013).

MEN'S HEALTH CONCERNS

Although health policies, campaigns, and community health organizations offer services for men, women's health is more often emphasized. Several barriers to men reaching their full health potential have been identified. Men do not participate in health care at the same level as women, apparently because of the traditional masculine gender role learned through socialization (Giorgianni et al, 2013). A study from researchers at Rutgers University found that men who held traditional beliefs about masculinity, such as toughness, bravery, self-reliant, and emotionally restrained, were less likely than women to seek medical help, more likely to choose a male provider, and less likely to be honest about their symptoms (in particular, minimizing their symptoms) (Himmelstein and Sanchez, 2016). Not only do these behaviors limit the opportunity to prevent disease through screening, health education, and counseling, but once they are diagnosed, management and treatment are more difficult.

Barriers such as these provide opportunities and challenges for the nurse. By recognizing bias and barriers in the health care system and realizing that something should be done, nurses can help reduce the bias and remove barriers to health for both genders. The nurse can develop strategies to get men involved in lifestyle changes that prevent illness. Health care providers can reach out to men and offer the guidance and knowledge to improve health. Nurses can actively participate in public policy development and implementation as well as encourage men to identify primary care providers and obtain a physical examination and the recommended screening tests.

Men who establish a working relationship with their health care provider and participate in the recommended screening tests may live healthier, happier, and longer lives. Refer to Box 20.5 for

---

BOX 20.5   Prevention Strategies for Adults

Dental Health
- Regular dental examinations
- Floss; brush with fluoride toothpaste

Health Screening
- Blood pressure
- Height and weight
- Nutritional screening (obesity)
- Lipid disorders (men 35 and older; women 45 and older)
- Papanicolaou (Pap) test (all sexually active women with a cervix)
- Colorectal cancer (adults 50 and older)
- Mammogram (women 40 and older)
- Osteoporosis (postmenopausal women 60 and older)
- Problem drinking
- Depression screening
- Tobacco use/tobacco-caused diseases
- Rubella serology or vaccination (women of childbearing age)
- Chlamydia (sexually active women age 25 and younger; women older than 25 with new/multiple sexual partners)
- Testicular cancer (symptomatic males)
- Coronary heart disease screening (electrocardiogram, exercise treadmill)
- Syphilis screening (for at-risk population only)
- Diabetes mellitus (adults with hypertension or hyperlipidemia)

Chemoprophylaxis
- Multivitamin, folic acid (women planning or capable of pregnancy)
- Aspirin prevention (adults at risk for coronary artery disease)

Immunizations
- Tetanus-diphtheria boosters
- Rubella (women of childbearing age)
- Pneumococcal vaccine (adults 65 and older)
- Influenza vaccine (adults 65 and older/at risk/annually)

---

a variety of screening tests with suggested frequencies. Health screenings, as well as other prevention strategies for adults, are regularly updated by the Agency for Healthcare Research and Quality (AHRQ). Some health screenings are clearly beneficial, and health care providers and researchers debate the benefit of other screening procedures. As a health care professional, it is important to keep up to date on current research and literature to identify the appropriate screenings for the specific population served.

The nurse can assume many roles to fulfill responsibilities to improve the health of men in the community. As an educator, the nurse provides the knowledge and skill for replacing unhealthy behaviors with a healthy lifestyle. As a client advocate, the nurse supports and interacts with those agencies to obtain the needed resources. The nurse acts as a change agent to assess needs and system influences, identify and set priorities, plan and implement programs for men, and evaluate results. Working within groups and communities, nurses can identify needs and priorities and develop interventions to reduce health risks and improve the health status not only of men, but also of their wives, mothers, daughters, and sisters and the communities in which they live.

Cancers Unique to Men

An estimated 180,890 new cases of prostate cancer were diagnosed in 2016 in the United States, with an estimated 26,120 resulting in deaths (ASC, 2016). The number of deaths from prostate cancer have been decreasing since the early 1990s, with improvement in screening methods and treatment (ASC, 2016). Health disparities are found with African American's mortality rate from prostate cancer being nearly twice as high as any other group (ACS, 2016). The ACS recommends men be informed about risks and possible benefits of prostate cancer screening. The information should be provided at age 50 for men at average risk for prostate cancer and age 45 for men at high risk, such as African American men and men who have had a father, brother, or son diagnosed with prostate cancer before age 65. Men who have had several of these family members diagnosed with prostate cancer at an early age should be informed about prostate screening at age 40 (ACS, 2016).

Two screening tests include the prostate-specific antigen (PSA) and the digital rectal examination (DRE). The PSA test is not accurate in terms of sensitivity or specificity. This blood test produces many false-positive results because many factors can elevate the PSA, such as infections, ejaculation, exercise, such as bike riding, and benign prostatic hyperplasia (BPH). The DRE is a procedure where the physician inserts a well-lubricated, gloved index finger into the rectum to palpate the prostate gland and examine the rectum for masses. The examiner is unable to palpate the anterior aspects of the prostate, reducing the accuracy of this examination. Men find this examination unpleasant and another reason for avoiding health care (ACS, 2016).

Testicular cancer is the most common solid tumor diagnosed in males between the ages of 15 and 40 years, with the peak incidence between the ages of 20 and 34 years. It is estimated that there were 8720 new cases of testicular cancer and 380 deaths in 2016 (National Cancer Institute [NCI], 2016).

However, testicular cancer is rare, and the 5-year survival rate by race was reported as 95.4% (NCI, 2016).

Most cases of testicular cancer are discovered accidentally by patients or their partners. Because painless testicular enlargement is commonly the first sign of testicular cancer, the testicular self-examination has traditionally been recommended for men. However, in 2011 the US Preventive Services Task Force (USPSTF) updated previously published guidelines that significantly altered that tradition for asymptomatic adolescent and adult males (USPSTF, 2014). The new guidelines recommend against screening by self-examination or clinical examination in asymptomatic adult or adolescent males due to insufficient evidence, low incidence rate, and high cure rate even with advanced testicular cancer (USPSTF, 2014).

Erectile Dysfunction

Erectile dysfunction (ED), also known as impotence, is the consistent inability to achieve or maintain an erection sufficient for satisfactory sexual performance. Up to 52% of men between the ages of 40 and 70 are affected by ED, and it is associated with decreased quality of life. ED can lead to withdrawal from intimacy, emotional stress, lower self-esteem, and avoidance of physical contact. The incidence of ED significantly increases with age, and 55% to 70% of men aged 77 to 79 years are sexually active (McMahon, 2014).

Although ED may be discussed more openly with health care providers since the increased publicity generated from the marketing of the medications for ED, many men are embarrassed and reluctant to discuss the subject. Men who respond positively to treatment for ED report significantly better quality of life. With this evidence of positive response, health care providers should be proactive in discussing ED with men.

In summary, regardless of the prevalence differences in the health problems described in this section between men and women, appropriate health care services must be provided, and men and women need to be encouraged equally to take advantage of these services.

HEALTH DISPARITIES AMONG SPECIAL GROUPS OF ADULTS

"A particular type of health difference that is closely linked with social or economic disadvantage. Health disparities adversely affect groups of people who have systematically experienced greater social and/or economic obstacles to health and/or a clean environment based on their racial or ethnic group; religion; socioeconomic status; gender; age; mental health; cognitive, sensory, or physical disability; sexual orientation; geographic location; or other characteristics historically linked to discrimination or exclusion" (National Partnership for Action [NPA], 2016). See Chapters 21, 22, and 23 for discussions of selected vulnerable groups who are at risk for health disparities.

Certain groups have been recognized as experiencing health disparities and have become a priority for policy efforts. Poverty is a strong and underlying current throughout all of the special groups. Selected groups will be discussed in this chapter to emphasize the importance of understanding and intervening in health disparities.

ADULTS OF COLOR

As a result of the 2010 Affordable Care Act, 20 million adult Americans have obtained health insurance, including 8.9 million white, 4 million Hispanic, and 3 million black adults ages 18 to 64 (AHRQ, 2016). As more Americans continue to obtain health insurance and use health care services, achievement of the National Quality Strategy aims of better, more affordable care for individuals and the community increasingly demands a focus on maintaining increased access to care and reducing health disparities that lead to unequal health outcomes (AHRQ, 2016). Although addressing these disparities is complex, the goal is to close the gap with regard to the health disparities in adults of color while at the same time preserving and respecting the richness and unique influences of various cultures. Nurses can advocate for culturally sensitive and gender-sensitive programs necessary in communities where adults of color may reside.

INCARCERATED ADULTS

There were 1,561,500 prisoners held by state and federal correctional authorities on December 31, 2014, a decrease of 1% or 15,400 from year-end 2013. The federal prison population decreased by 5300 inmates (down 2.5%) from 2013 to 2014; this was the second consecutive year of decline. However, the number of women in prison who were sentenced to more than 1 year increased by 1900 offenders (up 2%) in 2014 from 104,300 in 2013 to 106,200 in 2014. The decline in the Bureau of Prisons (BOP) population in 2014 was explained by 5% fewer admissions (down 2800) than in 2013 (US Department of Justice, Bureau of Justice Statistics [USDJ, BJS], 2015).

LESBIAN AND GAY ADULTS

Lesbian, gay, bisexual, and transgender (LGBT) adults represent a sometimes-hidden special population, in part because of the social stigma associated with homosexuality coupled with the fear of discrimination. Several studies have documented health disparities by sexual orientation in population-based data and have revealed differences in health between LGBT adults and their heterosexual counterparts, including higher risks of poor mental health, smoking, disability, and excessive drinking (Fredriksen-Goldsen et al, 2013).

ADULTS WITH PHYSICAL AND MENTAL DISABILITIES

Disability status is based on a person's ability to complete major life activities independently. Major life activities refer to self-care, receptive and expressive language, learning, mobility, self-direction, capacity for independent living, and financial sufficiency.

The Social Security Administration, which ultimately determines the individual's status for disability benefits, defines disability as "the inability to engage in any substantial gainful activity (SGA) by reason of any medically determinable physical or mental impairment(s), which can be expected to result in death or which has lasted or can be expected to last for a continuous period of not less than 12 months" (US Social Security Administration [USSSA], 2016, p 5). According to the Americans with Disabilities Act (ADA), the term *disability* means, with respect to an individual, (1) a physical or mental impairment that substantially limits one or more of the major life activities of such an individual, (2) a record of such an impairment, or (3) being regarded as having such an impairment. See http://ada.gov for more information on the ADA.

Nurses can develop an awareness of the many health-related issues facing adults with disabilities. In particular, care should be taken to recognize the physical barriers that prevent disabled adults from accessing health care, such as structures that are not accessible despite the ADA recommendations. Developing health promotion programs targeted at this vulnerable, high-risk group can assist in overall well-being.

FRAIL ELDERLY

One in seven of 13.1% of the U.S. population is an older American. The older population, defined as persons 65 years and older, comprised 43.1 million in 2012, and this was an increase of 7.6 million or 21% since 2002. Older women outnumber older men (USDDHS, 2013). In addition, the population of those 85 years and older is projected to increase. Minority persons make up 21% of the elderly population. Almost half (47%) of women age 75 and older live alone. Also, their major sources of income were Social Security, income from assets, private or government employee pensions, and earnings. Almost 3.9 million older persons were below the poverty level in 2012 (USDHHS, 2013).

One often overlooked concern of elders is that of abuse. Chapter 25 discusses violence in the community, including elder abuse. *Elder abuse* encompasses physical, psychological, financial, and social abuse, neglect, or violation of an individual's rights. Abuse consists of the following:
- The willful infliction of physical pain or injury
- Causing debilitating mental anguish and fear
- Theft or mismanagement of money or resources
- Unreasonable confinement or the deprivation of services

Neglect refers to a lack of services that are necessary for the physical and mental health of an individual by the individual or a caregiver. Older persons can make independent choices with which others may disagree. Their right to self-determination can be taken from them if they are declared incompetent. Exploitation is the illegal or improper use of a person or their resources for another's profit or advantage. During the assessment process, nurses need to be aware of conflicts between injuries and explanation of cause, dependency issues between client and caregiver, and substance abuse by the caregiver. Nearly all 50 states have enacted mandatory reporting laws and

have instituted protective service programs. The local social services agency or area agency on aging can help with information on reporting requirements.

A routine discussion of advance medical directives can help ease the difficult discussions faced by health care professionals, family, and clients. The nurse can assist an individual to complete a values history instrument. These instruments ask questions about specific wishes regarding different medical situations.

Legislated rights of the elderly include individualized care, freedom from discrimination, privacy, freedom from neglect and abuse, control of one's own funds, ability to sue, freedom from physical and chemical restraint, involvement in decision making, voting, access to community services, the right to raise grievances, obtain a will, enter into contracts, practice the religion of one's choice, and dispose of one's personal property.

Many older persons have at least one chronic condition, and many have multiple conditions, putting them at risk for experiencing frailty while living in a community setting. Frailty is a geriatric syndrome that places older adults at risk for adverse health outcomes, including falls, worsening disability, institutionalization, and death. Frailty is a complex state of impairment that signifies loss in areas of physical functioning, physiological resiliency, metabolism, and immune response.

The prevalence of frailty in the older population poses a major public health dilemma because the majority of this group will reside in a community setting, placing new demands on health care systems, family caregivers, and community resources. To improve the health the of frail elderly, community-based nursing programs need to address racial/ethnic and socioeconomic disparities.

FAMILY CAREGIVING

Eighty-five percent of all elderly people live in homes alone, with spouses or other family or friends. Female spouses represent the largest group of family caregivers. *Stress, strain,* and *burnout* are words that are used to reflect the negative effects of the family caregiver burden. Issues involve the work itself, past and present relationships, effect on others, and the caregivers' lifestyle and well-being. It is estimated that at least 5 million adults are providing direct care to an elderly relative at any given time, with another 44 to 45 million assuming some type of responsibility for an elderly relative. For many families the caregiving experience is a positive, rewarding, and fulfilling one. Nursing intervention can facilitate good health for older persons and their caregivers and contribute to meaningful family relationships during this period. Eliopoulos (2013) uses the acronym *TLC* to represent these interventions, as follows:

T = Training in care techniques, safe medication use, recognition of abnormalities, and available resources
L = Leaving the care situation periodically to obtain respite and relaxation and maintain normal living needs
C = Care for the caregiver through adequate sleep, rest, exercise, nutrition, socialization, solitude, support, financial aid, and health management

COMMUNITY-BASED MODELS FOR CARE OF ADULTS

The chronic care model (CCM) identifies the essential elements of a health care system that encourages high-quality chronic disease care. These elements are the community, the health system, self-management support, delivery system design, decision support, and clinical information systems. Evidence-based change concepts under each element, in combination, foster productive interactions between informed clients who take an active part in their care and providers with resources and expertise (Model Elements, 2014). The CCM continues to be implemented and evaluated today. Using electronic health records, provider reminders for key evidence-based care components, interprofessional teams communicating regularly, and community health classes to educate people with chronic diseases are ways the CCM is being implemented. A modification of the CCM to include health literacy was suggested by Koh et al (2013).

Knowledge of community resources is a fundamental part of caring for the adult with special needs in any community. The nurse assesses the need for and helps develop the resources. Every community has an area agency on aging that coordinates planning and delivery of needed services, and it can be a good resource for the nurse. Most communities have information and referral systems, as well as a public directory of services available.

COMMUNITY CARE SETTINGS

Senior Centers

Senior centers were developed in the early 1940s to provide social and recreational activities (Fig. 20.2). Many centers are multipurpose, offering recreation, education, counseling, therapies, hot meals, and case management, as well as health screening and education. Some even offer primary care services. Nurses have a unique opportunity to provide services to a

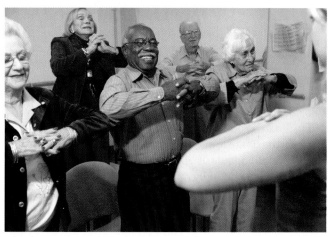

FIG. 20.2 Senior centers provide many valuable services, including social and recreational activities, exercise, and often nutritional services. (© 2012 Photos.com, a division of Getty Images. All rights reserved. Image 125557433.)

group of older persons who wish to remain independent in the community (Pardasani and Thompson, 2012).

Adult Day Health

Adult day health is for individuals whose mental or physical function requires them to obtain more health care and supervision. It serves as more of a medical model than the senior center, and often individuals return home to their caregivers at night. Some settings offer respite care for short-term overnight relief for caregivers. This provides caregivers the opportunity to work or have personal time during the day. Often, support groups for caregivers are offered by nurses (Fields et al, 2014).

Home Health and Hospice

Home health can be provided by multidisciplinary teams. Nurses provide individual and environmental assessments, direct skilled care and treatment, and short-term guidance and instruction. Nurses often function independently in the home and must rely on their own resources and knowledge to improvise and adapt care to meet the client's unique physical and social circumstances. They work closely with the family and other caregivers to provide necessary communication and continuity of care.

Hospice represents a philosophy of caring for and supporting life to its fullest until death occurs. The hospice team encourages the client and family to jointly make decisions to meet physical, emotional, spiritual, and comfort needs (see Chapter 30).

Assisted Living

Assisted living covers a wide variety of choices, from a single shared room to opulent independent living accommodations in a full-service, life-care community. The differences are related to the type and extent of the amenities provided and the contract signed for them. The role of the nurse varies depending on the philosophy and leadership of the management of the facility. The nurse generally provides assessment and interventions, medication review, education, and advocacy (Eliopoulos, 2013).

Long-Term Care and Rehabilitation

Each year, approximately 8 million people receive some type of long-term care service, such as nursing homes, adult day service centers, residential care communities, home health care, or hospice (Harris-Kojetin et al, 2013). About 70% of people 65 years old and older will need some type of long-term care during their lifetime, and over 40% will need care in a nursing home for some period of time (NIH Senior Health, 2015). In 2014 there were 1.4 million residents living in 15,6000 nursing home in the United States (NCHS, 2016a). Nursing homes provide a safe environment, special diets and activities, routine personal care, and the treatment and management of health care needs for those needing rehabilitation, as well as for those needing a permanent supportive residence. Rehabilitation is a combination of physical, occupational, psychological, and speech therapy to help debilitated persons maintain or recover their physical capacities. Rehabilitation is typically needed for older adults after a hip fracture, stroke, or prolonged illness that results in serious deconditioning (Eliopoulos, 2013).

Nursing homes and 24-hour skilled care at home are the most expensive types of long-term care, costing thousands of dollars a month, of which people rely on personal funds, government health insurance programs (such as Medicare and Medicaid), and private financing options (such as long-term care insurance) (NIH Senior Health, 2015). It is imperative that the care provided in long-term care facilities is of the highest quality. A recent study found that long-term care settings that utilized advanced practice nursing practitioners had several improvements in measures of health status and behaviors of the residents (including lower rates of depression, urinary incontinence, pressure ulcers, restraint use, and aggressive behaviors) and in family satisfaction (Donald et al, 2013).

> ## ▶▶ APPLYING CONTENT TO PRACTICE
>
> In this chapter, emphasis is placed on the community health needs of children, adolescents, and adults within the context of the family. The public health care functions of disease prevention, health promotion, and the three levels of health services are important. To meet the core public health competencies, nurses must learn how to assess children and adults using developmental principles to determine safety risks for injury and environmental health exposures. Policy and program development for the specific population is geared toward improving the built environment in which a child grows and in which adults live and educating on health promotion strategies. Nurses develop competencies in communication strategies to help families promote their health at home, in daycare centers, at schools, and at work. This chapter prepares nurses to provide comprehensive, developmentally appropriate education to families; deliver basic health care services in a holistic approach; and develop community programming to improve safety and environmental wellness for children and adults.

■ PRACTICE APPLICATION

Neighbors and the administrator of the senior high-rise residence where Mrs. Eldridge, a 79-year-old widow, lives reported her to the nurse who visited residents there. Mrs. Eldridge lives alone, and no one had been observed coming or going from her apartment recently. When Mrs. Eldridge was seen by her neighbors, she appeared self-neglected and did not appear to recognize her neighbors.

When the nurse made a visit to the apartment, Mrs. Eldridge answered the door. She was pleasant, but there was an odor of stale urine. The nurse validated the unkempt appearance of both Mrs. Eldridge and the apartment. Even though Mrs. Eldridge was hesitant and unsure in her answers, the history revealed medical problems. A son and daughter-in-law lived in the next county and phoned at least once a week; their number was taped to the table by the phone.

However, the son is an alcoholic, and the daughter-in-law has beginning symptoms of cardiovascular disease. Mrs. Eldridge's great-grandchild has asthma and is cared for by the son and daughter-in-law. Several pill bottles were observed on the kitchen counter with the names of a local physician and pharmacist.

The nurse noted that both Mrs. Eldridge and her clothes were dirty and that she moved without aids and appeared steady on her feet. The kitchen was littered with unwashed dishes and empty frozen-food boxes, which Mrs. Eldridge could not recall being bought or having been delivered. A billfold with several bills was lying open on the kitchen counter, as well as an uncashed Social Security check.

A. What should the nurse do about the situation she found?
   1. Call adult protective services and get an emergency order to put Mrs. Eldridge in a nursing home.
   2. Call Mrs. Eldridge's son and see if his mother can move in with him because she cannot take care of herself.
   3. Complete a physical and mental examination to first determine the cause of Mrs. Eldridge's situation.
   4. Call Mrs. Eldridge's pharmacist to see what medications she is taking.
   5. Call Mrs. Eldridge's son to discuss the situation with him and to make plans with him and his mother for her future.

B. What factors make this a difficult situation?
Answers can be found on the Evolve website.

■ REMEMBER THIS!

- Good nutrition is essential for healthy growth and development and influences disease prevention in later life. The adolescent population is at greatest risk for poor nutritional health.
- Immunizations are successful in the prevention of selected diseases. Barriers to immunizing children are cost and convenience.
- The family is critical to the growth and development of the child. Social support is one of the most powerful influences on successful parenting.
- Accidents and injuries are the major cause of health problems in the child and adolescent population. Most are preventable. Nurses have a major role in anticipatory guidance and prevention.

- Nurses are involved in strategies to meet the needs of the pediatric population in the community. Home-based service programs have been successful in providing care for at-risk populations. Children of homeless families are at risk for health problems, environmental dangers, and stress. Community programs to provide health care for the homeless may decrease those risks.
- The women's health movement was pivotal in bringing national recognition to women's health issues.
- Women have a longer life expectancy than men. However, women are more likely to have acute and chronic conditions that require them to use health services more than men.
- Women are known as the gatekeepers of health. Women make 75% of the health care decisions in American households.

- Women of color are statistically more likely to have poor health outcomes because of a poor understanding of health, lack of access to health care, and lifestyle practices.
- Smoking is a risk factor for some major health problems including lung cancer, heart disease, osteoporosis, and poor reproductive outcomes.
- Heart disease is the leading cause of death among women older than 50 years and the second leading cause of death among women 35 to 39 years of age.
- Cancer is the second leading cause of death for women.
- In response to the past lack of equality in health-related research and the provision of clinical care, there is now a major national focus on women's health issues.
- Men are physiologically the more vulnerable gender, demonstrated by shorter life span and a higher infant mortality.
- Life expectancy of men in the United States is one of the lowest in developed countries.
- Men engage in more risk-taking behaviors, such as physical challenges and illegal behaviors, than do women.

- Men tend to avoid diagnosis and treatment of illnesses that may result in serious health problems.
- The population 65 years of age and older in the United States is steadily growing, accompanied by an increase in chronic conditions, a greater demand for services, and strained health care budgets.
- Most older adults live in the community. The last few years of life often represent functional decline. Nurses strive to help elders maximize functional status and minimize costs through direct care and appropriate referral to community resources.
- Nurses address the chronic health concerns of elders with a focus on maintaining or improving self-care and preventing complications to maintain the highest possible quality of life.
- Assessing the elder incorporates physical, psychological, social, and spiritual domains. Individual and community-focused interventions involve all three levels of prevention through collaborative practice.
- Special at-risk populations in the community require nursing interventions at the primary, secondary, and tertiary levels.

EVOLVE WEBSITE

http://evolve.elsevier.com/Stanhope/foundations
- NCLEX® Review Questions
- Practice Application Answers

REFERENCES

Administration for Children and Families [ACF]: *About ACF*, Washington, DC, n.d., The Administration. Retrieved September 2016 from http://www.acf.hhs.gov/about.

Administration for Children and Families [ACF]: *Child Maltreatment Report, 2014*, Washington, DC, 2016, USDHHS. Available from http://www.acf.hhs.gov/programs/cb/research-data-technology/statistics-research/child-maltreatment.

Administration on Aging [AOA]: *About AoA*, Washington, DC, 2015, The Administration. Retrieved September 2016 from http://www.aoa.gov/AoARoot/About/index.aspx.

Agency for Healthcare Research and Quality [AHRQ]: *2015 national healthcare quality and disparities report and 5th update on the national quality strategy*, AHRQ Pub. No. 16-0015, Rockville, MD, 2016, AHRQ.

Alexander LL, LaRosa JH, Bader H, et al: *New dimensions in women's health*, ed 4, Boston, 2007, Jones and Bartlett.

American Academy of Child and Adolescent Psychiatry [AACAP]: *Facts for Families Guide*, 2015. Retrieved September 2016 from http://www.aacap.org/AACAP/Families_and_Youth/Facts_for_Families/FFF-Guide/FFF-Guide-Home.aspx.

American Academy of Pediatrics [AAP]: Policy statement: SIDS and other sleep-related infant deaths: expansion of recommendations for a safe infant sleeping environment, *Pediatrics* 135(4):e1105, 2011.

American Academy of Pediatrics [AAP]: *Pediatric environmental health*, ed 3, Elk Grove Village, IL, 2012, AAP.

American Academy of Pediatrics [AAP]: *Energy in energy out: finding the right balance for your children*, Elk Grove Village, IL, 2014, AAP, Product Code: HE50536.

American Cancer Society [ACS]: *Cancer facts and figures 2016*, Atlanta, GA, 2016, American Cancer Society.

American Diabetes Association [ADA]: *A Snapshot of diabetes in America*, 2014. Retrieved September 2016 from http://www.diabetes.org/diabetes-basics/statistics/cdc-infographic.html.

American Diabetes Association [ADA]: Standards of medical care in diabetes—2016, *Diabetes Care* 39(Suppl 1):S1–S106, 2016.

American Heart Association [AHA]: Heart disease and stroke statistics—2016 update, *Circulation* 133(4):447–454, 2016.

American Lung Association [ALA]: *Health effects of secondhand smoke*, 2016. Retrieved September 2016 from http://www.lung.org/stop-smoking/smoking-facts/health-effects-of-secondhand-smoke.html.

American Psychiatric Association: *Diagnostic and statistical manual of mental disorders*, ed 5, Arlington, VA, 2013, American Psychiatric Association Publishing.

American Sexual Health Association [ASHA]: *STDs/STIs*, 2016. Retrieved September 2016 from http://www.ashasexualhealth.org/stdsstis/.

Americans with Disabilities Act of 1990, PL 101-336, 1990.

Centers for Disease Control and Prevention [CDC]: *National Diabetes Statistics Report: estimates of diabetes and its burden in the United States*, Atlanta, GA, 2014, USDHHS, CDC.

Centers for Disease Control and Prevention [CDC]: *About Child and Teen BMI*, Atlanta, GA, 2015a, CDC. Retrieved September 2016 from https://www.cdc.gov/healthyweight/assessing/bmi/childrens_bmi/about_childrens_bmi.html.

Centers for Disease Control and Prevention [CDC]: Vital signs: disparities in nonsmokers' exposure to secondhand smoke—United States, 1999-2012. *Morbidity and Mortality Weekly Report* 64(4):103–108, 2015b.

Centers for Disease Control and Prevention [CDC]: *Gestational diabetes and pregnancy*, 2015c. Retrieved September 2016 from http://www.cdc.gov/pregnancy/diabetes-gestational.html.

Centers for Disease Control and Prevention [CDC]: *Ten leading causes of death and injury*, 2016a. Accessed through WISQARS Fatal Injury and Nonfatal Injury. Retrieved September 2016 from https://www.cdc.gov/injury/wisqars/leadingcauses.html.

Centers for Disease Control and Prevention [CDC]: *Child passenger safety: get the facts*, 2016b. Retrieved September 2016 from http://www.cdc.gov/motorvehiclesafety/child_passenger_safety/cps-factsheet.html.

Centers for Disease Control and Prevention [CDC]: *Contraception: how effective are birth control methods?* 2016c. Retrieved September 2016 from http://www.cdc.gov/reproductivehealth/contraception/index.htm.

Centers for Disease Control and Prevention, National Center for Injury Prevention and Control [CDC, NCIPC]: *National Action Plan for Child Injury Prevention*, Atlanta, GA, 2012, CDC, NCIPC.

Clement S, Schauman O, Graham T, et al: What is the impact of mental health-related stigma on help-seeking? A systematic review of quantitative and qualitative studies, *Psychol Med* 45(1):11–27, 2014.

DeNavas-Walt C, Proctor BD: *Income and poverty in the United States: 2014, US Census Bureau Current Population Reports P60-252*, Washington, DC, 2015, US Government Printing Office.

DeSisto CL, Kim SY, Sharma AJ: Prevalence estimates of gestational diabetes mellitus in the United States, pregnancy risk assessment monitoring system (PRAMS), 2007-2010, *Prev Chronic Dis* 11:130415, 2014.

Donald F, Martin-Misener R, Carter N, Donald EE, Kaasalainen S, Wickson-Griffiths A, Lloyd M, Akhtar-Danesh N, DiCenso A: A systematic review of the effectiveness of advanced practice nurses in long-term care, *J Advanced Nursing* 69(10):2148–2161, 2013.

Eliopoulos C: *Gerontological nursing*, ed 8, Philadelphia, 2013, Lippincott Williams, and Wilkins.

Fakhouri TH, Hughes JP, Brody DJ, et al: USDA characteristics and influential factors of food deserts, Economic Research Service, Economic Research Report Number 140, August 2013.

Federal Interagency Forum on Child and Family Statistics: *America's children in brief: key national indicators of well-being, 2016*, Washington, DC, 2016, US Government Printing Office.

Fields NL, Anderson KA, Dabelko-Schoeny H: The effectiveness of adult day services for older adults: a review of the literature from 2000-2011, *J Applied Gerontology* 33(2):130–163, 2014.

Flegal KM, Kruszon-Moran D, Carroll MD, et al: Trends in obesity among adults in the United States, 2005 to 2014, *JAMA* 315(21):284–2291, 2016.

Fredriksen-Goldsen K, Kim H, Barkan S, et al: Health disparities among lesbian, gay, and bisexual older adults: results from a population-based study, *Am J Public Health* 103(10):1802–1809, 2013. doi:10.2105/AJPH.2012.301110.

Furber G, Segal L, Leach M, Turnbull C, Procter N, Diamond M, Miller S, McGorry P: Preventing mental illness: closing the evidence-practice gap through workforce and services planning, *BMC Health Services Research* 15:283, 2015.

Garver W, Newmon S, Gonzales-Pacheco D, et al: The genetics of childhood obesity and interaction with dietary macronutrients, *Genes in Nutrition* 8:271–287, 2013.

Gindi RM, Jones LI: *Reasons for emergency room use among US children: National Health Interview Survey 2012, NCHS Data Brief, No. 160*, Rockville MD, 2014, US Department of Health and Human Services.

Giorgianni S, Porche D, Williams S, et al: Developing the discipline and practice of comprehensive men's health, *Am J Mens Health* 7(4):342–349, 2013. doi:10.1177/1557988313478649.

Goniewicz ML, Knysak J, Gawron M, et al: Levels of selected carcinogens and toxicants in vapour from electronic cigarettes, *Tob Control* 2013. doi:10.1136/tobaccocontrol-2012-050859.

Harris-Kojetin L, Sengupta M, Park-Lee E, Valverde R: Long-term care services in the United States: 2013 overview, *Vital Health Stat* 3(37):1–107, 2013.

Heron M: Deaths: leading causes for 2013, *National Vital Statistics Reports* 65(2):1–95, 2016.

Himmelstein MS, Sanchez DT: Masculinity in the doctor's office: masculinity, gendered doctor preference and doctor-patient communication, *Preventive Medicine* 84:34–40, 2016.

Hoelscher JM, Kirk S, Ritchie L, et al: Position of the Academy of Nutrition and Dietetics: interventions for the prevention and treatment of pediatric overweight and obesity, *J Acad Nutrit Dietetics* 113(10):1375–1394, 2013.

Hoover KW, Parsell BW, Leichliter JS, Habel MA, Tao G, Pearson WS, Gift TL: Continuing need for sexually transmitted disease clinics after the Affordable Care Act, *American Journal of Public Health* 105(Suppl 5):S690–S695, 2015.

Howlader N, Noone AM, Krapcho M, et al: editors: *SEER cancer statistics review, 1975-2013*, Bethesda, Md, 2016, National Cancer Institute. Retrieved September 2016 from http://seer.cancer.gov/csr/1975_2013/.

Kann L, Kinchen S, Shanklin SL, et al: Youth risk behavior surveillance Federal register, United States, 2013, *MMWR* 63(4):1–168, 2014.

Koh HK, Brach C, Harris LM, et al: A proposed 'Health Literate Care Model' would constitute a systems approach to improving patients' engagement in care, *Health Aff* 32(2):357–367, 2013.

March of Dimes: *Neural tube defects*, 2016. Retrieved September 2016 from http://www.marchofdimes.org/complications/neural-tube-defects.aspx.

Marco CA, Moskop JC, Schears RM, et al: The ethics of health care reform: impact on emergency medicine, *Academic Emergency Med* 19(4):461–468, 2012.

Martin A, Saunders DH, Shenkin SD, Sproute J: Lifestyle intervention for improving school achievement in overweight or obese children and adolescents, *Cochrane Database Syst Rev* 14(3):CD009728, 2014.

May AL, Kuklina EV, Yoon PW: Prevalence of cardiovascular disease risk factors among US adolescents 1999-2008, *Pediatrics* 129(6):1035–1041, 2012.

McKee C, Long L, Southward L, Walker B, McCown J: The role of parental misperception of child's body weight in childhood obesity, *Journal of Pediatric Nursing* 31:196–203, 2016.

McKenzie SK, Jenkin G, Collings S: Men's perspectives of common mental health problems: a metasynthesis of qualitative research, *International Journal of Men's Health Date* 15(91):80–104, 2016.

McMahon C: Erectile dysfunction, *Intern Med J* 44(1):18–26, 2014. doi:10.1111/imj.12325.

Model Elements: *Improving chronic illness care*, 2014. Retrieved September 2016 from http://www.improvingchroniccare.org/index.php?p=Model_Elementsands=18.

Morandi A, Maffeis C: Urogenital complications of obesity, *Best Pract Res Clin Endocrinol Metabolism* 27:209–218, 2013.

National Cancer Institute [NCI]: *SEER Stat Facts Sheets: Testis Cancer*, 2016. Retrieved September 2016 from http://seer.cancer.gov/statfacts/html/testis.html.

National Center for Chronic Disease Prevention and Health Promotion [NCCDPHP]: *Chronic diseases: the leading causes of death and disability in the United States*, Atlanta, GA, 2016, CDC. Retrieved September 2016 from http://www.cdc.gov/chronicdisease/overview/index.htm.

National Center for Health Statistics [NCHS]: *Health, United States, 2015: with special feature on racial and ethnic health disparities*, Hyattsville, MD, 2016a, NCHS.

National Center for Health Statistics [NCHS]: *FastStats – statistics by topic*, 2016b. Retrieved September 2016 from https://www.cdc.gov/nchs/fastats/default.htm.

National Highway Traffic Safety Administration [NHTSA]: *Traffic safety facts, 2014 data: occupant protection*, Washington, DC, 2016, US Department of Transportation, National Highway Traffic Safety Administration. Available at http://www-nrd.nhtsa.dot.gov/Pubs/812262.pdf.

National Institute of Arthritis and Musculoskeletal and Skin Diseases [NIAMSD]: *What is osteoporosis?* Bethesda, Md, 2014, National Institutes of Health. Retrieved September 2016 from http://www.niams.nih.gov/Health_Info/Bone/Osteoporosis/osteoporosis_ff.asp.

National Institute of Mental Health [NIMH]: *What are eating disorders?* Rockville, MD, 2014, USDHHS, National Institutes of Health.

National Institute of Mental Health, Substance Abuse and Mental Health Services Administration [NIMH, SAMHSA]: *Results from the 2012 national survey on drug use and health: mental health findings, NSDUH Series H-47, HHS Publication No. (SMA) 13-4805*, Rockville, MD, 2013, SAMHSA.

National Institute on Aging [NIA]: *Health and aging: hormones and menopause*, 2012. Retrieved September 2016 from https://www.nia.nih.gov/health/publication/hormones-and-menopause#what.

National Osteoporosis Foundation [NOF]: *Clinician's guide to prevention and treatment of osteoporosis*, Washington, DC, 2014, National Osteoporosis Foundation. Retrieved September 2016 from http://www.nof.org/professionals/pdfs/NOF_ClinicianGuide2009_v7.pdf.

National Partnership for Action [NPA]: *United States Department of Health and Human Services: Office of Minority Health*, Washington, DC, 2016, NPA. Retrieved September 2016 from http://minorityhealth.hhs.gov/npa/templates/browse.aspx?lvl=1andlvlid=34.

NIH Senior Health: *Long-term care*, 2015. Retrieved September 2016 from https://nihseniorhealth.gov/longtermcare/whatislongtermcare/01.html.

Papandreou D, Karabouta Z, Pantoleon A, et al: Investigation of anthropometric, biochemical and dietary parameters of obese children with and without non-alcoholic fatty liver disease, *Appetite*, 59:939–944, 2012.

Papoutsakis C, Priftis KN, Drakouli M, et al: Childhood overweight/obesity and asthma: is there a link? A systematic review of recent epidemiologic evidence, *J Acad Nutrition Dietetics* 113(1):77–105, 2013.

Pardasani M, Thompson P: Senior centers: innovative and emerging models, *J Applied Gerontology* 31(1):52–77, 2012.

Paulis WD, Silba S, Koes BW, et al: Overweight and obesity are associated with musculoskeletal complaints as early as childhood: a systematic review, *Obes Rev* 15:52–67, 2014.

Payne S: Address gender equality and gender equity? *Seminars in Reproductive Medicine* 33(1):53–60, 2015.

Perrin J, Anderson EL, Van Cleave J: Changing epidemiology of children's health – the rise in chronic conditions among infants, children, and youth can be met with continued health system innovations, *Health Affairs* 33(12):2099–2105, 2014.

Puhl RM, Peterson JL, Luedicke J: Weight-based victimization: bullying experiences of weight loss treatment-seeking youth, *Pediatrics* 131(e1):1–9, 2013.

Robinson L, Saisan J, Segal J: *Elder abuse and neglect: warning signs, risk factors, prevention, and reporting abuse*, 2016, Helpguide.org. Retrieved September 2016 from http://www.helpguide.org/articles/abuse/elder-abuse-and-neglect.htm.

Rogers B, Franke J, Jeras J, et al: The Family and Medical Leave Act: implications for occupational and environmental nursing, *Am Assoc Occup Health Nurses J* 57:239–250, 2009.

Temneanu OR, Trandafir MR, Purcarea MR: Type 2 diabetes mellitus in children and adolescents: a relatively new clinical problem within pediatric practice, *J Med and Life* 9(3):235–239, 2016.

Ting W, Huang C, Tu Y, et al: Association between weight status and depressive symptoms in adolescents: role of weight perceptions, weight concern, and dietary restraint, *Europ J Ped* 171:1247–1255, 2012.

US Consumer Product Safety Commission [USCPSC]: *Public playground safety handbook*, Bethesda, Md, 2010, USCPSC.

US Department of Agriculture [USDA]: *MyPlate Daily Checklist*, 2016. Retrieved September 2016 from https://www.choosemyplate.gov/MyPlate-Daily-Checklist.

US Department of Health and Human Services [USDHHS]: *2008 Physical activity guidelines for Americans*, Washington, DC, 2008, USDHHS. Retrieved September 2016 from https://health.gov/paguidelines/guidelines/.

US Department of Health and Human Services [USDHHS]: *Healthy People 2020*, Washington, DC, 2010, US Government Printing Office.

US Department of Health and Human Services, Administration on Aging [USDHHS, AOA]: *A profile of older Americans*, Washington, DC, 2013, USDHHS. Retrieved June 2017 from http://www.aoa.gov/aoaroot/aging_statistics/Profile/2011/docs/2011profile.pdf.

US Department of Justice, Bureau of Justice Statistics [USDJ, BJS]: *Prisoners in 2014*, 2015. Retrieved September 2016 from http://www.bjs.gov/index.cfm?ty=pbdetailandiid=5387.

US Preventive Services Task Force [USPSTF]: *Clinical summary: testicular cancer: screening, 2014*, 2014. Retrieved September 2016 from https://www.uspreventiveservicestaskforce.org/Page/Document/ClinicalSummaryFinal/testicular-cancer-screening.

US Social Security Administration [USSSA]: *2016 Red Book*, Baltimore, MD, 2016, SSA Office of Research. Retrieved September 2016 from https://www.ssa.gov/redbook/documents/TheRedBook2016.pdf.

Vollmer RL, Mobley AR: Parenting styles, feeding styles, and their influence on child obesogenic behaviors and body weight – a review, *Appetite* 71:232–241, 2013.

World Health Organization [WHO]: *World health statistics 2016: monitoring health for the SDGs*, Geneva, Switzerland, 2016, Publications of the World Health Organization. Available at http://www.who.int/whosis/indicatordefinitions/en/.

Xu J, Murphy SL, Kochanek KD, Bastian BA: Deaths: final data for 2013, *National Vital Statistics Reports* 64(2):1–119, 2016.

CHAPTER 21

Vulnerability and Vulnerable Populations: An Overview

Jeanette Lancaster

OBJECTIVES

After reading this chapter, the student should be able to:

1. Define the term *vulnerable populations,* and describe selected groups who are considered vulnerable.
2. Describe factors that led to the development of vulnerability in certain populations.
3. Examine ways in which public policies affect vulnerable populations and can reduce health disparities in these groups.
4. Examine the individual and social factors that contribute to vulnerability.
5. Describe strategies that nurses can use to improve the health status and eliminate the health disparities of vulnerable populations.

CHAPTER OUTLINE

Vulnerability: Definition and Influencing Factors
Factors Contributing to Vulnerability
    Social Determinants of Health
    Health Status
    Health Care of Veterans
Outcomes of Vulnerability

Public Policies Affecting Vulnerable Populations
Nursing Approaches to Care in the Community
    Levels of Prevention
    Assessment Issues
    Planning and Implementing Care for Vulnerable
      Populations

KEY TERMS

advocacy, 365
case management, 366
comprehensive services, 364
cumulative risks, 358
determinants of health, 360
disadvantaged, 359
disenfranchisement, 359

federal poverty guideline, 361
health disparities, 358
human capital, 359
linguistically appropriate health
   care, 365
poverty, 361
resilience, 358

risk, 358
social determinants of health, 359
social justice, 365
veterans, 362
vulnerability, 358
vulnerable populations, 358
wraparound services, 364

This chapter discusses the concept of vulnerability and the nursing roles in meeting the health needs of vulnerable populations. Selected populations groups that are at greater risk than others of poor health outcomes are described briefly in this chapter and in more detail in other chapters of the book. The relationship between health disparities, health equity, and vulnerability is described. A goal in the United States is to eliminate health disparities by expanding access to health care for vulnerable or at-risk populations. The document *Healthy People 2020* has as its mission having a society in which all people live long, healthy lives. Two of the four overarching goals of *Healthy People 2020* are to "achieve health equity, eliminate disparities, and improve the health of all groups; and create social and physical environments that promote good health for all." This chapter details the nurse's use of the nursing process with vulnerable population groups and presents case examples to identify how nurses can help individuals, families, groups, communities, and populations meet the goals of *Healthy People 2020* (US Department of Health and Human Services [USDHHS], 2010).

VULNERABILITY: DEFINITION AND INFLUENCING FACTORS

Vulnerability is defined as susceptibility to actual or potential stressors that may lead to an adverse effect. Vulnerability to poor health does not mean that some people have personal deficiencies. Rather, it results from the interacting effects of many internal and external factors over which people have little or no control. For example, a person may have some biological limitations, including genetic risks, that are made more severe by pollution, lead-based paint, excessive noise, or other external factors. **Vulnerable populations** are those groups who have an increased risk for developing adverse health outcomes.

As discussed in Chapter 9, **risk** is an epidemiological term that means some people have a higher probability than others of illness. In the epidemiological triangle, the agent, host, and environment interact to produce illness or poor health. The natural history of disease model explains how certain aspects of physiology and the environment, including personal habits, social environment, genetic factors, and physical environment, make it more likely that a person will develop particular health problems (Friss, 2010). For example, a smoker is at risk for developing lung cancer because cellular changes occur with smoking. However, not everyone who is at risk develops health problems; not all people who smoke develop lung cancer; and not all people who develop lung cancer have ever smoked. Some individuals are more likely than others to develop the health problems for which they are at risk. These people are more *vulnerable* than others. The web of causation model better explains what happens in these situations. A **vulnerable population** group is a subgroup of the population that is more likely to develop health problems as a result of exposure to risk or to have worse outcomes from these health problems than the rest of the population. That is, the interaction among many variables creates a more powerful combination of factors that predispose the person to illness. Vulnerable populations often experience multiple **cumulative risks,** and they are particularly sensitive to the effects of those risks. Risks come from environmental hazards (e.g., lead exposure from lead-based paint from peeling walls or paint used in toy manufacturing, melamine added to milk supplies), social hazards (e.g., crime, violence), personal behavior (e.g., diet, exercise habits, smoking), or biological or genetic makeup (e.g., congenital addiction, compromised immune status, mothers who contracted the Zika virus while pregnant). Members of vulnerable populations often have multiple illnesses, with each affecting the other. Genetics also plays a role in vulnerability and influences a person's resilience to

HOW GENETIC FACTORS INFLUENCE A PERSON'S VULNERABILITY TO HEALTH DISRUPTIONS

Some populations become vulnerable due to their genetic risks. An increasing amount of information is being learned about genetic influences on health. For this reason, public health nurses must be able to gather a comprehensive family history, identify family members at risk for genetically influenced factors, and help people make informed decisions about their health and become more resilient for the possible effects of genetics.

BOX 21.1 Vulnerable Population Groups of Special Concern to Nurses

- Poor and homeless persons
- Veterans
- Pregnant adolescents
- Migrant workers and immigrants
- Severely mentally ill individuals
- Substance abusers
- Abused individuals and victims of violence
- Persons with communicable disease and those at risk
- Persons who are human immunodeficiency virus–positive, have hepatitis B virus, or have a sexually transmitted disease

adverse socioeconomic conditions (Braveman and Gottlieb, 2014). Not all members of vulnerable populations succumb to the health risks that impinge on them. It is important to learn what factors help these people resist, or have **resilience** to, the effects of vulnerability.

Vulnerable individuals and families often have many risk factors. For example, nurses work with pregnant adolescents who are poor, have been abused, and are substance abusers. Nurses also work with substance abusers who test positive for human immunodeficiency virus (HIV) and for hepatitis B virus (HBV), as well as those who are severely mentally ill. Nurses who work in public health provide care to homeless and marginally housed individuals and families. They also provide care for migrant workers and immigrants. Any of these groups may be victimized by abuse and violence. Veterans, although not discussed in a later chapter, are often vulnerable to health care risks. Box 21.1 lists vulnerable population groups. Each of these groups is discussed in detail in Chapters 22 through 27. This chapter highlights some of the problems that the vulnerable populations just described have with access to care, quality and appropriateness of care, and health outcomes.

Vulnerable populations are more likely than the general population to suffer from health disparities. **Health disparities** refer to the wide variations in health services and health status among certain population groups. For more than two and a half decades, *Healthy People* has had an overarching goal of focusing on intervening in disparities. The goal in both *Healthy People 2000* and *Healthy People 2010* was to reduce health disparities. *Healthy People 2020* expanded the goal to aim to achieve health equity, eliminate disparities, and improve the health of all groups. *Healthy People 2020* defines health equity as attaining the highest possible level of health for all people and includes eliminating health disparities (USDHHS, 2010). Thirty-eight topic areas in *Healthy People 2020* emphasize access, chronic health problems, injury and violence prevention, environmental health, food safety, education and community-based programs, health communication, health information technologies, immunization and infectious diseases, and public health infrastructure, among others. These topic areas are discussed in chapters throughout the text.

As discussed in other chapters, *Healthy People 2020* is an implementation guide for all federal and most state health

♥ HEALTHY PEOPLE 2020
Objectives for Vulnerable Populations

Following are examples of objectives that nurses who work with vulnerable populations might want to note:

- **AHS-1:** Increase the proportion of persons with health insurance.
- **AHS-6:** Reduce the proportion of individuals who are unable to obtain or delay obtaining necessary medical care, dental care, or prescription medicines.
- **HIV-4:** Reduce the number of new HIV cases among adolescents and adults.
- **EMC-2.5:** Increase the proportion of parents with children under the age of 3 years whose doctors or other health care professionals talk with them about positive parenting practices.

From U.S. Department of Health and Human Services: *Healthy People 2020,* Washington DC, 2010, USDHHS. Retrieved April 10, 2016, from http://www.healthypeople.gov/.

initiatives. It is especially relevant to a discussion of vulnerable populations because these underserved and disadvantaged populations have fewer resources for promoting health and treating illness than does the average person in the United States. For example, a family or individual below the federal poverty line is considered disadvantaged in terms of access to economic resources. These groups are thought to be vulnerable because of the combination of risk factors, health status, and lack of resources needed to access health care and reduce risk factors.

There are health disparities in the cause of death by gender, age, race, socioeconomic, and other factors. For example, although the first and second leading causes of death in both males and females in 2013 were, respectively, heart disease and cancer, the third leading cause for males was unintentional injuries and for females was chronic lower respiratory disease. There are also differences related to age. For example, for younger age groups, external causes accounted for more deaths than they did for other age groups. For people ages 1 to 44, homicide and suicide were major causes of death, in contrast to those not being in the top 10 causes of death in people over 45 years. There are also variations in cause of death among racial groups. The National Vital Statistics Report differentiates race according to the following categories: white, black, American Indian or Alaska Native, and Asian and Pacific Islander (API). During 2014, the life expectancy increased for black males, Hispanic males and females, while it decreased for non-Hispanic white females. The 15 leading causes of death remained the same. Rates for the American Indian or Alaska Native and Asian or Pacific Islander populations should be interpreted with caution because of reporting problems regarding correct identification of race on both the death certificate and in population censuses and surveys (Kochanek, et al, 2016).

Race and ethnicity are not thought to be the causes of these disparities, although research is under way to determine biological susceptibilities by race, ethnicity, and gender. Rather, poverty and low educational levels are more likely to contribute to social conditions in which disparities develop. People who are poor often live in unsafe areas, work in stressful environments, have less access to healthful foods and opportunities for exercise, and are more likely to be uninsured or underinsured.

FACTORS CONTRIBUTING TO VULNERABILITY

Vulnerability results from the combined effects of limited resources. Limitations in physical resources, environmental resources, personal resources (or human capital), and biopsychosocial resources (e.g., the presence of illness, genetic predispositions) combine to cause vulnerability (Aday, 2001). Poverty, limited social support, and working in a hazardous environment are examples of limitations in physical and environmental resources. People with preexisting illnesses, such as those with communicable or infectious diseases or chronic illnesses such as cancer, heart disease, or chronic airway disease, have less physical ability to cope with stress than those without such physical problems. Human capital refers to all of the strengths, knowledge, and skills that enable a person to live a productive, happy life. People with little education have less human capital because their choices are more limited than those of people with higher levels of education.

Vulnerability has many aspects. It often comes from a feeling of lack of power, limited control, victimization, disadvantaged status, disenfranchisement, and health risks. Vulnerability can be reduced or reversed by increasing resilience. Useful nursing interventions to increase resilience include case finding, health education, care coordination, and policymaking related to improving health for vulnerable populations.

One aspect of vulnerability, disenfranchisement, refers to a feeling of separation from mainstream society. The person does not seem to have an emotional connection with any group in particular or with the larger society. Some groups such as the poor, the homeless, and migrant workers are "invisible" to society as a whole and tend to be forgotten in health and social planning. Vulnerable populations are at risk for disenfranchisement because their social supports are often weak, as are their linkages to formal community organizations such as churches, schools, and other types of social organizations. They also may have few informal sources of support, such as family, friends, and neighbors. In many ways, vulnerable groups have limited control over potential and actual health needs. In many communities, these groups are in the minority and disadvantaged because typical health planning focuses on the majority. Disadvantage also results from lack of resources that others may take for granted. Vulnerable population groups have limited social and economic resources with which to manage their health care. For example, women may endure domestic violence rather than risk losing a place for them and their children to live. Women who are among the working poor are more likely to become homeless when they leave an abusive partner. They may not be able to pay for a place to live when they lose their partner's income.

SOCIAL DETERMINANTS OF HEALTH

Social and economic factors contribute heavily to vulnerability. Social determinants of health are factors such as economic status, education, environmental factors, nutrition, stress, and prejudice that lead to resource constraints, poor health, and health risk (Lathrop, 2013; Wilensky and Satcher, 2009). Nursing interventions are designed to help vulnerable populations gain the resources needed for better health and reduction of risk factors.

From an international perspective, the World Health Organization (WHO, 2015) states that many factors in combination affect the health of individuals and communities. Specifically, "whether people are healthy or not is determined by their circumstances and environment." The WHO, consistent with *Healthy People 2020,* describes three overall determinants of health to be (1) the social and economic environment, (2) the physical environment, and (3) the person's individual characteristics and behaviors. The WHO also notes that individuals are unlikely to be able to directly control many of the determinants of health, and this is directly related to vulnerability. That is, when people experience adverse determinants of health that they cannot control, they are predisposed to becoming vulnerable. The WHO (2015) cites seven examples of factors that affect health. There are many more factors that affect health, as noted later in the *Healthy People 2020* document. The seven WHO factors are as follows (WHO, 2015, pp 1–2):

1. Income and social status: Higher income and social status are associated with better health.
2. Education: Low education is linked with poor health, more stress, and lower self-confidence.
3. Physical environment: Safe water and clean air; healthy workplaces; safer homes, communities, and roads; and good employment and working conditions, especially when the person has more control, all contribute to good health.
4. Social support networks: Family, friends, and community as well as culture, customs, traditions, and beliefs affect health.
5. Genetics, as well as personal behavior and coping skills, affect health.
6. Health services: Access and use of services affect health.
7. Gender: Men and women suffer from different types of diseases at different ages. See Fig. 21.1 for a street scene that depicts factors that could influence the determinants of health.

Healthy People 2020 (USDHHS, 2010) discusses the importance of social determinants of health by including "Create social and physical environments that promote good health for all" as one of the four overarching goals. This document explains that it is important to understand the relationship between how population groups experience "place" and the

effect that "place" has on the social determinants of health. This concept is consistent with an ecologic framework that examines the effect that people have on the environment and vice versa. *Healthy People 2020* lists 15 examples of social determinants of health: (1) availability of resources to meet daily needs; (2) access to educational, economic, and job opportunities; (3) access to health services; (4) quality of education and job training; (5) availability of community-based resources in support of community living and opportunities for recreation; (6) transportation options; (7) public safety; (8) social support; (9) social norms and attitudes; (10) exposure to crime, violence, and social disorder; (11) socioeconomic conditions; (12) residential segregation; (13) language/literacy; (14) access to mass media and emerging technologies; and (15) culture. This document also lists seven examples of physical determinants of health: (1) natural environment, such as green space and weather; (2) built environment, such as buildings, sidewalks, bike lanes, and roads; (3) worksites, schools, and recreational settings; (4) housing and community design; (5) exposure to toxic substances and other physical hazards; (6) physical barriers, especially for people with disabilities; and (7) aesthetic elements (USDHHS, 2010, pp 3–4). A useful diagram is also provided that depicts how the five key areas (determinants) of economic stability, education, social and community context, health and health care, and neighborhoods and the built environment serve as a framework for an approach to understanding the social determinants of health (USDHHS, 2010, p 4) (Fig. 21.2).

As mentioned, social status influences health in a variety of ways. First, the more wealth the person has, the more likely the person is to have access to better foods, more education, a safer community, recreation, and health care. These resources serve as protective barriers again chronic disease, injury, and premature mortality (Lathrop, 2013). Nursing interventions are

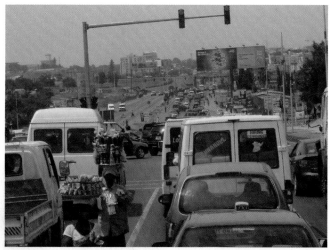

FIG. 21.1 Example of a street scene that could influence the determinants of health.

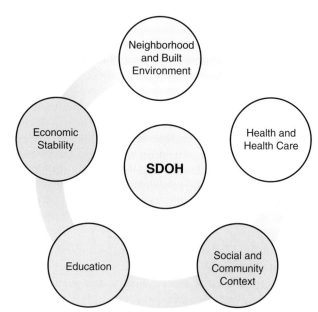

FIG. 21.2 Five key areas of social determinants of health as found in *Healthy People 2020.* (US Department of Health and Human Services: Social determinants of health. 2017. Retrieved February 2015 from http://www.healthypeople.gov/2020/topics-objectives/topic/social-determinants-health?topicid=39.)

designed to help vulnerable populations gain the resources needed for better health and reduction of risk factors.

Poverty is a primary cause of vulnerability, and it is a growing problem in the United States. The chronic stress of factors such as poverty, unemployment, and poor education can lead to maladaptive physical responses and disease (Lathrop, 2013). Poverty is a relative state. The federal definition of poverty is used to develop eligibility criteria for programs such as Medicaid and welfare assistance. In 2016 the federal poverty guideline for a family of four was $24,300 for all states except Hawaii and Alaska. Both Alaska and Hawaii have higher poverty guideline levels due to their higher cost of living (USDHHS, 2016). However, many people who earn just a little more than the federal poverty guideline are unable to pay for their living expenses but are ineligible for assistance programs.

People who do not have the financial resources to pay for medical care are considered medically indigent. They may be self-employed or work in small businesses and cannot afford health benefits. Other people have inadequate health insurance coverage. This may be either because the deductibles or copayments for their insurance are so high that they have to pay for most expenses or because few conditions or services are covered. In these situations, poverty in its relative sense causes vulnerability; uninsured and underinsured people are less likely to seek preventive health services because of the cost. They are then more likely to suffer the consequences of preventable illnesses. See Chapter 3, which discusses the health care and public health system, and Chapter 8, which discusses the economic influences on health care, for details about people who have health insurance and those who do not and what impact the Patient Protection and Affordable Care Act of 2010 has and will likely have on helping to insure more of these uninsured persons (Newhouse, 2010).

As discussed in Chapter 6, which discusses environmental health, people who are poor are more likely to live in hazardous environments that are overcrowded and have inadequate sanitation, work in high-risk jobs, have less nutritious diets, and have multiple stressors because they do not have the extra resources to manage unexpected crises and may not even have adequate resources to manage daily life. Poverty often reduces an individual's access to health care. In the developed countries of the world, this is more likely to be a problem for those just above the poverty line who are not eligible for public support, whereas in developing countries, poverty is correlated with decreased access to health care.

Education plays an important role in health status. Although education is related to income (Shi and Stevens, 2010), educational level seems to influence health separately. Higher levels of education may provide people with more information for making healthy lifestyle choices. More highly educated people are better able to make informed choices about health insurance and providers. Education also may influence perceptions of stressors and problem situations and give people more alternatives. Finally, education and language skills affect health literacy. Chapter 11 discusses health literacy and its effect on health. Also, pregnant teens, migrant workers, and homeless persons are often less likely to have adequate education, and this can influence their ability to access health care and to make healthy lifestyle choices.

Access to health care may be more limited for low socioeconomic groups. Barriers to access are policies and financial, geographic, or cultural features of health care that make services difficult to obtain or so unappealing that people do not wish to seek care. Examples include offering services only on weekdays without providing evening or weekend hours for working adults, being uninsured or underinsured, not having reasonably convenient or economical transportation, or providing services only in English and not in the population's primary language. Also, services for families may be offered in locations that make it difficult for people who do not have reliable forms of transportation. Removing these barriers by providing extended clinic hours, low-cost or free health services for people who are uninsured or underinsured, transportation, mobile vans, and professional interpreters helps improve access to care (Shi and Stevens, 2005). The interactions among multiple socioeconomic stressors make people more susceptible to risks than others with more financial resources, who may cope more effectively.

As discussed in Chapter 23, extreme poverty, in the form of homelessness or marginal housing, is related to risk for physical, dental, and mental health problems; food insecurity; and limited access to health care (Baggett et al, 2010). Those who are homeless or marginally housed have even fewer resources than poor people who have adequate housing. Homeless and marginally housed people must struggle with heavy demands as they try to manage daily life. These individuals and families do not have the advantage of consistent housing and must cope with finding a place to sleep at night and a place to stay during the day or moving frequently from one residence to another, as well as finding food, before even thinking about health care. Lack of access to nutritious food on a regular basis poses serious health problems (Borre et al 2010). Mental health problems can increase a person's vulnerability and lead to disability. They may result in high costs to society in the form of loss of productivity and treatment (Hudson et al, 2016). Adverse social and economic conditions contribute to the development of mental health problems; that is, poverty is often associated with depression, and persons who experience considerable stress may develop mental health problems. There is a growing gap between poor and richer children in the world's wealthiest countries, and this gap is at its highest level in three decades. Less advantaged children "do better in countries with well-established welfare systems and redistribution of income between the riches and the poorest" (Voice of America, 2016).

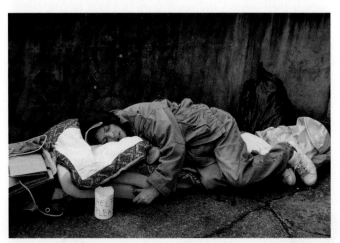

People who become homeless often once had a home and a family. (© 2012 Photos.com, a division of Getty Images. All rights reserved. Image #135090280.)

HEALTH STATUS

Age is related to vulnerability because people at both ends of the age continuum are often less able physiologically to adapt to stressors. For example, infants of substance-abusing mothers risk being born addicted and having severe physiological problems and developmental delays. Elderly individuals are more likely to develop active infections from communicable diseases such as the flu or pneumonia and generally have more difficulty recovering from infectious processes than do younger people because of the formers' less effective immune systems. Older people also may be more vulnerable to safety threats and loss of independence because of their age, multiple chronic illnesses, and impaired mobility. Chapter 24 discusses substance abuse, and Chapter 26 describes communicable disease risk.

Also, changes in normal physiology can predispose people to vulnerability. This may result from disease processes, such as in someone with single or multiple chronic diseases. As discussed in Chapter 27, HIV is a pathophysiological situation that increases vulnerability to opportunistic infections.

A person's life experiences, especially those early in life, influence vulnerability or resilience. For example, children who survive disasters may experience difficulties in later life if they do not receive adequate counseling. Higher levels of confidence in one's ability or internal locus of control appear to protect children (particularly adolescents) from the negative effects of disaster and trauma. Persons with an internal locus of control believe that they control their behavior and do not depend entirely on external people, events, or forces to control behavior. It is the person's perception of his or her level of personal control that influences the person's decisions. Persons with a high level of internal locus of control are more likely to participate in health screenings and take responsibility for their health. That is, they believe they can control to some extent their health outcomes. For example, a woman with a high internal locus of control would participate regularly in yoga and exercise classes to increase flexibility and build strength to preserve her bone and muscle tone. Vulnerable population groups often develop an external locus of control. They may believe that events are outside their control and result from bad luck or fate. People with an external locus of control have more difficulty taking action or seeking care for health problems. They may minimize the value of health promotion or illness prevention because they do not think they have control over their health destinies. Also, people who have been abused or have experienced chronic stress may have used up a lot of the reserves that others would normally have for coping with new forms of stress. Because mental and physical problems in adulthood are often associated with childhood stressors such as poverty and emotional deprivation, it is important to reduce or eliminate early health disparities (Hillemeier et al, 2013).

"Disability is an emerging field within public health; people with significant disabilities account for more than 12% of the US population" (Krahn et al 2015, p S198). Although there are many definitions of health disparities, what seems consistent in them is that they refer to differences in health outcomes at the population level; these differences appear to be associated with social, economic and environmental disadvantages. Similarly, the categories of people with disabilities are diverse; what is consistent is that they live with limitations of functioning, and this may lead to exclusion from full participation in their communities. Some of the issues related to the vulnerability of persons with a disability include:

1. When youths with disabilities or special health needs move from a pediatric to an adult care system, they may find that there are barriers with health systems not prepared to provide needed care for their complex needs.
2. Health expenditures tend to be high for this group.
3. Despite passage of the Americans with Disabilities Act, many health care facilities do not have accessible examination tables, mammography equipment, and weight scales, nor are their buildings architecturally accessible.
4. Disabled persons may also be at increased risk during a disaster.
5. Health care professionals may not be adequately prepared to provide needed care to persons with complex mental and/or physical health needs associated with a disability (Sullivan, 2015).

HEALTH CARE OF VETERANS

Other population groups that may be considered vulnerable include members of the military and their families, veterans, and persons with disabilities. "Military deployment can have a detrimental effect on both individual and family functioning" (Sullivan, 2015, p 89). Family members with a military service member have been found to be more susceptive to domestic violence and child maltreatment, and returning service members may have difficulty reconnecting with their families that have stayed at home. Specifically, children of deployed service members have been found to experience greater psychological difficulties, anxiety, school and peer problems, depression and suicidal ideation than children of nondeployed parents (Sullivan, 2015).

Never before in American history have so many people been engaged in warfare for such a long period of time. Veterans from past wars, World War II, Korea, Vietnam, Operations Desert Shield/Storm, and more recently those from service in Iraq and Afghanistan, are creating an enormous pool of Americans with health care issues and needs. The physical and psychological impact of both current and past wartime and military experiences has created a large population of veterans needing health care (Carlson, 2016). In the past, there have been large death rates due to combat. More recently due to increased triage, improved trauma treatment, and recovery strategies, more veterans are surviving and returning home with needs.

In 2014 there were 19.3 million veterans; of these, 1.6 million were female, 11.4 million were black, and 6.1 million were Hispanic (US Census Bureau, 2015). Stress from being deployed affected both the person serving and their families and significant others. For the service person, stress comes from "killing and watching friends die, personal danger, danger to others, danger of accidents; and need for constant vigilance related to difficulty determining who is the enemy" (Miltner et al, 2013, p. 46). Family members suffer from being left behind and having to cope with jobs, money, and missing their service member.

It is important for public health nurses to know about the health care issues and needs of veterans. First, learn how many veterans live in your area and where and how they live. That is, do they live with families or significant others? Or do they live alone in adequate housing, or are they homeless?

Many veterans suffer from posttraumatic stress disorder (PTSD) and major depression. Symptoms of PTSD may occur soon after the traumatic event or appear months or years later. They may also come and go. A good source of information for learning about PTSD is http://www.ptsd.va.gov/public/understanding_ptds/booklet.pdf. Major depression is characterized by at least 2 weeks of depressed mood or loss of interest or pleasure and by such symptoms as changes in appetite and weight, difficulty in thinking and concentrating, and thoughts of death or suicide. An evidence-based treatment found to be successful in helping persons with PTSD is cognitive behavioral therapy (CBT). This technique helps people learn skills to understand "how trauma changed their thoughts and feelings" (National Council for Behavioral Health, 2012, p. 7).

OUTCOMES OF VULNERABILITY

Outcomes of vulnerability may be negative, such as a lower health status than the rest of the population, or they may be positive with effective interventions. Vulnerable populations often have worse health outcomes than other people in terms of morbidity and mortality. These groups have a high prevalence of chronic illnesses, such as hypertension, and high levels of communicable diseases, including tuberculosis (TB), hepatitis B, and sexually transmitted diseases (STDs), as well as upper respiratory tract infections, including influenza. They also have higher mortality rates than the general population because of factors such as poor living conditions, diet, and health status, as well as crime and violence, including domestic violence.

There is often a cycle to vulnerability. That is, poor health creates stress as individuals and families try to manage health problems with inadequate resources. For example, if someone with acquired immunodeficiency syndrome (AIDS) develops one or more opportunistic infections and is either uninsured or underinsured, that person and the family and caregivers will have more difficulty managing than if the person had adequate insurance. Vulnerable populations often suffer many forms of stress. Sometimes when one problem is solved, another quickly emerges. This can lead to feelings of hopelessness, which result from an overwhelming sense of powerlessness and social isolation. For example, substance abusers who feel powerless over their addiction and who have isolated themselves from the people they care about may see no way to change their situation. Nursing interventions should include strategies that will increase resources or reduce health risks to decrease health disparities between vulnerable populations and populations with more advantages (Flaskerud and Winslow, 2010).

PUBLIC POLICIES AFFECTING VULNERABLE POPULATIONS

Three pieces of legislation have provided direct and indirect financial subsidies to certain vulnerable groups. The Social Security Act of 1935 created the largest federal support program in history for elderly and poor Americans. This act was intended to ensure a minimal level of support for people at risk for problems resulting from inadequate financial resources. This was accomplished by direct payments to eligible individuals. Later, the Social Security Act Amendments of 1965, Medicare and Medicaid, provided for the health care needs of older adults, the poor, and disabled people who might be vulnerable to impoverishment resulting from high medical bills or poor health status from inadequate access to health care. The Social Security Act and its Amendments created third-party health care payers at the federal and state levels. Title XXI of the Social Security Act, enacted in 1998, created the State Children's Health Insurance Program (SCHIP), which provides funds to insure currently uninsured children. The SCHIP program is jointly funded by the federal and state governments and administered by the states. Using broad federal guidelines, each state designs its own program, determines who is eligible for benefits, sets the payment levels, and decides on the administrative and operating procedures. President Obama signed the Children's Health Insurance Program Reauthorization Act of 2009 (CHIPRA). This legislation provided states with new funding, new program options, and a range of new incentives for covering children through Medicaid and the Children's Health Insurance Program (CHIP) (Centers for Medicare and Medicaid Services, 2009; CHIPRA, 2016). Although the uninsured rate among children is lower than in the past, many more children have coverage gaps throughout the year. Most of the uninsured children are eligible for either Medicaid and/or CHIP, but they may not be enrolled because they do not know about the program or the process of doing so is complex for them.

The Balanced Budget Act of 1997 also influenced the use of resources for providing health services. In an attempt to curb the rapid growth in spending on home health and financial fraud in that industry, the Health Care Financing Administration (HCFA) moved toward prospective payment for home health services. HCFA also set more stringent regulations about which services were reimbursed and for how long and limited access to care for certain vulnerable groups, such as frail elders, chronically ill individuals whose care is largely home based, and people who are HIV positive. The goal is to ensure that care is appropriate, rather than to limit access. Nurses and other health care providers must work closely with families to determine the kinds of services needed to foster self-care and the optimal timing of these services. The Balanced Budget Act of 1997 also reduced payments for services for Medicare beneficiaries, resulting in some providers choosing not to treat them. This means that people with major health needs (i.e., some chronically ill and the elderly) may have limited access to care. There are a variety of Medicare supplemental insurance plans, including those for prescription drugs, and the costs of the plans vary considerably depending on the level of coverage provided. Choosing the right supplemental plan is complex. Two useful sources of information about supplemental plans are the American Association of Retired Persons (see http://www.aarp.org) and http://www.Medicare.gov.

The Temporary Assistance for Needy Families (TANF) program replaced the previous Aid to Families with Dependent Children (AFDC) that was established by the Social Security Act of 1935 as a grant program to provide support to needy families. In TANF states receive block grants to design and implement programs that accomplish one of the TANF program purposes:

- Provide assistance to needy families so that children can be cared for in their homes.
- Reduce the dependency of needy parents by promoting job preparation, work, and marriage.
- Prevent and reduce the incidence of out-of-wedlock pregnancies.
- Encourage the formation and maintenance of two-parent families (see http://www.acf.hhs.gov. 2015).

Finally, one law focuses on the privacy and security of personal health information. The Health Insurance Portability and Accountability Act of 1996 (HIPAA) was intended to help people keep their health insurance when moving from one place to another. The Privacy Rule protects all "individually identifiable health information" (USDHHS, 2003) held or transmitted by a covered entity or its business associate in any form or media, whether electronic, paper, or oral. This information includes demographic data that related to the following:

- Person's past, present or future physical or mental health or condition,
- Provision of health care to the individual, or
- Past, present, or future payment for the provision of health care to the individual, which includes many common identifiers (e.g., name, address, birth date, Social Security number) (USDHHS, 2003, pp 3–4).

Ensuring the privacy and security of personal health information means that electronic and paper health records, case management, referrals, and physical space layouts (such as computer screen visibility and clinic registration sheets) must be managed to protect the client's privacy and safeguard the privacy of personal health information. In certain cases, health information for public health uses may be shared with appropriate public health agencies, such as in cases of suspected abuse or when investigating a communicable disease outbreak. As electronic health networks become more widely used, some provisions of this law may need to be updated (Greenberg et al, 2009).

Health care and its costs have been hotly debated in the United States for many years by both Congress and the public. Seemingly everyone wants comprehensive health care coverage, but the issue is who will pay for it. Will it be the government, the employer, the individual, or some combination of sources? See Chapters 3 (health care system), 7 (government, the law, and policy activism), and 8 (economic influences) for more detail on health care financing and the economics of health care. See also http://www.healthcare.gov/law/index.html and http://healthlawguide.aarp.org/. The chapters cited previously discuss the Affordable Care Act (ACA). However, it is important to note that the full intention of the ACA has not been realized. This act offers the promise to reduce disparities in health care, but the goal is yet to be realized. Not all states have expanded their Medicaid program for low-income children and families, and some have decided to develop their own programs. Interestingly, the states that have not yet chosen to expand Medicaid are home to the highest uninsured and poverty rates in the United States (Adepoju et al, 2015).

NURSING APPROACHES TO CARE IN THE COMMUNITY

There is a trend toward providing more comprehensive, family-centered services when treating vulnerable population groups. It is important to provide comprehensive, family-centered, "one-stop" services. Providing multiple services during a single clinic visit is an example of one-stop services. If social assistance and economic assistance are provided and included in interdisciplinary treatment plans, services can be more responsive to the combined effects of social and economic stressors on the health of special population groups. This situation is sometimes referred to as providing wraparound services, in which comprehensive health services are available and social and economic services are "wrapped around" these services. A newer approach is that of medical homes that "emphasize team-based, continuous, and holistic care across the care continuum" (Adepoju et al, 2015, p S665). Evidence on this approach is currently mixed as to its success. It has been found that the children most likely to benefit from a medical home are white children, and there is a quality gap in effective services provided between white and minority children. Another and seemingly more effective approach to provide coordinated services is that of accountable care organizations (ACOs). These organizations encourage physicians, hospitals, and allied health care providers to form networks and coordinate patient care. Traditionally, these programs have been part of Medicare, but there is beginning evidence of programs within Medicaid and private insurance plans (Adepoju et al, 2015).

It is helpful to provide comprehensive services in locations where people live and work, including schools, churches, neighborhoods, and workplaces. Comprehensive services are health services that focus on more than one health problem or concern. For example, some nurses use stationary or mobile outreach clinics to provide a wide array of health promotion, illness prevention, and illness management services in migrant camps, schools, and local communities. A single client visit may focus on an acute health problem such as influenza, but it also may include health education about diet and exercise, counseling for smoking cessation, and a follow-up appointment for immunizations once the influenza is over. The shift away from hospital-based care includes a renewed commitment to the public health services that vulnerable populations need to prevent illness and promote health, such as reductions in environmental hazards and violence and assurance of safe food and water. It is important to remember that referring clients to community agencies involves much more than simply making a phone call or completing a form. Nurses should make certain that the agency to which they refer a client is the right one to meet that client's needs. Nurses can do more harm than good by referring a stressed, discouraged client to an agency from which the client is not really eligible to receive services. Nurses should help the client learn how to get the most from the referral.

Nurses also focus on advocacy and social justice concerns. Advocacy refers to actions taken on behalf of another. Nurses may function as advocates for vulnerable populations by working for the passage and implementation of policies that lead to improved public health services for these populations. For example, a nurse may serve on a local coalition for uninsured people, and another may work to develop a plan for sharing the provision of free or low-cost health care by local health care organizations and providers.

Social justice includes the concepts of egalitarianism and equality. Braveman (2014, p 129) says that at the heart of social justice is "justice with respect to the treatment of more advantaged vs. less advantaged socioeconomic groups when it comes to health and health care." A society that subscribes to the concept of social justice is one that values equality and recognizes the worth of all members of that society. Such a society would provide humane care and social supports for all people. Nurses who function in advocacy roles and facilitate change in public policy are intervening to promote social justice. Nurses can be advocates for policy changes to improve social, economic, and environmental factors that predispose vulnerable populations to poor health. The overriding nursing goal for care of all people, including those who come from vulnerable populations, is to provide safe and quality care. See the Quality and Safety Education for Nurses (QSEN) box for information on quality care.

It is important for nurses to provide culturally and linguistically appropriate health care. Linguistically appropriate health care means communicating health-related information in the recipient's primary language when possible and always in a language the recipient can understand. It also means using words that the recipient can understand. The factors that predispose people to vulnerability and the outcomes of vulnerability create a cycle in which the outcomes reinforce the predisposing factors, leading to more negative outcomes. Unless the cycle is broken, it is difficult for vulnerable populations to improve their health. Nurses can identify areas in which they can work with vulnerable populations to break the cycle. The nursing process guides nurses in assessing vulnerable individuals, families, groups, and communities; developing nursing diagnoses of their strengths and needs; planning and implementing appropriate therapeutic nursing interventions in partnership with vulnerable clients; and evaluating the effectiveness of interventions.

QSEN FOCUS ON QUALITY AND SAFETY EDUCATION FOR NURSES

Targeted Competency: Quality Improvement—Use data to monitor the outcomes of care processes and use improvement methods to design and test changes to continuously improve the quality and safety of health care systems. Important aspects of quality improvement include:
- **Knowledge:** Explain the importance of variation and measurement in assessing quality of care.
- **Skills:** Use quality measures to understand performance.
- **Attitudes:** Value measurement and its role in good client care.

Quality Improvement Question:

Examine health statistics and demographic data in your geographic area to determine which vulnerable groups are predominant. Look on the web for examples of agencies you think provide services to these vulnerable groups. If the agency has a web page, read about the target population they serve, the types of services they provide, and how they are reimbursed for services. Learn about different agencies and share results during class. Based on your findings, identify gaps or overlaps in services provided to vulnerable groups in your community. Which data do these agencies collect to demonstrate the efficacy of their services? How could you deal with these gaps and overlaps to help clients receive needed services?

Prepared by Gail Armstrong, PhD, DNP, ACNS-BC, CNE, Associate Professor, University of Colorado College of Nursing.

In some situations, the nurse works with individual clients. The nurse also develops programs and policies for populations of vulnerable persons. In both examples, planning and implementing care for members of vulnerable populations involve partnerships between the nurse and client and build on careful assessment. Nurses need to avoid directing and controlling clients' care because this might interfere with their being able to establish a trusting relationship and may inadvertently foster a cycle of dependency and lack of personal health control. The most important initial step is for nurses to demonstrate they are trustworthy and dependable. For example, nurses who work in a community clinic for substance abusers must overcome any suspicion that clients may have of them and eliminate any fears clients may have of being manipulated.

Nurses working with vulnerable populations may fill numerous roles, including those listed in Box 21.2. They identify vulnerable individuals and families through outreach and case finding. They encourage vulnerable groups to obtain health services, and they develop programs that respond to their

BOX 21.2 Nursing Roles When Working with Vulnerable Population Groups
- Case finder
- Health educator
- Counselor
- Direct care provider
- Community assessor and developer
- Monitor and evaluator of care
- Case manager
- Advocate
- Health program planner
- Participant in developing health policies

needs. Nurses teach vulnerable individuals, families, and groups strategies to prevent illness and promote health. They counsel clients about ways to increase their sense of personal power and help them identify strengths and resources. They provide direct care to clients and families in a variety of settings, including storefront clinics, mobile clinics, shelters, homes, neighborhoods, worksites, churches, and schools.

Some examples of care to clients, families, and groups are: (1) a nurse in a mobile migrant clinic might administer a tetanus booster to a client who has been injured by a piece of farm machinery and may also check that client's blood pressure and cholesterol level during the same visit; (2) a home health nurse seeing a family referred by the courts for child abuse may weigh the child, conduct a nutritional assessment, and help the family learn how to manage anger and disciplinary problems; (3) a nurse working in a school-based clinic may lead a support group for pregnant adolescents and conduct a birthing class; and (4) a nurse may work with people being treated for TB to monitor drug treatment compliance and ensure that they complete their full course of therapy.

Public health nurses also serve as population health advocates and work with local, state, or national groups to develop and implement healthy public policy. They also collaborate with community members and serve as community assessors and developers, and they monitor and evaluate care and health programs. Nurses often function as case managers for vulnerable clients, making referrals and linking them to community services. Case management services are especially important for vulnerable persons because they often do not have the ability or resources to make their own arrangements. They may not be able to speak the language, or they may be unable to navigate the complex telephone systems that many agencies establish.

▶▶ APPLYING CONTENT TO PRACTICE

Generalist and staff public health nurses should have competencies in eight domains as defined by the Quad Council of Public Health Nursing Organizations (Swider et al, 2013). Each of the eight competencies is important in working with vulnerable populations. Public health nurses working with vulnerable populations should be able to analyze data and determine when a problem exists with an individual and within a vulnerable population group. They should be able to identify options for programs or policies that could be helpful to these populations and communicate their ideas and recommendations clearly. Public health nurses should be able to provide culturally competent interventions for individuals or for vulnerable populations. As an example, a public health nurse should be able to collect and analyze data related to the prevalence of violence among women in the community, identify key stakeholders, evaluate the cultural preferences of the population, work with others to develop a program to meet a defined need within this population, including preparation of a basic budget for the program, and ensure that the program is culturally appropriate for the population. The Council on Linkages between Academia and Public Health Practice (2014) published a similar list for public health professionals, including but not limited to public health nurses. This list includes an emphasis on evaluation and ongoing improvement of programs. In this example, the nurse would evaluate the program developed for women who are victims of violence and work with others to develop and implement quality improvements on a regular basis.

They also serve as advocates when they refer clients to other agencies, work with others to develop health programs, and influence legislation and health policies that affect vulnerable populations.

The nature of nurses' roles varies depending on whether the client is a single person, a family, or a group. For example, a nurse might teach an HIV-positive client about the need for prevention of opportunistic infections, may help a family with an HIV-positive member understand myths about transmission of HIV, or may work with a community group concerned about HIV transmission among students. In each case, the nurse teaches individuals how to prevent infectious and communicable diseases. The size of the group and the teaching method for each group differ.

Health education is often used in working with vulnerable populations. The nurse should teach members of populations with low educational levels what they need to do to promote health and prevent illness rather than directing health education to groups that the nurse *thinks* might be at high risk even though there is no evidence to support the perception. A new concern for nurses in public health is whether the populations with whom they work have adequate health literacy to benefit from health education. It may be necessary to collaborate with an educator, an interpreter, or an expert in health communications to design messages that vulnerable individuals and groups can understand and use. See Chapter 11, which describes health education and health literacy and the nursing roles with each topic.

LEVELS OF PREVENTION

Healthy People 2020 (USDHHS, 2010) objectives emphasize improving health by modifying the individual, social, and environmental determinants of health. One way to do this is for vulnerable individuals to have a primary care provider who both coordinates health services for them and provides their preventive services. This primary care provider may be an advanced-practice nurse or a primary care physician. Another approach is for a nurse to serve as a case manager for vulnerable clients and, again, coordinate services and provide illness prevention and health promotion services.

One example of primary prevention is to give influenza vaccinations to vulnerable populations who are immunocompromised (unless contraindicated). Secondary prevention is seen in conducting screening clinics for vulnerable populations. For example, nurses who work in homeless shelters, prisons, migrant camps, and substance abuse treatment facilities should know that these groups are at high risk for acquiring communicable diseases. Both clients and staff need routine screening for TB. Screening homeless adults and providing isoniazid to those who test positive for TB are examples of secondary prevention. An example of tertiary prevention is conducting a therapy group with the residents of a group home for severely mentally ill adults. Nurses who work with abused women to help them enhance their levels of self-esteem are also providing tertiary preventive activities.

LEVELS OF PREVENTION

Related to Vulnerable Populations

Primary Prevention
- Provide culturally and economically sensitive health teaching about balanced diet and exercise.
- Develop a portable immunization chart, such as a wallet card, that mobile population groups such as the homeless and migrant workers can carry with them.

Secondary Prevention
- Conduct screening clinics to assess for things such as obesity, diabetes, heart disease, or tuberculosis (TB).
- Develop a way for homeless individuals to read their TB skin test, if necessary, and to transfer the results back to the facility at which the skin test was administered.

Tertiary Prevention
- Develop community-based exercise programs for people identified as obese or who have increased blood pressure or increased blood sugar.
- Provide directly observed medication therapy for people with active TB.

ASSESSMENT ISSUES

Nurses who work with vulnerable populations need good assessment skills, current knowledge of available resources, and the ability to plan care based on client needs and receptivity to help. They also need to be able to show respect for the client. The How To box lists guidelines for assessing members of vulnerable population groups.

HOW TO Assess Members of Vulnerable Population Groups
Setting the Stage
- Create a comfortable, nonthreatening environment.
- Learn as much as you can about the culture of the clients you work with so that you will understand cultural practices and values that may influence their health care practices.
- Provide a culturally competent assessment by understanding the meaning of language and nonverbal behavior in the client's culture.
- Be sensitive to the fact that the individual or family you are assessing may have other priorities that are more important to them. These might include financial or legal problems. You may need to give them some tangible help with their most pressing priority before you will be able to address issues that are more traditionally thought of as health concerns.
- Collaborate with others as appropriate; you should not provide financial or legal advice. However, you should make sure to connect your client with someone who can and will help them.

Nursing History of an Individual or Family
- You may have only one opportunity to work with a vulnerable person or family. Try to complete a history that will provide all the essential information you need to help the individual or family on that day. This means that you will have to organize in your mind exactly what you need to ask. You should also understand why you need any information that you gather.
- It will help to use a comprehensive assessment form that has been modified to focus on the special needs of the vulnerable population group with whom you work. However, be flexible. With some clients, it will be both impractical and unethical to cover all questions on a comprehensive form. If you

know that you are likely to see the client again, ask the less-pressing questions at the next visit.
- Be sure to include questions about social support, economic status, resources for health care, developmental issues, current health problems, medications, and how the person or family manages their health status. Your goal is to obtain information that will enable you to provide family-centered care.
- Determine whether the individual has any condition that compromises his or her immune status, such as AIDS, or if the individual is undergoing therapy that would result in immunodeficiency, such as cancer chemotherapy.

Physical Examination or Home Assessment
- Again, complete as thorough a physical examination (on an individual) or home assessment as you can. Keep in mind that you should collect only data for which you have a use.
- Be alert for indications of physical abuse, substance use (e.g., needle marks, nasal abnormalities), or neglect (e.g., underweight, inadequate clothing).
- You can assess a family's living environment using good observational skills. Does the family live in an insect- or rat-infested environment? Do they have running water, functioning plumbing, electricity, and a telephone?
- Is perishable food left sitting out on tables and countertops? Are bed linens reasonably clean? Is paint peeling on the walls and ceilings? Is ventilation adequate? Is the temperature of the home adequate? Is the family exposed to raw sewage or animal waste? Is the home adjacent to a busy highway, possibly exposing the family to high noise levels and automobile exhaust?

Because members of vulnerable populations often experience multiple stressors, assessment must balance the need to be comprehensive while focusing only on information that the nurse needs and the client is willing to provide. Remember to ask questions about the client's perceptions of his or her *socioeconomic resources*, including identifying people who can provide support and financial resources. Support from other people may include information, caregiving, emotional support, and help with instrumental activities of daily living, such as transportation, shopping, and babysitting. Financial resources may include the extent to which the client can pay for health services and medications, as well as questions about eligibility for third-party payment. The nurse should ask the client about the perceived adequacy of both formal and informal support networks.

When possible, assessment should include an evaluation of clients' *preventive health needs*, including age-appropriate screening tests, such as immunization status, blood pressure, weight, serum cholesterol, Papanicolaou (Pap) smears, breast examinations, mammograms, prostate examinations, glaucoma screening, and dental evaluations. It may be necessary to make referrals for some of these tests. Assessment should also include preventive screening for physical health problems, for which certain vulnerable groups are at a particularly high risk. For example, people who are HIV positive should be evaluated regularly for T4 cell counts and common opportunistic infections, including TB and pneumonia. Intravenous drug users should be evaluated for HBV, including liver palpation and serum antigen tests as necessary. Alcoholic clients should also be asked about symptoms of liver disease and should be evaluated for jaundice and liver enlargement. Severely mentally ill clients should be assessed for the presence of tardive dyskinesia, indicating possible toxicity from their antipsychotic medications.

Vulnerable populations should be assessed for *congenital* and *genetic predisposition* to illness and either receive education and counseling as appropriate or be referred to other health professionals as necessary. For example, pregnant adolescents who are substance abusers should be referred to programs to help them quit using addictive substances during their pregnancies and, ideally, after delivery of their infants. Pregnant women older than 35 years should receive amniocentesis testing to determine whether genetic abnormalities exist in the fetus.

The nurse should also assess the amount of *stress* the person or family is having. Does the family have healthy coping skills and healthy family interaction? Are some family members able and willing to care for others? What is the level of mental health in each member? Also, are diet, exercise, and rest and sleep patterns conducive to good health?

The nurse should assess the *living environment* and *neighborhood surroundings* of vulnerable families and groups for environmental hazards such as lead-based paint, asbestos, water and air quality, industrial wastes, and the incidence of crime.

PLANNING AND IMPLEMENTING CARE FOR VULNERABLE POPULATIONS

Nurses who work in the community often have considerable involvement with vulnerable populations. The relationship with the client will depend on the nature of the contact. Some will be seen in clinics and others in homes, schools, and at work. Regardless of the setting, the following key nursing actions should be used:

- **Create a trusting environment.** Trust is essential because many of these individuals have previously been disappointed in their interactions with health care and social systems. It is important to follow through and do what you say you are going to do. If you do not know the answer to a question, the best reply is "I do not know, but I will try to find out."
- **Show respect, compassion, and concern.** Vulnerable people have been defeated again and again by life's circumstances. They may have reached a point at which they question whether they even deserve to get care. Listen carefully, because listening is a form of respect, as well as a way to gather information to plan care.
- **Do not make assumptions.** Assess each person and family. No two people or groups are alike.
- **Coordinate services and providers.** Getting health and social services is not always easy. Often people feel like they are traveling through a maze. In most communities a large number of useful services exist. People who need them simply may not know how to find them. For example, people may

need help finding a food bank or a free clinic or obtaining low-cost or free clothing through churches or in secondhand stores. Clients often need help in determining whether they meet the eligibility requirements. If gaps in service are found, nurses can work with others to try to get the needed services established.

- **Advocate for accessible health care services.** Vulnerable people have trouble getting access to services. Neighborhood clinics, mobile vans, and home visits can be valuable for them. Also, coordinating services at a central location is helpful. These multiservice centers can provide health care, social services, daycare, drug and alcohol recovery programs, and case management. When working with vulnerable populations, try to have as many services as possible available in a single location and at convenient times. This "one-stop shopping" approach to care delivery is helpful for populations experiencing multiple social, economic, and health-related stresses. Although it may seem difficult and costly to provide comprehensive services in one location, it may save money in the long run by preventing illness.
- **Focus on prevention.** Use every opportunity to teach about preventive health care. Primary prevention may include child and adult immunization and education about nutrition, foot care, safe sex, contraception, and the prevention of injuries or chronic illness. It also includes providing prophylactic antituberculosis drug therapy for HIV-positive people who live in homeless shelters or giving flu vaccine to people who are immunocompromised or older than 65 years of age. Secondary prevention would include screening for health problems such as TB, diabetes, hypertension, foot problems, anemia, or drug use or

---

CASE STUDY

Felicia is a 22-year-old single mother of three children whose primary source of income is Temporary Assistance for Needy Families (TANF). This program is designed to help needy families become self-sufficient. She is worried about the future because she will no longer be eligible for this funding by the end of the year. She has been unable to find a job that will pay enough for her to afford child care. Her friend Maria said that Felicia and her children can stay in Maria's trailer for a short time, but Felicia is afraid that her only choice after that will be a shelter.

Felicia recently took all three children with her to the health department because 15-month-old Hector needed immunizations. Felicia was also concerned about 5-year-old Martina, who had had a fever of 100° to 101° F on and off for the past month. Felicia and her friends in the trailer park think that some type of hazardous waste from the chemical plant adjacent to the park is making their children sick. Now that Martina was not feeling well, Felicia was particularly concerned. However, the health department nurse told her that no appointments were available that day and that she would need to bring Martina back to the clinic the next day. Felicia left discouraged because it was so difficult for her to get all three children ready and on the bus to go to the health department, not to mention the expense. She thought maybe Martina just had a cold and she would wait a little longer before bringing her back. However, she wanted to take care of Martina's problem before losing her medical card. Felicia is desperate to find a way to manage her money problems and take care of her children.

abuse. People who spend time in homeless shelters, substance abuse treatment facilities, and prisons often get communicable diseases such as influenza, TB, and methicillin-resistant *Staphylococcus aureus* (MRSA). Nurses who work in these facilities should plan regular influenza vaccination clinics and TB screening clinics. When planning these clinics, nurses should work with local physicians to develop signed protocols and should plan ahead for problems related to the transient nature of the population. For example, nurses should develop a way for homeless individuals to read their TB skin test if necessary and transfer the results back to the facility where the skin test was administered. It is helpful to develop a portable immunization chart, such as a wallet card, that mobile population groups such as the homeless and migrant workers can carry with them. A useful resource is the Prevention Status Reports (PSRs). The PSRs are a set of web-based, state-level (for all 50 states and the District of Columbia) reports that cite how states are using evidence-based policies and practices to address selected key health concerns in the United States. PSRs provide information on a state's status of dealing with problems related to the following areas: alcohol-related harms; food safety; healthcare-associated infections; heart disease and stroke; HIV; motor vehicle injuries; nutrition, physical activity, and obesity; prescription drug overdose; teen pregnancy; and tobacco use. They provide simple, easy-to-read, three-level ratings to show to what extent the state has policies or practices consistent with supporting evidence and/or expert recommendations. See http://www.cdd.gov/psr for more information (Centers for Disease Control and Prevention [CDC], n.d.).

- **Know when to "walk beside" the client and when to encourage the client to "walk ahead."** At times it is hard to know when to do something for people and when to teach or encourage them to do for themselves. Nursing actions range from providing encouragement and support to providing information and active intervention. It is important to assess for the presence of strength and the ability to problem solve, cope, and access services. For example, a local hospital might provide free mammograms for women who cannot pay. The nurse would need to decide whether to schedule the appointments for clients or to give them the information and encourage them to do the scheduling.
- **Know what resources are available.** Be familiar with community agencies that offer health and social services to vulnerable populations. Also follow up after you make a referral to make sure the client was able to obtain the needed help. Examples of agencies found in most communities are health departments, community mental health centers, voluntary organizations such as the American Red Cross, missions, shelters, soup kitchens, food banks, nurse-managed or free clinics, social service agencies such as the Salvation Army or Travelers' Aid, and church-sponsored health and social services.

- **Develop your own support network.** Working with vulnerable populations can be challenging, rewarding, and at times exhausting. Nurses need to find sources of support and strength. This can come from friends, colleagues, hobbies, exercise, poetry, music, and other sources.

In addition to the nursing actions described, the How To box summarizes goals and interventions and evaluates outcomes with vulnerable populations.

HOW TO Intervene with Vulnerable Populations

Goals

- Set reasonable goals based on the baseline data you collected. Focus on reducing disparities in health status among vulnerable populations.
- Work toward setting manageable goals with the client. Goals that seem unattainable may be discouraging.
- Set goals collaboratively with the client as a first step toward client empowerment.
- Set family-centered, culturally sensitive goals.

Interventions

- Set up outreach and case-finding programs to help increase access to health services by vulnerable populations.
- Do everything you can to minimize the "hassle factor" connected with the interventions you plan. Vulnerable groups do not have the extra energy, money, or time to cope with unnecessary waits, complicated treatment plans, or confusion. As your client's advocate, you should identify possible hassles and develop ways to avoid them. For example, this may include providing comprehensive services during a single encounter, rather than asking the client to return for multiple visits. Multiple visits for more specialized aspects of the client's needs, whether individual or family group, reinforce a perception that health care is fragmented and organized for the professional's convenience rather than that of the client.
- Work with clients to ensure that interventions are culturally sensitive and competent.
- Focus on teaching skills in health promotion and disease prevention. Also, teach clients how to be effective health care consumers. For example, role-play asking questions in a physician's office with a client.
- Help clients learn what to do if they cannot keep an appointment with a health care or social service professional.

Evaluating Outcomes

- It is often difficult for vulnerable clients to return for follow-up care. Help your client develop self-care strategies for evaluating outcomes. For example, teach homeless individuals how to read their own tuberculosis (TB) skin test, and give them a self-addressed, stamped card they can return by mail with the results.
- Remember to evaluate outcomes in terms of the goals you have mutually agreed on with the client. For example, one outcome for a homeless person receiving isoniazid therapy for TB might be that the person returns to the clinic daily for direct observation of compliance with the drug therapy.

In general, more agencies are needed that provide comprehensive services with nonrestrictive eligibility requirements. Communities often have many agencies that restrict eligibility to make it possible for more people to receive services. For example, shelters may prohibit people who have been drinking alcohol from staying overnight and limit the number of sequential nights a person can stay. Food banks usually limit the number of times a person can receive free food. Agencies are often specialized. For vulnerable individuals and families, this means that they must go to several agencies to obtain services for which they qualify and that meet their health needs. This is tiring, discouraging, and can be expensive, and people may forgo help because of these difficulties.

Nurses need to know about community agencies that offer various health and social services. It is important to follow up with the client after a referral to ensure that the desired outcomes were achieved. Sometimes excellent community resources may be available but prove impractical because of transportation or reimbursement issues. Nurses can identify these potential problems by following through with referrals, and they can also work with other team members to make referrals as convenient and realistic as possible. Although clients with social problems such as financial needs should be referred to social workers, it is useful for nurses to understand the close connections between health and social problems and know how to work effectively with other professionals. The following are examples of agency resources found in most communities:

- Health departments
- Community mental health centers
- American Red Cross and other voluntary organizations
- Food and clothing banks
- Missions and shelters
- Nurse-managed clinics
- Social service agencies such as Traveler's Aid and the Salvation Army
- Church-sponsored health and service assistance
- Free clinics and other community services

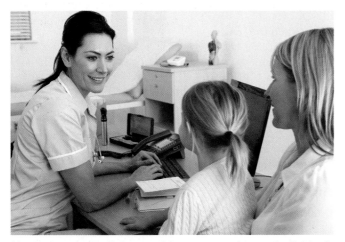

Nurse-managed clinics provide many services to individuals and families. (© 2012 Photos.com, a division of Getty Images. All rights reserved. Image #147727943.)

Nurses who work with vulnerable populations often need to coordinate services across multiple agencies for members of these groups. It is helpful to have a strong professional network of people who work in other agencies. Effective professional networks make it easier to coordinate care smoothly and in ways that do not add to clients' stress. Nurses can develop strong networks by participating in community coalitions and attending professional meetings. When making referrals to other agencies, a phone call can be a helpful way to obtain information that the client will need for the visit. When possible, having an interdisciplinary, interagency team plan of care for clients at high risk for health problems can be quite effective. It is crucial to obtain the clients' written and informed consent before engaging in this kind of planning because of confidentiality issues. The following list of tips can be helpful:

- Involve clients in making decisions about the kinds of services they will find beneficial and can use.
- Work with community coalitions to develop plans for service coordination for targeted vulnerable populations.
- Collaborate with legal counsel from the agencies involved in the coalitions to ensure that legal and ethical issues related to care coordination have been properly addressed. Examples of issues to address include privacy and security of clinical data and ensuring compliance with HIPAA, contractual provisions for coordinating care across agencies, and consent to treatment from multiple agencies.
- Develop policies and protocols for making referrals, following up on referrals, and ensuring that clients receiving care from multiple agencies experience the process as smooth and seamless.

HOW TO Use Case Management in Working with Vulnerable Populations

- Know available services and resources.
- Find out what is missing; look for creative solutions.
- Use your clinical skills.
- Develop long-term relationships with the families you serve.
- Strengthen the family's coping and survival skills and resourcefulness.
- Be the road map that guides the family to services, and help them get the services.
- Communicate with the family and the agencies that can help them.
- Work to change the environment and the policies that affect your clients.

Two other important categories of resources for vulnerable people are their own personal coping skills and sources of social support (Aday, 2001). These groups often are resourceful and creative in managing multiple stressors. Nurses can work with clients to help them identify their strengths and draw on those strengths when managing their health needs. Also, clients may be able to depend on informal support networks. Even though social isolation is a problem for many vulnerable clients, nurses should not assume they have no one who can or will help them. Case management involves linking clients with services and providing direct nursing services to them, including teaching, counseling, screening, and immunizing. Lillian Wald was the first case manager. She linked vulnerable families with various services to help them stay healthy (Buhler-Wilkerson, 1993). Nurses are often the link between personal health services and population-based health care. Linking, or brokering, health services is accomplished by making appropriate referrals and following up with clients to ensure that the desired outcomes from the referral were achieved. Nurses are effective case managers in community nursing clinics, health departments, hospitals, and various other health care agencies. Nurse case managers emphasize health promotion and illness prevention with vulnerable clients and focus on helping them avoid unnecessary hospitalization. Fig. 21.3 illustrates the coordination and brokering aspect of the nurse's role as case manager for vulnerable populations.

As can be seen, many of these nursing actions are in the realm of case management, in which the nurse makes referrals and links clients with other community services. In the case manager role, the nurse often is an advocate for the client or family. The nurse serves as an advocate when referring clients to other agencies, when working with others to develop health programs, and when trying to influence legislation and health policies that affect vulnerable population groups.

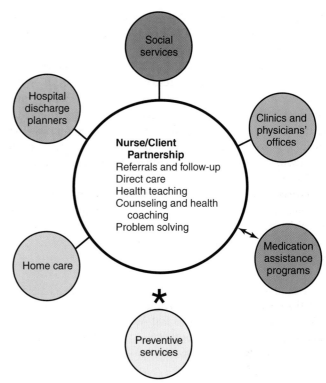

FIG. 21.3 The nurse as case manager for vulnerable populations.

PRACTICE APPLICATION

Ms. Green, a 46-year-old farm worker pregnant with her fifth child, has come to the clinic requesting treatment for swollen ankles. During your assessment, you learned that she had seen the nurse practitioner at the local health department 2 months ago. The nurse practitioner gave her some sample vitamins, but Ms. Green lost them. She has not received regular prenatal care and has no plans to do so. Her previous pregnancies were essentially normal, although she said she was "toxic" with her last child. She also said that her middle child was "not quite right." He is in the seventh grade at age 15. Ms. Green is 5 feet 2 inches tall, weighs 180 pounds, and has a blood pressure of 160/90. She has pitting edema of the ankles and a mild headache.

Ms. Green says that she usually takes chlorpromazine hydrochloride (Thorazine) but has run out of it and cannot afford to have her prescription refilled. She says that she has been in several mental hospitals in the past and that she has been more agitated lately and now has problems managing her daily activities. As her agitation grows, she says that she usually hears voices and this really makes her aggressive.

None of her children lives with her, and she has no plans for taking care of the infant. She thinks she will ask the child's father, a race-track worker, to help her because she usually travels around the country with him.

A. What additional information do you need to help you adequately assess Ms. Green's health status and current needs?

B. What nursing activities are suggested by her history, physical, and psychological descriptions?

Answers can be found on the Evolve website.

REMEMBER THIS!

- All countries have population subgroups that are more vulnerable to health threats than the general population is.
- Vulnerable populations are more likely to develop health problems as a result of exposure to risk or to have worse outcomes from those health problems than the population as a whole.
- Vulnerable populations are more sensitive to risk factors than those who are more resilient because they are often exposed to cumulative risk factors. These populations include poor or homeless persons, pregnant adolescents, migrant workers, severely mentally ill individuals, substance

abusers, abused individuals, people with communicable diseases, and people with sexually transmitted diseases.

- Factors leading to the growing number of poor people in the United States include reduced earnings, decreased availability of low-cost housing, more households headed by women, inadequate education, lack of marketable skills, welfare reform, and reduced Social Security payments to children.
- Poverty has a direct effect on health and well-being across the life span. Poor people have higher rates of chronic illness and infant morbidity and mortality, shorter life expectancy, and more complex health problems.

- Child poverty rates are twice as high as those for adults. Children who live in single-parent homes are twice as likely to be poor than those who live with both parents.
- The complex health problems of homeless people include the inability to obtain adequate rest, sleep, exercise, nutrition, and medication; exposure; infectious diseases; acute and chronic illness; infestations; and trauma and mental health problems.
- Health care is increasingly moving into the community. This began with deinstitutionalization of the severely mentally ill population and is continuing today as hospitals reduce inpatient stays. Vulnerable populations need a wide variety of services, and because these are often provided by multiple community agencies, nurses coordinate and manage the service needs of vulnerable groups.

- Socioeconomic problems, including poverty and social isolation, physiological and developmental aspects of age, poor health status, and highly stressful life experiences, predispose people to vulnerability. Vulnerability can become a cycle, with the predisposing factors leading to poor health outcomes, chronic stress, and hopelessness. These outcomes increase vulnerability.
- Nurses assess vulnerable individuals, families, and groups to determine which socioeconomic, physical, biological, psychological, and environmental factors are problematic for clients. They work as partners with vulnerable clients to identify client strengths and needs and develop intervention strategies designed to break the cycle of vulnerability.

EVOLVE WEBSITE

http://evolve.elsevier.com/Stanhope/foundations
- Case Study, with Questions and Answers
- NCLEX® Review Questions
- Practice Application Answers

REFERENCES

Aday LA: *At risk in America: the health and health care needs of vulnerable populations in the United States*, San Francisco, 2001, Jossey-Bass.

Adepoju OE, Preston MA, Gonzales G: Health care disparities in the post-Affordable Care Act era, *Am J Public Health* 105(Suppl 5):S665–S667, 2015.

Baggett TP, O'Connell JJ, Singer DE, et al: The unmet health care needs of homeless adults: a national study, *Am J Public Health* 100:1326–1333, 2010.

Borre K, Ertle L, Graff M: Working to eat: vulnerability, food insecurity, and obesity among migrant and seasonal farmworker families, *Am J Ind Med* 53:443–462, 2010.

Braveman P: What are health disparities and health equity? We need to be clear, *Public Health Rep* 129(Suppl 2):5–8, 2014.

Braveman P, Gottlieb L: The social determinants of health: it's time to consider the causes of the causes, *Public Health Rep* 129(Suppl 2):19–31, 2014.

Buhler-Wilkerson K: Bringing care to the people: Lillian Wald's legacy to public health nursing, *Am J Publ Health* 83:1778–1786, 1993.

Carlson J: Baccalaureate nursing faculty competencies and teaching strategies to enhance the care of the veteran population: Perspectives of Veterans Affairs Nursing Academy (VANA) faculty, *J Prof Nurs* 32(4):314–323, 2016.

Centers for Disease Control and Prevention: *Office for State, Tribal, Local and Territorial Support, PSR: Prevention Status Reports.* Retrieved December 2015 from http://www.cdc.gov/psr.

Centers for Medicare and Medicaid Services: *Children's Health Insurance Program Reauthorization (CHIPRA)*, Washington, DC, 2009, CMS. Retrieved March 21, 2013 from http://www.medicaid.gov/medicaid-chip-program-information/by-topics/childrens-health-insurance-program-chip/chipra.html.

CHIPRA: http://www.medicaid.gov/chip/chipra/chipra.htm. March 7, 2016. Retrieved April 9, 2016.

Council on Linkages between Academia and Public Health Practice. *Core competencies for public health professionals, Revised and adopted by the Council on Linkages between Academia and Public Health Practice*, Washington, DC, June 26, 2014, Public Health Foundation.

Flaskerud JH, Winslow BW: Vulnerable populations and ultimate responsibility, *Issues Ment Health Nurs* 31:298–299, 2010.

Friss RH: *Epidemiology 101 (essential public health)*, Sudbury, MA, 2010, Jones & Bartlett.

Greenberg MD, Ridgely MS, Hillestad RJ: Crossed wires: how yesterday's privacy rules might undercut tomorrow's nationwide health information network, *Health Aff* 28:450–452, 2009.

Hillemeier MM, Lanza ST, Landate NS, et al: Measuring early childhood health and health disparities: a new approach, *Matern Child Health J* 17:1852–1861, 2013.

Hudson DL, Kaphingst KA, Croston MA, Blanchard MS, Goodman MS: Estimates of mental health problems in a vulnerable population within a primary care setting, *J of Health Care for the Poor and Underserved* 27(2016):308–326.

Kochanek MA, Murphy SL, Xu J, Tejada-Vera B: Deaths: Final data for 2014, *National Vital Statistics Reports* 65(4):1–121, 2016.

Krahn GL, Walker SK, Correa De-Araujo R: Persons with disabilities as an unrecognized health disparity population, *Am J Public Health* 105(Suppl 2):S198–S2016, September 2, 2015.

Lathrop V: Nursing leadership in addressing the social determinants of health, *Policy Polit Nurse Pract* 14:41–47, 2013.

Miltner RS, Selleck CS, Moore RL, Patrician PA, Froelich KD, Eagerton GS, Harper DC: Equipping the nursing workforce to care for the unique needs of veterans and their families, *Nurse Leader* 11(5):45–48, October 2013.

National Council for Behavioral Health: *Meeting the behavioral health needs of veterans, author*. November 2012. Retrieved July 17, 2016, at http://www.thenationalcouncil.org/wp-content/uploads/2013/02/veternas-BH-Needs-reports.pdf.

Newhouse JP: Assessing health reform's impact on four key groups of Americans, *Health Aff* 29:1–11, 2010.

Schlein: L: UN: *Wealthy countries failing disadvantaged children*, April 13, 2016. http//:www.voanews.com/content/un-weathy-countries-failing-disadvanteages-children/3285173.html. Retrieved July 2016.

Shi L, Stevens GD: Vulnerability and unmet health care needs: the influence of multiple risk factors, *J Gen Intern Med* 20:148–154, 2005.

Shi L, Stevens GD: *Vulnerable populations in the United States*, San Francisco, 2010, Jossey-Bass.

Sullivan K: An application of family stress theory to clinical work with military families and other vulnerable populations, *Clin Soc Work J* 43:89–97, 2015.

Swider SM, Krothe J, Reyes D, Cravetz M: The Quad Council practice competencies for public health nursing, *Public Health Nursing* 30(6):519–536, 2013.

United States Census Bureau: *Newsroom, FFF: Veterans Day 2015: Nov 11, 2015, Release Number: CB15-FF.23.* Retrieved July 17, 2016 from http://www.census.gov.

US Department of Health and Human Services: Summary of the HIPAA privacy rule. Office for Civil Rights Privacy Brief. Last revised May 2003.

US Department of Health and Human Services: *Office of the Assistant Secretary for Planning and Evaluation: Aid to families with dependent children (AFDC) and temporary assistance for needy families (TANF)-overview.* 11/30/2009. Retrieved April 10, 2016 from http://www.census.gov/population/socdemo/statbriefs/whatAFDC.html.

US Department of Health and Human Services: *Healthy People 2020,* Washington, DC, 2010, USDHHS. Retrieved April 11, 2016 from http://www.healthypeople.gov/.

US Department of Health and Human Services: *Office of the Assistant Secretary for Planning and Evaluation. Poverty Guidelines,* January 25, 2016, Washington DC. See also the Federal Register notice of the 2016 poverty guidelines published January 25, 2016.

US Department of Health and Human Services: *Social determinants of health,* 2017. Retrieved February 2015 from http://www.healthypeople.gov/2020/topics-objectives/topic/social-determinants-health?topicid539.

Wilensky GR, Satcher D: Don't forget about the social determinants of health, *Health Aff* 28:w194–w198, 2009.

World Health Organization (WHO): *Health impact assessment (HIA): The determinants of health,* 2015. From http://www.who.int/hia/en/. Retrieved July 2016.

Rural Health and Migrant Health

Angeline Bushy, Marie Napolitano

OBJECTIVES

After reading this chapter, the student should be able to:

1. Compare and contrast definitions for *rural* and *urban*.
2. Describe the health status of rural populations on selected health measures.
3. Discuss access to service issues of rural underserved populations.
4. Define *migrant farmworker*, and discuss common health problems of this group and their families and the barriers they experience when seeking health care.
5. Explain the nursing role for serving persons in rural areas, including migrant farmworkers.

CHAPTER OUTLINE

Differences in Rural Versus Urban
Population Characteristics and Cultural Considerations
Health Status of Rural Residents
    Women's Health and Maternal and Infant Health
    Health of Children
    Mental Health
Occupational and Environmental Health Problems in Rural Areas
Rural Health Care Delivery Issues and Barriers to Care
Health of Minorities, Particularly Migrant Farmworkers
    Characteristics of Migrant Farmworkers

    Migrant Lifestyle
    Housing
    Issues in Migrant Health
    Other Specific Health Problems
    Children of Migrant Workers
Cultural Considerations in Migrant Health Care
    Nurse-Client Relationship
    Health: Values, Health Beliefs, and Practices
Nursing Care in Rural Environments
***Healthy People 2020:* Related to Rural Health**
    Use of Technology

KEY TERMS

documentation, 382
farm residency, 375
frontier, 378
genetic predisposition, 384
Health Professional Shortage Areas
    (HPSAs), 377

migrant farmworker, 379
Migrant Health Act, 383
migrant health center, 380
nonfarm residency, 375
pesticide exposure, 379
rural, 374

rural-urban continuum, 375
suburbs, 376
undocumented immigrant, 382
urban, 374

Access to health care is a national priority that remains unsolved. Access is a problem in rural areas, including farms that rely on migrant workers to harvest their crops, and in urban areas, especially in inner cities. This chapter discusses major issues surrounding health care delivery in rural environments. These issues may differ from those experienced by people living in urban or more populated areas. Recruiting and retraining qualified health care workers can be a problem in both rural and urban areas. One particular environment, that of the migrant worker, is discussed in detail because of the growing number of migrant workers and their unique health needs. Also, the role of the public health nurse in rural areas is discussed in this chapter.

Formal rural nursing began with the Red Cross Rural Nursing Service, which was organized in November 1912 (Bigbee and Crowder, 1985). Before that time, care of the sick in a small community was provided by informal social support systems. When self-care and family care were not effective in bringing about healing, women who had skills in helping others heal and who lived in the community provided care. Although the health needs of rural people are not all unique, they are different from those of urban populations. Scarcity of health care professionals, poverty, limited access to services, lack of knowledge, and social isolation have plagued many rural communities for generations. A major issue in the rural area is often the distance people must go to find health care services and providers. For migrant workers, a language barrier and cultural differences often exist between them and the farm owners, other area residents, and the health care providers.

DIFFERENCES IN RURAL VERSUS URBAN

Each of us has an idea as to what constitutes a rural as opposed to an urban residence. However, the distinctions are becoming blurred as people move further away from cities and towns into less-developed areas. *Rural* is defined generally either in terms of the geographic location and population density or the distance from (e.g., 20 miles) or the time needed (e.g., 30 minutes) to commute to an urban center. Other definitions link rural with farm residency and urban with nonfarm residency. Some consider rural to be a state of mind. For the more affluent, rural may bring to mind a recreational, retirement, or resort community located in the mountains or in lake country where people can relax and participate in outdoor activities, such as skiing, fishing, hiking, or hunting. For people with limited resources, rural may imply poor and/or crowded housing with lack of adequate facilities for water and sewage.

Just as each city has its own unique characteristics; there is no "typical rural town." For example, rural towns in Florida, Oregon, Alaska, Hawaii, and Idaho are different from one another and quite different from those in Vermont, Texas, Tennessee, Alabama, and California. Descriptions and definitions for rural areas are more subjective and relative than for urban areas.

For example, "small" communities with populations of more than 20,000 have some features that are found in cities. A person who lives in a community with fewer than 2000 people may consider a community with a population of 5000 to 10,000 to be a city. Although some communities may seem geographically remote on a map, the people who live there may not feel isolated. They may think they are within easy reach of services through telecommunication and dependable transportation, although extensive shopping facilities may be 50 to 100 miles from the family home, obstetrical care may be 150 miles away,

and nursing services in the district health department in an adjacent county may be 75 or more miles away.

Frequently used definitions to describe rural and urban and to differentiate between them are provided by several federal agencies (Cromartie and Parker, 2015). These definitions often fail to take into account the relative nature of ruralness. Rural and urban residencies are not opposing lifestyles. Rather, they are on a rural-urban continuum ranging from living on a remote farm, to a village or small town, to a larger town or city, to a large metropolitan area with a core inner city (Fig. 22.1).

Several federal agencies classify counties according to population density, specifically, metropolitan counties (84% of the total population area) and nonmetropolitan counties (16% of the total population area) (Cromartie and Parker, 2015). The terms *metropolitan* and *micropolitan statistical areas* (*metro* and *micro areas*) refer to geographic entities primarily used for collecting, tabulating, and publishing federal statistics. Core-based statistical area (CBSA) is a collective term for both metro and micro areas. A metro area contains a core urban area of 50,000 or more population. A micro area contains an urban core of at least 10,000 and less than 50,000 population. Each metro or micro area consists of one or more counties containing the core urban area. Likewise, adjacent counties have a high degree of social and economic integration (as measured by commuting to work) with its urban core.

Demographically, micro areas contain about 60% of the total nonmetro population, with an average of 43,000 people per county. In contrast, noncore counties, with no urban cluster of 10,000 or more residents, have on average about 14,000 residents. In general, lack of an urban core and low overall population density may place these counties at a disadvantage in efforts to expand and diversify their economic base. The designation of micro areas is an important step in recognizing nonmetro diversity. The term also provides a framework to understand population growth and economic restructuring in small towns and cities that have received less attention than metro areas. Nationally and regionally, many measures of health, health care use, and health care resources among rural

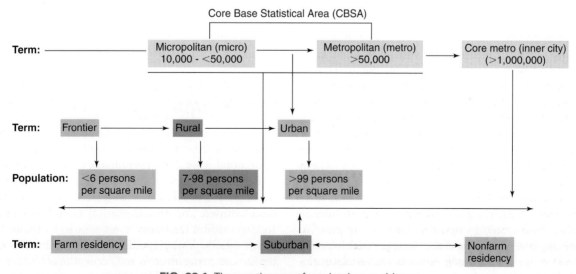

FIG. 22.1 The continuum of rural–urban residency.

populations vary by the level of urban influence in a particular region.

Micro areas typically share a residential preference for a small-town lifestyle—an ideal compromise between large, highly populated urban cities and sparsely populated rural settings. As information about these places makes its way into government data and publications alongside metro areas in the coming years, hopefully the notion of "micropolitan" will draw increased attention from policymakers and the business community.

The past decade has seen a population shift from urban to less-populated regions of the United States. The fastest growing rural counties are located in rural regions of the nation and along the edges of larger metropolitan counties. Demographers metaphorically refer to this demographic phenomenon as the "doughnut effect." That is to say, people are moving away from highly populated areas to outlying suburbs of urban centers. Most of the population growth has been in counties with a booming economy, with the geographic space to expand, and in Western and Southern states. Often people move to more rural areas to find more affordable housing. In this chapter, *rural* refers to areas having fewer than 99 persons per square mile and communities having 20,000 or fewer inhabitants.

POPULATION CHARACTERISTICS AND CULTURAL CONSIDERATIONS

Although regional variations exist, in general there are a higher proportion of whites in rural areas than in urban areas. Regional variations exist, and some rural counties have a large minority population. Demographically, rural communities have a higher proportion of residents younger than 18 years of age and older than 65 years of age and more residents who are married or widowed than their urban counterparts. Rural communities tend to include more residents who are married or widowed and have fewer years of formal education than their urban counterparts (USDA, 2013a). Comparing annual incomes with the standardized index established, more than one-fourth of rural Americans live in or near poverty, and nearly 40% of all rural children are impoverished. An important indicator of economic recovery is employment. The pace of employment increased in 2014 in rural areas. Rural areas continue to have loss of population (as workers move to more urban areas to find jobs), higher poverty rates, and lower educational levels than urban areas (Kusmin, 2015). However, there are exceptions to the outmigration from rural areas. Over 700 rural counties have added population between 2010 and 2014. These counties are concentrated in areas that offer a higher quality of life and are scenic, such as the Rocky Mountains or southern Appalachia, or in energy boom areas in the northern Great Plains (Kusmin, 2015).

As mentioned earlier in this chapter, poverty continues to be a problem in rural areas. The groups at highest risk are children, minority racial and ethnic groups, and single-parent families, especially those headed by a woman. Among racial minority groups, the Hispanic rate increased the most. See *Rural America at a Glance: 2015 edition* for details. Although the education level

BOX 22.1   Characteristics of Rural Life

- More space; greater distances between residents and services
- Cyclical or seasonal work and leisure activities
- Informal social and professional interactions
- Access to extended kinship systems
- Residents who are related or acquainted
- Lack of anonymity
- Challenges in maintaining confidentiality stemming from familiarity among residents
- Small (often family) enterprises, fewer large industries
- Economic orientation to land and nature (e.g., agriculture, mining, lumbering, fishing, marine related)
- More high-risk occupations
- Town as the center of trade
- Churches and schools as socialization centers
- Preference for interacting with locals (insiders)
- Mistrust of newcomers to the community (outsiders)

From Bushy A: The rural context and nursing practice. In Molinari D, Bushy A, editors: The rural nurse: transition to practice, New York, 2012, Springer, p 8.

of rural residents has increased, the number with college degrees remains far lower than for urban residents, and this gap has increased over time. It is not surprising that unemployment remains higher for people with the least education (Kusmin, 2015).

The working poor in rural areas are particularly at risk for being underinsured or uninsured. As mentioned earlier, about 16% or 50 million people live in rural areas. Populations in rural areas have different demographics than those in urban areas, and this affects their ability to take full advantage of the Affordable Care Act (ACA). Although many rural people fall in the target population for the ACA, low-to-moderate income families, they often live in states that are not currently implementing the Medicaid expansion. This means that they are disproportionally affected by state decisions about the implementation of the ACA. These individuals are more likely to fall below the poverty level and less likely to have insurance provided by an employer. " . . . many uninsured individuals under poverty will be left in a 'coverage gap' in which their incomes are above Medicaid eligibility levels but below eligibility levels for tax credits [for the purchase of health coverage]" (Newkirk and Damico, 2014, p 3).

For more discussion on characteristics of rural life, see Box 22.1.

HEALTH STATUS OF RURAL RESIDENTS

Despite the significant number of people who live in rural areas, their health problems and health behaviors are not fully understood. This section summarizes what is known about the overall health status of rural adults and children. The health status measures addressed are perceived health status, diagnosed chronic conditions, physical limitations, frequency of seeking medical treatment, usual source of care, maternal and infant health, children's health, mental health, minorities' health, and environmental and occupational health risks (Bolin and Bellamy, 2014; OSHA, 2013).

In general, people in rural areas have a poorer perception of their overall health and functional status than their urban counterparts. Rural residents older than 18 years of age assess their health status less favorably than do urban residents. Studies show that rural adults are less likely to engage in preventive behavior, which increases their exposure to risk. Specifically, they are more likely to smoke and report higher rates of alcohol use and obesity. They are less likely to engage in physical activity during leisure time, wear seat belts, have regular blood pressure checks, have Papanicolaou (Pap) smears, and do breast self-examinations. These behaviors then influence their overall health (Crosby et al, 2012; Blackwell, 2014).

In contrast to their urban counterparts, rural adults are more likely to have one or more of the following chronic conditions: heart disease, chronic obstructive pulmonary disease, hypertension, arthritis and rheumatism, diabetes, cardiovascular disease, and cancer. Nearly 50% of all rural adults have been diagnosed with at least one of these chronic conditions, in contrast to approximately 25% of nonrural adults. Also, the rate of diagnosed diabetes in rural adults is about 7 in 100 compared with 5 in 100 in nonrural residents. Rural adults are more likely to have cancer (about 7%) compared with urban adults (about 5%). Although most cases of acquired immunodeficiency syndrome (AIDS) are still found in urban areas, the rate is increasing in some rural populations (Smalley et al, 2012).

The percentage of rural adults who receive medical treatment for both life-threatening illnesses and degenerative or chronic conditions is higher than that of urban adults. Life-threatening conditions include malignant neoplasms, heart disease, cardiovascular problems, and liver disorders. Degenerative or chronic diseases include diabetes, kidney disease, arthritis, and chronic diseases of the circulatory, nervous, respiratory, and digestive systems. Rural residents have more chronic health problems than their urban counterparts (Bolin and Bellamy, 2014; Blackwell, 2014).

Rural adults tend to have an overall poorer health status and are less likely to seek medical care than urban adults. Maintaining independence is often more difficult because of the lack of services and staff. Home care services are especially helpful for rural people in that they often can prevent the need for institutionalization. Rural people typically want to remain in their homes as long as possible (Nelson and Gingerich, 2010). Not only are rural people less likely to seek medical care, but also there are fewer physicians from whom care can be sought. Ten percent of US physicians work in rural areas, whereas 25% of the population lives there. In addition, rural people are less likely to have employer-sponsored health insurance or prescription drug coverage. People living in rural areas have a greater risk than do their urban counterparts for being involved in an accident. Specifically, one-third of motor vehicle accidents and two-thirds of all deaths in motor vehicle accidents occur on rural roads. Likewise, rural people are twice as likely to die of unintentional injuries, and they have a significantly higher risk for gunshot deaths from hunting and other types of accidents (National Rural Health Association [NRHA], 2009). Also, because of the distances of a farm, ranch, or home from a town and also the likelihood of animals being a possible danger, guns may be more readily found in rural versus urban homes. Nurses can teach people how to prevent accidents, engage in safer and more healthful lifestyle behaviors, and reduce the risk for chronic health problems, and they can help them more effectively manage existing chronic conditions.

In general, a person who has a usual source of care is more likely to seek care when ill and to follow prescribed regimens. Rural adults are more likely than urban adults to identify a particular medical provider as their usual source of care. The providers most often seen by rural adults are general practitioners and advanced practice registered nurses (APRNs). In contrast, urban adults are more likely to seek care from a medical specialist. Nurses must be especially thorough in their health assessment of rural and migrant clients who may not receive regular care for chronic health conditions.

Traveling time or distance to ambulatory care services affects access to care for both rural and urban residents. For rural people, it may be the distance they must travel, and for urban people it may be not so much the distance but the amount of traffic they encounter. Both groups tend to wait the same amount of time once they arrive at the clinic or physician's office.

Often rural health care professionals live and practice in a particular community for decades, and they may provide care to people who live in several counties. One or two nurses in a county health department may offer a full range of services for all residents in a specified area, which may span more than 100 miles from one end of a county to the other. Consequently, rural physicians and nurses frequently report, "I provide care to individuals and families with all kinds of conditions, in all stages of life, and across several generations." In Health Professional Shortage Areas (HPSAs), a nurse practitioner or physician may provide services to people who live in several counties.

As mentioned earlier, managing a chronic illness is a particular challenge for people who live in rural areas. The challenges include dealing with the symptoms, a disability, complex medication schedules, getting adequate medical care, and adjusting to the changes brought on by the illness. Nursing faculty at Montana State University developed *My Health Companion (MHC)* to help rural women better understand and manage their chronic health conditions by using a paper personal health record. This tool provides a structure for tracking and maintaining health information and increasing health literacy. The researchers found that using the MHC helped women prepare for visits to multiple health care providers and have more satisfaction from the visits. The providers thought they were able to do a better job when the patients came with better preparation (Weinert et al, 2010).

Women's Health and Maternal and Infant Health

Despite conflicting reports, it seems that overall rural populations have higher infant and maternal morbidity rates, especially counties designated as HPSAs. These areas tend to have a high proportion of racial minorities, and fewer specialists, such as pediatricians, obstetricians, and gynecologists, are available to provide care to at-risk populations. There are extreme variations in pregnancy outcomes from one part of the country to another, and even within states. For example, in several counties located in the north-central and intermountain states, the pregnancy outcome is among the finest in the United States. However, in several other counties within those same states, the pregnancy outcome is among the worst. Particularly at risk are women who live on or near Indian reservations, female migrant workers, and African American women who live in rural counties of southeastern states (Bolin and Bellamy, 2014; Leipert et al, 2012).

Female victims of sexual assault are another at-risk group in rural areas. It is difficult to document the incidence of sexual assault in rural areas because of rural isolation and a higher likelihood that the person who is assaulted knows people in the community. For these reasons, it is thought that the rate is higher than in urban areas (Annan, 2011). Most assaults occur between a woman and someone she knows. Women may be hesitant to report the assault because people who know her may see her car parked at the site where she needs to make the report. Also, the woman may personally know the person(s) to whom the report is made and she would be embarrassed to reveal this incident (Annan, 2011). Because of the closeness of the population in terms of people knowing one another, confidentiality is often an issue in reports of sexual assault. Perpetrators are often family members, so the victim may not be believed or the victim may be threatened to remain silent about the incident.

CHECK YOUR PRACTICE

You work in a rural health clinic, and although you know many of the clients from seeing them at your children's school, at church, and other locations and events, you do not know Ms. Smith.
- She comes to the clinic complaining of vague pain in her abdomen and pelvic area.
- She seems quite anxious and reluctant to describe when her symptoms began.
- You suspect she may be a victim of a sexual assault.
- You know that rural women are concerned about confidentiality, and they also worry that they might see the health care provider in a setting outside the clinic and be embarrassed.
- What would you do?

Public health nurses appreciate the effects of socioeconomic factors, such as income level (poverty), education level, age, employment and unemployment patterns, and use of prenatal services, on pregnancy outcomes. There are other, less well-known determinants, such as environmental hazards, occupational risks, and the cultural meaning placed on childbearing and childrearing practices by a community. The effects of these multifaceted factors vary.

Health of Children

Some differences exist between rural and urban children younger than 6 years of age with respect to access to providers and use of services (Bolin and Bellamy, 2014). For example, urban children are less likely to have a usual provider but are more likely to see a pediatrician when they are ill, and rural adults and children are more likely to have a general practitioner as their regular caregiver. Children who work on farms and ranches are often exposed to noise, organic and inorganic dusts, and the hazards of working with farm equipment. Farm children learn how to work by modeling their parents, and some children may not use personal protective equipment. The highest rates of farmwork injuries occur in boys between 16 and 18 years of age. These injuries tend to result from using tractors, using all-terrain vehicles, working with cattle and horses, using farm hand-tools, dealing with barbed wire, and falling from heights, such as in a barn (Browning et al, 2003).

School nurses play an important role in the overall health status of children in the United States. The availability of school nurses in rural communities varies across regions. They tend to be scarce in frontier and rural areas of the United States because of (1) a shortage of health care professionals in the area and (2) fewer taxpayers and thus less income to support school nurses.

However, some creative approaches have enabled counties to provide better health care and school nursing services. For example, two or more counties may enter into a partnership in which they share the cost of a "district" health nurse. The nurse may be employed by the health department in one of the counties. Other counties have forged partnerships with an agency in an urban setting and contracted for specific health care services. In both of these situations, it is not unusual for the nurse to provide services to all children attending schools in the participating counties. In some frontier states, schools may be more than 100 miles apart and as many miles or more from the district health department office. Because of the number of schools and distances between them, the county nurse may be able to visit each school only once or maybe twice in a school term. Usually the nurse's visit is to update immunizations and perhaps to teach maturation classes to students in the upper grades.

Mental Health

Stress, stress-related conditions, and mental illness are prevalent among populations that have economic difficulties. When the economy in an area is depressed because of slowdowns in mining or lumbering; manufacturing; plant reductions or closings; or adverse weather that affects crops, workplaces, and homes, job losses follow. Economic recession contributes to a family's not having insurance or being underinsured or to their losing their home as a result of mortgage foreclosure. Often, even if mental health services are available and accessible, rural residents delay seeking care when they have an emotional problem until an emergency or a crisis arises. There appears to be a more persistent, endemic level of depression among rural residents. This prevalence may be related to the high rate of poverty, geographic isolation, and an insufficient number of mental health services. Depression may also contribute to the escalating incidence of accidents and suicides, especially among rural male adolescents and young men.

Like many of the indicators in the previous sections, reports on the incidence of domestic violence and alcohol, tobacco, and other drug use and abuse in rural populations are also conflicting. When people are related to one another or know each other well, they are less likely to report these behaviors. After a time, in small, tight-knit communities, destructive coping behaviors often come to be accepted as usual occurrences for a particular family. Family problems also may be ignored if formal social services and public health services are sparse or nonexistent and if the community does not trust the professionals who provide services within a local agency. In underserved rural areas, gaps exist in the continuum of mental health services, which, ideally, should include preventive education, anticipatory guidance, early intervention programs, crisis and acute care services, and follow-up care. As with other aspects of health care, nurses in rural areas play an important role in community education, case finding, advocacy, and case management of clients experiencing emotional problems and chronic mental health problems.

OCCUPATIONAL AND ENVIRONMENTAL HEALTH PROBLEMS IN RURAL AREAS

Four high-risk industries found primarily in rural areas are forestry, mining, marine-related fields, and agriculture. Associated health risks in these industries are machinery and vehicular accidents, trauma, some types of cancer, and allergies and respiratory conditions associated with repeated exposure to toxins, pesticides, and herbicides (NCHS, 2014; OSHA, 2013). Farming and ranching, often operated and owned by a family, may not fall under Occupational Safety and Health Administration (OSHA) guidelines, because they are considered small enterprises. Therefore safety standards are not enforceable. Workers' Compensation insurance usually is not available for the agriculture industry.

The most common health issues related to farmworkers are: (1) pesticide exposure; (2) heat and sun exposure; (3) hazardous tools and machinery; (4) infectious diseases; (5) musculoskeletal injuries; (6) respiratory illnesses; (7) skin disorders; and (8) eye injuries (National Center for Farmworker Health, 2013a).

Most of the North American food supply is treated with agricultural chemicals (i.e., pesticides), with the largest group being the organophosphate pesticides. These pesticides are known to be potential hazards. Farmworkers are exposed not only to the immediate effects of working in fields that are foggy or wet with pesticides but also to the unknown long-term effects of chronic exposure to agricultural chemicals. The farmworker's clothing and dwelling also can be major sources of cross-contamination for both the worker and his or her family. The Environmental Protection Agency (EPA) and OSHA require that farmworkers be given information about pesticide safety. However, migrant farmworkers may not receive this information, may get ineffectual training, or may not be able to read the educational information (Napolitano et al, 2002). Entire families may be at risk for pesticide exposure because of drift from nearby areas, not regularly washing their hands, and bringing contaminated clothes home.

Acute health effects of pesticide exposure include mild psychological and behavioral deficits, such as memory loss, difficulty with concentration, or mood changes; abdominal pain; nausea; vomiting; diarrhea; headache; malaise; skin rashes; and eye irritation. Acute severe pesticide poisoning can result in death. More chronic exposure may lead to long-term damage such as birth defects, cancers, blood disorders, neurological problems, and reproductive effects (NCFH, 2013a). See the How To box for information on how to recognize the signs and symptoms of pesticide exposure.

HOW TO Recognize the Signs and Symptoms of Pesticide Exposure

Signs and symptoms of pesticide exposure vary according to the amount and length of time of the exposure. The majority of body systems can be affected by pesticide exposure.

- Symptoms of acute poisoning include neuromuscular (i.e., headache, dizziness, confusion, irritability, twitching muscles, muscle weakness), respiratory (i.e., shortness of breath, difficulty breathing, nasal and pharyngeal irritation), and gastrointestinal (i.e., nausea, vomiting, diarrhea, stomach cramps).
- Symptoms of chronic exposure can be related to illnesses and conditions such as cancers, Parkinson-like symptoms, infertility or sterility, liver damage, and polyneuropathy and neurobehavioral problems.
- If symptoms of pesticide exposure are suspected, the nurse should develop a pesticide exposure history. A good example of an exposure form can be found at http://pesticide.umd.edu.

Working for hours in direct sunlight, in areas that may have high humidity can generate considerable body heat and can lead to heat stress. The signs and symptoms of heat exhaustion include heavy sweating; cold/pale/clammy skin; fast, weak pulse; nausea and vomiting; and fainting (NCFH, 2013a, p 3). An added danger is that pesticides are more readily absorbed through hot, sweaty skin than through cool skin. Accidents can occur from being struck by a vehicle or from hand tools, tractors, and other objects and equipment. Infectious diseases among this population are often caused by poor sanitation and crowded conditions. Farmworkers often bend, twist, carry heavy items and have repetitive motions during long work hours that can lead to musculoskeletal injuries. Farmworkers are often exposed to organic and mineral dusts, animal and plant dusts, toxic gases, molds, and other respiratory irritants. Those who perform the following tasks are at higher risk for respiratory illnesses (NCFH, 2013a, p 4):

- Working in dusty fields and buildings
- Handling hay
- Feeding or working with feedstuffs
- Working in corn silage
- Cleaning silos or grain bins
- Working around fishmeal, bird droppings, or dust from animal hair, fur, or feathers
- Applying fertilizers and pesticides

These same tasks and the environment in which the respiratory illnesses occur can also lead to skin disorders and eye injuries.

LEVELS OF PREVENTION
Related to Rural Health

Primary Prevention
Teach workers how to reduce exposure to pesticides.

Secondary Prevention
Conduct screening, such as urine testing for pesticide exposure.

Tertiary Prevention
Initiate treatment for the symptoms of pesticide exposure such as nausea, vomiting, and skin irritation.

RURAL HEALTH CARE DELIVERY ISSUES AND BARRIERS TO CARE

Although each rural community is unique, the experience of living in a rural area has several common characteristics (Bushy and Winters, 2013) (Box 22.2). Barriers to health care may be associated with whether services and professionals are available, affordable, accessible, or acceptable to rural consumers. Availability implies that health services exist and have the necessary personnel to provide essential services. Sparseness of population limits the number and array of health care services in a given geographic region. Therefore the cost of providing special services to a few people often is prohibitive, particularly in frontier states, where the number of physicians, nurses, and other types of health care providers is insufficient. Consequently, where services and personnel are scarce, they must be allocated wisely. Accessibility implies that a person has logistical access to needed services, as well as the ability to purchase them. Affordability is associated with both the availability and accessibility of care. It infers that services are of reasonable cost and that a family has sufficient resources to purchase them when they are needed. Acceptability of care means that a particular service is appropriate and offered in a manner that is congruent with the values of a target population. This can be hampered by both the

BOX 22.2   Barriers to Health Care in Rural Areas

- Lack of health care providers and services and great distances to obtain services
- Lack of personal transportation
- Unavailable public transportation
- Lack of telephone services
- Unavailable outreach services
- Inequitable reimbursement policies for providers
- Unpredictable weather or travel conditions
- Inability to pay for care or lack of health care insurance
- Lack of know-how to procure publicly funded entitlements and services
- Inadequate provider attitudes and understanding about rural populations
- Language barriers (caregivers are not linguistically competent)
- Care and services not culturally and linguistically appropriate

From Bushy A: The rural context and nursing practice. In Molinari D, Bushy A, editors: The rural nurse: transition to practice, New York, 2012, Springer, p 10.

client's cultural preference and the urban orientation of health professions.

Providers' attitudes, insights, and knowledge about rural populations are important. A demeaning attitude, lack of accurate knowledge about rural populations, or insensitivity about the rural lifestyle on the part of a nurse can cause difficulties in relating to those clients. Moreover, insensitivity generates mistrust, causing rural clients to view professionals as outsiders to the community. On the other hand, some professionals in rural practice express feelings of professional isolation and lack of community acceptance. To resolve these conflicting views, nursing faculty members can expose students to the rural environment with clinical experiences that include opportunities to provide care to clients in their natural (e.g., rural) setting to gain accurate insight about that particular community.

In developing community health programs that are available, accessible, affordable, and appropriate, nurses must design strategies and implement interventions that mesh with a client's belief system. This implies that a family and a community are actively involved in planning and delivering care for a member who needs it. Nurses must have an accurate perspective of rural clients. Although the importance of forming partnerships and ensuring mutual exchange seems obvious, most research about rural communities has been for policy or reimbursement purposes. Few empirical data are available about rural family systems in terms of their health beliefs, values, perception of illness, health care–seeking behaviors, and what constitutes appropriate care. Therefore nurses must be actively involved in conducting and implementing research on the nursing needs of rural populations to expand the profession's knowledge of this population and to provide services based on evidence.

Mobile health clinics are an effective method of health care delivery in rural areas. Often these clinics may be an outreach effort of a health center such as a migrant health center or another type of federally funded health center. They may be managed by nurses or by an interprofessional team. The goal is to take services to clients who need them and would have difficulty accessing the services in a stationary clinic, which might be some distance away or might not be open when the client could be away from work to seek care. Information about this valuable health care delivery format is available on the Mobile Health Clinics Association website (http://www.mobilehealthclinicsnetwork.org/).

HEALTH OF MINORITIES, PARTICULARLY MIGRANT FARMWORKERS
Characteristics of Migrant Farmworkers

Several at-risk minority groups in rural America have distinctive concerns (in particular, children, older adults, Native Americans, Native Alaskans, Native Hawaiians, migrant workers, African Americans, and the homeless) (Gamm et al, 2004). See Table 22.1 for further discussion on some of these groups. The rural homeless, for example, may be seasonal farmworkers or families whose farms were foreclosed. Sometimes the family may be allowed by law to continue living in the house on the farm they once owned. The family no longer has a means of

TABLE 22.1 Select Health Care Needs, Risks, and Conditions of Select Rural Aggregates

Rural Aggregates	Health Care Needs	Health Risks/Conditions
Farmers and ranchers	Advanced life support, emergency services Oral and dental care Obstetrical, perinatal, and pediatric services Mental and behavioral health services Agricultural health nurses Geriatric specialists	Agricultural chemicals and environmental hazards Dermatitis Stress, depression, and anxiety disorders Respiratory conditions (e.g., farmer's lung) Accidents (vehicular, machinery) Trauma-related chronic conditions Dental caries and loss Interpersonal and domestic violence
Native Americans	Advanced life support and emergency services Oral and dental care Obstetrical, perinatal, and pediatric services Mental and behavioral health services Culturally appropriate substance abuse treatment programs Epidemiologists Diabetes screening and educators Community health workers and education	Infectious diseases (e.g., hepatitis, tuberculosis) Sudden infant death syndrome (SIDS) Interpersonal and domestic violence Diabetes Alcohol and substance abuse Cirrhosis of the liver Vehicular accidents Hypothermic and environmental injuries Trauma-related injuries and chronic conditions Dental caries and loss
African Americans	Community nursing health promotion and screening services Diabetes screening and educators Hypertension screening and education Prenatal and perinatal health care services Oncology services (education, screening, follow-up interventions) HIV/AIDS prevention education, screening, and follow-up care Mental and behavioral health services	Diabetes Hypertension Sickle cell anemia Infectious diseases (e.g., hepatitis, HIV/AIDS) Cancer (e.g., prostate, breast) Dental caries and loss Depression Interpersonal and domestic violence
Migrant farmworkers	Environmental protection policies (e.g., safe drinking water, sanitation) Community nursing and migrant health services (primary, secondary, tertiary prevention) Diabetes screening and educators Hypertension screening and education Maternal and child services Oncology services (education, screening, follow-up interventions) Mental and behavioral health services	Infectious diseases (e.g., hepatitis, typhoid, tuberculosis, HIV/AIDS, STDs) Exposure effects of pesticides and herbicides Otitis media (children) Substance abuse (alcohol, recreational drugs, imported medicinal herbs) Dental caries and loss Interpersonal and domestic violence
Native Alaskans	Advanced life support and emergency care services Medical transport services Oral and dental care Obstetrical, perinatal, and pediatric services Mental and behavioral health services Culturally appropriate substance abuse treatment programs Epidemiologists Diabetes screening and educators	Infectious diseases (e.g., hepatitis, tuberculosis) Dental caries and loss Depression Interpersonal and domestic violence Environmental health risks (e.g., exposure to toxic substances, contaminants, hypothermia) Diabetes Alcohol and substance abuse Cirrhosis of the liver Vehicular accidents, trauma, and long-term chronic residual effects
Coal miners	Occupational Safety and Health Administration policy and standards Mental and behavioral health services Emergency and advanced life support services Occupational health nurses Grief counselors	Depression and substance abuse Occupational-related accidents and trauma Respiratory conditions (e.g., black lung, chronic obstructive pulmonary disease) Interpersonal and domestic violence

Meit, M, Knudson A, Gilbert T, et al: *The 2014 Update of the Rural-Urban Chartbook*. Accessed from the Rural Health Research Gateway at http://www.ruralhealthresearch.org/

livelihood and often remains hidden in the community, with insufficient income to purchase food or other necessary services.

Migrant and seasonal farmworkers are one example of an at-risk group. Migrant and seasonal farmworkers (MSFWs) are essential to the agricultural industry in the United States. Although the availability and affordability of food in the United States depend on these individuals, their economic status and social acceptance have not reflected the importance of their work. Estimates of the numbers of MSFWs in the United States vary, with the most commonly cited ranging between 2 and 3 million. Numbers vary because of differences in definition of migrants, different ways of estimating numbers, and difficulties in counting mobile populations. The majority of MSFWs are foreign born (70.7%) with 64.1% born in Mexico (NCFH, 2016). Other workers include Central Americans, African Americans, Jamaicans, Haitians, Laotians, and Thais. The composition of the migrant and seasonal population can vary from one area of the United States to another. Of the MSFWs, 52% have legal authorization to work in the United States. Less than 5% are in the United States as an H-2A guest worker (Villarejo, 2012). Thirty-one percent of foreign-born farmworkers have spent 20 or more years in the United States, and 29.4% have been in the United States for 10 to 19 years (NCFH, 2016).

Twenty eight percent said they could not speak English "at all" and nine percent said they could speak English "somewhat" (NCFH, 2016). The definition of a *migrant farmworker* may vary depending on the level of government agency and the type of service program. Federal statutes define a *migrant farmworker* as an individual whose principal employment within the past 24 months is in agriculture on a seasonal basis and who establishes for the purpose of such employment a temporary abode. Seasonal farmworkers work cyclically in agriculture but do not migrate. Although migrant and seasonal farmworkers make up two distinct populations, they do share many demographic, cultural, and occupational characteristics. Much of the information available on agricultural farmworkers does not distinguish between migrant and seasonal farmworkers.

Farmworkers who work in the United States are an average age of 37 years; 81% are older than 25 years of age, and 7.9% are between 22 and 24 years of age. Seventy-one percent are male, and 29% are female. Many migrants are American citizens or are authorized to work in the United States, but not all of them are documented workers. The majority of all farmworkers are not migratory (NCFH, 2016). The Office of Migrant Health of the U.S. Public Health Service defines a *migrant farmworker* as a person "whose principal employment is in agriculture on a seasonal basis, who has been so employed within the last 24 months, and who establishes for the purpose of such employment a temporary abode" (Office of the Federal Registrar, 1994, p 238). Seasonal farmworkers work cyclically in agriculture but do not migrate. Annually a large group of workers and their families (between 3 and 5 million) leave their homes to follow the crops. In many cases, migrant farmworkers coming into the United States for work settle in permanent locations after a period, seeking other types of employment.

EVIDENCE-BASED PRACTICE

Messias and colleagues (2015) described the difficulties that foreign-born individuals who are not documented immigrants have when they work in the United States. They note that being undocumented may not be a permanent state. People can change their status. For example, documented immigrants may let their visa expire and become undocumented, and people who arrive as undocumented immigrants may apply for and be granted permanent status.

Vulnerability and stress are common among undocumented immigrants. They often face a dangerous passage into the United States and once they arrive they may face rejection, stigmatization, and scapegoating. They constantly worry about potential or actual arrest or deportation. They may fear seeking help due to the worry about deportation if their status is apparent. Their challenges to getting health care are often due to language barriers, social and economic resources, restricted transportation and the distance to services, and fear and mistrust of the health care system. These barriers also lead them to use emergency services more often, which increases the cost of care.

Nurse Use

As the authors eloquently say, "Professional nursing ethics posit the fundamental expectation that nurses provide care of individuals, respecting each person's dignity and worth without regard for the nature of the health issue, social or economic status, or personal attributes or characteristics, including social, economic, or migration status," (p 92).

An area of growing interest is the difference between documented and undocumented immigrants. Approximately 28% of foreign-born residents in the United States are undocumented immigrants. These are "individuals who either entered or are currently residing in the country without valid immigration of residency documents" (Messias et al, 2015, p 86). In contrast, documentation "confers legal, social, and physical mobility and facilitates access to information, education, employment, services and legal protections" (Messias et al, 2015, p 87). See the Evidence-Based Practice box for further discussion of the implications of undocumented immigration on individual and population health in the United States.

Migrant Lifestyle

Migrant farmworkers often have an unpredictable and difficult lifestyle. Many must leave home each year and travel to distant locations to work. They may be uncertain about their work and housing. They may also feel isolated in new communities and lack adequate resources to meet their needs. All of these situations can lead to stress. The median pay for farmworkers is $20,090 per year or $9.66 per hour. The number of jobs in agriculture was expected to decline 6% between 2014 and 2016 (Bureau of Labor Statistics, 2016). Many of these workers send some of their earnings to family members in their country of origin. They rarely receive benefits such as Workers' Compensation, disability compensation, or health or retirement benefits.

Migrant farmworkers traditionally have followed one of three migratory streams: Eastern, originating in Florida; Midwestern, originating in Texas; and Western, originating in

California. However, as workers increasingly travel throughout the country seeking employment, these streams are becoming less distinct. Migrant farmworkers are employed in fruit and nut (29%), vegetable (27%), horticultural (24%), field (17%), and miscellaneous (2%) agricultural venues (NCFH, 2016). The cyclic nature of agricultural work and its dependence on weather and economic conditions results in considerable uncertainty for migrant farmworkers. These individuals and families leave their homes with the expectation of work at certain sites. Word of mouth from friends or family, newspaper announcements, or previous employment help determine their destinations. However, on arrival, migrant farmworkers may find that other workers have arrived first or that the crops are late, leaving the farmworkers unemployed.

Housing

When migrant workers reach a worksite, housing may not be available, it may be too expensive, or it may be in poor condition. Housing conditions vary among states and localities. Housing for migrant farmworkers may be in camps with cabins, trailers, or houses. Some even live in cars or tents if necessary. National data about the type and quality of housing occupied by farmworkers are limited; however, data indicate that the housing is generally crowded by federal standards (Culp and Umbarger, 2004). When housing costs are high, as many as 50 men may live in one house. In some cases, three or more families may share one house or mobile home. Much of the housing is substandard and lacks adequate sanitation and working appliances or may have severe structural defects (NCFH, 2012a). Many workers also support a home and family in their country of origin.

Housing may be located next to fields that have been sprayed by pesticides or where farm machinery is a danger to children. Poor-quality and crowded places of residence can contribute to health problems such as tuberculosis (TB), gastroenteritis, and hepatitis and to exposure to high levels of lead. Renting housing in rural areas is nearly impossible because of barriers such as high rent, substantial rental deposits, long-term leases, lack of credit, discrimination, and a lack of rental units. Federal programs provide some funds for farmworker housing, but they are insufficient to meet the demand. Increased funding and better coordination among agencies are needed, as is an increase in the availability of safe public housing.

Issues in Migrant Health

Poor and unsanitary working and housing conditions make farmworkers susceptible to health problems no longer seen as dangers to the general public or seen at a much lower rate. The agriculture industry is one of the most dangerous occupations in the United States. Although farmworkers have the same risks as other workers who deal with heavy equipment and do manual labor, they are also exposed to other hazards, including pesticide exposure, heat and sun exposure, skin disorders, infectious diseases, lung problems, hearing and vision disorders, and strained muscles and bones (NCFH,

2013a). In general, migrant workers have identified diabetes, poor dental health, obesity, and depression as major health problems (Cason, Snyder, and Jensen, 2004). The Migrant Health Act, signed in 1962, provides primary and supplemental health services to migrant workers and their families at 154 migrant health centers in 42 states. In 2014, of the 172 reporting grantees, migrant health centers served 814,178 people in the United States (Health Resources and Services Administration [HRSA], 2014). It is estimated that the number served by these clinics represents only a small proportion of migrant workers. Some of the reasons for lack of care are poverty of the workers, their constant mobility, language differences, and lack of transportation (Hoerster et al, 2011). Specifically, the following factors limit adequate provision of health care services:

- **Lack of knowledge about services.** Because of their isolation and lack of fluency in English, migrant farmworkers lack usual sources for information about available services, especially if they are not receiving public benefits.
- **Inability to afford care.** The Medicaid program, which is intended to serve the poor, often is not available to migrant farmworkers, especially undocumented workers. Workers may not remain in a geographic area long enough to be considered for benefits or may lose benefits when they relocate to a state with different eligibility standards. Their salaries may fluctuate monthly, making them ineligible for periods. If they do not work, they are not paid, so many avoid taking time off to get care.
- **Affordable Care Act or health insurance subsidies.** Although it is difficult to determine numbers, many farmworkers do not receive employer-mandated health coverage or subsidies because of the small farm exemption and the exclusion of seasonal workers who are employed less than 120 days in the employer's tax year. Undocumented workers are excluded from any employer and individual insurance mandates. Only 47% of farmworkers report being covered by employer-provided health insurance, and 57% do not receive any type of need-based or contribution-based public assistance, while 43% **do (NCFH, 2016).**
- **Availability of services.** Immigrants are treated differently depending on whether they were in the United States before the welfare reform legislation of 1966, and depending on the category of their immigration status. Each state determines whether to fill any part of the service's gap to immigrants. As a result, many legal immigrants and unauthorized immigrants are ineligible for services such as Supplemental Security Income (SSI) and the Supplemental Nutrition Assistance Program (SNAP; food stamps).
- **Transportation.** Health care services may be located far from work or home. Transportation may be unavailable, unreliable, or expensive. Many migrant farmworkers do not have access to vehicles. Privacy is compromised when migrant workers depend on employers to provide transportation to clinics (Napolitano, 2008).
- **Hours of services.** Many health services are available only during work hours; therefore, seeking health care leads to lost earnings.

- **Mobility and tracking.** Although migrant families move from job to job, their health care records typically do not go with them. This leads to fragmented services in areas such as treatment for TB, chronic illness management, and immunizations. For example, health departments are known to dispense medications for TB on a monthly basis. Adequate treatment for TB requires 6 to 12 months of medication. When migrant farmworkers move, they must independently seek out new health services to continue their medications. The Migrant Clinicians Network (MCN) TB tracking program makes available to a farmworker's current provider any previous provider information that was entered into the program. This tracking helps maintain continuity of TB care for a mobile population (MCN, 2016).
- **Language barriers.** As discussed in Chapter 5, the inability to speak English presents many barriers to getting adequate health care. Often, immigrant adults speak primarily the language of their native country. They may not be able to read or write in English. They also may be embarrassed to admit this lack, so they nod or say yes, when their understanding of what is being said is minimal. Although children may be more competent in English, the adults may prefer that children not know about their health needs or conditions. It is important for the nurse to verify whether clients understand what they are being asked or told. Because the majority of seasonal farmworkers are primarily Spanish speakers, the recruitment and retention of bicultural and bilingual health care provider staff are important priorities.
- **Discrimination.** Although migrant farmworkers and their families bring revenue into the community, they are often perceived as poor, uneducated, transient, and ethnically different. These perceptions foster attitudes and acts of discrimination against them.
- **Documentation.** Unauthorized individuals fear that getting services in a federally funded or state-funded clinic may lead to discovery and deportation.
- **Cultural aspects of health care.** See the later discussion of cultural considerations in migrant health care.

Other Specific Health Problems

Dental disease is one of the most common health problems for farmworkers of all ages. Farmworkers may not have dental insurance. They may have long travel times to get dental care, have language problems, and be in an area where there is a shortage of dental providers. Mexican Americans have higher rates of tooth decay and periodontal disease than non-Hispanic whites, and their children are not spared from oral health problems (NCFH, 2013b).

The incidence of TB is estimated to be higher in migrant farmworkers than in the general population, and they are more likely to die of the disease. The majority of migrant farmworkers are foreign-born and Hispanic. MSFWs are at increased risk for TB because of higher rates in their countries of origin, crowded living conditions, and malnutrition (NCFH, 2013c).

It is difficult to obtain accurate data about the incidence of HIV and AIDS for migrant farmworkers. According to the NCFH report, estimates range from 2.6% to 13%. In 2009, there were 7347 new HIV diagnoses and 6719 AIDS diagnoses among Hispanics. Latinos are disproportionately affected by HIV. In 2009 Latinos represented only 16% of the US population and 20% of new HIV infections (NCFH, 2011a). The risk factors for contracting HIV are similar to those for TB among migrant workers: poverty, low income, substandard housing, limited access to health care, limited English competence, mobile lifestyle, and social isolation. Other risk factors include having unprotected sex with prostitutes or men, injection drug use, and tattooing (NCFH, 2011a).

Depression and stress are areas of concern for adult migrants, and this may be related to isolation, economic hardship, their legal status, poor living conditions, and weather conditions that interrupt their work (MCH, 2008). They may also experience stress due to having to adjust to a new culture, low self-esteem, discrimination, frequent mobility, long work hours, and limited or nonexistent benefits (NCFH, 2013d). Migrant women are at risk for significant anxiety caused by their duties and responsibilities. In addition to working all day under the same conditions as the men, the women then return home to cook, clean, and take care of the children. Unfortunately, an unknown number of these women experience domestic violence, which is a major health problem with significant physical, emotional, and psychological consequences. Female farmworkers, especially the undocumented, are a vulnerable population who often suffer harassment and sexual abuse. This abuse is so common that many of the women think that it is part of the job (Human Rights Watch, 2012).

Farmworkers may be vulnerable to developing type 2 diabetes mellitus due to factors such as poverty, stress, cultural and dietary practices, long-term exposure to certain pesticides, and genetic predispositions. Although the total prevalence of type 1 and type 2 diabetes among farmworkers is not known, it appears higher among Hispanics of all ages (NCFH, 2014). Diabetes and tuberculosis may also interact similar to how HIV/AIDS and TB interact. When both conditions are present, they produce more severe effects, and that makes management and treatment more complex (NCFH, 2014).

Children of Migrant Workers

Migrant farmworker parents want a better future for their children. In fact, this strong desire is often the catalyst that causes many farmworkers to leave their country of origin. These children often appear to the outsider as happy, outgoing, and inquisitive. On the surface, they may look like children from any other aggregate. However, they often suffer from health care deficits, including malnutrition (e.g., vitamin A, iron), infectious diseases (e.g., upper respiratory tract infection, gastroenteritis), dental caries (caused by prolonged use of the bottle, bottle propping, limited access to fluoride or dental care), inadequate immunization status, pesticide exposure, injuries, overcrowding and exposure to lead in poor housing conditions, and disruption of their social and school life.

In many instances, it is difficult to determine the exact age of children in migrant communities. Children as young as 12 years of age may work to help support their family. The Fair Labor Standards Act of 1938 states that the minimum age that a child can work in agriculture is 14 years; the age is 16 years in other industries. Children 12 to 13 years of age can work on a farm with the parents' consent or if the parent works on the same farm. Children younger than 12 years of age can work on a farm with fewer than seven full-time workers (Davis, 2001). Workers younger than 18 years of age are likely found in larger numbers in states that have the highest numbers of adult farmworkers. These states are California, Florida, North Carolina, Texas, Oregon, and Washington (NCFH, November 2012). Federal law does not protect children from overworking or regulate the time of day they work. Hence some children work before they go to school or work late into the evening, which interferes with their ability to do homework and get adequate rest.

Migrant children, as young as 8 years of age, may stay home to care for younger children. The Migrant Head Start Program is a safe, healthy, and educative option for children 6 months to 5 years of age. However, inadequate funding results in lack of services for all migrant children. The Migrant Education Program is a state and nationally sponsored summer school program for farmworkers' children older than 5 years of age. However, this program is not available to all eligible migrant youth. Although the threats to youth from working on farms are similar to those for adults, the most common are as follows (NCFH, November 2012):

- Working with heavy machinery, equipment and tools such as knives, chainsaws, tall ladders, and tractors or trucks
- Repetitive motion injuries resulting from bending at the waist, kneeling, reaching, and holding things in awkward positions
- Pressure to work fast without taking breaks and often despite an injury
- Heat and sun stress
- Pesticides

CULTURAL CONSIDERATIONS IN MIGRANT HEALTH CARE

As discussed in Chapter 5, to provide culturally competent care to migrant farmworkers, nurses need to appreciate and understand the cultural backgrounds of these individuals. Because the majority of migrant farmworkers are of Mexican descent, this section focuses on Mexican cultures. Although certain health beliefs and practices have been identified with the Mexican culture, the nurse must remember that beliefs and practices differ among regions and localities of a country and among individuals. Mexico is a multicultural country; therefore, the cultural backgrounds of Mexican immigrants vary, depending on their place of origin. Many indigenous groups in Mexico speak their regional dialect. Mexican immigrants may or may not be able to read, understand, or speak Spanish. Mexican immigrants who are less educated, with fewer economic resources, and from the rural areas tend to possess more traditional beliefs and practices.

Folk medicine, traditional, or alternative health practices are observed by the majority of the Mexican population while they are in Mexico (NCFH, 2011b). Many will continue to use folk medicine when they work in the United States. The practice of folk medicine is not unique to farmworkers or people from Mexico; people around the world use alternative medicines in addition to or instead of Western, or allopathic, medicine. It is important to know what folk medicine practices clients use so you can determine whether they interfere with the allopathic medical practices that client uses. See the section later in the chapter discussing health values, health beliefs, and health practices for more detail about folk health practices.

Nurse-Client Relationship

The nurse is considered an authority figure who should respect (respeto) the individual, be able to relate to the individual (personalismo), and maintain the individual's dignity (dignidad). Mexican individuals prefer polite, nonconfrontational relationships with others (simpatia). At times, because of simpatia, individuals and families may appear to understand what is being said to them (by nodding their heads) when in actuality they do not understand. The nurse should take measures to validate the understanding of these individuals. Mexicans expect to talk about personal matters (chit-chat) for the first few minutes of an encounter. They expect the nurse not to appear rushed and to be a good listener. Humor is appreciated, and touching as a caring gesture is seen as a positive behavior.

Mexican clients may not seek care with health care professionals first. Rather, they may have consulted with knowledgeable individuals in their family or community (the popular arena of care) or with folk healers (the traditional arena of care). Examples of the members of the popular arena are the señora, or wise older woman living in the community, one's grandmother (la abuela), and the local parish priest.

Health: Values, Beliefs, and Practices

Family, in general, is a significant component of a Mexican individual's health care and social support system. The woman in the household is considered the caretaker, whereas the man is considered the major decision maker. However, Mexican women in certain families have significant influence over most matters, including health decisions. Grandmothers and sisters are highly significant to the wife in the immediate family. They provide advice, care, and support. Even though they communicate regularly with their family in Mexico, they may not have a support system in the United States.

Love of their children, rather than concern for their own health, may encourage migrant parents to adopt healthier lifestyles. One example is when the parents of a child with asthma choose to stop smoking (Napolitano, 2008). In Oregon, when asked if they protected themselves from pesticide exposure, Mexican migrant parents responded negatively in general. However, they were willing to change their behaviors if, as a result, their children would be protected from pesticides (Napolitano et al, 2002).

The Mexican client may be more willing to follow the advice of another Mexican individual with a similar health problem than the advice of the health care professional. When health care providers fail to take into account the client's culture and ways of living, the client is likely to ignore the information and turn to friends and family for information. Although the majority of Mexican immigrants may identify themselves as Catholics, many Mexican individuals belong to other churches. The individual's religion may influence his or her health practices, such as birth control; however, the nurse cannot assume that a Catholic, for example, will not use some method of birth control.

In the Mexican culture, health may be considered a gift from God. Another common perception of health is that a healthy person is one who can continue to work and maintain daily activities independent of symptoms or diagnosed diseases. A person may miss a clinic appointment if he or she is able to work that day. Mexican immigrants may believe that illness is a punishment from God and think this is why therapies have not cured them. This more commonly occurs with chronic illnesses. Four common folk illnesses that a nurse may encounter with the Mexican client are (1) mal de ojo (evil eye), (2) susto (fright), (3) empacho (indigestion), and (4) caida de mollera (fallen fontanel). Symptoms and treatments may vary depending on the individual's or family's place of origin in Mexico. Other cultural beliefs relate to hot-cold balance, pregnancy, and postpartum behaviors (cuarentena).

When experiencing a folk illness, the traditional Mexican individual would prefer to seek care with a folk healer. The more common healers are the curanderos, herbalistas, and espiritualistas. The most commonly used herbs are manzanilla (chamomile), yerba buena (peppermint), aloe vera, nopales (cactus), and epazote.

QSEN FOCUS ON QUALITY AND SAFETY EDUCATION FOR NURSES

Targeted Competency: Patient-Centered Care—Recognize the client or designee as the source of control and full partner in providing compassionate and coordinated care (interventions) based on respect for the client's preferences, values, and needs.

Important aspects of client-centered interventions include:

- **Knowledge:** Discuss principles of effective communication.
- **Skills:** Assess own level of communication skill in encounters with clients and families.
- **Attitudes:** Value continuous improvement of own communication and conflict resolution skills.

Client-Centered Care Question

To provide client-centered care, it is important to not only be able to communicate with the person(s) but also to understand their cultural perspectives that influence their health care practices. If you are caring for clients who live in migrant farmworker camps and you observe that they are allowing their children to work several hours both before and after they go to school, how would you approach this situation?

- Would you begin by speaking with the parents?
- Would you speak with the person who owns or manages the farm?
- Describe your approach to the client(s) for whom you provide care.
- At what point would you consider involving community resources? If you choose this route, what resources would you consider?

CASE STUDY

Public health nurse Lynn Smith received a referral to visit 19-year-old primipara, Conchita Garcia, who was near term yet had not received prenatal care. Ms. Smith planned a home visit immediately. Having recently come from Mexico, Ms. Garcia was living in a clean, sparsely furnished apartment with other newly immigrated men and the father of her baby. Rapport was quickly established with the client, because Ms. Smith was fluent in Spanish.

Ms. Garcia knew little about the birthing process, so the nurse explained vaginal and cesarean births. Ms. Smith taught her the signs of labor, as well as complications that would merit a visit to the hospital or clinic. Ms. Garcia's physical assessment was normal. Ms. Smith then assessed whether the home environment would be safe for the baby and noted that the young family had bought infant clothes and a crib. The next day, Ms. Garcia gave birth to a healthy baby girl in the hospital.

During the second home visit, the nurse completed a newborn assessment on a well-hydrated, normal newborn that weighed a couple of ounces less than her birth weight. Ms. Garcia reported that the child would not latch on for breastfeeding but denied giving the child formula. The mother's breasts were moderately engorged, and she was feeding the baby breast milk she had pumped. Being far from family, especially female support, Ms. Garcia did not know how to breastfeed well, but she and the baby's father had made good use of the pump and filled bottles with her breast milk. Ms. Smith spent most of the visit teaching breastfeeding techniques.

There was a Band-Aid on the infant's umbilicus. Despite Ms. Smith's warning that the Band-Aid might not allow the umbilicus to dry and fall off, the Band-Aid was always present on each subsequent visit, even after healing was complete; the parents believed the Band-Aid would prevent a protruding umbilicus in later years. (Another tradition in some Hispanic cultures is to put a coin or a piece of thread over the umbilicus.)

Ms. Smith made referrals for postnatal and newborn health care so that the family would have health care at home, avoiding inappropriate use of the emergency department. Because another pregnancy soon would not be optimal, Ms. Smith explained birth control methods that could be used until the mother's postnatal visit. Ms. Garcia's isolation was a concern because she could not drive or speak English, so the nurse suggested attending a church of the family's religious denomination that had a service in Spanish each Sunday and a thriving congregation known to be supportive of young families in need. The health department enrolled the mother and baby in the Special Supplemental Nutrition Program for Women, Infants and Children (WIC), a federal nutrition program for low-income pregnant or breastfeeding mothers and their children younger than 5 years of age. Ms. Smith continued to visit the family, giving anticipatory guidance on the child's needs and advocating for them in the health care system while they learned English and got settled in a new country.

Created by Deborah C. Conway, Assistant Professor, School of Nursing, University of Virginia.

NURSING CARE IN RURAL ENVIRONMENTS

Rural people, including migrant and seasonal farmworkers, often develop independent and creative ways to cope because of the distance, isolation, and sparse resources they encounter. They may prefer to seek help first through their informal networks, such as neighbors, extended family, church, and civic clubs, before seeking a professional's care. Nurses describe some interesting differences when they work in rural areas versus urban ones. The boundaries between one's home and work roles may blur in nurses who go to the same church, shop at the same stores, and have children in the same schools as their clients. Thus many, if not all, clients are personally known as neighbors, as friends of an immediate family member, or perhaps part of one's extended family. There are, then, both social informality and a corresponding lack of anonymity in a small town. Some rural nurses say, "I never really feel like I am off duty because everybody in the county knows me through my work." In part, this may be because nurses are highly regarded by the community and viewed by local people as experts on health and illness. Residents may ask health-related questions and recommendations about physicians when they see the nurse (who may be a neighbor, friend, or relative) in a grocery store, at a service station, during a basketball game, or at church functions. Nurses in rural areas may also be expected to, in general, know something about everything, and this can be a demanding expectation. Some of the challenges of rural practice are professional isolation, limited opportunities for continuing education, lack of other kinds of health care personnel or professionals with whom one can interact, heavy workloads, the ability to function well in several clinical areas, lack of anonymity, and, for some, a restricted social life (Bushy, 2012). Many nurses value the close relationships with clients and co-workers, along with the diverse clinical experiences that evolve from caring for clients of all ages who have a variety of health problems, caring for clients for long periods (in some cases, across several generations), opportunities for professional development, greater autonomy, and the pleasures of living in a rural area. The nurse can often keep a finger on the pulse of the community by staying active in local political, social, religious, and employment activities that affect their clients. The nurse can be a catalyst for change, act as a community educator, and know how to find resources and services (Box 22.3).

Nurses working in rural areas, including those working with migrant farmworkers, can use many public health nursing skills. One of the first and most important is that of prevention. Given the barriers to receiving health care in rural areas, the ideal situation is to prevent health disruptions whenever possible. Case management and community-oriented primary health care (COPHC) are two effective models used to address some of those deficits and resolve rural health disparities. The steps of the COPHC process are as follows:

1. Define and characterize the community.
2. Identify the community's health problems.

BOX 22.3 Characteristics of Nursing Practice in Rural Areas

- Variety and diversity in clinical experiences
- Broader and expanding scope of practice
- Generalist skills with specialty knowledge of crises assessment and management across disciplines and specialties
- Flexibility and creativity in delivering care
- Sparse resources (i.e., materials, professionals, equipment, fiscal)
- Professional or personal isolation
- Greater independence and autonomy
- Role overlap with other disciplines
- Slower pace
- Lack of anonymity
- Increased opportunity for informal interactions with clients and co-workers
- Opportunity for client follow-up on discharge in informal community settings
- Discharge planning allowing for integration of formal and informal resources
- Care for clients across the life span
- Exposure to clients with a full range of conditions and diagnoses
- Status in the community (viewed as prestigious)
- Viewed as a professional role model
- Opportunity for community involvement and informal health education

From Bushy A: The rural context and nursing practice. In Molinari D, Bushy A, editors: The rural nurse: transition to practice, New York, 2012, Springer, p 12.

3. Develop or modify health care services in response to the community's identified needs.
4. Monitor and evaluate program process and client outcomes.

The "Clinical Application" section later in this chapter demonstrates how nursing case management can allow an older adult resident to stay at home in a rural environment if adequate supports can be provided. Outcomes are often remarkably different when case management is used. Additional information on case management is found in Chapter 13. The need for nursing services in the community varies by community. However, there is a prevailing need in most rural areas for the following:

- School nurses
- Family planning services
- Prenatal care
- Care for individuals with AIDS and their families
- Emergency care services
- Children with special needs, including those who are physically and mentally challenged
- Mental health services
- Services for older adults (especially frail older adults and those with Alzheimer's disease), such as adult daycare, hospice care, respite care, homemaker services, and meal deliveries to older adults who remain at home

Providing a continuum of care has been hindered by the closure of many small hospitals in the past two decades and the possible continuation of this trend. Several associations, government agencies, and academic programs provide excellent resources for nurses who work in rural areas. See Box 22.4 for some suggested resources.

BOX 22.4 Resources for Nurses In Providing Services to Farmworkers, Especially Migrant and Seasonal Farmworkers

1. **National Center for Farmworker Health, Inc. (NCFH):** The NCFH offers vast resources available for both professionals and clients. For professionals, they offer fact sheets on farmworkers, demographics, human immunodeficiency virus and acquired immunodeficiency syndrome, maternal and child health, child labor, occupational health, oral health, tuberculosis, indigenous farmworkers, and folk medicine. These fact sheets are updated periodically and rely on many sources to provide succinct and easy-to-read information.

   The NCFH has developed a series of client health tips. These tips are in both English and Spanish and are distributed in print and electronically to organizations that wish to provide them to clients. They began this service in 2004, and each year the NFCH publishes on four to six topics. Selected topics are nutrition, facts about skin cancer, obesity and children, back pain, and domestic violence. Each Health Tip has photos to supplement the easy-to-read text material. Visit http://www.ncfh.org.

2. **Centers for Disease Control and Prevention (CDC):** The CDC has a national program (Racial and Ethnic Approaches to Community Health [REACH]) designed to eliminate racial and ethnic disparities in health. The REACH program is one in which the CDC partners with grantees in local areas to establish community-based programs and culturally appropriate interventions to eliminate health disparities among minority groups. In 2012, approximately $32 million was devoted to that effort. Although REACH is not targeted to rural areas, many of the partner communities are located in rural areas. Also, many of the successful interventions in urban areas can be used effectively in rural areas. See *Family & Community Health* supplement to Volume 34, No. IS, 2011 for a description of REACH exemplar programs. Visit http://www.cdc.gov/reach/ for their resource library and publications.

3. **The Health Resources and Services Administration within the U.S. Department of Health and Human Services (USDHHS):** The HRSA has a section on rural health that provides a range of resources. Visit http://www.hrsa.gov/ruralhealth.

4. **National Rural Health Association (NRHA):** The NRHA has resources on rural health (visit http://www.ruralhealthweb.org), and the School of Rural Public Health at Texas A&M Health Sciences has "Your Community's Emergency Preparedness Planning: Get Involved" at the e-mail address USACenter@srph.tamhsc.edu.

HEALTHY PEOPLE 2020: RELATED TO RURAL HEALTH

The goals of Healthy People 2020 have important implications for nurses who work with rural and migrant populations. Many objectives are relevant to these groups. It is especially important when working in rural areas and with migrant and seasonal farmworker populations to engage the community, including the public, private, and voluntary sectors, to achieve agreed-upon local objectives in planning ways to implement the Healthy People 2020 objectives.

When implementing the objectives of Healthy People 2020, consider rural factors, such as sparse population, geographic remoteness, scarce resources, personnel shortages, and physical, emotional, and social isolation. Remember that members of the community must be involved in developing the plan and assume some ownership for it. Consider how to use resources such as mobile health clinics and outreach programs of federally and privately funded clinics and the area health departments to achieve the goals of reducing health disparities and providing quality care. The How To box describes ways to build community partnerships.

♥ *HEALTHY PEOPLE 2020*

The following selected objectives pertain to residents of both rural and urban areas, including migrant workers:

- **AHS-3:** Increase the proportion of persons with a usual primary care provider.
- **MHMD-9:** Increase the proportion of adults with mental disorders who receive treatment.
- **IVP-1:** Reduce fatal and nonfatal injuries.
- **OSH-3:** Reduce the rate of injury and illness cases involving days away from work because of overexertion or repetitive motion.

U.S. Department of Health and Human Services: Healthy People 2020, Washington, DC, 2012, USDHHS. Retrieved May 2016 from http://www.healthypeople.gov.

HOW TO Build Professional, Community, and Client Partnerships

1. Gain the local perspective.
2. Assess the degree of public awareness and support for the cause.
3. Identify special interest groups.
4. List existing services to avoid duplication of programs.
5. Note real and potential barriers to existing resources and services.
6. Generate a list of potential community volunteers and professionals who are willing to assist with the project.
7. Create awareness among target groups of a particular program (e.g., individuals, families, seniors, church and recreation groups, health care professionals, law enforcement personnel, and members of other religious, service, and civic clubs).
8. Identify potential funding sources to implement the program.
9. Establish the community's health care priority list, and involve large numbers of community members in considering and selecting their health care options.
10. Incorporate business principles in marketing the program.
11. Measure the health care system's local economic impact.
12. Educate residents about the important role the local health care system plays in the economic infrastructure of the community and the consequences of a system failure.
13. Develop local leadership and support for the community's health care system through training and providing experience in decision making.

Use of Technology

Technology has great potential for connecting rural public health providers and consumers with resources outside their community, as well as with keeping in touch with them. For example, some nurses use text or e-mail messages to stay in close touch with clients and help them remember the details of their health maintenance plan. Being able to keep in touch in these ways requires that the clients have a cell phone and know how to text and that they have a computer and know how to use e-mail. The concept of telehealth is an expansion of the term telemedicine. Essentially, telemedicine more narrowly focuses on the curative aspect of health care, whereas telehealth encompasses preventive, promotive, and curative aspects of health care and can include delivery of education and information to a more distant site. Telehealth uses a variety of technology solutions such as health care providers communicating by e-mail with clients, ordering medications from a pharmacy, consulting with other health care providers, or accessing advanced or continuing education offered by a university located some distance from the receiving site. More specifically, telecommunication technology could be as simple as nurses in two or more different public health settings consulting over the telephone or via computer video conferencing to coordinate local health fairs or as complex as nurse scholars collaborating with international peers on a community health–focused research project or a medical specialist located at a health science center completing complex robotic surgical technology on a client who is located in another country. Regardless of the practice setting, the nurse must be computer literate and be proficient in using the communication technology available in that community. Increasingly, the Internet is linking nurses in rural public health practice with nursing colleagues, educators, and researchers in urban-based academic settings, thereby addressing often-cited concerns associated with professional isolation.

> ## APPLYING CONTENT TO PRACTICE
>
> As discussed, practice in rural areas relies on excellent nursing and public health skills in assessment, communication, cultural competency, problem solving, coalition building, coordination, and policy development, among others. Documents that guide the practice include the American Nurses Association Standards of Nursing Practice, the core competencies as identified by the Council on Linkages between Academic and Public Health Practice (2010), and the Quad Council Public Health Nursing Competencies (Swider et al, 2013). As one example of the congruence, consider assessment. The Council on Linkages' Core Competency of "Assess the health status of populations and their related determinants of health and illness" under their analytic assessment skills is then elaborated on by the Quad Council as a public health nursing skill of "Conducts comprehensive, in-depth system/organizational assessment as it relates to population health" (p 525). The relationship among these three sets of standards continues through all phases of the public health care provision process.

CLINICAL APPLICATION

Ethyl Lewis, a 73-year-old widow, was diagnosed more than 10 years ago with progressive Parkinson's disease. Her husband of more than 40 years died suddenly 3 years ago after a serious stroke. Her two married daughters live in California and Illinois. Her small Midwestern town has 1000 residents, and the nearest health care agency is 100 miles away. Her 75-year-old widowed sister, Suzanna Ames, also lives in town. Their brother, Bill Jones, (71 years of age) has recently entered the county nursing home located in a town 20 miles away. Despite her physical rigidity and ataxia, Ms. Lewis manages to live alone in her two-bedroom home with her dog and cat. She insists that she will not relinquish her private, independent lifestyle as her brother has. Yet within this past year she has been hospitalized three times—for a bad chest cold, for a bladder infection, and after a neighbor found her lying unconscious in the garden. Her doctor says that this last episode was related to "a heart problem."

After discharge, a home-health nurse, Liz Moore, was assigned as her case manager. Ms. Moore's office is based at the County Senior Center near the nursing home where her brother is a resident. He is also one of the clients whom the nurse checks on weekly. She provides outreach services to all of the residents in the county who are referred by a large home-health agency in the city. As a case manager, she works closely with the hospital's discharge planners to arrange a continuum of care for clients in the two-county area. Her activities include coordinating formal and informal services for clients, including nutrition, hydration, pharmacological care, personal care, homemaker services, and routine activities, such as writing checks, home maintenance, and emergency backup services.

A. Describe the nursing roles that the nurse assumes in coordinating a continuum of care for Ethyl in terms of nutrition, transportation, and health care.

B. Identify formal health care and support resources that can be accessed for Ms. Lewis.

C. Identify informal support resources that can be used to ensure that Ms. Lewis is safe.

D. Identify three outcomes that have been achieved by using nursing care management.

E. Select a rural community in your geographic area. Create hypothetical situations or select real clients with real health problems (e.g., an older adult with Alzheimer's disease, a middle-aged person with cancer requiring end-of-life care, a child who is dependent on technology as a result of a farm accident). Prepare a list of services and referral agencies in that community that could be used to develop a continuum of care for each of these cases. How are these the same as or different from the case described in this chapter?

Answers can be found on the Evolve website.

REMEMBER THIS!

- Rural environments are diverse and different from those in urban areas.
- The health status of rural populations varies, depending on genetic, social, environmental, economic, and political factors.
- The incidence of working poor in rural America is higher than in more populated areas.
- Rural adults 18 years of age and older are in poorer health than their urban counterparts; nearly 50% have been diagnosed with at least one major chronic condition. However,

they average one less physician visit each year than their healthier urban counterparts.

- Approximately 26% of rural families live below the poverty level; more than 40% of all rural children younger than 18 years of age live in poverty.
- A migrant farmworker is a laborer whose principal employment involves traveling from place to place planting or harvesting agricultural products and living in temporary housing situations.
- An estimated 3 to 5 million migrant farmworkers are in the United States. These numbers are controversial because of the inconsistency in defining farmworkers and limitations in obtaining data.
- The life expectancy of the migrant farmworker is 49 years, in contrast to 75 years for other U.S. residents.
- Health problems of migrant farmworkers are linked to their work environment, limited access to health services and education, and lack of economic opportunities.
- Migrant farmworkers are faced with uncertainty regarding work and housing, inadequate wages, unsafe working conditions, and lack of enforcement regarding legislation for field sanitation and safety regulations.

- Farmworkers are exposed not only to the immediate effects in the fields (foggy or wet with pesticides) but also to unknown long-term effects of chronic exposure to pesticides.
- When harvesting is completed, the migrant farmworker becomes simultaneously homeless and unemployed. Forced migration to find employment leaves little time or energy to seek out and improve living standards. Many of them return to their country of origin after the growing season ends.
- Children of migrant farmworkers may need to work for the family's economic survival.
- Nurses must consider the belief systems and lifestyles of a rural population when assessing, planning, implementing, and evaluating community services.
- Barriers to rural health care include the lack of availability, affordability, accessibility, and acceptability of services.
- Partnership models, in particular community health primary health care, are effective models to provide a comprehensive continuum of care in environments with scarce resources.
- Technology offers many options for providing care to people who live in rural areas.

EVOLVE WEBSITE

http://evolve.elsevier.com/Stanhope/foundations
- Case Study, with Questions and Answers
- NCLEX® Review Questions
- Practice Application Answers

REFERENCES

Annan SL: "It's not just a job. This is where we live. This is our backyard": the experiences of expert legal and advocate providers with sexually assaulted women in rural areas, *J Am Psychiatric Nurs Assoc* 17:139–147, 2011.

Bigbee J, Crowder E: The Red Cross Rural Nursing Service: an innovation of public health nursing delivery, *Public Health Nurs* 2:109–121, 1985.

Blackwell, DL, Lucas JW, Clarke TC: Summary health statistics for U.S. adults: National Health Interview Survey. 2012. *National Center for Health Stat* 10(260), 2014.

Bolin J, Bellamy G: *Rural Healthy People: 2020*, 2014, Southwest Rural Health Research Center, Texas A&M Health Science Center, School of Rural Public Health. Retrieved May 2016 from http://www.sph.tamhsc.edu/srhrc/doc/rhp2020.pdf.

Browning SR, Westneat SC, Donnelly C, et al: Agricultural tasks and injuries among Kentucky farm children: results of the farm family health and hazard surveillance project, *South Med J* 96:1203–1212, 2003.

Bureau of Labor Statistics, U.S. Department of Labor: *Occupational Outlook Handbook, 2016–17 Edition, Agricultural Workers.* Retrieved December 17, 2015 from http://www.bls.gov/ooh/farming-fishing-and-forestry/agricultural-workers.htm.

Bushy A: The rural context and nursing practice. In Molinari D, Bushy A, editors: *The rural nurse: transition to practice*, New York, 2012, Springer, pp 3–23.

Bushy A, Winters C: Nursing workforce development, clinical practice, research and nursing theory: Connecting the dots.

In Winters C, editor: *Rural health: best practices and preventive modes*, New York, NY, 2013, Springer.

Cason K, Synder A, Jensen L: *The health and nutrition of Hispanic and seasonal farmworker*, Harrisburg, Pa, 2004, The Center for Rural Pennsylvania.

Council on Linkages Between Academic and Public Health Practice: *Core competencies for public health professionals*, Washington DC, 2010, Public Health Foundation/Health Resources and Service Administration.

Cromartie J, Parker T: *What is rural?* 2015. United States Department of Agriculture. Retrieved May 2016 from https://www.ers.usda.gov/topics/rural-economy-population/rural-classifications/what-is-rural.aspx.

Crosby R, Wendell M, Vanderpool R, et al: *Rural populations and health: determinants, disparities and solutions*, Hoboken, NJ, 2012, Wiley.

Culp K, Umbarger M: Seasonal and migrant agricultural workers, *AAOHN J* 52:383–390, 2004.

Davis S: *Child labor, migrant health issues*, Monograph Series, Buda Texas, October 2001, National Center for Farmworker Health.

Gamm LD, Hutchinson LL, Dabney B, et al: *Rural Healthy People 2010: a companion document to Healthy People 2010*, vol 3, College Station, Tex, 2004, Texas A&M University System Health Science Center, School of Rural Public Health, Southwest Rural Health Research Center.

Health Resources and Services Administration: *2014 Health center data, national migrant health centers program grantee data*, Washington, DC, 2014, HRSA. Retrieved Mary 2016 from http://bphc.hrsa.gov/healthcenterdata.

Hoerster KD, Mayer JA, Gabbard S, et al: Impact of individual-, environmental-, and policy-level factors on health care utilization among US farmworkers, *Am J Public Health* 101:685–692, 2011.

Human Rights Watch: *Cultivating fear: the vulnerability of immigrant farmworkers in the U.S. to sexual violence and sexual harassment*, 2012. Retrieved May 2016 from http:/www.hrw.org.

Kusmin L: *Rural America at a glance: 2015 edition*. Retrieved November 2015 from https://www.ers.usda.gov/publications/pub-details/?pubid=44016.

Leipert B, Leach B, Thurston W, editors: *Rural women's health*, Toronto, 2012, University of Toronto.

Meit, M, Knudson A, Gilbert T, et al: *The 2014 Update of the Rural-Urban Chartbook*. Accessed from the Rural Health Research Gateway at http://www.ruralhealthresearch.org/

Messias DKF, McEwen MM, Clark L: The impact and implications of undocumented immigration on individual and collective health in the United States, *Nurs Outlook* 23:86–94, 2015.

Migrant Clinicians Network: *Tuberculosis*, 2016. Retrieved July 2016 from www.migrantclinician.org.

Napolitano M: Migrant health issues. In Stanhope M, Lancaster J, editors: *Public health nursing: population-centered health care in the community*, St. Louis, 2008, Mosby.

Napolitano M, Lasarev M, Beltran M, et al: Un lugar seguro para sus niños: development and evaluation of a pesticide education video, *J Immigr Health* 4:135–145, 2002.

National Center for Farmworker Health: *Maternal & child health fact sheet*, Buda, Tex, 2009, NCFH. Retrieved May 2016 from www.ncfh.org.

National Center for Farmworker Health: *HIV/AIDS farmworker factsheet*, Buda, Tex, 2011a, NCFH. Retrieved May 2016 from http://www.ncfh.org.

National Center for Farmworker Health: *Folk medicine and traditional healing*, Buda, Tex, 2011b, NCFH. Retrieved Mar 2016 from http://www.ncfh.org.

National Center for Farmworker Health: *Facts about farmworkers*, Buda, Tex, 2012a, NCFH. Retrieved May 2016 from http://www.ncfh.org.

National Center for Farmworker Health: *Child labor*, Buda, Tex, 2012b, NCFH. Retrieved May 2016 from http://www.ncfh.org.

National Center for Farmworker Health: *Occupational safety and health*, Buda, Tex, 2013a, NCFR. Retrieved May 2016 from www.ncfh.org.

National Center for Farmworker Health: *Oral health*, Buda, Tex, 2013b, NCFH. Retrieved May 2016 from http://www.ncfh.org.

National Center for Farmworker Health: *Tuberculosis*, Buda, Tex, 2013c, NCFH. Retrieved May 2016 from http://www.ncfh.org.

National Center for Farmworker Health: *Farmworkers and mental health*, Buda, Tex, 2013d, Retrieved July 2016 from http://www.ncfh.org.

National Center for Farmworker Health: *Diabetes*, Buda, Tex, 2014, Retrieved July 2016 from http://www.ncfh.org.

National Center for Farmworker Health: *Demographics*, Buda, Tex, 2016, NCFH. Retrieved May 2016 from http://www.ncfh.org.

National Rural Health Association: *What's different about rural health care?* Washington, DC, 2007–2009, NRHA. Retrieved May 2016 from http://www.ruralhealthweb.org.

Nelson JA, Gingerich BS: Rural health: access to care and services, *Home Health Care Manag Pract* 22:339–343, 2010.

Newkirk VR, Damico A: *The Affordable Care Act and insurance coverage in rural areas*, May 2014, The Kaiser Commission on Medicaid and the Uninsured, Issue Brief.

Occupational Safety and Health Administration: *Safety and health topics: agricultural operations*, Washington, DC, 2013, OSHA. Retrieved May 2016 from https://www.osha.gov/dsg/topics/agriculturaloperation/index.html.

Smalley K, Warren J, Rainer J, editors: *Rural mental health issues, policies, and practices*, New York, 2012, Springer.

Swider SM, Krothe J, Reyes D, Cravetz M: The Quad Council practice competencies for public health nursing, *Public Health Nurs* 30:519–536, 2013.

U.S. Department of Health and Human Services: *Healthy People 2020*, Washington, DC, 2012, USDHHS. Retrieved May 2016 from https://www.healthypeople.gov.

Villarego D: *Health related inequities among hired farm workers and the resurgence of labor-intensive agriculture*, Troy, Mich, 2012. Kresge Foundation.

Weinert C, Cudney S, Kinion E: Development of My Health Companion© to enhance self-care management of chronic health conditions in rural dwellers, *Public Health Nurs* 27:263–269, 2010.

23 | CHAPTER

Poverty, Homelessness, Teen Pregnancy, and Mental Illness

Dyan A. Aretakis, Ann Connor, Anita Thompson-Heisterman

OBJECTIVES

After reading this chapter, the student should be able to:

1. Describe the social, political, cultural, and environmental factors that influence poverty.
2. Discuss the effects of poverty on the health and well-being of individuals, families, and communities.
3. Discuss how being homeless affects the health and well-being of individuals, families, and communities.
4. Describe the ways in which teen pregnancies affect the baby, the parents, and their families.
5. Develop nursing interventions for the prevention of pregnancy problems that at-risk adolescents might experience.
6. Explain the extent of the problem of patients who have mental illness or who are at risk for mental illness.
7. Explain nursing interventions for poor and homeless people, pregnant teens and their significant others, and individuals who are mentally ill or at risk for mental illness.

CHAPTER OUTLINE

Attitudes, Beliefs, and Media Communication About Vulnerable Groups
Poverty: Definition and Description
  Poverty and Health: Effects Across the Life Span
Homelessness: Understanding the Concept
  Effects of Homelessness on Health
  Homelessness and At-Risk Populations
Trends in Adolescent Sexual Behavior and Pregnancy
  Background Factors
  Sexual Activity, Use of Birth Control, and Peer and Partner Pressure

Other Factors
Young Men and Paternity
Early Identification of the Pregnant Teen
Special Issues in Caring for the Pregnant Teen
Mental Illness in the United States
  Deinstitutionalization
  At-Risk Populations for Mental Illness
Levels of Prevention and the Nurse
Role of the Nurse

KEY TERMS

abortion, 402
adoption, 402
consumer price index (CPI), 394
crisis poverty, 397
cultural attitudes, 393
deinstitutionalization, 406
Federal Income Poverty Guidelines, 393
gynecological age, 403

homeless persons, 397
low birth weight, 402
mental health, 404
mental illness, 405
neighborhood poverty, 394
noncustodial parents, 395
paternity, 401
persistent poverty, 394
poverty, 393

sexual debut, 400
sexual victimization, 400
Supplemental Nutrition Program for Women, Infants, and Children (WIC), 394
Stewart B. McKinney Homeless Assistance Act of 1994, 396
Temporary Assistance to Needy Families (TANF), 393

Four groups of people who represent members of vulnerable populations—the poor, the homeless, pregnant teens, and those who are mentally ill—present complex nursing needs. In a society that values self-reliance, individual responsibility, and personal accountability, members of these vulnerable groups may not get the understanding and respect they deserve. Nurses need to understand their own beliefs about these groups as well as the issues surrounding the clients' illness or personal situation. To be able to interact effectively with these groups it is important for the nurse to identify health care needs, barriers to care, and essential health care services for each of these groups and, in some instances, for their families, as well.

This chapter describes the many ways that poverty, homelessness, teen pregnancy, and mental illness affect the health status of individuals, families, and communities and contains effective nursing intervention strategies for these groups.

ATTITUDES, BELIEFS, AND MEDIA COMMUNICATION ABOUT VULNERABLE GROUPS

Cultural attitudes are the beliefs and perspectives that a society values. Perspectives on individual responsibility for health and well-being are influenced by prevailing cultural attitudes. The media communicate thoughts and attitudes through literature, film, art, television, newspapers, and the Internet. Media images of persons on welfare or who are homeless, pregnant, or mentally ill are influenced by cultural attitudes and values. For example, criminals in films and television programs may be portrayed as poor, seriously mentally ill, or drug users. In recent years, as a result of the economic downturn, the concept of who is poor and who is or might become homeless has changed. Many individuals and families who have been able to take care of themselves have suffered economic setbacks because of job losses and the subsequent loss of homes, health insurance, and other essential resources.

These questions have no easy answers. However, nurses' behaviors in these situations influence their relationships with their clients. It is important for nurses to value individuals, promote health, respect and restore human dignity, and improve the quality of life of individuals, families, and aggregates. Nursing care needs to be multidimensional and include consideration of biological, psychological, social, cultural, environmental, economic, and spiritual factors. Conflicts in values, beliefs, and perceptions may arise when nurses work with persons from different social, cultural, and economic backgrounds. A lack of agreement between the professional's and the client's perceptions of need can lead to misunderstanding and conflict. When clients do not understand what they are being told or when they disagree, they may not follow the prescribed treatment protocol; the nurse may then inaccurately interpret the client's behavior as resistance, lack of cooperation, or noncompliance.

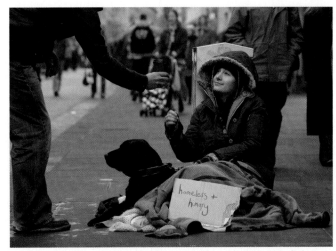

Many women, young and old, as well as those with children, are becoming homeless. (Copyright © 2013 Thinkstock. All rights reserved. Image # 79166814.)

POVERTY: DEFINITION AND DESCRIPTION

In 2014, there were 46.7 (14.8%) million Americans living in poverty. Neither these numbers nor the rate were significantly different than in 2013. In 2014 the poverty rate for children under the age of 18 years was 21.2%; for people between the ages of 18 and 64, the rate was 13.5%, and for people over 65 years, the rate was 10% (DeNavas-Walt et al, 2015). The 2016 poverty guideline for a family of four was $24,300 (excluding Alaska and Hawaii, which have higher rates that are adjusted for the cost of living in this areas) (US Department of Health and Human Services [USDHHS], 2016). The poverty guidelines are used to determine whether a family is eligible for public programs (and in some instances private program eligibility). It is thought that families need about twice as much as the federal poverty level to meet their basic needs. See Chapter 21 for a discussion of poverty in relation to vulnerability.

People who live in poverty are not a homogenous group; therefore, be sure to listen to and learn about each person. In general, poverty refers to having insufficient resources to meet basic living expenses. These expenses include food, shelter, clothing, transportation, and health care. People who are poor are more likely to live in dangerous environments, be underemployed or unemployed or work at high-risk jobs, eat less nutritious foods, and have many stressors.

For many years, income level was used as the criterion that determines whether someone is poor. Although income continues to be the measurement of choice, the federal poverty guidelines have been renamed the federal income guidelines.

The federal government uses two terms to discuss poverty: *poverty thresholds* and *poverty guidelines*. The Poverty Threshold Guidelines are issued by the US Bureau of the Census and used primarily for statistical purposes. The Federal Income Poverty Guidelines are issued by the USDHHS and are used to determine whether a person or family is financially eligible for assistance or services under a particular federal program. Income is also a qualifying factor for a variety of programs, such as federal housing subsidies; Temporary Assistance to Needy

TABLE 23.1 Poverty Guidelines for the 48 Contiguous States and the District of Columbia, 2016*

Size of Family Unit	Income Guideline ($)
1	11,880
2	16,020
3	20,160
4	24,300
5	28,440
6	32,580
7	36,730
8	40,890
8 or more	Add $5,200 per person

From *Federal Register*, January 25, 2016, p 2.
*The poverty guideline is higher for Alaska and Hawaii.

Families (TANF), formerly called *Aid to Families with Dependent Children (AFDC)*; medical assistance; food stamps; the Supplemental Nutrition Program for Women, Infants, and Children (WIC); and Head Start. The federal income guidelines are updated annually to be consistent with the consumer price index (CPI). The CPI is a measure of the average change over time in the prices paid by households for fixed market basket of consumer goods and services including housing, electricity, food, clothing, fuels, health care, transportation, and other goods and services required for day-to-day living (US Bureau of Labor Statistics, 2015).

Many people who earn slightly more than the government-defined income levels (Table 23.1) are unable to meet their living expenses and are not eligible for government assistance programs. In a family of four, for example, whose annual income is considered above the defined income level of $24,300 the adult family members would not qualify for Medicaid in some states. The terms *persistent poverty* and *neighborhood poverty* are used to describe types of poverty. Persistent poverty refers to individuals and families who remain poor for long periods and who pass poverty on to their descendants. Neighborhood poverty refers to geographically defined areas of high poverty, characterized by dilapidated housing and high levels of unemployment. For nurses, the most significant factor is being able to accept and respect clients and attempt to understand how their life situations influence their health and well-being. Being poor is one variable that must be measured against the presence of other variables that may increase or decrease the negative effects of poverty.

It was not until 1964 that the Social Security Administration established the income level of the official poverty line. Individuals and families with incomes below the federal poverty line were considered to be living in poverty. In 1965 the Medicare amendments to the Social Security Act were passed. Policy changes during the 1980s led to an emphasis on defense spending rather than on social programs. A series of events in the 1980s, such as the visibility of the homeless and the media attention on an underclass of individuals, seemed to blame the person for being poor. During the 1990s, record numbers of people received welfare benefits. In 1996 a bill creating the

TANF program was enacted. This welfare reform legislation replaced the AFDC program with a program of temporary welfare benefits. Under TANF, people are provided with benefits for a limited time and are required to find jobs and/or to enroll in job-training programs. Low-income workers often do not earn enough money to cover the costs of everyday living. Some get help from government programs, including food stamps, WIC, and child care subsidies. However as mentioned, these supports may not fully meet the most basic needs of the low-income working family.

The causes of poverty are complex and interrelated. The following factors affect the growing number of poor persons in the United States:

- Decreased earnings
- Increased unemployment rates
- Changes in retirement benefits, particularly when companies move, close, or file for bankruptcy protection and eliminate or reduce retirement benefits
- Changes in the labor force
- Increase in female-headed households
- Inadequate education and job skills
- Inadequate antipoverty programs and welfare benefits
- Weak enforcement of child support statutes
- Dwindling Social Security payments to children
- Increased numbers of children born to single women
- Outsourcing of American jobs
- Trade deficits, debt, and involvement in wars

As the fiscal characteristics of most industrialized nations have changed from industrial economies to service economies, job opportunities have increasingly excluded workers who do not have at least a high school education. Many manufacturing jobs do not pay sufficient salary to support a family, and many jobs have been moved to foreign countries where lower wages can be paid than in the United States. Also, many jobs at the lower end of the pay scale do not include health care or retirement benefits.

POVERTY AND HEALTH: EFFECTS ACROSS THE LIFE SPAN

Poverty directly affects health and well-being, resulting in the following:

- Higher rates of chronic illness
- Higher infant morbidity and mortality
- Shorter life expectancy
- More complex health problems
- More significant complications and physical limitations resulting from the higher incidence of chronic disease, such as asthma, diabetes, and hypertension
- Hospitalization rates greater than those for persons with higher incomes

These poor health outcomes are often secondary to barriers that impede access to health care, such as an inability to pay for health care, lack of insurance, geographic location, language, inability to find a health care provider, transportation difficulties, inconvenient clinic hours, and negative attitudes of health care providers toward poor clients. Access to health care is especially difficult for the working poor. Many employers, especially those paying low or minimum wage, do not provide health care insurance for their employees. Persons working for these employers are ineligible for most public health insurance programs, and they are often unable to obtain affordable health care. The Affordable Health Care Act has positively influenced some, but not all of these obstacles to getting adequate health insurance.

Poverty, while presenting a significant obstacle to health across the life span, has an especially negative effect on *women of childbearing age.* Women living in poverty have lower levels of physical functioning and higher reported levels of bodily discomfort than women in higher socioeconomic groups. Minority women are disproportionally affected by diabetes, hypertension, overweight and obesity, asthma, HIV/AIDS, and sexually transmitted diseases (STDs). Women living in rural areas face additional barriers. They may have less income, education, and socioeconomic status and live in areas with fewer providers (USDHHS, Health Resources and Services Administration, 2012).

Poverty among children in the United States has risen in all racial and ethnic groups and in all geographic settings. Any decrease in social support services increases the number of children living in poverty or near poverty. Young children are at highest risk for the effects of poverty (Box 23.1), especially lack of adequate nutrition and brain development, exposure to environmental toxins, trauma, abuse, and lower quality daily care (Children's Defense Fund, 2014).

Poverty has significant effects on *adolescent women.* Poor teens are four times more likely than nonpoor teens to have below-average academic skills. Regardless of their race, poor teens are nearly three times more likely to drop out of school as their nonpoor counterparts. Teenage women who are poor and who have below-average skills are more likely to have children than nonpoor teenage women. Poor pregnant women are more likely than other women to receive late or no prenatal care and to deliver low-birth-weight babies, premature babies, or babies with birth defects (National Center for Children in Poverty [NCCP], 2014).

Under current federal law, noncustodial parents are required to provide financial support to their children. Current child support policies are designed to provide financial security to children, prevent single-parent families from entering the welfare system, help single-parent families get off welfare as quickly as possible, and decrease welfare expenditures. Individual states are responsible for locating nonsupporting custodial parents, establishing paternity, and enforcing financial responsibility. In most states, government involvement in locating noncustodial parents begins when the custodial parent applies for TANF. There are complications in that many parents were never married and have intermittent work histories.

Although the term *deadbeat dad* was created for fathers who do not contribute to the financial support of their children, noncustodial mothers are equally responsible under the law to provide for the economic well-being of their children. Thus the term *deadbeat parent* is more gender-sensitive and appropriate.

In 2014 an estimated 10% of *older adults* (i.e., $\geq$ 65 years) lived in poverty (DeNavas-Walt et al, 2015). This is not statistically different from the rates in 2013. Poverty rates for this age group are lower, largely because of improvements in Social Security and the Supplemental Security Income (SSI) program. See the Social Security website for information about eligibility for SSI for children, survivors, retirees, and people with a disability (http://www.ssa.gov/). Poverty hits some groups more than others. Over 25 million Americans 60 years and older are economically insecure. They struggle with rising housing and health care bills, inadequate nutrition, lack of access to transportation, reduced savings, and job loss. For example, in 2014, 3 million households with a senior over 65 years had food insecurity, and only 41% of older adults eligible for the Supplemental Nutrition Assistance Program were enrolled (National Council on Aging, n.d.). People who are poor want to be treated like everyone else. It is important not to judge people who cannot pay their bills because many complex factors lead to this situation. People may be unable to pay for their medications but are embarrassed to admit this, so asking a direction question such as "Will you be able to purchase your medication?" may enable the person to acknowledge this problem and seek assistance. It is also important to learn about programs in the community that can be of assistance with medication, food, and other necessities such as utility bills. Examples might be food banks, churches, or clothing centers.

Poverty affects both urban and rural communities. Several characteristics describe poor communities. For example, poorer neighborhoods may have more minority residents and single-parent families, higher rates of unemployment, and lower wage rates. These residents are also more likely to be victims of crime, substance abuse, and racial discrimination. Differences in quality and level of education also exist. Health care is less available to residents of poor neighborhoods. Housing conditions in some areas are deplorable, with many families living in run-down shacks or condemned apartment buildings. People who live in poverty are often exposed to environmental hazards, such as inadequate heating and cooling, exposure to rain and snow, inadequate water and plumbing, and the presence of pests and other vermin. These neighborhoods often lack

BOX 23.1 Effects of Poverty on the Health of Children

- Higher rates of prematurity, low birth weight, and birth defects
- Higher infant mortality rates
- Increased incidence of chronic disease
- Increased incidence of traumatic death and injuries
- Increased incidence of nutritional deficits
- Increased incidence of growth restriction and developmental delays
- Increased incidence of iron deficiency anemia
- Increased incidence of elevated blood lead levels
- Increased incidence of infections
- Increased risk for homelessness
- Decreased opportunities for education, income, and occupation

safe areas for exercise, play, after-school, or other beneficial programs. They also tend to be targets for drug and alcohol advertising and the presence of liquor stores, where paychecks may be cashed (Robert Wood Johnson Foundation, 2014). Poverty and homelessness are linked in that poor people are often unable to pay for housing, food, child care, health care, and education.

HOMELESSNESS: UNDERSTANDING THE CONCEPT

Poverty can lead to homelessness. Homelessness, like poverty, is a complex concept. Although people who have never been homeless cannot truly understand what it means to be homeless, nurses can increase their sensitivity toward homeless clients by examining their own personal beliefs, values, and knowledge of homelessness. The questions in the How To box can aid in reflection and value clarification. Some homeless people find lodging in shelters or with family or friends. Others are less fortunate and live inside only sporadically; at other times they live on the streets.

HOW TO Evaluate the Concept of Homelessness

- What is it like to live on the streets?
- What issues might confront a young mother and her children inside a homeless shelter?
- How is it that people are so poor that they have no place to go?
- What really causes homelessness?
- How do you respond to the person on the street asking for money to buy a sandwich or catch a bus?
- How is your response different (or not) when a young mother with children asks you for money?
- How do you react to the smell of urine in a stairwell or elevator?

Poverty and homelessness are affected by the employment rate. When companies close, downsize, or relocate, workers often go long periods without a steady income. Unemployed people often lose their homes and may need to move from the home where they and their family have connections with friends and organizations such as schools, places of worship, or social organizations. Many families move first to rental sites, and some may become unable to afford the rent and move in with family or friends or become homeless. They may also lose their vehicles and become much less able to get to work, school, and appointments.

People who live on the street are the poorest of the poor, and they may be viewed as faceless, nameless, invisible, and inaudible entities. It is important for nurses to respect the individuality of all clients, including those who are homeless. People become homeless for many reasons, and there is no one set of circumstances or patterns that leads to and sustains homelessness.

Consider the situation of Mary Jones and her children, Sam and Julie, ages 6 and 8 years, respectively, and discuss with one or more of your classmates the kinds of nursing interventions that might assist this family.

CASE EXAMPLE

Ms. Jones, a single mother, was able for several years to maintain an apartment, have an older-model car, and purchase an adequate amount of food for her children. She worked for a cleaning service, and although the pay was not especially good, she worked regular hours and had health insurance for her children. She hurt her back at work, and when her workers' compensation payments expired, she found herself unable to afford her rent or keep her car. She was able to stay in a shelter at night with her children, and they were all able to have breakfast and dinner there and take regular showers. By living at the shelter from approximately sunset to sunrise, she was able to get her children to school, and she looked for work that would not aggravate her injured back.

Imagine what the life of the Jones family is now in contrast to the time when they had a home and a car. What are the most pressing issues this family faces? What options do you think are available to the family to improve their living situation? How would you respond if Ms. Jones or one of the children approached you on the street and asked you for money to buy food? Identify services and resources in your community that would help Ms. Jones if she lived there. For example, are there job training programs? Is there other assistance for which she would qualify?

As illustrated by the case of Mary Jones, the typical sheltered family is made up of a single mother with two or three children; they are most likely to be people of color, and the mothers typically do not have a high school diploma and have poor job skills and limited work options that pay a livable wage. The mothers have often been victims of domestic violence, and they often have more medical, mental health, and substance abuse problems than women who are housed (Bassuk, 2010).

According to the Stewart B. McKinney Homeless Assistance Act of 1994, people are considered homeless in the following cases (National Coalition for the Homeless, 2014):

1. Lacks a fixed, regular, and adequate night-time residence and
2. Has a primary night-time residency that is:
   A. A supervised publicly or privately operated shelter designed to provide temporary living accommodation
   B. An institution that provides a temporary residence for individuals intended to be institutionalized
   C. A public or private place not designed for, or ordinarily used as, a regular sleeping accommodation for human beings.

This definition generally refers to persons who are homeless on the streets, in shelters, or face eviction within 1 week. The two primary ways to determine the number of people who are homeless are:

1. Point-in-time counts
2. Period prevalence counts, which examine the number of people who are homeless over a given period of time.

Both methods undercount the homeless because they fail to visit many locations where homeless people stay (National Coalition for the Homeless, 2014). It is hard to know exactly how many people are homeless. On a given night in January

2015 it was estimated that 564,708 people were homeless. This means that they were sleeping outside, in an emergency shelter, or in a transitional housing program (National Alliance to End Homelessness, 2016). Accuracy is complicated by the following several factors:

- Homeless persons are often hard to locate because many sleep in boxcars, on roofs of buildings, in doorways, or under freeways. Others stay temporarily with relatives.
- Once located, many homeless persons refuse to be interviewed or deliberately hide the fact that they are homeless.
- Some persons experience short intervals of homelessness or have intermittent homeless episodes. They are harder to identify at any specific time.
- It is difficult to generalize from one location to another. For example, the patterns of homelessness differ in large versus small cities and in urban versus rural areas.

The concept of homelessness includes two broad categories, crisis poverty and persistent poverty. In crisis poverty the lives of those involved are marked by hardship and struggle. For them, homelessness is often transient or episodic, and they may have brief stays in shelters or other temporary accommodations. In the second category, persistent poverty, those affected are typically chronically homeless, and many of them have mental or physical disabilities. A person who is chronically homeless typically has been homeless for more than a year or has had four episodes of homelessness in the last 3 years (National Coalition for the Homeless, 2014). Physical and mental disabilities often coexist with alcohol and other drug abuse, severe mental illness, other chronic health problems, or chronic family difficulties. People in this group tend to be older, lack money and family support, and they need economic help, rehabilitation, and ongoing support. This group is often identified with homelessness in the United States.

Many homeless people previously had homes and managed to survive on limited incomes. Today's homeless include people of every age, sex, ethnic group, and family type. They are both rural and urban people. Surprisingly, the single homeless tend to be younger and better educated than stereotypes would suggest. Many are long-standing residents of their communities and have some history of job success. More single men are homeless than women. Families with children are the fastest-growing segment of the homeless population, with the numbers higher in rural areas. Other groups who live in poverty and are found in the homeless population are victims of domestic violence, veterans, and persons suffering from addiction. The Substance Abuse and Mental Health Services Administration (SAMHSA) has launched a Homelessness Resource Center website. The site is designed to support persons working to improve the lives of individuals who are homeless and also have mental health conditions, substance use disorders, and histories of trauma. The site is http://www.homeless.samhsa.gov. See also http://www.va.gov/homeless/ for information about help for veterans. The Veteran's Administration has also worked to reduce homelessness of veterans.

As mentioned in the previous Case Example, many homeless people sleep at night in shelters but must leave during the day. This means that during the day if they do not attend school or are not looking for work, they may sit or stand on the street, in parks, alleys, shopping centers, or libraries and in places such as trash bins or cardboard boxes or under loading docks at industrial sites. They may also seek shelter in public buildings, such as train and bus stations. Those who do not sleep in shelters may sleep in single-room-occupancy hotels, all-night movie theaters, abandoned buildings, and vehicles.

EFFECTS OF HOMELESSNESS ON HEALTH

Homelessness is correlated with poor health outcomes. The prevalence of illness in homeless people is estimated to be as high as 55%, and the average life expectancy of a homeless person in the United States is 44 years in contrast to 78 years for the general population (Gerber, 2013). Homeless people are exposed to the elements, crowded and unsanitary living conditions, malnutrition, lack of sleep and stress. Health care is usually crisis oriented and sought in emergency departments, and those who access health care have a hard time following prescribed regimens. For example, an insulin-dependent diabetic man who lives on the street may sleep in a shelter. His ability to get adequate rest and exercise, take insulin on a schedule, eat regular meals, or follow a prescribed diet is virtually impossible. How does someone purchase an antibiotic without money? How is a child treated for scabies and lice when there are no bathing facilities? How does an older adult with peripheral vascular disease elevate his legs when he must be out of the shelter at 7 AM and on the streets all day? These health problems are often directly related to poor access to preventive health care services. Homeless people devote a large portion of their time trying to survive. Health promotion activities are a luxury for them, not a part of their daily lives. *Healthy People 2020* has goals to increase awareness and use of preventive health services (see *Healthy People 2020* box), but this is difficult for the homeless.

Homeless people often have the following health problems:
- Hypothermia and heat-related illnesses
- Infestations and poor skin integrity
- Peripheral vascular disease and hypertension
- Diabetes and nutritional deficits
- Respiratory infections and chronic obstructive pulmonary diseases
- Tuberculosis (TB)
- HIV/AIDS
- Trauma
- Mental illness
- Use and abuse of tobacco, alcohol, and illicit drugs

Homeless persons are on their feet for many hours and often sleep in positions that compromise their peripheral circulation. Hypertension is exacerbated by high rates of alcohol abuse and the high sodium content of foods served in fast-food restaurants, shelters, and other meal sites. Crowded living conditions put homeless persons at risk for exposure to viruses and bacteria that cause pneumonia and TB. AIDS is also a growing concern among the homeless population because of conditions associated with homelessness. A disproportionately high proportion of homeless people suffer from substance abuse disorders. Many of them inject drugs intravenously, and may share or reuse needles; others engage in sexual practices that put them at risk. It is often difficult for the homeless person to adequately treat diseases, including HIV, because of cost and the complex treatment regimen (National Alliance to End Homelessness, 2014). Trauma is a major cause of death and disability for homeless people. Major trauma includes gunshot or stab wounds, head trauma, suicide attempts, and fractures. Minor trauma includes bruises, abrasions, concussions, sprains, puncture wounds, eye injuries, and cellulitis. Also, homeless people do not have access to dental care, places to bathe, and nutritious food, which makes it important for nursing assessments to consider teeth, skin, and feet.

In addition to its effects on physical health, homelessness also affects psychological, social, and spiritual well-being. Becoming homeless means more than losing a home or a regular place to sleep and eat; it also means losing friends, personal possessions, and familiar surroundings. Homeless persons live in chaos, confusion, and fear. Many describe experiencing loss of dignity, low self-esteem, lack of social support, and generalized despair.

HOMELESSNESS AND AT-RISK POPULATIONS

Being homeless affects health across the life span. Imagine the effect of homelessness on pregnancy, childhood, adolescence, or older adulthood; each group has different needs. Nurses must be aware of the unique needs of homeless clients at every age.

Homeless pregnant women are at high risk for complex health problems. Richards et al (2011), in studying homeless pregnant women in 31 states, found them to be younger, unmarried, uninsured, less educated, and less likely to initiate and sustain breastfeeding and to have fewer prenatal and well-child visits than other pregnant women. Outcomes for homeless pregnant women are significantly poorer than for pregnant women in the general population. Pregnant homeless women present several challenges. They have higher rates of sexually transmitted infections (STIs), higher incidences of addiction to drugs and alcohol, poorer nutritional status, more kidney and bladder infections, and poorer birth outcomes (e.g., lower birth weight, preterm labor). Although homeless women who are pregnant are at increased risk for complications of pregnancy, they have less access to prenatal care (Merrill et al, 2011).

The health problems of homeless children, although similar to those of poor children, often have more serious consequences. Homeless children have poorer health than children in the general population, and they experience more symptoms of acute illness, such as fever, ear infection, diarrhea, and asthma, than their housed counterparts. Homeless children living on the streets in urban areas are at greatest risk for poor health as a result of poor nutrition, inconsistent health care, high levels of anxiety, and an inability to practice good health behaviors. Homeless children also experience higher rates of school absenteeism, academic failure, depression, and emotional and behavioral maladjustments. They change schools often, which affects them and the school. They lose their sense of place, friends, pets, possessions, and sometimes their families. There is little stability in their lives. The stress of homelessness can be manifested in behaviors such as withdrawal, depression, anxiety, aggression, regression, and self-mutilation. Homeless children may have delayed communication, more mental health problems, and histories of abuse. They also typically witness more violence than their housed counterparts and are less likely to have attended school regularly (Gerber, 2013).

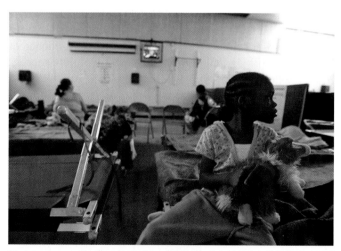

Living in a shelter can be difficult for both children and adults. (Courtesy Federal Emergency Management Agency/ Andrea Booher. Image #40530.)

EVIDENCE-BASED PRACTICE

A qualitative descriptive study using a narrative content analysis was used to explore the perceptions of homeless women about their experience in a homeless shelter–based garden project. The women planted and cared for a vegetable garden and prepared and ate their produce. The project lasted 4 weeks, and data were gathered in semistructured interviews.

Nurse Use
The findings indicated that the gardening experience interrupted the participants' negative ruminations, offering stress relief and elements of social inclusion and self-actualization. Gardening is an inexpensive and positive intervention for promoting mental wellness in a population that has a high incidence of mental illness and distress. Also, if the garden is productive, the participants can eat and share with others the results of their work.

Grabbe L, Ball J, Goldstein A: Gardening for the mental well-being of homeless women. *J Holistic Nurs* 31:258-266, 2013.

Homeless adolescents living on the streets exhibit greater risk-taking behaviors, including earlier onset of sexual activity. They also have poorer health status and decreased access to health care than do teens in the general population. They are at high risk for contracting serious communicable diseases, such as AIDS and hepatitis B, and are more likely to use alcohol and illicit substances. Homeless teens often have histories of runaway behavior, physical abuse, and sexual abuse. Once on the streets, many homeless adolescents exchange sex for food, clothing, and shelter. In addition to the increased risk for STDs and other serious communicable diseases, homeless adolescent girls who exchange sex for survival are at high risk for unintended pregnancy.

Homeless older adults are the most vulnerable of the impoverished older-adult population. They have lived in long-standing poverty, have fewer supportive relationships, and are likely to have become homeless as a result of catastrophic events. Life expectancy for homeless older adults is significantly lower than for older housed adults. The average life expectancy for someone who is homeless is 44 years (Gerber, 2013). Permanent physical deformities, often secondary to poor or absent medical care, are common among homeless older adults. They often suffer from untreated chronic conditions, including TB, hypertension, arthritis, cardiovascular disease, injuries, malnutrition, poor oral health, and hypothermia. As with younger homeless persons, older adults who are homeless must focus their energy on survival, leaving little time for health promotion activities (van den Berk-Clark and McGuire, 2013).

Homelessness has a negative effect on the health of persons across the life span. Nurses need to identify the precursors to homelessness; anticipate the effects of homelessness on physical, emotional, and spiritual well-being; and learn about resources to assist the homeless.

TRENDS IN ADOLESCENT SEXUAL BEHAVIOR AND PREGNANCY

Teen pregnancy is a public health concern because of its significant effect on communities. Female teens in the United States have higher rates of pregnancy than in other developed countries. Teens in the United States are twice as likely to give birth compared with teens in Canada and ten times as likely as teens in Switzerland. Racial and ethnic minority groups have higher rates of teen pregnancy than their nonminority peers. In 2010 the teen pregnancy rate for African Americans was nearly twice that of white teens (Danawi et al, 2016). Although some specific risk factors are discussed here, there are four social determinants of health that influence teen pregnancy rates: (1) income, (2) education, (3) social support networks, and (4) living environment (Danawi et al, 2016). These four social determinants are discussed for a variety of populations in Chapter 21 in regard to contributing factors to vulnerability.

Resources to support the special needs of pregnant teenagers are decreasing, and there are high costs associated with sustaining young families. There have been some improvements in teen risk behaviors and some worsening of others. High school students report a significant involvement in sexual intercourse. The Youth Risk Behavior Surveillance System monitors six categories of health-risk behaviors among youth and young adults. One of these categories relates to sexual behaviors that contribute to unintended pregnancy and STDs. Nationwide, in 2014 to 2015, 41.2% of students reported in the Youth Risk Behavior Surveillance study that they had sexual intercourse, and 11.5% said they had had sexual intercourse with four or more persons during their life (Kann et al, 2016). Other health issues associated with the teen years are use of alcohol and marijuana; mental health issues, including feeling sad and hopeless; and behaviors that place teenagers at risk for chronic illnesses and the leading causes of morbidity and mortality, including cardiovascular disease, cancer, and diabetes. Further, according to this study, 13.9% were obese, and 16.0% were overweight (Kann et al, 2016). Two-thirds of the teens who become pregnant are 18 to 19 years of age.

On a more positive note, today's teens have more ambitious goals than ever before, and most say that they want to remain in school and complete a 2- or 4-year college program. Also, at present, teens report being involved in their communities and volunteering at least occasionally. Teens say that religion is important to them, even though fewer than half of all teens regularly attend religious services. Since the late 1990s, teens have increased their use of media and technology; social networking is popular among this group, and most teens have cell phones and take advantage of the many functions available on their phones (Stewart and Kaye, 2012).

Teenagers who become pregnant often get caught in a cycle of poverty and school failure. They often have limited life options, and some become homeless. In addition to the goals listed in the box earlier in the chapter, *Healthy People 2020* (USDHHS, 2010) includes goals to reduce pregnancy rates among adolescent females (FP-8) and increase the proportion of adolescents aged 17 years and under who have never had sexual intercourse (FP-9).

BACKGROUND FACTORS

The majority of today's teens say they have received some formal sex education and have been taught to say no to sex, about sexually transmitted disease, and how to prevent HIV/AIDS. They do say they would like more information about abstinence and contraception (Stewart and Kaye, 2012). Many adults have difficulty understanding why young people would jeopardize their careers and personal potential by becoming pregnant during the teen years. Adolescents, however, do not view the world in the same way as adults do. Teens often feel invincible and may not recognize the risk related to their behaviors or anticipate the consequences. That is, they may not believe that sexual activity will lead to pregnancy. When teens become pregnant, many do not think they will experience any negative effects on their lives. Many think they are unique and different and that everything will work out fine. The developmental changes of adolescence, coupled with potential background disadvantages, can magnify the problems facing the pregnant and parenting teen. Pregnant teens often express the unrealistic attitude that they can do it all—school, work, parenting, and socializing.

Of teens that report having sex, the majority say they wish they had waited longer, and especially the young women in this group say that the sexual experience was unwanted. One in 10 teens say they have experienced date violence (Stewart and Kaye, 2012). Several factors that often contribute to pregnancy are discussed next.

SEXUAL ACTIVITY, USE OF BIRTH CONTROL, AND PEER AND PARTNER PRESSURE

The sexual debut, or first experience with intercourse, for a teen affects pregnancy risk. In the 2015 Youth Risk Behavior Surveillance survey, among the currently sexually active high school students, 56.5% had used a condom during their last sexual intercourse. Also, since the earliest survey the prevalence of most health-risk behaviors among youth have decreased including current sexual behavior (Kann et al, 2016). A *Healthy People 2020* goal is to increase the proportion of adolescents who have never engaged in sexual intercourse by age 17. Although more teens have begun using birth control in the past 10 years, there still is concern. *Healthy People 2020* addresses this concern with goals to increase the proportion of 15- to 19-year-olds who use condoms and a hormonal contraceptive and to increase the proportion of teens who receive reproductive health information through formal instruction and from parents or guardians (USDHHS, 2010).

Teens have many myths that contribute to poor use of birth control, such as believing you cannot get pregnant the first time, and some teens have incorrect knowledge about a woman's fertile time. Failure to use birth control can also reflect teens' embarrassment in discussing this practice with partners, friends, parents, and health care providers and the obstacles they encounter finding facilities that provide confidential and affordable birth control.

The earlier the sexual debut, the less likely a birth control method will be used, because younger teens have less knowledge and skill related to sexuality and birth control. School-based sex education can come too late or not at all. Birth control is usually discussed in the secondary-school curriculum, but this could be 8th grade in one school district and 10th grade in another;

school curricula are not standardized. Younger teens may falsely believe that they are too young to purchase birth control methods such as condoms. Confidential reproductive health care services may be available for teens, but problems are still associated with transportation, school absences, and costs of care that ultimately restrict access to these services.

Great improvement in overall contraceptive use has occurred. The current recommendation for greatest protection against pregnancy and sexually transmitted infections (STIs) is the use of a hormonal contraceptive, preferably long-acting reversible contraception (LARC), and a condom, referred to as dual protection. In 2012 the American College of Obstetricians and Gynecologists strongly recommended the use of LARC methods-intrauterine devices and contraceptive implants. These methods are reversible and have the highest rates of continuation and prevention of pregnancy, rapid repeat pregnancy, and abortion in young women (American College of Obstetricians and Gynecologists, 2012).

The use of alcohol and other substances is common among adolescents and can influence sexual activity and unplanned pregnancies. Teens are influenced by peers, partners, and parents. They are more likely to be sexually active if their friends are sexually active (Wisnieski et al, 2013). Both young men and young women may think that allowing a pregnancy to happen verifies one's love and commitment for the other. In addition, young men from socioeconomically disadvantaged backgrounds may be more likely to say that fathering a child would make them feel more manly, and they are less likely to use an effective contraceptive (Heavey et al, 2008). An online support site for parents, Onetoughjob.org, offers suggestions to parents in six major categories. One of the categories, "parenting tips sorted by age," has a section on teens, which contains 20 articles. One of the articles is "Talking to Your Teen About Sex and Sexuality." Within this section, the following tips are offered:
- It's never too soon.
- Incorporate your own values.
- Listen closely.
- Educate yourself.
- Talk about what you see and hear.
- Talk with your teen about sexual orientation.

It is important to also understand that infants may go through withdrawal if their mothers took addictive substances while pregnant. The most common drugs used by pregnant mothers are methadone, buprenorphine, opioids, benzodiazepines, barbiturates, alcohol, heroin, and marijuana. Neonatal abstinence syndrome will increase as teen mothers continue to use addictive substances (Nelson, 2013). Nurses can teach, coach, and support parents in learning how to talk with their children directly and provide useful, factual information.

OTHER FACTORS

A history of sexual victimization, family structure, and parental behaviors can influence teen pregnancy. These teens are more likely to have been sexually abused during their lifetime, with rates recorded as high as 60% to 70% (Finer and Philbin, 2013). Adolescent girls with a history of sexual abuse are at risk for earlier initiation of voluntary sexual intercourse, are less likely to use birth control, are more likely to use drugs and alcohol at first intercourse, and are more likely to have older sexual partners. The youngest women are more likely to experience coercive sex (65% of women who had intercourse before age 14 reported that it was involuntary) (Child Trends Data Bank, 2013). Young women may also become pregnant as a result of forced sexual intercourse. A history of sexual victimization will influence a young woman's ability to exert control over future sexual experiences, which will affect the use of birth control and rejection of unwanted sexual experiences. All of these factors contribute to an increased risk for becoming pregnant (Miller et al, 2010). Also, young women who have experienced a lifetime of economic, social, and psychological deprivation may think a baby will bring joy into an otherwise bleak existence. Some mistakenly think that a baby can provide the love and attention their families have not provided.

Family structure can influence adolescent sexual behavior and pregnancy. Adolescents raised in single-parent families are more likely to have intercourse and to give birth than those raised in two-parent families. Parenting styles can influence a young woman's risk for early sexual experiences and pregnancy. Parents who are extremely demanding and controlling or neglectful and who have low expectations are least successful in instilling parental values in their children. Parents who have high demands for their children to act maturely and who offer warmth and understanding with parental rules have children more likely to exhibit appropriate social behavior and to delay early sexual experiences and pregnancy. Children of parents who are neglectful are the most sexually experienced, followed by children of parents who are very strict. Furthermore, parents who discuss birth control, sexuality, and pregnancy with their children can positively influence delay of sexual initiation and effective birth control use. Parents who do not communicate about sexuality with their teens may find them more at risk for sexual permissiveness and pregnancy (Bersamin et al, 2008).

YOUNG MEN AND PATERNITY

Although there have been declines in the number of pregnant female teens in recent years, there are few data about the numbers for teen males. About 9% have become fathers before the age of 20; two-thirds were ages 18 to 19 years when they fathered their first child, and one-third were younger than 18 years. These are conservative numbers because not all of the males are aware that a partner became pregnant, nor do they always know the outcome of the pregnancy. Teen fathers face special challenges because of their own social problems, including delinquency, alcohol or substance use, school problems, and limited future plans or ability to provide support. Paternity, or fatherhood, is legally established at the time of the birth for a married teen. It is more difficult to establish paternity among nonmarried couples. Some of the difficulty lies in the complexity of the specific state system for young men to acknowledge paternity. In some states, a young man may have to work with the judicial system outside of the hospital after the birth, and if he is younger than 18 years, he may need to involve his parents.

Some young couples do not attempt to establish paternity and prefer a verbal promise of assistance for the teen mother and child. Although a verbal commitment may be acceptable when the child is born, the mother may become more inclined to pursue the establishment of paternity later when the relationship ends or for reasons related to financial, social, or emotional needs of the child. Young women who receive state or federal assistance (e.g., TANF, Medicaid) may be asked to name the child's father so the judicial process can be used to establish paternity.

Young men's reactions to learning that their partner is pregnant vary. The reaction often depends on the nature of the relationship before the pregnancy. Many young men will accompany the young woman to a health care center for pregnancy diagnosis and counseling and prenatal visits and will attend the delivery. They may also choose to be involved with their children regardless of changes in their relationships with the teen mother. It is not unusual for a young man to be excluded or even rejected by the young woman's family (usually her mother). He may then begin to act as though he is disinterested when he may really feel that he cannot provide resources for his child or does not know how to take care of the child. Mothers who report less social support from their child's father are more apt to be unhappy and distressed in the parenting role and consequently more at risk for abuse of the child (Savio Beers and Hollo, 2009) (Fig. 23.1).

Nurses can acknowledge and support the young man as he develops in the role of father. His involvement can positively affect his child's development and provide greater personal satisfaction for himself and greater role satisfaction for the young mother. The immediate concerns revolve around his financial responsibility, living arrangements, relationship issues, school, and work. The families of both teen parents can help clarify these issues and identify roles and responsibilities.

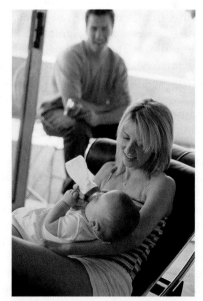

FIG. 23.1 It is important to include both the teen mother and the father in teaching about child development. (© 2012 Photos.com, a division of Getty Images. All rights reserved. Image #77280263.)

EARLY IDENTIFICATION OF THE PREGNANT TEEN

Some teens delay getting pregnancy services because they do not recognize signs such as breast tenderness and a late period. Most young women, however, suspect pregnancy as soon as a period is late. These young women may still delay seeking care because they falsely hope that the pregnancy will just go away. A teen also may delay seeking care to keep the pregnancy a secret from family members, who may be angry, disappointed, or force her into a decision she does not want to make, or because she does not want to have a gynecological examination.

Pay attention to subtle cues that a teenager may offer about sexuality and pregnancy concerns, such as questions about fertile periods or requests for confirmation that you need not miss a period to be pregnant. Once the nurse identifies the specific concern, he or she should then provide information about how and when to obtain pregnancy testing. The nurse should determine how a teenager would react to the possible pregnancy before completing the test. If the test is negative, the nurse should assess whether the young woman would consider birth control counseling to prevent pregnancy. A follow-up visit is important after a negative test result, to determine whether retesting is necessary or if another problem exists.

If the pregnancy test result is positive, the next step is to perform a physical examination and pregnancy counseling. It is useful to do both at the same time so that the counseling is consistent with the findings of the examination. The purpose of the examination is to assess the duration and well-being of the pregnancy, as well as to test for STDs. Pregnancy counseling should include the following:

*   Information on adoption, abortion, and childrearing
*   Assessment of support systems for the young woman
*   Identification of the immediate concerns she might have

The availability of affordable abortion services up to 13 weeks of gestation varies from community to community. Similarly, second-trimester services may be available locally or involve extensive travel and cost. The nurse should be knowledgeable about abortion services and provide information or refer the pregnant teenager to a pregnancy counseling service that can assist.

The pregnant teenager needs information about adoption, such as current policies among agencies that allow continued contact with the adopting family. Also, church organizations, private attorneys, and social service agencies provide a variety of adoption services with which the nurse should be familiar.

Pregnancy counseling requires that the nurse and young woman explore strengths and weaknesses for personal care and responsibility during pregnancy and parenting. Young women vary in their interest in including the partner or their parents in this discussion. It is important to discuss education and career plans, family finances and qualifications for outside assistance, and personal values about pregnancy and parenting at this time in their life. It may be difficult to focus on counseling in any depth at the time of the initial pregnancy testing results. A follow-up visit is usually more productive and should be arranged as soon as possible.

As decisions are made about the course of the pregnancy, the nurse is instrumental in referral to appropriate programs such as WIC, Medicaid, and prenatal services. The young woman and her family also need to know about expected costs of care and, if there is a family insurance policy, whether it will cover the pregnancy-related expenses of a dependent child. For those without insurance, the family can apply for Medicaid or determine whether local facilities offer indigent care programs (e.g., Hill-Burton programs for assistance with hospital expenses). The nurse can also begin prenatal education and counseling on nutrition, substance abuse and use, exercise, and special medical concerns.

SPECIAL ISSUES IN CARING FOR THE PREGNANT TEEN

Pregnant teenagers are considered high-risk obstetrical clients. Pregnancy complications can result from poverty, late entry into prenatal care, sporadic prenatal care, and limited self-care knowledge. Teens are more likely to get no prenatal care or to begin the care later in the pregnancy than their older counterparts. Barriers are the real or perceived costs of care, denial of the pregnancy, fear of telling their parents, transportation, dislike of the care provided, or the attitude of the providers (Aruda et al, 2010; Neinstein, 2008). Teens are more likely than adult women to deliver infants weighing less than 5.5 pounds or to deliver before 37 weeks of gestation. These low-birth-weight and premature infants are at greater risk for death in the first year of life and are more at risk for long-term physical, emotional, and cognitive problems, including autism (Schendel and Bhasin, 2008). For example, low-birth-weight and premature infants can be more difficult to feed and soothe. This challenges the limited skills of the young mother and can further strain relations with other members of the household, who may not know how to offer support or assistance. The risk for low-birth-weight infants and premature births can be reduced if the teen gets early and regular prenatal care. After the pregnancy, nursing supervision is important to ensure that the mother and infant care is appropriate and that everyone in the home is coping adequately with the strain of a small infant. Nursing interventions through education and early identification of problems may dramatically alter the course of the pregnancy and the birth outcome.

Violence

Teens are more likely to experience violence during their pregnancies than adult women. Age may be a factor in their greater vulnerability to potential perpetrators, who include partners, family members, and other acquaintances. Violence in pregnancy has been associated with an increased risk for substance abuse, poor compliance with prenatal care, and poor birth outcome. In the case of partner violence, young women may be protective of their partners because of fear or helplessness. Eliciting this history from an adolescent is not easy. The nurse must ask about violence at each visit. Frequent routine assessments are more revealing than a single inquiry at the first prenatal visit. Violence that begins in pregnancy may continue for several years after, with increasing severity. Variations by ethnicity have also been observed during this postpartum period; intimate partner violence may peak at 3 months postpartum among African American and Hispanic/Latino new mothers and at 18 months for white mothers (Harrykissoon et al, 2002). The nurse should look for physical signs of abuse, as well as for controlling or intrusive partner behavior (Guillery et al, 2012).

Nutrition

The nutritional needs of a pregnant teenager are especially important. First, the teen lifestyle does not lend itself to overall good nutrition. Fast foods, frequent snacking, and hectic social schedules limit nutritious food choices. Snacks, which account for approximately a third of a teen's daily caloric intake, tend to be high in fat, sugar, and sodium and limited in essential vitamins and minerals. Second, the nutritive needs of both pregnancy and the concurrent adolescent growth spurt require the adolescent to change her diet substantially. The growing teen must increase caloric nutrients to meet individual growth needs as well as allow for adequate fetal growth. Third, poor eating patterns of the teen and her current growth requirement may leave her with limited reserves of essential vitamins and minerals when the pregnancy begins. The nurse can assess the pregnant teenager's current eating pattern and provide creative guidance. For example, protein can be increased at fast-food establishments by ordering milkshakes instead of soft drinks, and cheeseburgers or broiled chicken sandwiches can be ordered instead of hamburgers. Healthy eating is very important during pregnancy, and this is especially true for vegetarians. It is recommended that vegetarian pregnant women need to consume the following daily portions: dark green vegetables (1–2); other vegetables and fruits (4–5); bean and soy products (3–4); whole grains (6); and nuts, seeds, and wheat germ (1–2) (Penney and Miller, 2008). Although these recommendations are for all women, they may need to be modified to specific teens depending on the teen's size and health status.

The recommended nutritional needs of the adolescent may depend on the **gynecological age** of the teen—that is, the number of years between her chronological age and her age at menarche, as well as her chronological age. Young women with a gynecological age of 2 or fewer years or those younger than 16 years may

have increased nutrient requirements because of their own growth. Furthermore, the younger and still-growing teen may compete nutritionally with the fetus. Fetuses may show evidence of slower growth in young women (Stang et al, 2005). The nurse, in collaboration with a nutritionist, can determine the nutritional needs of the pregnant teenager so that education can be tailored appropriately. Table 23.2 describes adolescent nutritional needs in pregnancy.

Weight gain during pregnancy is one of the strongest predictors of infant birth weight. Although precise weight gain goals in adolescence are controversial, pregnant adolescents who gain 25 to 35 pounds have the lowest incidence of low-birth-weight babies. Younger teen mothers (i.e., ages 13–16 years), because of their own growth demands, may need to gain more weight than older teen mothers (i.e., ≥17 years) to have a baby of the same birth weight. Teenagers who begin the pregnancy at a normal weight should be counseled to begin weight gain in the first trimester and to average gains of 1 pound per week for the second and third trimesters (Stang et al, 2005). Be alert to the teens' views about weight gain. Family support of the pregnant teen can influence adequate weight gain and good nutrition during the pregnancy. Nutrition education should emphasize what causes weight gain and how fetal growth will benefit. Gaining weight beyond the recommendations raises the risk for infants to be hypoglycemic, to be large for gestational age, and to have a low Apgar score, seizures, and polycythemia (American Dietetic Association, 2008).

Iron deficiency is the most common nutritional problem among both pregnant and nonpregnant adolescent females. The adolescent may begin a pregnancy with low or absent iron stores because of heavy menstrual periods, a previous pregnancy, growth demands, poor iron intake, or substance abuse. The increased maternal plasma volume and increased fetal demands for iron (especially in the third trimester) can further compromise the adolescent. Iron deficiency in pregnancy may contribute to increased prematurity, low birth weight, postpartum hemorrhage, maternal headaches, dizziness, shortness of breath, and so on (Stang et al, 2005). The nurse can reinforce the need for the teen to take prenatal vitamins during pregnancy and after the baby's birth. Vitamins

TABLE 23.2   Adolescent Nutritional Needs During Pregnancy

Nutrient	Daily Requirement During Pregnancy*	Food Source
Calcium	1300 mg (decrease to 1000 mg for 19-year-olds)	Macaroni and cheese; Taco Bell chili cheese burrito; pizza; McDonald's Big Mac; puddings, low-fat milk, yogurt; also, fortified juices, dried fruits, tofu, almonds, kale, sesame seeds, breakfast bars
Iron	30 mg (recommendation is for 30 mg elemental iron as daily supplement)	Meats, dried beans and peas, dark green leafy vegetables, whole grains, fortified cereal, dried fruits, nuts
Zinc	15 mg	Seafood, meats, eggs, legumes, whole grains
Folate (folic acid)	0.6 mg (prenatal vitamins contain 0.4–1.0 mg of folic acid)	Green leafy vegetables, liver, breakfast cereals, orange juice, asparagus, broccoli, beets
Vitamin A	800 mcg	Dark yellow and green vegetables, fruits
Vitamin B6	2.2 mg	Chicken, fish, liver, pork, eggs
Vitamin D	5 mcg	Fortified milk products and cereals
Protein	85–90 g	Lean meats, fish, low-fat dairy products, nuts, seeds

Modified from Earhart, M: What are the nutritional needs of the pregnant teens? Retrieved from Livestrong.com on July 5, 2013. Livestrong.com is the official partner of the Livestrong Foundation.
*Higher ranges are especially important for the younger pregnant teen.

should contain 30 to 60 mg elemental iron daily. The nurse should educate the teen about iron-rich foods and foods that promote iron absorption, such as those containing vitamin C.

Infant Care

Many adolescents have cared for babies and small children and feel confident and competent. Few teens are ever prepared, however, for the reality of 24-hour care of an infant. The nurse can help prepare the teen for the transition to motherhood while she is still pregnant. The trend toward early discharge from the hospital has made prenatal preparation even more important. The nurse can enlist the support of the teen's parents in education about infant care and stimulation. Young fathers-to-be would benefit from this education as well. Adolescents may not know how to communicate with an infant or know about their growth and development, or they may have unrealistic expectations about their children's development (Ryan-Krause et al, 2009). For example, they may expect their children to feed themselves at an early age or think that their children's behavior is more difficult than an adult mother might think. These skills can be taught and may prevent the child from later developing academic or behavioral problems.

Abusive parenting is more likely to occur when the parents have limited knowledge about normal child development or when they cannot adequately empathize with a child's needs. Younger teens are at risk for being unable to understand what their infant or child needs. This frustration may be exhibited as abusive behavior toward the child. Teens who exhibit more psychological distress or lack social supports should also be continuously assessed for risk for child abuse (Lee, 2009).

After the birth of the baby, the nurse should observe how the mother responds to infant cues for basic needs and distress. Specific techniques that the new mother can be instructed to use in early child care are listed in the How To box. Parenting

---

HOW TO **Promote Interactions Between the Teen Mother and Her Baby**

The nurse can make the following suggestions to the teen mother:

- Make eye contact with your baby. Position your face 8 to 10 inches from your baby's face, and smile.
- Talk to your baby often. Use simple sentences, but try to avoid baby talk. Allow time for your baby to "answer." This will help your baby acquire language and communication skills.
- Babies often enjoy when you sing to them, and this may help soothe them during a difficult time or help them fall asleep. Experiment with different songs and melodies to see which your baby seems to like.
- Babies at this age cannot be spoiled. Instead, when babies are held and cuddled, they feel secure and loved.
- Babies cry for many reasons and for no reason at all. If your baby has a clean diaper, has recently been fed, and is safe and secure, he or she may just need to cry for a few minutes. What works to calm your baby may be different from that for other babies you have known. You can try rocking, gentle reassuring words, soft music, or quiet.
- Make feeding times pleasant for both of you. Do not prop the bottle in your baby's mouth. Instead, you should sit comfortably, hold your baby in your arms, and offer the bottle or breast.
- When babies are awake, they love to play. They enjoy taking walks and looking at brightly colored objects or pictures and toys that make noises, such as rattles and musical toys.

---

education should begin as early as possible. Adolescents who feel competent as parents have higher self-esteem, which in turn positively influences their relationship with their child. Recognizing these good parenting skills and providing positive feedback help a young mother gain confidence in her role (Ryan-Krause et al, 2009).

Schooling and Educational Needs

Teen parents may have had limited school success before the pregnancy. In addition, the demands of pregnancy and parenting may make completing high school difficult or impossible. Returning to school may reduce the possibility of a closely spaced second birth, which would pose both physical and emotional stresses for the teen. Federal legislation passed in 1975 prohibits schools from excluding students because they are pregnant. Instead it is important to keep the pregnant adolescent in school during the pregnancy and to have her return as soon as possible after the birth. Several factors may positively influence a young woman's return to school. These include her parents' level of education and marital stability, small family size, whether there have been reading materials at home, whether her mother is employed, and whether the young woman is African American.

It may be hard to find affordable quality child care. Young women who have pregnancy complications may choose home instruction. The availability of home education depends on state board of education regulations. If the teen returns to school, be sure to discuss these needs: (1) using the bathroom frequently, (2) carrying and drinking more fluids or eating more snacks to relieve nausea, (3) climbing stairs and carrying heavy book bags, and (4) fitting comfortably behind stationary desks. Schools that are committed to keeping students enrolled are generally helpful and will assist in accommodating special needs.

A useful example of a program to reduce teenage pregnancy was implemented in New Britain, Connecticut as part of the National Campaign to Prevent Teen Pregnancy. This program has applicability for nurses who work with youth in the community. Their goal was to keep young people in school rather than focusing on sex education. Since it began in 1993, only 3 of about 200 boys and girls who have participated in the multiyear, intensive after-school program have become pregnant or fathered a child. The motto of the program—"Diplomas Before Diapers"—is displayed on the walls and on T-shirts. Students spend time developing basic work skills and academics. The philosophy of the program is that college is the only sure way to achieve success in their community, which has lost many of its factory jobs that paid adequate wages (Isaacs and Colby, 2008). They spent 1 hour per week only on discussions about sex education.

▌MENTAL ILLNESS IN THE UNITED STATES

Mental health and illness can be viewed as a continuum. **Mental health** is defined in *Healthy People 2020* (USDHHS,

2010) as being able to engage in productive activities and fulfilling relationships with other people, to adapt to change, and to cope with adversity. Mental health is an integral part of personal well-being, of both family and interpersonal relationships, and of contributions to community or society. Mental disorders are conditions characterized by alterations in thinking, mood, or behavior associated with distress or impaired functioning. Mental illness refers collectively to all diagnosable mental disorders. Severe mental disorders are determined by diagnoses and criteria that include the degree of functional disability (American Psychiatric Association, 2013). Mental disorders occur across the life span and affect persons of all races, cultures, sexes, and educational and socioeconomic groups. They are common in the United States and internationally.

The Center for Behavioral Health Statistics and Quality of the Substance Abuse and Mental Health Services Administration (SAMHSA) of the USDHHS provides annual estimates of any mental illness (AMI) and serious mental illness (SMI) for adults aged 18 or older. "An adult with AMI was defined as having any mental, behavioral, or emotional disorder in that past year that met DSM-IV criteria (excluding developmental disorders and SUDs)." Adults with AMI were defined as having SMI if they had any mental, behavioral, or emotional disorder that substantially interfered with or limited one or more major life activities (Center for Behavioral Health Statistics and Quality, 2015, p 28). In 2014 an estimated 43.6 million adults aged 18 or older had AMI in the United States, and an estimated 9.8 million adults in this age range had SMI. The age groups with the higher percentage of AMI were 18 to 25 (20.1%) and 26 to 49 (20.4%). Also, in 2014 there were an estimated 15.7 million (6.6% of adults 18 or older) had at least one major depression episode (MDE), and 10.2 million (4.3%) had an MDE with severe impairment. In the same year 11.4% of youth from 12 to 17 years (2.8 million) had an MDE during the past year. The percentage of MDE in this age group was about three times higher for female adolescents than for male adolescents (SAMHSA, 2015). Of these adolescents, 41.2% received treatment for depression, and there was no significant difference in males and females for receiving treatment. The issue of mental impairment is more serious when there is a co-occurrence with substance use.

Alzheimer's disease, the primary cause of dementia, is increasing. In 2016 an estimated 5.4 million Americans had Alzheimer's disease. This number includes 5.2 million people 65 years or older and approximately 200,000 who are under 65 years (early onset Alzheimer's disease) and creates a major health burden for individuals and families (Alzheimer's Association, 2016). The number of cases doubles every 5 years of age past age 60 and is becoming a public health crisis as the Baby Boom generation ages. Affective disorders include major depression and manic-depressive or bipolar illness. Although bipolar illness affects a small proportion of the population, major depression is pervasive and is the leading cause of disability among adults ages 15 to 44. Anxiety disorders—including panic disorder, obsessive-compulsive disorder, posttraumatic

stress disorder (PTSD), and phobias—are prevalent, affecting 18% of American adults each year. Mental disorders can also be a secondary problem among people with other disabilities. Depression and anxiety, for example, occur more frequently among people with disabilities (National Institute of Mental Health [NIMH], 2013).

The impact of mental illness on overall health and productivity in the United States and throughout the world is often underrecognized. In the United States mental illness causes about the same amount of disability as heart disease and cancer. Mental health disorders such as depression are among the 20 leading causes of death worldwide (World Health Organization [WHO], 2014). Depression is the leading cause of years of productivity loss because of disability. Despite the prevalence of mental illness, only one-third of persons with a mental disorder obtain help for their illness in any part of the health care system, and the majority of persons with mental disorders do not receive any specialty mental health care. The WHO reports that there is a sizable global burden of mental health, substance abuse, and neurological diseases at 14%, and in recognition of the lack of resources, the WHO launched a mental health global action program (mhGAP) to begin to address the needs (WHO, 2016). The WHO poster "No Health Without Mental Health" describes the need to integrate physical and mental health services. It is important for nurses to recognize and provide health services for those with mental disorders in a variety of nontraditional community settings.

In addition to diagnosable mental conditions, there is growing awareness and concern about the public health burden of stress, especially after terrorist attacks around the world; natural disasters such as hurricanes, earthquakes, nuclear plant meltdowns, and major fires; and human-made disasters, the wars in Iraq and Afghanistan, and the effects of the economic crisis. Strengthening the public health sector to respond to these events involves developing community mental health responses, as well as addressing physical health concerns. Community mental health nurses (CMHNs) play an important role in identifying stressful events, assessing stress responses, educating communities, and intervening to prevent or alleviate disability and disease resulting from stress.

Although every person is vulnerable to stressful life events and may develop mental health problems, those with chronic and persistent mental illness have numerous problems. Mental illness is misunderstood, and those who suffer from it often experience stigma and lack of social support that is critical to health. Persons with mental illness are often identified by the illness as a "schizophrenic" instead of a person with the illness. The onset of the disruptive symptoms of schizophrenia often occurs just as young persons are attempting to finish schooling and develop a career, shattering lives and driving many into a lifetime of underemployment, poverty, and lack of access to adequate health services, housing, and social supports. Many accessible and coordinated services are needed to enable people with chronic mental illness to live in the community, yet these often are not available. Despite the inadequacy of resources, advances have been made in the treatment of mental illness. Two movements have influenced treatment advances: consumer advocacy and better understanding of the neurobiology of mental illness (May, 2011; Pandya and Jan Myrick, 2013). Naturally, the financing of mental health services affects access to care and influences treatment. The system known as managed care had a significant impact on service delivery for the past 25 years, and passage of mental health parity and national health care reform through the Patient Protection and Affordable Health Care Act will influence mental health care in the future (Mechanic, 2012; Pearlman, 2013). It takes many accessible and coordinated services to enable people with chronic mental illness to stay in the community, and these services are not always available. The following descriptions of several key issues and populations at high risk for mental illness illustrate the scope of this public health concern.

DEINSTITUTIONALIZATION

Deinstitutionalization involved moving many people from state psychiatric hospitals to communities. The cost of institutional care was perhaps the main reason for the movement; other influences included the discovery of psychotropic medications and civil rights activism (Boyd, 2011). The goal of deinstitutionalization was to improve the quality of life for people with mental disorders by providing services in the communities in which they lived rather than in large institutions. To change the locus of care, large hospital wards were closed, and persons with severe mental disorders were returned to the community to live. Many were discharged to the care of family members; others went to nursing homes. Still others were placed in apartments or other types of adult housing; some of these were supervised settings, and others were not.

Not surprisingly, the community-based services were not often in place when persons were released to the community, and continuity of care became a problem. Deinstitutionalization was noble in conception yet bankrupt in implementation. For example, families were not prepared for the treatment responsibilities they had to assume, and few mental health systems offered them education and support programs. Although many older adult clients were admitted to nursing homes and personal care settings, education programs were seldom available for staff. The staff often lacked the skills necessary to treat persons with mental disorders. In addition, some clients found themselves in independent settings such as rooming houses and single-room occupancy hotels with little or no supervision, and others were placed in jails and prisons. These types of issues prompted additional legislation and advocacy efforts.

The development of community mental health centers (CMHCs) was based partially on the principle that persons with mental disorders had a right to treatment in the least restrictive environment (Boyd, 2011). Although CMHCs were less restrictive than institutions, they lacked necessary services. For example, people with severe mental disorders require daily monitoring or hospitalization during acute

episodes of illness. Even though hospital services were available, many individuals expressed their rights to refuse treatment and resisted admission. Also, transitional care after discharge for those who were admitted to hospitals was not available in most communities. With the repeal of the Mental Health Systems Act in 1980, federal leadership was reduced, and costs were shifted back to the states from the federal government. This further impeded the implementation and provision of community mental health services. State systems of mental health services developed in varied ways and were often inadequate. In 1990 the Americans with Disabilities Act (ADA) was passed. The ADA mandated that individuals with mental and physical disabilities not be discriminated against and be brought into the mainstream of American life through access to employment and public services (Boyd, 2011). History reveals that past legislation promoted the rights of persons with mental disorders, but litigation was also responsible for the lack of growth, if not the decline, in community mental health services.

AT-RISK POPULATIONS FOR MENTAL ILLNESS
Children and Adolescents

Healthy People 2020 objectives aim to increase the number of children screened and treated for mental health problems. Children are at risk for disruption of normal development by biological, environmental, and psychosocial factors that impair their mental health, interfere with education and social interactions, and keep them from realizing their full potential as adults (USDHHS, 2010). For example, children may become depressed after a loss or may develop behavior problems from abuse or neglect. Examples of environmental factors include crowded living conditions, violence, separation from parents, and lack of consistent caregivers. Exposure to community violence was related to significant stress and depression in children. Depression, anxiety, and attention deficit disorders are often diagnosed in children, and intellectual disabilities, Down syndrome, and autism are examples of chronic disorders. These problems affect growth and development and influence mental health during adolescence.

Suicide was the 10th leading cause of death for all ages in 2013 (Centers for Disease Control and Prevention [CDC], 2015). Also, an estimated 1.3 million people 18 years or older attempted suicide in that year, and 8% of students in grades 9 to 12 attempted suicide. Males take their lives about four times more often than do females, yet females are more likely to have suicidal thoughts than are males are. Firearms are the most common method of suicide among males, and poisoning among females. Two of the *Healthy People 2020* objectives relate to reducing the rate of suicides and reducing adolescent suicide attempts. Some of the risk factors for both adolescents and adults include prior suicide attempts, stressful life events, and access to lethal methods. In addition to depression and substance abuse, adolescent problems include conduct disorders and eating disorders.

Effective services for children, particularly for those with serious emotional disturbances, depends on promoting collaboration across critical areas of support, including schools, families, social services, health, mental health, and juvenile justice. Better services and collaboration for children with serious emotional disturbance and their families will result in greater school retention, decreased contact with the juvenile justice system, increased stability of living arrangements, and improved educational, emotional, and behavioral development. Children and adolescents require a variety of mental health services, including crisis intervention and both short-term and long-term counseling. Nurses working in community settings, well-child clinics, and home health can help offset this problem through prevention and education and by including parents in program planning. Because many children and adolescents lack services or access to them, community mental health assessment activities are essential. Assessment activities include identifying types of programs available or lacking in places in which children and adolescents spend time. Assessments should be performed in schools and in homes of clients, as well as in daycare centers, churches, and organizations that plan and guide age-specific play and entertainment programs. Assessment data are essential for planning and developing programs that address mental health problems prevalent from the prenatal period through adolescence. Preventing problems during these developmental periods can reduce mental health problems in adulthood. Areas that should be considered include children and adolescents who engage in physical fights and bullying. *Healthy People 2020* includes objectives on both reducing youth fighting and youth bullying. Families, schools, religious and community organizations, and the media are important influences on the way children and youth view violence, and education and role modeling are important aspects of prevention.

Adults

Stress contributes to adults' mental health status. Sources of stress include multiple role responsibilities, job insecurity, lack of or diminishing resources, and unstable relationships. These and other conditions can undermine mental health and contribute to serious mental illness, depression, anxiety disorders, and substance abuse. Objectives of *Healthy People 2020* are aimed at helping adults access treatment to decrease associated human and economic costs and to reduce rates of suicide.

At some time or another, almost all adults will experience a tragic or unexpected loss, a serious setback, or a time of profound sadness, grief, or distress. Major depressive disorder, however, differs both in intensity and duration from normal sadness or grief. Depression disrupts relationships and the ability to function and can be fatal. In terms of suicide, the diagnosable mental disorder is most likely to be depression. Other risk factors include prior suicide attempts, stressful life events, and access to lethal methods. Also, domestic violence can lead to PTSD and major depression among women. Available medications and psychological treatment can help 80% of those with depression, yet only a few seek help. Those with depression are more likely to visit a physician for some other reason, and the mental health condition may not be noted. Therefore it is important that nurses in all settings recognize and screen for depression.

Anxiety disorders are common both in the United States and elsewhere. An alarming 18% of the population will experience an anxiety disorder, many with overlapping substance abuse disorders (NIMH, 2013). Anxiety disorders may have an early onset and are characterized by recurrent episodes of illness and periods of disability.

The lifetime rates of co-occurrence of mental disorders and addictive disorders are high. About one in four persons in the United States has a mental disorder in the course of a year. Individuals with co-occurring disorders are more likely to experience a chronic course and to use more services than are those with either type of disorder alone, yet the services are often fragmented, and treatment occurs in different segments of the system (NIMH, 2013).

How can nurses intervene? The general medical sector, including primary care clinics, hospitals, and nursing homes, has long been identified as the initial point of contact for many adults with mental disorders; for some, these providers may be the only source of mental health services. Early detection and intervention for mental health problems can be increased if persons seeking primary care are assessed for mental health problems. Nurses are in an ideal position to assess and detect mental health problems. They conduct comprehensive biopsychosocial assessments and are often the professionals whom clients trust most with sensitive information. The use of screening tools for depression, anxiety, substance abuse, and cognitive impairment can assist in early detection and intervention for mental health problems. Suicide can be prevented in many cases by early recognition and treatment of mental disorders and by preventive interventions that focus on risk factors. Thus reduction in access to lethal methods and recognition and treatment of mental and substance abuse disorders are among the most promising approaches to suicide prevention. Nurses, long respected as community health providers, can work with legislators to develop measures to limit access to weapons such as handguns.

Adults with Serious Mental Illness

Objectives of *Healthy People 2020* that address tertiary prevention and are targeted to persons with serious mental illness are to reduce the proportion of homeless adults who have serious mental illness, to increase their employment, and to decrease the number of adults with mental disorders who are incarcerated. Brief hospital stays and inadequate community resources have resulted in an increased number of persons with serious mental illness living on the streets or in jail. Many of the persons in jail actually suffer from a mental illness. Some people arrested for nonviolent crimes could be better served if diverted from the jail system to a community-based mental health treatment program with linkage to mental health services. About half of the homeless persons in the United States have a serious mental illness or a substance abuse problem, and on any given night 60,000 are veterans (National Coalition for Homeless Veterans, 2014). Many people with severe mental disorders live in poverty because they lack the ability to earn or maintain a suitable standard of living. Even people who live with family caregivers or in supervised housing are at risk for inadequate

CASE STUDY

Two-year-old twins Reba and Tracy have had an eventful childhood. Their 16-year-old mother, Sheri, started prenatal care late in her pregnancy and delivered them at 35 weeks of gestation; they were small for gestational age. Sheri and the baby's father, Jeb, who was 21, had dropped out of high school; he used illegal drugs. The twins left the hospital at 2 weeks of age to live with Sheri at the Salvation Army apartments. Sheri's erratic and hostile behavior was impossible for her parents to tolerate. Her father was on disability compensation for extreme hypertension, and his elderly, bedridden mother lived in the mobile home as well.

Sheri, Jeb, and the twins were evicted from the Salvation Army when Sheri was found to be using drugs, so they moved in with some other young friends. By the time the twins were 15 months old, they showed clear signs of developmental delay. Tracy seemed not to see well, and Reba did not walk yet. Neither of the twins spoke an intelligible word, and neither was up to date on immunizations. With Sheri's permission, public health nurse Gina Smith talked with Sheri's parents about taking custody of the twins so that they might get the stability and care they needed. The grandparents agreed, and Sheri looked relieved when she moved the girls in with her parents. Sheri returned to living with friends.

Ms. Smith assessed the safety of the grandparents' mobile home for toddlers. She reviewed the normal milestones the girls should be attaining and taught the grandparents games they could play that would help the girls progress in their speech. She brought children's books from the local Book Buddies program for them to look at together. Normal nutritional needs for toddlers were reviewed. Within months the girls started talking and gaining weight. Tracy got glasses, and Reba got physical therapy to help her learn to walk. With the help of the nurse and their grandparents, the twins began to thrive. Are there other actions that the nurse could take to provide comprehensive care to the grandparents who have now become the caregivers for these young twins?

Created by Deborah C. Conway. Assistant Professor, School of Nursing, University of Virginia.

services because the long-term care they require frequently depletes human and fiscal resources. Rehabilitation services, intensive case management, and persistent patient outreach and engagement strategies have been shown to be effective in helping persons with serious mental illness and in lowering rates of hospitalization (Cook et al, 2009).

Nurses can provide important case management services, coordinate resources for consumers, and function as important members of assertive community treatment programs, which provide continuous assistance to persons with mental illness. Nurses by philosophy and training promote independent living and provide support and encouragement for persons to achieve a maximal level of wellness and function. Nurses recognize the importance of the mental health benefits of meaningful work that improves self-esteem and independence. Nursing interventions can be provided in shelters, soup kitchens, and other places in which homeless persons receive food and protection. In providing these nursing interventions, consider the nutritional value of the meals served in the shelters and soup kitchens. Would the food be appropriate for a person with diabetes, hypertension, or another chronic disease? If the person being housed in a shelter is mentally ill and needs to take medication regularly, will that be possible in terms of getting the medication and keeping it in a safe place?

Older Adults

In the United States the number of adult 65 years and older is projected to reach 72.1 million by 2030, up from 40.3 million in 2010. During this time, the ethnic, racial, and cultural makeup of this group will become more diverse. The mental health and substance use (MH/SU) needs of this population often occur with other health problems, and this complicates treatment. The most prevalent of these conditions are depressive disorders and dementia-related behavioral and psychiatric symptoms. Compounding the problem is the fact that older people metabolize alcohol and drugs differently than their younger counterparts, and commonly used medications may alter physical or mental health problems and increase the person's risk for overdose. Although many older people maintain highly functional lives, others have mental health deficits associated with normal sensory losses related to aging, failing physical health, difficulty performing activities of daily living, and social deprivation or isolation. Life changes related to work roles and retirement often result in reduced social contacts and support. Other losses are associated with the death of a spouse, other family members, or friends. Reduced social networks and contacts brought about by these life events can influence mood and contribute to serious states of depression. However, depression is not a normal part of aging. Given the losses of family, friends, and possibly their health that older individuals experience, it is important to differentiate between grief and major depression.

The depression rate among older adults is half that of younger people, but the presence of a physical or chronic illness increases rates of depression. Depression rates for older adults in nursing homes range from 15% to 25%. As previously mentioned, in the United States, men between the ages of 65 and 74 are in the highest risk category for suicide; men account for 80% of all suicides of those older than age 65; the highest rate is in men over 85 years of age (NIMH, 2013). Alzheimer's disease and vascular conditions can cause a severe loss of mental abilities with behavioral manifestations. Nearly half of those older than 85 years of age have symptoms of cognitive impairment. All of these conditions affect the mental health status of individuals and their family caregivers.

Older adults, because they may depend on others for care, are at risk for abuse and neglect. Healthy aging activities such as physical activity and establishing social networks improve the mental health of older adults. Older adults underuse the mental health system and are more likely to be seen in primary care or be recipients of care in institutions. The nurse can reach them by organizing health promotion programs through senior centers or other community-based settings. Home health care nurses can assess and intervene to protect those at risk for abuse and neglect, and mental health nurses can provide stress management education for nursing home staff. Stress management for caregivers and respite daycare programs for an older adult family member can increase coping and prevent abuse. Nurses can advocate with health authorities and localities to increase awareness of the importance of meeting the mental health needs of this growing population.

Most family caregivers are women who care for a spouse, an aging parent, or a child with a long-term disabling illness. These caregivers are also at risk for health disruption. The impact of caregiving has been studied in persons who care for those with chronic illness and in families of persons with schizophrenia. Caregivers of persons with severely disabling mental disorders often have their mental health threatened by lack of social support, the stigma of the disease, and chronic strain. During stressful life events such as these, it is important for caregivers to know how to manage the many competing demands in their lives.

Activities to improve the mental health status of adults include public education programs, prevention approaches, and providing mental health services in primary care. Specific approaches to reduce stress include the use of community support groups, education about lifestyle management, and worksite programs. Nevertheless, most programs currently available for adults, families, and caregivers with health problems primarily monitor or restore health rather than prevent problems. Therefore the nurse can refer family caregivers and others to organizations such as the local Alliance for the Mentally Ill for group support services. In addition, many national organizations designed for groups with specific problems have local chapters or information that can be accessed on the Internet (Box 23.2). Some state activities expand mental health services to include older adults, and *Healthy People 2020* aims to increase cultural competence within the mental health system.

Cultural Diversity

As discussed in Chapter 5, health care providers need to understand the cultural differences among the various populations they serve. In particular, nurses need to know how various groups in the United States perceive mental health and mental illness and treatment services. These factors affect whether people seek mental health care, how they describe their symptoms,

the duration of care, and the outcomes of the care received. Research has shown that various populations use mental health services differently. They may not seek mental health services in the formal system, they may drop out of care, or they may seek care at much later stages of illness, driving the service costs higher. Although all socioeconomic and cultural groups have mental health problems, low-income groups are at greater risk because they often lack resources for meeting basic physical and mental health needs.

The predominant minority populations in the United States are Hispanics, African Americans, Asian and Pacific Islander Americans, and Native Americans, including Native Alaskans. There is a great deal of diversity among these groups, as well as within each of these groups, because they are comprised of subgroups with unique cultural differences. Therefore it is important to avoid simplification and overgeneralization in discussions about the characteristics and problems of minorities. It is increasingly important to have competent interpreters if the health care provider does not speak the language of the patient or the family. Also, it is critical to conduct community assessments to determine unique characteristics and factors that contribute to mental health needs within specific aggregates of the population. The information presented here is intended to stimulate thinking and awareness for developing nursing activities in individual communities. Community assessments that include data about specific populations from organized agencies such as the Indian Health Service are important because assessment data guide the nurses' activities during all steps of the nursing process. Nurses working within broad-based coalitions of consumers, families, other providers, and community leaders can help achieve the goals of accessible, culturally sensitive, and quality mental health services for all of our people.

BOX 23.2 Examples of Sources of Information and Help for People With Mental Illness and Mental Health Problems

- National Alliance for the Mentally Ill: http://www.nami.org
- Alcoholics Anonymous: http://www.aa.org
- Al-Anon: http://www.a-anon.alateen.org
- Alzheimer's Association: http://www.alz.org/index.asp
- American Anorexia/Bulimia Association: http://www.anad.org
- American Association of Suicidology: http://www.suicidology.org
- Anxiety Disorders Association of America: http://www.adaa.org
- Attention Deficit Information Network: http://www.ishcc.org/MA/Needham/attention-deficit—information-network-inc
- Children and Adults with Attention Deficit Disorder: http://www.chadd.org
- Depression and Bipolar Support Alliance: http://www.dbsalliance.org/site/PageServer?pagename=home
- Gamblers Anonymous: http://www.gamblersanonymous.org
- National Center for Post-Traumatic Stress Disorder: http://www.ncptsd.va.gov
- National Center for Learning Disabilities: http://www.ncld.org
- Obsessive-Compulsive Foundation: http://www.ocfoundation.org
- Overeaters Anonymous: http://www.oa.org
- Schizophrenics Anonymous: http://www.sardaa.org/schizophrenics-anonymous

---

LEVELS OF PREVENTION AND THE NURSE

It is important for nurses to understand levels of prevention related to poverty, homelessness, teen pregnancy, and mental illness. Nurses can influence political and social policies and programs such as those for affordable housing, community outreach services, preventive health services, and other assistance programs for their clients. It is difficult to separate services for these high-risk groups into primary, secondary, and tertiary levels of prevention because interventions can be assigned to more than one level. Affordable housing, for example, may qualify as primary prevention, but it could also be an important secondary or tertiary preventive intervention.

Examples of primary preventive services include affordable housing, housing subsidies, effective job-training programs, employer incentives, preventive health care services, multisystem case management, birth control services, safe-sex education, needle exchange programs, parent education, and counseling programs. As primary prevention for mental health problems, nurses can provide education about stress reduction techniques to seniors attending a health fair. They also can form networks with other health professionals to educate policymakers and the public about the value of these preventive services.

LEVELS OF PREVENTION

Related to Community Mental Health

Primary Prevention: Prevent Disability
- Educate populations about mental health issues.
- Teach stress reduction techniques.
- Support and provide prenatal education.
- Provide support to caregivers.

Secondary Prevention: Limit Disability
- Conduct screenings to detect mental health disorders.
- Provide mental health interventions after stressful events.

Tertiary Prevention: Reduce Disability
- Provide health promotion activities to persons with serious and persistent mental illness.
- Promote support group participation for those with mental health disabilities.
- Advocate for rehabilitation and recovery services.

These programs could provide health education and other forms of care to strengthen community residents and consequently prevent many devastating sequelae.

Secondary preventive activities are aimed at reducing the prevalence or pathological nature of a condition. They involve early diagnosis, prompt treatment, and limitation of disability. For example, these services might target persons on the verge of becoming high risk because of the threat of homelessness, as well as those who are newly homeless.

Examples include supportive and emergency housing, targeted case management, housing subsidies, soup kitchens and meal sites, and comprehensive physical and mental health services. Nurses can work with homeless and near-homeless aggregates to provide education about existing services and strategies for influencing public policy that will provide more comprehensive services for homeless and near-homeless persons. Screening members of a community for depression during National Depression Screening Day is an example of secondary prevention.

Tertiary prevention efforts attempt to restore and enhance functioning. On a community level, these might include support of affordable housing, promotion of psychosocial rehabilitation programs, and involvement in advocacy groups for the mentally ill or homeless population. Tertiary prevention of homelessness includes comprehensive case management, physical and mental health services, emergency shelter housing, needle exchange programs, and drug and alcohol treatment. It is important to know about the social and political environment in which problems occur. Nurses can influence politicians and other policymakers at the federal, state, and local levels about the plight of vulnerable populations in their community.

ROLE OF THE NURSE

Nurses have a critical role in the delivery of health care to poor, homeless, mentally ill, and other high-risk people. To be effective, nurses need strong physical and psychosocial assessment skills, current knowledge of available resources, and an ability

QSEN FOCUS ON QUALITY AND SAFETY EDUCATION FOR NURSES

Targeted Competency: Client-Centered Care—Recognize the client or designee as the source of control and full partner in providing compassionate and coordinated care based on respect for client's preferences, values, and needs.

Important aspects of client-centered care include the following:
- **Knowledge:** Describe how diverse cultural, ethnic, and social backgrounds function as sources of client, family, and community values.
- **Skills:** Provide client-centered care with sensitivity and respect for the diversity of human experience.
- **Attitudes:** Recognize personally held attitudes about working with clients from different ethnic, cultural, and social backgrounds.

Client-Centered Care Question:

Self-awareness is a key component of providing authentic, genuine client-centered care. To clarify their own values and perspectives about poverty, nurses should ask themselves the following questions about poverty and persons living in poverty:
- What do I believe to be true about being poor?
- What do I personally know about being poor?
- How have family and friends influenced my ideas about being poor?
- Have I ever personally been poor?
- How have media images of poor persons helped shape our images of poverty and poor persons?
- What do I feel when I see a hungry child? A hungry adult?
- Do I believe that people are poor because they just do not want to work? Or do I believe that society has a significant influence on one's becoming poor?
- What really causes poverty?
- What do I really think can be done to prevent poverty and homelessness?

Prepared by Gail Armstrong, PhD, DNP, ACNS-BC, CNE, Associate Professor, University of Colorado College of Nursing.

to convey respect, dignity, and value to each person. Nurses need to be able to work with their clients to promote, maintain, and restore health. Nurses must be prepared to look at the whole picture: the person, the family, and the community interacting with the environment. The assessment may take place in the home or in a community site. Visiting in the home provides a great deal of useful information about the family, their resources, support systems, and knowledge of common housekeeping and health issues.

For example, the nurse should assess the adequacy of heating and cooling, water, cleanliness, cooking facilities, food storage, sleeping arrangements, and safety issues such as loose rugs, fire extinguishers, and fire alarms. The following strategies are important to consider when working with at-risk individuals, families, and aggregates:
- **Create a trusting environment.** Trust is essential to the development of a therapeutic relationship. Many clients and families have been disappointed by their interactions with health care and social systems; they are now mistrustful and see little hope for change. By following through and doing what they say they will do, nurses can establish trusting relationships with clients. If the answer to a question is unknown, an appropriate response might be, "I don't know the answer, but I will try to find out. Let me make a few phone calls, and I will let you know Friday." Reliability helps build the foundation for a trusting relationship.

- **Show respect, compassion, and concern.** High-risk clients are defeated so often by life's circumstances that they may feel they do not deserve attention. Listen carefully, and empathize with clients to help them believe they are worthy of care. Health and social service workers may not always treat clients with respect and dignity. Because clients respond well to nursing interactions that demonstrate respect, it is helpful to use reflective statements that convey acceptance and understanding of their situation.
- **Do not make assumptions.** A comprehensive and holistic assessment is crucial to identifying underlying needs. Just because a young mother with three preschool children misses a clinic appointment does not mean that she does not care about the health of her children; she may not have transportation, one child may be sick, or she may be sick. Find out the reason for the absence, and help solve the problem.
- **Coordinate a network of services and providers.** The multiple and complex needs of high-risk clients make working with them challenging. Many services exist, but often the people who could benefit are unaware of their existence. Developing a coordinated network of providers involves conducting a thorough assessment of the service area to identify available federal, state, and local services. Where are the food banks? Where can you get clothing? What programs are available in the local churches and schools? How do people access these services? What are the eligibility requirements? How helpful are the people who work at the service agencies? What service is provided to eligible individuals and families? Specifically, four types of programs in the community have the strongest evidence of encouraging pregnancy prevention: HIV and sexuality education programs with a life skills component; clinic-based programs with a focus on sexual behavior; service learning programs that include both volunteer work and classroom discussions about the service; and programs that are multifaceted and have youth development components, health care services, and close relationships with staff. Nurses can identify these services and help link families with appropriate resources (see the How To box). In addition, a thorough assessment of available services in a nurse's service area can identify significant gaps in essential services. Once these gaps are identified, nurses serving as case managers can work with other health care providers and with community members to advocate for necessary services (Caldwell et al, 2010).
- **Advocate for accessible health care services.** Poverty, homelessness, teen pregnancy, and mental illness can create barriers that prevent access to health care services. Nurses can advocate for accessible and convenient locations of health care services. Neighborhood clinics, mobile vans, and home visits can bring health care to people unable to access care. Coordinating services at a central location often improves client compliance because it reduces the stress of getting to multiple places. Many shelters and transitional housing units have clinics on site. These multiservice centers provide health care, social services, daycare, drug and alcohol recovery programs, and comprehensive case management.

HOW TO Apply Case Management Strategies
- Determine available services and resources.
- Determine missing resources, and develop creative solutions for service deficiencies.
- Integrate and use clinical skills.
- Establish long-term therapeutic relationships with families.
- Enhance the family's personal coping skills, survival skills, and resourcefulness.
- Facilitate service delivery on behalf of the family.
- Guide the family toward the use of appropriate community resources.
- Communicate and collaborate with professionals from multiple service systems.
- Advocate for the development of creative solutions.
- Participate in policy analysis and political activism.
- Manipulate and modify the environment as needed.
- Connect with local, state, and federal legislators.

- **Focus on prevention.** Nurses can use every opportunity to provide preventive care and health teaching. Important health promotion (primary prevention) topics include child and adult immunization and education regarding sound nutrition, foot care, safe sex, contraception, and prevention of chronic illness. Screening for health problems such as TB, diabetes, hypertension, foot problems, and anemia is an important form of secondary prevention. Know what other screening and health promotion services are available in the target area, such as nutrition programs, job-training programs, educational programs, housing programs, and legal services. All of these services may be included in a comprehensive plan of care. Younger sisters of pregnant teens are twice as likely to become pregnant themselves. Thus health teaching about sexuality issues when seeing the teens in the home or clinic can increase their knowledge and awareness.
- **Know when to walk beside the client and when to encourage the client to walk ahead.** This area is often difficult for the nurse to implement. Nursing interventions range from extensive care activities to minimal support. At times, nursing actions include providing encouragement and support or providing information. At other times, nurses may actually call a pediatrician to set up an appointment for a sick child and may call again to see that the appointment was kept. Nurses assess for the presence of strengths, problem-solving ability, and coping ability of an individual or family while providing information on where and how to gain access to services. For example, a local hospital may provide free mammograms for uninsured women. Women who qualify for this free service may not take advantage of it because they are afraid they may have breast cancer. Nurses can find out about this important service, inform the women of the service, teach them about the importance of preventive care, and assess and deal with fear and anxiety. The challenge for the nurse becomes choosing whether to schedule the appointments for the women or simply provide them with a referral sheet, knowing that many will not follow through. The choice is not clear, but the goal is to

make a needed screening intervention available without taking away the woman's right to decide what to do for herself.

- **Develop a network of support for yourself.** Caring for high-risk populations is challenging, rewarding, and at times exhausting. It is important to find a source of personal strength, renewal, and hope. The people you encounter are often looking to you to maintain hope and provide encouragement. Discover for yourself what restores and encourages you. For some nurses it is poetry, music, painting, or weaving. For others it is a walk in a peaceful place, a weekend retreat, a good run, a workout at the gym, or meeting with other nurses who are engaged in the same work. Be attentive to your own needs, and create the time and space to restore your spirit.

> ## APPLYING CONTENT TO PRACTICE
>
> This chapter describes the role of the nurse who works with persons who are poor or who may be homeless, have serious mental illness, or be a teen parent. With each population, the role is diverse and complex and relies on basic nursing knowledge, as well as specific knowledge about the population. Providing effective nursing care in the community draws on many of the recommendations of nursing and public health groups. For example, the core competencies adopted by the Council on Linkages Between Academia and Public Health Practice (2010) include those related to assessment, policy development and program-planning skills, communication and cultural competency skills, and involvement with the community to provide services effectively. Swider et al on behalf of the Quad Council of Public Nursing Organizations (2013) further develop these skills and make clear application to nursing practice. Also, the American Nurses Association, American Psychiatric Nurses' Association, and International Society of Psychiatric-Mental Health Nurses (2007) scope and standards of practice identify specific nursing competencies by specialty area.

PRACTICE APPLICATION

A local youth-serving agency requested the assistance of a nurse in community health, Kristen Moore, in the implementation of a new high school–based program for pregnant and parenting teen girls. The primary goal of the program was to keep these teens in school through graduation. The secondary goal was to provide knowledge and skills about healthy pregnancy, labor and delivery, and parenting. After delivery, students enrolled in this program were paid for school attendance, and this money could be used to defray the costs of child care.

A nurse in community health was the ideal choice to conduct the educational sessions. The group met weekly during the lunch hour. The curriculum that was developed had topics ranging from early pregnancy through the toddler years. Occasionally, Ms. Moore brought in outside speakers such as a labor and delivery nurse or an early intervention specialist.

She also met individually with each enrolled student to provide case management services. Ideally, she would ensure that each student had a health care provider for prenatal care, that each was visited at home by a nurse in community health, that each had enrolled in WIC and Medicaid, if eligible,

and that both the pregnant teen and her partner knew about other parenting and support groups.

One educational session that was particularly interesting was the discussion about the postpartum period—the 6 weeks after delivery. There were many lively discussions about labor experiences, as well as some emotional discussions about the reality of coming home with a baby and changes in the relationship with the new mothers' male partner. Many girls benefited from understanding the normalcy of postpartum blues, but one young woman recognized that she had a more serious and persistent depression and privately approached the nurse for assistance.

At the end of the first school year, the dropout rate for pregnant and parenting teens had been reduced by half, and preterm labor rates had also declined. The local school board and the local youth-serving agency joined together to provide financial support to continue this program for an additional 2 years. Ms. Moore was asked to expand the educational programs and interventions she had developed.

What are some directions in which the nurse could expand the program? List four.
Answers can be found on the Evolve website.

REMEMBER THIS!

- Poverty and homelessness affect the health status of people.
- To understand poverty, homelessness, teen pregnancy, and mental illness, consider your personal beliefs and attitudes, clients' perceptions of their condition, and the social, political, cultural, and environmental factors that influence the client's situation.
- The definition of poverty varies depending on the source consulted. The federal government defines poverty on the basis of income, family size, age of the head of household, and number of children younger than 18 years. Those who are poor insist that poverty has less to do with income and more to do with a lack of family, friends, love, and support.
- Factors leading to the growing number of poor persons in the United States include decreased earnings, diminishing availability of low-cost housing, increases in the number of households headed by women (women's incomes are traditionally lower than men's), inadequate education, lack of marketable job skills, welfare reform, and reduced Social Security payments to children.
- Poverty has a direct effect on health and well-being across the life span. Poor persons have higher rates of chronic illness, higher infant morbidity and mortality, shorter life expectancy, and more complex health problems.
- At present, the following groups often constitute the homeless in both rural and urban areas: families, single mothers, single women, recently unemployed persons, substance abusers, adolescent runaways, mentally ill individuals, and single men.

- Factors contributing to homelessness include an increase in the number of persons living in poverty, diminishing availability of low-cost housing, increased unemployment, substance abuse, lack of treatment facilities for mentally ill persons, domestic violence, and family situations causing children to run away.
- The complex health problems of homeless persons include inability to get adequate rest, exercise, and nutrition; exposure; infectious diseases; acute and chronic illness; infestations; trauma; and mental health problems.
- The provision of reproductive health care services to teens requires sensitivity to the special needs of this age group, including knowing about state laws concerning confidentiality and services for birth control, pregnancy, abortion, and adoption.
- Factors such as a history of sexual victimization, family dysfunction, substance use, and failure to use birth control can influence whether a young woman becomes pregnant.

- Adolescents, especially those who become pregnant, have special nutritional needs.
- The pregnant teen will need support during and after the pregnancy from the family and friends and from the father of the baby.
- Prevalence rates for mental health problems are high, and people are at risk for threats to mental health at all ages across the life span.
- Low-income and minority groups are often at increased risk for mental illness because they may lack access to services.
- Nurses have a critical role in the delivery of care to persons who are high risk. Nurses bring to each client encounter the ability to assess the client in context and intervene in ways that restore, maintain, or promote health.

ⓔ EVOLVE WEBSITE

http://evolve.elsevier.com/Stanhope/foundations
- Case Study, with Questions and Answers
- NCLEX® Review Questions
- Practice Application Answers

REFERENCES

Alzheimer's Association: *Alzheimer's disease facts and figures 2016*, Retrieved August 2016 at http://www.ALZ.org/fact/overview/asp.

American College of Obstetricians and Gynecologists: Committee opinion no. 539. Adolescents and long acting reversible contraception: implants and intrauterine devices, *Obstet Gynecol* 120:983–988, 2012.

American Dietetic Association Report: Position of the American Dietetic Association: nutrition and lifestyle for a healthy pregnancy outcome, *J Am Dietet Assoc* 108:553–561, 2008.

American Nurses Association, American Psychiatric Nurses' Association, International Society of Psychiatric-Mental Health Nurses: *Scope and standards of psychiatric-mental health nursing*, Washington, DC, 2007, American Nurses Publishing.

American Psychiatric Association: *Diagnostic and statistical manual of mental disorders*, ed 5, Washington, DC, 2013, APA.

Aruda M, Wadicor K, Frese L, et al: Early pregnancy in adolescents: diagnosis, assessment, options, counseling, and referral, *J Pediatr Health Care* 24:4–13, 2010.

Bassuk EL: Ending child homelessness in America, *Am J Orthopsychiatry* 80:496–504, 2010.

Bersamin M, Todd M, Fisher DA, et al: Parenting practices and adolescent sexual behavior: a longitudinal study, *J Marriage Fam* 70:97–112, 2008.

Boyd MA: Social change and mental health. In Boyd MA, editor: *Psychiatric nursing: contemporary practice*, ed 4, Philadelphia, 2011, Lippincott Williams & Wilkins.

Caldwell BA, Sclafani M, Swarbrick M, et al: Psychiatric nursing practice and the recovery model of care, *J Psychosoc Nurs Ment Health Serv* 48:42–48, 2010.

Center for Behavioral Health Statistics and Quality: *Behavioral trends in the United States: Results from the 2014 National Survey on Drug Use and Health* (HHS Publication No SMA 15-4927, NSDUH Series H-50), 2015. Retrieved August 2016 from http://www.samhsa.gov/data/.

Centers for Disease Control and Prevention: Suicide: *Facts at a Glance*, 2015. Retrieved August 2016 from http://www.cdc.gov/violenceprevention.

Child Trends Data Bank: *Statutory rape: sex between young teens and older individuals*, Washington, DC, 2013, Child Trends.

Children's Defense Fund: *The State of America's Children 2014 Report*, 2014. Retrieved August 2016 from http://www.childrendefense.org.

Cook JA, Copeland ME, Hamilton MM, et al: Initial outcomes of a mental illness self-management program based on wellness recovery action planning, *Psychiatr Serv* 60(2):246–249, 2009.

Council on Linkages Between Academic and Public Health Practice: *Core competencies for public health professionals*, Washington, DC, 2010, Public Health Foundation, Health Resources and Services Administration.

Danawi H, Bryant Z, Hasbini T: Targeting unintended teen pregnancy in the US International, *Journal of Childbirth Education* 31(1):28–31, January 2016.

DeNavas-Walt C, Proctor D, Smith JC: *Income and poverty, in the United States: 2014, Report Number P60–252*, Washington, DC, 2015, US Government Printing Office.

Earhart M: *What are the nutritional needs of the pregnant teens?* August 13, 2015. Retrieved from Livestrong.com on June 18, 2017.

Finer LB, Philbin JM: Sexual initiation, contraceptive use and pregnancy among young adolescents, *Pediatrics* 131:886–891, 2013.

Gerber L: Bringing home effective nursing care for the homeless, *Nursing* 43:32–38, 2013.

Grabbe L, Ball J, Goldstein A: Gardening for the mental well-being of homeless women, *J Holistic Nurs* 31:258–266, 2013.

Guillery ME, Benzies KM, Mannion C, et al: Postpartum nurses' perceptions of barriers to screening for intimate partner violence: a cross-sectional survey, *BMC Nurs* 11(2):1–8, 2012.

Harrykissoon SD, Rickert VI, Wiemann CW: Prevalence and patterns of intimate partner violence among adolescent mothers during the postpartum period, *Arch Pediatr Adolesc Med* 156:325, 2002.

Heavey EJ, Moysich KB, Hyland A, et al: Female adolescents' perceptions of male partners' pregnancy desire, *J Midwifery Women's Health* 53:338–344, 2008.

Kann L, McManus T, Harris WA, et al: Youth risk behavior surveillance—United States, 2015, *MMWR* 65(6):1, June 10, 2016.

Lee Y: Early motherhood and harsh parenting: the role of human, social and cultural capital, *Child Abuse Negl* 33:625–637, 2009.

May A: Experience-dependent structural plasticity in the adult human brain, *Trends Cogn Sci* 15:475–482, 2011.

Mechanic D: Seizing opportunities under the Affordable Care Act for transforming the mental and behavioral health system, *Health Aff* 31:376–382, 2012.

Merrill RM, Richards R, Sloan A: Prenatal maternal stress and physical abuse among homeless women and infant health outcomes in the United States, *Epidemiol Res Int* 2011:2011. Retrieved August 2016 from http://www/dx/doi.org/10.1155/2011/467265.

National Alliance to End Homelessness: *Homelessness: snapshot of homelessness*, Washington, DC, 2014. http://www.Endhomelessness.org.

National Alliance to End Homelessness: *The State of Homelessness in America*, Washington, DC, 2016. http://www.Endhomelessness.org.

National Center for Children in Poverty (NCCP): *Basic factors about low-income children: children under 18 years (fact sheet)*, 2014. Retrieved August 2016 from http://www.nccp.org.

National Coalition for Homeless Veterans: *Background and statistics*, 2014. Retrieved August 2016 from http://www.nchv.org.

National Coalition for the Homeless: *Homelessness in America*, 2014. Retrieved August 2016 from http://www.Nationalhomeless.org/abouthomelessness/.

National Council on Aging: *Economic security: fact sheet*, n.d., Retrieved August 2016 from http://www.mcoa.org.

National Institute of Mental Health: *The numbers count: mental disorders in America*, Bethesda, MD, 2013, NIMH. Retrieved August 2012 from http://www.nimh.nih.gov/health/publications/.

Neinstein LS, editor: *Adolescent health care*, ed 5, Philadelphia, 2008, Lippincott Williams and Wilkins.

Nelson MM: Neonatal abstinence syndrome: The nurse's role, *International Journal of Childbirth Education* 28(1):38–42, January 2013.

One tough job.org: *Talking to your teen about sex and sexuality*. Retrieved June 2013 from http://www.onetoughjob.org/tips/teens/talking-to-your-teens-about-sex-and-sexuality.

Pandya A, Jan Myrick K: Wellness recovery program: a model of self-advocacy for people living with mental illness, *J Psychiatr Pract* 19:242–246, 2013.

Pearlman SA: The Patient Protection and Affordable Health Care Act: impact on mental health services demand and provider availability, *J Am Psychiatric Nurses Assoc* 19:327–334, 2013.

Penny DS, Miller KG: Nutritional counseling for vegetarians during pregnancy and lactation, *J Midwifery Women's Health* 53:37–44, 2008.

Richards R, Merrill RM, Baksh L: Health behaviors and infant health outcomes in homeless pregnant women in the United States, *Pediatrics* 128:438–446, 2011.

Robert Wood Johnson Foundation: *Neighborhoods and health: exploring the social determinants of health* (Issue Brief 38), 2014.

Ryan-Krause P, Meadows-Oliver M, Sadler L, et al: Developmental status of children of teen mothers: contrasting objective assessments with maternal reports, *J Pediatr Health Care* 23:303–309, 2009.

Savio Beers LA, Hollo RE: Approaching the adolescent-headed family: a review of teen parenting, *Curr Probl Pediatr Adolesc Health Care* 39:216–233, 2009.

Schendel D, Bhasin TK: Birth weight and gestational age characteristics of children with autism, including a comparison with other developmental disabilities, *Pediatrics* 121:1155–1161, 2008.

Stang J, Story M, Feldman S: Nutrition in adolescent pregnancy, *Int J Childbirth Educ* 20:4–11, 2005.

Stewart A, Kaye K: *Freeze frame 2012: a snapshot of America's teens*, Washington, DC, 2012, National Campaign to Prevent Teen and Unplanned Pregnancy.

Substance Abuse and Mental Health Services Administration: *Behavioral Health Barometer: United States, 2015*. HHS Publication No. SMA-16-Bar0-2015. Rockville, MD, 2015, Substance Abuse and Mental Health Services Administration.

Swider SM, Krothe J, Reyes D, Cravetz M: The Quad Council practice competencies for public health nursing, *Public Health Nursing* 30(6):519–536, 2013.

US Bureau of Labor Statistics: *Consumer price index*, Washington, DC, 2015, US Department of Labor.

US Department of Health and Human Services: *Healthy People 2020*, Washington, DC, 2010, US Government Printing Office.

U. S. Department of Health and Human Services: *Poverty Guidelines, 1/25/2016*. Washington DC, 2016, Office of the Federal Register.

US Department of Health and Human Services: *Poverty Guidelines*, Washington, DC, January 25, 2016, Office of the Federal Register.

US Department of Health and Human Services, Health Resources and Services Administration: *Women's Health USA 2012*, Washington, DC, 2012, US Government Printing Office.

Van den Berk-Clark, McGuire J: Elderly homeless veterans in Los Angeles: Chronicity and precipitants of homelessness, *Am J Public Health* 103(Suppl 2):S232–S238, 2013.

Wisnieski D, Sieving RE, Garwick AW: Influence of peers on young adolescent females' romantic decisions, *Am J Health Educ* 44:32–40, 2013.

World Health Organization: *10 facts on the state of global health*, 2014. Retrieved August 2016 at http://www.who.int.

World Health Organization: *Mental health. mhGAP Programme expands to include scalable psychological interventions*, May 20, 2016. Retrieved August 2016 from http://www.who.int.

CHAPTER 24

Alcohol, Tobacco, and Other Drug Problems in the Community

Mary Lynn Mathre

OBJECTIVES

After reading this chapter, the student should be able to:

1. Describe attitudes about alcohol, tobacco, and other drug problems.
2. Differentiate among these terms: *substance use, abuse, dependence,* and *addiction.*
3. Discuss the differences among the major psychoactive drug categories of depressants, stimulants, marijuana, hallucinogens, and inhalants.
4. Explain the role of the nurse in primary, secondary, and tertiary prevention of alcohol, tobacco, and other drug problems as it relates to individual clients and their families.
5. Explain the effect of substance abuse on the community and on people within the community.

CHAPTER OUTLINE

Scope of the Problem
  Definitions
Psychoactive Drugs
  Alcohol
  Tobacco
  Electronic Nicotine Delivery Systems
  Caffeine
Illicit Drug Use
  Opioids
  Cocaine
  Amphetamines and Methamphetamine
  Marijuana
  Street Drugs Commonly Used
Predisposing and Contributing Factors
  Genetic Factors in Addiction

Primary Prevention and the Role of the Nurse
  Drug Education
Secondary Prevention and the Role of the Nurse
  Assessing for Alcohol, Tobacco, and Other Drug
    Problems
  Drug Testing
  High-Risk Groups
  Codependency and Family Involvement
Tertiary Prevention and the Role of the Nurse
  Detoxification
  Addiction Treatment
  Smoking Cessation Programs
  Support Groups
The Nurse's Role

KEY TERMS

addiction treatment, 428
alcohol, 417
Alcoholics Anonymous (AA), 429
alcoholism, 417
amphetamines, 421
blood alcohol concentration
    (BAC), 418
brief interventions, 429
cocaine, 421
codependency, 427
denial, 425
depressants, 417
detoxification, 428

drug addiction, 417
drug dependence, 417
electronic cigarettes (e-cigarettes),
    419
enabling, 427
energy drinks, 417
fetal alcohol syndrome (FAS), 427
genetics, 418
harm reduction, 416
heroin, 421
injection drug users (IDUs), 427
mainstream smoke, 419
marijuana, 422

methamphetamines, 421
opioids, 421
polysubstance use or abuse, 424
psychoactive drugs, 417
secondhand smoke, 419
set, 422
setting, 422
sidestream smoke, 419
stimulants, 417
substance abuse, 417
tolerance, 418
vaping, 420
withdrawal, 417

Substance abuse is the leading national health problem, causing more deaths, illnesses, and disabilities than any other health condition. Considerable death and disability are caused by the use of alcohol, tobacco, and illicit drugs. The substance abuser not only is at risk for personal health problems but also may be a threat to the health and safety of family members, coworkers, and other members of the community. Substance abuse and addiction affect all ages, races, sexes, and segments of society. *Healthy People 2020* (US Department of Health and Human Services [USDHHS], 2010a) in collaboration with the Institute of Medicine have identified 12 key topics, 24 key objectives, and 24 leading indicators that are essential to the health needs of the nation (Institute of Medicine, 2011). Substance abuse, one of the top 10 indicators, affects individuals, families, and communities, and the effects are cumulative. Some of the problems that *Healthy People 2020* states are caused by substance abuse include teenage pregnancy, human immunodeficiency virus (HIV) infection, acquired immunodeficiency syndrome (AIDS), other sexually transmitted diseases (STDs), domestic violence, child abuse, motor vehicle crashes, physical fights, crime, homicide, and suicide (USDHHS, 2010a). Similarly, tobacco use is a significant health risk in that cancer, heart disease, and the lung diseases of emphysema, bronchitis, and chronic airway obstruction are associated with tobacco use. Additionally, premature birth, low birth weight, stillbirth, and infant death are associated with tobacco use (USDHHS, 2010a). New forms of substance use include e-cigarettes and the increasing use of opioids.

The newer phrase *alcohol, tobacco, and other drug (ATOD) problems,* rather than *substance abuse,* reminds us that alcohol and tobacco represent the major drugs of abuse when discussing substance abuse, drug addiction, or chemical dependency. The term *ATOD* will be used primarily in the chapter.

SCOPE OF THE PROBLEM

As mentioned previously, substance or ATOD abuse and addiction can cause multiple health problems for individuals. Factors that contribute to the substance abuse problem include lack of knowledge about the use of drugs, the labeling of certain drugs (i.e., alcohol, nicotine, and caffeine) as nondrugs, lack of quality control of illegal drugs, law enforcement rather than prevention and treatment of the abuse of and addictions to ATODs, and drug laws that label certain drug users as criminals, which encourages negative attitudes and stigma toward these persons. Evidence also points to a relationship between genetic factors and ATOD dependence (Dick and Agrawal, 2008).

Every culture has beliefs and attitudes toward ATOD. These attitudes are influenced by the way society categorizes drugs as either "good" or "bad." In the United States, good drugs are over-the-counter (OTC) drugs or drugs prescribed by a health care provider, although this makes them no less problematic or addictive. "Bad drugs" are the illegal drugs, and persons who use these drugs are considered criminals regardless of whether the drug has caused any problems. Americans rely heavily on prescription and OTC drugs to relieve (or mask) anxiety, tension, fatigue, and physical or emotional pain. Rather than

learning nonmedicinal methods of coping, many people choose the "quick fix" and take pills to deal with their problems or negative feelings. Addicted persons are often viewed as immoral, weak-willed, or irresponsible, and others often think they should try harder to help themselves. Although alcoholism was recognized as a disease by the American Medical Association in 1954, and drug addiction was recognized as a disease some years later, much of the public and many health care professionals do not consider alcoholics and addicted persons to be ill and in need of health care.

In many cultures, people with ATOD problems are treated through the criminal justice system. As one example, the United States is having an epidemic of drug overdose deaths, with the biggest offenders being opioid pain relievers and heroin (Rudd et al, 2016). However, a newer approach, the **harm reduction** model, is a public health approach to ATOD problems. The early countries to use this approach were Great Britain, the Netherlands, Germany, Switzerland, and Australia. Increased interest and momentum are spreading throughout Europe and Canada. This public health model recognizes the following:

- Addiction is a health problem.
- Any psychoactive drug can be abused.
- Accurate information can help people make responsible decisions about drug use.
- People who have ATOD problems can be helped.

This approach accepts that psychoactive drug use is endemic, and it focuses on pragmatic interventions, especially education, to reduce the adverse consequences of drug use and get treatment for addicted persons. The United States has already taken a harm reduction approach with tobacco and alcohol. Educational campaigns are used to inform the public about the health risks of tobacco use. Warnings have appeared on tobacco product labels since 1967 as a result of the Surgeon General's 1966 report on the dangers of smoking. In 1971 a ban on television and radio cigarette advertising was imposed. Cigarette smoking has decreased since that time. Smoking is on the decline among 12- to 17-year-olds. "Tobacco smoking is the leading cause of preventable disease and death in the United States" (Jama et al, 2015, p 1233). The number of adults in the United States who smoke declined from 20.9% in 2005 to 16.8% in 2014. Likewise, cigarette smoking among youth has declined in recent years, but the use of other tobacco products has increased, especially the use of electronic cigarettes and hookahs. The habit of smoking typically begins by the age of 18 (Centers for Disease Control and Prevention [CDC], 2016).

It is important to continue educating people about the dangers of smoking and of alcohol and other drug abuse and to establish guidelines for safe alcohol use. Nurses need to know about the new forms of smoking that deliver tobacco's toxic effects. Nurses need to identify the causes of various health problems and plan realistic, nonjudgmental, holistic, and positive actions. The harm reduction model can be used effectively for ATOD problems. To develop a therapeutic attitude, the nurse must realize that any drug can be abused, that anyone may develop drug dependence, and that drug addiction can be successfully treated.

DEFINITIONS

The terms *drug use* and *drug abuse* have virtually lost their usefulness because the public and government have narrowed the term *drug* to include only illegal drugs rather than including prescription, OTC, and legal recreational drugs. The current phrase *alcohol, tobacco, and other drugs* (ATOD) reminds us that the leading drug problems involve alcohol and tobacco and that new forms of abuse are being tried by youth and adults. The term *substance* broadens the scope to include alcohol, tobacco, legal drugs, and even foods and substances such as bath salts. Substance abuse is the use of any substance that threatens a person's health or impairs social or economic functioning. This definition is more objective and universal than the government's definition of drug abuse, which is the use of a drug without a prescription or any use of an illegal drug. Although any drug or food can be abused, this chapter focuses on psychoactive drugs—drugs that affect mood, perception, and thought.

Drug dependence and drug addiction are often used interchangeably, but they are not synonymous. Drug dependence is a state of neuroadaptation (a physiological change in the central nervous system [CNS] and alterations in other systems caused by the chronic, regular administration of a drug). People who are dependent on drugs must continue using them to prevent symptoms of withdrawal. For example, when a person is given an opiate such as morphine on a regular basis for pain management, the morphine needs to be gradually tapered rather than abruptly stopped, to prevent symptoms of withdrawal. Drug dependence is both psychological and physical. Psychological dependence includes feelings of satisfaction and a desire to repeat the drug experience or to avoid the discomfort of not having the drug. Craving and compulsion are part of this dependence. Physical dependence is seen when there is an abstinence effect. This effect results in physical changes that are uncomfortable.

Drug addiction is a pattern of abuse characterized by an overwhelming preoccupation with the use (compulsive use) of a drug and securing its supply and a high tendency to relapse if the drug is removed. Addicts may be both physically and psychologically dependent on a drug, and there may be a risk for harm and the need to stop drug use.

Alcoholism is addiction to the drug called *alcohol*. Alcoholism and drug addiction are recognized as illnesses under a biopsychosocial model. Simply stated, the disease concept of addiction and alcoholism identifies them as chronic and progressive diseases in which a person's use of a drug or drugs continues despite problems it causes in any area of life—physical, emotional, social, economic, or spiritual.

PSYCHOACTIVE DRUGS

Although any drug can be abused, ATOD abuse and addiction problems generally involve psychoactive drugs. These drugs, which can alter emotions, are used for enjoyment in social and recreational settings and for personal use to self-medicate physical or emotional discomfort. Psychoactive drugs are divided into categories according to their effect on the CNS and the general feelings or experiences the drugs may induce. The Internet or a pharmacology text can provide detailed information on these drug categories (e.g., depressants, stimulants, hallucinogens). Often, if persons cannot obtain their drug of choice, another drug from the same category will be substituted. For example, a person who cannot drink alcohol may begin using a benzodiazepine as an alternative because both are CNS depressants.

Depressants lower the body's overall energy level, reduce sensitivity to outside stimulation, and, in high doses, induce sleep. Low doses of depressants may produce a feeling of stimulation caused by initial sedation of the inhibitory centers in the brain. In general, depressants decrease heart rate, respiration rate, muscular coordination, and energy while dulling the senses. Higher doses lead to coma and, if the vital functions shut down, death. Major categories include alcohol, barbiturates, benzodiazepines, and opioids. This chapter discusses alcohol and heroin.

People use stimulants to feel more alert or energetic. These drugs activate or excite the nervous system. An increase in alertness and energy results as the stimulant causes the nerve fibers to release noradrenaline and other stimulating neurotransmitters. However, these drugs do not give the person more energy; they only make the body expend its own energy sooner and in greater quantities than it normally would. Stimulants can be useful and have few negative effects if used carefully and appropriately. The body must be allowed time to replenish itself after use of a stimulant. The cost for the "high" is the "down" state after the use of a stimulant—a feeling of sleepiness, laziness, mental fatigue, and possibly depression. Many persons abusing stimulants begin a vicious cycle of avoiding the down feeling by taking another dose. They then become physically dependent on the stimulant to function. Common stimulants include nicotine, cocaine, caffeine, and amphetamines. There is a growing public health issue related to the use of energy drinks by children, adolescents, and young adults. Energy drinks are "beverages that contain caffeine, taurine, vitamins, herbal supplements, and sugar or sweeteners and are marketed to improve energy, weight loss, stamina, athletic performance, and concentration" (Seifert et al, 2011, p 512). The sale of energy drinks is growing greatly. Caffeine is their main ingredient, and they are different from sports drinks and vitamin waters. Caffeine causes coronary and cerebral vasoconstriction, relaxes smooth muscle, stimulates skeletal muscle, has cardiac effects, and reduces insulin sensitivity (Seifert et al, 2011). On the basis of an extensive review, Seifert et al found that energy drinks have no therapeutic value and may put some children at risk for serious adverse health effects due to the high levels of caffeine. It should be noted that manufacturers claim that energy drinks are nutritional supplements, which shields them from the caffeine limits imposed on sodas and the safety testing and labeling required of pharmaceuticals (2011, p 522).

ALCOHOL

Alcohol (ethyl alcohol, or ethanol) is the oldest and most widely used psychoactive drug in the world. In the *National Survey on Drug Use and Health—2014,* about two-thirds of people 12 years and older reported that they drank alcohol in the past 12 months. There were 139.7 million persons 12 years or older who were past month alcohol drinkers and 163 million were heavy users. Underage alcohol use (12–20 years) and binge and heavy use among young adults (18–25 years) have declined over time but still remain a concern because in 2014 more than one-third of young adults were binge alcohol users, and about 1 in 10 were heavy alcohol users (Center for Behavioral Health Statistics and Quality, 2015). Because motor vehicle accidents are the leading causes of death among youths and young adults (16–25 years) in the United States, there is public health concern about driving while under the influence of alcohol, marijuana, or the combination of them. The rate of driving under the influence of alcohol alone and alcohol and marijuana combined has declined among persons aged 16 to 20 and 21 to 25 years. However, these data cannot be accepted as totally valid because no standard measurement exists for measuring marijuana-related driving impairment (Alejandro et al, 2015). Genetics and personal characteristics do influence the development of alcohol use disorders (O'Connor, 2016). Research demonstrates that genes are responsible for about half of the risk for abuse of alcohol (National Institute on Alcohol Abuse and Alcoholism [NIAAA], n.d.). According to the NIAAA (n.d.), "Multiple genes play in a role in a person's risk for developing alcoholism." Some genes increase a person's risk, and some decrease the risk. As an example, some people of Asian descent carry a gene variant that alters the rate at which they metabolize alcohol. This may cause symptoms such as flushing, nausea, and rapid heartbeat when they drink (NIAAA, n.d.)

Alcohol abuse costs billions of dollars in lost productivity, property damage, medical expenses from alcohol-related illnesses and accidents, family disruptions, alcohol-related violence, and neglect or abuse of children. Chronic alcohol abuse has multiple metabolic and physiological effects on all organ systems. People who use excessive amounts of alcohol may also not eat an adequate diet and then may develop vitamin and other nutritional deficiencies. In additional to the nutritional effects of low folate, iron and niacin levels, there may be gastrointestinal disturbances of the esophagus and stomach that can lead to inflammation and cancer. The liver and pancreas may be affected as well. Cardiovascular disturbances include cardiac dysrhythmias, cardiomyopathy, hypertension, atherosclerosis, and blood dyscrasias. CNS problems include depression, sleep disturbances, memory loss, organic brain syndrome, Wernicke-Korsakoff syndrome, and alcohol withdrawal syndrome. Neuromuscular problems include myopathy and peripheral neuropathy. There may be effects to the reproductive organs including decreased sex drive and, in men, enlarged breasts, smooth skin, and shrinking of the testes (O'Connor, 2016). Females who drink during pregnancy may have neonates with fetal alcohol syndrome (FAS) or fetal alcohol effects. Some of the metabolic disturbances include hypokalemia, hypomagnesemia, and ketoacidosis. Living in a household where one or both parents abuse alcohol can have significant effects on the children and their development, learning, and socialization.

Blood alcohol concentration (BAC) is determined by the concentration of alcohol in the drink, the rate of drinking, the rate of absorption (slower in the presence of food), the rate of metabolism, and a person's weight and sex. The amount of alcohol the liver can metabolize per hour is equal to about 0.25 oz of whiskey, 4 oz of wine, or 12 oz of beer. Tolerance will develop with chronic consumption, and a person can reach a high BAC with minimal CNS effects. Women are more affected by alcohol than men because women have less alcohol dehydrogenase activity than men (except for males with chronic alcoholism). Because this enzyme detoxifies alcohol, a deficiency results in a higher bioavailability of alcohol. Consequently, females suffer the long-term effects of alcohol intake at much lower doses in a shorter time span. Women also tend to have smaller body sizes than men. Alcohol use in moderation may provide health benefits by providing mild relaxation and lowering the serum cholesterol. Stott et al (2008), in their study of 3000 women between the ages of 70 and 82 years, found that the moderate consumption of alcohol resulted in better mental acuity and slower cognitive decline. Controlled drinking organizations such as Moderation Management (see http://www.moderation.org) provide guidelines for persons who want to have alcohol in their lives.

TOBACCO

As mentioned, tobacco smoking is the foremost preventable cause of death in the United States resulting in about 480,000 premature deaths and more than $300 billion in direct health care costs and losses in productivity (Jamal et al, 2015). Cigarette smoking is declining in the United States; however, it remains a public health problem due to the morbidity and premature mortality that it causes.

Nicotine, the active ingredient in the tobacco plant, is a toxic drug. To protect itself, the body quickly develops tolerance to the nicotine. If a person smokes regularly, tolerance to nicotine develops within hours, in contrast to days for heroin or months for alcohol. Pipes and cigars are less hazardous than cigarettes because the harsher smoke discourages deep inhalation. However, pipes and cigars increase the risk for cancer of the lips, mouth, and throat. There are large economic costs associated with the use of tobacco because of the diseases related to its use.

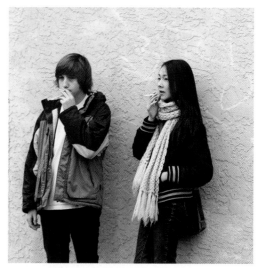

Cigarette smoking poses many health risks. (© 2012 Photos.com, a division of Getty Images. All rights reserved. Image #137167089.)

Smoke can be inhaled directly by the smoker (mainstream smoke), or it can enter the atmosphere from the lighted end of the cigarette and be inhaled by others in the vicinity (sidestream smoke or secondhand smoke). Secondhand smoke contains higher concentrations of toxic and carcinogenic compounds than mainstream smoke. According to *Healthy People 2020*, all exposure to secondhand smoke has a risk. Secondhand smoke causes heart disease and lung cancer in adults and health problems in infants and children, including severe asthma attacks, respiratory infections, ear infections, and sudden infant death syndrome (SIDS) (USDHHS, 2010a). Smoking bans are being adopted to reduce the discomfort and health hazards among nonsmokers. See Fig. 24.1 for the health consequences causally linked to smoking and exposure to secondhand smoke.

Nicotine is also used as chewing tobacco or snuff. Marketed as "smokeless tobacco," a wad is put in the mouth, and the nicotine is absorbed sublingually. Higher doses of nicotine are delivered in the smokeless forms because the nicotine is not destroyed by heat. Nevertheless, this form is less addictive because nicotine enters the bloodstream less directly.

ELECTRONIC NICOTINE DELIVERY SYSTEMS

This topic, because of its growing popularity, deserves its own section in the text. Electronic cigarettes (e-cigarettes) are battery-operated products that deliver an aerosol by heating a solution generally containing nicotine in propylene glycol or glycerol with flavoring agents. They are marketed as a smoking cessation tool and an alternative to cigarettes. In 2014, 12.6% of adults had tried an e-cigarette at least once, with men more likely than women to try them. The age group most likely to try e-cigarettes (20%) is individuals between the ages of 18 and 24 years. Non-Hispanic American Indian or Alaska Native (AIAN) adults (20.2%) and non-Hispanic white adults (14.8%) were more likely than Hispanic (8.6%), non-Hispanic black (7.1%), and non-Hispanic Asian (6.2%) adults to have ever tried e-cigarettes. Nicotine use among young people, including e-cigarette use, is dangerous (Singh et al, 2016). Some of the current data about users of e-cigarettes are as follows:

- Current cigarette smokers and recent former smokers (quit smoking within the past year) were more likely to

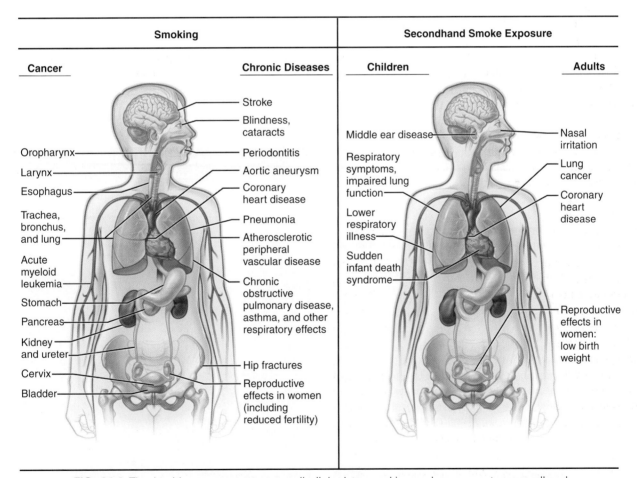

FIG. 24.1 The health consequences causally linked to smoking and exposure to secondhand smoke. (From US Department of Health and Human Services: How tobacco smoke causes disease: the biology and behavioral basis for smoking-attributable disease: a report of the Surgeon General. Atlanta, GA, 2010b, US Department of Health and Human Services, Centers for Disease Control and Prevention, National Center for Chronic Disease Prevention and Health Promotion, Office on Smoking and Health. Retrieved November 2012 from http://www.surgeongeneral.gov/library/reports/tobaccosmoke/executivesummary.pdf.)

use e-cigarettes than long-term former smokers (quit smoking more than 1 year ago) and adults who had never smoked.

- Current smokers who had tried to quit in the past year were more likely to use e-cigarettes than those who had not tried to quit.
- Among adults who had never smoked cigarettes, young adults aged 18 to 24 were more likely than older adults to have tried e-cigarettes (Schoenborn and Gindi, 2015, pp 3–5).
- Approximately 7 out of 10 US middle and high school students saw or heard e-cigarette advertisements in 2014 (Singh et al 2016).

Remember that nicotine is a potent toxin, and the refill liquids for e-cigarettes have high nicotine concentrations. Because e-cigarettes do not contain tobacco, they are not subject to US tobacco laws and US Food and Drug Administration (FDA) regulations. The components include an indicator light, rechargeable battery, vaporizer unit, cartridge, and mouthpiece (Carr, 2014).

People who use e-cigarettes do not consider that they are smoking. Instead, they say they are vaping. Vaping users often have their own customs, traditions, and language. You can activate the e-cigarette device by pressing a button that "heats and aerosolizes the liquid in the cartridge containing a liquid, creating a vapor" (Antolin and Barkley, 2015, p 60). The vapor is sent into the lungs and exhaled as a fine mist that can expose others to nicotine. According to Britton et al (2014), the eight primary health risks of e-cigarettes are as follows:

- Addiction to nicotine
- Progression to smoking traditional cigarettes
- Lung damage
- Unsafe handling of the parts of the e-cigarette
- Appeal to youth
- Potentially changing social norms, making tobacco smoking more acceptable
- Poisoning in children
- Secondhand exposure to the vapor

Nurses have a key role to play in assessing for the use of e-cigarettes. They can then offer advice about the risks of smoking and vaping. For this reason, it is important that nurses have current information in an area that is changing rapidly.

CAFFEINE

Caffeine is one of the most widely used psychoactive drugs in the world. Caffeine is found in coffee, tea, chocolate, soft drinks, and various medications (Table 24.1). Moderate doses of caffeine, from 100 to 300 mg per day, increase mental alertness and probably have little negative effect on health. Higher doses can lead to insomnia, irritability, tremulousness, anxiety, cardiac dysrhythmias, gastrointestinal (GI) disturbances, and headaches. Regular use of high doses can lead to physical dependence, and the withdrawal symptoms may include headaches, slowness, and occasional depression (Mayo Clinic Staff, 2009). Treating afternoon headaches with analgesics containing caffeine may in reality be preventing a withdrawal symptom from heavy morning coffee consumption. As discussed previously, the caffeine in energy drinks poses a major problem for youth users.

EVIDENCE-BASED PRACTICE

Carr did a thorough review of the facts, perceptions, and marketing messages of the rapidly growing e-cigarette industry. She noted that few studies have been published that document the safety of or the health risks from the use of e-cigarettes. Because they do not contain tobacco, they are not subject to the US tobacco laws or the US Food and Drug Administration (FDA) regulations. Because of the lack of regulation, the amount of nicotine in e-cigarettes can vary. Also, there is no age limit to those who can buy e-cigarettes, and they are sold online, as well as in a variety of retail sites. Carr found that by late 2013, there were over 300 brands of e-cigarettes being manufactured, with China being the largest producer and Johnson Creek, a US company, being second in revenue from the production of e-cigarettes. In summary, e-cigarettes are readily available, reasonably inexpensive, unregulated, and possibly dangerous to one's health.

Nurse Use

Nurses, who are considered reliable sources of information, need to be informed about e-cigarettes and the potential dangers associated with them. The goal is to teach patients, families, caregivers, and community members about e-cigarettes. This means that nurses will need to continually educate themselves about e-cigarettes because the research is growing, as is their use.

Carr RE: E-cigarettes: Facts, perceptions, and marketing messages, *Clin J Oncology* 2014, (Feb 18):1: 112-116.

TABLE 24.1 Caffeine Content in Commonly Consumed Substances		
Drink/Food/Supplement	**Amount of Drink/Food**	**Amount of Caffeine (mg)**
SoBe No Fear	8 oz	83
Monster energy drink	16 oz	160
Rockstar energy drink	8 oz	80
Red Bull energy drink	8.3 oz	80
Jolt cola	12 oz	72
Mountain Dew	12 oz	55
Coca-Cola	12 oz	34
Diet Coke	12 oz	45
Pepsi	12 oz	38
7-Up	12 oz	0
Brewed coffee (drip method)	5 oz	115*
Iced tea	12 oz	70*
Cocoa beverage	5 oz	4*
Chocolate milk beverage	8 oz	5*
Dark chocolate	1 oz	20*
Milk chocolate	1 oz	6*
Jolt gum	1 stick	33
Cold relief medication	1 tablet	30*
Vivarin	1 tablet	200
Excedrin (Extra Strength)	2 tablets	130

From US Food and Drug Administration, National Soft Drink Association, Center for Science in the Public Interest. Retrieved July 2010 from http://kidshealth.org/teen/drug_alcohol/drugs/caffeine.html#.
*Denotes average amount of caffeine.

ILLICIT DRUG USE

In 2014, 27.0 million Americans 12 years of age and older reported the use of an illicit drug in the past 30 days. This represents an increase over the period from 2002. Illicit drug use continues to be driven by marijuana and nonmedical prescription pain relievers. Men had higher rates of illicit drug dependence than women, and American Indians and Alaska Natives have the highest rates followed by African Americans. The lowest rates are found in Asian Americans. More than 50% of people 12 years and older who used pain relievers for nonmedical reasons got them from a friend or relative (Center for Behavioral Health Statistics and Quality, 2015).

The following section discusses specific information on selected illicit drugs.

OPIOIDS

There is an epidemic in the United States of poisoning deaths from drug overdose, including a 200% increase since 2000 of deaths due to opioids, such as opioid pain relievers and heroin. "Natural and semisynthetic opioids, which include the most commonly prescribed opioid pain relievers, oxycodone and hydrocodone, continue to be involved in more overdose deaths than by other opioid type" (Rudd et al, 2016, p 1379).

Heroin is one of the opioids. Opioids include the natural drugs found in the opium poppy, namely *opium, morphine,* and *codeine.* Opioids are synthetic drugs, such as heroin (semisynthetic), meperidine, methadone, oxycodone, and propoxyphene; they mimic the effects of the natural opiates. The effectiveness of opioids for pain relief is being questioned. Previously, they were by far the most effective drugs for pain relief. Some studies have demonstrated that their use for chronic pain may worsen pain and functioning by increasing pain perception (Frieden and Houry, 2016). Even though there may be benefits to pain relief with the use of opioids, the risks of addiction and overdose must be considered. The CDC has issued a guideline about opioid prescribing that emphasizes patient care and safety. The CDC used a rigorous system process to develop the guidelines. The guidelines were based on three key principles: (1) "nonopioid therapy is preferred for chronic pain outside the context of active cancer, palliative, or end-of-life care," and nonpharmacological therapies can ameliorate chronic pain while posing substantially less risk to patients (e.g., exercise, weight loss, psychological therapies such as cognitive behavioral therapy, interventions to improve sleep, and certain procedures); (2) when using opioids, use the lowest possible dose; and (3) exercise caution, and monitor patients closely (Frieden and Houry, 2016, pp 2–3).

Heroin is the opioid that is used most often for recreational purposes and is the strongest of the opioids. Others include codeine (low potential for dependence), oxycodone (alone and in various combinations, e.g., with acetaminophen), meperidine, morphine, pentazocine, and hydromorphone (O'Connor, 2016).

COCAINE

Cocaine is an expensive way to get high; it has powerful effects on the brain, heart, and emotions. Many users become addicted, and even occasional users run the risk of sudden death. Cocaine is a purified extract from the coca shrub found on the eastern slopes of the Andes region of South America. There are two main forms: (1) powdered, which dissolves in water and can be snorted or injected; and (2) crack, which is made by a chemical process that leaves it in a "freebase" form that is smoked. Young men between the ages of 18 and 25 are the biggest users of cocaine.

Cocaine users often describe a feeling of being "high," which includes an increased sense of energy and alertness, an elevated mood, and a feeling of supremacy. Other people feel irritable, paranoid, restless, and anxious. Signs of cocaine use include dilated pupils; high levels of energy and activity; and excited, exuberant speech. The immediate effects wear off in 30 to 120 minutes. In addition to effects on the brain, heart, and emotions, there can be effects on the lungs and respiratory system, GI tract, kidneys, and sexual function. After regular cocaine use for a period of time, withdrawal systems can include depression and anxiety, fatigue, difficulty concentrating, inability to feel pleasure, an increasing craving for the drug, and physical symptoms such as aches, pains, tremors, and chills (WebMD, 2016).

AMPHETAMINES AND METHAMPHETAMINES

Amphetamines are a class of stimulants similar to cocaine, but the effects last longer, and the drugs are cheaper. Amphetamines have a chemical structure similar to that of adrenaline and noradrenaline and are generally used to decrease fatigue, increase mental alertness, suppress appetite, and create a sense of wellbeing. They are popular among people who need to stay awake for long hours to work or study. They can be taken as pills, injected, snorted, or smoked. When taken intravenously, they quickly induce an intense euphoric feeling (a "rush"). The user may speed for several days (go on a "speed run") and then fall into a deep sleep for 18 or more hours ("crash"). They cause an elevation in mood, increased wakefulness, alertness, concentration, intensified physical performance, and a feeling of wellbeing; they typically cause erectile dysfunction in men while enhancing sexual desire. Use is often associated with unsafe sexual practices, including exposure to STDs and HIV. Users are prone to accidents because the drug produces a state of excitement and grandiosity, and their usual danger warning signals do not work effectively.

Methamphetamines (meth) is an easy-to-make street drug that users swallow, smoke, snort, or inject. Like amphetamines, meth is a stimulant that creates an immediate high that fades quickly. Because of the fading, users may take the substance frequently, and this can lead to addiction. The physical effects are similar to those of cocaine and amphetamines. They include increased breathing, rapid heart rate, high blood pressure, and increased body temperature; with repeated use, meth users often lose weight, get skin sores, and have dental issues. Injecting the drug has all the same effects as any other drug injection (WebMD, 2015).

MARIJUANA

Marijuana (*Cannabis sativa* or *Cannabis indica*) is the most widely used illicit drug in the United States. In contrast to the other psychoactive drugs, marijuana has little toxicity and is one of the safest therapeutic agents known ("Marijuana," 2013). Psychological dependence can occur with chronic use, but little is known about any potential physical dependence. However, because of its illegal status, there is no quality control, and a user may consume contaminated marijuana. Users enjoy a mild euphoria, a relaxed feeling, and an intensity of sensory perceptions. Some call the effect a dreamy state of consciousness in which ideas seem disconnected, unanticipated, and free-flowing. Time, color, and spatial perceptions may be altered ("Marijuana," 2013). Side effects include dry and reddened eyes, increased appetite, dry mouth, drowsiness, and mild tachycardia. Adverse reactions include anxiety, disorientation, and paranoia.

The greatest physical concern for chronic users is possible damage to the respiratory tract from smoking the drug. For chronic users, tolerance and physical dependence can develop; however, the withdrawal symptoms are benign. Addiction can occur for some chronic users and is difficult to treat because the progression tends to be subtle. Despite its beneficial effects, especially in treating pain, the only legal access to this medicine was through the US Food and Drug Administration's (FDA's) Compassionate Investigational New Drug Program. This program was closed in 1992. In response to this complete prohibition, some health care organizations support access to this medication through formal resolutions, including several state nurses associations, the American Nurses Association, and the American Public Health Association. Several states and Washington, DC, have passed laws, and other states have laws under consideration, allowing patients to use marijuana as medicine under the recommendation of their physician. As more states legalize the use of marijuana for both medical and recreational reasons, there is every reason to think the quality of the product will improve.

STREET DRUGS COMMONLY USED

There are a variety of street drugs that are currently being used. Examples include bath salts, ecstasy, flakka, krokodil, LSD, mushrooms, salvia, and spice in addition to the ones described in this chapter: cocaine, heroin, marijuana, and methamphetamines. Bath salts are a crystalline powder that can be swallowed, inhaled, or injected and that is highly addictive. They contain man-made stimulants, cathinones, which are similar to amphetamines. They increase dopamine levels and can create feelings of euphoria. They can also have serious health and behavioral effects. Flakka is, like bath salts, a synthetic cathinone that can be eaten, snorted, injected, or used in e-cigarettes. Although it has a stimulant effect, it can also lead to paranoia, hallucinations, and violence or self-harm. Ecstasy is a man-made stimulant and hallucinogen that can be snorted or injected into a vein. It increases levels of chemicals in the brain, such as serotonin, dopamine, and norepinephrine, that alter mood and make the person feel more connected to others. When the drug wears off, it can lead to confusion, depression, anxiety, and sleep problems. Krokodil is widely used in Russia and is an opioid drug type that is injected into the bloodstream, with rapid effects. LSD is a hallucinogen that became popular in the 1960s, and it causes people to see, hear, and feel things that seem, but are not, real. Certain types of mushrooms can be eaten, brewed in tea, or added to food to give users a high. Salvia is an herb in the mint family that is also a hallucinogen. Their active ingredient is psilocybin, and it is a hallucinogen.

PREDISPOSING AND CONTRIBUTING FACTORS

In addition to the specific drug being used, two other major variables influence the particular drug experience: set and setting. To understand various patterns of drug use and abuse by individuals, all three factors (i.e., drug, set, and setting) should be considered.

Set refers to the individual using the drug, as well as that person's expectations, including unconscious expectations, about the drug being used. A person's current health may alter a drug's effects from one day to the next. Some people are genetically predisposed to alcoholism or other drug addiction, and their chemical makeup is such that simply consuming the drug triggers the disease process. Persons with underlying mood disorders or other mental illness may try to self-medicate with psychoactive drugs. Sometimes their choice of drug exacerbates their symptoms; for example, a depressed person might consume alcohol and become more depressed.

Setting is the influence of the physical, social, and cultural environment within which the use occurs. Social conditions influence the use of drugs. The fast pace of life, competition at school or in the workplace, and the pressure to accumulate material possessions are daily stressors. The advertising of pharmaceutical, alcohol, and tobacco companies entices people to use their products to feel and sleep better, to have more energy, or just as a "treat." Often people think that most of life's problems can be solved quickly and easily through the use of a drug. For some people, many of life's opportunities may seem out of reach. Rather than seeking relief through medical care, the use of psychoactive drugs may offer a way to numb the pain or escape from a hopeless reality. They also rely on alcohol or illicit drugs, which are more readily available. For some, dealing in illicit drugs may appear to be the only way to avoid a future of poverty and unemployment.

GENETIC FACTORS IN ADDICTION

Dependence on alcohol and other drugs often co-occurs. Evidence indicates that both disorders are, at least partially, influenced by genetic factors. Twin studies have been used to support this co-occurrence. Specifically, "a finding that the correlation between alcohol dependence in twin 1 and drug dependence in twin 2 is higher for identical (i.e. monozygotic) twins, who share 100% of their genes than for fraternal (i.e. dizygotic) twins, who share on average only 50% of their genes, indicates that shared genes influence the risk of both alcohol and drug dependence" (Dick and Agrawal, 2008). It is complex to identify exactly which genes are likely to contribute to a person's susceptibility to alcohol and/or drug dependence. Environment is also a contributing factor. Some research indicates that addiction is 50% due to genetic factors and 50% to poor coping skills. Also, children of addicts are eight times more likely to develop addiction than children of nonaddicts (Addictions and Recovery.org, 2016). The NIAAA has been funding the Collaborative Studies on Genetics of Alcoholism since 1989. The goal of these studies is to identify the specific genes that influence alcoholism (NIAAA, n.d.).

PRIMARY PREVENTION AND THE ROLE OF THE NURSE

Harm reduction, a primary care approach to substance abuse, focuses on health promotion and disease prevention. Primary prevention for ATOD problems includes (1) the promotion of healthy lifestyles and resiliency factors and (2) education about drugs and guidelines for their use. Nurses can be effective in teaching, promoting, and facilitating people in choosing healthy options rather than reliance on drugs. This may entail adding these health-promoting actions to the use of prescription drugs or complementary remedies if the latter are consistent with the recommendations of the health care provider.

Specifically, you can teach clients to be assertive in their relationships with others and how to make better decisions by looking carefully at the pros and cons of each option and the related consequences. People may turn to medications, especially psychoactive drugs, when they experience persistent health problems such as difficulty sleeping, muscle tension, lack of energy, chronic stress, and mood swings. Nurses can help clients understand that medications may mask problems rather than solve them.

CHECK YOUR PRACTICE

You are working with a group of 18-year-old males who have recently completed a drug rehabilitation program. Your goal is to help them learn a new set of coping strategies other than the use of recreational drugs. Looking back at Chapter 11, which discusses health promotion, what would be some of the stress reduction strategies you would recommend? Are any of these strategies that you have tried for stress in your own life? You know that lack of sleep, improper diet, and lack of exercise contribute to many health complaints and may cause significant stress. Your goal is to provide stress-relieving strategies as an alternative to drug usage. Assisting clients to balance their need for rest, nutrition, and exercise on a daily basis can reduce these complaints. Nurses can provide useful information to groups, assisting in the development of community recreational resources or facilitating stress reduction, relaxation, or exercise groups. Nurses can help people learn about drug-free community activities. The How To box lists community activities in which the nurse may become involved.

Lack of educational opportunities, job training, or both can contribute to socioeconomic stress and poor self-esteem, which can lead to drug use to escape the situation. Nurses can help clients identify community resources and solve problems to meet basic needs rather than avoid them. In addition to decreasing risk factors associated with ATOD problems, it is important to increase protective or resiliency factors. Prevention guidelines to teach parents and teachers how to increase resiliency in youths include the following strategies:

- Help them develop an increased sense of responsibility for their own success.
- Help them identify their talents.
- Motivate them to dedicate their lives to helping society rather than believing that their only purpose in life is to be consumers.
- Provide realistic appraisals and feedback, stress multicultural competence, and encourage and value education and skills training.
- Increase cooperative solutions to problems rather than competitive or aggressive solutions.

HOW TO Set Up Community-Based Activities Aimed at Substance Abuse Prevention

- Increase involvement and pride in school activities.
- Organize student assistant programs (students helping students).
- Organize a Students Against Drunk Driving (SADD) chapter.
- Mobilize parental awareness and action groups (e.g., Mothers Against Drunk Driving [MADD]).
- Increase the availability of recreational facilities.
- Encourage parental commitment to nondrinking parties.
- Encourage religious institutions to convey nonuse messages and provide activities associated with nonuse.
- Curtail media messages that glamorize drug and alcohol use.
- Support and reinforce anti–drug use peer-pressure skills.
- Provide general health screenings, including for alcohol, tobacco, and other drug use.
- Collaborate with community leaders to solve problems related to crime, housing, jobs, and access to health care.

These skills also apply to adults. The objectives in *Healthy People 2020* provide guidance for ways to decrease the reliance on alcohol, drugs, and tobacco (USDHHS, 2010a).

DRUG EDUCATION

ATOD problems include more than abuse of psychoactive drugs. Today more than 450,000 different drugs and drug combinations are available, and prescription drugs are involved in almost 60% of all drug-related emergency room visits and 70% of all drug-related deaths. Nurses know about medication administration, the possible dangers of indiscriminate drug use, and the inability of drugs to cure all problems. Nurses can influence the health of clients by destroying the myth of good drugs versus bad drugs.

This means (1) teaching clients that no drug is completely safe and that any drug can be abused, (2) helping persons learn how to make informed decisions about their drug use to minimize potential harm, and (3) teaching them to always tell their health care provider what supplements they are taking.

Drug technology is growing, yet the public receives little information about how to safely use this technology. Harm reduction as a goal recognizes that people consume drugs and that they need to know about the use of drugs and risks involved to make decisions about their drug use. Drug education should begin on an individual basis by reviewing the client's prescription medications. Because a physician or nurse practitioner has prescribed the medication, clients often presume little risk is involved.

Is the client aware of any untoward interactions this drug may have with other drugs being used or with food? A common occurrence with drug users is taking drugs from different categories together or at different times to regulate how they feel. This practice is known as **polysubstance use or abuse.** For example, a person may drink alcohol when snorting cocaine to "take the edge off"; or some intravenous drug users combine cocaine with heroin (speedball) for similar reasons. Polysubstance use can cause drug interactions that can have addictive, synergistic, or antagonistic effects. Indiscriminate polysubstance abuse may lead to serious physiological consequences and can be complicated for the health care professional to assess and treat. It is important to encourage clients to ask questions about their drug use. The following list in the How To box has six key pieces of information that clients should obtain before taking a drug or medication to decrease the possible harm from unsafe medication consumption.

HOW TO Determine the Relative Safety of a Drug for Personal or Client Use

Before using a drug or medication, always determine the following:
- The chemical in the drug
- How and where the drug works in the body
- The correct dosage
- If there might be drug interactions, including those with herbal remedies
- If there are potential allergic reactions
- If there might be drug tolerance or if the drug might lead to physical dependence*

---

*__Caution:__ Approximately 10% of the population may suffer from the disease of addiction. For them, responsible use of psychoactive drugs is limited because of their disease. They need to notify their physician of the addiction if the use of psychoactive medicines is being considered as treatment.

Nurses can identify references and community resources available to provide the necessary information, and they can clarify the information. User-friendly reference texts and online resources are available that describe drug interactions among medications, other drugs (including alcohol, tobacco,

 LEVELS OF PREVENTION

Related to Abuse of Alcohol, Tobacco, and Other Drugs (Substance Abuse)

Primary Prevention
Provide community education to teach healthy lifestyles; focus on how to resist getting involved in the use of alcohol, tobacco, or drugs.

Secondary Prevention
Institute early detection programs in schools, the workplace, and other areas in which people gather to determine the presence of substance abuse.

Tertiary Prevention
Develop programs to help people reduce or end substance abuse.

---

marijuana, and cocaine), and other substances (food and beverages, including energy drinks) and that serve as excellent guides for nurses and their clients. See http://www.drugdigest.org for more information. Clients should learn about and ask questions about their prescription medications and self-administered OTC products, including supplements, herbal remedies, and recreational drugs. This does not mean that nurses should encourage other drug use, but rather that the potential harm from self-medication can be reduced if clients have the necessary information to make more informed decisions. (See the Levels of Prevention box.)

Parents should seek information about their use of medications so they can act as role models for their children. It can be confusing for children and adolescents to be told to "just say no" to drugs when they see their parents or drug advertisements try to "quick fix" every health complaint, feeling of stress, anxiety, or depression with a medication. The simple "just say no" approach does not help young people for several reasons. First, children are naturally curious, and drug experimentation is often a part of normal development. Second, children from dysfunctional homes may use drugs to get attention or to escape an intolerable environment. And finally, the "just say no" approach does not address the powerful influence of peer pressure ("Marijuana," 2013).

Drug education has moved into the school curriculum with Project DARE (Drug Abuse Resistance Education), the most widely used school-based drug-use prevention program in the United States. This program uses law enforcement officers to teach the material, but recent studies find that it is less effective than other interactive prevention programs and may even result in increased drug use (Pan and Bai, 2009). Basic ATOD prevention programs for young people should combine efforts to increase resiliency factors with drug education. Nurses can serve as educators or as advisors to the school systems or community groups to ensure that all of these areas are addressed. Role playing is useful in teaching many of these skills.

Targeted Competency: Informatics—Use information and technology to communicate, manage knowledge, mitigate error, and support decision making. Important aspects of informatics include the following:

- **Knowledge:** Identify essential information that must be available in a common database to support client care.
- **Skills:** Use information management tools to monitor outcomes of care processes.
- **Attitudes:** Value technologies that support clinical decision making, error prevention, and care coordination

Informatics Question:

You are taking over the role of school nurse at a large regional high school. There has been a recent tragedy involving a senior from this high school drinking and driving with friends in the car, resulting in one student death and significant injury to the driver and another passenger. You have been asked to address the use of alcohol, tobacco, and other drugs (ATOD) at this high school.

1. What data will you collect to assess the scope of the ATOD problem at this school?
2. Who might be some key informants to interview? What information might they provide that would not be clear from quantitative statistics?
3. You decide that an alcohol and drug education class is needed in your school. What data should you gather to track over time to assess the effectiveness of this intervention?

SECONDARY PREVENTION AND THE ROLE OF THE NURSE

To identify substance abuse and plan appropriate interventions, nurses must assess each client individually. When drug abuse, dependence, or addiction is identified, the nurse assists clients to understand the connection between their drug-use patterns and the negative consequences on their health, their families, and the community.

ASSESSING FOR ALCOHOL, TOBACCO, AND OTHER DRUG PROBLEMS

The NIAAA published a clinician's guide for assessing health problems related to drinking. This free booklet, entitled "Helping Patients Who Drink Too Much: A Clinician's Guide," is available at http://www.niaaa.nih.gov/guide. Self-assessment tools are available online at http://www.alcoholscreening.org and http://www.drugscreening.org. These screening tools are based on the Alcohol, Smoking, and Substance Involvement Screening Test (ASSIST) developed by the World Health Organization and allow takers to get immediate anonymous feedback.

During health assessment, the nurse assesses for substance abuse problems, including both self-medication practices and recreational drug use. Thus all relevant drug use history is collected and aids in the assessment of drug use patterns. Note any changes in drug use patterns over time. After obtaining a medication history, follow-up questions can determine whether problems exist. The following are examples:

- If using a prescription drug, is the client following the directions correctly?

- Has the client increased the dosage or frequency above the prescription level?
- Is the person using any prescribed psychoactive drugs? If yes, for how long, and what is the dosage?

When assessing self-medication and recreational or social drug-use patterns, determine the reason the person uses the drug. Some underlying health problems (e.g., pain, stress, weight, insomnia) may be relieved by nonpharmaceutical interventions. The amount, frequency, and duration of use and the route of administration of each drug should be determined. To establish the presence of a substance abuse problem, determine whether the drug use is causing any negative health consequences or problems with relationships, employment, finances, or the legal system. The How To box lists examples of questions to ask to determine the presence of socioeconomic problems that are often secondary to substance abuse. If a pattern of chronic, regular, and frequent use of a drug exists, nurses should assess for a history of withdrawal symptoms to determine whether there is physical dependence on the drug. A progression in drug use patterns and related problems warns about the possibility of addiction. Denial is a primary symptom of addiction. Methods of denial include the following:

- Lying about use
- Minimizing use patterns
- Blaming or rationalizing
- Intellectualizing
- Changing the subject
- Using anger or humor
- "Going with the flow" (i.e., agreeing that a problem exists, stating the behavior will change, but not demonstrating any behavior changes)

A problem should be suspected if the client becomes defensive or exhibits other behavior indicating denial when asked about alcohol or other drug use.

HOW TO **Assess Socioeconomic Problems Resulting from Substance Abuse**

If the client admits to use of alcohol, tobacco, or other drugs, ask the following questions:

- Do your parents, spouse, or friends worry or complain about your drinking or using drugs?
- Has a family member asked for help for your drinking or using drugs?
- Have you neglected family obligations as a result of drinking or using drugs?
- Have you missed work and/or does your boss complain about your drinking or using drugs?
- Do you drink or use drugs before or during work?
- Have you ever been fired or quit a job because of drinking or using drugs?
- Have you ever been charged with driving under the influence (DUI) or being drunk in public (DIP)?
- Have you ever had any other legal problems related to drinking and using drugs, such as assault and battery, breaking and entering, or theft?
- Have you had any accidents while intoxicated, such as falls, burns, or motor vehicle accidents?
- Have you spent your money on alcohol or other drugs instead of paying your bills (e.g., telephone, electricity, rent)?

DRUG TESTING

During the 1980s, preemployment or random drug testing in the workplace gained popularity. You can test for drugs by examining a person's urine, blood, saliva, breath (alcohol), or hair. Urine testing, the most common method, indicates only past use of certain drugs, not intoxication. You can identify a person who has used a certain drug in the recent past, but urine testing does not determine the degree of intoxication and extent of performance impairment. Also, most drug-related problems in the workplace are related to alcohol, and alcohol is not always included in a urine drug screen. When is drug testing appropriate? Drug testing that follows documented impairment may help substantiate the cause of the impairment and serve as a backup rather than the primary screening method. It is also useful for recovering addicts. Part of their treatment is to abstain from psychoactive drug use; therefore, a urine test yielding positive results for a drug indicates a relapse.

Blood, breath, and saliva drug tests can indicate current use and amount. Any of these tests can help determine alcohol intoxication, and they are often used to substantiate suspected impairment. A serum drug screen can be useful when overdose is suspected to determine the specific drug ingested. The testing of hair is gaining attention because the results can provide a long history of drug use patterns.

Alcohol and other drug testing should be used as a clinical and public health tool but not for harassment and punishment. For example, approximately 40% to 50% of people who are seen in trauma centers were drinking at the time of their injuries. Hence, it is recommended that breath alcohol testing be routinely done for persons admitted to the emergency department for traumatic injuries (Physicians and Lawyers for National Drug Policy, 2008).

Employee assistance programs (EAPs) are a beneficial service in many work settings. Often a sizable number of EAP clients have substance use problems because most adults with these problems are employed. EAP programs can identify health problems among employees and offer counseling or referral to other health care providers as necessary. Such programs provide early identification of and intervention for substance abuse problems; they also offer services to employees to reduce stress and provide health care or counseling so that they may prevent substance abuse problems from developing. Nurses frequently develop and run these programs.

HIGH-RISK GROUPS

Identifying high-risk groups helps nurses design programs to meet specific needs and mobilize community resources.

Adolescents

The younger a person is when beginning intensive experimentation with drugs, the more likely dependence will develop. Underage drinking is seen as the most serious drug problem for youth in the United States. In 2014, 22.8% of underage people were current alcohol users, 13.8% were binge alcohol users, and 3.4% were heavy alcohol users (Center for Behavioral

 HEALTHY PEOPLE 2020

Objectives Related to Substance Abuse

- **SA-2:** Increase the proportion of adolescents never using substances.
- **TU-3:** Reduce initiation of tobacco use among children, adolescents, and young adults.
- **TU-11:** Reduce the proportion of nonsmokers exposed to secondhand smoke.

US Department of Health and Human Services: *Healthy People 2020*, Washington, DC, 2010a, US Government Printing Office.

Health Statistics and Quality, 2015). The most common illicit drug use at present is the use of marijuana and the nonmedical use of prescription pain relievers. The estimated use of marijuana was higher in 2014 than between 2002 and 2009 for young adults between 18 and 25 years.

Heavy drug use during adolescence can interfere with normal development. Note that *Healthy People 2020* objectives SA-2 and TU-3 reduce initiation of the use of tobacco, alcohol, and other drugs (see the *Healthy People 2020* box). Family-related factors (e.g., genetics, family stress, parenting styles, child victimization) may be the greatest variable that influences substance abuse among adolescents. The co-occurrence with psychiatric disorders (especially mood disorders) and behavioral problems is also associated with substance abuse among adolescents, leaving peer pressure as a less influential factor. Research suggests that successful social influence–based prevention programs may be driven by their ability to foster social norms that reduce an adolescent's social motivation to begin using ATOD.

Older Adults

Worldwide, the number of older people is increasing. Alcohol abuse, and its associated disorders in the elderly, is a common and underrecognized occurrence. The disorders associated with the use of ATOD are a major cause of physical and psychological health problems. The social and physical changes that often accompany aging may increase a person's vulnerability to substance abuse. For example, the loss of loved ones, retirement, illness, lower levels of achievement, lack of mobility, having to move from one's home, juggling many roles, and being tired or sleep deprived may cause people to seek illicit drugs or self-medicate for anxiety and depression. This age group consumes more prescribed and OTC medications than any other age group. See the free public education brochure "As You Age . . . A Guide to Aging, Medicines and Alcohol" at http://www.asyouage.samhsa.gov/material/ (retrieved May 2016). The increased use of prescription drugs and alcohol causes slowed metabolic turnover of drugs, age-related organ changes, enhanced drug sensitivities, and a tendency to use drugs over long periods. A frequent use of multiple drugs contributes to greater negative consequences from drug use among older adults. Alcohol abuse may not be identified because its effects on cognitive abilities may mimic changes associated with normal aging or degenerative brain disease. Also, depression may be simply attributed to more frequent losses rather than the depressant effects of alcohol, and the older adult may subsequently receive medical treatment for depression rather than alcoholism.

Injection Drug Users

In addition to the problem of addiction, injection drug users (IDUs) (i.e., those who self-administer intravenously or subcutaneously) are at risk for other health complications. Intravenous administration of drugs always carries a greater risk for overdose because the drug goes directly into the bloodstream. With illicit drugs, the danger is increased because the exact dosage is unknown. In addition, the drug may be contaminated with other chemicals, such as sugar, starch, or quinine, and these ingredients can cause negative consequences. Often IDUs make their own solution for intravenous administration, and any particles present can result in complications from emboli.

Addicted persons often share needles. Contaminated needles can transmit hepatitis C and HIV infection and other bloodborne diseases. Using dirty needles or having poor administration techniques may lead to infections and abscesses. Despite their overall decline, IDUs continue to represent a substantial proportion of persons with new HIV diagnoses, with the highest number in 2015 among whites (CDC, 2017). Abstinence is ideal but unrealistic for many addicts. Using the harm reduction model, the nurse should provide education on cleaning needles with bleach between uses and on needle exchange programs to decrease the spread of the virus. Studies indicate that needle exchange programs have not increased injection drug abuse but have increased the number of people entering treatment programs (Knox, 2012).

Drug Use During Pregnancy

Most drugs can negatively affect a fetus. Thus the use of any drug during pregnancy should be discouraged unless medically necessary. *Healthy People 2020* objectives address this issue under the Maternal, Infant and Child Health topic area. Several objectives have recommendations to improve the health of infants, such as reduce the occurrence of fetal alcohol syndrome (FAS) in MICH-25 and increase abstinence from alcohol, cigarettes, and illicit drugs among pregnant women in MICH-11. FAS is considered the leading preventable birth defect, causing mental and behavioral impairment. Heavy drinking is becoming less of a problem for pregnant women; tobacco remains the most significant problem (Substance Abuse and Mental Health Services Administration [SAMHSA], 2013). Symptoms of depression and anxiety are often prevalent during pregnancy and influence a woman's decision to use alcohol or other substances. In some states, pregnant women who are using illicit drugs are reported to child protective services because of the potential harm to the fetus.

Despite the increased focus on drug abuse interventions, many pregnant women with drug problems do not receive the help they need. This may be a result of ignorance, poverty, lack of concern for the fetus, lack of available services, and fear of the consequences of revealing drug use. The fear of criminal prosecution may push addicted women farther away from the health care system, cause them to conceal their drug use from medical providers, and cause them to avoid the critical treatment and medical care they need (Brady and Ashley, 2005).

Use of Illicit Drugs

The strategy of "just say no" to drugs is both simplistic and misleading. Indiscriminate use of "good" drugs has caused more health problems from adverse reactions, drug interactions, dependence, addiction, and overdoses than use of "bad" drugs. However, the war on drugs focuses on illicit drugs and punishes illicit drug users. The black market associated with illicit drug use puts otherwise law-abiding citizens in close contact with criminals, prevents any quality control of the drugs, increases the risk for AIDS and hepatitis secondary to needle sharing, and hinders health care professionals' accessibility to the abuser or addict. Lack of quality control (i.e., unknown strength and purity) can cause unexpected overdoses or secondary effects of the impurities; for example, a synthetic analog of fentanyl (3-methylfentanyl) marketed as "heroin" is 6000 times as potent as morphine. Unsafe administration (contaminated needles) leads to local and systemic infections. The high cost of drugs on the black market leads to crime to support the addiction. In 2013 the highest rate of illicit drug use was among 18- to 20-years-olds, with marijuana being the most used drug (Center for Behavioral Health and Quality, 2015). See *Behavioral Health Trends in the United States: Results From the 2014 National Health Survey on Drug Use and Health* for details on specific drug use among various age groups (Center for Behavioral Health and Quality, 2015).

CODEPENDENCY AND FAMILY INVOLVEMENT

Drug addiction is often a family disease. One in four Americans experiences family problems related to alcohol abuse. People close to the addicted person often develop unhealthy coping mechanisms to continue the relationship. This behavior is known as codependency, a stress-induced preoccupation with the addicted person's life, leading to extreme dependence and excessive concern for the addict. Strict rules typically develop in a codependent family to maintain the relationships, such as don't talk, don't feel, don't trust, don't lose control, and don't seek help from outside the family.

Codependents try to meet the addicted person's needs at the expense of their own. Codependency may underlie medical complaints and emotional stress seen by health care providers such as ulcers, skin disorders, migraine headaches, chronic colds, and backaches. When the addicted person refuses to admit the problem, the family continues to adapt to emotionally survive the stress of the addict's irrational, inconsistent, and unpredictable behavior. Family members consequently develop roles that tend to be gross exaggerations of normal family roles, and they cling irrationally to these roles, even when they are no longer functional. One of the most significant roles a family member may assume is that of an enabler. Enabling is the act of shielding or preventing the addict from experiencing the consequences of the addiction. As a result, the addict does not always understand the cost of the addiction and thus is "enabled" to continue to use. Although codependency and enabling are closely related, a person does not have to be codependent to enable. Anyone can be an enabler—a police officer, a supervisor or coworker, and even a drug treatment counselor. Health care professionals can be enablers when they fail to address the negative health consequences of drug use with the addicted person.

The nurse can help families recognize the problem of addiction and help them confront the addicted member in a caring manner. Regardless of whether the addicted family member is agreeable to treatment, family members should be given guidance about the resources and services available to help them cope more effectively. The nurse can help identify treatment options, counseling assistance, financial assistance, support services, and (if necessary) legal services for the family members. Children of ATOD abusers or addicts are themselves at a greater risk for developing an addiction and must be targeted for primary prevention. A useful website is the National Institute on Drug Abuse at http://www.drugabuse.gov. See the Drug Facts series, which covers a range of topics, including prescription and OTC medications, spice (synthetic marijuana), and commonly abused prescription drugs.

TERTIARY PREVENTION AND THE ROLE OF THE NURSE

The nurse is in a key position to help the addicted person and his or her family. The nurse's knowledge of community resources and how to mobilize them can significantly influence the quality of care clients receive.

DETOXIFICATION

Detoxification is the clearing of one or more drugs from the person's body and managing the withdrawal symptoms. Depending on the particular drug and the degree of dependence, the time required may range from a few days to several weeks. Because withdrawal symptoms vary (depending on the drug used) and range from uncomfortable to life-threatening, the setting for and management of withdrawal depends on the drug used. Stimulants or opiates may produce withdrawal symptoms that are uncomfortable but not life-threatening. Detoxification from these drugs does not require direct medical supervision, but medical management of the withdrawal symptoms increases the comfort level. On the other hand, drugs such as alcohol, benzodiazepines, and barbiturates can produce life-threatening withdrawal symptoms. These clients should be under close medical supervision during detoxification and should receive medical management of the withdrawal symptoms to ensure a safe withdrawal. Of those who develop delirium tremens from alcohol withdrawal, 15% may not survive despite medical management; therefore close medical management is initiated as the blood alcohol level begins to fall. A general rule in detoxification management is to wean the person off the drug by gradually reducing the dosage and frequency of administration. Thus a person with chronic alcoholism could be safely detoxified by a gradual reduction in alcohol consumption. In practice, however, the switch to another drug,

usually a benzodiazepine, often offers a safer withdrawal from alcohol as well as an abrupt end to the intoxication from the drug of choice. For example, chlordiazepoxide (Librium) is commonly used for alcohol detoxification. Outpatient or home detoxification for persons requiring medical detoxification for alcohol withdrawal can be a cost-effective treatment. Nurses can monitor and evaluate the client's health status in the home environment to reduce the risk for medical complications related to alcohol withdrawal and to provide encouragement and support for the client to complete the detoxification.

ADDICTION TREATMENT

Addiction treatment differs from the management of negative health consequences of chronic drug abuse, overdose, and detoxification. Addiction treatment focuses on the addiction process. The goal is to help clients view addiction as a chronic disease and assist them to make lifestyle changes to halt progression of the disease. According to the disease theory, addicted persons are not responsible for the symptoms of their disease; they are, however, responsible for treating their disease. People 12 years of age and older seek treatment for addictions.

Most treatment facilities are multidisciplinary because the intervention strategies require a wide range of approaches. Their programs involve interactions among the addict, family, culture, and community. Strategies include medical management, education, counseling, vocational rehabilitation, stress management, and support services. The key to effective treatment is to match individual clients with the interventions most appropriate for them.

For those addicted individuals unwilling or unable to completely abstain from psychoactive drugs, other medications can assist them in abstaining from their drug of choice. Methadone maintenance programs are used to treat heroin and other opioid addictions. Methadone, when administered in moderate or high daily doses, produces a cross-tolerance to other opioids, thereby blocking their effects and decreasing the craving for heroin. The advantages of methadone are that it is long acting and effective orally, does not produce a "high," is inexpensive, and has few known side effects. The oral use of methadone offers a solution to the danger of the spread of HIV infection and other blood-borne infections that commonly occur among needle-sharing addicts. Although not recognized as a cure for heroin (or other opiate) addiction, methadone maintenance is a harm reduction intervention because it reduces deviant behavior and introduces addicted persons to the health care system (Volkow et al, 2014).

Recovery from addiction requires a lifetime commitment and may include periods of relapse. The addicted person must realize that modern medicine has not found a cure for addiction; therefore returning to drug use may ultimately reactivate the disease process.

Long-term residential programs, also called *halfway houses*, can help ease the person recovering from an addiction back into society. These facilities provide continued support and counseling in a structured environment for persons needing long-term

Ryan Swabbs, MSN, works at a drug rehabilitation center and provides individual and group counseling for clients who are in the process of controlling or stopping their drug addiction. Tonya Lamburg is a 16-year-old mother of a 2-year-old son who currently lives with his grandmother. Ms. Lamburg entered the drug rehabilitation center with the goal of ending her problem with the use of alcohol and cocaine. Mr. Swabbs is assigned to her case.

At their first meeting, Mr. Swabbs assesses Ms. Lamburg's level of drug abuse and readiness for change. Ms. Lamburg has been at the center for 1 week and has not used any drugs since checking in. She said that she has repeatedly tried to quit alcohol and cocaine "cold turkey" but started to feel "bad and shaky" and went back to using to stop the withdrawal symptoms. "I have no money. I cannot pay for food for my baby. Everything goes to pay for booze or to get high," said Ms. Lamburg. "I dropped out of school when I got pregnant. Everywhere I try to work I get fired. I decided to get help when I saw my baby get into my coke stash. I do not want my boy to die. I do not want to die." If you were the nurse working with Ms. Lamburg, what steps would you take to help her succeed in meeting her goal of becoming drug-free? What would your first goal be? Depending on her response, what might your next steps be?

assistance in adjusting to a drug-free lifestyle. The residents are expected to secure employment and take responsibility in managing their financial obligations.

Outpatient programs are similar in the education and counseling offered, but they allow the clients to live at home and continue to work while undergoing treatment. This method is effective for persons in the earlier stages of addiction who feel confident that they can abstain from drug use and who have established a strong support network.

Most programs include family counseling and education. In addition, specific programs address the needs of various populations such as adolescents, women during pregnancy, specific ethnic groups, gays and lesbians, and health care professionals.

SMOKING CESSATION PROGRAMS

Nearly 35 million Americans try to quit smoking each year. Fewer than 10% of those who try to quit on their own are able to stop for a year; those who use an intervention are more likely to be successful. Interventions that involve medications and behavioral treatments appear most promising (USDHHS, 2014). For example, nicotine replacement therapy can be used to help smokers withdraw from nicotine while focusing their efforts on breaking the psychological craving or habit. Four types of nicotine replacement products are available: nicotine gum and skin patches are available OTC, and nicotine nasal spray and inhalers are available by prescription. These products are about equally effective and can almost double the chances of successfully quitting. Other treatments include smoking cessation clinics, hypnosis, and acupuncture. The most effective way to get people to stop smoking and prevent relapse involves multiple interventions and continuous reinforcement, and most smokers require several attempts at cessation before they

are successful. Many resources are available on smoking cessation and support groups.

SUPPORT GROUPS

The founding of Alcoholics Anonymous (AA) in 1935 began a strong movement of peer support to treat a chronic illness. AA groups have developed around the world. Their success has led to the development of other support groups such as the following:
- Narcotics Anonymous (NA) for persons with narcotic addiction
- Pills Anonymous for persons with polydrug addictions
- Overeaters Anonymous
- Gamblers Anonymous

AA and NA help addicted people develop a daily program of recovery and reinforce the recovery process. The fellowship, support, and encouragement among AA members provide a vital social network for the person recovering from an addiction.

Al-Anon and Alateen are similar self-help programs for spouses, parents, children, or others involved in a painful relationship with an alcoholic (Nar-Anon for those in relationships with persons with narcotic addictions). Al-Anon family groups are available to anyone who has been affected by involvement with an alcoholic person. The purposes of Alateen include providing a forum for adolescents to discuss family stressors, learn coping skills from one another, and gain support and encouragement from knowledgeable peers. Adult Children of Alcoholics (ACOA) groups are also available in most areas to address the recovery of adults who grew up in alcoholic homes and are still carrying the scars and retaining dysfunctional behaviors.

For some persons, the AA program places too much emphasis on a higher power or focuses too much on the negative consequences of past drinking. Women for Sobriety focuses on rebuilding self-esteem, a core issue for many women with alcoholic problems. See http://www.womenforsobriety.org for additional information.

THE NURSE'S ROLE

Many people with alcoholism and drug addiction become lost in the health care system. If satisfactory care is not provided in one agency or the waiting list is months long, the person may give up rather than seeking alternative sources of care. The nurse who knows the client's history, environment, and support systems and the local treatment programs can offer guidance to the most effective treatment modality. See the Center for Substance Abuse Treatment information on the Substance Abuse and Mental Health Services Administration website at http://www.samhsa.gov for a variety of print and video materials for professionals on helping persons with substance abuse problems. Brief interventions by health care professionals who are not treatment experts can be effective in helping ATOD abusers and addicted persons change their risky behavior. Brief interventions may convince the ATOD abuser to reduce substance consumption or follow through with a treatment referral (SAMHSA, 2011). Box 24.1 describes six elements commonly included in brief interventions, using the acronym FRAMES.

BOX 24.1 Brief Interventions Using the FRAMES Acronym

- **Feedback.** Provide the client direct feedback about the potential or actual personal risk or impairment related to drug use.
- **Responsibility.** Emphasize personal responsibility for change.
- **Advice.** Provide clear advice to change risky behavior.
- **Menu.** Provide a menu of options or choices for changing behavior.
- **Empathy.** Provide a warm, reflective, empathetic, and understanding approach.
- **Self-efficacy.** Provide encouragement and belief in the client's ability to change.

Modified from Bien TH, Miller WR, Tonigan JS: Brief interventions for alcohol problems: a review, *Addictions* 88:315, 1993.

BOX 24-2 Stages of Change

Precontemplation
At this stage, the person does not intend to change in the foreseeable future. The person is often unaware of any problem. Resistance to recognizing or modifying a problem is the hallmark of precontemplation.

Contemplation
At this stage, the individual is aware that a problem exists and is seriously thinking about overcoming it but has not yet made a commitment to take action. The nurse can encourage the individual to weigh the pros and cons of the problem and the solution to the problem.

Preparation
Preparation was originally referred to as decision making. At this stage, the individual is prepared for action and may reduce the problem behavior but has not yet taken effective action (e.g., cuts down amount of smoking but does not abstain).

Action
At this stage, the individual modifies the behavior, experiences, or environment to overcome the problem. The action requires considerable time and energy. Modification of the target behavior to an acceptable criterion and significant overt efforts to change are the hallmarks of action.

Maintenance
In this stage, the individual works to prevent relapse and consolidate the gains attained during action. Stabilizing behavior change and avoiding relapse are the hallmarks of maintenance.

Modified from DiClemente CC, Schlundt D, Gemmell L: Readiness and stages of change in addiction treatment, *Am J Addictions* 13:103-120, 2004

Strategies used with clients can vary depending on their readiness for change. Understanding the stages of change listed in Box 24.2 and recognizing which stage a client is in are important factors for determining which interventions and programs may be most helpful to the client (DiClemente et al, 2004). After the client has received treatment, the nurse can coordinate aftercare referrals and follow up on the client's progress. The nurse can provide additional support in the home as the client and family adjust to changing roles and the stress involved with such changes. The nurse can support addicted persons who have relapsed by reminding them that relapses may well occur but that they and their families can continue to work toward recovery and an improved quality of life.

▷▷ APPLYING CONTENT TO PRACTICE

Using the tools of primary, secondary, and tertiary prevention with individuals, families, and communities for whom alcohol and other drug use is an issue incorporates both public health and public health nursing guidelines and competencies. Specifically, the core competencies of the Council on Linkages Between Academia and Public Health Practice (2010) begin by identifying the analytic and assessment skills needed by public health professionals. The 12 skills in this competency category are used in providing services to the population described in this chapter. For example, you begin by assessing the "health status of populations and their related determinants of health and stress." You next move to skill 2, which is describing the "characteristics of a population-based health problem." These competencies are described through a set of eight domains. Each domain can be used with populations dealing with alcohol and other drug problems.

Similarly, the Intervention Wheel has many applications with this population. The Intervention Wheel specifies that "Interventions are actions that PHNs take on behalf of individuals, families, and systems, and communities to improve or protect health status" (Council on Linkages, 2010, p 1). This tool outlines 17 public health interventions. All 17 of these interventions have applications with the populations described in this chapter. For example, case finding, referral and follow-up, health teaching, counseling, and policy development and enforcement are selected examples of ways in which public health nurses intervene in serving a vulnerable population with alcohol-related and drug-related problems.

▮ PRACTICE APPLICATION

Jane Doe, RN, is a home health case manager in a large, low-income housing area in her local community. She designs care plans and coordinates health care services for clients who need health care at home. She makes the initial visits to determine the level and frequency of care needed and then acts as supervisor of the volunteers and aides who perform most of the day-to-day care. Single-parent families are the norm, and drug dealing is commonplace in this housing area.

Ms. Doe made a home visit to Anne Smith, a 26-year-old mother of three who takes care of her 62-year-old maternal grandfather, Mr. Jones, who is recovering from cardiac bypass surgery. Mr. Jones has a history of smoking two packs per day for almost

40 years. Since his surgery, he has decreased to one pack per day, but he refuses to quit. He had a history of alcohol dependence, reportedly consuming up to a fifth of liquor per day, and a history of withdrawal seizures. Four years ago, Mr. Jones went through alcohol detoxification, but he refused to stay at the facility for continued treatment, stating he could stay sober on his own. Since that time he has had several binge episodes, but Ms. Smith says he has not been drinking since the surgery. A widower for 5 years, Mr. Jones now lives with his granddaughter and her children.

Ms. Smith is a widow and has two sons, ages 3 and 9 years, and a daughter, age 5 years. The oldest son's father is an alcoholic who is currently incarcerated for manslaughter while driving under the influence of alcohol, and the father of her two youngest children was killed by a stray bullet in a cocaine bust 3 years ago. She and her husband had smoked crack cocaine for several months, but both stopped when she became pregnant with their youngest child and remained cocaine-free. She has been angry at the system and frightened of police officers ever since the drug raid in which her husband was killed. Other residents were also hurt, and less than $500 worth of cocaine was found three apartments away from hers.

Ms. Smith does not consume alcohol, but she smokes one to two packs of cigarettes per day. She quit smoking during her pregnancies but restarted soon after each birth.

A. What type of interventions can the nurse provide for Mr. Jones regarding his smoking?

B. How can the nurse help Ms. Smith cope with the potential risk for Mr. Jones continuing to drink when he progresses to more independence?
C. How can Ms. Doe help Ms. Smith with her cigarette smoking?
D. Knowing that there is a genetic link to alcoholism and being aware of the high rate of drug problems in the housing area, how can Ms. Doe help prevent Ms. Smith and her children from developing substance abuse problems?
E. Which are the most significant problems related to the drug laws, and what can Ms. Doe do to help make the environment safer and more nurturing?

Answers can be found on the Evolve website.

REMEMBER THIS!

- Substance abuse is the leading national health problem, linked to numerous forms of morbidity and mortality.
- Harm reduction is a new approach to ATOD problems; it deals with substance abuse primarily as a health problem rather than a criminal problem.
- All persons have ideas, opinions, and attitudes about drugs that influence their actions.
- Social conditions such as a fast-paced life, excessive stress, and the availability of drugs influence the incidence of substance abuse.
- New forms of substance abuse are growing, including the use of electronic cigarettes and energy drinks. Nurses need to be familiar with these substances and their effects.
- Primary prevention for substance abuse includes education about drugs and guidelines for use, as well as the promotion of healthy alternatives to drug use either for recreation or to relieve stress.

- Nurses can play a key role in developing community prevention programs.
- Secondary prevention depends heavily on careful assessment of the client's use of drugs. Such assessment should be part of all basic health assessments.
- High-risk groups include pregnant women, young people, older adults, intravenous drug users, and illicit drug users.
- Drug addiction is often a family problem, not merely an individual problem.
- Codependency describes a companion illness to the addiction of one person in which the codependent member is addicted to the addicted person.
- Brief interventions by a nurse can be as effective as treatment.
- Nurses are in ideal roles to assist with tertiary prevention for both the addicted person and the family.

EVOLVE WEBSITE
http://evolve.elsevier.com/Stanhope/foundations
- Case Study, with Questions and Answers
- NCLEX® Review Questions
- Practice Application Answers

REFERENCES

Addictions and Recovery.org: *The genetics of addiction*, June 18, 2017, Author.
Alejandro A, Mattson ME, Lyerla R: Driving under the influence of alcohol, marijuana, and alcohol and marijuana combined among persons aged 16-25 years-United States, 2002-2014. *Morbidity and Mortality Weekly Report* 64(48):1325–1329, 2015.
Antolin VM, Barkley TW: Electronic cigarettes: what nurses need to know. *Nursing* 45(11):60–64, 2015.
Bien TH, Miller WR, Tonigan JS: Brief interventions for alcohol problems: a review, *Addictions* 88:315, 1993.
Brady TM, Ashley OS, editors: *Women in substance abuse treatment: results from the Alcohol and Drug Services Study (ADSS). USDHHS*

Pub no. SMA 04-3968, Analytic Series A-26, Rockville, Md, 2005, Substance Abuse and Mental Health Services Administration, Office of Applied Studies.
Britton J, Bogdanovica I, Ashcroft R, McNeill A: Electronic cigarettes, smoking and population health, *Clin Med* 14(4):334–337, 2014.
Carr ER: E-cigarettes: Facts, perception, and marketing messages, *Clin J Oncology* 18(1):112–116, Feb 2014.
Center for Behavioral Health Statistics and Quality: *Behavioral health trends in the United States: Results from the 2014 National Survey on Drug Use and Health (HHS Publication No. SMA15-4927, HSDUH Series H-50)*, 2015. Retrieved May 2016 from http://www.samhsa.gov/data/.
Centers for Disease Control and Prevention: *HIV and Injection Drug Use*, 2017, Available at http://www.cdc.gov. Accessed June 18, 2017.
Centers for Disease Control and Prevention: *Youth and tobacco use*, 2016. Available at http://www.cdc.gov. Accessed June 18, 2017.
Council on Linkages Between Academic and Public Health Practice: *Core competencies for public health professionals*, Washington, DC, 2010, Public Health Foundation, Health Resources and Services Administration.
Dick DM, Agrawal A: The genetics of alcohol and other drug dependence, *Alcohol Research and Health* 31(2):111–118, 2008.

DiClemente CC, Schlundt D, Gemmell L: Readiness and stages of change in addiction treatment, *Am J Addictions* 13:103–120, 2004.

Frieden TR, Houry D: Reducing the risks of relief-the CDC Opioid-prescribing guideline, *N Engl J of Med* downloaded from nejm.org on March 29, 2016. Vol 374:1501–1504, April 21, 2016.

Institute of Medicine: *Leading health indicators for Healthy People 2020* [letter report], Washington, DC, 2011, IOM. Retrieved May 2016 from http://www.iom.nationalacademiesorg/hmd/~/media/files/Report . . . .

Jamal A, Homa DM, O'Connor E, Babb SD, Caraballo RS, Singh T, Hu SS, King BA: Current cigarette smoking among adults-United States, 2005-2014, *Morbidity and Mortality Weekly Review (MMWR)* 64(44):1233–1240, November 13, 2015.

Knox R: Needle exchanges often overlooked in AIDS fight, *Health News from NPR* July 24, 2012. Available at http://www.npr.org/blogs/health/2012/07/24/157283038/needle-exchanges-often-overlooked-in-aids-fight. Accessed June 16, 2014.

Marijuana: *The Merck manual*, January 2016. Retrieved June 18, 2017 from http://www.merckmanual.

Mayo Clinic Staff: *Caffeine: how much is too much?* Rochester, MN, March 2009, Mayo Clinic. Retrieved July 2012 from http://www.mayoclinic.com/health/caffeine/NU00600/METHOD print.

National Institute on Alcohol Abuse and Alcoholism: *Genetics of alcohol use disorder*. Retrieved June 18, 2017 from https://www.niaaa.nih.gov/alcohol-health/overview-alcohol-consumption/alcohol-use-disorders/genetics-alcohol-use-disorders.

O'Connor PG: *Merck Manual Consumer Version*, 2016. Retrieved May 2016 from http://www.merckmanual.

Pan W, Bai H: A multivariate approach to a meta-analytic review of the effectiveness of the D.A.R.E. program, *Int J Environ Res Public Health* 61(1):267–277, 2009.

Physicians and Lawyers for National Drug Policy: *Policy priorities: summary*, 2008. Retrieved August 2012 from http://www.plndp.org/Policy_Priorities/Summary.html.

Rudd RA, Aleshire N, Zibbell JE, Gladden RM: Increases in drug and opioid overdose death-United States, 2000-2014, *Morbidity and Mortality Weekly Report (MMWR)* 64(50):1378–1382, January 1, 2016.

Schoenborn CA, Gindi RM: *Electronic cigarette use among adults: United States, 2014, NCHS Data Brief No. 217*, Hyattsville MD, October 2015, Centers for Disease Control and Prevention.

Seifert SM, Schaechter JL, Hershorin EG, Lipshultz SE: Health effects of energy drinks on children, adolescents, and young adults, *Pediatrics* published online February 14, 2011. http://www.content/early/2011/02/14/peds.2009-3592.

Singh R, Marynak K, Arrazola RA, Cox S, Rolle IV, King BA: Vital signs: exposure to electronic cigarette advertising among middle school and high school students-United States, 2014, *Morbidity and Mortality Weekly Report (MMWR)* 64(Early Release):1–6, January 5, 2016.

Stott DG, Falconer A, Kerr GD, et al: Does low to moderate alcohol intake protect against cognitive decline in older people? *J Am Geriatric Soc* 56:2217–2224, 2008.

Substance Abuse and Mental Health Services Administration: *Screening, Brief Intervention and referral to Treatment (SBIBT) in Behavioral Healthcare*, January 4, 2011. Available at http://bigsbirteducation.webs.com/SMIRTwhitepaper.pdf. Accessed June 25, 2014.

US Department of Health and Human Services: *Healthy People 2020*, Washington, DC, 2010a, US Government Printing Office.

US Department of Health and Human Services: *How tobacco smoke causes disease: the biology and behavioral basis for smoking-attributable disease: a report of the Surgeon General*, Atlanta, GA, 2010b, US Department of Health and Human Services, Centers for Disease Control and Prevention, National Center for Chronic Disease Prevention and Health Promotion, Office on Smoking and Health. Retrieved November 2012 from http://www.surgeongeneral.gov/library/reports/tobaccosmoke/executivesummary.pdf.

US Department of Health and Human Services: *The health consequences of smoking—50 years of progress: a report of the Surgeon General*, Atlanta, GA, 2014, USDHHS, CDC, National Center for Chronic Disease Prevention and Health Promotion.

US Food and Drug Administration, National Soft Drink Association: *Center for Science in the Public Interest*. Retrieved July 2010 from http://kidshealth.org/teen/drug_alcohol/drugs/caffeine.html#.

Volkow ND, Frieden TR, Hyde PS, et al: Medical-assisted therapies-tackling the opioid overdose epidemic. *N Engl J Med* 370:2063–2066, 2014.

WebMD: *Street drugs: know the facts and risks*. Reviewed July 15, 2015 by William Blahd MD. Retrieved May 2016 from http://www.webmd.com.

WebMD: *Cocaine and its effects*. Reviewed January 16, 2016 by Joseph Goldberg MD. http://www.webmd.com. Retrieved May 2016.

CHAPTER 25

Violence and Human Abuse

Erika Metzler Sawin, Jacquelyn C. Campbell, Jeanne Alhusen,
Rosa Gonzales-Guarda, Tina Bloom

OBJECTIVES

After reading this chapter, the student should be able to:

1. Discuss the scope of the problem of violence in American communities, and describe at least three factors in most communities that encourage violence and human abuse.
2. Identify common predictors of potential child abuse and indicators of its presence.
3. Define the four general types of child abuse: neglect, physical, emotional, and sexual.
4. Discuss the dynamics and signs of female abuse by male partners.
5. Describe the growing community health problem of elder abuse.
6. Analyze the nursing role in working with survivors of violence.
7. Discuss forensic nursing and its relationship to public health nursing.

CHAPTER OUTLINE

Social and Community Factors Influencing Violence
  Work
  Education
  Media
  Organized Religion
  Population
  Community Facilities
Violence against Individuals or Oneself
  Homicide
  Assault
  Sexual Violence and Rape
  Suicide
Family Violence and Abuse
  Development of Abusive Patterns
  Types of Family Violence
  Abuse of Older Adults
Nursing Interventions

KEY TERMS

assault, 437
child abuse, 443
child neglect, 444
elder abuse, 440
emotional abuse, 443
emotional neglect, 444
family violence, 440
forensic nursing, 439
homicide, 436
incest, 444
intimate partner violence (IPV), 445
neglect, 441
physical abuse, 441
physical neglect, 444
rape, 437
sexual abuse, 441
sexual assault nurse examiner, 439
sexual violence, 437
spouse abuse, 441
suicide, 439
violence, 434
wife abuse, 445

The word violence comes from the Latin *violare*, meaning to violate, injure, or rape. Violence is a public health problem that has both emotional and physical effects. The United States, like many other countries, has a sizable problem with violence. Some societies are basically nonviolent, and for them violence is not a significant health problem. It remains unclear if violence stems from an innate aggressive drive or is a learned behavior. What is clear is that learned behavior, social norms, and community actions can influence the types and levels of violence. It is important to understand the conditions that can lead to aggression and violence and, conversely, what keeps them in check and promotes nonviolent conflict resolution.

Violence is a concern for nurses. Significant mortality and morbidity result from violence. Public health nurses regularly see the evidence of violence and the effect on individuals and families. Nurses often care for the victims, the perpetrators, and those who witness physical and psychological violence. The more types and instances of violence that are experienced or witnessed, the more negative are the effects on health

(Musicant, 2011). Nurses also can take an active role in the development of public policy, resources, and community responses to violence.

Violence is generally defined as those nonaccidental acts, interpersonal or intrapersonal, that result in physical or psychological injury to one or more persons. Violent behavior is predictable and thus preventable, especially with community action. To make progress in reducing health inequities and improve health for people who live in communities with significant levels of violence, there needs to be organized and inclusive community efforts to prevent violence (Musicant, 2011).

The Centers for Disease Control and Prevention (CDC) has many training resources available on its website. For example, there are fact sheets related to understanding teen dating violence, elder maltreatment, intimate partner violence (IPV), child maltreatment, and bullying, to name only a few examples. Visit http://www.cdc.gov/ViolencePrevention/index.html for guides and information. In 2014 the World Health Organization (WHO) published its "Global Status Report on Violence Prevention," which is the first report of its kind to assess national efforts that address interpersonal violence, namely child maltreatment, youth violence, intimate partner and sexual violence, and elder abuse worldwide (WHO, 2014a).

Based on models developed in the 1980s, communities are developing a coordinated response in which multiple agencies work together to assist with preventing IPV. In addition to the criminal justice system, advocates for women, health care providers, and employers are encouraged to learn about and assist their employees with issues of IPV (Pennington-Zoellner, 2009). All of these community programs have the same goal: to decrease the incidence and prevalence of violence in our communities. Violence is a major cause of premature mortality and life-long disability, and violence-related morbidity is a significant factor in health care costs. To guide prevention of violence, a section of the Healthy People 2020 objectives is devoted to violence.

This chapter examines violence as a public health problem and discusses how nurses can help individuals, families, groups, and communities prevent, cope with, and reduce violence and abuse. Nurses work with clients in many settings, including the home. Because they are in key positions to detect and intervene in community and family violence, nurses

---

♥ *HEALTHY PEOPLE 2020*

Objectives for Reducing Violence

- **IVP-29:** Reduce homicides.
- **IVP-30:** Reduce firearm-related deaths.
- **IVP-35:** Reduce bullying among adolescents.
- **IVP-37:** Reduce child maltreatment deaths.
- **IVP-39:** Reduce violence by current or former intimate partners.
- **IVP-40:** Reduce sexual violence.
- **IVP-42:** Reduce children's exposure to violence.

---

need to understand how community-level influences can affect all types of violence. Nurses are often considered the "first responders" when it comes to recognizing and dealing with violence (Trossman, 2009).

SOCIAL AND COMMUNITY FACTORS INFLUENCING VIOLENCE

Many factors in a community can support or minimize violence. Changing social conditions, multiple demands on people, economic conditions, and social institutions influence the level of violence and human abuse. The following discussion of selected social conditions describes factors that influence violent behavior.

Work

Productive and paid work is an expectation in mainstream American society. Work can be fulfilling and contribute to a sense of well-being; it also can be frustrating and unfulfilling, contributing to stress that may lead to aggression and violence. Some people are frustrated by jobs that are repetitive, are boring, and lack stimulation. Others may report to supervisors whom they neither like nor respect and who are verbally abusive or demeaning. Workers may go home feeling physically and psychologically drained. They may have difficulty separating feelings generated at work from those at home. For example, a father arrives home feeling tired, angry, and generally inadequate because of a series of reprimands from his boss. Soon after he sits down, his 4-year-old son runs through the house pretending to fly a toy airplane. After about three loud trips past his father, who keeps shouting for the child to be quiet and go outside, the boy hits the father in the head with the airplane. The father could hit the boy out of frustration and anger.

People hesitate to give up jobs, even if they are frustrating, boring, or stressful. This is particularly true in times of economic downturns when jobs are scarce and competition for them is keen. Family needs may necessitate that these persons keep the hated job. People feel trapped and may resent those who depend on them. This frustration and resentment may contribute to violent behavior. Unemployment is also associated with violence both within and outside the home and is associated with domestic violence (Capaldi et al, 2012). The inability to secure or keep a job may lead to feelings of inadequacy, guilt, boredom, dissatisfaction, and frustration. Young minority men have the highest rates of unemployment in the United States, ranging up to 50%, even in times of economic prosperity (U.S. Department of Labor, 2014). This group also has the highest rate of violence. They may feel oppressed or discriminated against, and their lack of opportunities for jobs may encourage anger and violence. Most analyses conclude that the differential rates of violence between African Americans and whites in the United States have more to do with economic realities, such as poverty, unemployment, and overcrowding, than with race (Cho, 2012).

Education

In recent years, schools have assumed many responsibilities traditionally assigned to the family. Schools teach sexual development, discipline children, and often serve as a haven where children are fed and given the developmental support needed. Large classes often mean that teachers spend more time and energy monitoring and disciplining children than challenging and stimulating them to learn. In large classes, children who do not conform to expected behaviors are often isolated. The nonconforming child may be removed from the classroom because there is little or no time to help the child learn alternative ways of behavior.

Some schools and parents may use spanking as a form of discipline. Such punishment only reinforces the child's tendency to strike out at others. Schools are often places in which the stressors and frustrations that can contribute to violence are abundant, and violence is learned rather than discouraged. School violence is a subset of youth violence and can include bullying, slapping, punching, and using weapons.

One of these forms of youth violence, bullying, is especially important in that it can occur in person or through technology. Bullying includes attack or intimidation with the intent to cause fear, distress, or harm; there is typically an imbalance of power between the bully and the victim, and there are repeated attacks or intimidation between the same children over time (CDC, 2015a). Some of the factors associated with a higher likelihood that a child will bully are impulsivity or poor self-control, harsh parenting by caregivers, and an accepting attitude toward violence. In contrast, some of the factors that may be associated with a higher likelihood of being the victim of a bully are having trouble-making friends, having poor self-esteem, and being quiet and lacking in assertiveness (CDC, 2015a). Bullying can have devastating effects on the health of the victim and result in physical injury; social and emotional distress, including depression and anxiety; psychosomatic complaints; and poor school adjustment (CDC, 2015a) and can lead to self-harm (Hamm, 2015). Cyberbullying, an intentional form of hostile electronic communication, takes place constantly. It often leads to depression, isolation, and absenteeism. Many schools and parent groups are targeting bullying behavior on a larger scale by focusing on peer groups and population-based interventions (Ayers et al, 2012).

Schools can be a powerful contributor to nonviolence. Classes can help adolescents learn peaceful conflict resolution and help young children deal with the threat of sexual abuse and issues of date rape (Regan, 2010). Parents can be advised of the availability of such programs, and school boards should be urged to adopt them into the curriculum. The CDC recommends four approaches for addressing problems like school violence (CDC, 2015b):
- Improve student supervision
- Use existing school rules and management structure to provide consequences for bullying
- Have a whole-school antibullying policy
- Promote cooperation between school staff and parents, as well as among varied professionals

Media

The media can influence the occurrence of both violence and caring, compassionate behaviors. Television programs and print articles can inform and increase public awareness about family violence. Programs that raise the social awareness of IPV may play a role in reducing violence in interpersonal relationships (Regan, 2010). The efforts may include online social marketing and public service announcements that discuss health and social care resources (Best, 2014). Abused women and rape victims benefit from media attention, which tends to decrease the stigma of such victimization and publicize available services. Also, media are used to publicize services.

Conversely, many toys and video games depict violence. Children and youth are often skilled at video and computer gaming, and these games can depict positive qualities such as friendship, honor, pride, and happiness, as well as aggression, pain, and fear. Research on violent television and films, video games, social media, and music demonstrates that media violence can increase the likelihood of aggressive and violent behavior, both short-and long-term (Anderson et al, 2003, Patton et al, 2014). A recent systematic review demonstrates a relationship between online social media and interpersonal violence (Patton et al, 2014).

Mass media is thought to be one of many possible influences on the development of aggressive or violent behavior. Violent adults and adolescents were often violent children. Therefore it is important to identify factors that are important influences on children, including media violence, and acknowledge their ability to possibly contribute to the development of violent behaviors.

Communities, including schools, parent-teacher organizations, and religious organizations, should teach parents and children how to be informed and healthy media consumers. Parents and caregivers must monitor what media reaches their children. Parents need quality tools to assist them to monitor and then modify their children's media habits. Violence prevention researchers should work with media researchers to create and disseminate solutions to social and public health problems.

Organized Religion

Churches meet many human needs, including the need for stimulation, a sense of value, belonging, closeness, and worth, as well as the need for power. Religion generally teaches nonviolent conflict resolution. Churches, clergy, and members of church groups often provide positive role models and reinforce peaceful behavior. Historically, a seemingly contradictory relationship exists between abuse and religion. For example, many religious groups uphold the philosophy of "spare the rod, spoil the child." Also, some faiths support the victimization of women or spouses when they disapprove of divorce. Family members may stay together, although they are at emotional or physical war with one another, because of religious commitments (Knickmeyer et al, 2010).

Although churches have been slow to recognize domestic violence, some changes are taking place. Male domination over women has become a major issue of discussion in some church groups, whereas in other groups women continue to be blamed for the abuse they sustain. Clergy need to be taught about the nature and dynamics of violence in the family, about religious messages and the potential for support, and about the need for collaboration between the church and advocates for the prevention of domestic violence.

Population

A community's structure and population can influence the potential for violence. For example, when people are poor and live in crowded conditions, the potential for tension and violence is greater. High–population-density communities can positively or negatively influence violence. Those with a sense of cohesiveness may have a lower crime rate than areas of similar size that lack social and cultural groups to support unity among members. Bonds formed within church groups, clubs, and professional organizations can promote harmony. In such groups, members can talk about stressors rather than responding with violence. For example, residents of public housing often form neighborhood associations to deal with common residential situations. Tension can be released in a productive way via projects carried out by the association.

Some residents of high-population areas feel powerless and helpless rather than cohesive. Low-paying jobs and a lack of jobs can lead to feelings of inadequacy, despair, and social alienation. Social alienation and exclusion from opportunities can lead to decreased social cohesion and increased violence (Beyer et al, 2015). Fear and apathy may cause community residents to withdraw from social contact. Withdrawal can foster crime because many residents assume someone else will report suspicious behavior or they fear reprisals for such reports.

Youths may deal with feelings of powerlessness by forming gangs. Poverty and lack of education appear to be the overriding risk factors. Some of these young adults try to deal with their feelings by engaging in crime against people and property to release frustration. In many cities, these gangs are highly destructive. Through community mobilization efforts, primary prevention programs have been implemented that deal with youth disenfranchisement and gang violence (Pitts, 2009).

Some high-population areas are characterized by a sense of confusion, resulting in disintegration and disorganization. These areas often have transient populations who have limited physical or emotional investment in the community. Lack of community concern allows crime and violence to go unchecked and may become a norm for the area. As crime increases, residents who are able to do so often leave the area. This increases community disintegration because the residents who leave are often the most capable members of the population.

The potential for violence may increase among highly diverse populations. Differences in age, socioeconomic status, ethnicity, religion, citizenship, acculturation, or other cultural characteristics can disrupt community stability. Highly divergent groups may not communicate effectively and may neither accept nor understand one another. These groups can become hostile and antagonistic toward other groups. Each may see the other as different and not belonging. The alienated group may become the focal point for the others' frustrations, anger, and fears. Racism, classism, and heterosexism are examples of major causes of community disintegration resulting in a vicious cycle of dishonesty, distrust, and hate.

Community Facilities

Communities provide a large range of resources and facilities to residents. Some are more desirable places to live, work, and raise families and have facilities that can reduce the potential for crime and violence. Recreational facilities such as playgrounds, parks, swimming pools, movie theaters, and tennis, basketball and other sport courts provide socially acceptable outlets for a variety of feelings, including aggression. These facilities are resources the residents can use for exercise, release of tension and stress, and for pleasure, personal enrichment, and group development. Spectator sports, such as football, baseball, basketball, soccer, or hockey, also allow community members to express feelings of anger and frustration. However, watching physically aggressive sports can encourage violence when players hit or shove one another. Familiarity with factors contributing to a community's violence or potential for violence enables nurses to recognize them and intervene accordingly.

VIOLENCE AGAINST INDIVIDUALS OR ONESELF

The potential for violence against individuals (e.g., murder, robbery, rape, assault) or oneself (e.g., suicide) is directly related to the level of violence in the community. Persons living in areas with high rates of crime and violence are more likely to become victims than those in more peaceful areas. The major categories of violence addressed in this chapter are described in terms of the scope of the problem in the United States and the underlying dynamics.

Homicide

Homicide is defined as a death resulting from the use of force against another person when a preponderance of evidence indicates that force was intentional (Parks, 2014). Although homicide rates have decreased over the last 20 years, homicide rates in the United States are alarming. Homicide is the second leading cause of death for young African American women 15 to 34 years of age and for young Native American women 20 to 34 years of age and is the fourth, third, and fifth leading causes of death for white women 15 to 19, 20 to 24, and 25 to 34 years of age, respectively (Parks, 2014). Young black males 10 to 24 years of age have a higher rate of homicide (51 per 100,000) than both young Hispanic American males (13.5 per 100,000) and non-Hispanic white males (2.9 per 100,000) (CDC, 2012). These statistics do not account for the significant morbidity associated with interpersonal violence. For every person who dies as a result of violence, many more are injured and suffer lasting physical, sexual, and mental health sequelae. As the WHO has reported, when interpersonal violence results in large numbers of deaths, the issue is a significant public health concern necessitating attention from researchers, policy makers, health care providers, and the public (Krug et al, 2002).

Homicide is increasing the most among adolescents, but even among very young children in the United States homicide occurs at an alarming rate; homicide is one of the top five leading causes of death for children and youth between 1 and 14 years of age (CDC, 2014a). The majority of homicides of children are perpetrated by parents. Homicides committed by intimate partners account for 14% of all US homicides, and 70% of those victims were female (Smith et al, 2014).

Strangers cause only 15% of male and 9% of female homicides in the United States (Catalano et al, 2009). When strangers are involved, many of the deaths are related to the use of illegal substances. Most homicides are committed during an argument by a friend, acquaintance, or family member. Prevention of homicide is an issue for both the public health system and the criminal justice system.

An alarming aspect of family homicide is that children may witness the murder or find the body of a family member (Lysell et al, 2016). No automatic follow-up or counseling of these children occurs through the criminal justice or mental health system in most communities. These children are at great risk for mental disorder, self-harm, substance use, and completed suicide if older than 18 years of age (Lysell et al, 2016).

The underlying dynamics of homicide within families vary greatly from those of other murders. Women are nine times more likely to be killed by an intimate partner than a stranger. The intimate partner may be a husband, boyfriend, same-sex partner, or ex-partner (Campbell et al, 2007). The top risk factor for intimate partner homicide (IPH) is previous domestic violence; other risk factors are access to guns, estrangement, threats to kill and threats with a weapon, nonfatal strangulation, and a stepchild in the home if the victim is a female (Campbell et al, 2007). Other risk factors are violent crime convictions in general and major mental disorder (Lysell et al, 2016).

Thus prevention of family homicide involves working with abusive families. In a study of IPH of women, 75% of the women who were killed by a husband, boyfriend, or ex-partner had been seen in a health care setting during the year before the homicide (Nannini et al, 2008). Nurses have a duty to warn family members of the possibility of homicide when severe abuse is present, just as they warn them of the hazards of

smoking. Other nursing care issues are discussed further in the section on family violence and abuse.

Assault

The death toll from violence is staggering, yet the physical injuries and emotional costs of assault are equally important issues in both the acute health care system and the community. Violent crime rates, including simple and aggravated assault, robbery, and rape or sexual assault, have remained steady, at a rate of 20.1 per 1000. This is much lower than earlier rates of 78 per 1000 in 1993 (Truman & Langston, 2015). Aggravated assault is reported to police more often than simple assault or rape, but all assault types are underreported (Truman & Langston, 2015). The greatest risk factor for an individual's victimization through violence is age, and youths are at significantly higher risk. Whereas more males than females are victims of homicide and assault, women are more likely to be victimized by a relative, especially a male partner. Both females (50%) and males (44%) suffer injuries as victims of intimate partner violence (Catalano, 2013). Sometimes the difference between a homicide and an assault is only the response time and the quality of emergency transport and treatment facilities. The same community measures used to address homicide can be used to combat assault. Also, nurses often see assaulted persons in home health care with long-term health problems such as head injuries, spinal cord injuries, and stomas from abdominal gunshot wounds. In addition to physical care, nurses must address the emotional trauma of a violent attack. They can help victims talk through their traumatic experience to try to make some sense of the violence and refer them for further counseling if anxiety, sleeping problems, or depression persists after the assault.

Sexual Violence and Rape

Sexual violence is forcing a person to take part in a sexual act when the person does not consent, and includes rape (attempted and completed), sexual coercion, being made to penetrate a perpetrator, unwanted sexual contact experiences, and unwanted sexual noncontact experiences (e.g. being flashed or made to view sexually explicit media) (Breiding et al, 2014). In 2010 the CDC's National Center for Injury Prevention and Control began the National Intimate Partner and Sexual Violence Survey, in which they interviewed 9086 women and 7421 men. Their report presents information about several types of violence that have not been measured in a national survey, including expressive aggression, coercive control, and control of reproductive or sexual health (Black et al, 2011). From these interviews, they learned that nearly 1 in 5 black women (22.0%), 1 in 5 white women (18.8%), 1 in 7 Hispanic women (14.6%), and 1 in 71 men (1.4%) in the United States have been raped at some time in their lives. Over one-fourth of American Indian and Alaska Native women reported being raped at some time in their lives. Over one-half of the female victims were raped by an intimate partner, and 40.8% were raped by an acquaintance. For male victims, over one-half were raped by an acquaintance and 15.1% by a stranger. The first rape for most of the female victims occurred before 25 years of age, and 27.8%

of male victims were raped when they were 10 years of age or younger (Black et al, 2011). These numbers underestimate the extent of the problem because many cases are never reported. Victims may be ashamed, embarrassed, or afraid. They may think they will not be believed. Victim reporting of rape has improved. Hospital personnel, emergency personnel, and police have better protocols for victims of rape. Even though the collection of information leading to prosecution is emphasized, the protocols try to ensure respectful and supportive treatment for victims. However, although about 80% of female victims of IPV are treated in US hospitals, most are not identified as abuse victims, even though it is known that routine questioning can identify victims who do not volunteer information about IPV. Rhodes and colleagues found that the "vast majority of police-identified female IPV victims are using the ED for health care, but they are unlikely to be identified or receive intervention for IPV in the ED setting" (2011, p 898).

Rape on college campuses has some unique characteristics, such that the White House established the Task Force to Protect Students from Sexual Assault in 2014 (Krebs et al, 2016). Sexual assault prevention is a discussion in freshman orientation at most if not all universities. However, freshmen are busy adjusting to life away from home, classes, and new friends, and they often do not pay close attention to the safety measures they are being taught. Also, the availability of alcohol compounds the situation. Primary prevention is the first step. That is, teach people they need to be aware, to understand what they are seeing and experiencing, and to take steps toward maintaining their safety. In fact, one in four college women will be a victim of sexual assault; of these assaults, 60% will be perpetrated by an acquaintance of the victim, heavy episodic drinking will increase the chance of being raped eight-fold (One in Four USA, 2016), and fewer than 5% of all incidents will be brought to the attention of administrators or authorities. Nonheterosexual students are more likely to be victimized than heterosexual students (Krebs et al, 2016). Many colleges and universities advocate bystander education, which teaches peers not to look at women as victims and men as perpetrators but rather to consider each person a bystander who has a responsibility to ensure the safety of persons in his or her community. Bystander education has application in all settings in which sexual assault could occur, not just on college campuses. Women on college campuses often underreport allegations of rape because of issues of confidentiality and fear of being discredited (Krebs et al, 2016).

Sexual violence can affect health by causing both physical injuries and emotional harm. Physical injuries can be cuts, scratches, bruises, or welts or more serious injuries such as broken bones, internal bleeding, chronic pain, stomach problems, sexually transmitted diseases (STDs), unwanted pregnancies, and head trauma. The emotional pain can lead to trauma symptoms such as flashbacks, panic attacks, trouble sleeping, eating disorders, and depression (Black et al, 2011). Victims may engage in negative health behaviors such as smoking, abusing alcohol or drugs, or engaging in risky sexual behaviors.

Also be alert for signs of date and marital rape. Rape victims seldom offer sensitive information unless you specifically ask

for it and make it clear that confidentiality will be upheld (WHO, 2014c). Dating violence includes rape, physical violence, and stalking, and can take place in person or electronically such as by texting or posting sexual pictures of a partner online (CDC, 2016a). Teen victims of dating violence are more likely to be depressed and do poorly in school. They may take part in unhealthy behaviors such as using drugs and alcohol and have eating disorders, or consider or attempt suicide (CDC, 2016a).

For reported rapes, cities constitute higher risk areas than do rural areas, and the hours between 8 pm and 2 am, the weekends, and the summer are the most critical times. In about 50% of rapes, the victim and the offender meet on the street, whereas in other cases the rapist either enters the victim's home or somehow entices or forces the victim to accompany him. The majority of rapists are known to the victim.

Prevention of rape, like that of other forms of human abuse, requires a broad-based community focus for educating both the community as a whole and key groups such as police, health care providers, educators, and social workers. Prevention should begin early by promoting healthy, respectful relationships in families so that children learn that interactions should be based on respect and trust and conflict resolution should occur without using violence. These same forms of communication should be reinforced in schools and social organizations. It is also important to address the beliefs, attitudes, and messages that are sent that may condone sexual violence, stalking, and IPV. Violence should be recognized as being deep-rooted, and as having social and economic causes (CDC, 2014b).

It is also important to be aware of cultural differences related to sexual violence, including rape. Cultural and social norms influence behavior, including violence. For example, the use of violence to solve conflicts or as part of childrearing can be a risk factor for interpersonal violence. Children learn to accept the use of violence when they see corporal punishment, violence in the family, or violence in the media or other settings. Examples of cultural and social norms that support violence would include beliefs that men have a right to control or discipline women through physical means, which can lead to IPV and sexual exploitation of girls. Other factors would be the belief that violence is a private affair, which might prevent the victims from speaking out (WHO, 2014a). Also, societies that tolerate higher rates of acute alcohol intoxication report stronger associations between alcohol use and violence than societies in which alcohol is used more moderately. Some specific examples of culture-specific norms that affect sexual violence include (1) child maltreatment when female children are valued less in society than males (Peru), (2) when children in general have a low status in society and within the family (Guatemala), (3) when genital mutilation is practiced (Nigeria or Sudan), or when child marriage is acceptable. In terms of sexual violence, some examples of cultural norms are: (1) sex is a man's right in marriage (Pakistan); (2) girls are responsible for controlling a man's sexual urges (South Africa); (3) sexual violence such as rape is perceived as shameful for the victims and they do not disclose the act (United States), or (4) reporting youth violence of bullying is unacceptable (United Kingdom). See the "Global

Status Report on Violence Prevention" (WHO, 2014a) for many more examples of cultural and social norms that support violence and examples of ways to change these norms.

A first step in intervening in the incidence of rape and treatment of rape survivors is to change and clarify misconceptions about rape and victims of rape. Rape is a crime of violence, not a crime of passion. The underlying issues are hostility, power, and control rather than sexual desire. The defining issue is lack of consent of the victim. When a woman or man refuses any sexual activity, that refusal means "no." People have the right to change their mind, even when they seemed initially agreeable. Pressure from physical contact, threats, or deliberate inducement of drug or alcohol intoxication is a violation of the law. The myths that women say "no" to sex when they really mean "yes" and that the victims of rape are culpable because of the way they dress or act must end. On college campuses, attitudes toward acquaintance or date rape are slow to change. Also, one of the risk factors for teen dating violence that applies to instances on college campuses is the use of alcohol.

People react to rape differently, depending on their personality, past experiences, background, and support received after the trauma. Some cry, shout, or discuss the experience. Others withdraw and are afraid to discuss the attack. During the immediate and follow-up stages, victims may blame themselves for what has happened. When working with rape victims, help them identify the issues behind self-blame. Fault should not be placed on survivors; they should be taught to take control, learn assertiveness, and think they can take specific actions to prevent future rapes. Survivors need to talk about what happened and to express their feelings and fears in a nonjudgmental atmosphere. Nonjudgmental listening is important. In any psychological trauma, the right to privacy and confidentiality is crucial. Victims should be given privacy, respect, and assurance of confidentiality; told about health care procedures conducted immediately after the rape; given a complete physical examination by a trained nurse examiner (i.e., sexual assault or forensic nurse examiner); and linked with proper resources for ease of reporting. Other suggestions for sexual violence prevention are outlined in "STOP SV: A Technical Package to Prevent Sexual Violence" (Basile et al, 2016).

When a person is admitted to a hospital with traumatic injuries, the person should be evaluated to determine the forensic nature of the injuries (Sheridan and Nash, 2009). Nurses often provide continuous care once the victim enters the health care system. Because many victims deny the event once the initial crisis has passed, a single-session debriefing should be completed during the initial examination. Specially trained providers should conduct the physical assessment, examination, and debriefing. In most states, nurses trained in sexual assault examination (**sexual assault nurse examiner** [SANE] nurses, a subspecialty of **forensic nursing**) perform the physical examination in the emergency department to gather evidence (e.g., hair samples, skin fragments beneath the victim's fingernails, evidence from pelvic examinations using colposcopy) for criminal prosecution of sexual assault. This crucial nursing intervention often takes time and allows the nurse to begin communication with the victim (Campbell et al, 2011). Nurses' evidence is credible

and effective in court proceedings (Campbell, 2014). These nurses often have experience in emergency and trauma services and can analyze wound patterns and the physiological response to injury. The nurse who works in the forensic area often provides a key link between the investigative process, health care, and the court (Campbell et al, 2014). Campbell and colleagues (2014) wrote a toolkit that outlines how SANE nurses can work within their communities to increase sexual assault reporting by victims, a historically challenging issue.

There are specific actions that nurses should take when they work with victims. It is essential that they carefully collect evidence in a systematic manner. For example, when cutting the shirt off a person who has been shot in the chest, be sure to avoid cutting through the bullet hole in the shirt. Instead, cut to the side of the hole to protect the point of origin of the bullet for later criminal investigation. The most common types of evidence are clothing, bullets, bloodstains, hairs, fibers, and small pieces of material, such as fragments of metal, glass, paint, and wood. Also, DNA provides key information in the analysis of sexual assault. When nurses treat victims of rape, it is important to do so in a manner that preserves evidence for the victim.

Rape is a situational crisis for which advance preparation is rarely possible. Therefore nurses need to help victims cope with the stress and disruption of their lives caused by the attack. Counseling focuses on the crisis and the fears, feelings, and issues involved. Nurses can help survivors learn how to regroup personal forces. If posttraumatic stress disorder (PTSD) has developed, professional psychological or psychiatric treatment is indicated.

Many rape victims need follow-up mental health services to help them cope with the short-term and long-term effects of the crisis. The time after a rape is one of disequilibrium, psychological breakdown, and reorganization of attitudes about the safety of the world. Common, everyday tasks often tax a person's resources. Many individuals forget or fail to keep appointments. Nurses can make appropriate referrals and obtain permission from the victim to remain in contact through telephone conversations, which allows for ongoing assessment of the victim's needs and opportunities to intervene when needed.

The best way to prevent sexual violence is to stop it before it begins. The CDC advocates strategies such as (1) promoting social norms that protect against violence; (2) teaching skills to prevent sexual violence; (3) providing opportunities to empower girls and women; (4) creating protective environments; and (5) supporting victims/survivors to lessen harm (Basile et al, 2016). The CDC also uses the following four-step approach to address public health problems such as sexual violence:
1. Define the problem.
2. Identify risk and protective factors.
3. Develop and test prevention strategies.
4. Ensure widespread adoption (CDC, 2014c).

Suicide

According to the National Violent Death Reporting System, **suicide** accounted for 38,364 deaths in 2012, which averages 105 suicides per day (CDC, 2015c). Suicide is the 10th leading cause of death in the United States. The most frequent ways in which violent deaths occur are by firearms, hanging, strangulation and suffocation, or poisoning. Precipitating factors are IPV and mental or physical health problems. The risk for death by suicide is greater than for death by homicide. Rates of completed suicide are higher for men, especially American Indian and Alaska Natives, military personnel, middle-aged men, and rural residents (CDC, 2015c; American Foundation for Suicide Prevention, 2016). Affluent and educated people often have higher rates of suicide than do the economically and educationally disadvantaged, except for Native Alaskan and American Indian populations, who are often poor and yet commit suicide in alarming numbers. The presence of a gun in the home is an important risk factor for both suicide and homicide (Miller & Hemenway, 2008).

Suicides take a high toll on individuals, families, and communities. Suicide is the second leading cause of death among young people 10 to 34 years of age (CDC, 2014a). Men are 3.5 times more likely to die by suicide than females. For young adults between 15 and 24 years of age, there are approximately 100 to 200 attempts for every completed suicide (American Foundation for Suicide Prevention, 2016). Over 800 000 people die due to suicide per year. There are indications that for each adult who died of suicide there may have been more than 20 others attempting suicide (WHO, 2014b).

Leading risk factors for suicide are mental health, unintended pregnancy, and STD, especially HIV (Eaton et al, 2010). More young females (22.4%) than males (11.6%) have seriously considered suicide, and the prevalence is highest in Hispanic adolescent females (26%) (Kann et al, 2014). An important risk factor for actual and attempted suicide in adult women is IPV.

Leading risk factors for suicide are depression and other mental disorders, substance abuse disorders, and intimate partner problems. Other risk factors include a prior suicide attempt, a family history of suicide, mental disorder, substance abuse or violence, firearms in the home, incarceration, and exposure to the suicidal behavior of others, that is, family, peers, or media figures (CDC, 2015c).

Nurses can aid in reducing suicide and in caring for victims, at the community, family, and individual level. On a community level, nurses can be involved in a coordinated response for suicide prevention and the care of people who attempt suicide. Nurses can assist in developing policies and protocols for suicide prevention across the life span. Care may focus on family members and friends of suicide victims. Survivors often feel angry toward the dead person, yet may turn the anger inward. Likewise, survivors often question their own liability for the death. The impact of suicide can affect family, friends, co-workers, and the community. Survivors may find it hard to deal with their feelings toward the dead person. It may be difficult for them to concentrate, and they may limit their social activities because their friends and family may be unable to talk about the suicide. Nurses can help survivors cope with the trauma of the loss and make referrals to a counselor or support groups.

FAMILY VIOLENCE AND ABUSE

Family violence, including sexual, emotional, and physical abuse, causes significant injury and death. These three forms tend to occur together as part of a system of coercive control.

Generally, family violence is violence of the most powerful against the least powerful. IPV is directed primarily toward women in heterosexual relationships (although they may physically fight back). Although the rate of serious intimate partner violence has declined 72% for females and 64% for males, IPV is nonetheless a serious problem in the United States, and includes injury and sexual violence (Catalano, 2013). Dynamics related to power and control caused by race, gender expression, ability, immigration status, age, and class are methods of control in same-sex IPV (Walters et al, 2013). Approximately 26% of gay males have been physically or sexually assaulted or stalked.

Recognizing the battered child or spouse in the emergency department is relatively simple after the fact. It is unfortunate that by the time medical care is sought, serious physical and emotional damage may have already occurred. Nurses are in a key position to predict and deal with abusive tendencies. By understanding factors contributing to the development of abusive behaviors, nurses can identify abuse-prone families and can assist them to describe their abuse in a nonthreatening environment.

Development of Abusive Patterns

To help abusive families, nurses need to understand that the factors that characterize people who become involved in family violence include upbringing, living conditions, and increased stress. Of these factors, the one most predictably present is previous exposure to some form of violence. As children, abusers were often beaten or saw siblings or parents beaten. They learned that violence is a way to manage conflict. Both men and women who witnessed abuse as children were more likely to abuse their children. Financial solvency and support tended to decrease the incidence of child abuse (Zimmerman & Mercy, 2010). Childhood physical punishment teaches children to use violent conflict resolution as an adult. A child may learn to associate love with violence because a parent is usually the first person to hit a child. Children may think that those who love them also are those who hit them. The moral rightness of hitting other family members thus may be established when physical punishment is used to train children, especially when it is used more than occasionally. These experiences predispose children ultimately to use violence with their own children.

As well as having a history of child abuse themselves, people who become abusers tend to have hostile personality styles and be verbally aggressive. They often learn these behaviors from their own childhood experiences. Their parents may have set unrealistic goals, and when the children failed to perform accordingly, they were criticized, demeaned, punished, and denied affection. Additionally, parents who are at risk for child abuse tend to be young, single, have many children who are dependent on them, substance abuse issues, mental health problems, and low income (Fortson et al, 2016). These children grow up feeling unloved and worthless. They may want a child of their own so that they will feel love.

To protect themselves from feelings of worthlessness and fear of rejection, abused children form a protective shell and may become hostile and distrustful of others. The behavior of potential abusers reflects a low tolerance for frustration, emotional instability, and the onset of aggressive feelings with minimal provocation. Because of their emotional insecurity, they often depend on a child or spouse to meet their needs of feeling valued and secure. When their needs are not met by others, they become overly critical. Critical, resentful behavior and unrealistic expectations of others lead to a vicious cycle. The more critical these people become, the more they are rejected and alienated from others. Abusive individuals often think the target of their hostility is "out to get" them. For example, a parent might think or say that an infant deliberately kept him or her awake all night. We know that infants do not intentionally keep parents awake. Rather, infants cry and fret for a reason of their own, not to annoy and inconvenience others.

A perceived or actual crisis may precede an abusive incident. Because a crisis reinforces feelings of inadequacy and low self-esteem, multiple events may occur in a short time to precipitate abusive patterns. Unemployment, marital strains, or an unplanned pregnancy can set off violence. The daily hassles of raising young children, especially in an economically strained household, intensify an already stressed atmosphere for which an unexpected and difficult event provokes violence. Stressful life events, poverty, and the number of small children in the home are often associated with family violence. Crowded living conditions can precipitate abuse. Several people living in a small space increases tensions and reduces privacy. Tempers flare as a result of the constant stimulation from others.

Social isolation reduces social support and can decrease a family's ability to cope with stress and lead to abuse. The problem may be intensified if a violent family member tries to keep the family isolated to escape detection. Therefore, if a family misses clinic or home visit appointments, nurses need to consider the possibility of abuse. Nurses can encourage involvement in community activities and can help neighbors reach out to one another to help prevent abuse.

Frequent moves disrupt social support systems, are associated with an increased stress level, and tend to isolate people, at least briefly. Mobility can have a serious negative effect on the abuse-prone family. These families do not readily initiate new relationships. They rely on the family for support. Resources may be unfamiliar or inaccessible to them. Because frequent moving may be both a risk factor for abuse and a sign of an abusive family trying to avoid detection, nurses should assess such families carefully for abuse.

Types of Family Violence

Family violence may not be limited to one family member; thus, nurses who detect child abuse should also suspect other forms of family violence. When older adult parents report that their (now adult) child was abused or has a history of violence toward others, the nurse should recognize the potential for elder abuse. Physical abuse of women may be accompanied by sexual abuse, both inside and outside the marital relationship. Severe wife abusers may commit other acts of violence, especially child abuse. Also, when one child is abused, others may be physically, sexually, or emotionally abused. Families who are verbally aggressive in conflict resolution (e.g., using name calling, belittling,

screaming, yelling) are more likely to be physically abusive. Although the various forms of family violence are discussed separately, they should not be thought of as totally separate phenomena. No member of the family is guaranteed immunity from abuse and neglect. Spouse abuse, child abuse, elder abuse, serious violence among siblings, and mutual abuse by members all occur. Although these examples are not inclusive, they demonstrate the scope of family violence. Remember that abuse is about power and control. Emotional abuse and controlling behaviors often occur before physical abuse. Box 25.1 lists ways in which abusers can control and intimidate those whom they abuse. Remember that no one deserves to be treated this way.

Child Abuse

A national survey estimated that in 2014 there were approximately 702,000 unique reports of children and adolescents who were subjected to neglect, medical neglect, physical and sexual abuse, or emotional maltreatment (U.S. Department of Health and Human

---

BOX 25.1 Abuse is About Power and Control

All of these actions are unhealthy, and some are illegal.

Isolation: The abuser keeps you:
- Away from seeing friends and family
- From going to work or school
- In an overly protective relationship and is jealous and possessive
- From using the car or otherwise traveling freely on your own

Threats: The abuser threatens to:
- Hurt or kill you or your family or friends
- Take your children away
- Report you to welfare or immigration authorities
- Hurt himself or herself

Intimidation: The abuser:
- Insults you, puts you down, calls you names, or humiliates you in front of others
- Interrupts when you speak
- Stalks or harasses you or tries to make you think you are crazy

Using children: The abuser:
- Calls you a bad parent or tries to turn others against you
- Uses others, especially children, to deliver nasty messages to you
- Harasses with threats about custody, visitation, or family court orders

Being cruel: The abuser:
- Denies you food, sleep, or medical care
- Abuses or kills your pets
- Destroys your things such as clothes, photos, heirlooms, or other valued items

Withholds support: The abuser:
- Takes your money, fails to give you adequate money, or makes you account for everything you buy
- Denies you access to bank accounts or credit cards

Sexual abuse: The abuser:
- Withholds sex or affection
- Prevents you from using birth control or condoms to protect against sexually transmitted diseases
- Forces you to engage in sexual acts

Modified from Health Bulletin: Domestic violence and abuse. Health Ment Hyg News 2:10, 2003, New York City Department of Health and Mental Hygiene.

Services, Administration for Children and Families [USDHHS ACF], 2016). This number represents 9.4 victims per 1000 children. Of these children, 78% were victims of neglect; 18% were victims of physical abuse; 9% were sexually abused; and the remaining children were psychologically maltreated or medically neglected (CDC, 2014d). There were 1640 fatalities caused by abuse in 2012. This is probably a conservative figure, because only the most severe cases are reported. Except for sexual abuse, which is four times as high for girls as for boys, victims are equally distributed among male and female children. The age group with the largest increase in cases is children younger than 1 year of age (USDHHS ACF, 2016). Child abuse tends to increase when there is increased family stress, especially during economic crunches. Babies are at risk for suffering brain injury when an adult, often feeling overwhelmed, violently shakes the baby, whose muscles are too weak to hold his or her head steady, thereby exposing the brain to injury (CDC, 2016b). In 2012, 54% of perpetrators were women and 45% of perpetrators were men (CDC, 2014d).

Many children are exposed to violence, not only as victims, but also as witnesses (Child Trends Data Bank, 2016). Children witnessing domestic violence may experience PTSD and exhibit aggressive behavior (Kletter et al, 2009). Also, children living in homes in which violence takes place between their parents are more likely to be abused themselves. Risk factors for children who are abused include parental factors such as limited family economic resources, lack of social support, parental domestic violence, and problems with substance abuse. Some of the risk factors are identified in Box 25.2. Children who witness parental domestic violence may react differently according to their age, level of development, and sex; their reactions are influenced by the severity and frequency of the abuse witnessed (Kelly et al, 2010).

The presence of child abuse signifies ineffective family functioning. Abusive parents who recognize their problem are often reluctant to seek assistance because of the stigma attached to being considered a child abuser. Children may be victims of abuse because they are small and relatively powerless. In many families, only one child is abused. Parents may identify with this particular child and be especially critical of the child's behavior. In some cases, the child may have certain qualities, such as looking like a relative, being handicapped, trying to resist the violence, or being particularly bright and capable or strong willed, that provoke the parent. Often, in families in which child abuse occurs, there is an explicit or covert threat to children other than the one who is most severely abused. Thus other children may have conflicting feelings of both guilt and relief, and the targeted child is often coerced into silence by threats toward the sibling(s).

Parents with low social support, a tendency toward depression, multiple economic stressors, and a history of abuse are at risk for abusing their children (Fortson et al, 2016). Abusive parents often have unrealistic expectations of a child's developmental abilities. They tend to have little involvement with and show minimal warmth toward their child (Child Welfare Information Gateway, 2013a). Parents who abuse their children use physical discipline more frequently, often in the form of physical punishment, and verbal abuse (Wilkins et al, 2014). The nurse must teach normal parental behavior and also address the underlying emotional needs of the parents. They need to teach forms of parental control other than physical punishment. These parents often experience pain and poor emotional stability and need intervention as much as their children. The How To box lists some of the behavioral indicators of potentially abusive parents.

BOX 25.2 Determining Risk Factors for Child Abuse

Ask the following questions or observe the following behaviors to determine whether risk factors are present.

1. Are the parents unemployed?
2. Do the parents have the financial resources to care for a child?
3. Is there a support network that is willing to offer assistance?
4. Do one or both parents have a history of child abuse?
5. Is a parent a victim or perpetrator of intimate partner violence?
6. Do the parents have knowledge about child development?
7. Do one or both parents have problems with substance abuse?
8. Are the parents overly critical of the child?
9. Are the parents communicative with each other and the nurse?
10. Does the mother of the child seem frightened of her partner?
11. Does the child suffer from recurrent injuries or unexplained illnesses?

Data from Rodriguez CM: Personal contextual characteristics and cognitions: predicting child abuse potential and disciplinary style. J Interpers Viol 25:315–335, 2010; U.S. Department of Health & Human Services, Administration for Children and Families, Administration on Children, Youth and Families, Children's Bureau: *Child maltreatment 2014,* Retrieved from http://www.acf.hhs.gov/programs/cb/research-data-technology/statistics-research/child-maltreatment, 2016; Zimmerman F, Mercy JA: A better start: child maltreatment prevention as a public health priority. Zero to Three 30:4–10, 2010.

HOW TO Identify Potentially Abusive Parents

The following characteristics in couples expecting a child constitute warning signs of actual or potential abuse:

- Denial of the reality of the pregnancy, for example, refusal to talk about the impending birth or to think of a name for the child
- An obvious concern or fear that the baby will not meet some predetermined standard, for example, sex, hair color, temperament, or resemblance to family members
- Failure to follow through on the desire for an abortion
- An initial decision to place the child for adoption and a change of mind
- Rejection of the mother by the father of the baby
- Family experiencing stress and numerous crises so that the birth of a child may be the last straw
- Initial and unresolved negative feelings about having a child
- Lack of support for the new parents
- Isolation from friends, neighbors, or family
- Parental evidence of poor impulse control or fear of losing control
- Contradictory history
- Appearance of detachment
- Appearance of misusing drugs or alcohol
- Shopping for hospitals or health care providers
- Unrealistic expectations of the child
- Verbal, physical, or sexual abuse of the mother by the father, especially during pregnancy
- Child is not the biological offspring of the husband or the mother's current boyfriend
- Excessive talk of needing to "discipline" children and plans to use harsh physical punishment to enforce discipline

As nurse Marie Mason was preparing to visit a newborn and her mother, Vicki Jones, she was told that two other children had been removed from Ms. Jones's care in the past by Child Protective Services. During the initial visit and all other visits, Ms. Mason would unclothe the baby and assess her growth and development, as well as look for bruises or abrasions. Ms. Mason gained the mother's trust during her weekly visits, and for the first month thought all was progressing well. The father of the baby, Max, was often present, and he appeared to care for the child. Although the grandmother lived in the apartment at night, she spent her days at a treatment center for the mentally ill.

When the infant was 2 months of age, the nurse noticed that Ms. Jones did not support the infant's head despite her explanations that the baby needed that. Also, the mother advanced the baby's diet to include pureed canned fruits and meats, well ahead of what had been advised. Ms. Jones, who had type 2 diabetes mellitus, also ate erratically and failed to test her own blood sugars. She was overweight but said she had been losing weight because she was only eating take-out Chinese food once a day. Ms. Mason set small goals with Ms. Jones each week, such as adding an easy nutritious breakfast to her diet and testing her blood sugar at least once per day.

When the baby was 3 months of age, Ms. Jones told Ms. Mason that she had told Max not to come back because he had spoken harshly of her mother. On further questioning, she said that she was afraid Max would hurt her and that he had slapped her on occasion. There was also a new man who seemed to be living in the house and was clearly fond of Ms. Jones and her child.

Created by Deborah C. Conway, Assistant Professor, School of Nursing, University of Virginia.

CHECK YOUR PRACTICE

The case study illustrates many of the signs of a potentially abusive pattern. Looking back at the case, note that the nurse did the following: carefully examined the baby during each visit to detect any signs of abuse; used role modeling to demonstrate how to hold the baby and to show that babies are to be held in a careful way; and helped the mother set small goals for her own diet to maintain her diabetes in better control. What else did the nurse do that had a positive effect? Although signs of active abuse were not noted in the case, there were signs of neglect as a result of limited knowledge. What could the nurse do in future visits to help this family not become abusive? What community resources might be considered, such as parenting classes or groups for mothers? Are there role models for good parenting who live near Ms. Jones who might be lay helpers with this family?

When child abuse is discovered, the child is often placed in a foster home. Unfortunately, quality foster care is not available for all abused children. Abused children generally want to return to their parents, and most agencies try to keep natural families together as long as it is safe for the child. Nurses often monitor a family in which a formerly abused child is returned from foster care. Keen judgment and close collaboration with social services are essential. The nurse must ensure the safety of the child while working with the parents in an empathetic way. The nurse's goal is to enhance their parenting skills, not to be viewed as yet another watchdog. Remember also that abusive parents may try to replace a child who has been removed by the courts because of abuse. This is a normal response to the grief of losing a child. Rather than regarding another pregnancy as a sign of continued poor judgment or pathological behavior, the pregnancy can be perceived by the nurse as an opportunity for intensive intervention to prevent the abuse of the expected child. Generally, the parents are eager to avoid further problems if they are enlisted as partners in the project.

Indicators of child abuse. Nurses need to recognize the physical and behavioral indicators of abuse and neglect. Child abuse ranges from violent physical attacks to passive neglect. The children suffer physical injuries, including cuts, bruises, burns, and broken bones; they may also be beaten, burned, kicked, or shook. Passive neglect may result in malnutrition or other problems. Abuse is not limited to physical maltreatment but includes emotional abuse such as yelling at or continually demeaning, shaming, rejecting, withholding love from, threatening, and criticizing the child. Maltreatment can cause stress that can disrupt early brain development and, at extreme levels, can affect the development of the nervous and immune systems. Abused children are then at higher risk for adult health problems, including alcoholism, depression, substance abuse, eating disorders, obesity, sexual proximity, smoking, suicide, and some chronic diseases (Child Welfare Information Gateway, 2013b; CDC, 2016c).

Children at risk for child maltreatment are those who (1) come from a family in which IPV is present—these children are at greater risk for physical and psychological abuse and child neglect (Fletcher, 2010; USHHS ACF, 2016); (2) are younger than 4 years of age—these children are at the greatest risk for severe injury and death; (3) live in communities with a high level of violence that accepts child abuse; and (4) live in families with great stress, such as from substance abuse, poverty, and chronic illness, and who do not have nearby friends or relatives who can provide support and assistance (CDC, 2014d).

Emotional abuse involves extreme debasement of feelings and may result in the child feeling inadequate, inept, uncared for, and worthless. Victims of emotional abuse learn to hide their feelings to avoid incurring additional scorn. They may act out by performing poorly in school, becoming truant, and being hostile and aggressive. Children who are abused or who witness domestic violence can suffer developmentally; adolescents may run away from home as a direct result of domestic violence, abuse substances, or become depressed (Fletcher, 2010; Ford et al, 2010; Rodriguez, 2010; Child Welfare Information Gateway, 2013b).

Physical symptoms of stress from physical, sexual, or emotional abuse may include hyperactivity, withdrawal, overeating, dermatological problems, vague physical complaints, and exacerbation of stress-related physical problems, such as asthma, stuttering, enuresis (bladder incontinence), and encopresis (bowel incontinence). Sadly, bedwetting is often a trigger for further abuse, which creates a particularly vicious cycle. When a child displays physical symptoms without clear physiological origin, ruling out the possibility of abuse should be part of the nurse's assessment process.

HOW TO **Recognize Actual or Potential Child Abuse**

Be alert to the following:

- An unexplained injury
- Skin: Burns, old or recent scars, ecchymosis, soft tissue swelling, human bites
- Fractures: Recent or older ones that have healed
- Subdural hematomas
- Trauma to genitalia
- Whiplash (caused by shaking small children)
- Dehydration or malnourishment without obvious cause
- Provision of inappropriate food or drugs (e.g., alcohol, tobacco, medication prescribed for someone else, foods not appropriate for the child's age)
- Evidence of general poor care: Poor hygiene, dirty clothes, unkempt hair, dirty nails
- Unusual fear of the nurse and others
- Considered to be a "bad" child
- Inappropriate dress for the season or weather conditions
- Reports or shows evidence of sexual abuse
- Injuries not mentioned in the history
- Seems to need to take care of the parent and speak for the parent
- Maternal depression
- Maladjustment of older siblings
- Current or history of intimate partner violence in the home

---

Child Neglect

Neglect is the failure to meet a child's basic needs, including those for housing, food, clothing, education, and access to health care (Child Welfare Information Gateway, 2013a). The two categories of child neglect are physical and emotional. Physical neglect is defined as failure to provide adequate food, proper clothing, shelter, hygiene, or necessary medical care. Physical neglect is most often associated with extreme poverty. In contrast, emotional neglect is the omission of basic nurturing, acceptance, and caring essential for healthy personal development. These children are largely ignored or in many cases treated as nonpersons. Such neglect usually affects the development of self-esteem. It is difficult for a neglected child to feel a great deal of self-worth because the parents have not demonstrated that they value the child. Neglect is more difficult to assess and evaluate than abuse because it is subtle and may go unnoticed. It is not directly related to poverty and occurs across the socioeconomic spectrum of families. Astute observations of children, their homes, and the way in which they relate to their caregivers can provide clues of neglect.

Sexual Abuse

Child abuse also includes sexual abuse. Approximately 1 in 4 female children and 1 in 6 male children in the United States will experience some form of sexual abuse by the time they are 18 years of age. Teenagers are three and a half times more likely than the general population to experience rape (attempted or completed) or sexual assault (U.S. Department of Justice, NSOPW, no date). The exact prevalence is difficult to obtain because not all children have the cognitive ability to describe these experiences. This abuse ranges from unwanted

sexual touching to intercourse. 69% of teen sexual assaults occur in the victim's home, and the majority of childhood sexual abuse is perpetrated by someone the child knows and trusts; 81% of the perpetrators are parents (USDHHS ACF, 2016; U.S. Department of Justice, NSOPW, no date). Although sexual abuse is perpetrated by all categories of caregivers, a child's risk for abuse is higher with stepparents or nonrelated caregivers. Adults whom children and parents are inclined to trust, such as coaches, scout leaders, priests, and other church workers, have been reported sexual abusers. The long-term effects of sexual abuse include depression, sexual disturbances, and substance abuse (Child Welfare Information Gateway, 2013b).

Parents who are physically abusive and those who are sexually abusive share many of the same characteristics such as unhappiness, loneliness, and rigidity. However, sexually abused boys have a higher risk for being perpetrators of IPV and youth violence as they get older (Child Welfare Information Gateway, 2013b).

Father-daughter incest is the type of intrafamilial sexual abuse most often reported. Although mother-son incest takes place, the incidence remains small. Many cases of parental incest go unreported because victims fear punishment, abandonment, rejection, or family disruption if they acknowledge the problem. Incest occurs in all races, religious groups, and socioeconomic classes. Although incest is receiving greater attention because of mandatory reporting laws, too often its incidence remains a family secret.

Because nurses are often involved in helping women deal with the aftermath of incest, it is crucial to understand the typical patterns and the long-term implications. In a typical pattern of paternal incest, the daughter involved is usually about 9 years of age at the onset and is often the oldest or only daughter. The father or stepfather seldom uses physical force. He most likely relies on threats, bribes, intimidation, or misrepresentation of moral standards, or he exploits the daughter's need for human affection.

Nurses must be aware of the incidence, signs and symptoms, and psychological and physical trauma of incest. Symptoms of sexual abuse include difficulty walking or sitting, changes in appetite, bizarre or inappropriate sexual knowledge or behavior, and somatic symptoms of headaches, eating and sleeping disorders, menstrual problems, and gastrointestinal distress (Child Welfare Information Gateway, 2013a). Other symptoms include difficulties in social situations, especially in forming and maintaining close relationships with men, and behavioral symptoms such as substance abuse and sexual dysfunction. Children often try to avoid or escape the abusive behavior. Avoidance can take the form of either behavioral or mental reactions, such as dressing to cover one's body or pretending that the abuse is not taking place. The child can escape either physically by running away or emotionally by withdrawing into other activities (Child Welfare Information Gateway, 2013a).

Adolescents may display inappropriate sexual activity or truancy or may run away from home. Running away is usually considered a sign of delinquency; however, an adolescent who runs away may be using a healthy response to a violent family situation. Therefore the assessment should include a thorough inquiry about sexual and physical abuse at home and an appropriate physical examination. It is also important to remember that absence of physical evidence does not mean that sexual violence such as rape did not occur (WHO, 2015).

Intimate Partner Abuse

Most domestic violence is committed by men against women. However, men also abuse male partners, and women abuse male partners and female partners. The rates of violence against intimate partners is between 2 and 3 per 1000, and has declined since the 1990s (Catalano, 2013). From 2002 to 2011, a greater percentage of female (13%) than male (5%) intimate partner victimizations resulted in serious injury (e.g., internal injury, unconsciousness, broken bones); an average of 18% of females and 11% of males were medically treated for injuries sustained during intimate partner violent victimizations (Catalano, 2013). Intimate partner sexual assault and rape are used as a form of power and control to intimidate and demean victims (National Coalition Against Domestic Violence, 2017). Neither the term wife abuse nor the term spouse abuse takes into account violence in dating or cohabiting relationships or violence in same-sex relationships. Intimate partner violence (IPV) is defined as threatened, attempted, or completed physical, sexual, or emotional abuse by a current or former intimate partner. Within the realm of emotional or psychological abuse is financial abuse. The partner may be a spouse, ex-spouse, current or former boyfriend or girlfriend, or a dating partner (Breiding et al, 2015). Intimate partners can be of the same or opposite sex, and the incidence of violence in same-sex relationships is considered the same as in heterosexual relationships (Walters et al, 2013). The abuse of female partners has the most serious community health ramifications because of the greater prevalence, the greater potential for homicide (Campbell, 2007), the effects on the children in the household, and the more serious long-term emotional and physical consequences (American College of Obstetricians and Gynecologists [ACOG], 2012).

Victims of child abuse and individuals who saw their mothers being battered are at risk for using violence toward an intimate partner, whether one is male or female. However, using evidence of a violent childhood to identify women at risk for abuse is less useful, because abuse cannot be predicted on the basis of characteristics of the individual woman. The violent background of an abusive male, combined with his tendencies to be possessive, controlling, and extremely jealous, is most predictive of abuse (CDC, 2014e). Substance abuse is also associated with battering, although it cannot be said to cause the violence.

Signs of abuse. Battered women often have bruises and lacerations of the face, head, and trunk of the body. Attacks are often carefully inflicted on parts of the body that can easily be disguised by clothing, such as breasts, abdomen, upper thighs, and back (Sheridan and Nash, 2009; World Health Organization, 2013). Ranging from physical restraint to murder, the American College of Obstetricians and Gynecologists (ACOG) (2012) lists these forms of physical abuse: hitting, kicking, punching, slapping, strangling, shaking, confining, burning, freezing, pushing, tripping, scratching, cutting, biting, pinching, throwing things, or hiding medications. Emotional, psychological, and verbal abuse include coercion, manipulation, isolation, intimidation, mocking or criticizing, humiliating, lying, screaming, threatening, or using menacing forms of nonverbal behavior (ACOG, 2012). Financial abuse is seen when a partner limits the other person's access to money as a method of control.

Once abused, women tend to exhibit low self-esteem and depression (Humphreys and Campbell, 2010). Few are able to come right out and ask for help, which means that the nurse needs to communicate honestly, openly, and with sensitivity. Complete any screening in a quiet, private setting; do not ask anyone who accompanies the woman to translate or explain; it is best to have no one else present during the interview; and remember that any person accompanying the victim might be an abuser (WHO, 2014a).

When a woman has a black eye or bruises about the mouth ask "Who hit you?" rather than "What happened to you?" The latter implies that the nurse is neither knowledgeable nor comfortable with violence, and this may prompt the woman to fabricate a more acceptable cause of her injury.

Abused women have more physical health problems than other women, specifically chronic headaches, palpitations, sleep and appetite disturbances, chronic pelvic pain, urinary frequency and/or urgency, irritable bowel syndrome and other abdominal symptoms, sexual dysfunction, and recurrent vaginal infections (ACOG, 2012). Ask, "When did this happen?" Also ask, "Where did this happen?" Write up what the person actually said using quotation marks, and make note of grooming, posture, and mannerisms (WHO, 2015).

Abuse as a process. Ford-Gilboe et al (2011) identified a process of response to battering in which the woman's emotional and behavioral reactions change. Initially she tries to minimize the seriousness of the situation. The violence usually starts with a slight shove in the middle of a heated argument. Most couples argue and disagree, and some fight. When there is any physical aggression, both the man and the woman tend to blame the incident on something external such as a particularly stressful day at work or drinking too much. The male partner usually apologizes for the incident, and as with any problem in a relationship, the couple tries to improve the situation. Although marital counseling may be useful at this early stage, it is generally contraindicated at all other stages because of the risk to the woman's safety. Unfortunately, abuse tends to escalate in frequency and severity over time, and the man's remorse tends to lessen. The risk is such that women who try to leave an abusive relationship are at significant risk for homicide (Campbell, 2007).

Because women often feel responsible for the success of a relationship, they may try to change their behavior to end the violence. They may even blame themselves for infuriating their spouse. Women who blame themselves for provoking the abuse are more likely to have low self-esteem and be depressed than those who do not blame themselves. Some women experience a moral conflict between their need to leave an abusive relationship and their sense that it is their responsibility to maintain the relationship (Black et al, 2011; WHO, 2013). Women find that no matter what they do, the violence continues. During this period, the woman tries to hide the violence because of the stigma attached. She tries to placate her spouse and feels she is losing her sense of self. She is often concerned about her children, whether she leaves or stays. Some women literally fear for their lives and those of their children. She fears that her partner will try to kill her, the children, or both if she attempts to leave. This fear may be justified. She may kill herself or her abuser to escape because she sees no other way out (Campbell, 2007). Because of the severity of the abuse, a woman may flee to a shelter to obtain physical safety for herself and her children (WHO, 2013). As a woman tries to leave, the risk for homicide increases. Thirty-nine percent of homicides of women in the United States are committed by an intimate partner (Catalano, 2013). Often the woman thinks she will die if she stays or leaves the relationship. A nurse encountering a family in which there is severe abuse needs to consider the safety of the woman and her children as the priority. The woman will need an order of protection, a legal document specifically designed to keep the abuser away from her. The abuser may ignore the order of protection. The woman will also need help in getting to a safe place, such as a wife abuse shelter in a location that the abuser cannot find. At the very least, the woman must design a carefully thought-out plan for escape and arrange for a neighbor or an adolescent child to call the police when another violent episode occurs.

Short-term help for women in abusive relationships can often be found. Many women, however, have identified a dearth of long-term and family-oriented services. Unfortunately, financial constraints sometimes factor into the decision-making process of whether to remain in abusive relationships. The high cost of attorney fees to obtain equitable divorces or child custody is a factor many women face when leaving these relationships.

An alternative to ending the relationship is for the male partner to attend a program for batterers. These programs are most effective if they are court mandated and if the perpetrator's underlying values about women are addressed, as well as his violence, and if the perpetrator is held accountable (Black, 2011; CDC 2014e). Abused women need affirmation, support, reassurances of the normalcy of their responses, accurate information about shelters and legal resources, and brainstorming about possible solutions. These needs can be met by other women in similar situations and by professionals such as nurses. Women should not be pushed into actions that they are not ready to take (WHO, 2014c). Also consider cultural factors that influence the way in which women respond to IPV, and use this information to

design the intervention (Belknap & VandeVusse, 2010; Ward & Wood, 2009).

After the abusive relationship has ended, a period of recovery ensues. This includes a normal grief response for the relationship that has ended and a search for meaning in the experience. Thus a formerly battered woman who is feeling depressed and lonely after the relationship has ended is exhibiting a normal response for which support is needed.

Nurses need to assess for intimate sexual abuse in which the battered woman is forced into sexual encounters. Often women who have come to emergency departments because of abuse have also been sexually abused. These women are at risk for STDs and mental health problems (ACOG, 2012; CDC, 2015d). Therefore like intimate partner violence in the past, marital rape remains a private issue. There is also an alarming incidence of date rape, the dynamics of which may parallel marital rape. Adolescent boys are more likely to perpetrate sexual dating violence than are girls. Young women who have been victims of dating violence experience low self-esteem, depression, anger, irritability, and physical health problems (CDC, 2016a).

To assess for sexual assault, the question "Have you ever been forced into sex you did not wish to participate in?" should be used in all nursing assessments to see if marital rape, date rape, or rape of a male has occurred (WHO, 2014c).

HOW TO **Assess for Intimate Partner Violence**

Ask the following questions:
- Is somebody hurting you?
- You seem frightened of your partner. Has he hurt you?
- Did someone you know do this to you?

Battering during pregnancy has serious implications for the health of both women and their children. Approximately 3% to 8% of pregnant women are physically battered during pregnancy, with a larger proportion (20%) of adolescents abused during pregnancy than adult women. Although abuse during pregnancy occurs across ethnic groups, Puerto Rican, white, and African American women experience a significantly higher severity of abuse than Hispanic women from Mexico or Central America (Bloom et al, 2010). These women are at risk for spontaneous abortion, premature delivery, delivery of low–birth-weight infants, substance abuse during pregnancy, and depression (ACOG, 2012). Abuse before pregnancy often precedes abuse during pregnancy. A man's control of contraception, a form of abusive controlling, may lead to unintended pregnancy and subsequent abuse. In addition, a man's refusal to use a condom places a woman at an increased risk for STDs, including infection with HIV (ACOG, 2012). Infants whose mothers were battered are often at high risk for child abuse. All pregnant women should be assessed for abuse at each prenatal care visit, and postpartum home visits should include assessment for child abuse and partner abuse.

Abuse of Older Adults

Elder abuse is growing as a form of family violence. Like spouse abuse and child abuse, most cases of elder abuse go unreported because the elder is afraid to tell police, friends, or family about the violence (CDC, 2016d). As with other forms of human abuse, elder maltreatment can be physical when the person is hit, kicked, pushed, slapped, or burned or sexual when the elder is forced to take part in a sexual act against his or her will or when the elder cannot consent. Emotional abuse includes behaviors to demean or affect the elder's self-esteem, such as name calling, scaring, embarrassing, destroying property, or not letting the person see family or friends. Neglect occurs when the basic needs for food, housing, clothing, and medical care are not met, and in abandonment the caregiver leaves the elder and no longer provides care for him or her. In financial abuse, the elder's money, property, or assets are misused (Hall et al, 2016). Elders also may be abused by the following actions of caregivers:

- Rough handling that can lead to bruises and bleeding into body tissues because of the fragility of elders' skin and vascular systems. It is often difficult to determine whether the injuries of elders result from abuse, falls, or other natural causes. Careful assessment through both observation and discussion can help determine the cause of injuries.
- Imposing unrealistic toileting demands.
- Ignoring special needs and previous living patterns.
- Giving food that they cannot chew or swallow or that is contraindicated because of dietary restrictions or social or cultural preferences.

- Giving medication to induce confusion or drowsiness so that the elders will be less troublesome, will need less care, or will allow others to gain control of their financial and personal resources.

The most common form of psychological abuse is rejection or simply ignoring older adults, indicating that they are worthless and useless to others. Elders may subsequently regress and become increasingly dependent on others, who tend to resent the imposition and demands on their time and lifestyles. The pattern becomes cyclical; as the person becomes more regressed, the level of dependence increases. Furthermore, the past accomplishments and present abilities of the older person may not be consistently acknowledged, causing the person to feel even less capable. Indicators of actual or potential older adult abuse are listed in the How to box.

HOW TO Identify Potential or Actual Older Adult Abuse

Be alert to the following:
- Financial mismanagement
- Withdrawal and passivity
- Depression
- Unexplained or repeated physical injuries
- Untreated health problems such as decubitus ulcers
- Poor nutrition
- Unexplained genital infections
- Physical neglect and unmet basic needs
- Social isolation
- Rejection of assistance by caregiver
- Lack of compliance to health regimens

From Hall JE, Karch DL, Crosby AE: Elder abuse surveillance: uniform definitions and recommended core data elements for use in elder abuse surveillance, version 1.0. Atlanta, Ga, 2016, National Center for Injury Prevention and Control, Centers for Disease Control and Prevention; Post LA, Page C, Conner T, et al: Elder abuse in long-term care: types, patterns, and risk factors. *Res Aging* 32:323–348, 2010; Acierno R, Hernandez MA, Amstadter AB, et al: Prevalence and correlates of emotional, physical, sexual, and financial abuse and potential neglect in the National Elder Mistreatment Study. *Am J Public Health* 100:292–297, 2010.

There are several precipitating factors for elder abuse. The elder may be a physical, emotional, or financial burden on the caregiver, leading to frustration and resentment. Or the elder may have previously been the abuser. The abuser may be an acquaintance, close or extended family member, caregiver, or stranger (Acierno et al, 2010; CDC, 2014f). Children who have lived in abusive households learn that behavior. All elders should be assessed for abuse. This is especially true for confused and frail elders. These illnesses place a high burden on the caregiver, with subsequent caregiver depression. Living with and providing care to a confused elder is difficult. The around-the-clock tasks often exhaust family members. In addition, clients with Alzheimer's disease may become verbally and even physically aggressive as a result of their illness, which may trigger retaliatory violence. Family stress increases as members work harder to fulfill their other responsibilities in addition to meeting the needs of the elder.

When families plan to care for an older family member at home, nurses must help them fully evaluate that decision and prepare for the stressors that will be involved. A plan for regular respite care is essential. Strategies for the primary and secondary prevention of elder abuse include victim support groups, senior advocacy volunteer programs, and training for providers working with elders.

Elderly people need to retain as much autonomy and decision-making ability as possible. Nurses have many ways to detect elder abuse, and they have the skills and responsibility for discovering it, giving treatment, and making referrals. Many families who care for elderly members exhaust their resources and coping ability. Nurses can help them find new sources of support and aid.

NURSING INTERVENTIONS

Primary prevention begins with a community approach that incorporates strategies from criminal justice, education, social services, community advocacy, and public health to prevent violence. Some communities have used the following:

- School-based curricula that teach children and youth how to cope with anger, stress, and frustration and that also teach communication and mediation skills.
- Family programs that teach parents how to deal with their children more effectively.
- Preschool programs that develop intellectual and social skills.
- Public education programs that educate communities about different forms of violence and ways to get help and intervene.
- Nurse home visitation programs with families at risk that aim to prevent child abuse and neglect.
- Lobbying for passage of legislation to outlaw physical punishment in schools and marital rape.

Strong community sanctions against violence in the home, as well as high levels of community cohesion, can reduce levels of abuse (CDC, 2014f; Wilkins et al, 2014). Neighbors can watch what is happening and work together to address problems in other families; this is not an invasion of privacy but a sign of community cohesiveness. Nurses can work with advocate groups to make sure police deal with assault within marriage as swiftly, surely, and severely as assault between strangers. Nurses can encourage others to intervene when they see children beaten in a grocery store, notice that an elder is not being properly cared for, see a neighborhood bully beat up his classmates, or hear a neighbor hitting his wife.

Second, people can take measures to reduce their vulnerability to violence by improving the physical security of their homes and learning personal defense measures. Nurses can encourage people to keep windows and doors locked, trim shrubs around their homes, and keep lights on during high-crime periods. Many neighborhoods organize crime watch programs and post signs to that effect. Other signs indicate that certain homes will assist children who need help; these homes are identified by the sign of a hand, usually posted in a window. Other neighbors informally agree to monitor one another's

property and safety. Also, many law enforcement agencies evaluate homes for security and teach individual or neighborhood safety programs. Individuals install home security systems, participate in personal defense programs such as judo or karate, and purchase firearms for their protection.

Unfortunately, handguns are far more likely to kill family members than intruders (Hahn et al, 2005). Firearm accidents are a leading cause of death for young children, and handguns kept in the home are easy to use in moments of extreme anger with other family members or in extreme depression. The majority of homicides between family members and most suicides involve a handgun. Nursing assessments should include a question about guns kept in the home. The family should be made aware of the risk that a handgun holds for family members. If the family thinks that keeping a gun is necessary, safety measures should be taught, such as keeping the gun unloaded and in a locked compartment, keeping the ammunition separate from the gun and also locked away, and instructing children about the dangers of firearms. Lobbying for handgun-control laws is a primary prevention effort that can significantly decrease the rate of death and serious injury caused by handguns in the United States.

Identification of risk factors is an important part of primary prevention used by nurses who work with clients in a variety of settings. Although abuse cannot be predicted with certainty, several factors influence the onset and support the continuation of abusive patterns. Factors to include in an assessment for individual or family violence, or for potential family violence, are illustrated in Fig. 25.1. Factors to be included when assessing a community for violence are shown in Box 25.3.

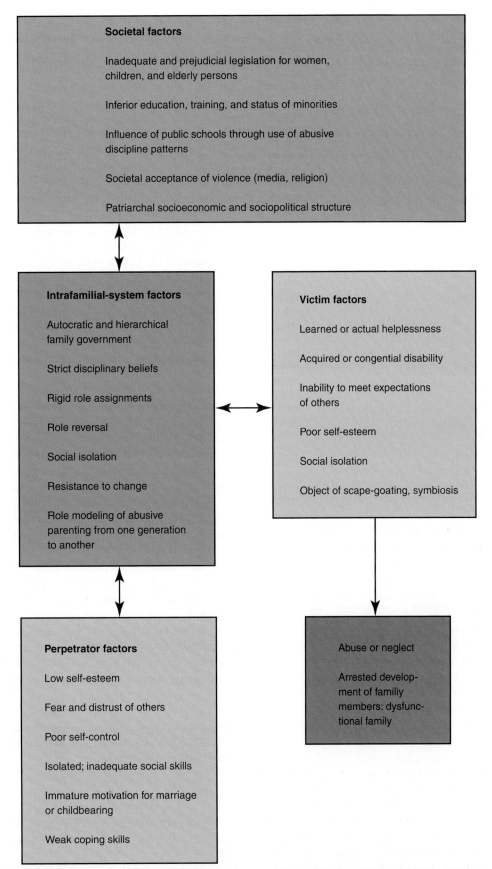

FIG. 25.1 Factors to include when assessing an individual's or family's potential for violence.

BOX 25.3 Assessing for Violence in a Community Context

Individual Factors

- Signs of physical abuse (e.g., abrasions, contusions, burns)
- Physical symptoms related to emotional distress
- Developmental and behavioral difficulties
- Presence of physical disability
- Social isolation
- Decreased role performance within the family and on the job or decreased school-related activities
- Mental health problems such as depression, low self-esteem, and anxiety
- Fear of intimacy with others
- Substance abuse

Familial Factors

- Economic stressors
- Presence of some form of family violence
- Poor communication
- Problems with childrearing
- Lack of family cohesion
- Recurrent familial conflict
- Lack of social support networks
- Poor social integration into the community
- Multiple changes of residence
- Access to guns
- Homelessness

Community Characteristics

- High crime rate
- High levels of unemployment
- Lack of neighborhood resources and support systems
- Lack of community cohesiveness

BOX 25.4 Prevention Strategies for Violence

Individual and Family Levels

- Assess during routine examination (secondary)
- Assess for marital discord (secondary)
- Educate on developmental stages and the needs of children (primary)
- Counsel for at-risk parents (secondary)
- Teach parenting techniques (primary)
- Assist with controlling anger (secondary)
- Treat for substance abuse (tertiary)
- Teach stress-reduction techniques (primary)

Community Level

- Develop policy
- Conduct community resource mapping
- Collaborate with the community to develop systematic responses to violence
- Develop a media campaign
- Develop resources such as transition housing and shelters

As seen in the Levels of Prevention box and in Box 25.4, primary prevention of violence can take place through community, family, and individual interventions. Nurses, in their work in schools, community groups, employee groups, daycare centers, and other community institutions, can foster healthy developmental patterns and identify signs of potential abuse. Nurses may participate in media campaigns that identify risk factors for abuse or in developing after-school programs and late-night programs to support youth in using their energies toward positive goals and developing a constructive support network. Nurses can strengthen families by teaching parenting skills such as diapering, feeding, quieting, holding, rocking, and nonphysical disciplining. They can serve as role models during visits with the family and demonstrate by their actions positive behaviors toward the children. There are many contributing factors to violence, which makes it important that public health professionals understand the root causes of violence, be able listen to the community and bring the community together to learn about the problem and develop an action plan, use data to determine the extent of the problem, and evaluate progress (Musicant, 2011; Wilkins et al, 2014).

When abuse occurs, nurses can initiate secondary prevention measures to reduce or terminate further abuse. Both developmental and situational crises present opportunities for abusive situations to develop. Nurses can help form groups to assist battered women. They can be primary leaders in the development of assessment practices in the health care arena. The development of training programs for health care providers can be an effective step toward identifying and respectfully treating victims of violence. Nurses can work closely with shelters in identifying the needs of individuals who seek sanctuary from abusive situations. On a family level, nurses can help family members discuss problems and seek ways to deal with the tension that led to the abusive situations. Injured persons must be temporarily or permanently placed in a safe location. Secondary preventive measures are most useful when potential abusers recognize their tendency to be abusive and seek help. For children, there is often a need for 24-hour child protection services or caregivers who can take care of the child until the acute family or individual crisis is resolved. Respite care is extremely important in families with frail elderly family members. Telephone crisis lines can be used to provide immediate emergency assistance to families.

Effective communication with abusive families is important. Typically, these families do not want to discuss their problems, and many are embarrassed to be involved in an abusive situation. Often feelings of guilt are present. Effective communication must be preceded by an attitude of acceptance. It

🔲 LEVELS OF PREVENTION

Related to Violence

Primary Prevention
Strengthen the individual and family by teaching parenting skills.

Secondary Prevention
Reduce or end abuse by early screening; teach families how to deal with stress and how to have fun and enjoy recreation.

Tertiary Prevention
When signs of abuse are evident, refer the client to appropriate community organizations.

is often difficult for nurses to value the worth of an individual who willfully abuses another. The behavior, not the person, must be condemned.

In addition, not all families know how to have fun. Nurses can assess how much recreation is integrated into the family's lifestyle. Through community assessment, nurses know what resources and facilities are available and how much they cost. Families may need counseling about the value of recreation and play in reducing tension and appropriately channeling aggressive impulses.

Although it may be difficult to form a trusting relationship with abusive families, nurses can engage in tertiary prevention by acting as a case manager and coordinating the other agencies and activities involved. Principles of giving care to families who are experiencing violence include the following:

- Intolerance for violence
- Respect and caring for all family members
- Safety as the first priority
- Absolute honesty
- Empowerment

Abusers frequently fear they will be condemned for their actions, so it is often difficult to make and maintain contact with abusive families. Although nurses convey an attitude of caring and concern for them, families may doubt the sincerity of this concern. They may avoid being home at the scheduled visit time because of fear of the consequences of the visit or an inability to believe that anyone really wants to help them. If the victim is a child, parents may fear that the nurse will try to remove the child. Nurses are mandatory reporters of child abuse, even when only suspected, in all states. They are also mandatory reporters of elder abuse and abuse of other physically and cognitively dependent adults, as well as of felony assaults of anyone in most states. The mandatory reporting laws also protect reporters from legal action on cases that are never substantiated. Even so, physicians and nurses are sometimes reluctant to report abuse. They may be more willing to report abuse in a poor family than in a middle-class one, or they may think that an older adult or child is better off at home than in a nursing home or foster home. Referral to protective service agencies is a way to get help, rather than an automatic step toward removal of the victim or toward criminal justice action. Families should be included in any reporting so they can have input. Absolute honesty about what will be reported to officials, what the family can expect, what the nurse is entering into records, and what the nurse is feeling is essential.

To further assist the family, the nurse needs to recognize and capitalize on the violent family's strengths, as well as to assess and deal with its problems. The nurse must use a nurse-family

BOX 25.5 Common Community Services

- Child protective services
- Child abuse prevention programs
- Adult protective services
- Parents Anonymous
- Wife abuse shelter
- Program for children of battered women
- Community support group
- 24-Hour hotline for crisis intervention or counseling. These crisis hotlines may offer a variety of counseling services or only target one type of crisis. They are available at national and local levels. For example, in Maryland the House of Ruth offers services for domestic violence (http://www.hruth.org); in Buffalo and Erie County in New York, Crisis Services (http://crisisservices.org) offers counseling for rape and domestic violence, suicide prevention, homelessness, mental health, and trauma; and the National Suicide Prevention Lifeline (https://suicidepreventionlifeline.org/) is nationwide at 800-273-TALK.
- Legal advocacy or information
- State coalition against domestic violence
- Batterer treatment
- Victim assistance programs
- Sexual assault programs

partnership rather than a paternalistic or authoritarian approach. Families often can generate many of their own solutions, which tend to be more culturally appropriate and individualized than those the nurse generates in isolation. Victims of direct attacks need information about their options and resources and reassurance that abuse is unfortunately rather common and that they are not alone in their dilemma. They also need reassurance that their responses are normal and that they do not deserve to be abused. Continued support for their decisions must be coupled with nursing actions to ensure their safety.

Referral is an important component of tertiary prevention. Nurses should know about available community resources for abuse victims and perpetrators. Examples of community resources are listed in Box 25.5. If attitudes and resources are inadequate, it is often helpful to work with local radio and television stations and newspapers to provide information about the nature and extent of human abuse as a community health problem. This also helps acquaint people with available services and resources. Frequently, people do not seek services early in an abusive situation because they simply do not know what is available to them. Ideally, a program or plan for abused people begins with a needs assessment to identify potential clients and to determine how to effectively serve this group. Nurses can help get programs started and provide public education.

CLINICAL APPLICATION

Mrs. Smith, a 75-year-old bedridden woman, consistently became rude and combative when her daughter, Mary, attempted to bathe her and change her clothes each morning. During a home visit, Mary told the nurse, Mrs. Jones, that she had gotten so frustrated with her mother on the previous morning that she had hit her. Mary felt terrible about her behavior. She stressed that her mother's incontinence made it essential that she be kept clean; her clothes had to be changed every day for her own safety and physical well-being.

A. How should Mrs. Jones respond to this disclosure?

B. What specific nursing actions should be taken?

C. What ongoing services does the nurse need to provide?

Answers can be found on the Evolve website.

REMEMBER THIS!

- Violence and human abuse are not new phenomena, but they are growing community health concerns.
- People in communities across the United States are frustrated by increasing levels of violence.
- Nurses can evaluate and intervene in community and family violence.
- To intervene effectively, nurses must understand the dynamics of violence and human abuse.
- Factors influencing social and community violence include changing social conditions, economic conditions, population density, community facilities, and institutions within a community, such as organized religion, education, the mass communication media, and work.
- Violence and abuse of family members can happen to any family member: spouse, elder, child, or physically or mentally compromised person.
- People who abuse family members were often abused themselves; they react poorly to real or perceived crises. Other factors that characterize the abuser are the way the person was raised and the unique character of that person. Cultural factors should be considered when abuse is suspected.
- Child abuse can be physical, emotional, or sexual. Incest is a common and particularly destructive form of child abuse.
- Spouse abuse is usually wife abuse. It involves physical, emotional, and frequently, sexual abuse within a context of coercive control. It usually increases in severity and frequency and can escalate to homicide of either partner.
- Nurses can identify potential victims of family abuse because they see clients in a variety of settings, such as schools, businesses, homes, and clinics. Treatment of family abuse includes primary, secondary, and tertiary prevention and therapeutic intervention.

WHAT WOULD YOU DO?

1. Read in the local newspaper or online to determine what are the most common forms of violence in your community. Based on what you learn, what would be a beneficial form of primary prevention that public health nurses could implement?
2. If you learned, after a careful assessment of your community, that family violence is a significant community health problem, what plan of action could you take to intervene? Remember that the goal is to promote health. Outline a plan of action with objectives, timetables, implementation strategies, and evaluation plans for intervening in family violence in your community.
3. What resources are available in your community for victims of violence?
   a. Interview a person who works in an agency that seeks to aid victims of violence.
   b. What is the role of the agency? Do its services seem adequate? Who is eligible? Is there a waiting list? What is the fee scale? Is the care culturally competent?

ⓔ EVOLVE WEBSITE

http://evolve.elsevier.com/Stanhope/foundations
- Case Study, with Questions and Answers
- NCLEX® Review Questions
- Practice Application Answers

REFERENCES

Acierno R, Hernandez MA, Amstadter AB, et al: Prevalence and correlates of emotional, physical, sexual, and financial abuse and potential neglect in the United States: The National Elder Mistreatment Study, *Am J Public Health* 100:292–297, 2010.

American College of Obstetricians and Gynecologists: Intimate partner violence, Committee opinion No. 518, *Obstet Gynecol* 119:412–417, 2012.

American Public Health Association: *10 Essential public health services,* Washington, DC, 2016, APHA. Retrieved July 2016 from http://www.apha.org/about-apha/centers-and-programs/quality-improvement-initiatives/national-public-health-performance-standards-program/10-essential-public-health-services.

American Foundation for Suicide Prevention: *Suicide Statistics,* 2015. Retrieved July 2016 from https://afsp.org/about-suicide/suicide-statistics.

Anderson CA, Berkowitz L, Donnerstein E, et al: The influence of media violence on youth, *Psychol Sci Public Interest* 4:81–110, 2003.

Ayers SL, Wagaman MA, Geiger JM, Bermudez-Parsai M, Herberg EC: Examining school-based bullying interventions using multi-level discrete time hazard modeling, *Prev Sci* 13:539–550, 2012.

Basile KC, DeGue S, Jones K, et al: *STOP SV: A technical package to prevent sexual violence,* Atlanta, Ga, 2016, National Center for Injury Prevention and Control, Centers for Disease Control and Prevention.

Belknap RA, VandeVusse L: Listening sessions with Latinas: documenting life contexts and creating connections, *Public Health Nurs* 27:337–346, 2010.

Best P, Manktelow R, Taylor B: Online communication, social media and adolescent wellbeing: A systematic narrative review, *Child Youth Serv Rev* 41:27–36, 2014.

Beyer K, Wallis AB, Hamberger LK: Neighborhood environment and intimate partner violence: a systematic review, *Trauma Violence Abuse* 16:16–47, 2015.

Black MC, Basile KC, Breiding MJ, et al: *The national intimate partner and sexual violence survey (NISVS): 2010 summary report,* Atlanta, 2011, National Center for Injury Prevention and Control, Centers for Disease Control and Prevention.

Bloom T, Bullock L, Sharps PW, et al: Intimate partner violence during pregnancy. In Humphreys J, Campbell JC, editors: *Family violence and nursing practice,* ed 2, New York, 2010, Springer, pp 279–398.

Breiding MJ, Smith SG, Basile KC, et al: Prevalence and characteristics of sexual violence, stalking, and intimate partner violence victimization: National Intimate Partner and Sexual Violence Survey, United States, 2011, *MMWR* 63:1–18, 2014.

Breiding MJ, Basile KC, Smith SG, et al: *Intimate partner violence surveillance: uniform definitions and recommended data elements, version 2.0*, Atlanta, Ga, 2015, National Center for Injury Prevention and Control, Centers for Disease Control and Prevention. Retrieved July 2016 from http://www.cdc.gov/violenceprevention/pdf/intimatepartnerviolence.pdf.

Campbell JC: *Assessing dangerousness: violence by batterers and child abusers*, ed 2, New York, 2007, Springer.

Campbell JC, Glass N, Sharps PW, et al: Intimate partner homicide: review and implications of research and policy, *Trauma Violence Abuse* 8:246–269, 2007.

Campbell R, Greeson M, Patterson D: Defining the boundaries: How sexual assault nurse examiners (SANEs) balance patient care and law enforcement collaboration, *J Forensic Nurs* 7:7–26, 2011.

Campbell R, Townsend SM, Shaw J, et al: Evaluating the legal impact of sexual assault nurse examiner programs: An empirically validated toolkit for practitioners, *J Forensic Nurs* 10:208–216, 2014.

Capaldi DM, Knoble NB, Shortt JW, Kim HK: A systematic review of risk factors for intimate partner violence, *Partner Abuse* 3: 231–280, 2012.

Catalano S, Smith E, Snyder H, Rand M: *Female victims of violence, U.S. Department of Justice, Office of Justice Programs, Bureau of Justice Statistics Selected Findings* (NCJ 228356), Washington, DC, 2009, USDOJ. Retrieved August 2016 from http//bjs.gov/content/pub/pdf/fvv.pdf.

Catalano S: *Intimate partner violence: attributes of victimization, 1993-2011*, Washington, DC, 2013, Bureau of Justice Statistics. Retrieved July 2016 from http://www.bjs.gov/content/pub/pdf/ipvav9311.pdf.

Centers for Disease Control and Prevention: *Youth violence: facts at a glance, 2012*, Atlanta, Ga, 2012. Retrieved July 2016 from http://www.cdc.gov/violenceprevention/pdf/yv-datasheet-a.pdf.

Centers for Disease Control and Prevention: *Ten leading causes of death by age group, United States, 2014*. Atlanta, 2014a. Retrieved July 2016 from http://www.cdc.gov/injury/wisqars/pdf/leading_causes_of_death_by_age_group_2014-a.pdf.

Centers for Disease Control and Prevention: *Youth violence: Facts at a glance, 2014*, Atlanta, Ga, 2014b. Retrieved July 2016 from http://www.cdc.gov/violenceprevention/pdf/yv-factsheet-a.pdf.

Centers for Disease Control and Prevention: *Understanding Sexual violence*, Atlanta, Ga, 2014c. Retrieved July 2016 from http://www.cdc.gov/violenceprevention/pdf/sv-factsheet.pdf.

Centers for Disease Control and Prevention: *Child maltreatment: facts at a glance*, Atlanta, Ga, 2014d. Retrieved July 2016 from http://www.cdc.gov/violenceprevention/pdf/childmaltreatment-facts-at-a-glance.pdf.

Centers for Disease Control and Prevention: *Intimate partner violence fact sheet*. Atlanta, Ga, 2014e. Retrieved August 10, 2017 from https://www.cdc.gov/violenceprevention/pdf/ipv-factsheet.pdf.

Centers for Disease Control and Prevention: *Elder abuse: risk and protective factors*, Atlanta, Ga, 2014f. Retrieved July 2016 from https://www.cdc.gov/violenceprevention/elderabuse/riskprotectivefactors.html.

Centers for Disease Control and Prevention: *Understanding bullying: fact sheet*, Atlanta, Ga, 2015a, CDC. Retrieved July 2016 from http://www.cdc.gov/violenceprevention/pdf/bullying_factsheet.pdf.

Centers for Disease Control and Prevention: *School violence: fact sheet*, Atlanta, Ga, 2015b, CDC. Retrieved August 2016 from http://www.cdc.gov/violenceprevention/pdf/School_Violence_Fact_Sheet-a.pdf.

Centers for Disease Control and Prevention: *Understanding suicide*, Atlanta, Ga, 2015c. Retrieved July 2016 from http://www.cdc.gov/violenceprevention/pdf/suicide_factsheet-a.pdf.

Centers for Disease Control and Prevention: *Intimate partner violence: consequences*, Atlanta, Ga, 2015d. Retrieved July 2016 from http://www.cdc.gov/violenceprevention/intimatepartnerviolence/consequences.html.

Centers for Disease Control and Prevention: *Understanding teen dating violence fact sheet*, Atlanta, Ga, 2016a. Retrieved July 2016 from http://www.cdc.gov/violenceprevention/pdf/teen-dating-violence-factsheet-a.pdf.

Centers for Disease Control and Prevention: *Preventing abusive head trauma in children*, Atlanta, Ga, 2016b. Retrieved July 2016 from http://www.cdc.gov/violenceprevention/childmaltreatment/abusive-head-trauma.html.

Centers for Disease Control and Prevention: *Child abuse and neglect*, Atlanta, Ga, 2016c. Retrieved July 2016 from http://www.cdc.gov/ViolencePrevention/childmaltreatment/consequences.html.

Centers for Disease Control and Prevention: *Understanding elder abuse fact sheet*, Atlanta, Ga, 2016d. Retrieved August 10, 2017 from https://www.cdc.gov/violenceprevention/elderabuse/index/html.

Child Welfare Information Gateway: *What is child abuse and neglect? Recognizing the signs and symptoms*, Washington, DC: U.S. Department of Health and Human Services, Children's Bureau, 2013a.

Child Welfare Information Gateway: *Long term consequences of child abuse and neglect*, Washington, DC, 2013b, U.S. Department of Health and Human Services, Children's Bureau.

Child Trends Data Bank: *Children's exposure to violence: Indicators on children and youth*, 2016. Retrieved July 2016 from http://www.childtrends.org/wp-content/uploads/2016/05/118_Exposure_to_Violence.pdf.

Cho G: Racial differences in the prevalence of intimate partner violence against women and associated factors, *J Interpersonal Violence* 27:344–363, 2012.

Eaton DK, Kann L, Kinchen S, et al: Youth risk behavior surveillance: United States, 2009, *MMWR Surveill Summ* 59:1–42, 2010.

Fletcher J: The effects of intimate partner violence on health in young adulthood in the United States, *Soc Sci Med* 70:130–135, 2010.

Ford-Gilboe M, Varcoe C, Wuest J, Merritt-Gray M: Intimate partner violence and nursing practice. In Humphreys J, Campbell JC, editors: *Intimate partner violence and nursing practice*, New York, 2011, Springer, pp 115–153.

Ford JD, Elhai JD, Connor DF, et al: Poly-victimization and risk of posttraumatic, depressive, and substance use disorders and involvement in delinquency in a national sample of adolescents. *J Adolesc Health* 46:545–552, 2010.

Fortson BL, Klevens J, Merrick MT, et al: *Preventing child abuse and neglect: A technical package for policy, norm, and programmatic activities*, Atlanta, Ga, 2016, National Center for Injury Prevention and Control, Centers for Disease Control and Prevention.

Gonzalez-Guarda RM, Ferranti D, Halstead V, Ilias VM: Experiences with dating violence and help seeking among hispanic females in their late adolescence, *Issues Mental Health Nurs* 37:229–238, 2016.

Hahn RA, Bilukha O, Crosby A, et al: Firearms laws and the reduction of violence: a systematic review, *Am J Prev Med* 28:40–71, 2005.

Hall, JE, Karch, DL, Crosby AE: *Elder abuse surveillance: uniform definitions and recommended core data elements for use in elder abuse surveillance, version 1.0*, Atlanta, Ga, 2016, National Center for Injury Prevention and Control, Centers for Disease Control and Prevention.

Hamm MP, Newton AS, Chisholm A, et al: Prevalence and effect of cyberbullying on children and young people: a scoping review of social media studies, *JAMA Pediatr* 169:770–777, 2015.

Health Bulletin: Domestic violence and abuse, *Health Ment Hyg News* 2:10, 2003.

Humphreys JC, Campbell JC: *Family violence and nursing practice,* New York, 2010, Springer.

Kann L, Kinchen S, Shanklin SL, et al: Youth risk behavior surveillance—United States, 2013, *MMWR Surveill Summ* 63:1–168, 2014.

Kelly UA, Gonzalez-Guarda RM, Taylor J: Theories of intimate partner violence. In Humphreys J, Campbell JC, editors: *Intimate partner violence and nursing practice,* ed 2, New York, 2010, Springer, pp 253–278.

Kletter H, Weems CF, Carrion VG: Guilt and posttraumatic stress symptoms in child victims of interpersonal violence, *Clin Child Psychol Psychiatry* 14:71–83, 2009.

Knickmeyer N, Levitt H, Horne SG: Putting on the Sunday best: the silencing of battered women within Christian faith communities, *Fem Psychol* 20:94–113, 2010.

Krebs C, Lindquist C, Berzofsky M, et al: *Campus Climate Survey Validation Study final technical report,* Washington, DC, January 2016, Bureau of Justice Statistics. R&DP-2015:04, NCJ 249545.

Krug EG, Dahlberg LL, Mercy JA, et al: *World report on violence and health,* Geneva, Switzerland, 2002, World Health Organization.

Lysell, H, Dahlin M, Langstrom N, et al: Killing the mother of one's child: Psychiatric risk factors among male perpetrators and offspring consequences, *J Clin Psychiatry* 77:342–347, 2016.

McCabe BE, Gonzalez-Guarda RM, Peragallo NP, Mitrani VB: Mechanisms of partner violence reduction in a group HIV-risk intervention for Hispanic women, *J Interpers Violence* 31:2316–2337, 2016.

Miller M, Hemenway D: Guns and suicide in the United States, *N Engl J Med* 359:989–991, 2008.

Musicant G: A call to action: preventing community violence, *Public Health Nurs* 28:295–298, 2011.

Nannini A, Lazar J, Berg C, et al: Physical injuries reported on hospital visits for assault during the pregnancy-associated period, *Nurs Res* 57:144–149, 2008.

National Coalition Against Domestic Violence, Domestic violence and sexual assault, 2017. Retrieved August 10, 2017 from http://ncadv.org/files/Domestic%20and%20Abuse%20NCADV.pdf.

One in Four USA: *Sexual assault statistics.* Retrieved July 2016 from http://www.oneinfourusa.org/statistics.php.

Parks SE, Johnson LL, McDaniel DD, et al: Surveillance for violent deaths—National Violent Death Reporting System, 16 States, 2010, *MMWR Surveill Summ* 63:1–33, 2014.

Patton DU, Hong JS, Ranney M, et al: Social media as a vector for youth violence: A review of the literature, *Comput Human Behav* 35:548–553, 2014.

Pennington-Zoellner K: Expanding "community" in the community response to intimate partner violence, *J Fam Viol* 24:539–545, 2009.

Pitts J: Youth gangs, ethnicity and the politics of estrangement, *Youth Policy* 102:101–113, 2009.

Post LA, Page C, Conner T, et al: Elder abuse in long-term care: types, patterns, and risk factors, *Res Aging* 32:323–348, 2010.

Regan ME: Implementation and evaluation of a youth violence prevention program for adolescents, *J Sch Nurs* 25:27–33, 2010.

Rhodes VK, Kothari CL, Dichter M, et al: Intimate partner violence identification and response: time for a change in strategy, *J Gen Intern Med* 26:894–899, 2011.

Rodriguez CM: Personal contextual characteristics and cognitions: predicting child abuse potential and disciplinary style, *J Interpers Viol* 25:315–335, 2010.

Sheridan DJ, Nash KR: Acute injury patterns of intimate partner violence victims, *Trauma Violence Abuse* 8:281–289, 2009.

Smith SG, Fowler KA, Niolon PH: Intimate partner homicide and corollary victims in 16 states: National Violent Death Reporting System, 2003–2009, *Am J Public Health* 104:461–466, 2014.

Swider SM, Krothe J, Reyes D, et al: The Quad Council practice competencies for public health nursing, *Public Health Nurs* 30:519–536, 2013.

Trossman S: Issues up close: ending the cycle, *Am Nurse Today* 4:26–28, 2009.

Truman JL, Langston L: *Criminal victimization 2014,* Washington, DC, August 2015, Bureau of Justice Statistics. NCJ 248973.

U.S. Department of Health and Human Services: *Healthy People 2020 Objectives,* Washington, DC, 2010, Office of Disease Prevention and Health Promotion, USDHHS.

U.S. Department of Health and Human Services, Administration for Children and Families, Administration on Children, Youth and Families, Children's Bureau: *Child maltreatment 2014,* January 26, 2016. Retrieved August 10, 2017 from http://www.acf.hhs.gov/programs/cb/research-data-technology/statistics-research/child-maltreatment.

U.S. Department of Justice, NSOPW: *Raising awareness about sexual abuse: facts and statistics,* no date. Retrieved August 2016 from https://www.nsopw.gov/en/Education/FactsStatistics.

U.S. Department of Labor, Bureau of Labor Statistics: *Demographics,* Washington, DC, 2014. Retrieved July 2016 from http://www.bls.gov/opub/reports/race-and-ethnicity/archive/labor-force-characteristics-by-race-and-ethnicity-2014.pdf.

Walters ML, Chen J, Breiding MJ: *The National Intimate Partner and Sexual Violence Survey (NISVS): 2010 Findings on Victimization by Sexual Orientation,* Atlanta, Ga, 2013, National Center for Injury Prevention and Control, Division of Violence Prevention, Centers for Disease Control and Prevention.

Ward C, Wood A: Intimate partner violence: NP role in assessment, *Am J Nurs Pract* 13:9–15, 2009.

Wilkins N, Tsao B, Hertz M, et al: *Connecting the dots: an overview of the links among multiple forms of violence,* Atlanta, Ga, 2014, National Center for Injury Prevention and Control, Centers for Disease Control and Prevention. Oakland, Calif: Prevention Institute.

World Health Organization: *Responding to intimate partner violence and sexual violence against women: WHO clinical and policy guidelines,* Geneva, Switzerland, 2013, WHO. Retrieved July 2016 from http://apps.who.int/iris/bitstream/10665/85240/1/9789241548595_eng.pdf?ua=1.

World Health Organization: *Global status report on violence prevention 2014,* Geneva, Switzerland, 2014a, WHO. Retrieved July 2016 from www.who.int/violence_injury_prevention/violence/status_report/2014.

World Health Organization: *Preventing suicide: A global imperative,* Geneva, Switzerland, 2014b, WHO. Retrieved July 2016 from http://www.who.int/mental_health/suicide-prevention/world_report_2014/en/.

World Health Organization: *Health care for women subjected to intimate partner violence or sexual violence,* Geneva, Switzerland, 2014c, WHO. Retrieved July 2016 from http://apps.who.int/iris/bitstream/10665/136101/1/WHO_RHR_14.26_eng.pdf?ua=1.

World Health Organization: *Strengthening the medico-legal response to sexual violence,* Geneva, Switzerland, 2015, WHO. Retrieved July 2016 from http://apps.who.int/iris/bitstream/10665/197498/1/WHO_RHR_15.24_eng.pdf?ua=1.

Zimmerman F, Mercy JA: A better start: child maltreatment prevention as a public health priority, *Zero to Three* 30:4–10, 2010.

CHAPTER 26

Infectious Disease Prevention and Control

Francisco S. Sy and Susan C. Long-Marin

OBJECTIVES

After reading this chapter, the student should be able to:

1. Discuss the current effect and threats of infectious diseases on individuals, families, communities, and society.
2. Explain how the elements of the epidemiological triangle interact to cause infectious diseases.
3. Provide examples of infectious disease control interventions at the three levels of public health prevention.
4. Explain the multisystem approach to the control of communicable diseases.
5. Discuss the factors contributing to newly emerging or reemerging infectious diseases.
6. Discuss the illnesses most likely to be associated with the intentional release of a biological agent.
7. Discuss issues related to obtaining and maintaining appropriate levels of immunization against vaccine-preventable diseases.
8. Describe issues and agents associated with foodborne illness and appropriate prevention measures.

CHAPTER OUTLINE

Historical and Current Perspectives
Transmission of Communicable Diseases
  Agent, Host, and Environment
  Modes of Transmission
  Disease Development
  Disease Spectrum
Surveillance of Communicable Diseases
  Surveillance for Agents of Bioterrorism
  List of Reportable Diseases
Emerging Infectious Diseases
  Emergence Factors
Prevention and Control of Communicable Diseases
  Primary, Secondary, and Tertiary Prevention
Agents of Bioterrorism
  Anthrax
  Smallpox
Vaccine-Preventable Diseases
  Routine Childhood Immunization Schedule
  Measles
  Rubella

  Pertussis
  Influenza
Foodborne and Waterborne Diseases
  Salmonellosis
  Escherichia coli O157:H7
  Waterborne Disease Outbreaks and Pathogens
Vector-Borne Diseases and Zoonoses
  Lyme Disease
  Rocky Mountain Spotted Fever
  Zika Virus
  Zoonoses
Parasitic Diseases
  Intestinal Parasitic Infections
  Parasitic Opportunistic Infections
Diseases of Travelers
  Malaria
  Foodborne and Waterborne Diseases
  Diarrheal Diseases
Health Care–Acquired Infections

KEY TERMS

acquired immunity, 458
active immunization, 458
agent, 458
anthrax, 464
common vehicle, 459
communicable diseases, 458
communicable period, 459

disease, 459
Ebola virus, 461
elimination, 462
emerging infectious diseases, 461
endemic, 460
environment, 459
epidemic, 460

epidemiological triangle, 458
eradication, 462
health care–acquired infections (HAIs), 475
herd immunity, 459
horizontal transmission, 459
host, 458

Continued

455

KEY TERMS—cont'd

incubation period, 459	passive immunization, 458	surveillance, 460
infection, 459	resistance, 458	vaccines, 465
infectiousness, 459	severe acute respiratory syndrome	vectors, 459
natural immunity, 458	(SARS), 457	vertical transmission, 459
pandemic, 460	smallpox, 464	Zika virus, 471

Worldwide concern about infectious diseases has grown, and new and reemerging diseases have developed. Migration can increase the spread of infectious diseases when people move from one place to another and bring their diseases, levels of immunity and resistance to diseases, and the viruses or bacteria they may harbor that have not emerged as diseases in them. The topic is complex and includes the study of a wide range and variety of organisms and the pathological conditions they may cause, as well as their diagnosis, treatment, prevention, and control. The topic also requires a global perspective, as evidenced in the recent outbreaks of the Ebola and Zika viruses. This chapter presents an overview of the communicable diseases with which nurses working in the community deal most often. Diseases are grouped according to descriptive category (by mode of transmission or means of prevention) rather than by individual organism (e.g., *Escherichia coli*) or taxonomic group (e.g., viral, parasitic). A detailed discussion of sexually transmitted diseases or infections (STDs or STIs), human immunodeficiency virus (HIV), acquired immunodeficiency syndrome (AIDS), viral hepatitis, and tuberculosis (TB) is provided in Chapter 27. Although not all infectious diseases are directly transferred from person to person, the terms *infectious diseases* and *communicable diseases* are used interchangeably throughout this chapter.

HISTORICAL AND CURRENT PERSPECTIVES

In 1900, communicable diseases were the leading causes of death in the United States. Since that time, improved sanitation and nutrition, the discovery of antibiotics, and the development of vaccines has ended some epidemics such as diphtheria and typhoid fever and greatly reduced the incidence of others such as tuberculosis (TB). In 1900 TB was the second leading cause of death. Contrast that number to the 555 deaths in 2013 (Centers for Disease Control and Prevention [CDC], 2015a). As people live longer, chronic diseases—heart disease, cancer, and stroke—have replaced infectious diseases as the leading causes of death in the United States. Infectious diseases, however, have not vanished. They are still the leading cause of death worldwide among children and adolescents, and the second leading cause overall, killing an estimated 8 million people a year (World Health Organization [WHO] 2014). Organisms once susceptible to antibiotics are becoming increasingly drug resistant; this may result in vulnerability to diseases previously thought to no longer be a threat. And in the 21st century, infectious diseases have become a means of terrorism.

New killers are emerging, and old familiar diseases are taking on different, more virulent characteristics. Consider the following developments. The identification of infectious agents causing Lyme disease and ehrlichiosis has led to two new tick-borne diseases. Ehrlichiosis is a bacterial illness transmitted by ticks that causes flulike symptoms and is common in the spring and summer when people are likely to come in contact with ticks. The symptoms range from mild body aches to severe fever and appear within 1 to 2 weeks after the tick bite. This illness can be effectively treated with antibiotics if treatment begins quickly. Lyme disease is caused when infected blacklegged ticks carrying the bacterium *Borrelia burgdorferi* bite a person. The symptoms are fever, headache, fatigue, and a characteristic rash called *erythema migrans*. If untreated, the effects of Lyme disease are more serious than those of ehrlichiosis in that they can affect joints, the heart, and the nervous system. In both diseases, the best prevention is to use insect repellant, remove the tick promptly, and use pesticides in tick-infested areas. There is a more extensive discussion of Lyme disease later in the chapter.

In the summer of 1993, in the southwestern United States, healthy young adults were stricken with a mysterious and unknown but often fatal respiratory disease that is now known as hantavirus pulmonary syndrome. In 1994 a severe invasive strain of *Streptococcus pyogenes* group A, called by the press the "flesh-eating" bacteria, was identified. This devastating disease occurs when bacteria enter a wound such as from an insect bite, burn, or cut and lead to necrotizing fasciitis, which results in death in one of four affected persons (see information on necrotizing fasciitis at http://www.WebMD). Consumption of improperly cooked hamburgers and unpasteurized apple juice contaminated with a highly toxic strain of *E. coli*, O157:H7, caused illness and death in children across the country. In 1996, 10 states had outbreaks of diarrheal disease traced to imported fresh berries. The implicated organism in these outbreaks is *Cyclospora cayetanensis* (a coccidian parasite). A person becomes infected when consuming food or water contaminated with the parasite, and the symptoms can last from 2 days to 2 weeks. It is important to be cautious about this parasite when traveling to other countries.

Also in 1996 the fear that "mad cow disease" (bovine spongiform encephalopathy [BSE]) could be transferred to humans through beef consumption led to the slaughter of thousands of British cattle and a ban on the international sale of British beef. Although not seen in the United States until 2003 when a BSE case was imported from Canada, BSE has been reported in many countries, including several in Europe, as well as in Japan, Canada, and Israel.

Vancomycin-resistant *Staphylococcus aureus* (VRSA) was reported in 1997; previously, vancomycin had been considered the only effective antibiotic against methicillin-resistant *Staphylococcus aureus* (MRSA). MRSA is increasingly a problem for people who acquire the bacteria in the hospital, and there is a growing incidence of community-acquired MRSA. These latter outbreaks are associated with (but not limited to) places in which people share facilities, such as locker rooms, prisons, and other close bathing areas.

Ebola hemorrhagic fever, a sporadic but highly fatal virus unknown to most people 30 years ago, emerged in 2002 in Gabon and the Republic of the Congo and reemerged in 2014 in Guinea, Liberia, and Sierra Leone. A small number of cases of Ebola emerged in other countries in West Africa. An air traveler brought a case to the United States, and a small number of nurses and other health care workers who went to help treat Ebola in West Africa contracted the disease. By January 2015, there were 8650 reported deaths due to this epidemic. The majority of cases of Ebola and deaths were in Guinea, Liberia, and Sierra Leone (CDC, 2015b). Ebola virus is spread through direct contact with blood or body fluids and can enter the person's body through broken skin or unprotected mucous membranes. This virus can also be spread through needlesticks by needles that are contaminated with the virus, infected fruit bats or primates, and possibly from contact with semen from a man who has recovered from Ebola (CDC, 2015c).

And in 1999 the first Western Hemisphere activity of West Nile virus (WNV), a mosquito-transmitted illness that can affect livestock, birds, and humans, occurred in New York City. By 2002, WNV, believed to be carried by infected birds and possibly mosquitoes in cargo containers, had spread across the United States as far west as California and was reported in Canada and Central America as well. Any person with a febrile or acute neurological illness who has recently been exposed to mosquitoes, blood transfusion, or organ transplantation should be evaluated for WNV. Most symptomatic persons have an acute febrile illness that can include headache, weakness, myalgia, or arthralgia; gastrointestinal symptoms and a transient maculopapular rash are also often observed (CDC, 2015d). Both Ebola and WNV are discussed in more detail later in the chapter.

Also, in early 2003, severe acute respiratory syndrome (SARS), a previously unknown disease of undetermined etiology and no definitive treatment, emerged with major outbreaks in China, Hong Kong, Taiwan, Vietnam, Singapore, and Canada, with additional cases reported from 20 locations around the world. This syndrome ended as suddenly as it had begun, with only a few cases being reported since 2003.

In the 21st century, foodborne infections again have made headlines as *E. coli*–infected spinach sickened and killed individuals across the United States. In 2008 tomatoes were blamed for a nationwide outbreak of salmonellosis but were ruled innocent when the green chilies that accompanied them in salsa were found to be the actual culprit. *Salmonella* again made the news as contaminated peanut butter forced recalls across the United States, sickened hundreds, and resulted in several deaths. Even chocolate chip cookie dough was not safe; a national recall in 2009 followed the discovery that people had been sickened after eating raw dough contaminated with *E. coli*. Perhaps the most publicized infectious disease event of 2009 was the advent of a new strain of flu, novel influenza A H1N1. First reported from Mexico and rapidly acquired by travelers to that country, H1N1 spread quickly across the world, causing the WHO to declare a pandemic and stimulate the race for a vaccine. During the 2013 to 2014 flu season in the United States, H1N1 became a predominant strain, primarily affecting young and middle-aged people. In 2012 the Middle Eastern respiratory syndrome coronavirus, or MERS-CoV, similar to SARS, appeared in the Arabian Peninsula and affected people there and those who traveled there. The reservoir for this disease is unknown but appears to be associated with camels.

Worldwide, the leading causes of deaths from infectious diseases are respiratory infections, diarrheal diseases, HIV/AIDS, TB, malaria, meningitis, pertussis, measles, hepatitis B, and other infectious diseases (Fauci and Morens, 2012). Infections are unpredictable and can have an explosive global effect as people move around the world. Most infectious diseases are caused by a single agent that often can be affected by general disease control measures such as sanitation, chemical disinfection, hand washing, or vector control, as well as specific medical measures such as vaccination or antimicrobial treatment. See the How To box in the section of the chapter on prevention and control of communicable diseases for ways to prevent infection transmission at home. Fauci and Morens (2012) emphasize ways to prevent contracting an infectious disease when they say, "Infectious diseases are acquired specifically and directly as a result of our behaviors and lifestyles" (p 455). They point out that we contract infectious diseases from social gatherings, travel and transportation, sexual activity, occupational exposures, sports and recreational activities, what we eat and drink, our pets, the environment, and even from people in hospitals.

Infectious diseases are expensive. Foodborne illnesses alone are estimated to cost $77.7 billion annually in the United States (Scharff, 2012). In 2011 the CDC listed "Ten great public health achievements—worldwide, 2001-2010." The 10 achievements, not in rank order, are (1) reductions in child mortality, (2) reductions in vaccine-preventable diseases, (3) access to safe water and sanitation, (4) malaria prevention and control, (5) prevention and control of HIV/AIDS, (6) tuberculosis control, (7) control of neglected tropical diseases, (8) tobacco control, (9) increased awareness and response for improving global road safety, and (10) improved preparedness and response to global health threats. The first seven relate to control of infectious diseases (CDC, 2011).

Because of the morbidity (rate of an illness or abnormal quality), mortality (rate of death), and associated cost of infectious diseases, the national health promotion and disease prevention goals outlined in *Healthy People 2020* list objectives for reducing the incidence of these illnesses in the section on Immunization & Infectious Disease (see the *Healthy People 2020* box). Objectives for reducing salmonellosis and other foodborne infections are found in the section on Food Safety, and an objective for reducing malaria cases reported in the United States may be seen under Global Health. Although infectious diseases are not currently the leading causes of death in the United States, they continue to present varied, multiple, and complex challenges to all health care providers. Nurses must know about these diseases to effectively participate in diagnosis, treatment, prevention, and control.

HEALTHY PEOPLE 2020

Selected Objectives Related to Immunization and Infectious Diseases

- **IID-1:** Reduce, eliminate, or maintain elimination of cases of vaccine-preventable diseases.
- **IID-4:** Reduce invasive pneumococcal infections.
- **IID-24:** Reduce chronic hepatitis B virus infections in infants and young children (perinatal infections).
- **IID-27:** Increase the percentage of persons aware they have a chronic hepatitis C infection.

From U.S. Department of Health and Human Services: *Healthy People 2020*, Washington, DC, 2010, U.S. Government Printing Office.

TRANSMISSION OF COMMUNICABLE DISEASES

AGENT, HOST, AND ENVIRONMENT

The transmission of communicable diseases depends on the successful interaction of the infectious agent, the host, and the environment. These three factors make up the epidemiological triangle (Fig. 26.1), as discussed in Chapter 9 (epidemiology). Changes in the characteristics of any of the factors may result in disease transmission. Consider the following examples. Not only may antibiotic therapy eliminate a specific pathological agent but it also may alter the balance of normally occurring organisms in the body. As a result, one of these agents overruns another and disease, such as a yeast infection, occurs. HIV performs its deadly work not by directly poisoning the host but by destroying the host's immune reaction to other disease-producing agents. Individuals living in the temperate climate of the United States do not contract malaria at home, but they may become infected if they change their environment by traveling to a climate in which malaria-carrying mosquitoes thrive. As these examples illustrate, the balance among agent, host, and environment is often precarious and may be unintentionally disrupted. The potential results of such disruption require attention as advances in science and technology, destruction of natural habitats, natural disasters, explosive population growth, political instability, and a worldwide transportation network combine to alter the balance among the environment, people, and the agents that produce disease.

Agent Factor

Four main categories of infectious agents can cause infection or disease: bacteria, fungi, parasites, and viruses. The individual agent may be described by its ability to cause disease and by the nature and the severity of the disease. *Infectivity, pathogenicity, virulence, toxicity, invasiveness,* and *antigenicity,* terms commonly used to characterize infectious agents, are defined in Box 26.1.

Host Factor

A human or animal host can harbor an infectious agent. The characteristics of the host that may influence the spread of disease are host resistance, immunity, herd immunity, and infectiousness of the host. Resistance is the ability of the host to withstand infection, and it may involve natural or acquired immunity.

Natural immunity refers to species-determined, innate resistance to an infectious agent. For example, opossums rarely contract rabies. Acquired immunity is the resistance acquired by a host as a result of previous natural exposure to an infectious agent. Having measles once protects against future infection. Acquired immunity may be induced by active or passive immunization. Active immunization refers to the immunization of an individual by administration of an antigen (infectious agent or vaccine) and is usually characterized by the presence of an antibody produced by the individual host. Vaccinating children against childhood diseases is an example of inducing active immunity. Passive immunization refers to immunization through the transfer of a specific antibody from an immunized individual to a nonimmunized individual, such as the transfer of antibody from mother to infant or by administration of an antibody-containing preparation (i.e., immunoglobulin or antiserum). Passive immunity from immunoglobulin is almost immediate but short-lived. It is often induced as a stopgap measure until active immunity has time to develop after vaccination. Examples of commonly used immunoglobulins include those for hepatitis A, rabies, and tetanus.

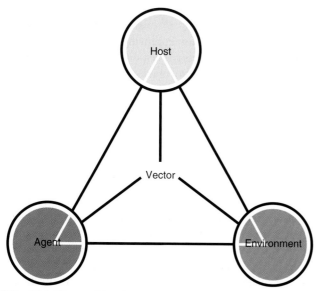

FIG. 26.1 The epidemiological triangle of disease. (From Gordis L: *Epidemiology*, Philadelphia, 1996, Saunders.)

BOX 26.1   Six Characteristics of an Infectious Agent

- **Infectivity:** The ability to enter and multiply in the host
- **Pathogenicity:** The ability to produce a specific clinical reaction after infection occurs
- **Virulence:** The ability to produce a severe pathological reaction
- **Toxicity:** The ability to produce a poisonous reaction
- **Invasiveness:** The ability to penetrate and spread throughout a tissue
- **Antigenicity:** The ability to stimulate an immunological response

Herd immunity refers to the immunity of a group or community. It is the resistance of a group of people to invasion and spread of an infectious agent. Herd immunity is based on the resistance of a high proportion of individual members of a group to infection. It is the basis for increasing immunization coverage for vaccine-preventable diseases. Higher immunization coverage will lead to greater herd immunity, which in turn will block the further spread of the disease.

Infectiousness is a measure of the potential ability of an infected host to transmit the infection to other hosts. It reflects the relative ease with which the infectious agent is transmitted to others. Individuals with measles are extremely infectious; the virus spreads readily on airborne droplets. A person with Lyme disease cannot spread the disease to other people (although the infected tick can).

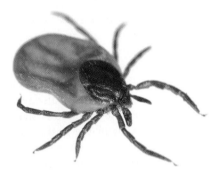

Ticks are a common cause of Lyme disease. (© 2012 Photos.com, a division of Getty Images. All rights reserved. Image #136602031.)

Environment Factor

The environment refers to the physical, biological, social, and cultural factors that are external to the human host. These environmental factors facilitate the transmission of an infectious agent from an infected host to other susceptible hosts. Reduction in communicable disease risk can be achieved by altering these environmental factors. Using mosquito nets and repellents to avoid bug bites, avoiding having even small amounts of standing water that can breed mosquitos, installing sewage systems to prevent fecal contamination of water supplies, and washing utensils after contact with raw meat to reduce bacterial contamination are all examples of altering the environment to prevent disease.

MODES OF TRANSMISSION

Infectious diseases can be transmitted horizontally or vertically. Vertical transmission occurs when the infection is passed from parent to offspring via sperm, placenta, milk, or contact in the vaginal canal at birth. Examples of vertical transmission are transplacental transmission of HIV and syphilis. Horizontal transmission is the person-to-person spread of infection through one or more of the following four routes: direct or indirect contact, common vehicle, airborne, or vector-borne.

Most STDs are spread by direct sexual contact. Enterobiasis, or pinworm infection, can be acquired through direct contact or indirect contact with contaminated objects such as toys, clothing, and bedding. A growing problem of horizontal transmission is that of bedbugs, which are often found in bedding and other soft surfaces. Common vehicle refers to transportation of the infectious agent from an infected host to a susceptible host via food, water, milk, blood, serum, saliva, or plasma. Hepatitis A can be transmitted through contaminated food and water; hepatitis B can be transmitted through contaminated blood. Legionellosis and TB are both spread via contaminated droplets in the air. Vectors are arthropods such as ticks and mosquitoes or other invertebrates such as snails that can transmit the infectious agent by biting or depositing the infective material near the host.

DISEASE DEVELOPMENT

Exposure to an infectious agent does not always lead to an infection. Similarly, infection does not always lead to disease. Infection depends on the infective dose, the infectivity of the infectious agent, and the immunocompetence of the host. It is important to differentiate infection and disease, as clearly illustrated by the HIV/AIDS epidemic. Infection refers to the entry, development, and multiplication of the infectious agent in the susceptible host. Disease is one of the possible outcomes of infection, and it may indicate a physiological dysfunction or pathological reaction. An individual who tests positive for HIV is infected, but if that person shows no clinical signs, the individual is not diseased. Similarly, an individual who tests positive for HIV and also exhibits clinical signs of AIDS is both infected and diseased.

Incubation period and communicable period are not synonymous. Incubation period is the time interval between invasion by an infectious agent and the first appearance of signs and symptoms of the disease. The incubation periods of infectious diseases vary from between 2 and 4 hours for staphylococcal food poisoning to between 10 and 15 years for AIDS (HIV stage III). Communicable period is the interval during which an infectious agent may be transferred directly or indirectly from an infected person to another person. The period of communicability for influenza is 3 to 5 days after the clinical onset of symptoms. Hepatitis B–infected persons are infectious many weeks before the onset of the first symptoms and remain infective during the acute phase and chronic carrier state, which may persist for life.

DISEASE SPECTRUM

Persons with infectious diseases may exhibit a broad spectrum of disease ranging from subclinical infection to severe and fatal disease. Those with subclinical or nonapparent infections are important from the public health point of view because they are a source of infection but may not be receiving the care that those with clinical disease are receiving. They should be targeted for early diagnosis and treatment. Those with clinical disease may exhibit localized or systemic symptoms and mild to severe illness. The final outcome of a disease may be recovery, death, or something in between, including a carrier state, complications requiring an extended hospital stay, or disability requiring rehabilitation.

At the community level, the disease may occur in endemic, epidemic, or pandemic proportion. Endemic refers to the constant presence of a disease within a geographic area or a population. Pertussis is endemic in the United States. Epidemic refers to the occurrence of a disease in a community or region in excess of normal expectancy. Although people tend to associate large numbers with epidemics, even one case can be termed *epidemic* if the disease is considered to have been eliminated from that area. For example, one case of polio, a disease that is considered to have been eliminated from the United States, would be considered epidemic. Pandemic refers to an epidemic that occurs worldwide and affects large populations. HIV/AIDS is both epidemic and pandemic because the number of cases is growing rapidly across various regions of the world. SARS and novel influenza A H1N1 are both emerging infectious diseases and are responsible for recent pandemics.

SURVEILLANCE OF COMMUNICABLE DISEASES

When conducting surveillance, you gather the *who, when, where,* and *what;* these elements are then used to answer *why.* A good surveillance system systematically collects, organizes, and analyzes current, accurate, and complete data for a defined disease condition. The resulting information is promptly released to those who need it for effective planning, implementation, and evaluation of disease prevention and control programs. Infectious disease surveillance incorporates and analyzes data from a variety of sources. Box 26.2 lists 10 commonly used data elements.

SURVEILLANCE FOR AGENTS OF BIOTERRORISM

Since September 11, 2001, greater emphasis has been placed on surveillance for any disease that might be associated with the intentional release of a biological agent. The concern is that because of the interval between exposure and disease, a covert release may go unrecognized and without response for some

---

BOX 26.2   10 Basic Elements of Surveillance

1. Mortality registration
2. Morbidity reporting
3. Epidemic reporting
4. Epidemic field investigation
5. Laboratory reporting
6. Individual case investigation
7. Surveys
8. Usage of biological agents and drugs
9. Distribution of animal reservoirs and vectors
10. Demographic and environmental data

---

time if the resulting outbreak closely resembles a naturally occurring one. Health care providers need to be alert to (1) temporal or geographic clustering of illnesses (e.g., people who attended the same public gathering or visited the same location), especially those with clinical signs that resemble an infectious disease outbreak—previously healthy people with unexplained fever accompanied by sepsis, pneumonia, respiratory failure, rash, or flaccid paralysis; (2) an unusual age distribution for a common disease (e.g., chickenpox-like disease in adults without a child source case); and (3) a large number of cases of acute flaccid paralysis, such as that seen in *Clostridium botulinum* intoxication. Although more active infectious disease surveillance is being encouraged because of the potential for bioterrorism, the positive benefit is increased surveillance for other communicable diseases as well.

Because of the heightened concern about possible bioterrorist attacks, various sorts of syndromic surveillance systems have been developed by public health agencies across the country. Syndromic surveillance systems use existing health data in real time to provide immediate analysis and feedback to those charged with investigation and follow-up of potential outbreaks. These systems incorporate factors such as the previously mentioned temporal and geographic clustering and unusual age distributions with groups of disease symptoms or syndromes (e.g., flaccid paralysis, respiratory signs, skin rashes, gastrointestinal symptoms) with the goal of detecting early signs of diseases that could result from a bioterrorism-related attack. Syndromic surveillance systems may include tracking emergency department visits sorted by syndrome symptoms, as well as other indicators of illness, including school absenteeism and sales of selected over-the-counter medications. In recent years, the tracking of cold medicines used to make crystal methamphetamine has received considerable attention. Nurses are frequently involved at different levels of the surveillance system. They collect data, make diagnoses, investigate and report cases, and provide information to the general public. Nurses may investigate sources and contacts in outbreaks of pertussis in school settings or shigellosis in daycare; TB testing and contact tracing; collecting and reporting information about notifiable communicable diseases; and providing morbidity and mortality statistics to those who request them, including the media, the public, service planners, and grant writers. See Chapter 15 for a complete discussion of surveillance and outbreak investigation.

LIST OF REPORTABLE DISEASES

States rather than the federal government mandate requirements for disease reporting. Notifiable or reportable diseases are those in which regular, frequent, and timely information about each case is needed for the prevention and control of the disease. The list of reportable diseases varies by state. State health departments, on a voluntary basis, report cases of selected diseases to the Centers for Disease Control and Prevention (CDC) in Atlanta, Georgia. The CDC updates these diseases conditions annually, and the list can be found under the heading of *Nationally notifiable infectious* diseases on the CDC website. See also Chapter 15: Surveillance and Outbreak Investigation for this list.

EMERGING INFECTIOUS DISEASES

EMERGENCE FACTORS

Emerging infectious diseases are those in which the incidence has actually increased in the past two decades or has the potential to increase in the near future. These emerging diseases may include new or known infectious diseases. Consider the following examples. Ebola virus was identified in 1976 when sporadic outbreaks occurred in Sudan and Zaire. Ebola virus is a mysterious killer with a high mortality rate, has no known treatment, and has no recognized reservoir in nature. It appears to be transmitted through direct contact with bodily secretions and can be contained once cases are identified. It is not clear why outbreaks occur. The CDC has current information on the Ebola virus and its fellow virus Marburg.

West Nile virus (WNV) was first identified in Uganda in 1937. There are two lineages: one in Africa that seems to be enzootic (i.e., related to animals in a particular vicinity) and that does not result in severe human illness and a second associated with clinical human encephalitis that has been seen in Africa, Asia, India, Europe, and now North America. How WNV first arrived in the United States is not known, but the answer most likely involves infected birds or mosquitoes. Because the virus is new in this country and the outbreak of 2002 caused many deaths, WNV has gained a great deal of media attention. However, for the majority of people, infection with WNV has no clinical signs or only mild flulike symptoms. In a small percentage of individuals—usually the young, the old, and the immunocompromised—a more severe, potentially fatal encephalitis may develop. After first appearing in New York City in 1999, the virus spent several years quietly spreading up and down the East Coast without remarkable morbidity or mortality. This situation changed abruptly in the summer of 2002 when WNV was reported across the country and was accompanied by significant avian, equine, and human mortality. By the fall of 2002, more than 3000 human cases with more than 180 deaths had been recorded, and WNV has been reported in most states. These periodic outbreaks appeared to result from a complex interaction of multiple factors, including weather—hot, dry summers followed by rain, which influences mosquito breeding sites and population growth. The number of WNV cases increased significantly in 2012, and the cause seemed to be the unusually hot weather in many parts of the United States. Because the ecology of WNV is not fully understood, the future pattern and nature of the virus in this country are uncertain; preventing human infection will continue to be a challenge for the foreseeable future. Currently, an equine vaccine exists, and work is under way in developing vaccines for both birds and humans. The best way to prevent WNV is to avoid mosquito bites by using insect repellents when outside; wearing long sleeves and long pants from dawn to dusk; avoiding standing water in open containers, including flower pots, buckets, or children's pools; installing or repairing window and door

TABLE 26.1 Factors That Can Influence the Emergence of New Infectious Diseases

Categories	Specific Examples
Societal events	Economic impoverishment, war or civil conflict, population growth and migration, urban decay
Health care	New medical devices, organ or tissue transplantation, drugs causing immunosuppression, widespread use of antibiotics
Food production	Globalization of food supplies, changes in food processing and packaging
Human behavior	Sexual behavior, drug use, travel, diet, outdoor recreation, use of child-care facilities
Environment	Deforestation or reforestation, changes in water ecosystems, flood or drought, famine, global changes (e.g., warming)
Public health	Curtailment or reduction in prevention programs, inadequate communicable disease infrastructure surveillance, lack of trained personnel (epidemiologists, laboratory scientists, vector and rodent control specialists)
Microbial adaptation	Changes in virulence and toxin production, development of drug resistance, microbes as cofactors in chronic diseases

From Centers for Disease Control and Prevention: Addressing emerging infectious disease threats: a prevention strategy for the United States (Executive Summary), *MMWR* 43 (No. RR-5):1-16, 1994.

screens and using air conditioning when possible. Visit the CDC website on WNV for more information.

Several factors, operating singly or in combination, can influence the emergence of these diseases (Table 26.1) (CDC, 1994). Except for microbial adaptation and changes made by the infectious agent, such as those likely in the emergence of *E. coli* O157:H7, most of the emergence factors are consequences of activities and behavior of the human hosts and environmental changes such as deforestation, urbanization, and industrialization. The rise in households with two working parents has increased the number of children in daycare, and with this shift has come an increase in diarrheal diseases such as shigellosis. Changing sexual behavior and illegal drug use influence the spread of HIV/AIDS and other STDs. Before the use of large air-conditioning systems with cooling towers, legionellosis was virtually unknown. Modern transportation systems closely and quickly connect regions of the world that for centuries had little contact. Insects and animals, as well as humans, may carry disease between continents via ships and planes. Immigrants, legal and illegal, as well as travelers, bring with them a variety of known and potentially unknown diseases. To prevent and control these emerging diseases, effective ways to educate people and change their behavior and to develop effective drugs and vaccines must be developed. Also, current surveillance systems must be strengthened and expanded to improve the detection and tracking of these diseases. The list of emerging infectious diseases changes as has been seen in the last few years. The best source of current information will be the latest edition of Heymann DL, editor: *Control of Communicable Diseases Manual* or the CDC. Examples include the various infectious diseases previously mentioned in Table 26.2.

TABLE 26.2   Examples of Emerging Infectious Diseases

Infectious Agent	Diseases/Symptoms	Mode of Transmission	Causes of Emergence
Borrelia burgdorferi	Lyme disease: rash, fever, arthritis, neurological and cardiac abnormalities	Bite of infective *Ixodes* tick	Increase in deer and human populations in wooded areas
Cryptosporidium	Cryptosporidiosis; infection of epithelial cells in gastrointestinal and respiratory tracts	Fecal–oral, person-to-person, waterborne	Development near watershed areas; immunosuppression
Ebola-Marburg viruses	Fulminant, high mortality, hemorrhagic fever	Direct contact with infected blood, organs, secretions, and semen	Unknown, likely human invasion of virus ecological niche
Escherichia coli O157:H7	Hemorrhagic colitis; thrombocytopenia; hemolytic uremic syndrome	Ingestion of contaminated food, especially undercooked beef and raw milk	Likely caused by a new pathogen
Hantavirus	Hemorrhagic fever with renal syndrome; pulmonary syndrome	Inhalation of aerosolized rodent urine and feces	Human invasion of virus ecological niche
Human immunodeficiency virus (HIV-1)	HIV infection; AIDS (HIV stage III); severe immune dysfunction, opportunistic infections	Sexual contact with or exposure to blood or tissues of infected persons; perinatal	Urbanization; lifestyle changes; drug use; international travel; transfusions; transplant
Human papillomavirus (HPV)	Skin and mucous membrane lesions (warts); strongly linked to cancer of the cervix and penis	Direct sexual contact, contact with contaminated surfaces	Newly recognized; changes in sexual lifestyle
Influenza A H1N1 virus (novel, pandemic)	Influenza: fever, cough, headache, myalgia, prostration, possibly gastrointestinal signs	Person-to-person, airborne (droplet), and contact (direct and indirect)	Antigenic shift
Influenza A H5N1 virus (novel, avian)	Influenza: fever, cough, headache, myalgia, prostration	Direct contact with infected poultry or birds; limited person-to-person transmission	Antigenic shift
Legionella pneumophila	Legionnaires' disease: malaise, myalgia, fever, headache, respiratory illness	Air cooling systems, water supplies	Recognition in an epidemic situation
Pneumocystis jiroveci	Acute pneumonia	Unknown; possibly airborne or reactivation of latent infection	Immunosuppression
SARS	Severe and acute pneumonia	Person-to-person, airborne (droplet) and direct and indirect contact with respiratory secretions and other bodily fluid	Unknown; newly recognized coronavirus; possible animal transmission into Chinese population
West Nile virus	No clinical signs to mild flulike symptoms to fatal neuroinvasive disease	Bite of infected mosquitoes; infected birds serve as reservoirs	International travel and commerce

Based on information from Heymann DL, editor: *Control of communicable diseases manual*, ed 20, Washington, DC, 2014, American Public Health Association; Fauci AS, Touchette NA, Folkers GK: Emerging infectious diseases: a 10-year perspective from the National Institute of Allergy and Infectious Diseases, *Emerg Infect Dis* 11(4):519-525, 2005.

CASE STUDY

Li Ming emigrated to America from Tibet with her father and brother after her mother's death. During a trip to the emergency room with a fever, hemoptysis, and cough, she was diagnosed with drug-resistant tuberculosis and placed in directly observed therapy (DOT), which meant a nurse from the local health department had to witness her ingesting her medication daily. Ms. Ming found taking the medication to be a big problem; swallowing the pills caused her to gag. She was embarrassed to have to take them in front of a nurse, and that made the whole situation even harder. Fortunately, all the rest of the family had negative purified protein derivative (PPD) skin tests and needed to be tested only periodically.

Ms. Ming was thin but not emaciated. She spoke English well enough to communicate with the nurse, Rachel Jones, who told her she could take her time swallowing the medication. They chatted each day about Ms. Ming's life in Tibet and her adjustment to America. Ms. Ming worked in a beauty salon washing hair. Although she was 25 years old, her father did not want her to date, and so she never had.

Ms. Jones worked to decrease Ms. Ming's anxiety. She taught Ms. Ming some relaxation exercises that Ms. Ming was able to use. During the first week of visits it took about an hour for the pills to be ingested. A month later the pill taking was down to 15 minutes and she no longer gagged. How can you apply what Ms. Jones did with Ms. Ming to get her to take her medication and to reduce her anxiety to other patients for whom you provide care? Were there other actions that Ms. Jones might have taken with this patient? How can you apply this case in the community?

Created by Deborah C. Conway, Assistant Professor, School of Nursing, University of Virginia.

PREVENTION AND CONTROL OF COMMUNICABLE DISEASES

Communicable disease can be prevented and controlled. The goal of prevention and control programs is to reduce the prevalence of a disease to a level at which it no longer poses a major public health problem. In some cases, diseases may even be eliminated or eradicated. The goal of elimination is to remove a disease from a large geographic area such as a country or region of the world. Eradication is the irreversible termination of all transmission of infection by extermination of the infectious agents worldwide. The World Health Assembly officially declared the global eradication of smallpox in 1980. After the successful eradication of smallpox, the eradication of other communicable diseases became a realistic challenge. The Americas were certified to be polio-free in 1994. Because of the devastating effects of polio, the WHO partnered with national governments, Rotary International, the CDC and the United Nations Children Fund (UNICEF) in the Global Polio Eradication Initiative. This initiative has worked tirelessly to immunize people against polio. Ways to prevent infectious disease in homes are listed in the How To box.

> **HOW TO Prevent Infectious Disease in Your Home**
> - Wash your hands (often and for at least 20 seconds with warm water).
> - Routinely clean and disinfect surfaces (bathroom and kitchen).
> - Handle and prepare food safely (separate and do not cross-contaminate one food with another).
> - Get immunized.
> - Use antibiotics appropriately.
> - Be careful with pets.
> - Avoid contact with wild animals.

From Centers for Disease Control and Prevention: *An ounce of prevention keeps the germs away: seven keys to a safer healthier home*, Atlanta, n.d., CDC. Retrieved June 2016 from http://www.cdc.gov/ounceofprevention

PRIMARY, SECONDARY, AND TERTIARY PREVENTION

As discussed in previous chapters, the three levels of prevention in public health are *primary, secondary,* and *tertiary.* In the prevention and control of infectious disease, primary prevention seeks to reduce the incidence of disease by preventing it before it happens, and in this, governments often provide assistance. Many interventions at the primary level, such as federally supplied vaccines and "no shots, no school" immunization laws, are population based because of public health mandate. Nurses deliver many childhood immunizations in public and community health settings, check immunization records in daycare facilities, and monitor immunization records in schools. Nurses often provide the teaching necessary to prevent communicable diseases.

The goal of secondary prevention is to prevent the spread of disease once it occurs. These activities center on rapid identification of potential contacts of a reported case. Contacts may be (1) identified as new cases and treated or (2) determined to be possibly exposed but not diseased and appropriately treated with prophylaxis. Public health disease control laws assist in secondary prevention because they require investigation and prevention measures for individuals affected by a communicable disease report or outbreak. These laws can extend to the entire community if the exposure potential appears great enough (i.e., an outbreak of smallpox or epidemic influenza). Nurses perform much of the communicable disease surveillance and control work in this country and are often responsible for reporting cases so that transmission can be reduced. Also, nurses perform much of the screening, such as for TB, HIV, and STDs (or STIs). Education can be both primary and secondary prevention.

Nurses who work in clinics, home health, schools, and other sites provide tertiary prevention care that is designed to reduce complications and disabilities through treatment and rehabilitation. This care may include helping people recover and return to their previous or a new level of health, as well as aspects of

LEVELS OF PREVENTION
Related to Infectious Disease Interventions

Primary Prevention
Goal: To prevent the occurrence of disease
- Educate about safe food-handling practices in the home.

Secondary Prevention
Goal: To prevent the spread of disease
- Immediately evaluate the possible source of any foodborne outbreak.

Tertiary Prevention
Goal: To reduce complications and disabilities through treatment and rehabilitation
- Immediately treat any foodborne infection.

primary and secondary care to prevent the continuation of the infectious disease and its further spread. Include family in all aspects of prevention, including tertiary, to help develop a treatment plan for the affected person and to prevent transmission of the disease.

Effective control of communicable diseases requires a multisystem approach. The primary goals and examples of such an approach include the following:
1. Improving host resistance to infectious agents and other environmental hazards, such as by improved hygiene, nutrition, physical fitness, and immunization coverage and providing drugs for prevention and treatment, as well as aids for improved mental health. In some locales, trash accumulates, dead animals are on the sides of roads, and standing water is a breeding ground for mosquitos.
2. Improve safety of the environment, such as by improved sanitation, clean water, and clean air; teaching proper cooking and storage of food; and control of vectors and animal reservoir hosts.
3. Improve public health systems by increasing access to health care and appropriate and timely health education and improving surveillance and reporting.
4. Facilitate social and political change to ensure better health for all people, such as by individual, group, and community action and legislation.
See the Levels of Prevention box.

AGENTS OF BIOTERRORISM

Both the attacks of September 11, 2001, and the subsequent anthrax attacks demonstrated the possibilities for the intentional release of a biological agent, or bioterrorism. The CDC suggests that the biological agents most likely to be employed in a bioterrorist attack are those that both have the potential for high mortality and can be easily disseminated, with the results of major public panic and social disruption. The diseases and infectious agents of highest concern are anthrax (*Bacillus anthracis*), plague (*Yersinia pestis*), smallpox (*Variola major*), botulism (*Clostridium botulinum*), tularemia (*Francisella tularensis),* and selected hemorrhagic viruses (Filoviridae and Arenaviridae). Visit the CDC Emergency Preparedness and Response website (http://www.bt.cdc.gov/) for more information.

ANTHRAX

Until the fall of 2001, anthrax was more commonly a concern of veterinarians and military strategists than the general public. After September 11, 2001, the news of deaths caused by letters deliberately contaminated with anthrax and sent through the postal service profoundly changed our view of this infectious disease. Anthrax is an acute disease caused by the spore-forming bacterium *Bacillus anthracis*. It is found naturally in soil and often affects domestic and wild animals. It is not spread from human to human but typically from handling products from infected animals or eating undercooked meat from affected animals (CDC, 2015e).

Anthrax is an organism that perpetuates itself by forming spores. A spore is a cell that is dormant but may come to life under the right conditions, such as when animals dying from anthrax suffer terminal hemorrhage, and infected blood comes into contact with the air; the bacillus organism then turns into spores. These spores are highly resistant to disinfection and environmental destruction and may remain in contaminated soil for many years. There are three types of anthrax, as follows (CDC, 2006):

1. Cutaneous, in which the first symptom is a small sore that develops into a blister that then develops into a skin ulcer with a black area in the center. The sore, blister, and ulcer do not hurt.
2. Gastrointestinal, with symptoms of nausea, loss of appetite, bloody diarrhea, and fever, followed by stomach pain.
3. Respiratory, or inhalational, which has cold or flu symptoms and can lead to cough, chest discomfort, shortness of breath, tiredness, and muscle aches.

Symptoms often appear within 7 days of coming in contact with the bacterium. Treatment for a person who is exposed but not yet sick generally includes an antibiotic combined with anthrax vaccine; treatment for a person after infection is usually a 60-day course of antibiotics. Success depends on the type of anthrax and how soon treatment begins.

Because of factors such as the ability to become an aerosol, resistance to environmental degradation, and a high fatality rate, inhalational anthrax is considered to have an extremely high potential for being the single greatest biological warfare threat (Fauci et al, 2008). Any threat of anthrax should be reported to the Federal Bureau of Investigation and to local and state health departments. Anthrax is most often found in the agricultural regions of Central and South America, sub-Saharan Africa, central and southwestern Asia, southern and eastern Europe, and the Caribbean (CDC, 2015e). The people who are most at risk are those who handle animal products, veterinarians, livestock producers, travelers, laboratory professionals, mail handlers, military personnel, and response workers who may be exposed during a bioterrorism attack involving anthrax spores (CDC, 2015f).

SMALLPOX

Formerly a disease found worldwide, smallpox has been considered eradicated since 1979. The last known natural death from smallpox occurred in Somalia in 1977. The United States stopped routinely immunizing for smallpox in 1982. The only documented existing virus sources are located in freezers at the CDC in Atlanta and a research institute in Novosibirsk, Russia. Controversy exists over the destruction of these viral stocks, and despite an earlier call by the WHO for destruction in 2002, this date has been postponed to allow for additional research needed should clandestine supplies fall into terrorist hands.

Smallpox could be a leading candidate as an agent of bioterrorism. Susceptibility is 100% in the unvaccinated (those vaccinated before 1982 are not considered protected, although they may possess some immunity), and the fatality rate is estimated at 20% to 40% or higher. Vaccinia vaccine, the immunizing agent for smallpox, is available through the CDC and is effective even after exposure. A second-generation vaccinia vaccine, the immunizing agent for smallpox that was licensed by the U.S. Food and Drug Administration in 2007, is available through the CDC and can be effective even several days after exposure. Because of the potential for bioterrorism and the fact that many health care providers have never seen this disease, it is important to become familiar with the clinical and epidemiological features of smallpox and how it is differentiated from chickenpox (see the How To box).

Despite the availability of a vaccine, chickenpox is still a common disease of childhood and may be seen in susceptible adults as well. Although many health care providers are familiar with chickenpox, most have never seen a case of smallpox. Because of the potential for smallpox to be used as a bioweapon,

---

HOW TO Distinguish Chickenpox from Smallpox

Chickenpox (Varicella)	Smallpox (Historical Variola Major)
Sudden onset with slight fever and mild constitutional symptoms (both may be more severe in adults)	Sudden onset of fever, prostration, severe body aches, and occasional abdominal pain and vomiting, as in influenza
Rash is present at onset	Clear-cut prodromal illness; rash follows 2–4 days after fever begins decreasing
Rash progression is maculopapular for a few hours, vesicular for 3–4 days, followed by granular scabs	Progression is macular, papular, vesicular, and pustular, followed by crusted scabs that fall off after 3–4 weeks if client survives
Rash is "centrifugal," with lesions most abundant on the trunk or areas of the body usually covered by clothing	Rash is "centripetal," with lesions most abundant on the face and extremities
Lesions appear in "crops" and can be at various stages in the same area of the body	Lesions are all at same stage in all areas
Vesicles are superficial and collapse on puncture; mild scarring may occur	Vesicles are deep-seated and do not collapse on puncture; pitting and scarring are common

From Heymann, DL, editor: *Control of communicable diseases manual*, ed 19, Washington, DC, 2008, American Public Health Association; and Henderson DA: Smallpox: clinical and epidemiologic features, *Emerg Infect Dis* 5:537-539, 1999.

the CDC suggests that nurses and other practitioners familiarize themselves with the differences in presentation between the two diseases. The rash pattern for each disease is distinctive, but it has been observed that in the first 2 to 3 days of development, the two may be indistinguishable. Infectious disease texts and posters provide a pictorial description. If a smallpox infection is suspected, the local health department should be notified immediately.

VACCINE-PREVENTABLE DISEASE

Vaccines are one of the most effective methods of preventing and controlling communicable diseases. The smallpox vaccine, which left distinctive scars on so many shoulders, is no longer in general use because the smallpox virus has been declared totally eradicated from the world's population. Despite threats of bioterrorism, there are no plans to reintroduce universal smallpox immunization with the existing vaccine because of potential side effects. Diseases such as polio, diphtheria, pertussis, and measles, which previously occurred in epidemic proportions, are now controlled by routine childhood immunization. They have not, however, been eradicated, so children need to be immunized against these diseases. In the United States "no shots, no school" legislation has resulted in the immunization of most children by the time they enter school. However, many infants and toddlers, the group most vulnerable to these potentially severe diseases, do not receive scheduled immunizations on time despite the availability of free vaccines. Surveys show that inner-city children from minority and ethnic groups are particularly at risk for incomplete immunization. Children from religious communities whose beliefs prohibit immunization and children with parents who have philosophical objections to immunization may receive no protection at all. Studies also show low levels of vaccination against pneumonia in senior citizens and lower levels of influenza coverage in adults from minority and ethnic groups. Research also suggests that adolescents have lower rates of coverage than children or adults, perhaps because they do not as frequently access preventive care. *Healthy People 2020* includes several objectives about obtaining and maintaining appropriate levels of immunization in all age groups. (Additional information on vaccine-preventable diseases may be found at the CDC website: http://www.cdc.gov/vaccines/.)

Because many children receive their immunizations at public health departments, nurses play a major role in increasing immunization coverage of infants and toddlers. Nurses track children known to be at risk for underimmunization and call or send reminders to their parents. They help avoid missed immunization opportunities by checking the immunization status of every young child encountered, whether the clinic or home visit is related to immunization or not. In addition, they organize immunization outreach activities in the community that deliver immunization services; provide answers to parents' questions and concerns about immunization; and educate parents about why immunizations are needed, about inappropriate contraindications to immunization, and about the importance of completing the immunization schedule on time.

EVIDENCE-BASED PRACTICE

Because they are too young to be fully immunized, infants under 6 months of age are at greatest risk for complications and death from pertussis. New mothers, fathers, caretakers, and close contacts to the infant are frequently the source of infection, leading to the concept of cocooning the infant against pertussis through immunizing individuals who have close contact with the baby. In examining ways to increase Tdap (tetanus, reduced diphtheria, acellular pertussis) uptake in new mothers, researchers looked at two hospitals with zero postpartum Tdap immunization rates. One followed standard procedures and the other instituted a standing order for new mothers to receive Tdap before discharge. Implementing the standing orders raised the zero starting rate to 69%. At the hospital that followed standard procedures, the rate of postpartum Tdap immunization remained at zero. Since this study, the Advisory Committee on Immunization Practices has updated its recommendation to say women should receive Tdap, if they have not already, toward the end of their second trimester or during their third trimester of pregnancy. However, even with this new recommendation, studies find only a small percentage of unimmunized pregnant women receive a Tdap vaccination (LABioMed, 2014).

Nurse Use

The adult public has been slow to embrace Tdap. One reason may be a lack of awareness of the availability of the vaccine and/or of the importance it plays in keeping infants safe. There are a variety of ways to approach this issue, starting with consumer awareness and provider education and advocacy. This study shows how a change in standard practice within an institution had a dramatic effect on Tdap immunization in postpartum mothers. Whether Tdap or other issues that require attention, nurses manage clinics and take leadership roles in hospitals, physicians' offices, health departments, and safety-net health services, which puts them in a position to both assess where there are opportunities for intervention and to change practice to address important public health concerns.

ROUTINE CHILDHOOD IMMUNIZATION SCHEDULE

The CDC regularly publishes the recommended immunization schedule for children ages 1 to 6 years and for children ages 7 to 18 as well as for adults (CDC, 2016a). The recommended vaccine schedule is complex and changes, so consult the CDC website for current information. Other useful sites related to immunization schedules and requirements are those of the American Academy of Pediatrics (http://www.aap.org) and the American Academy of Family Physicians (http://www.aafp.org). Because most of these vaccines require three or four doses, they ideally should begin when an infant is 2 months old to achieve recommended immunization levels by 2 years of age. Additional doses may be required before a child enters school and at adolescence or on entering college. Booster doses of tetanus should be given every 10 years.

MEASLES

Measles is an acute, highly contagious respiratory disease that although considered a childhood illness can occur in adolescents and young adults. Symptoms include fever, runny nose, sneezing, cough, a rash all over the body, and small white spots on the inside of the cheek (Koplik spots). Measles is caused by the rubeola virus and is spread through the air by breathing, coughing, or sneezing. The contagious nature, combined with the fact that people are most contagious before they know they are infected, makes measles a disease that can spread rapidly. Infection with measles confers lifelong immunity (Heymann, 2014).

Measles was declared eliminated in the United States in 2000, and it is rare in North and South America because of the high level of vaccination. However, in 2014, 667 cases were reported to the CDC; 289 cases were reported in 2015; and from January 2 to April 29, 2016, 10 people in 4 states reported having measles (CDC, 2016b). The WHO estimated that 20 million people are affected annually, with over 100,000 deaths—mostly children under the age of 5. The good news is that with the launch of the Measles and Rubella Initiative in 2001, global measles deaths have decreased by 78% worldwide from 652,400 deaths in 2000 to 122,000 deaths in 2012 (WHO, 2014). However, it still kills about 200,000 people worldwide. Measles is still common in some parts of Europe, Asia, the Pacific, and Africa. People going to these countries need to have current measles vaccinations. Many of the cases of measles in the United States are related to children whose families do not believe in vaccination, to travelers who visit the United States, and to U.S. citizens who travel with their children to countries where measles is still prevalent.

Healthy People 2020 calls for the sustained elimination of indigenous cases of vaccine-preventable disease. Efforts to meet this goal will require (1) rapid detection of cases and implementation of appropriate outbreak control measures, (2) achievement and maintenance of high levels of vaccination coverage among preschool-aged children in all geographic regions, (3) continued implementation and enforcement of the two-dose schedule among young adults, (4) the determination of the source of all outbreaks and sporadic infections, and (5) cooperation among countries in measles control efforts. Nurses receive reports of cases, investigate them, initiate control measures for outbreaks, and use every opportunity to immunize adolescents and young adults who lack documentation of two doses of measles vaccine. Nurses who work in regions in which undocumented residents are common, where groups obtain exemption from immunization on religious grounds, where preschool coverage is low, or where international visitors are frequent need to be especially alert for cases of measles and the need for prompt outbreak control among particularly susceptible populations.

RUBELLA

The rubella (German measles) virus causes a mild febrile disease characterized by enlarged lymph nodes and a fine, pink rash that is often difficult to distinguish from those of measles or scarlet fever. In contrast to measles, rubella is only moderately contagious. Transmission is through inhalation of or direct contact with infected droplets from respiratory tract secretions of infected persons. Children may show few or no symptoms, and adults usually experience several days of low-grade fever, headache, malaise, runny nose, and conjunctivitis before the rash appears. Many infections occur without a rash (Heymann, 2014).

Since the introduction of a vaccine in 1969, cases of rubella in the United States have dropped greatly. This decrease has changed the epidemiology of the disease. Although still considered a childhood illness, rubella can occur in adolescents and young adults. Pregnant women are at particular risk in that rubella infection can cause intrauterine death, spontaneous abortion, and congenital anomalies (known as congenital rubella syndrome [CRS]) in the baby, including deafness, cataracts, heart defects, mental retardation, and liver and spleen damage. Unimmunized immigrants do not necessarily import disease, but their unimmunized status leaves them vulnerable to infection once they arrive. Eliminating rubella and CRS will require many of the same efforts discussed for other vaccine-preventable diseases, including achievement and maintenance of high rates of immunization among children; ensuring vaccination among women of childbearing age, especially those who are foreign-born; continued aggressive surveillance; and rapid response to outbreaks. Rubella was considered eliminated from the United States in 2014. Today fewer than 10 people in the United States have rubella, although it is a problem in other parts of the world. Since 2012, it appears that all cases of rubella in the United States were infected while outside the United States (CDC, 2016c).

PERTUSSIS

Pertussis (whooping cough) begins as a mild upper respiratory tract infection that progresses to an irritating cough and in 1 to 2 weeks may become paroxysmal (a series of repeated violent coughs). The repeated coughs occur without intervening breaths and can be followed by a characteristic inspiratory "whoop" sound. Pertussis is caused by the bacterium *Bordetella pertussis* and is transmitted via an airborne route through contact with infected droplets. It is highly contagious and is considered endemic in the United States. Vaccination against pertussis, delivered in combination with diphtheria and tetanus, is a part of the routine childhood immunization schedule. Treatment of infected individuals with antibiotics such as erythromycin may shorten the period of communicability but does not relieve symptoms unless given early in the course of the infection. Prophylactic treatment with antibiotics is recommended for family members and close contacts of infected individuals, regardless of immunization status and age, if there is a child in the house under the age of 1 year or a woman in the last 3 weeks of pregnancy or to prevent ongoing transmission within the family (Heymann, 2014).

Pertussis in children, especially those younger than 6 months, is attributed to being too young to have received the first three of the five doses of vaccine recommended by 6 years of age. Cases in older children also result largely from inadequate or underimmunization. In adolescents and adults with histories of complete immunization, cases are thought to be the result of waning immunity. Natural infection with pertussis results in permanent immunity. A schedule of five doses of DTaP (diphtheria, tetanus, acellular pertussis) is given to infants until they are 6 years of age. A dose of Tdap is recommended for children at age 11 or 12 and can be given to children as young as 7 years if they missed one or more of the childhood doses of DTaP. People 19 years of age and older should get a booster dose of Td every 10 years. Adults under 65 years of age who have never gotten Tdap should get one dose of Tdap as their next booster, and adults 65 and older who expect to have close contact with a baby younger than 12 months of age should get a dose of Tdap to help protect the baby from pertussis. Pertussis can cause serious illness in babies, children, teens, and adults and can be life-threatening especially in babies (CDC, 2015g).

Nurses may expect periodic outbreaks of pertussis because of its cyclical nature. Working with the community to maintain the highest possible levels of immunization coverage can minimize these occurrences. Because of the contagious nature of pertussis, nurses play a major role in limiting transmission during outbreaks by ensuring appropriate treatment of family members, classmates, and other close contacts.

INFLUENZA

Influenza (flu) is a viral respiratory infection often indistinguishable from the common cold or other respiratory diseases. Transmission is airborne and through direct contact with infected droplets. Unlike many viruses that do not survive long in the environment, the flu virus may survive for many hours in dried mucus. Outbreaks are common in the winter and early spring in areas in which people gather indoors, such as in schools and nursing homes. Gastrointestinal and respiratory symptoms are common. Because symptoms do not always follow a characteristic pattern, many viral diseases that are not influenza are often called *flu*. The most important factors to note about influenza are its epidemic nature and the mortality that may result from pulmonary complications, especially in older adults and children under 2 years of age.

QSEN FOCUS ON QUALITY AND SAFETY EDUCATION FOR NURSES

Targeted Competency: Safety—Minimizes risk for harm to clients and providers through both system effectiveness and individual performance. Important aspects of safety include the following:

- **Knowledge:** Discuss potential and actual impact of national client safety resources, initiatives, and regulations
- **Skills:** Use national client safety resources for own professional development and to focus attention on safety in care settings
- **Attitudes:** Value relationship between national safety campaigns and implementation in local practices and practice settings

Safety Question:

Pertussis has become an increasing infectious disease concern.

- Look into local statistics around pertussis occurrence. Has there been an increased occurrence of pertussis over the last 5 years?
- How do your local statistics compare to national statistics for pertussis from the Centers for Disease Control and Prevention?
- What might be some systems approaches to educating your community about the risk for pertussis?
- What might be some systems approaches to providing pertussis vaccinations to the appropriate populations?
- What data points will you want to track to assess whether your interventions have been effective?

Prepared by Gail Armstrong, DNP, ACNS-BC, CNE, Associate Professor, University of Colorado Denver College of Nursing.

There are three types of influenza viruses: A, B, and C. Type A is usually responsible for large epidemics, whereas outbreaks from type B are more regionalized; type C epidemics are less common and usually result in only mild illness. Influenza viruses often change in the nature of their surface appearance or their antigenic makeup. Types B and C are fairly stable viruses, but type A changes constantly. Minor antigenic changes are referred to as *antigenic drift,* and they result in yearly epidemics and regional outbreaks. Major changes such as the emergence of new subtypes are called *antigenic shift;* these occur only with type A viruses. Antigenic shift and drift lead to epidemic outbreaks every few years and pandemic outbreaks every 10 to 40 years, as seen with novel influenza A H1N1 in 2009 and influenza now in A H3N2, which is associated with interacting with pigs and attendance at state fairs.

The preparation of influenza vaccine each year is based on the best possible prediction of what type and variant of the virus will be most prevalent that year. Because of the changing nature of the virus, yearly immunization is necessary and in the United States is given in early fall before the flu season begins. The flu season in the United States can range from October to March. The CDC recommends an annual flu vaccine for everyone 6 months of age and older, and people should be vaccinated as soon as the vaccine becomes available (CDC, 2016d). Specifically, if vaccine were available, immunization for seasonal flu is especially recommended for children ages 6 months to 19 years, pregnant women, people 50 years of age and older, people of any age with certain chronic medical conditions, people who live in nursing homes and other long-term care facilities, and people who live with or care for those at risk for complications from flu. During 2015 the vaccine did not effectively protect against influenza due to a variation in the virus that was unpredicted.

The use of influenza antiviral drugs should be considered in the nonimmunized or groups at high risk for complications. Antiviral drugs are prescription medicines that fight flu in the body. They are not sold over the counter, and they are not a substitute for the flu vaccine. These drugs can lessen symptoms and shorten the time a person is sick with the flu; they also can prevent serious flu complications such as pneumonia. The CDC annually publishes Recommendations for Influenza Antiviral Medications.

Healthy People 2020 recommends increasing the proportion of the population vaccinated annually against influenza and pneumococcal disease. Nurses often spearhead influenza immunization campaigns that target older adults. Examples include conducting flu clinics at polling places during elections or at community centers and churches during "senior vaccination Sundays." Inhabitants of nursing homes and residences for older adults are at risk because influenza can spread rapidly with severe consequences through such living arrangements. As with children, nurses should check immunization history and encourage immunization for every older adult encountered in a clinic or home visit. When nurses get immunized against influenza, they are protecting not only themselves but their patients, and they are serving as role models for health promotion and disease prevention.

Antiviral agents can reduce the severity and duration of illness, and these drugs must be taken under a physician's prescription. Prevention of this virus requires the same precautionary measures as those of many other communicable diseases, including the following:

- Wash hands properly or use alcohol-based hand rub, especially after you cough or sneeze.
- Avoid touching your mouth, nose, or eyes.
- Cover your mouth when you cough or sneeze, and do not spit.
- Do not go to work or school if you develop influenza symptoms.
- If you develop flulike symptoms, stay home for 7 days after the symptoms begin or until you have been symptom-free for 24 hours. (CDC, 2009)

FOODBORNE AND WATERBORNE DISEASES

Protecting a nation's food supply from contamination by all virulent microbes is complex, costly, and time consuming. However, much foodborne illness, regardless of causal organism, can be prevented by simple changes in food preparation, handling, and storage to destroy or denature contaminants and prevent their further spread. Because these measures are so important in preventing foodborne disease, *Healthy People 2020* includes an objective directed toward food safety, and the WHO has developed *Five Keys to Safer Food*, which replaces and simplifies the *Ten Golden Rules for Safe Food Preparation*, which was developed in the early 1990s (Box 26.3).

Foodborne illness, often called "food poisoning," can be categorized as either a food infection or food intoxication. Food infection results from bacterial, viral, or parasitic infection of food and includes salmonellosis, hepatitis A, and trichinosis. Food intoxication results from toxins produced by bacterial growth, chemical contaminants (heavy metals), and a variety of disease-producing substances found naturally in certain foods such as mushrooms and some seafood. Examples of food intoxications are botulism, mercury poisoning, and paralytic shellfish poisoning. Table 26.3 presents some of the most common agents of food intoxication, their incubation period, source, symptoms, and pathology. Although it is not a hard-and-fast rule, food infections are associated with incubation periods of 12 hours to several days after ingestion of the infected food, whereas food intoxications become obvious within minutes to hours after ingestion. Some botulism is a clear exception to this rule, with an incubation period of a week or more in adults. The expression *ptomaine poisoning,* often used when discussing foodborne illness, does not refer to a specific causal organism.

The spectrum of foodborne illness is constantly changing, and foodborne illnesses affect people of all socioeconomic levels, races, sexes, ages, occupations, educations, and areas of residence. The very young, old, and debilitated are the most susceptible and have the highest burden of morbidity and mortality. FoodNet is a CDC sentinel surveillance system targeting 10 state health departments. FoodNet is a collaborative effort among the CDC, the U.S. Department of Agriculture (USDA), and the U.S. Food and Drug Administration (FDA).

BOX 26.3 Five Keys To Safer Food

1. Keep clean.
   - Wash your hands before handling food and often during food preparation.
   - Wash your hands after going to the toilet.
   - Wash and sanitize all surfaces and equipment used for food preparation.
   - Protect kitchen areas and food from insects, pests, and other animals.
2. Separate raw and cooked.
   - Separate raw meat, poultry, and seafood from other foods.
   - Use separate equipment and utensils, such as knives and cutting boards, for handling raw foods.
   - Store food in containers to avoid contact between raw and prepared foods.
3. Cook thoroughly.
   - Cook food thoroughly, especially meat, poultry, eggs, and seafood.
   - Bring foods such as soups and stews to boiling to make sure that they reach 70° C (158° F). For meat and poultry, make sure that juices are clear, not pink. Ideally use a thermometer.
4. Keep food at safe temperatures.
   - Do not leave cooked food at room temperature for more than 2 hours.
   - Refrigerate promptly all cooked and perishable food (preferably below 5° C [41° F]).
   - Keep cooked food piping hot (more than 60° C [140° F]) before serving.
   - Do not store food too long even in the refrigerator.
   - Do not thaw frozen food at room temperature.
5. Use safe water and raw materials.
   - Use safe water or treat it to make it safe.
   - Select fresh and wholesome foods.
   - Choose foods processed for safety, such as pasteurized milk.
   - Wash fruits and vegetables, especially if eaten raw.
   - Do not use food beyond its expiration date.

From World Health Organization: *Five keys to safer food,* Geneva, n.d., WHO. Retrieved August 2012 from http://www.who.int/foodsafety/publications/consumer/en/5keys_en.pdf

The surveillance includes 15% of the U.S. population. FoodNet collects data on the following pathogens: *Salmonella, Campylobacter, Shigella, Cryptosporidium, Cyclospora, Listeria, E. coli,* and *Yersinia* (Huang et al, 2016). Confirmed foodborne outbreaks are reported by states to the CDC through the Foodborne Disease Outbreak Surveillance System. In 2015 FoodNet received reports of 20,107 confirmed cases, 4531 hospitalizations, and 77 deaths.

In recent years, publicity has surrounded foodborne outbreaks affecting people nationwide. Examples include the illness and, in some cases, deaths of individuals after eating fresh spinach contaminated with a virulent strain of *E. coli;* peanut butter infected with salmonella; cans of corned beef, chili, and beef stew pulled from grocery shelves because of possible botulism; and a warning not to eat fresh tomatoes for fear of contracting an unusual strain of *Salmonella,* although the actual culprit turned out to be chili peppers. Although the young, the old, and the debilitated are most susceptible, anyone can acquire a foodborne illness. However, a new, particularly susceptible population is emerging as the adult population ages and chronic diseases (e.g., AIDS) and advanced medical treatment (e.g., chemotherapy, organ transplants) result in growing numbers of immunosuppressed individuals. At the same time, centralized food processing draws from multiple producers and

TABLE 26.3 Commonly Encountered Food Intoxications

Causal Agent	Incubation Period	Duration	Clinical Presentation	Associated Food
Staphylococcus aureus	30 min–7 hr	1–2 days	Sudden onset of nausea, cramps, vomiting, and prostration, often accompanied by diarrhea; rarely fatal	All foods, especially those likely to come into contact with food-handlers' hands that may be contaminated from infections of the eyes and skin
Clostridium perfringens (strain A)	6–24 hr	1 day or less	Sudden onset of colic and diarrhea, maybe nausea; vomiting and fever unusual; rarely fatal	Inadequately heated meats or stews; food contaminated by soil or feces becomes infective when improper storage or reheating allows multiplication of organism
Vibrio parahaemolyticus	4–96 hr	1–7 days	Watery diarrhea and abdominal cramps; sometimes nausea, vomiting, fever, and headache; rarely fatal	Raw or inadequately cooked seafood; period of time at room temperature usually required for multiplication of organisms
Clostridium botulinum	12–36 hr; sometimes days	Slow recovery; could be months	Central nervous system signs; blurred vision, difficulty in swallowing and dry mouth, followed by descending symmetrical flaccid paralysis of an alert person; "floppy baby" in infant; fatality <15% with antitoxin and respiratory support	Home-canned fruits and vegetables that have not been preserved with adequate heating; infants have become infected from ingesting honey

Data from Heymann DL, editor: *Control of communicable diseases manual,* ed 18, Washington, DC, 2008, American Public Health Association.

suppliers outside the country, as well as within, and marketing through widespread distribution networks increases the potential for any contamination to result in a large-scale foodborne outbreak, compounding the difficulty in attempting to trace the source. Public health officials think the reported cases of foodborne illness vastly underrepresent the true number of cases and that this number is likely to increase.

SALMONELLOSIS

Salmonellosis is a bacterial disease characterized by a sudden onset of headache, abdominal pain, diarrhea, nausea, sometimes vomiting, and almost always fever. Onset is typically within 48 hours of ingestion, but the clinical signs are impossible to distinguish from those of other causes of gastrointestinal distress. Diarrhea and lack of appetite may last several days, and dehydration may be severe. Although morbidity can be significant, death is uncommon except among infants, older adults, and the debilitated. The rate of infection is highest among infants and small children. It is estimated that only a small proportion of cases is recognized clinically and that only 1% of clinical cases are reported. The number of *Salmonella* infections yearly may actually number in the millions (Heymann, 2014).

Outbreaks occur commonly in restaurants, hospitals, nursing homes, and institutions for children. The transmission route is eating food that comes from an infected animal or food contaminated by feces of an infected animal or person. Meat, poultry, and eggs are the foods most often associated with *Salmonella* outbreaks. However, recently regional and national outbreaks have resulted from vegetables (e.g., lettuce, green onions, tomatoes, chili peppers) and peanut butter. Animals are

the common reservoir for the various *Salmonella* serotypes, although infected humans also may fill this role. Animals are more likely to be chronic carriers. In 2016 there were seven multistate outbreaks linked to live poultry in backyard flocks (CDC, 2016e). *Salmonella* carriers include reptiles such as iguanas, pet turtles, poultry, cattle, swine, rodents, dogs, and cats. Person-to-person transmission is an important consideration in daycare and institutional settings.

ESCHERICHIA COLI O157:H7

E. coli O157:H7 belongs to the enterohemorrhagic category of *E. coli* serotypes that produce a strong cytotoxin called a Shiga toxin and are collectively known as Shiga toxin–producing *E. coli* (STEC). *E. coli* serotypes in this group can cause a potentially fatal hemorrhagic colitis. This pathogen was first described in humans in 1992 after two outbreaks of illness were associated with eating hamburgers from a fast-food restaurant chain. Undercooked hamburger and chicken has been implicated in several outbreaks, as have beef, alfalfa sprouts, melons, lettuce, unpasteurized milk and apple cider, municipal water, jalapenos, uncooked spinach, ready to eat salads, lettuce, cheese, prepackaged cookie dough, pizza, flour, and tacos (CDC, 2014). There is often person-to-person transmission in daycare centers, homes, and institutions. Outbreaks also have been associated with petting zoos. Infection with *E. coli* O157:H7 causes bloody diarrhea, abdominal cramps, and, infrequently, fever. Children and older adults are at highest risk for clinical disease and complications. Hemolytic-uremic syndrome is seen in about 15% of cases among children and a smaller number of adults and may result in acute renal failure. The case fatality rate can be as high as 5% (Heymann, 2014).

Hamburger is often involved in outbreaks because the grinding process exposes pathogens on the surface of the whole meat to the interior of the ground meat, effectively mixing the once-exterior bacteria thoroughly throughout the hamburger so that searing the surface no longer suffices to kill all bacteria. Tracking the contamination is complicated by the fact that hamburger is often made of meat ground from several sources. The best protection against this pathogen, as with most foodborne agents, is to thoroughly cook food before eating it.

WATERBORNE DISEASE OUTBREAKS AND PATHOGENS

Waterborne pathogens usually enter water supplies through animal or human fecal contamination and often cause enteric disease. They include viruses, bacteria, and protozoans. Hepatitis A virus is probably the best known waterborne viral agent, although other viruses may be transmitted by this route (i.e., enteroviruses, rotaviruses, paramyxoviruses). The most important waterborne bacterial diseases are cholera, typhoid fever, and bacillary dysentery. However, other *Salmonella* types, *Shigella*, *Vibrio*, and *Campylobacter* species and various coliform bacteria, including *E. coli* O157:H7, may be transmitted in the same manner. In the past, the most important waterborne protozoans have been *Entamoeba histolytica* (amebic dysentery) and *Giardia lamblia*, but outbreaks of cryptosporidiosis in municipal water have called attention to the importance of protecting sources of water. Protozoans do not respond to traditional chlorine treatment as do enteric and coliform bacteria, and their small size requires special filtration. *Giardia* is often an issue for U.S. citizens who travel to other countries and have no immunity from the protozoans in those countries. *Giardia* is a microscopic parasite passed via stool and can survive for weeks or months. It can be contracted by swallowing water while swimming, drinking water or ice made from infected sources, eating foods prepared in infected water, or having contact with someone with giardiasis. The symptoms include diarrhea, gas, greasy stools that can float, stomach or abdominal cramps, upset stomach, nausea, and dehydration. It may last 2 to 6 weeks. The treatment is to drink fluids and get medication (CDC, 2015h).

The CDC defines an outbreak of waterborne disease as an incident in which two or more persons experience similar illness after consuming water that epidemiological evidence implicates as the source of that illness. Only a single incident is required in cases of chemical contamination. The CDC and the Environmental Protection Agency (EPA) maintain a collaborative surveillance program for collection and periodic reporting of data on the occurrence and causes of waterborne disease outbreaks.

VECTOR-BORNE DISEASE AND ZOONOSES

In vector-borne diseases the infectious agent is transmitted by a carrier, or vector, usually an arthropod (i.e., mosquito, tick, fly), either biologically or mechanically. With *biological transmission,* the vector is necessary for the infectious agent to develop. For example, mosquitoes can carry malaria. *Mechanical transmission* occurs when an insect contacts the infectious agent with its legs or mouthparts and carries it to the host. For example, flies and cockroaches may contaminate food or cooking utensils.

Vector-borne diseases typically involve zoonotic cycles and require an animal host or reservoir. Vector-borne diseases commonly found in the United States are those associated with ticks, such as Lyme disease *(Borrelia burgdorferi)*, ehrlichiosis *(Ehrlichia)*, anaplasmosis *(Anaplasma phagocytophilum)*, and Rocky Mountain spotted fever *(Rickettsia rickettsii)*. Nurses who work with large immigrant populations or with international travelers may encounter malaria and dengue fever, both carried by mosquitoes. WNV is an example of endemic mosquito-borne viral diseases, which include St. Louis, LaCrosse, and western and eastern equine encephalitis. Plague *(Yersinia pestis)* is carried by fleas of wild rodents. More rarely seen are babesiosis *(Babesia microti)*, tularemia *(Francisella tularensis)*, and Q fever *(Coxiella burnetii)*, all associated with ticks.

LYME DISEASE

Parents in Lyme, Connecticut, concerned about the unusual incidence of juvenile rheumatoid arthritis in their children, were the first to bring attention to this tick-borne infection that now bears their town's name. First described in 1975, Lyme disease became a nationally notifiable disease in 1991. Lyme disease typically occurs in summer during tick season, and it has been reported throughout the United States, with 95% of cases concentrated in rural and suburban areas of the northeast, mid-Atlantic, and north-central states, especially Wisconsin and Minnesota. The causative agent, the spirochete *B. burgdorferi,* was identified in 1982. Lyme disease is transmitted by ixodid ticks that are associated with white-tailed deer *(Odocoileus virginianus)* and the white-footed mouse *(Peromyscus leucopus)*.

Clinically, Lyme disease is divided into three stages. Stage I is characterized by erythema chronicum migrans, a distinctive skin lesion often called a *bull's-eye lesion* because it begins as a red area at the site of the tick attachment that spreads outward in a ringlike fashion as the center clears. About 70% to 80% of infected persons develop this lesion 3 to 30 days after a tick bite. The skin lesion may be accompanied or preceded by fever, fatigue, malaise, headache, muscle pains, and a stiff neck, as well as tender and enlarged lymph nodes and migratory joint pain. The lesion can reach 12 inches in diameter (CDC, 2015i). Most clients diagnosed in this early stage respond well to 10 to 14 days of oral tetracycline or penicillin.

If not treated during the first stage, Lyme disease can progress to stage II, which may include additional skin lesions, headache, and neurological and cardiac abnormalities. Clients who progress to stage III have recurrent attacks of arthritis and arthralgia, especially in the knees, which may begin months to years after the initial lesion. The clinical diagnosis of classic Lyme disease with the distinctive skin lesion is straightforward. Illness without the lesion is more difficult to diagnose because serological tests are more accurate in stages II and III than in stage I (Heymann, 2014). See the CDC's "Signs and Symptoms of Untreated Lyme Disease" for a good description (CDC, 2015i).

Measures for preventing exposure to ticks include reducing tick populations, avoiding tick-infested areas, wearing protective clothing when outdoors (i.e., long sleeves and long pants tucked into socks), using repellants, and immediately inspecting for and removing ticks when returning indoors. Ticks require a prolonged period of attachment (6–48 hours) before they start blood-feeding on the host; prompt tick discovery and removal can help prevent transmission of disease. When outdoors, permethrin sprayed on clothing and tick repellents containing 20% to 30% diethyltoluamide (DEET) can offer effective protection; use of DEET should be avoided in children younger than 2 years because of reports of significant toxicity, including skin irritation, anaphylaxis, and seizures. Read more about tick-associated diseases at the CDC website: http://www.cdc.gov/ticks/.

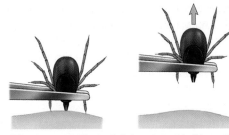

FIG. 26.2 The progression of tick removal. (From Centers for Disease Control and Prevention: Tick Removal. https://www.cdc.gov/ticks/removing_a_tick.html)

tick-borne infection. RMSF responds readily to treatment with tetracycline. A definitive diagnosis can be made with paired serum titers. Because early treatment is important in decreasing morbidity and mortality, treatment should be started in response to clinical and epidemiological considerations rather than waiting for laboratory confirmation (Heymann, 2014).

CHECK YOUR PRACTICE

A client was bitten by a tick while working in his tree-covered lawn comes to see you who. He knew it was important to remove the tick in the correct manner. You know exactly how to correctly remove the tick. You remove the tick while simultaneously teaching the client how to do this if he ever gets another tick bite. The steps that you follow are:

1. Use fine-tipped tweezers to grasp the tick as close to the skin's surface as possible.
2. Pull upward with steady, even pressure. Do not twist or jerk the tick because this could cause the mouthparts to break off and remain in the skin. Should you break the mouthparts, remove them with tweezers. If you cannot remove them, leave them alone, and let the area heal.
3. After removing the tick, thoroughly clean the bite area and your hands with rubbing alcohol, an iodine scrub, or soap and water.
4. Dispose of the live tick by putting it in alcohol, placing in a sealed bag/container, wrapping it tightly with tape, or flushing it down the toilet.
5. Never crush a tick with your fingers.
6. If you develop a rash or fever within several weeks after removing the tick, see a health care professional. (CDC, 2015j)

ROCKY MOUNTAIN SPOTTED FEVER

Contrary to its name, Rocky Mountain spotted fever (RMSF) is seldom seen in the Rocky Mountains and most commonly occurs in the southeast, Oklahoma, Kansas, and Missouri. The infectious agent is *R. rickettsii*. The tick vector varies according to geographic region. The dog tick (Fig. 26.2), *Dermacentor variabilis,* is the vector in the eastern and southern United States. RMSF is not transmitted from person to person. It is thought that one attack confers lifelong immunity.

Clinical signs include a sudden onset of moderate to high fever, severe headache, chills, deep muscle pain, and malaise. About 50% of cases experience a rash on the extremities that spreads to most of the body. Many cases of what has been referred to as "spotless" RMSF may actually be caused by recently identified forms of human ehrlichiosis, another

ZIKA VIRUS

Zika virus infection is the most recent of four unexpected arthropod-borne viral infections in the Western Hemisphere in the past 20 years. First there was dengue, then West Nile Virus and chikungunya, and now Zika. This latest virus first emerged in Uganda in 1947. It is transmitted by Aedes mosquitoes (Fauci and Morens, 2016). The virus emerged in the Bahia region of Brazil and moved to several other countries fairly rapidly. It came to the United States via persons who traveled to or moved from areas with active Zika virus transmission. Most Zika virus infections are asymptomatic or cause only mild clinical symptoms. Persons with clinical symptoms may have fever, rash, muscle aches, eye pain, prostration, and maculopapular rash. Symptoms typically last for several days to 1 week. There have been documented cases of Guillain-Barre syndrome. The most serious effect is for pregnant women, whose babies may be born with microcephaly (Fauci and Morens, 2016; Dasgupta et al, 2016).

Currently there is no vaccine to prevent the Zika virus and no specific antiviral treatment. The only way to prevent the virus is by avoiding areas where there is transmission of the virus or carefully following steps to not be bitten by mosquitos. Prevention from being bitten by mosquitos includes the following: using air conditioning or having window and door screens, wearing long sleeves and pants, using permethrin-treated clothing and gear, and using insect repellents (Staples et al 2016). It is also important to empty or cover any container that can hold water, such as tires, buckets, flower pots, and bird baths, and repair leaks or taps on septic tanks. Mosquito repellents should be reapplied every 2 or so hours, and it is best to use one that the CDC recommends, such as DEET, picaridin, oil of lemon, eucalyptus, or IR3535. Some excellent resources for learning about repellants include the CDC Yellow Book (Chapter 2 on traveler's health), as well as the sites that deal with insect repellants.

In 2016, Zika virus infection became a nationally notifiable disease (Walker et al, 2016). Nurses and other health care providers need to educate clients, especially pregnant women and people who live in areas where the Zika virus has been identified, about ways to avoid the virus.

ZOONOSES

A zoonosis is an infection transmitted from a vertebrate animal to a human under natural conditions. Zoonotic diseases can by caused by viruses, bacteria, parasites, and fungi. They are common diseases. The agents that cause zoonoses do not need humans to maintain their life cycles; infected humans have simply somehow managed to get in their way. Means of transmission include animal bites (bats and rabies), inhalation (rodent excrement and hantavirus), ingestion (milk and listeriosis), direct contact (rabbit carcasses and tularemia), and arthropod intermediates. This last transmission route means that some vector-borne diseases also may be zoonoses. For example, white-tailed deer harbor ticks that can carry Lyme disease, and rats and ground squirrels may be infected with fleas that can transmit plague. Other than vector-borne diseases, some of the more common zoonoses in the United States include toxoplasmosis (*Toxoplasma gondii*), cat-scratch disease (*Bartonella henselae*), brucellosis (*Brucella* species), listeriosis (*Listeria monocytogenes*), salmonellosis (*Salmonella* serotypes), and rabies (family Rhabdoviridae, genus *Lyssavirus*). Many of the more recent emerging infections such as avian influenza A H5N1, WNV, monkeypox, hantavirus pulmonary syndrome, and variant Creutzfeldt-Jakob disease are zoonoses. Children under 5 years should not own reptiles, such as turtles, or amphibians, such as frogs. Pregnant women should avoid contact with pet rodents. They should avoid adopting or handling stray cats to avoid getting toxoplasmosis. Immune-compromised persons and persons with HIV infection or AIDS should be careful when choosing pets and should talk with a veterinarian or health care provider before making a decision (CDC, 2014a).

Rabies (Hydrophobia)

Rabies, one of the most feared of human diseases, has the highest case fatality rate of any known human infection—essentially 100%. To date, fewer than 10 cases of human survival from clinical rabies have been reported, and only two have not had a history of preexposure or postexposure prophylaxis. Most dogs are vaccinated for rabies, and thus, the major carriers are raccoons, skunks, foxes, coyotes, and bats (CDC, 2012). When the virus spreads from wild to domestic animals, cats may be involved.

Rabies is transmitted to humans by introducing virus-carrying saliva into the body, usually via an animal bite or scratch. Transmission may also occur if infected saliva comes into contact with a fresh cut or intact mucous membranes. Rabies is found in neural tissue and is not transmitted via blood, urine, or feces. Airborne transmission has been documented in caves with infected bat colonies. Transmission from human to human is theoretically possible but has been documented only in the case of organ transplants harvested from individuals who died of undiagnosed rabies. Guidelines for organ donation exist to

minimize this possibility (Heymann, 2014). The best protection against rabies remains vaccinating domestic animals—dogs, cats, cattle, and horses. If a person is bitten, clean the bite wound thoroughly with soap and water and immediately consult a physician. Suspicion of rabies should exist if the bite is from a wild animal or an unprovoked attack from a domestic animal. Even when there is no suspicion of rabies, a physician should be contacted because tetanus or antibiotic prophylaxis may be indicated.

No successful treatment exists for rabies once symptoms appear, but if given promptly and as directed, postexposure prophylaxis with human rabies immunoglobulin and rabies vaccine can prevent development of the disease. Three products are licensed for use as rabies vaccine in the United States: human diploid cell vaccine (HDCV), rabies vaccine adsorbed (RVA), and purified chick embryo cell culture vaccine (PCECV). Only HDCV and PCECV are available for use in the United States (CDC, 2008). In 2010 the previously recommended series of five 1-mL doses injected into the deltoid muscle was changed to four (CDC, 2010). Reactions to the vaccine are fewer and less serious than with previously used vaccines. Individuals who deal frequently with animals, such as zookeepers, laboratory workers, and veterinarians, may choose to receive the vaccine as preexposure prophylaxis. The decision to administer the vaccine to a bite victim depends on the circumstances of the bite and is made on an individual basis.

Recommendations for providing postexposure prophylaxis treatment are provided by the Advisory Committee for Recommendations on Immunization Practices and are available through local public health officials or the CDC. In general, cats and dogs that have bitten someone and have verified rabies vaccinations are confined for 10 days for observation. Treatment is initiated only if signs of rabies are observed during this period. If the animal is known or suspected to be rabid, treatment begins immediately. If the animal is unknown to the victim and escapes, public health officials should be consulted for help in deciding whether treatment is indicated. With wild animal bites, treatment is begun immediately. With bites from livestock, rodents, and rabbits, treatment is considered on an individual basis. Postexposure prophylaxis consists of a dose of human rabies immune globulin and rabies vaccine given on the day of exposure a dose is then given again on days 3, 7, and 14 (CDC, 2016f). A health care professional and the local health department can guide clients through the process of rabies postexposure vaccinations. See also http://www.cdc.gov/rabies.

PARASITIC DISEASES

Parasitical diseases are more prevalent in developing countries than in the United States because of tropical climates and inadequate prevention and control measures. A lack of cheap and effective drugs, poor sanitation, and a scarcity of funding lead to high reinfection rates even when control programs are attempted. Parasites are classified into four groups (Table 26.4): nematodes (roundworms), cestodes (tapeworms), trematodes (flukes), and protozoa (single-celled

TABLE 26.4 Examples of Diseases Resulting from Endoparasitic Infection by Category

Category	Parasite	Disease
Cestodes	*Taenia saginata, Taenia solium*	Beef tapeworm, pork tapeworm
Nematodes	*Ancylostoma, Necator*	Ancylostomiasis, necatoriasis (hookworm)
Intestinal	*Ascaris, Toxocara*	Ascariasis, toxocariasis (roundworm)
	Enterobius vermicularis	Enterobiasis (pinworm)
	Trichuris trichiura	Trichuriasis (whipworm)
Blood/Tissue	*Dracunculiasis medinensis*	Guinea worm
	Onchocerca volvulus	Onchocerciasis (river blindness)
	Wuchereria bancrofti	Lymphatic filariasis (elephantiasis)
Trematodes	*Schistosoma* sp.	Schistosomiasis (snail fever)
Protozoans	*Entamoeba histolytica*	Amebiasis
	Giardia lamblia	Giardiasis
	Leishmania spp.	Leishmaniasis
	Plasmodium spp.	Malaria
	Toxoplasma gondii	Toxoplasmosis
	Trichomonas vaginalis	Trichomoniasis
	Trypanosoma spp.	African sleeping sickness, Chagas' disease

Based on information from Heymann DL, editor: *Control of communicable diseases manual*, ed 20, Washington, DC, 2014, American Public Health Association.

animals). Nematodes, cestodes, and trematodes are all referred to as *helminths*. Nurses and other health professionals should be aware of the growing numbers of reported parasitic infections in the United States.

INTESTINAL PARASITIC INFECTIONS

Enterobiasis (pinworm) is the most common helminthic infection in the United States. Pinworm infection is seen most often among children and is most prevalent in crowded and institutional settings. Pinworms resemble small pieces of white thread and can be seen with the naked eye. Diagnosis is usually accomplished by pressing cellophane tape to the perianal region early in the morning. Treatment with oral vermicides results in a cure rate of 90% to 100%. The opportunities for widespread indigenous transmission of these intestinal parasites are reduced because of improved sanitary conditions in this country. Effective drug treatment is available for these intestinal parasitic infections.

Cryptosporidiosis is caused by a microscopic parasite that causes this diarrheal disease. Both the parasite and the disease are called crypto. Although the disease is spread in many ways, the most common is via water both drinking and recreational water. The groups most at risk are children in daycare, childcare workers, parents of infected children, international travelers, people who drink unfiltered, untreated water. The symptoms include watery diarrhea, stomach cramps or pain, dehydration, nausea,

vomiting, fever, and weight loss. The symptoms can last 1 to 2 weeks. Nitazoxanide has been approved by the FDA for the treatment of persons with a healthy immune system (CDC, 2015k).

PARASITIC OPPORTUNISTIC INFECTIONS

Opportunistic infections (OIs) are those more frequent or more severe in individuals immunocompromised by HIV infection. Before the introduction of routine prophylactic treatment and potent-combination, highly active antiretroviral therapies (ARTs), OIs were the leading cause of illness and death in this group. Some of the protozoan parasitic OIs seen in clients with HIV disease and others who are immunocompromised include *Pneumocystis jiroveci* pneumonia (PCP), cryptosporidiosis, microsporidiosis, and isosporiasis, all producing diarrheal disease and transmitted by fecal–oral contact, as well as toxoplasmosis. With the advent of ARTs, the incidence of OIs in American clients with HIV disease has dropped dramatically. Isosporiasis was always rare, but the rates for cryptosporidiosis and microsporidiosis also have declined markedly. Although no longer seen with the frequency of the past, toxoplasmosis and PCP have not disappeared. They are more likely to appear in individuals unaware of their HIV disease or without good access to health care. Guidelines for prevention and treatment of OIs are regularly updated by the Panel on Opportunistic Infections in HIV-Infected Adults and Adolescents representing opinion from the CDC, the National Institutes of Health, and the HIV Medicine Association of the Infectious Diseases Society of America. See http://aidsinfor.nih.gov.

Toxoplasma gondii is a coccidial organism harbored by cats infected by ingesting other infected animals. Although rodents, ruminants, swine, poultry, and other birds may have infective organisms in their muscle tissue, only cats carry this parasite in their intestinal tract, allowing the excretion of infected eggs. People contract the disease through contact with infected cat feces or eating improperly cooked meat. In most healthy people, toxoplasmosis produces a mild to inapparent infection, but in immunodeficient individuals, the disease may, in addition to rash and skeletal muscle involvement, result in cerebritis, pneumonia, chorioretinitis, myocarditis, or death. CNS infection is common with HIV disease. Because toxoplasmosis is not a nationally reportable disease, it is not possible to get accurate numbers of cases. However, toxoplasmosis is the leading cause of deaths resulting from foodborne illnesses in the United States. Correct diagnosis by nurses and other health care workers leads to appropriate treatment and client education for preventing and controlling parasitic infections. The diagnosis of parasitic diseases is based on history of travel, characteristic clinical signs and symptoms, and the use of appropriate laboratory tests to confirm the clinical diagnosis. It is important to know what specimens to collect, how and when to collect them, and what laboratory techniques to use to establish a correct diagnosis. Effective drug treatment is available for most parasitic diseases. The high cost of the drugs, drug resistance, and toxicity are some of the common therapeutic problems. Measures for prevention and control of parasitic diseases include early diagnosis and treatment, improved personal hygiene, safer sex practices, community health education, vector control, and improvements in sanitary control of food, water, and waste disposal.

DISEASES OF TRAVELERS

Individuals traveling outside the United States should take precautions against diseases to which they may be exposed. The specific diseases and precautions depend on the individual's health status, the travel destination, the reason for travel, and the length of travel. Persons who plan to travel in remote regions for an extended period may need to consider rare diseases and take special precautions that would not apply to the average traveler. The health department and travel clinics in other settings can provide specific health information and recommendations for the area in question.

On returning from visits to exotic places, travelers may bring back an unplanned souvenir in the form of disease. Therefore a history of travel should always be closely considered. Even the apparently healthy returned traveler, especially one who was in a tropical country for some time, should undergo routine screening to rule out acquired infections. Likewise, refugees and immigrants may arrive with infectious disease problems ranging from helminthic infections to diseases of major public health significance, such as tuberculosis, malaria, cholera, HIV disease, and hepatitis. Nurses may find themselves dealing with these diseases because refugees and immigrants, especially the undocumented, are often treated through the public health system. The CDC offers current information for both medical professionals and travelers at its Travelers' Health webpage, including the Yellow Book, *CDC Health Information for International Travel.* Go to http://www.cdc.gov and type in "travelers' health" to access the Yellow Book and many other useful resources.

MALARIA

Caused by the blood-borne parasite *Plasmodium* that infects the *Anopheles* mosquito, malaria is a potentially fatal disease characterized by regular cycles of high fever, flulike illness, and shaking chills. Transmission is through the bite of an infected mosquito into a person. The word *malaria* is based on an association between the illness and the "bad air" of the marshes in which the mosquitoes breed. Malaria is an old disease that first appears in recorded history in 1700 BCE in China. Malaria was considered eliminated from the United States in the 1950s with approximately 1500 to 2000 cases annually in the United States and largely affecting travelers and immigrants. In 2015 there were an estimated 214 million cases worldwide with about 438,000 deaths; children in Africa were the most affected. No vaccine is available to protect against this disease, and there is some resistance to both the drugs used to treat malaria and the insecticides that are used in malaria control (CDC, 2016g).

Malaria prevention depends on protection against mosquitoes and appropriate chemoprophylaxis. Drug resistance is an increasing problem in combating malaria. Of the four causes of human malaria, *Plasmodium ovale* and *Plasmodium vivax*

result in disease that can progress to relapsing malaria, and *P. vivax* is increasingly drug resistant. *Plasmodium falciparum* causes the most serious malarial infection and is highly drug resistant. Thus decisions about antimalarial drugs must be tailored individually on the basis of the type of malaria in the specific area of the country to be visited, the purpose of the trip, and the length of the visit. The CDC and the WHO publish guides on the status of malaria and recommendations for prophylaxis on a country-by-country basis. At this time, no one drug or drug combination is known to be safe and efficacious in preventing all types of malaria. Antimalarials are generally started a week to several weeks before leaving the United States and are continued for 4 to 6 weeks after returning. Despite appropriate prophylaxis, malaria may still be contracted. Travelers should seek immediate medical care if they exhibit symptoms of cyclical fever and chills up to 1 year after returning home. Immigrants and visitors from areas in which malaria is endemic may become clinically ill after entering this country. Visit the CDC malaria homepage at http://www.cdc.gov/malaria for more useful information about malaria.

FOODBORNE AND WATERBORNE DISEASES

Considerable foodborne disease abroad and at home can be avoided if a person eats thoroughly cooked foods prepared with reasonable hygiene. Eating foods from street vendors may not be a good idea. Trichinosis, tapeworms, and fluke infections, as well as bacterial infections, result from eating raw or undercooked meats. Raw vegetables may be a source of bacterial, viral, helminthic, or protozoal infection if they have been grown with or washed in contaminated water. Fruits that can be peeled immediately before eating, such as bananas, are less likely to be a source of infection. Dairy products should be pasteurized and appropriately refrigerated.

Water in many areas of the world is not potable (safe to drink), and drinking this water can lead to infection with a variety of protozoal, viral, and bacterial agents, including *Entamoeba, Giardia, Cryptosporidium,* and various coliform bacteria, and also can lead to hepatitis and cholera. Unless traveling in an area in which the piped water is known to be safe, only boiled water (boiled for 1 minute), bottled water, or water purified with iodine or chlorine compounds should be consumed. Ice should be avoided because freezing does not inactivate these agents. If the water is questionable, choose coffee or tea made with boiled water, carbonated beverages without ice, beer, wine, or canned fruit juices.

DIARRHEAL DISEASES

Travelers often suffer from diarrhea, and names such as *Montezuma's revenge, turista,* and *Colorado quickstep* are used to describe these bouts of intestinal upset. Some of these diarrheas do not have infectious causes and result from stress, fatigue, schedule changes, and eating unfamiliar foods. Acute infectious diarrheas are usually of viral or bacterial origin. *E. coli* probably causes more cases of traveler's diarrhea than all other infective agents combined. Protozoan-induced diarrheas, such as those resulting from *Entamoeba* and *Giardia,* are less likely to be acute, and they more commonly present once the traveler returns home. Travelers need to pay special attention to what they eat and drink. Often the culprit is food that is washed in unclean water. Read more about traveler's health at the CDC website: http://www.cdc.gov/travel.

HEALTH CARE–ACQUIRED INFECTIONS

Previously referred to as nosocomial infections, health care–acquired infections (HAIs) are infections acquired during hospitalization or developed within a hospital setting. They may involve clients, health care workers, visitors, or anyone who has contact with a hospital. Invasive diagnostic and surgical procedures, broad-spectrum antibiotics, and immunosuppressive drugs, along with the original underlying illness, leave hospitalized clients particularly vulnerable to exposure to virulent infectious agents from other clients and indigenous hospital flora from health care staff. In this setting, the simple act of performing hand hygiene before approaching every client becomes critical. Although progress has been made in preventing some infection types, work needs to be done. About 1 in 25 hospital patients has at least one HAI on any given day (CDC, 2016h). The CDC maintains the National Healthcare Safety Network, a voluntary, Internet-based surveillance system managed by the Division of Healthcare Quality Promotion at the CDC, to provide national data on the epidemiology of HAIs in the United States. See http://ww.cdc.gov/hai for more information about how to prevent HAIs and antibiotic resistance.

Infection control practitioners play a key role in hospital infection surveillance and control programs. Without a qualified and well-trained person in this position, the infection control program is ineffective. The majority of infection control practitioners are nurses. Their common job titles are *infection control nurse, infection control coordinator,* and *nurse epidemiologist.*

▶ APPLYING CONTENT TO PRACTICE

Public health involves the prevention of disease, promotion of health, and protection against hazards that threaten the health of the community, as reflected in the public health logo and summed up in the mission "assuring conditions in which people can be healthy." The three core functions of public health in achieving this mission as defined in 1988 by the Institute of Medicine in Recommendations for the Future of Public Health are *Assessment, Policy Development,* and *Assurance.* These three have been further divided into the "Ten Essential Services of Public Health" as a means of evaluating the effectiveness of public health efforts.

This chapter presents communicable diseases that commonly challenge the health of a community as well as prevention and control roles for public health nurses. Examples of some of the "Essential Services" under which these roles fall are presented by core function.

Assessment: (1) Monitor health/identify problems, and (2) diagnose and investigate health problems. Examples include surveillance, investigation, and identification of reportable communicable disease cases. **Policy Development:** (3) Inform, educate, and empower, and (4) mobilize community partnerships. Examples include evaluating immunization status, explaining the reason for immunizations and how to comply with the immunization schedule, organizing community partners to provide immunizations and documentation through a registry, and mounting a community campaign to inform the community of the importance of age-appropriate immunization. **Assurance:** (5) Enforce laws and regulations, and (6) link to services and provide care. Examples include assuring compliance with communicable disease control laws through treatment or prophylaxis for exposure to reportable diseases, excluding diseased students from daycare or school, and linking individuals without insurance to follow-up care for communicable disease treatment or exposure.

■ PRACTICE APPLICATION

The rising numbers of foreign-born residents in communities that did not previously have large immigrant populations provide a challenge to those involved with communicable disease control, especially in outbreak situations. Language barriers, specific cultural practices, travel to and from their home country, and undocumented status all contribute to opportunities for infection and present obstacles to prevention and control. It is common for diseases such as TB, brucellosis, measles, hepatitis B, Zika virus, and parasitic infections to originate in other countries and be diagnosed only after arrival of the person in the United States. People coming from countries without, with newly established, or with poorly enforced vaccination programs may be unimmunized. These people are particularly susceptible to infection in outbreak situations. For example, many people coming from Latin America have not been immunized against rubella. Differences in cultural practices can lead to outbreaks of foodborne illness. Listeriosis outbreaks have been traced to the use of unpasteurized milk in cottage industry cheese production.

In the face of a single infectious disease report or an outbreak situation, when working with communities whose members speak little English, it is vital (1) to have a means of communication, (2) to be able to provide a culturally appropriate message, and (3) to have an established level of trust. Ideally, these requirements are addressed before an outbreak occurs, allowing a prompt and efficient response when immediate action is needed.

A. What would be a useful first step in building trust with a largely non–English-speaking immigrant community?
  1. Hold a health fair in the community.
  2. Provide incentives to use health department services.
  3. Identify trusted community leaders, such as religious leaders, and ask for their help in developing a plan.
  4. Distribute a brochure in the target community's language.
B. What might best encourage undocumented residents to respond to a request to be immunized during an outbreak situation?
  5. Use an already established public health program to provide interpreter services, making it clear that proof of immigration status is not required for services.
  6. Place a request in the newspaper in the language of the targeted individuals.

7. Involve trusted community leaders in making the request.
8. Explain the severity of the consequences of lack of immunization.

C. What means of communication would work best when targeting largely non–English-speaking communities of recent immigrants?

9. Publish newspaper articles in the target language.
10. Request radio announcements in the target language.
11. Post fliers in the target language in the community.
12. Enlist trusted community leaders to make announcements.

D. How would public health officials best go about developing information to effectively reach a largely non–English-speaking community of recent immigrants?

13. Use the services of the local university communications department.
14. Ask community leaders to work with translators and prevention specialists to develop messages using their own words.
15. Hire a professional to translate an existing well-developed English-language brochure.
16. Use brochures provided by the state health department.

Answers can be found on the Evolve website.

▮ REMEMBER THIS!

- The burden of infectious diseases is high in both human and economic terms. Preventing these diseases must be given high priority in our present health care system.
- The successful interaction of the infectious agent, host, and environment is necessary for disease transmission. Knowledge of the characteristics of each of these three factors is important in understanding the transmission, prevention, and control of these diseases.
- Effective intervention measures at the individual and community levels must be aimed at breaking the chain linking the agent, host, and environment. An integrated approach focused on all three factors simultaneously is an ideal goal to strive for but may not be feasible for all diseases.
- Health care professionals must constantly be aware of vulnerability to threats posed by emerging infectious diseases. Most of the factors causing the emergence of these diseases are influenced by human activities and behavior.
- Communicable diseases are preventable. Preventing infection through primary prevention activities is the most cost-effective public health strategy.
- Health care professionals must always apply infection control principles and procedures in the work environment. They should strictly practice the universal blood and body fluid precautions strategy to prevent transmission of HIV and other blood-borne pathogens.

- Effective control of communicable diseases requires the use of a multisystem approach focusing on improving host resistance, improving the safety of the environment, improving public health systems, and facilitating social and political changes to ensure health for all people.
- Communicable disease prevention and control programs must move beyond providing drug treatment and vaccines. Health promotion and education aimed at changing individual and community behavior must be emphasized.
- Nurses play a key role in all aspects of prevention and control of communicable diseases. Close cooperation with other members of the interdisciplinary health care team must be maintained. Mobilizing community participation is essential to successful implementation of programs.
- The successful global eradication of smallpox proved the feasibility of the eradication of communicable diseases. As professionals and concerned citizens of the global village, health care workers must support the current global eradication campaigns against poliomyelitis and dracunculiasis. The latter disease is also known as guinea worm disease and is caused by drinking unfiltered water containing small crustaceans infected with larvae of *D. medinesis*. See this CDC website for more information: http://www.dpd.cdc.gov/dpdx/HTML/.
- New diseases occur and old diseases reoccur. This was seen most recently in the emergence of the Zika virus, which first emerged in Uganda in 1947, then reemerged in 2016 in Brazil.

ⓔ EVOLVE WEBSITE

http://evolve.elsevier.com/Stanhope/foundations
- Case Study, with Questions and Answers
- NCLEX® Review Questions
- Practice Application Answers

REFERENCES

Centers for Disease Control and Prevention: *An ounce of prevention keeps the germs away: seven keys to a safer healthier home*, Atlanta, n.d., CDC. Retrieved June 2016 from http://www.cdc.gov/ounceofprevention/.

Centers for Disease Control and Prevention: *Addressing emerging infectious disease threats: a prevention strategy for the U.S.*, Atlanta, GA, 1994, CDC.

Centers for Disease Control and Prevention: *Anthrax: what you need to know*, Atlanta, GA, 2006, CDC. Retrieved August 2012 from http://www.bt.cdc.gov/agent/anthrax/needtoknow.asp.

Centers for Disease Control and Prevention: Human rabies prevention: United States, 2008, *MMWR Morb Mortal Wkly Rep* 57(RR03):1–26, 28, 2008.

Centers for Disease Control and Prevention: *2009 H1N1 flu: situation update*, Atlanta, GA, 2009, CDC. Retrieved April 11, 5, 2013 from http://www.cdc.gov/h1n1flu/update.htm.

Centers for Disease Control and Prevention: Use of a reduced (4-dose) vaccine schedule for postexposure prophylaxis to prevent human rabies: recommendations of the Advisory Committee on Immunization Practices, *MMWR Morb Mortal Wkly Rep Recomm Rep* 59:1–9, 2010.

Centers for Disease Control and Prevention: Ten great public health achievements: worldwide, 2001-2010, *MMWR Morb Mortal Wkly Rep* 60:814–818, 2011.

Centers for Disease Control and Prevention: *What are the signs and symptoms of rabies?* Atlanta, GA, 2012, CDC. Retrieved August 2012 from http://www.cdc.gov/rabies/symptoms.index.html.

Centers for Disease Control and Prevention: *Healthy pets and people*, 2014a. http://www.cdc.gov/zoonotic/gi/index.html.

Centers for Disease Control and Prevention: *Reports of selected E. coli outbreak investigations*, Atlanta, GA, 2014b, CDC. Retrieved July 2, 2016 from http://www.cdc.gov/ecoli.

Centers for Disease Control and Prevention: *Trends in tuberculosis, 2014, fact sheet*, 2015a. Retrieved July 2, 2016 from http://www.cdc.gov.tb.

Centers for Disease Control and Prevention: *Ebola virus disease*, Atlanta, GA, 2015b, CDC. Retrieved July 20016 from http://www.cdc.gov/vhf/ebola/.

Centers for Disease Control and Prevention: *Ebola transmission*, Atlanta, GA, 2015c, CDC. Retrieved July 2016 from http://www.ebola/transmission/index.html.

Centers for Disease Control and Prevention: *West Nile Virus: Preliminary maps and data for 2015*, Atlanta, GA, 2015d, CDC. Retrieved July 2016 from http://www.cdc.gov.westnile/index.html.

Centers for Disease Control and Prevention: *Anthrax: Basic information*, Atlanta, GA, 2015e, CDC. Retrieved July 2016 from http://www.cdc.gov/anthrax/bioterrorism/index.html.

Centers for Disease Control and Prevention: *Anthrax: who is at risk*, Atlanta, GA, 2015f, CDC. Retrieved July 2016 from http://www.cdc.gov/anthrax/bioterrorism/index.html.

Centers for Disease Control and Prevention: *Pertussis: Fast facts*, Atlanta, GA, 2015g, CDC. Retrieved July 2016 from http://www.cdc.gov/pertussis.

Centers for Disease Control and Prevention: *Giardia: General information*, Atlanta, GA, 2015h, CDC. Retrieved July 2016 from http://www.cdc.gov/parasites/giardia.

Centers for Disease Control and Prevention: *Signs and symptoms of Lyme Disease*, Atlanta, GA, 2015i, CDC. Retrieved July 2016 from http://www.cdc.gov/lyme/index.html.

Centers for Disease Control and Prevention: *Tick removal and testing*, Atlanta, GA, 2015j, CDC. Retrieved July 2016 from http//www.cdc.gov/lyme/removal/index.html.

Centers for Disease Control and Prevention: *Cryptosporidiosis: General information for the public*, Atlanta, GA, 2015k, CDC. Retrieved July 2016 from http://www.cdc.gov/parasites/crypto.

Centers for Disease Control and Prevention: *Recommended immunization schedule for persons aged 0 through 18 years-United States, 2016*, Atlanta, GA, 2016a, CDC. Retrieved July 2016 from http://www.cdc.gov/vaccines/schedules/downloads/child/0-18yrs-schedule.pdf.

Centers for Disease Control and Prevention: *Measles cases and outbreaks*, Atlanta, GA, 2016b, CDC. Retrieved July 2016 from http://www.cdc.gov/measles/cases-outbreaks.html.

Centers for Disease Control and Prevention: *Rubella in the U.S.*, Atlanta, GA, 2016c, CDC. Retrieved July 2016 from http://www.cdc.gov/rubella/about/index.html.

Centers for Disease Control and Prevention: *What you should know for the 2015-2016 influenza season*, Atlanta, GA, 2016d, CDC. Retrieved July 2016 from http://www.cdc.gov/flu/about/season/flu-season-2015-2016.htm.

Centers for Disease Control and Prevention: *Seven multistate outbreaks of human salmonella infections linked to live poultry in backyard flocks*, Atlanta, GA, 2016e, CDC. Retrieved July 2016 from http://www.cdc.gov/salmonella/live-poultry-05-16/index.html.

Centers for Disease Control and Prevention: *What care will I receive?* Atlanta, GA, 2016f, CDC. Retrieved July 2016 from http://www.cdc.gov/rabies.

Centers for Disease Control and Prevention: *Malaria facts*, Atlanta, GA, 2016g, CDC. Retrieved July 2016 from http://www.cdc.gov/malaria.

Centers for Disease Control and Prevention: *HAI data and statistics*, Atlanta, GA, 2016h, CDC. Retrieved July 2016 from http://www.cdc.gov/hai.

Dasgupta S, Reagan-Steiner S, Goodenough D, et al: Patterns in Zika virus testing and infection, by report of symptoms and pregnancy status-United States, January 3-March 5, 2016, *Morb Mort Wkly Rep* 65(15):395–399, April 22, 2016.

Fauci AS, Braunwald E, Kasper DK, et al: *Harrison's principles of international medicine*, ed 17, Columbus, OH, 2008, McGraw-Hill.

Fauci, AS, Morens DM: The perpetual challenge of infectious disease, *N Engl J Med* 366:454–461, 2012.

Fauci AS, Morens DM: Zika virus in the Americas-yet another arbovirus threat, *N Engl J Med* January 13, 2016. Published online at NEJM.org.

Fauci AS, Touchette NA, Folkers GK: Emerging infectious diseases: a 10-year perspective from the National Institute of Allergy and Infectious Diseases, *Emerg Infect Dis* 11:519–525, 2005.

Gordis L: *Epidemiology*, Philadelphia, 1996, Saunders.

Henderson DA: Smallpox: clinical and epidemiologic features, *Emerg Infect Dis* 5:537–539, 1999.

Heymann DL, editor: *Control of communicable diseases manual*, ed 19, Washington, DC, 2008, American Public Health Association.

Heymann DL, editor: *Control of communicable diseases manual*, ed 20, Washington, DC, 2014, American Public Health Association.

Huang JY, Henao OL, Griffin PM, et al: Centers for Disease Control and Prevention (CDC). Infection with pathogens transmitted commonly through food and the effect of increasing use of culture-independent diagnostic tests on surveillance-foodborne diseases active surveillance network, 10 U.S. Sites, 2012-2015, *MMWR Morb Mortal Wkly Rep* 15(65):368–371, April 2016.

LABioMed (Los Angeles Biomedical Research Institute at Harbor-UCLA Medical Center): *Changes in hospital orders increase pertussis immunization rates*, 2014, Science Daily. Retrieved May 2014 from http://www.sciencedaily.com/releases/2014/03/140305110923.

Scharff RL: Economic burden from health losses due to foodborne illness in the United States, *J Food Prot* 75(1):123–131, 2012.

Staples JE, Sziuban EJ, Fishcher M, et al: Interim guidelines for the evaluation and testing of infants with possible congenital Zika virus infection-United States, 2016, *MMWR MorB Mortal Wkly Rep* Early Release/Vol 65:1–5, January 26, 2016.

U.S. Department of Health and Human Services: *Healthy People 2020*, Washington, DC, 2010, U.S. Government Printing Office.

Walker WL, Lindsey NP, Lehman JA, et al: Zika Virus Disease Cases-50 States and the District of Columbia, January 1-July 31, 2016, *MMWR Morb Mortal Wkly Repo* 65:983–986, 2016.

Wenzel RP: Control of communicable diseases: overview. In Wallace RB, editor: *Public health and preventive medicine*, ed 14, Stamford CT, 1998, Appleton & Lange.

World Health Organization: *Five keys to safer food*, Geneva, n.d., WHO. Retrieved August 2012 from http://www.who.int/food-safety/publications/consumer/en/5keys_en.pdf.

World Health Organization: *Measles, Fact Sheet No. 286. WHO Media Center*, Geneva, Reviewed 2016, WHO. Retrieved July 2016 from http://www.who.int/mediacentre/factsheets/fs286/en/.

HIV Infection, Hepatitis, Tuberculosis, and Sexually Transmitted Diseases

Erika Metzler Sawin and Patty J. Hale

OBJECTIVES

After reading this chapter, the student should be able to:

1. Describe the natural history of human immunodeficiency virus (HIV) infection, and plan appropriate client education at each stage.
2. Discuss the clinical signs of HIV, hepatitis, and sexually transmitted diseases (STDs).
3. Describe the scope of the problem with HIV, STDs, hepatitis, and tuberculosis (TB), and identify groups that are at greatest risk.
4. Analyze behaviors that place people at risk for contracting selected communicable diseases.
5. Describe nursing actions to prevent these diseases and care for people who experience these diseases.

CHAPTER OUTLINE

Human Immunodeficiency Virus Infection
  Natural History of Human Immunodeficiency Virus Infection
  Transmission
  Epidemiology and Surveillance of Human Immunodeficiency Virus and Acquired Immunodeficiency Syndrome
  Human Immunodeficiency Virus Testing
  Caring for Clients with Acquired Immunodeficiency Syndrome in the Community
Sexually Transmitted Diseases
  Gonorrhea
  Syphilis
  Chlamydia

Herpes Simplex Virus 2 (Genital Herpes)
Human Papillomavirus Infection
Hepatitis
  Hepatitis A Virus
  Hepatitis B Virus
  Hepatitis C Virus
Tuberculosis
Nurse's Role in Providing Preventive Care for Communicable Diseases
  Primary Prevention
  Secondary Prevention
  Tertiary Prevention

KEY TERMS

acquired immunodeficiency syndrome (AIDS), 478
chlamydia, 485
directly observed therapy (DOT), 490
genital herpes, 486
genital warts, 486
gonorrhea, 482
hepatitis A virus (HAV), 487

hepatitis B virus (HBV), 487
hepatitis C virus (HCV), 489
HIV antibody test, 481
human immunodeficiency virus (HIV), 478
human papillomavirus (HPV), 486
incidence, 493
incubation period, 479
injection drug use, 481

nongonococcal urethritis (NGU), 485
partner notification, 494
pelvic inflammatory disease (PID), 482
sexually transmitted diseases (STDs), 478
syphilis, 485
tuberculosis (TB), 489

Knowledge about the risk for communicable diseases changes often as some diseases become resistant to methods of treatment, new diseases emerge, new treatments are developed, and some diseases increase in the number of people affected and others show a decline. Concern about infectious diseases prompted the development of standards for sexually transmitted diseases (STDs), human immunodeficiency virus (HIV) and acquired immunodeficiency syndrome (AIDS), hepatitis, and tuberculosis (TB) in the *Healthy People 2020* report. The *Healthy People 2020* box lists objectives related to HIV, hepatitis, and STDs. Because these diseases are often acquired through behaviors that can be avoided or changed, nursing actions focus particularly on disease prevention. Prevention can take the form of vaccine administration (as for hepatitis A and hepatitis B), early detection (for TB), or teaching clients about abstinence or safer sex. Individuals who live with these chronic infections can transmit them to others. This chapter describes selected communicable diseases and their nursing management, including primary, secondary, and tertiary prevention. STDs are also called sexually transmitted infections (STIs), because many times the infections are asymptomatic. In this chapter, the term *STDs* will be used.

HUMAN IMMUNODEFICIENCY VIRUS INFECTION

In a July 2012 article in the *New England Journal of Medicine,* authors Havlir and Beyrer (2012) question whether we are seeing the "beginning of the end of AIDS." This is a disease that has grown rapidly since the June 5, 1981 issue of the *Morbidity and Mortality Weekly Report* published by the Centers for Disease Control and Prevention (CDC) reported on five cases of *Pneumocystis carinii* pneumonia in healthy young men in Los Angeles, California. These cases became the first recognized reports of AIDS in the United States. Since then, HIV/AIDS has become one of the world's greatest public health challenges. HIV infection and AIDS have had a major political, social, and financial impact on society. The economic costs include the costs of the medication, the cost of lost wages, and the disruption that the disease causes to individuals and families. The lifetime costs of HIV care are enormous. The Ryan White HIV/AIDS Treatment Extension Act of 2009, previously the Ryan White Comprehensive AIDS Resource Emergency Act of 1990, provides services for persons with HIV infection (US Department of Health and Human Services [USDHHS], n.d.). This program provides funds for health care in the geographic areas with the largest number of AIDS cases. Health services that are covered include emergency services, services for early intervention and care (sometimes including coverage of health insurance), and drug reimbursement programs for HIV-infected individuals. The AIDS Drug Assistance Programs (ADAPs) are awards that pay for medications on the basis of the estimated number of persons living with AIDS in the individual state (USDHHS, Health Resources and Services Administration, 2014).

NATURAL HISTORY OF HUMAN IMMUNODEFICIENCY VIRUS INFECTION

The natural history of HIV includes the following three stages (Buttaro et al, 2013):
1. The primary infection (within about 1 month of contracting the virus)
2. Clinical latency, a period with no obvious symptoms
3. A final stage of symptomatic disease

When HIV enters the body, it can cause a mononucleosis-like syndrome referred to as a *primary infection* that can last for a few weeks. This may go unrecognized. Initially the body's CD4 white blood cell count drops for a brief time when the virus is most plentiful in the body. The immune system increases antibody production in response to this initial infection, which is a self-limiting illness. The symptoms are lymphadenopathy, myalgia, sore throat, lethargy, rash, and fever (CDC, 2016a). An antibody test at this stage is usually negative, so it is often not recognized as HIV.

After approximately 6 weeks to 3 months, HIV antibodies appear in the blood. Although most antibodies serve a protective role, HIV antibodies do not. Their presence does help in the detection of HIV infection because tests show their presence in the bloodstream.

During this prolonged incubation period, clients experience a gradual deterioration of the immune system and can transmit the virus to others. The use of highly active antiretroviral therapy (HAART) has greatly increased the survival time of persons with HIV/AIDS. The USDHHS Panel on Antiretroviral Guidelines for Adults and Adolescents updated recommendations for practitioners caring for persons with HIV infection in 2016. Topics covered in both the previous guidelines and the updated one include baseline evaluation, treatment goals, indications for beginning HAART, choosing initial therapy in HAART-naive patients, drugs or combinations to be avoided, managing adverse effects and drug interactions, managing treatment failure, and HAART-related considerations for specific populations, including HIV in older patients in the most recent guidelines (USDHHS, 2016b).

Acquired immunodeficiency syndrome (AIDS, a.k.a HIV Stage 3) is the last stage on the long continuum of HIV infection and may result from damage caused by HIV, secondary cancers, or opportunistic organisms. AIDS is defined as a disabling or life-threatening illness caused by HIV; it is diagnosed in a person with a CD4+ T-lymphocyte count of less than 200/mL with or without documented HIV infection (CDC, 2014a).

Many of the AIDS-related opportunistic infections are caused by microorganisms that are commonly present in healthy individuals but do not cause disease in persons with an intact immune system. These microorganisms increase in persons with HIV/AIDS as a result of a weakened immune system. Bacteria, fungi, viruses, or protozoa can cause opportunistic infections. The most common opportunistic diseases are *Pneumocystis jiroveci* (formerly *carinii*) pneumonia and oral candidiasis; other diseases are pulmonary TB, invasive cervical cancer, and recurrent pneumonia. TB can spread rapidly among immunosuppressed individuals. Thus HIV-infected individuals

Targeted Competency: Evidence-Based Practice (EBP)—Integrate best current evidence with clinical expertise and client/family preferences and values for delivery of optimal care.
- **Knowledge:** Explain the role of evidence in determining best clinical practice.
- **Skills:** Locate evidence reports related to clinical practice topics and guidelines.
- **Attitudes:** Value the concept of EBP as integral to determining best clinical practice.

Client-Centered Care Question:
Evidence supports the fact that some medications previously effective in treating sexually transmitted diseases (STDs) no longer are effective. If you learned that

a colleague was planning to use a treatment that is no longer considered effective to treat a specific STD, what would you do to ensure that the care the client receives is based on current evidence?

Answer:
With your colleague, collect current treatment guidelines information about that specific STD. The first place that you might look would be the Centers for Disease Control guidelines for that disease. The National Institutes of Health is also helpful. For example, you might look at HIV Treatment Guidelines for Adults and Adolescents Updated (2016) to find out what is the most effective antiretroviral therapy (ART) for the treatment of HIV infection. See https://aidsinfo.nih.gov/guidelines.

must be carefully screened for TB and deemed noninfectious before admission to such settings as long-term care facilities, correctional facilities, and drug treatment facilities.

TRANSMISSION

HIV is transmitted through exposure to blood, semen, transplanted organs, vaginal secretions, and breast milk (Heymann, 2015). It is not transmitted through casual contact such as touching or hugging someone who has HIV infection. Also, HIV is not transmitted by insects, coughing, sneezing, touching office equipment, or sitting next to or eating with someone who has HIV infection. The modes of transmission are listed in Box 27.1. Rare transmission methods include accidental needlestick injury, organ transplants, and blood transfusions (Heymann, 2015).

Potential blood and tissue donors are interviewed to screen for a history of high-risk activities, and they are screened with the HIV antibody test. Blood or tissue is not used from individuals who have a history of high-risk behavior or who are HIV infected. In addition to being screened, coagulation factors used to treat hemophilia and other blood disorders are made safe through heat treatments to inactivate the virus. Screening has significantly reduced the risk for transmission of HIV by blood products and organ donations. The presence of an STD infection such as chlamydia or gonorrhea increases the risk for HIV infection, and HIV may also increase the risk for other STDs. This may result from

any of the following: open lesions providing a portal of entry for pathogens; STDs decreasing the host's immune status, resulting in a rapid progression of HIV infection; and HIV changing the natural history of STDs or the effectiveness of medications used in treating STDs (Heymann, 2015).

Nurses can educate people about the modes of transmission and can be role models for how to behave toward and provide supportive care for those with HIV infection. An understanding of how transmission does and does not occur will help family and community members feel more comfortable in relating to and caring for persons with HIV.

EPIDEMIOLOGY AND SURVEILLANCE OF HUMAN IMMUNODEFICIENCY VIRUS AND ACQUIRED IMMUNODEFICIENCY SYNDROME

Nurses must identify the trends of HIV infection in the populations they serve so they can screen clients who may be at risk and adequately plan prevention programs and illness care resources. For example, knowing that AIDS disproportionately affects minorities assists the nurse to set priorities and plan services for these groups. Factors such as geographic location, age, and ethnic distribution are tracked to more effectively target programs. Worldwide, 36.7 million persons live with HIV infection (UNAIDS, 2016a), and 25.5 million live in sub-Saharan Africa (UNAIDS, 2016b). Seventeen million people with HIV are able to access antiretroviral therapy, and this number increased significantly since 2010, when only 7.5 million people were accessing therapy (UNAIDS, 2016a).

The CDC estimates that 1.2 million people in the United States are living with HIV infection, and about 1 in 8 of these people are unaware of their infection. Forty-four percent of people who are unaware of their infection are between 13 and 24 years of age. Although new HIV diagnosis in general has declined 19%, young black gay and bisexual men are the most affected, with an 87% increase in diagnosis, which is a slight (2%) decline since 2010 (CDC, 2016b). The largest number of new HIV infections in 2014 (29,418) was in men who had sex with other men (MSM), and this was followed by heterosexual transmission (10,527). See Fig. 27.1 for the number of new HIV infections by population group in 2014.

BOX 27.1   Modes of Transmission of Human Immunodeficiency Virus

Human immunodeficiency virus can be transmitted in the following ways:
- Sexual contact, involving the exchange of body fluids, with an infected person
- Sharing or reusing needles, syringes, or other equipment used to prepare injectable drugs
- Perinatal transmission from an infected mother to her fetus during pregnancy or delivery or to an infant when breastfeeding
- Transfusions or other exposure to HIV-contaminated blood or blood products, organs, or semen

From Heymann D: *Control of communicable diseases manual,* Washington, DC, 2015, American Public Health Association.

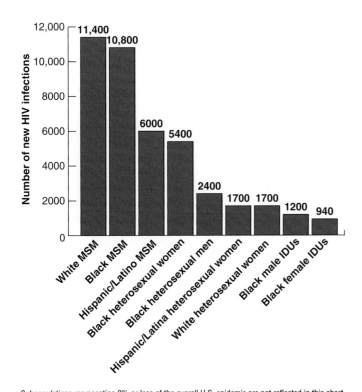

Subpopulations representing 2% or less of the overall U.S. epidemic are not reflected in this chart.

FIG. 27.1 Estimates of new HIV infections in the United States, 2009, for the most-affected subpopulations (Centers for Disease Control and Prevention: *HIV in the United States: at a glance,* Atlanta, GA, 2012c, CDC. Retrieved August 2012 from http://www.cdc.gov/nchhstp/newsroom/docs/Hiv-infections-2006-2009.pdf.)

Heterosexuals accounted for 24% of the estimated new HIV cases in 2014. HIV infections in women are primarily due to heterosexual contact or injection drug use. In 2014 women accounted for 20% of new HIV infections, and injection drug users (IDUs) represented 6% of new HIV cases. African Americans experience the most severe burden of HIV in that they represented 12% of the US population and an estimated 44% of new HIV cases in 2014, and Hispanic/Latinos represented 17% of the population in 2014 and 23% of new HIV cases (CDC, 2015a, 2016b). Although persons over 50 years of age continue to represent a relatively small proportion of new infections, those who have unprotected sex, consume alcohol, or inject drugs are at higher risk for contracting HIV/AIDS than younger people with the same lifestyle characteristics. Aging brings a decline in the immune response and decreased organ reserves, which slows the person's ability to deal with risk factors for HIV/AIDS (National Institute on Aging, 2015). Also, the geographic distribution of HIV infections is more concentrated in urban areas. The distribution of pediatric HIV infection has fallen dramatically because of prenatal care that includes HIV testing, antiretroviral therapy for the mother, and cesarean delivery.

HUMAN IMMUNODEFICIENCY VIRUS TESTING

The HIV antibody test is the most commonly used screening test for determining infection. This test does just as its name implies: it does not reveal whether an individual has

symptomatic AIDS, nor does it isolate the virus. It does indicate the presence of the antibody to HIV. The most commonly used form of this test is the enzyme-linked immunosorbent assay (EIA). The EIA effectively screens blood and other donor products. To minimize false-positive results, a confirmatory test, the Western blot, is used to verify the results. False-negative results may also occur after infection and before antibodies are produced. Sometimes referred to as the window period, this can last from 6 weeks to 3 months.

Rapid HIV antibody testing using oral fluid samples (e.g., OraQuick, Home Access HIV-1 Test System) is 99.5% accurate and provides results within 20 minutes, allowing immediate results to be given (US Preventive Services Task Force [USPSTF] 2013; CDC, 2016c). In addition to the rapid results, this test may appeal to persons who fear having their blood drawn. If the test is positive, it requires a second specific confirmatory test.

Routine voluntary HIV testing is recommended for all adults ages 15 to 65 (USPSTF, 2013). Voluntary screening programs for HIV may be either confidential or anonymous; the process for each is unique. Confidential testing involves reporting by identifying the person's name and other identifying information; this information is considered protected by confidentiality. With anonymous testing, the client is given an identification code number that is attached to all records of the test results and is not linked to the person's name and address (CDC, 2016c). Demographic data such as the person's sex, age, and race may be collected, but there is no record of the client's name and associated identifying information. An advantage of anonymous testing may be that it increases the number of people who are willing to be tested because many of those at risk are engaged in illegal activities. The anonymity eliminates their concern about the possibility of arrest or discrimination. However, anonymous testing does not allow for follow-up if the test is positive because the client's name and address are not available.

CARING FOR CLIENTS WITH ACQUIRED IMMUNODEFICIENCY SYNDROME IN THE COMMUNITY

Because AIDS is a chronic disease, affected individuals continue to live and work in the community. They have bouts of illness interspersed with periods of wellness in which they are able to return to school or work. When they are ill, much of their care is provided in the home. The nurse teaches families and significant others about personal care and hygiene, medication administration, Standard Precautions to ensure infection control, and healthy lifestyle behaviors such as adequate rest, balanced nutrition, and exercise. It is essential that clients adhere to their HAART regimen because administration must be consistent to be effective (Heymann, 2015).

The Americans with Disabilities Act of 1990 and other laws protect persons with HIV/AIDS against discrimination in housing, at work, and in other public situations (US Department of Justice, 2012). Policies regarding school and worksite attendance have been developed by most states and localities on the basis of these laws.

Nurses can rely on these policies to provide direction for the community's response when an individual develops HIV infection. Nursing actions include the following:

- Identifying resources such as social and financial support services
- Interpreting school and work policies
- Assisting employers by educating managers about how to deal with ill or infected workers to reduce the risk of breaching confidentiality or wrongful actions such as termination

HIV-infected children should attend school because the benefits of attendance far outweigh the risks for transmitting or acquiring infections. None of the cases of HIV infection in the United States have been transmitted in a school setting. An interdisciplinary team made up of the child's physician, public health personnel, the child's parent or guardian, and the nurse should make decisions about educational and care needs. Individual decisions about risk to the infected child or others should be based on the behavior, neurological development, and physical condition of the child. Attendance may be inadvisable if cases of childhood infections, such as chickenpox or measles, are in the school, because the immunosuppressed child is at greater risk for suffering complications. Alternative arrangements, such as homebound instruction, might be instituted if a child is unable to control body secretions or displays biting behavior.

A growing number of services are available for persons with HIV/AIDS. Voluntary and faith-based groups, such as community organizations or AIDS support organizations, are available in some localities to address their many needs. Services include counseling, support groups, legal aid, personal care services, housing programs, and community education programs. Nurses collaborate with workers from community organizations in the client's home and may advise these groups in their supportive work. The federal government and many organizations have established toll-free numbers and websites to provide information. Eliminating HIV/AIDS is complex and beyond the scope of one group or agency. Public health partnerships that bring together public and private persons and groups as well as greater access to mandatory HIV testing will be essential. Prevention messages should be culturally appropriate and should talk about the role alcohol and drug abuse play in HIV risk. An additional strategy focuses on improved monitoring of HIV infections to refine the targeting and delivery of efforts at prevention (CDC, 2011).

Considerable work has been done and progress is being made in finding effective methods to prevent and treat HIV. Preexposure prophylaxis, or PrEP, is a new HIV prevention method for people who do not have the infection but would like to reduce their risk for becoming infected. PrEP requires taking a pill to prevent the HIV virus from getting into the body. It has been shown to be effective for people at very high risk for HIV infection through sex; the results about its effectiveness with injection drug users are not yet available. This prevention method requires strict adherence to taking the medication and having regular HIV testing; it is also used in combination with other HIV prevention methods rather than in isolation (CDC, 2012a; US Public Health Service, 2014). In 2012 the US Food and Drug Administration (FDA) approved the use of Truvada, a drug produced by Gilead Sciences Inc. This drug is a combination of two antiretroviral medications used to treat HIV—tenofovir disoproxil fumarate and emtricitabine (US FDA, 2012). In addition to strictly adhering to the medication protocol, the person must first be tested to make sure he or she is HIV negative.

SEXUALLY TRANSMITTED DISEASES

STDs are a major public health challenge in the United States. The numbers of new cases of gonorrhea are declining, whereas others, such as herpes simplex and chlamydia, continue to increase. Chlamydia is the most commonly reported infectious disease, and gonorrhea is the second most common. The common STDs listed in Table 27.1 are grouped according to their having either a bacterial or viral cause. The bacterial infections include gonorrhea, syphilis, and chlamydia. Most of these infections are cured with antibiotics. The exceptions are the newly emerging antibiotic-resistant strains of gonorrhea. In contrast, STDs caused by viruses cannot be cured. These are chronic diseases leading to a lifetime of symptom management and infection control. The viral infections include herpes simplex virus and human papillomavirus (HPV), also referred to as *genital warts*. The hepatitis A and hepatitis B viruses, which may also be transmitted via sexual activity, are discussed in the section of this chapter on hepatitis.

GONORRHEA

Gonorrhea is the second most commonly reported infectious disease in the United States, and the CDC estimates that about 820,000 Americans are infected annually. Fewer than half of these cases are detected and reported to the CDC (CDC, 2015b). *Neisseria gonorrheae* is a gram-negative intracellular diplococcal bacterium that infects the mucous membranes of the genitourinary tract, rectum, and pharynx. Gonorrhea can be transmitted by having vaginal, anal, or oral sex with a person who has the disease. It can be transmitted via fluids even if a male does not ejaculate. It can also be spread from an untreated mother to the infant during childbirth. Gonorrhea is identified as either uncomplicated or complicated. Uncomplicated gonorrhea refers to limited cervical or urethral infection. Complicated gonorrhea includes salpingitis, epididymitis, systemic gonococcal infection, and gonococcal meningitis. The signs and symptoms of infection in males are purulent and copious urethral discharge and dysuria. An estimated 10% to 20% of males are asymptomatic. Symptoms in males are typically significant enough for the person to seek treatment. These symptoms include a burning sensation when urinating or a white, yellow, or green discharge from the penis. Some men may get swollen or painful testicles. In men, gonorrhea can cause epididymitis, a painful condition of the testicles that if untreated can lead to infertility. In contrast, symptoms in women are often asymptomatic and may be confused with a bladder or vaginal infection (CDC, 2015b). Treatment may not be sought, and this could allow the disease to continue to spread and possibly not be detected until pelvic inflammatory disease (PID) occurs. In women, infection with *N. gonorrheae* is a major cause of PID, ectopic pregnancy, and infertility. Untreated gonorrhea can increase a person's risk for acquiring or transmitting HIV (CDC, 2015c).

When gonococcal infection is asymptomatic and treatment is sought, it can continue to be spread to others through sexual

TABLE 27.1   Summary of Sexually Transmitted Diseases

Disease and Pathogen	Incubation	Signs and Symptoms	Diagnosis	Treatment	Nursing Implications
Bacterial					
Chlamydia: *Chlamydia trachomatis*	3–21 days	Male: None or nongonococcal urethritis (NGU); painful urination and urethral discharge; epididymitis Female: None or mucopurulent cervicitis (MPC), vaginal discharge; if untreated, progresses to symptoms of pelvic inflammatory disease (PID); diffuse abdominal pain, fever, chills	Tissue culture; Gram stain of endocervical or urethral discharge: presence of PMNs without gram-negative intracellular diplococci suggests NGU	One of the following treatments: Doxycycline 100 mg PO twice/day × 7 days; an inexpensive drug azithromycin 1 g PO × 1 in a single dose or use one of these alternatives: erythromycin, ofloxacin, or levofloxacin	Refer partners of past 60 days; counsel client to use condoms and to avoid sex until therapy is complete and symptoms are gone in both client and partners; medication teaching Annual screening recommended for all sexually active women under 25 years of age and women over 25 years if new or multiple sexual partners
Gonorrhea: *Neisseria gonorrheae*	3–21 days	Male: Urethritis, purulent discharge, painful urination, urinary frequency; epididymitis Female: None, or symptoms of PID	Culture and nucleic acid amplification test (NAAT) Culture of endocervical (women) or urethral (male)	Ceftriaxone 250 mg IM in a single dose PLUS azithromycin 1 g orally in a single dose	Refer partners of past 60 days; return for evaluation if symptoms persist; counsel client to use therapy until complete and symptoms are gone in both client and partners; medication teaching Counsel to be tested for HIV; screen all partners of the past 3 months; reexamine the client at 3 and 6 months
Syphilis: *Treponema pallidum*	10–90 days	Primary: Ulcer or chancre Usually single, painless chancre; if untreated, heals in a few weeks	Visualization of pathogen on darkfield microscopic examination; tests to determine *T. pallidum* directly from lesion exudate or tissue	Penicillin G 2.4 million units, IM in a single dose Penicillin G administered parenterally is the preferred drug for treating all stages of syphilis and is the only documented therapy for syphilis during pregnancy If penicillin allergy (for nonpregnant or HIV-infected individuals): doxycycline 100 mg PO twice/day × 14 days OR tetracycline 500 mg four times/day × 14 days, but data to support these alternatives is limited	
	6 wk–6 mo	Secondary: skin rash, mucocutaneous lesions, and lymphadenopathy	Clinical signs of secondary syphilis	Penicillin G, administered parenterally, is the preferred drug for treating persons in all stages of syphilis The preparation used (i.e., benzathine, aqueous procaine, or aqueous crystalline), dosage, and length of treatment depend on the stage and clinical manifestations of the disease	
	Within 1 yr of infection	Early latency: Asymptomatic; infectious lesions may recur	Persons can receive a diagnosis of early latent syphilis if, during the year preceding the diagnosis, they had (1) a documented seroconversion or a sustained (>2 week) fourfold or greater increase in nontreponemal test titers; (2) unequivocal symptoms of primary or secondary syphilis; or (3) a sex partner documented to have primary, secondary, or early latent syphilis	Early latent: Benzathine penicillin G 2.4 million units IM once	Primary goal is to prevent complications and to make sure that transmission from pregnant woman to fetus does not occur
	After 1 yr from date of infection	Late latency: Asymptomatic; noninfectious except to fetus of pregnant women	Lumbar puncture, CSF cell count, protein level determination, and VDRL	Penicillin G 7.2 million units total in three doses of 2.4 million units each at 1-week intervals In general, penicillins are prescribed in varying doses depending on diagnosis	

Continued

TABLE 27.1 Summary of Sexually Transmitted Diseases—cont'd

Disease and Pathogen	Incubation	Signs and Symptoms	Diagnosis	Treatment	Nursing Implications
	Late active: 2–40 yr 20–30 yr 10–30 yr	Gummas of skin, bone, mucous membranes, heart, liver Cardiovascular involvement: aortic aneurysm, aortic valve insufficiency Does NOT refer to neurosyphilis	CSF examination	Penicillin G 7.2 million units total in three doses of 2.4 million units each at 1-week intervals	HIV education and counseling; partner referral for evaluation; medication education; assessment and referral Men who have sex with men should be tested annually for HIV, chlamydia, syphilis, and gonorrhea
Viral Human immunodeficiency virus (HIV)	4–6 wk	*Possible:* Acute mononucleosis-like illness (lymphadenopathy, fever, rash, joint and muscle pain, sore throat)	Laboratory-based immunoassay, which if repeatedly reactive is followed by a supplemental test (e.g., an HIV-1/ HIV-2 antibody differentiation assay, Western blot, or indirect immunofluorescence assay) However, available HIV laboratory antigen/antibody immunoassays detect HIV infection earlier than these supplemental tests *HIV antibody test:* EIA or the Western blot test; OraSure (new test, SmithKline Beecham)—an oral HIV-1 antibody testing system—test results in about 3 days	Prophylactic administration of zidovudine (ZDV) immediately after exposure may prevent seroconversion Postexposure prophylaxis (PEP) should begin as soon as possible Choice of antiviral drug therapy is made based on toxicity and drug resistance Combinations of drugs are considered such as zidovudine (ZDV) and 3TC Drug selection is complicated and evolving Preexposure prophylaxis (PrEP) was approved in 2012, consisting of daily tenofovir disoproxil fumarate plus emtricitabine (TDF/FTC), for use among sexually active, at-risk adults	
	Seroconversion: 6 wk–3 mo	Appearance of HIV antibody	$CD4^+$ T-lymphocyte count of less than 200/mcl with documented HIV infection, or diagnosis with clinical manifestations of AIDS as defined by the CDC		
	HIV Stage 3/ AIDS: month to years	*Opportunistic diseases:* Most commonly *Pneumocystis jiroveci* pneumonia, oral candidiasis, Kaposi's sarcoma		Symptomatic infection: start ZDV 20 mg every 8 hours; alternatives to ZDV: didanosine (ddI), stavudine (d4t), zalcitabine (ddC), and a combination of ZDV and ddI; additional treatments are necessary for opportunistic infections	
Genital warts: human papillomavirus (HPV)	4–6 wk most common; up to 9 mo	Often subclinical infection; painless lesions near vaginal openings, anus, shaft of penis, vagina, cervix; lesions are textured, cauliflower appearance; may remain unchanged over time	Visual inspection for lesions; Pap smear; hybrid capture 2 HPV DNA test; colposcopy: HPV tests for women >30 years undergoing cervical cancer screening	No cure; one-third of lesions will disappear without topical treatment *Patient-applied:* topical podofilox 0.5% or imiquimod 5% cream *Provider administered:* trichloroacetic acid (TCA) and bichloroacetic acid (BCA) 80%–90%—repeat weekly if needed; cryotherapy with liquid nitrogen, laser, or surgical removal	Warts and surrounding tissues contain HPV, so removal of warts does not completely eradicate the virus; examination of partners is not necessary because treatment is only symptomatic; condom use may reduce transmission; medication application
Genital herpes: herpes simplex virus 2 (HSV-2)	2–20 days; average, 6 days	Vesicles, painful ulceration of penis, vagina, labia, perineum, or anus; lesions last 5–6 wk, and recurrence is common; may be asymptomatic	Presence of vesicles; cell culture and polymerase chain reaction (PCR) viral culture is obtained only when lesions are present and before they have scabbed over	No cure; treatment may be episodic or suppressive for frequent recurrence *Episodic treatment for 1st episode:* acyclovir 400 mg three times orally/day × 7–10 days, or acyclovir 200 mg orally five times/day × 7–10 days, or valacyclovir 1 g PO daily × 7–10 days, or famciclovir 250 mg orally three times × 7-10 days Regimen is similar for recurrent genital herpes	Refer partners for evaluation; teach clients about the likelihood of recurrent episodes and the ability to transmit to others even if asymptomatic; condom use; annual Pap smear

From Centers for Disease Control and Prevention: Sexually transmitted diseases treatment guidelines, 2015c. MMWR Morb Mortal Wkly Rep 64(RR3):1-137.
AIDS, acquired immunodeficiency syndrome; *CDC,* Centers for Disease Control and Prevention; *CSF,* cerebrospinal fluid; *EIA,* enzyme-linked immunosorbent assay; *IM,* intramuscularly; *PMN:* polymorphonuclear leukocytes; *PO,* orally; *VDRL,* Venereal Disease Research Laboratory (test).

activity. Some individuals, even when symptomatic, continue to be sexually active and infect others. As a result of increasing drug resistance, treatment of gonorrhea is becoming more complex. The 2015 CDC guidelines for treatment recommend that a single intramuscular dose of ceftriaxone 250 mg IM be used in combination with azithromycin 1 g orally (CDC, 2015c).

Because gonorrhea is now resistant to many of the previously effective drugs it is important that cases be detected and treated early. The CDC encourages all health care providers to (1) obtain a sexual history, (2) treat all patients diagnosed with gonorrhea promptly using CDC guidelines, (3) make every effort to evaluate and treat all of the patient's sex partners for the past 60 days, (4) obtain cultures to test for decreased susceptibility from any patients with suspected or documented gonorrhea treatment failures, and (5) report any suspected treatment failure to local or state public health officials within 24 hours to try to recognize promptly any potential resistance (CDC, 2015b).

SYPHILIS

Syphilis, caused by *Treponema pallidum,* infects moist mucosal or cutaneous membranes and is spread through direct contact, usually by sexual contact or from mother to fetus. Syphilis is passed from one person to another by direct contact with a syphilis sore. These sores are generally on the external genitals or in the vagina, anus, or in the rectum. Pregnant women can pass the disease on to their babies. Many people do not have symptoms for years after being infected. Syphilis is dramatically on the rise; the number of cases increased by 15.1% from 2013 to 2014 (CDC, 2015d). The highest rates are among MSM; however, in recent years the number of cases in women has been increasing.

The clinical signs of syphilis are divided into primary, secondary, and tertiary infections. Latency, a period when the person is symptom-free but has serological evidence, may occur early or late in the infection. If latency occurs in the first year of infection, it is called early latency, in contrast to late latency, which occurs after year 1. During latency, relapse can occur.

The first stage is called *primary syphilis.* When the disease is acquired sexually, the bacteria produce infection in the form of a chancre at the site of entry. The chancre is usually firm, round, small, and painless. The lesion begins as a macula, progresses to a papule, and later ulcerates. If left untreated, this chancre persists for 3 to 6 weeks and then heals spontaneously (Heymann, 2015). However, if the infection is not adequately treated, it progresses to the secondary stage.

Secondary syphilis occurs when the organism enters the lymph system and spreads throughout the body (Fig. 27.2). Signs include skin rash on one or more areas of the body that do not cause itching. Other symptoms may include fever, swollen lymph glands, sore throat, patchy hair loss, headaches, weight loss, muscle aches, and fatigue. The signs and symptoms will go away with or without treatment; without treatment, the infection will move to latent and possibly late stages of the disease (CDC, 2016d).

Tertiary, late, or *latent syphilis* can lead to damage to internal organs, including the brain, nerves, eyes, heart, blood vessels, liver, bones, and joints. Signs and symptoms of late-stage syphilis include the development of lesions of the bones, skin,

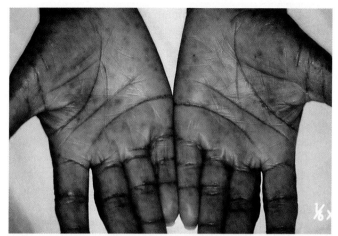

FIG. 27.2 Example of a secondary palmar rash. (Courtesy Centers for Disease Control and Prevention, Public Health Image Library [PHIL] ID 3476. Source: CDC/Dr. M.F. Rein.) (Centers for Disease Control and Prevention: *Syphilis: CDC fact sheet,* Atlanta, 2012d, CDC. Retrieved September 2012 from http://www.cdc.gov/std/syphilis/stdfact-syphilis.htm.)

and mucous membranes, known as *gummas,* difficulty coordinating muscle movements, paralysis, numbness, gradual blindness, and dementia. The damage can lead to death.

In *congenital syphilis,* syphilis is transmitted transplacentally and, if untreated, can lead to serious problems within a few weeks. Untreated syphilis can cause premature stillbirth, blindness, deafness, facial abnormalities, crippling, or death. Signs include jaundice, skin rash, hepatosplenomegaly, and pseudoparalysis of an extremity. Treatment of syphilis for adults consists of penicillin G given intramuscularly (CDC, 2015c).

CHLAMYDIA

Chlamydia infection, caused by the bacterium *Chlamydia trachomatis,* infects the genitourinary tract and rectum of adults and causes conjunctivitis and pneumonia in neonates. Transmission occurs when mucopurulent discharge from infected sites, such as the cervix or urethra, comes into contact with the mucous membranes of a noninfected person. Because the cervix of teenage girls and young women is not fully matured and may be more susceptive to infection, they are an especially high-risk group if they are sexually active. Like gonorrhea, the infection is asymptomatic in men in as many as 90% of cases and in women in as many as 70% to 95% of cases and is called a "silent" disease (Heymann, 2015; CDC, 2016e). If symptoms do appear, they typically do so within 1 to 3 weeks after exposure. If left untreated, chlamydia can result in PID. When chlamydia infection is present, symptoms in women include dysuria, urinary frequency, and purulent vaginal discharge. If the infection spreads from the cervix to the fallopian tubes, some women may have no symptoms, and others have lower abdominal pain, low back pain, nausea, fever, pain during intercourse, or bleeding between menstrual periods. In men the urethra is the most common site of infection, resulting in nongonococcal urethritis (NGU). The symptoms of NGU are dysuria and urethral discharge. Epididymitis is a possible complication.

Chlamydia is the most common reportable infectious disease in the United States. It is estimated that 1 out of every 20 women ages 14 to 24 has chlamydia. In 2012 over 1.4 million chlamydia infections were reported to the CDC from the 50 states and the District of Columbia (CDC, 2016e). There is considerable underreporting because most people with this infection are unaware of it and are not tested. It is estimated that 2.86 million infections occur annually in the United States, and women are often reinfected if their sex partners are not treated (CDC, 2016e). Because it causes PID, ectopic pregnancy, infertility, and neonatal complications, chlamydia infection is a major focus of preventive efforts. Rates of chlamydia have increased in recent years, partly because of improved diagnosis and reporting. Risk factors that positively correlate with chlamydial infection are age of less than 25 years, multiple sexual partners, and a history of infection with other STDs (CDC, 2016e). Chlamydia can be treated and cured with antibiotics. The most commonly used treatment is a single dose of azithromycin or a week of doxycycline (twice daily) (CDC, 2015c). All sex partners should be evaluated, tested, and treated. This infection can be prevented by abstaining from sexual contact or by being in a long-term relationship with a partner who is not infected. Latex male condoms, when used consistently and correctly, can reduce the risk for transmission. The CDC recommends annual chlamydia testing of all sexually active women 25 years or younger and older women with risk factors for the infection and testing of all pregnant women.

HERPES SIMPLEX VIRUS 2 (GENITAL HERPES)

Herpes viruses infect genital and nongenital sites. Herpes simplex virus 1 (HSV-1) primarily causes nongenital lesions such as cold sores that may appear on the lip or mouth. Herpes simplex virus 2 (HSV-2) is the primary cause of genital herpes. Genital herpes affects about one in six people in the United States in the age range of 14 to 49 years. Like other viral STDs, there is no cure for HSV-2 infection, and it is considered a chronic disease. The virus is transmitted through direct exposure and infects the genitalia and surrounding skin. After the initial infection, the virus remains latent in the sacral nerve of the central nervous system and may reactivate periodically with or without visible vesicles (CDC, 2015e).

Signs and symptoms of HSV-2 infection range from no symptoms to mild symptoms to painful lesions or blisters around the genitals, rectum, or mouth. The blisters break and leave painful sores that may take 2 to 4 weeks to heal. The first episode is typically longer and is usually characterized by more lesions than seen in subsequent episodes. Lesions may occur on the vulva, vagina, upper thighs, buttocks, and penis and have an average duration of 11 days. The vesicles can cause itching and pain and may be accompanied by dysuria or rectal pain. Although the ability to pass the infection to others is higher with active lesions, some individuals can spread the virus even when they are asymptomatic. Many people experience a prodromal phase. This may include a mild, tingling sensation up to 48 hours before eruption or shooting pains in the buttocks, legs, or hips (Heymann, 2015; American Sexual Health Association, 2016).

If a person with genital herpes touches the lesions and then touches another body part, the infection may be transferred, which is especially problematic if the infection is transferred to the eyes. Also, genital herpes can cause sores on skin or mucous membrane breaks; when the sores come into contract with the breaks during sex, they can increase the risk for the transmission of HIV if either partner is HIV infected. The consequences of HSV-2 are of particular concern for women and their children. Genital herpes infection can lead to miscarriage or premature birth, and the infection can be passed from mother to child, leading to a fatal infection. The clinical infection in infants may present as liver disease, encephalitis, or infection limited to the skin, eyes, or mouth (Heymann, 2015). A pregnant woman who has active lesions at the time of giving birth should have a cesarean delivery before the rupture of amniotic membranes to avoid fetal contact with the herpetic lesions, whereas those who have no clinical evidence of herpes lesions should be delivered vaginally. A small number of infants are infected in utero.

HUMAN PAPILLOMAVIRUS INFECTION

Genital human papillomavirus (HPV) is an STD that can lead to genital warts, cervical cancer, and other HPV-related cancers. Most people with HPV are asymptomatic, and in 90% of the cases the body's immune system clears HPV naturally within 2 years. HPV is transmitted through genital contact, often during vaginal or anal sex. HPV can cause normal cells on infected skin to turn abnormal. The changes are usually not detected; in most cases, the body fights off HPV naturally, and the infected cells return to normal. However, when the body does not fight off HPV, the infection can cause visible changes that result in genital warts or cancer. Warts can develop within weeks or months after being infected; cancer often takes years to develop.

Genital warts are most commonly found on the penis and scrotum in men and the vulva, labia, vagina, and cervix in women. The warts may appear as a small bump or a group of bumps in the genital areas. They can be small or large, raised or flat, and may have what is sometimes described as a cauliflower appearance. They may be difficult to visualize, so careful examination is required. HPV is common in young sexually active women (CDC, 2016f). As with genital herpes, it is hard to know the actual prevalence because this is not a reported disease, and many infections are subclinical.

There are several ways to prevent contracting HPV. Vaccines can protect both males and females against some of the most common types of HPV. These vaccines are given in three shots, and all three must be taken. The vaccines are most effective when given at 11 or 12 years of age. HPV vaccines are available to protect females against the types of HPV that can cause cervical cancer. Gardasil also protects against most genital warts, and Gardasil has been found to protect against anal, vaginal, and vulvar cancers. If individuals did not get the vaccine at the earlier age, they can still be vaccinated up to age 26 for females or age 21 for males (CDC, 2016f). In 2015 use of the 9-valent HPV vaccination (FGardasil-9) was approved as one of three approved HPV immunizations, in addition to Cervarix and Gardasil (CDC, 2015f). Condoms may also lower the risk, but they are not entirely effective because they do not cover all the possible areas that could be infected (CDC, 2013).

Complications of HPV infection are especially serious for women. The link between HPV infection and cervical cancer has been established and is associated with specific types of the virus. Papanicolaou (Pap) smears are important because they allow for microscopic examination of cells to detect HPV and tumors. The tumors often can be surgically removed if found early (Heymann, 2015). HPV infection is exacerbated in both pregnancy and immune-related disorders, which are believed to result from a decrease in cell-mediated immune functioning. HPV may infect the fetus during pregnancy and can result in a laryngeal papilloma that can obstruct the infant's airway. Genital warts may enlarge and become friable during pregnancy, and therefore surgical removal may be recommended.

HEPATITIS

Viral hepatitis refers to a group of infections that primarily affect the liver. These infections have similar clinical presentations but different causes and characteristics. Brief profiles of the types of hepatitis are presented in Table 27.2.

HEPATITIS A VIRUS

Hepatitis A virus (HAV) is most often transmitted through the fecal–oral route. Sources may be water, food, or sexual contact. The virus level in the feces appears to peak 1 to 2 weeks before symptoms appear, making individuals highly contagious before they realize they are ill (Heymann, 2015). Although there has been a vaccine for this disease since 1995, hepatitis A infection remains one of the most frequently reported vaccine-preventable diseases. Persons most at risk for HAV infection are travelers to countries with high rates of infection, children living in areas with high rates of infection, injection drug users, MSM, and persons with clotting disorders or chronic liver disease.

Hepatitis A is found worldwide. In developing countries where sanitation is inadequate, epidemics are not common because most adults are immune from childhood infection. In countries with improved sanitation, outbreaks are common in daycare centers whose staff must change diapers, among household and sexual contacts of infected individuals, and among travelers to countries where hepatitis A is endemic. In many outbreaks, one individual is the source of an infection that may become community-wide. In other cases, hepatitis A is spread through food contaminated by an infected food-handler, contaminated produce, or contaminated water. The source of infection may never be identified in many outbreaks (Heymann, 2015).

The clinical course of hepatitis A ranges from mild to severe and may entail a prolonged convalescence. Onset is usually acute, with fever, nausea, lack of appetite, malaise, and abdominal discomfort, followed after several days by jaundice. Because the clinical presentation for all types of hepatitis is identical, hepatitis A diagnosis must be serologically confirmed or meet the clinical case definition and occur in a person who has an epidemiological link to a person with hepatitis A (CDC, 2016g). Good sanitation and personal hygiene are the best means of preventing infection. People who travel often or for long periods in countries in which the disease is endemic should have the HAV vaccine. Candidates for immunoglobulin administration and vaccine after exposure to HAV are listed in Box 27.2 (Heymann, 2015; CDC, 2016h).

HEPATITIS B VIRUS

The number of new cases of hepatitis B virus (HBV) in the United States has been decreasing as a result of the use of HBV vaccine. The groups with the highest prevalence are injection drug users, persons with STDs or multiple sex partners, immigrants and

TABLE 27.2	**Viral Hepatitis Profiles**		
	Hepatitis A	**Hepatitis B**	**Hepatitis C**
Incubation period	Average, 28 days; range, 15–50 days	Average, 90 days; range, 60–150 days	Average, 45 days; range, 14–180 days
Mode of transmission	Fecal–oral, contaminated food/water, sexual	Blood-borne, sexual, perinatal	Primarily blood-borne; also sexual and perinatal
Incidence	Reported in the United States in 2014: 1,239–estimated 2,500	Reported acute cases in the United States in 2014: 2,953; estimated new cases in 2014: 19,200 Chronic hepatitis B in the United States ranges from 850,000–2.2. million	Estimated 30,500 new cases/yr in United States in 2014; reported in the United States in 2014: 2,194 Chronic hepatitis C incidence in the United States estimated at 3.5 million.
Chronic carrier state?	No	Yes, 5% of adult cases; 90% of infants; 25%–50% of children aged 1–5 years	Yes, 75%–85% or more of cases
Diagnosis	Serological test (anti-HAV), viral isolation	Serological tests (e.g., HBsAg), viral isolation	Serological tests (anti-HCV)
Sequelae	No chronic infection	Chronic liver disease; liver cancer	Chronic liver disease; liver cancer
Vaccine availability	Yes, vaccination of all children at 1 year, children in areas of high disease rates recommended; travelers to endemic regions; men who have sex with men; injection and noninjection drug users	Yes, vaccination of infants recommended; all children who have not been already immunized; individuals with exposure risks; men who have sex with men; people with end-stage renal disease, people with HIV infection	No
Control and prevention	Good hygiene (e.g., hand washing); proper sanitation	Preexposure vaccination; reduce exposure risk behaviors	Screening of blood/organ donors; reduce exposure risk behaviors

HAV, hepatitis A virus; *HBsAg,* hepatitis B surface antigen; *HBV,* hepatitis B virus; *HCV,* hepatitis C virus.
Centers for Disease Control and Prevention: *Viral hepatitis surveillance 2014,* Atlanta, GA, 2014b, CDC. Retrieved August 2016 from: http://www.cdc.gov/hepatitis/statistics/2014surveillance/pdfs/2014hepsurveillancerpt.pdf

---

BOX 27.2   Recommendations for Administration of Hepatitis A Vaccine

- Are traveling to countries where hepatitis A is common
- Are a man who has sex with other men
- Use illegal drugs
- Have a chronic liver disease such as hepatitis B or hepatitis C
- Are being treated with clotting-factor concentrates
- Work with hepatitis A–infected animals or in a hepatitis A research laboratory
- Expect to have close personal contact with an international adoptee from a country where hepatitis A is common

Centers for Disease Control and Prevention: *Hepatitis A vaccine: what you need to know,* Atlanta, GA, 2016h, CDC. Retrieved August 2016 from: http://www.cdc.gov/vaccines/hcp/vis/vis-statements/hep-a.pdf

refugees and their descendants who came from areas where there is a high endemic rate of HBV, health care workers, clients on hemodialysis, and inmates of long-term correctional institutions.

HBV is spread through blood and body fluids and, like HIV, is referred to as a *blood-borne pathogen*. It has the same transmission properties as HIV, and thus, individuals should take the same precautions to prevent the spread of both HIV and HBV. A major difference is that HBV remains alive outside the body for a longer time than HIV and thus has greater infectivity. The virus can survive for at least 1 week dried at room temperature on environmental surfaces, and therefore infection control measures are paramount in preventing transmission from client to client (Heymann, 2015).

Infection with HBV results in either acute or chronic HBV infection. The acute infection is self-limited, and individuals develop an antibody to the virus and successfully eliminate the virus from the body. They subsequently have lifelong immunity against the virus. Symptoms range from mild, flulike symptoms to a more severe response that includes jaundice, extreme lethargy, nausea, fever, and joint pain. Any of these more severe symptoms may result in hospitalization. A second possible outcome from infection is chronic HBV infection, which more likely occurs in persons with immunodeficiency (Heymann, 2015). These individuals cannot rid their bodies of the virus and remain lifelong carriers of the hepatitis B surface antigen (HBsAg). As carriers, they can transmit the HBV to others.

CASE STUDY 27-1

Hepatitis

On Friday afternoon, Jane Brown, the nurse epidemiologist at the Bertrand County Health Department, had just finished her last influenza vaccine clinic for the season. She sat down at her desk to respond to telephone and e-mail messages. She found a voice-mail message that Dr. Smith, a local physician, left earlier in the day to report two cases of acute hepatitis B infection. Dr. Smith said both of these patients were elderly and lived in an assisted living facility. He stated that he would fax a copy of the reportable disease form and the laboratory results to the health department that day. He said that he was calling not only to report the infections but to seek direction on what to advise the facility.

Ms. Brown read the form Dr. Smith had faxed and confirmed that both patients are in their 80s, live at the same address, and have laboratory evidence of acute hepatitis B infection. She is puzzled by the report because she has never seen an acute case of hepatitis B in an elderly person in the past. In fact, she has only had three reported cases of acute hepatitis B infection in the 5 years she has been at the health department: one in an infant, another in a health care worker who had a needlestick injury, and the other in a 40-year-old man with a history of intravenous drug use.

Ms. Brown called the physician to discuss the report and gather additional information about the cases. She learned that the physician had left for the day, but she spoke with his nurse, Sally Johnson. Ms. Johnson said that both patients were seen the prior week for complaints of nausea, lethargy, and weight loss, and one had yellowing of the skin. Based on their presenting symptoms Dr. Smith decided to perform a hepatitis B and C panel and draw blood to evaluate their liver enzymes. The hepatitis C antibody results were negative, but the liver enzymes were elevated and the hepatitis B surface antigen was positive, along with the hepatitis B core immunoglobulin M. The remaining markers were negative. The patients have no known history of exposure to hepatitis B, drug abuse, or multiple sex partners, and both have lived in the facility for over 5 years. Ms. Brown explains to the nurse that this is an unusual event and that she will launch an investigation to try to identify the source of transmission and help the assisted living facility effectively manage the residents. She called the facility immediately to set up a meeting with the administrator that evening.

CHECK YOUR PRACTICE

1. Which term describes the system the physician used to collect, organize, and report disease information?
   A. Screening
   B. Surveillance
   C. Distribution
   D. Rate adjustment
2. What data source would *not* be useful to the nurse epidemiologist in this situation?
   A. Medical records
   B. Facility staff (administrator, nurse supervisor, nursing staff, housekeeping)
   C. Policy and procedure manuals
   D. Food history
   E. Medication administration log

In analyzing the data, Ms. Brown identifies commonalities among the two patients. She learns that both patients live in the same unit, eat in the same dining hall, are diabetic, and receive blood glucose monitoring. Ms. Brown knows that the hepatitis B virus can be transmitted by blood, so she decides to observe the nurse performing glucose monitoring. She sees that the nurse used a penlet device to secure the lancets that are used on the residents and that all residents have their own glucometer. The nurse uses a separate lancet for each patient, but the same penlet is used on each resident. Ms. Brown also observes dried blood on the lancet. Based on this observation, she decides to test all of the diabetic residents for hepatitis B infection.

3. What level of prevention is the nurse exercising in this situation?
   A. Primary
   B. Secondary
   C. Tertiary
   D. None

Ms. Brown reviews the hepatitis B testing results and learns that one patient has chronic hepatitis B infection and three other patients have had the infection in the past but are no longer infected. She recommends hepatitis B vaccine for all of the residents and staff who are susceptible to the infection.

4. Immunizations represent what level of prevention?
   A. Primary
   B. Secondary
   C. Tertiary
   D. None

Case prepared by Mary Beth White-Comstock, MSN, RN, CIC.

They may develop hepatic carcinoma or chronic active hepatitis. The signs and symptoms of chronic hepatitis B include anorexia, fatigue, abdominal discomfort, hepatomegaly, and jaundice (Heymann, 2015).

HBV infection can be prevented by immunization, prevention of nosocomial occupational exposure, and prevention of sexual and injection drug use exposure. Vaccination is recommended for persons with occupational risk, such as health care workers, and for children. Protection from HBV consists of a series of three intramuscular injections, with the second and third doses administered 1 and 6 months after the first (Heymann, 2015). Testing continues to be recommended for pregnant women, infants born to HBsAg-positive mothers, household contacts and sexual partners of HBV-infected persons, individuals who may be exposed to blood or body builds that are contaminated (e.g., a needlestick injury in a health care worker), or persons infected with HIV (CDC, 2015g). The CDC published new testing guidelines in 2008 that recommend testing for HBsAg for persons born in geographic regions with HBsAg prevalence of 2% or greater, persons born in the United States who were not vaccinated as infants and whose parents came from geographic regions with HBsAg prevalence of 8% or greater, injection drug users, MSM, persons with elevated alanine aminotransferase and aspartate aminotransferase (ALT/AST) of unknown cause, and persons with selected medical conditions who need immunosuppressive therapy (CDC, 2015g). All pregnant women should be tested for HBsAg, and if the mother is positive, newborns require hepatitis B immunoglobulin in addition to the hepatitis B vaccine at within 12 hours of delivery, and then at 1 and 6 months thereafter (CDC, 2016i). In instances in which the person is not protected by vaccination and is exposed to HBV, hepatitis B immunoglobulin is given as soon as possible (within 24 days is optimal) and the HBV vaccine started (CDC, 2016i).

In 1992, the Occupational Safety and Health Administration (OSHA) released *Occupational Exposure to Bloodborne Pathogens* (OSHA, n.d.), the standard that mandates specific activities to protect workers from HBV and other blood-borne pathogens. This was revised in 2000, titled the Needlestick Safety and Prevention Act, and is a regulation that prescribes safeguards to protect workers against health hazards related to blood-borne pathogens (OSHA, no date). Potential exposures for health care workers are needlestick injuries and mucous membrane splashes. The OSHA standard requires employers to identify the risk for blood exposure to various employees. If employees perform work that involves potential exposure to the body fluids of other people, employers are mandated to offer the HBV vaccine to the employee at the employer's expense and to offer annual educational programs on preventing HBV and HIV exposure in the workplace. Employees have the right to refuse the vaccine.

HEPATITIS C VIRUS

Hepatitis C virus (HCV) infection is the most common chronic blood-borne infection in the United States (CDC, 2015h). HCV is transmitted when blood or body fluids of an infected person enter an uninfected person. Today most people are infected with hepatitis C by sharing needles or other equipment to inject drugs. Those groups at highest risk include health care workers and emergency personnel who are accidentally exposed, infants of infected mothers, and injection drug users who share needles or other drug use equipment. Risk is greatest for persons exposed to infected blood. Others at risk include clients on hemodialysis (from dialysis equipment shared with infected persons) and recipients of donor organs and blood products before 1992 (CDC, 2015h).

An estimated 2.7 to 3.9 million people in the United States have chronic hepatitis C, and most do not know they have the infection due to underascertainment and underreporting. Annually about 30,500 people in the United States become acutely infected with hepatitis C. The clinical signs of hepatitis C may be so mild that an infected individual does not seek medical attention. The incubation period ranges from 2 weeks to 6 months. Clients may experience fatigue and other nonspecific symptoms. Acute hepatitis C is a short-term illness that occurs about 6 months after exposure; of those with the acute disease, approximately 15% to 25% have the disease clear without treatment, and about 75% to 85% develop chronic or lifelong infection. Chronic hepatitis C can lead to liver damage, cirrhosis, liver failure, or liver cancer (CDC, 2015i).

Hepatitis C virus (HCV) treatment has evolved substantially since the introduction of HCV protease inhibitor therapies in 2011, and new drugs with different mechanisms of action have become and continue to become available. For more information about currently approved FDA therapies to treat hepatitis C, please visit http://www.hepatitisc.uw.edu/page/treatment/drugs. (CDC, 2015h).

Primary prevention of HCV infection includes screening of blood products and donor organs and tissue; risk reduction counseling and services, including obtaining a history of injection drug use; and infection control practices. Secondary prevention strategies include testing of high-risk individuals, including those who currently inject drugs or injected drugs in the past, have HIV infection, have abnormal liver tests or liver disease, received blood or an organ transplant before 1992, are on hemodialysis, and have been exposed to blood on the job through a needlestick or injury with a sharp object (CDC, 2015h).

TUBERCULOSIS

Tuberculosis (TB) is a mycobacterial disease caused by *Mycobacterium tuberculosis*. Transmission usually occurs through exposure to the tubercle bacilli in airborne droplets from persons with pulmonary tuberculosis who talk, cough, or sneeze. Common symptoms are cough, fever, hemoptysis, chest pains, fatigue, and weight loss. The incubation period is 4 to 12 weeks. The most critical period for development of clinical disease is the first 6 to 12 months after infection. About 5% of those initially infected may develop pulmonary tuberculosis or extrapulmonary involvement. The infection in about 95% of those initially infected becomes latent, but in about 10% of otherwise healthy individuals, it may be reactivated later in life. The chance of reactivation of latent infections increases in immunocompromised persons, substance abusers, underweight and undernourished persons, and persons with diabetes, silicosis, or gastrectomies (Heymann, 2015).

The World Health Organization (WHO) estimates that one-third of the world's population has latent TB, meaning that individuals are infected with TB bacteria but they are not yet ill, nor can they transmit the disease (WHO, 2016). Worldwide, low- and middle-income countries account for 95% of TB deaths. The incidence of TB infection in Africa reflects the incidence of infection with HIV because HIV-infected individuals are 20 to 30 times more likely to contract TB (WHO, 2016). The rate of cases of TB has declined annually since 1993. In 2014 the TB case rate for US-born persons was 2.96 cases per 100,000 persons. This compares to 7.4 cases per 100,000 in 1993 (CDC, 2016j). The rate declined for foreign-born persons living in the United States, although not as much as for US-born persons. Between 2007 and 2011, the countries of origin of foreign-born persons in the United States with TB were Mexico, the Philippines, India, Vietnam, and China (CDC, 2015j).

To prevent TB, the CDC works with public health agencies in other countries to improve screening and reporting of cases and to improve treatment strategies (Fig. 27.3). This includes coordination of treatment for infected individuals who migrate to the United States. This coordination is particularly significant between Mexico and the United States.

The most effective tuberculin skin test (TST) is the Mantoux test. The TST, previously referred to as purified protein derivative (PPD) test, is used for initial screening. It can be followed by chest radiography for persons with a positive skin reaction and pulmonary symptoms. Persons who are immunosuppressed by drugs or who have diseases such as advanced tuberculosis, AIDS, or measles may not have the ability to mount an immune response to the TST, so the result may be a false-negative skin test reaction resulting from anergy (nonreaction). A second issue with the TST is that a positive result may come from an earlier TST boosting the person's ability to respond to the infection and not from a recent infection. Therefore it is difficult to determine whether the infection is old or recent. A blood test (in vitro gamma release interferon assays [IVGRA]) is available and is

increasingly used for providing clinical care (Buttaro, 2013; CDC 2016k). One example is the QuantiFERON-TB blood test to detect *M. tuberculosis* infection. Diagnosis can also be made through stained sputum smears and other body fluids to determine the presence of acid-fast bacilli (for presumptive diagnosis) and culture of the tubercle bacilli for definitive diagnosis. The How To box describes how to read a TST.

HOW TO Perform a Tuberculin Skin Test

Apply and Read the Tuberculin Skin Test (TST)
- For the Mantoux test, inject 0.1 mL containing 5 tuberculin units of purified protein derivative tuberculin.
- Read the reaction 48 to 72 hours after injection.
- Measure only induration.
- Record results in millimeters.

Interpret the TST
The test is positive if the induration is ≥5 mm in the following:
- Immunosuppressed clients
- Persons known to have human immunodeficiency virus (HIV) infection
- Persons whose chest radiograph is suggestive of previous tuberculosis (TB) that was untreated
- Close contacts of a person with infectious TB
- Organ transplant recipients

Test is positive if the induration is ≥10 mm in the following:
- Persons with certain medical conditions, such as diabetes, alcoholism, or drug abuse
- Persons who inject drugs (if HIV negative)
- Foreign-born persons from areas where TB is common
- Children under 4 years of age
- Residents and staff of long-term care facilities, jails, and prisons

Test is positive if the induration is ≥15 mm in the following:
- All persons more than 4 years of age with no risk factors for TB

From Heymann D: *Control of communicable diseases manual,* Washington DC, 2015, American Public Health Association; Centers for Disease Control and Prevention (CDC): Mantoux Tuberculin Skin Test: Facilitator Guide, 2003. Available at: http://www.cdc.gov/tb/education/mantoux/images/mantoux.pdf.

Clients with TB should be treated promptly with the appropriate combination of multiple antimicrobial drugs. Effective drug regimens used in the United States include isoniazid, rifampin, ethambutol (EMB), and pyrazinamide (PZA) (CDC, treatment, 2016l). Treatment regimens for persons with active symptomatic infection may be different from the regimens used for persons with latent TB infection or with HIV (CDC, 2016l). Treatment failure may be due to clients' poor adherence in taking the medication, which can result in drug resistance. Nurses usually administer TSTs and provide education on the importance of compliance to long-term therapy. They also may be involved in directly observed therapy (DOT) and contact investigations of cases in the community.

Clients with TB should be treated promptly with the appropriate combination of multiple antimicrobial drugs. Effective drug regimens used in the United States include isoniazid (INH), rifampin, and pyrazinamide. Multidrug-resistant TB (MDR-TB) refers to a type of TB that does not respond to the best drugs, INH and rifampin. Resistance can develop when

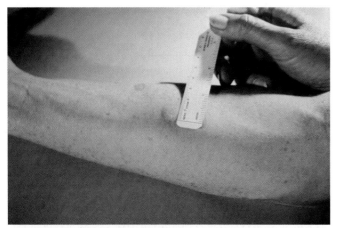

FIG. 27.3 Testing for tuberculosis infection. (Courtesy Centers for Disease Control and Prevention, Public Health Image Library [PHIL] ID 3752. Source: CDC/Donald Kopanoff.)

CASE STUDY 27-2

TB Screening in a Homeless Population

Jill Miles is the nurse epidemiologist for the Warren County Health Department. Part of Ms. Miles's role at the health department is to administer tuberculosis (TB) screening to at-risk populations and to track TB cases seen in the county. Ms. Miles has identified the homeless population in Warren County as a high-risk population for TB.

Ms. Miles has already implemented a TB education program at the homeless shelter. Every other month, she goes to the shelter and teaches a class about TB—what it is, who is at risk, and why to get a TB screening test. Furthermore, every person who wishes to stay at the shelter must receive a TB screening test.

Yesterday, the homeless shelter contacted Ms. Miles and reported that one of the men staying at the shelter tested positive for active TB, but they now cannot find him. The shelter director suspects the man has left to work at one of the rural farms that offer temporary work, but he does not know which farm.

Ms. Miles talks to the men at the shelter who spoke with the client. She learns that the client, José, is in his 30s and speaks only Spanish. The friends give Ms. Miles some leads of possible farms to which José may have gone. Ms. Miles calls the farms and speaks to the farm managers. Luckily, Ms. Miles discovers one of the farm managers had recently been at the shelter to recruit workers. She visits the farm and, through interviewing the newly hired men, finds José, the missing person with active TB. Because of José's transient lifestyle, Ms. Miles decides to enroll him in directly observed therapy (DOT) for TB treatment. DOT will provide a hotel room and meals for him while he receives TB treatment.

there is poor client adherence in taking the medication or when the wrong drug is prescribed (CDC, 2016l). Nurses administer TSTs and provide education on the importance of compliance to long-term therapy. They also may be involved in DOT and contact investigations of cases in the community.

NURSE'S ROLE IN PROVIDING PREVENTIVE CARE FOR COMMUNICABLE DISEASES

From prevention to treatment, the nurse functions as a counselor, educator, advocate, case manager, and primary care provider. Appropriate interventions for primary, secondary, and tertiary prevention are reviewed. In primary prevention, the nursing process is used to care for clients with communicable diseases. Nurses are in an ideal position to affect the outcomes of communicable diseases, and their influence begins with primary prevention.

PRIMARY PREVENTION

Primary prevention aims to keep people healthy and avoid the onset of disease. First, assess for risk behavior and provide relevant intervention through education on how to avoid infection, mostly through healthy behaviors. To assess the risk for acquiring an infection, obtain a history that focuses on potential exposure, which varies with the specific organism being studied and its mode of transmission. The questions to be asked can be especially challenging with clients who have an STD. The nurse should obtain a sexual and injection drug use history for clients and their partners. The sexual history provides information that leads to the need for specific diagnostic tests, treatment

approaches, and partner notification. It also facilitates evaluation of risk factors and is necessary for the nurse to be able to provide relevant education for the client's lifestyle. A thorough sexual history requires obtaining personal and sensitive information. Ask about the types of relationships, the number of sexual partners and encounters, and the types of sexual behaviors practiced. The confidential nature of the information and how it will be used should be shared with the client to establish open communication and goal-directed interaction. Most clients feel uneasy disclosing such personal information. The nurse can ease this discomfort by remaining supportive and open during the interview to facilitate honesty about intimate activities. The nurse serves as a model for discussing sensitive information in a candid manner. When discussing precautions, use direct and simple language to describe specific behaviors. This encourages the client to openly discuss sexuality during this interaction and with future partners.

Nurses who are uncomfortable discussing topics such as sexual behavior or sexual orientation are likely to avoid assessing risk behaviors with the client and therefore may compromise data collection. Nurses can gain confidence in conducting sexual risk assessments by understanding their own values and feelings about sexuality and realizing that the purpose of the interaction is to improve the client's health. The nurse's comfort in discussing sexual behavior can be improved by using role-playing to practice assessments of sexual and intravenous drug use behavior and by contracting with clients to make behavior changes.

Identifying the number of sexual partners and partners who are injection drug users and the number of contacts with these partners provides information about the client's risk. The chance of exposure decreases as the number of partners decreases, so people in mutually monogamous relationships are at low risk for acquiring STDs. You can obtain this information by asking, "How many sex (or drug) partners have you had over the past 6 months?" It is important to avoid basing assumptions about the

LEVELS OF PREVENTION

Related to Nursing Interventions

Primary Prevention
- Provide community education about prevention of communicable diseases to well populations.
- Vaccinate for hepatitis A virus (HAV) or hepatitis B virus (HBV).
- Provide community outreach for education and needle exchange.

Secondary Prevention
- Administer purified protein derivative (PPD).
- Test and counsel for human immunodeficiency virus (HIV).
- Notify partners and trace contacts.

Tertiary Prevention
- Educate caregivers of persons with HIV about Standard Precautions.
- Maintain long-term directly observed therapy (DOT) for tuberculosis treatment.
- Identify community resources for providing supportive care (e.g., funds for purchasing medications).
- Set up support groups for persons with herpes simplex virus 2.

sexual partner or partners on the client's sex, age, ethnicity, or any other factor. Stereotypes and assumptions about who people are and what they do are common problems that keep interviewers from asking the questions that lead to obtaining useful information. For example, it should not be taken for granted that if a man is homosexual, he always has more than one partner. Be aware also that the long incubation of HIV and the subclinical phase of many STDs lead some monogamous individuals to assume erroneously that they are not at risk.

It is important to determine whether the person has sexual contact with men, women, or both. This information can be obtained simply by asking. This lets the client know that the nurse is open to hearing about these behaviors, and thus, the nurse is more likely to obtain information that is relevant to sexual practices and risk. Women who are exclusively lesbian are at low risk for acquiring STDs, but bisexual women may transmit STDs between male and female partners. In addition, it is possible for men to have sexual contact with other men and not label themselves as homosexual. Therefore education to

EVIDENCE-BASED PRACTICE

Vaccination to prevent transmission of human papillomavirus (HPV) has been recommended for several years for young men as well as women, with primary vaccination recommended for boys at 11 to 12 years and secondary vaccination to catch those never vaccinated through age 26. There is an emphasis on vaccination because half of new HPV infections occur in young people between the ages of 15 and 24.

In this study, nurse researchers surveyed 735 male college students (ages 18–25) who were sexually active (previously or currently) with men, women, or both and examined their vaccination rates, personal perceptions of risk for sexually transmitted infections, and barriers to vaccination. Researchers collected both quantitative and qualitative data from the student participants, consisting of demographic data, vaccination rates, data about sexual practices, and qualitative data about perspectives on the HPV vaccination, such as why they had not received it or why they may not have completed the three-dose vaccination.

The researchers found that although the student participants engaged in risky sexual practices such as a high number of lifetime sexual partners (mean 6.3) and over half either never using condoms (10%) or sometimes using condoms (41%), 93% of participants did not view themselves as being at risk for sexually transmitted infections. Multivariate analysis revealed that participants who always wore condoms were more likely to have received the vaccine, and the older the participant was, the less likely he was to have received the vaccine.

Quantitative data about the HPV vaccination focused on barriers to obtaining the vaccine, such as cost and inconvenience. Many participants had not heard of either HPV itself or the vaccine or did not know that men could get the vaccine. The male participants also did not know about the link between oropharyngeal cancer and HPV for men, and only some participants knew about the link between cervical cancer and HPV for women.

Nurse Use

This study highlights the importance of education and awareness about HPV and the HPV vaccination for both men and women. Nurses can play a large role in information dissemination and the vaccination promotion effort.

Data from: Fontenot HB, Fantasia HC, Charyk A, et al: Human papillomavirus (HPV) risk factors, vaccination patterns, and vaccine perceptions among a sample of male college students. *Journal of American College Health* 62(3):186–192, 2014. DOI:10.1080/07448481.2013.872649.

reduce risk that is aimed at homosexual men will not be heeded by men who do not see themselves as homosexual. In such situations the nurse can ask, "When was the last time you had sex with another man?"

Certain sexual practices are more likely to result in exposure to and transmission of STDs. Dangerous sexual activities include unprotected anal or vaginal intercourse, oral–anal contact, and insertion of finger or fist into the rectum. These practices introduce a high risk for transmission of enteric organisms or result in physical trauma during sexual encounters. The nurse can obtain information about sexual encounters by asking, "Can you tell me the kinds of sexual practices in which you engage? This will help determine what risks you may have and the type of tests we should do." Clients who engage in genital–anal, oral–anal, or oral–genital contact will need throat and rectal cultures for some STDs, as well as cervical and urethral cultures.

Drug use is linked to STD transmission in several ways. Drugs such as alcohol put people at risk because these drugs can lower inhibitions and impair judgment about engaging in risky behaviors. Addictions to drugs may cause individuals to acquire the drug or money to purchase the drug through sexual favors. This increases both the frequency of sexual contacts and the chances of contracting STDs. Thus the nurse should obtain information on the type and frequency of drug use and the presence of risk behaviors. The administration of vaccines to prevent infection such as for hepatitis A and hepatitis C is an example of primary prevention.

Interventions to prevent infection are aimed at preventing specific infections. These interventions can take several forms and include, for example, education on how to prevent infection or the availability of vaccines. For example, on the basis of the information obtained in the sexual history and risk assessment just described, the nurse can identify specific education and counseling needs of the client. The nursing interventions focus on contracting with clients to change behavior and reduce their risk in regard to sexual practice.

Safer Sex

Sexual abstinence is the best way to prevent STDs. However, for many people sexual abstinence is not realistic, and teaching how to make sexual behavior safer is critical. Safer sexual behavior includes masturbation, dry kissing, touching, fantasy, and vaginal and oral sex with a condom.

If used correctly and consistently, condoms can prevent both pregnancy and most STDs because they prevent the exchange of body fluids during sexual activity. Condom failure may occur from incorrect use rather than condom breakage. Thus information about proper use of condoms and how to communicate with a partner is also necessary. The nurse has many opportunities to convey this information during counseling. Condom use may be viewed as inconvenient, as messy, or as decreasing sensation. Consuming alcohol may accompany sexual activity and decrease condom use. Nurses can use role-playing to help clients gain skill in discussing safer sex by role modeling and by practicing communication skills.

Female condoms can also be a barrier to body fluid contact and therefore protect against pregnancy and STDs. The main advantage of the female condom is that its use is controlled by the woman. Because it is made of polyurethane, it is also useful if a latex sensitivity develops to regular male condoms. Symptoms of latex allergy include penile, vaginal, or rectal itching or swelling after use of a male condom or diaphragm. The female condom consists of a sheath over two rings, with one closed end that fits over the cervix. The condoms are often free at public health clinics, or cost ranges from $2.50 to $5.00 per condom.

Clients should understand that it is important to know the risk behavior of their sexual partners, including a history of injection drug use and STDs, bisexuality, and any current symptoms. This is because each sexual partner is potentially exposed to all the STDs of all the persons with whom the other partner has been sexually active.

Drug Use

Injection drug use is risky because the potential for injecting blood-borne pathogens, such as HIV and HBV, exists when needles and syringes are shared. During injection drug use, small quantities of drugs are repeatedly injected. Blood is withdrawn into the syringe and is then injected back into the user's vein. Individuals should be advised against using injectable drugs and sharing needles, syringes, or other drug paraphernalia. If equipment is shared, it should be in contact with full-strength bleach for 30 seconds and then rinsed with water several times to prevent injecting bleach (CDC, 2016m). People who inject drugs are difficult to reach for health care services. Effective outreach programs include using community peers, increasing accessibility of drug treatment programs combined with HIV testing and counseling, and long-term repeat contacts after completion of the program.

Community Outreach, Education, and Evaluation

Because of the illegal nature of injectable drugs and the poverty associated with HIV, many people at risk have neither the inclination nor the resources to seek health care. Nurses may work to establish programs within communities because the opportunities for counseling on the prevention of HIV and other STDs are increased by bringing services into the neighborhoods of those at risk. Workers go into communities to disseminate information on safer sex, drug treatment programs, and discontinuation of drug use or safer drug use practices (e.g., using new needles and syringes with each injection). Some programs provide sterile needles and syringes, condoms, and literature about anonymous test sites.

Using primary prevention, nurses can educate healthy groups about prevention of communicable diseases. Information about modes of transmission, testing, availability of vaccines, and early symptoms can be provided to groups in the community and can help prevent the spread of STDs and HIV. Effective and convenient places to hold these educational sessions include schools, businesses, and churches. When talking with groups about HIV infection, be sure to discuss the following:

- The number of people infected with HIV and the number who are living with AIDS
- Modes of transmission of the virus
- How to prevent infection

- Testing services
- Common symptoms of illness
- Providing a compassionate response to those affected
- Available community resources
- Content about other STDs because the mode of transmission (sexual contact) is the same
- Information on these diseases, including the distribution, incidence, and consequences of the infection for individuals and society

Evaluation is based on whether risky behavior has changed to safe behavior and, ultimately, whether illness is prevented. Condom use is evaluated for consistency of use if the client is sexually active. Other behaviors, such as abstinence or monogamy, can be evaluated for their implementation. At the community level, behavioral surveys can be done to measure reported condom use and condom sales, and measures of disease incidence and prevalence can be calculated to evaluate the effectiveness of intervention.

SECONDARY PREVENTION

Secondary prevention includes screening for diseases to ensure their early identification and treatment and follow-up with contacts to prevent further spread. In general, client teaching and counseling should include education about preventing self-reinfection, managing symptoms, and preventing the infection of others. HIV screening is recommended for all patients in health care settings unless the patient declines testing. Persons at high risk should be tested annually.

This includes people with one or more of the following: a history of STDs; multiple sex partners; injection drug use; a history of intercourse without using a condom; a history of intercourse with someone who has another partner; a history of sex with a prostitute; men with a history of homosexual or bisexual activity; and a history of being a sexual partner to anyone in one of these groups.

If HIV infection is discovered before the onset of symptoms, the disease process and CD4 lymphocyte counts or viral loads can be monitored early. In addition, prophylactic therapy with antibiotics or antiretroviral therapy may be started and may delay the onset of symptomatic illness. Thus testing enables clients to benefit from early detection and treatment, as well as risk-reduction education.

Human Immunodeficiency Virus Test Counseling

Persons who have a negative test should be counseled about risk reduction activities to prevent any future transmission. Clients should understand that the test may not be truly negative because it does not reveal infections that may have been acquired within the several weeks before the test. As noted earlier, evidence of HIV antibody takes from 6 to 12 weeks. Clients must be aware of the ways viral transmission occurs, and how to avoid infection.

All clients who are antibody positive should be counseled about the need to reduce their risks and notify partners. If the client is unwilling or hesitant to notify past partners, partner notification (or contact tracing, as will be described) is often

> ### » APPLYING CONTENT TO PRACTICE

This chapter emphasizes the epidemiology and prevention of selected communicable diseases, as well as the public health nursing services provided to clients. The Council on Linkages Domains and Core Competencies are addressed through activities in caring for clients with communicable diseases. Examples of how these eight domains are used in providing nursing care to clients with communicable disease are as follows:

Domain 1, Analytic Assessment Skills, is achieved through the review of the incidence and prevalence rates of communicable diseases to determine population health status.

Domain 3, Communication Skills, is applied when public health nurses teach how to prevent and treat infections.

Domain 4, Cultural Competency Skills, is met through understanding the various social and behavioral factors that make health care acceptable to diverse populations.

Council on Linkages Between Academic and Public Health Practice: *Core competencies for public health professionals,* Washington, DC, 2014. Public Health Foundation/Health Resource and Services Administration.

done by the nurse. Clients should seek treatment from their primary health care provider so that physical evaluation can be performed and, if indicated, antiviral or other therapies begun.

Psychosocial counseling is indicated when positive HIV test results precipitate acute anxiety, depression, or suicidal ideation. The client should be informed about available counseling services. The person should be cautioned to consider carefully who should be informed of the test results. Many individuals have told others about their HIV-positive test, only to experience isolation and discrimination. Plans for the future should be explored, and clients should be advised to avoid stress, drugs, and infections to maintain optimal health.

Partner Notification and Contact Tracing

Partner notification, also known as *contact tracing,* is an example of a population-level intervention aimed at controlling communicable diseases. Partner notification programs usually occur in conjunction with reportable disease requirements and are carried out by most health departments. It involves confidentially identifying and notifying exposed individuals of clients who are found to have reportable diseases. This could result in, for example, family members and close contacts of individuals with TB being given a TST, which may be administered in the home.

Individuals diagnosed with a reportable STD are asked to provide the names and locations of all partners so these individuals can be informed of their exposure and obtain the necessary treatment. Clients may be encouraged to notify their partners and to encourage them to seek treatment. If the client agrees to do so, suggestions on how to tell partners and how to deal with possible reactions may be explored. In some instances, clients may feel more comfortable if the nurse notifies those who are exposed. If clients contact their partners about possible infection, the nurse contacts health care providers or clinics to verify examination of exposed partners.

If the client prefers not to participate in notifying partners, the nurse contacts them—often by a home visit—and counsels them to seek evaluation and treatment. The client is offered literature regarding treatment, risk reduction, and the clinic's location and hours of operation. The identity of the infected client who names sexual and injection drug–using partners cannot be revealed. Maintaining confidentiality is critical with all STDs but particularly with HIV, because discrimination may still occur.

TERTIARY PREVENTION

Tertiary prevention can apply to many of the chronic viral STDs and TB. For viral STDs, much of this effort focuses on managing symptoms and maintaining psychosocial support. Many clients report feeling contaminated and thus feel lower self-worth. Support groups may be available to help clients cope with chronic STDs, such as genital herpes or genital warts.

Directly Observed Therapy

In DOT programs for TB medication, nurses observe and document individual clients taking their TB drugs. When clients prematurely stop taking TB medications, there is a risk for the TB becoming resistant to the medications. This can affect an entire community of people who are susceptible to this airborne disease. Health professionals share in the responsibility of adhering to treatment, and DOT ensures that TB-infected clients have adequate medication. Thus DOT programs are aimed at the population level to prevent antibiotic resistance in the community and to ensure effective treatment at the individual level. Many health departments have DOT home health programs to ensure adequate treatment. DOT short course (DOTS) is a variation applied in specific countries of the world to combat multidrug-resistant TB (WHO, 2010; CDC, 2012b).

The management of AIDS in the home may include monitoring physical status and referring the family to additional care services for maintaining the client in the home. Case management is important in all phases of HIV infection. It is especially important to ensure that clients have adequate services to meet their needs. This may include ensuring that medication can be obtained through identifying funding resources, maintaining infection control standards, reducing risk behaviors, identifying sources of respite care for caretakers, or referring clients for home or hospice care. Nursing interventions include teaching families about managing symptomatic illness by preventing deteriorating conditions such as diarrhea, skin breakdown, and inadequate nutrition.

Standard Precautions

It is important to teach caregivers about infection control in the home. Clients, families, friends, and others may express concerns about the transmission of diseases. Whereas fear may be expressed by some, others who are caring for loved ones with communicable and infectious diseases may not take adequate precautions, such as wearing of gloves, because of concern about appearing as though they do not want to touch a loved one.

Standard precautions must be taught to caregivers in the home setting. All blood and articles soiled with body fluids must be handled as if they were infectious or contaminated by blood-borne pathogens. Gloves should be worn whenever hands might touch nonintact skin, mucous membranes, blood, or other fluids. A mask, goggles, and gown should also be worn if there is potential for splashing or spraying of infectious material during any care. All protective equipment should be worn only once and then disposed of. If the skin or mucous membranes of the caregiver come in contact with body fluids, the skin should be washed with soap and water, and the mucous membranes should be flushed with water as soon as possible after the exposure. Thorough handwashing with soap and water—a major infection control measure—should be conducted whenever hands become contaminated and whenever gloves or other protective equipment (e.g., mask, gown) is removed. Soiled clothing or linen should be washed in a washing machine filled with hot water, using bleach as an additive, and dried on the hot-air cycle of a dryer.

PRACTICE APPLICATION

Yvonne Jackson is a 20-year-old woman who visits the Hopetown City Health Department's maternity clinic. Examination reveals she is at 14 weeks' gestation. She is single but has been in a steady relationship for the past 6 months with Phil. She states that she has no other children. The HIV test is routinely performed during the initial prenatal visit. The results are positive.

Yvonne is shocked and emotionally distraught about the positive test results. Understanding that Yvonne will not be able to concentrate on all of the questions and information that need to be covered, the nurse sets priorities regarding essential information to obtain and provide during this visit.

A. List the relevant factors to consider on the basis of this information.

B. What questions do you need to ask with regard to controlling the spread of HIV to others?

C. What information is most important to give to Yvonne at this time?

D. What follow-up does the nurse need to arrange for Yvonne?

Answers can be found on the Evolve website.

REMEMBER THIS!

- Nearly all communicable diseases discussed in this chapter are preventable because they are transmitted through specific, known behaviors.
- Sexually transmitted diseases (STDs) are among the most serious public health problems in the United States. Not only is there an increased incidence of drug-resistant gonococcal infection, but other STDs, such as human papillomavirus (HPV, genital warts), human immunodeficiency virus (HIV), and herpes simplex virus (HSV) (genital herpes), are associated with cancer.
- STDs affect certain groups in greater numbers. Factors associated with risk include being younger than 25 years, being a member of a minority group, residing in an urban setting, being impoverished, and using crack cocaine.
- It is important for nurses to educate clients about ways to prevent communicable diseases.
- Many STDs do not produce symptoms in clients.
- Aside from death, the most serious complications caused by STDs are pelvic inflammatory disease, infertility, ectopic pregnancy, neonatal morbidity and mortality, and neoplasia.

- Hepatitis A is often silent in children, and children are a significant source of infection to others.
- The emergence of multidrug-resistant TB has prompted the use of directly observed therapy (DOT) in the United States and other countries to ensure adherence to drug treatment regimens.
- Early detection of communicable diseases is important because it results in early treatment and prevention of additional transmission to others. Treatment includes effective medications, stress reduction, and proper nutrition.
- Partner notification, or contact tracing, is done by identifying, contacting, and ensuring evaluation and treatment of persons exposed to sexual and injectable drug–using partners. Contact tracing is also conducted for tuberculosis (TB) and hepatitis A virus (HAV).
- Most of the care (both home and outpatient) that is provided for HIV is done within the community setting, which reduces direct health care costs but increases the need for financial support of home and community health services.

Ⓔ EVOLVE WEBSITE

http://evolve.elsevier.com/Stanhope/foundations
- Case Study, with Questions and Answers
- NCLEX® Review Questions
- Practice Application Answers

REFERENCES

American Sexual Health Association: *Herpes signs and symptoms*, Research Triangle Park, NC, 2016, ASHA. http://www.ashasexualhealth.org/stdsstis/herpes/signs-symptoms/. Accessed June 19, 2017.

Buttaro T, Trybulski J, Polgar Bailey P, et al: *Primary care: a collaborative practice*, ed 4, St Louis, MO, 2013, Mosby.

Centers for Disease Control and Prevention (CDC): *Mantoux tuberculin skin test: facilitator guide*, 2003. Available at http://www.cdc.gov/tb/education/mantoux/images/mantoux.pdf.

Centers for Disease Control and Prevention: Thirty years of HIV/AIDS: United States, 1981-2011, *MMWR Morb Mortal Wkly Rep* 60(21):689, 2011.

Centers for Disease Control and Prevention: *PrEP: a new tool for HIV prevention—CDC fact sheet*, Atlanta, GA, August 2012a, CDC. Retrieved August 2016 from http://www.cdc.gov/hiv/pdf/prevention_PrEP_factsheet.pdf.

Centers for Disease Control and Prevention: *Menu of suggested provisions for state tuberculosis prevention and control laws*, 2012b. Available at http://www.cdc.gov/tb/programs/Laws/menu/treatment.htm#2. Accessed August 15, 2016.

Centers for Disease Control and Prevention: *HIV in the United States: at a glance*, Atlanta, GA, 2012c, CDC. Retrieved August 2012 from http://www.cdc.gov/nchhstp/newsroom/docs/Hiv-infections-2006-2009.pdf.

Centers for Disease Control and Prevention: *Syphilis: CDC fact sheet*, Atlanta, GA, 2012d, CDC. Retrieved September 2012 from http://www.cdc.gov/std/syphilis/stdfact-syphilis.htm.

Centers for Disease Control and Prevention: *Condom fact sheet in brief*, Atlanta, GA, 2013, CDC. Retrieved August 2016 from http://www.cdc.gov/condomeffectiveness/brief.html.

Centers for Disease Control and Prevention: Revised surveillance case definition for HIV infection: United States, 2014, *MMWR Morb Mortal Wkly Rep* 63(RR03):1–10, 2014a. Retrieved August 2016 from http://www.cdc.gov/mmwr/pdf/rr/rr6303.pdf.

Centers for Disease Control and Prevention: *Viral hepatitis surveillance 2014*, Atlanta, GA, 2014b, CDC. Retrieved August 2016 from http://www.cdc.gov/hepatitis/statistics/2014surveillance/pdfs/2014hepsurveillancerpt.pdf.

Centers for Disease Control and Prevention: *HIV Surveillance Report, 2014; vol. 26*, Atlanta, GA, 2015a, CDC. http://www.cdc.gov/hiv/library/reports/surveillance. Accessed June 19, 2017.

Centers for Disease Control and Prevention: *Gonorrhea: CDC fact sheet (detailed version)*, Atlanta, GA, 2015b, CDC. Retrieved June 19, 2017 from http://www.cdc.gov/std/gonorrhea/stdfact-gonorrhea-detailed.htm.

Centers for Disease Control and Prevention: Sexually transmitted diseases treatment guidelines, 2015, *MMWR Morb Mortal Wkly Rep* 64(RR3):1–137, Atlanta, GA, 2015c.

Centers for Disease Control and Prevention: *Sexually Transmitted Disease Surveillance 2014*, Atlanta, 2015d, US Department of Health and Human Services. Retrieved August 2016 from http://www.cdc.gov/std/stats14/surv-2014-print.pdf.

Centers for Disease Control and Prevention: *Genital herpes: CDC fact sheet, detailed version*, Atlanta, GA, 2015e, CDC. Retrieved August 2016 from http://www.cdc.gov/std/herpes/stdfact-herpes-detailed.htm.

Centers for Disease Control and Prevention: Use of 9-valent Human Papilloma Virus (HPV) vaccine: Updated HPV Vaccination Recommendations of the Advisory Committee on Immunizations Practices: Atlanta, GA, CDC, *MMWR* 64(11): 300–304, 2015f.

Centers for Disease Control and Prevention: *Viral hepatitis: testing and public health management of persons with chronic hepatitis B virus infection*, Atlanta, GA, 2015g, CDC. Retrieved August 2016 from http://www.cdc.gov/hepatitis/HBV/testingchronic.htm.

Centers for Disease Control and Prevention: *Hepatitis C FAQs for health professionals, overview and statistics*, Atlanta, GA, 2015h, CDC. Retrieved August 2016 from http://www.cdc.gov/hepatitis/hcv/hcvfaq.htm#section1.

Centers for Disease Control and Prevention: *Hepatitis C: how likely is hepatitis C to become chronic?* Atlanta, GA, 2015i, CDC. Retrieved August 2016 from http://www.cdc.gov/hepatitis/hcv/hcvfaq.htm#a8.

Centers for Disease Control and Prevention: *Reported Tuberculosis in the United States, 2014*, Atlanta, GA, 2015j, CDC. Retrieved August 2016 from http://www.cdc.gov/tb/statistics/reports/2014/default.htm.

Centers for Disease Control and Prevention: *About HIV/ AIDS—How do I know if I have HIV?* Atlanta, GA, 2016a. CDC. Retrieved June 19, 2017 from http://www.cdc.gov/hiv/basics/whatishiv.html.

Centers for Disease Control and Prevention: *HIV in the United States: at a glance*, Atlanta, 2016b, CDC. Retrieved August 2016 from http://www.cdc.gov/hiv/statistics/overview/ataglance.html.

Centers for Disease Control and Prevention: *Testing: HIV Basics/HIV/ AIDS*, 2016c, CDC. Available at http://www.cdc.gov/hiv/basics/testing.html. Accessed June 19, 2017.

Centers for Disease Control and Prevention: *Syphilis: CDC fact sheet (detailed version)*, Atlanta, GA, 2016d, CDC. Retrieved August 2016 from http://www.cdc.gov/std/syphilis/stdfact-syphilis-detailed.htm.

Centers for Disease Control and Prevention: *Chlamydia: CDC fact sheet (detailed version)*, Atlanta, GA, 2016e, CDC. Retrieved August 2016 from http://www.cdc.gov/std/chlamydia/stdfact-chlamydia-detailed.htm.

Centers for Disease Control and Prevention: *Genital HPV infection: CDC fact sheet*, Atlanta, GA, 2016f, CDC. Retrieved August 2016 from http://www.cdc.gov/std/hpv/stdfact-hpv.htm.

Centers for Disease Control and Prevention: *Viral hepatitis A: overview and statistics*, Atlanta, GA, 2016g, CDC. Retrieved August 2016 from http://www.cdc.gov/hepatitis/hav/havfaq.htm#general.

Centers for Disease Control and Prevention: *Hepatitis A vaccine: What you need to know*, Atlanta, GA, 2016h, CDC. Retrieved August 2016 from http://www.cdc.gov/vaccines/hcp/vis/vis-statements/hep-a.pdf.

Centers for Disease Control and Prevention: *Vaccines and immunizations: immunization schedule*, Atlanta, GA, 2016i, CDC. Retrieved August 2016 from http://www.cdc.gov/vaccines/schedules/index.html.

Centers for Disease Control and Prevention: *Basic TB facts*, Atlanta, GA, 2016j, CDC. Available at http://www.cdc.gov/TB/topic/basics/default.htm. Accessed June 19, 2017.

Centers for Disease Control and Prevention: *Testing for Tuberculosis, 2016*, Atlanta, GA, 2016k, CDC. Available at http://www.cdc.gov/tb/publications/factsheets/testing/TB_testing.htm. Accessed August, 2016.

Centers for Disease Control and Prevention: *Treatment for TB disease*, Atlanta, GA, 2016l, CDC. Retrieved June 19, 2017 from http://www.cdc.gov/tb/topic/treatment/tbdisease.htm.

Centers for Disease Control and Prevention: *HIV Prevention, 2016*, Atlanta, GA, 2016m, CDC. Available at http://www.cdc.gov/hiv/basics/prevention.html. Accessed August, 2016.

Council on Linkages Between Academic and Public Health Practice: *Core competencies for public health professionals*, Washington, DC, 2014, Public Health Foundation/Health Resource and Services Administration.

Fontenot HB, Fantasia HC, Charyk A, et al: Human papillomavirus (HPV) risk factors, vaccination patterns, and vaccine perceptions among a sample of male college students, *Journal of American College Health* 62(3):186–192, 2014. DOI: 10.1080/07448481.2013.872649.

Havlir D, Beyrer C: The beginning of the end of AIDS? *N Engl J Med* 367:685–687, 2012.

Heymann D: *Control of communicable diseases manual*, ed 20, Washington, DC, 2015, American Public Health Association.

National Institute on Aging: *Age Page: HIV, AIDS, and Older People*, Washington, DC, 2015. Retrieved August 2016 from https://www.nia.nih.gov/health/publication/hiv-aids-and-older-people.

Occupational Safety and Health Administration (OSHA): *Bloodborne pathogens and needlestick prevention*, n.d. Retrieved August 2016 from https://www.osha.gov/SLTC/bloodbornepathogens/standards.html.

UNAIDS: *Global AIDS Update 2016: UNAIDS fact sheet*, Geneva, 2016a, UNAIDS. Retrieved August 2016 from http://www.unaids.org/sites/default/files/media_asset/UNAIDS_FactSheet_en.pdf.

UNAIDS: *Global AIDS Update 2016*, Geneva, 2016b, UNAIDS. Retrieved August 2016 from http://www.unaids.org/sites/default/files/media_asset/global-AIDS-update-2016_en.pdf.

US Department of Health and Human Services: *About the Ryan White HIV/AIDS program: legislation*. Washington, DC, n.d., USDHHS. Retrieved August 2016 from http://hab.hrsa.gov/abouthab/legislation.html.

US Department of Health and Human Services: *Healthy People 2020*, Washington, DC, 2016a, US Government Printing Office. Retrieved August 2016 from https://www.healthypeople.gov/2020/topics-objectives.

US Department of Health and Human Services: *Guidelines for the use of antiretroviral agents in HIV-1-infected adults and adolescents*, Washington, DC, 2016b, USDHHS. Retrieved September 2016 from https://aidsinfo.nih.gov/contentfiles/lvguidelines/adultandadolescentgl.pdf.

US Department of Health and Human Services (USDHHS), Health Resources and Services Administration: *The HIV/AIDS Program: Part B-AIDS Drug Assistance Program*, Washington, DC, 2014, USDHHS. Available at http://hab.hrsa.gov/abouthab/partbdrug.html. Accessed August 15, 2016.

US Department of Justice: *Questions and answers: The Americans with Disabilities Act and persons with HIV/AIDS*, Washington, DC, 2012, USDJ. Retrieved August, 2016 from https://www.ada.gov/aids/ada_q&a_aids.pdf.

US Food and Drug Administration: *FDA approves first medication to reduce HIV risk*, Washington, DC, 2012, US FDA. Retrieved August 2016 from http://www.fda.gov/ForConsumers/ConsumerUpdates/ucm311821.htm.

US Preventive Services Task Force (USPSTF): *Screening for HIV: US Preventive Services Task Force Recommendation Statement*, 2013. Available at http://www.uspreventiveservicestaskforce.org/uspstf13/hiv/hivfinalrs.pdf. Accessed June 19, 2017.

US Public Health Service: *Pre-exposure prophylaxis for the prevention of HIV infection in the United States*, 2014. http://www.cdc.gov/hiv/pdf/PrEPguidelines2014.pdf.

World Health Organization (WHO): *The Stop TB Strategy*, Geneva, 2010, WHO Press. Available at http://www.who.int/tb/publications/2010/strategy_en.pdf?ua=1. Accessed June 19, 2017.

World Health Organization: *Tuberculosis: fact sheet*, Geneva, 2016, WHO. Retrieved August 2016 from http://www.who.int/mediacentre/factsheets/fs104/en/index.html.

28 | CHAPTER

Nursing Practice at the Local, State, and National Levels in Public Health

Lois Davis

OBJECTIVES

After reading this chapter, the student should be able to:

1. Define public health, public health system, public health nursing, and local, state, and national roles.
2. Identify trends in public health nursing.
3. Describe examples of public health nursing roles.
4. Assess the emerging public health issues that specifically affect public health nursing.
5. Describe the principles of partnerships.
6. Identify educational preparation of public health nurses and competencies necessary to practice.

CHAPTER OUTLINE

Roles of Local, State, and Federal Public Health Agencies
History and Trends of Public Health
Scope, Standards, and Roles of Nursing in Public Health
Issues and Trends in Public Health Nursing

Education and Knowledge Requirements for Public Health Nurses
National Health Objectives
Functions of Public Health Nurses

KEY TERMS

advocate, 505
assessor, 506
case manager, 505
disaster responders, 507
educator, 506
federal public health agencies, 499

incident commander, 507
local public health agencies, 499
outreach workers, 500
primary caregivers, 506
public health, 499
public health nurses, 501

public health programs, 498
referral resource, 506
role model, 506
state public health agency, 499

All of public health involves partnerships. Public health programs are designed with the goal of improving a population's health status. They go beyond the administration of health care to include the following:

- Community health assessment
- Community level interventions
- Analysis of health statistics
- Public education
- Outreach
- Case management
- Advocacy

- Recordkeeping
- Professional education for providers
- Disease surveillance and investigation
- Emergency preparedness and response
- Compliance with regulations for some institutions, agencies, and school systems
- Follow-up of population health problems
  The following are examples requiring follow-up care:
- Persons with active, untreated tuberculosis
- Pregnant women who have not kept prenatal visits
- Parents of underimmunized children

  Public health programs are frequently implemented by the development of partnerships or coalitions with other providers, agencies, and groups in the location being served. Nurses are involved in these activities in various ways depending on the public

The authors wish to thank Diane V. Downing for her previous contributions to this chapter.

BOX 28.1   Principles of Partnership

Community-Campus Partnerships for Health (CCPH) involved its members and partners in developing the following "principles of good practice" for community partnerships:

- The Partnership forms to serve a specific purpose and may take on new goals over time.
- The Partnership agrees upon mission, values, goals, measurable outcomes and processes for accountability.
- The relationship between partners in the Partnership is characterized by mutual trust, respect, genuineness, and commitment.
- The Partnership builds upon identified strengths and assets, but also works to address needs and increase capacity of all partners.
- The Partnership balances power among partners and enables resources among partners to be shared.
- Partners make clear and open communication an ongoing priority in the Partnership by striving to understand each other's needs and self-interests and developing a common language.
- Principles and processes for the Partnership are established with the input and agreement of all partners, especially for decision making and conflict resolution.
- There is feedback among all stakeholders in the Partnership, with the goal of continuously improving the Partnership and its outcomes.
- Partners share the benefits of the Partnership's accomplishments.
- Partnerships can dissolve, and when they do, need to plan a process for closure.
- Partnerships consider the nature of the environment within which they exist as a principle of their design, evaluation, and sustainability.
- The Partnership values multiple kinds of knowledge and life experiences.

From Community-Campus Partnerships for Health (CCPH) Board of Directors: *Position Statement of Authentic Partnerships. Community-Campus Partnerships for Health,* 2013. Available at https://ccph.memberclicks.net/principles-of-partnership. Accessed May 13, 2015.

health agency (local, state, federal) and the identified needs. The Community-Campus Partnerships for Health (CCPH) defines partnerships as "a close mutual cooperation between parties having common interests, responsibilities, privileges and power" (CCPH Board of Directors, 2013). A nurse may be the facilitator of the partnership or a member of the partnership representing the agency for which he or she works. Box 28.1 explains the principles of partnerships.

Public health is not a branch of medicine; it is an organized community approach designed to prevent disease, promote health, and protect populations. It works across many disciplines and is based on the scientific core of epidemiology (Institute of Medicine [IOM], 1988, 2003; Friis and Sellers, 2013). Nurses in public health work with multidisciplinary teams of people both within the public health areas and in other human services agencies. A critical partnership that shapes public health in the United States is the interaction of local, state, and federal agencies.

ROLES OF LOCAL, STATE, AND FEDERAL PUBLIC HEALTH AGENCIES

In the United States the local–state–federal partnership includes federal agencies, the state and territorial public health agencies, and the 3200 local public health agencies. The interaction of these agencies is critical to effectively use precious resources—financial and personnel—and protect and promote the health of populations. Nurses working in all of these agencies work together to identify, develop, and implement interventions that will improve and maintain the nation's health.

Federal public health agencies develop regulations that implement policies formulated by Congress and provide a significant amount of funding to state and territorial health agencies to do the following (IOM, 1988, 2003):

- Provide public health activities
- Survey the nation's health status and health needs
- Set practices and standards
- Provide expertise that facilitates evidence-based practice
- Coordinate public health activities that cross state lines
- Support health services research

The US Department of Health and Human Services (USDHHS) and the Environmental Protection Agency are the federal agencies that most influence public health activities at the state and local levels. The USDHHS includes the Centers for Disease Control and Prevention (CDC); the Health Resources and Services Administration; the Agency for Healthcare, Research, and Quality; and the US Food and Drug Administration. The USDHHS is the agency that facilitates development of the nation's *Healthy People* objectives (USDHHS, 2010).

Each of the states and territories has a single identified official **state public health agency** that is managed by a state health commissioner. The structure of state public health agencies varies. Some states require that the state health commissioner be a physician. A growing number of states do not limit the position to physicians, but rather require specific public health experience. California, Maryland, Iowa, Oregon, Washington, and Michigan are examples of states that focus on public health experience as a requirement for the state health commissioner position. This allows for the appointments of nurses and other professionals to this position. State public health agencies are responsible for monitoring health status and enforcing laws and regulations that protect and improve the public's health. These agencies receive funding from federal agencies for the implementation of public health interventions. The following are examples:

- Communicable disease programs
- Maternal and child health programs
- Chronic disease prevention programs
- Injury prevention programs

The agencies distribute federal and state funds to the local public health agencies to implement programs at the community level, and they provide oversight and consultation for local public health agencies. State health agencies also delegate some public health powers, such as the power to quarantine, to local health officers.

Local public health agencies have responsibilities that vary depending on the locality, but they are the agencies that are responsible for implementing and enforcing local, state, and federal public health codes and ordinances and providing essential public health programs to a community. The goal of the local public health department is to safeguard the public's health and improve the community's health status. The health department's authority is delegated by the state for specific functions (Box 28.2). As with state health departments, some states require that local

BOX 28.2 Local Public Health Agency Functions

The following are selected standards by selected essential public health services performed by local public health agencies:

Essential Public Health Service 1: Monitor Health Status to Identify Community Health Problems
- Obtain data that provide information on the community's health.
- Develop relationships with local providers and others in the community who have information on reportable diseases and other conditions of public health interest and facilitate information exchange.
- Conduct or contribute expertise to periodic community health assessments in order to develop a comprehensive picture of the public's health.
- Integrate data with other health assessment and data collection efforts conducted by the public health system.
- Analyze data to identify trends and population health risks.

Essential Public Health Service 4: Mobilize Community Partnerships to Identify and Solve Health Problems
- Engage the local public health system in an ongoing, strategic, community-driven, comprehensive planning process to identify, prioritize, and solve public health problems; establish public health goals; and evaluate success in meeting the goals.
- Promote the community's understanding of, and advocacy for, policies and activities that will improve the public's health.
- Develop partnerships to generate interest in and support for improved community health status, including new and emerging public health issues.

Essential Public Health Service 7: Link People to Needed Personal Health Services and Ensure the Provision of Health Care When Otherwise Unavailable
- Engage the community to identify gaps in culturally competent, appropriate, and equitable personal health services, including preventive and health promotion services, and develop strategies to close the gaps.
- Support and implement strategies to increase access to care and establish systems of personal health services, including preventive and health promotion services, in partnership with the community.
- Link individuals to available, accessible personal health care providers.

From National Association of County and City Health Officials: *Operational definition of a functional local health department*, 2014. Available at http://www.naccho.org. Accessed August 23, 2014.

health directors be physicians, whereas others focus on public health experience. For example, public health nurses in Maryland, Washington, Wisconsin, and California hold local health director positions. The duties of local health departments vary depending on the state and local public health codes and ordinances and the responsibilities assigned by the state and local governments. Usually, the local public health department provides for the administration, regulatory oversight, public health, and environmental services for a geographic area.

The majority of local, state, and federal public health agencies will be involved in the following:
- Collecting and analyzing vital statistics
- Providing health education and information to the population served
- Receiving reports about and investigating and controlling communicable diseases
- Protecting the environment to reduce the risk to health

- Providing some health services to particular populations at risk or with limited access to care (local public health agencies, guided by state and federal policies and goals and community needs)
- Planning for and responding to natural and human-made disasters and emergencies
- Identifying public health problems for at-risk and high-risk populations
- Conducting community assessments to identify community assets and gaps
- Partnering with other organizations to develop and implement responses to identified public health concerns

Nurses in public health work for local, state, and federal agencies. They work in partnership with each other, other public health staff, other governmental agencies, and the community to fulfill the functions of providing some health services to individuals, families, and groups who may have limited access to health care. They also engage in case finding to identify persons at risk for disease and those being lost to the health care system.

Other public health agency staffs include the following:
- Physicians
- Nutritionists
- Environmental health professionals
- Health educators
- Various laboratory workers
- Epidemiologists
- Health planners
- Paraprofessional home visitors
- Outreach workers

Examples of community-based organizations include the following:
- The United Way
- The American Red Cross
- Free clinics
- Head Start programs
- Daycare centers
- Community health centers
- Hospitals
- Senior centers
- Advocacy groups
- Churches
- Academic institutions
- Businesses

Other government agencies include the fire and emergency services department, law enforcement agencies, schools, parks and recreation departments, and elected officials. Changes in local, state, and federal governments affect public health services, and nursing has to develop strategies for dealing with these changes. To meet the changing needs of a community, nurses must identify public health concerns and work in programs to provide needed services.

HISTORY AND TRENDS OF PUBLIC HEALTH

A person born today can expect to live 30 years longer than a person born in 1900. Medical care accounts for 5 years of that increase, but public health is responsible for the additional 25 years through prevention efforts brought about by changes in social policies, community actions, and individual and group changes in behavior (USDHHS, 2010). Historically, nurses working in public health were valued by and important to society and functioned in an autonomous setting. They worked with populations and in settings that were not of interest to other health care disciplines or groups. Much public health service was delivered to the poor and to women and children, who did not have political power or voice. During the course of the 20th century, public health responsibilities expanded beyond communicable disease prevention, occupational health, and environmental health programs to include reproductive health, chronic disease prevention, and injury prevention activities.

As a result of Medicaid managed care, many public health agencies were no longer providing personal health care services. Public health agencies began to shift emphasis from a focus on primary health care services to a focus on core public health activities such as the investigation and control of diseases and injuries, community health assessment, community health planning, and involvement in environmental health activities. As the 20th century came to a close, genetics, newly emerging communicable diseases, preventing bioterrorism and violence, and handling and disposing of hazardous waste were emerging as additional public health issues (CDC, 2011; Schneider, 2017).

The Institute of Medicine (IOM, 2003) identified the following seven priorities for public health in the 21st century:
- Understand and emphasize the broad determinants of health.
- Develop a policy focus on population health.
- Strengthen the public health infrastructure.
- Build partnerships.
- Develop systems of accountability.
- Emphasize evidence-based practice.
- Enhance communication.

Public health activities at the beginning of the 21st century were shaped by the September 11, 2001, airplane attacks on the World Trade Center and the Pentagon and the plane crash into a field in Pennsylvania, in which thousands were murdered. However, public health activities at the federal, state, and local levels were even more dramatically affected by a series of anthrax exposures that occurred shortly after the airplane attacks. In addition to anthrax exposures in Florida and New York, a month after the plane attacks, thousands of workers at the Brentwood Post Office and the Senate Building in Washington, D.C., were exposed to an especially virulent strain of anthrax from a contaminated letter. The anthrax exposures alerted policymakers to the weakening public health infrastructure required to respond to bioterrorism events.

By the end of the 20th century, resources for communicable disease services had decreased as surveillance and containment activities and protection of water and food supplies produced decreasing rates of communicable disease. As the 21st century arrived, nurses in public health were faced with issues such as unprecedented influenza, tetanus, and childhood vaccine shortages and emerging infections that competed with bioterrorism activities for resources. As an example, in 2009 an outbreak of H1N1 occurred in the United States that led to President Barack

Obama declaring the outbreak a national emergency, and in 2015 and 2016 the emergence of the Ebola and Zika viruses in the United States alerted the public to how ill-prepared the country was to deal with public health concerns.

During the 20th century, public health nurses were a major force in the nation, achieving immunization rates that accounted for the dramatic decrease in measles. In 1996 nearly 900,000 fewer cases of measles were reported than in 1941 (Turnock, 2015). However, the general public was not informed about how this immunization activity was accomplished or about its effect on improving health and lowering health care cost. For public health services to receive adequate funding, it is necessary for the public and the government to be aware of the benefits provided to a community by nurses. A prime example of emerging infectious diseases in the 21st century is severe acute respiratory syndrome (SARS), caused by a virus, which brought illness and death to many in 2003. The disease spread quickly from China to other countries, being transported by airline passengers traveling internationally. The same means of transportation is a prime cause of other infectious diseases such as the Ebola and Zika viruses.

SCOPE, STANDARDS, AND ROLES OF NURSING IN PUBLIC HEALTH

In 1920, C. E. A. Winslow defined public health as "the science and art of preventing disease, prolonging life and promoting health and efficiency through organized community effort" (Turnock, 2015, p 11). This definition is still used in public health textbooks because it focuses on the relationship between social conditions and health across all levels of society. Nursing practice in public health focuses on the individuals, families, and groups in areas in which nurses live, work, and play. Nurses educated as public health nurses work with communities and populations.

Additional knowledge, skills, and aptitudes are necessary for a nurse to go beyond focusing on the health needs of the individual to focusing on the health needs of populations (see Chapter 1). This additional knowledge distinguishes the public health nurse from other nurses who are practicing in the community setting.

A variety of settings and a diversity of perspectives are available to nurses interested in developing a career in public health. Nurses working at the federal, state, and local levels integrate community involvement and knowledge about the entire population with clinical understandings of the health and illness experiences of individuals and families in the population. They translate and articulate the health and illness experiences of diverse, often vulnerable individuals and families in the population to health planners and policymakers, and they help members of the community voice their problems and aspirations. Nurses are knowledgeable about multiple strategies for intervention, focusing primarily on those for the family and the individual. They translate knowledge from the health and social sciences to individuals and population groups through targeted interventions, programs, and advocacy. Nurses are directly engaged in the interdisciplinary activities of the core public health functions of assessment, assurance, and policy development. In any setting, the role of the nurse focuses on the prevention of illness, injury, or disability and on the promotion and maintenance of the health of populations (American Nurses Association, 2013; American Public Health Association, Public Health Nursing Section, 2013; Public Health Nursing Section, 2001).

Public health nurses deliver services within the framework of ever-constricting resources coupled with emerging and complex public health issues. This requires the efficient, equitable, and evidence-based use of resources. The National Public Health Performance Standards Program (CDC, 2015), a federal, state, and local partnership, has developed evaluation instruments that can be used to collect and analyze data on the programs provided through state and local public health systems. The instruments link with the 10 essential services of public health that define the core functions of public health (see Chapter 1).

Nurses make a significant difference in improving the health of a community by monitoring and assessing critical health status indicators such as the following:

- Immunization levels
- Communicable diseases
- Infant mortality

On the basis of their assessment and in partnership with the community, nurses advocate for evidence-based interventions to respond to negative health status indicators. Nurses provide the link for people who need personal health services and ensure health care when it is needed and not available elsewhere (USDHHS, 2010).

A shift in the focus of public health from being the primary care provider of last resort to developing partnerships to meet the health promotion and disease prevention needs of populations in a community has raised concerns about available health care for the uninsured and underinsured. The nurses' role in this ongoing shift in health care delivery is still being developed for many agencies. Nurses retain responsibility for ensuring that all populations have access to affordable, quality health care services. They accomplish this by the following:

- Providing clinical preventive services to certain high-risk populations
- Establishing programs and services to meet special needs
- Recommending clinical care and other services to clients and their families in clinics, homes, and the community
- Providing referrals through community links to needed care
- Participating in community provider coalitions and meetings to educate others and identify service centers for community populations
- Providing clinical surveillance and identification of communicable disease

Levels of Prevention

Related to Nurses in Public Health

Primary Prevention
- Partnering with the community to conduct a community health assessment to identify community assets and gaps
- Partnering with the community to develop programs that target root causes, with a focus on primary prevention in response to identified gaps
- Providing information about safe-sex practices
- Educating daycare center personnel and families about the dangers of lead-based paint
- Educating daycare center personnel, school staff, and the general community about the importance of hand hygiene to prevent transmission of communicable diseases
- Inspecting daycare centers, nursing homes, and hospitals to ensure client safety and quality of care
- Providing immunizations
- Advocating for issues such as mandatory seat-belt legislation, smoke-free environments, and universal access to health care
- Providing no-charge infant car seats accompanied by classes in the use of safety seats
- Identifying environmental hazards such as housing quality, playground safety, pedestrian safety, and product safety hazards and working with the community and policymakers to mitigate the identified hazards
- Developing social networking interventions to modify community norms related to sexual risk behaviors, condom use, and abstinence
- Controlling mosquito larva through treatment in areas frequented by populations 55 years of age and over
- Working with communities to develop citizen emergency preparedness plans

Secondary Prevention
- Identifying and treating clients in a sexually transmitted disease (STD) clinic
- Identifying and treating clients with tuberculosis (TB) infection and disease in a TB clinic
- Providing directly observed therapy (DOT) for clients with active TB
- Conducting contacting and tracing for individuals exposed to a client with an active case of TB or an STD
- Conducting lead-screening activities for children
- Conducting ongoing disease surveillance for communicable diseases and implementing control measures when an outbreak is identified
- Implementing screening programs for genetic disorders and metabolic deficiencies in newborns; breast, cervical, and testicular cancer; diabetes; hypertension; and sensory impairments in children and ensuring follow-up services for clients with positive results
- Conducting syndromic surveillance to ensure early identification of victims in an influenza epidemic or bioterrorism event
- Providing low-cost antibiotics for treatment of Lyme disease
- Conducting enhanced surveillance for novel influenza virus infection among travelers with severe unexplained respiratory illness returning from affected countries
- Establishing mass dispensing clinics for antibiotic distribution in response to a bioterrorism event or influenza pandemic

Tertiary Prevention
- Providing case management services that link clients with chronic illnesses to health care and community support services
- Providing case management services that link clients with serious mental illnesses to mental health and community support services
- Educating at rehabilitation centers to help clients with stroke optimize their functioning.
- Establishing an alternative treatment site for victims of a smallpox epidemic

From US Department of Health and Human Services: *Healthy People 2020: National Health Promotion and Disease Prevention Objectives, 2010.* Available @ www.healthypeople.gov. Accessed May 13, 2015

Case management at the community level is a renewed effort in nursing. Through case management activities, nurses link persons with needed health care providers (see Chapter 13).

Uninsured individuals seek services on a sliding payment scale from sources such as university clinics, public hospital clinics, neighborhood health centers, or one of the variety of free clinics. Nurses serve as a bridge between these populations and the resource needs for this at-risk group by approaching health care providers on behalf of individuals seeking medical or health services and keeping the needs of this population on the political agenda. Frequently, low-income populations or populations with multiple chronic illnesses lack the knowledge and skills to negotiate the complex health care system. This population needs the following:

- Education and training in identifying their problems
- Approaches to self-care
- Illness prevention strategies
- Lifestyle choices that will have an effect on their health

The nurse understands the barriers these populations confront, such as transportation and difficulty understanding and following health care provider instructions.

Although vulnerable populations have always benefited from nursing services, the populations that are most acutely in need of public health services have changed dramatically over the past two decades. Of particular concern are the number of young women and their partners who are substance abusers and have risky behaviors that put their pregnancy or children at high risk for injury or abuse. Nurses at the federal, state, and local levels have developed innovative, collaborative approaches to prepare staff to work effectively with this population.

The population and public health are benefiting from the passing of the Affordable Care Act (2010). The Affordable Care Act provides for the Prevention Fund for an expanded and sustained national investment in prevention and public health programs that will improve health and help restrain the rate of growth in private- and public-sector health care costs. The law provides for many preventive services to be free so that health care issues can be caught early or totally prevented. The senior members of the population and children receive free preventive services, Medicaid coverage has been expanded, and more access to home health and community services is available (USDHHS, 2014).

ISSUES AND TRENDS IN PUBLIC HEALTH NURSING

The discovery and development of antibiotics in the 1940s, coupled with immunization programs and improvements in sanitation, contributed to the decrease in infectious disease–related morbidity and mortality during the 20th century (CDC, 2011; Rosen, 2015). Twenty-first-century issues facing nurses in public health include the following:

- Increasing rates of drug resistance to community-acquired pathogens
- Social issues such as welfare reform
- Racial and ethnic disparities in health outcomes
- Behaviorally influenced issues (e.g., chronic diseases, violence in society, substance abuse)
- Emergency preparedness activities

- Emerging infections
- Unequal access to health care

Nurses must keep abreast of the issues that affect all of society. Assessments need to be changed to include the factors that affect the populations they serve.

For example, a major 21st-century public health challenge is emerging infections resulting from drug-resistant organisms. The widespread, often inappropriate use of antimicrobial drugs has resulted in a loss of effectiveness for some community-acquired infections such as gonorrhea, pneumococcal infections, and tuberculosis (TB), and increasing rates of drug resistance in community-acquired pathogens such as *Streptococcus pneumonia, Escherichia coli,* and *Salmonella* species (World Health Organization [WHO], 2014). The nurse can influence this trend by objecting to inappropriate use of antibiotics by providers and educating individuals, families, health care providers, and the community about the dangers of misuse and overuse of antibiotics.

Social issues such as welfare and health insurance reform will influence a population's ability to obtain preventive health services either because of providers not accepting government-sponsored health care coverage or because the low-wage jobs they take do not allow time off for health care.

When child care is an issue for the welfare mother returning to work, effects on the individual, family, community, and population must be considered. Nurses assess the problem and determine what is wrong with a system that forces parents to go to work so they can be removed from welfare rolls but does not provide for child care. The question to be answered by a nurse is: What will it take to change the system?

Partnerships and collaboration among groups are much more powerful in making change than the individual client and nurse working alone. As another example, the depressed, nonfunctional mother in need of counseling is a significant public health concern because the needs of the mother, children, and family are not being met. Frequently, the problem may not be obvious to the health professional who sees this woman for the first time. Nurses have special preparation to help them both identify the individual's problem and look at its effects on the broader community. In this example, consider the following:

- The children may grow to be adults with mental health problems.
- The mental health services of the community services will need to be able to handle the increase in this population.
- Children may become violent adults, resulting in a need for more correction facilities.
- Mothers may need additional mental health services.
- Children may be absent from school often and may not be able to contribute to society.
- Adults may be nonproductive in the workplace because absence from school leads to lack of skills.

Often, one problem of the single individual places great burdens on the community.

Healthy People 2020 includes objectives to address racial and ethnic disparities in health outcomes (USDHHS, 2010). The IOM (2002) reports that disparities in health care treatment account for some of the gaps in health outcomes between racial and ethnic groups. This report found that minority groups receive lower-quality health care than Caucasian people, regardless of insurance status, income, and severity of the condition. This report is supported by the National Healthcare Quality and Disparities Report (Agency for Healthcare Research and Quality, 2015). The report indicates that access to health care did not improve for most racial and ethnic groups in the years 2002 through 2008, leading up to enactment of the Patient Protection and Affordable Care Act of 2010. The data contained in the National Healthcare Disparities Report and the companion National Healthcare Quality Report predate the Patient Protection and Affordable Care Act; however, some provisions in the new health care law are improving health care quality and addressing health care disparities. The USDHHS Action Plan to Reduce Health Disparities, announced in April 2011, outlines goals and actions to reduce health disparities among racial and ethnic minorities, building on important efforts made possible by the Patient Protection and Affordable Care Act and other ongoing initiatives.

Nurses work as case managers and at the policy level to promote equal access to health care, including health literature and spoken services that reflect the community in which the services are being delivered. The nurse working directly as a case manager or in a clinic setting can promote culturally and linguistically appropriate services by partnering with other community agencies, such as interpreter services. Equal access to health care can be facilitated by identifying and alerting the community to gaps in services available in the community. For example, some communities may appear to have an adequate number of pediatricians to meet the community's needs. However, a community assessment may reveal that the community is home to a high number of children who rely on Medicaid as payment for services or to families whose primary language is not English. Matching this information with the pediatrician population may reveal that none of the pediatricians accept Medicaid as payment for services or that they all deliver services in English only.

EDUCATION AND KNOWLEDGE REQUIREMENTS FOR PUBLIC HEALTH NURSES

The Association of Community Health Nursing Educators states that the educational preparation of public health nurses should be at least a baccalaureate degree. Those who have associate degrees are encouraged to seek further degrees because of the increasing complexity of better care delivery in public health.

The Council on Linkages Between Academia and Public Health Practice (2001, 2010, 2014) examined a decade of work to identify a list of core public health competencies that represent a set of skills, knowledge, and attitudes necessary for the broad practice of public health. They capture the crosscutting competencies necessary for all disciplines that work in public health, including nurses, physicians, environmental health specialists, health educators, and epidemiologists. The competencies are applied (at the three skill levels of *aware,* *knowledgeable,* and *proficient*) to three job categories of entry level, supervisors/managers, and senior managers/CEOs. For more information on the list of core competencies by job category and skill level, see Appendix C.3. In addition to having the core public health competencies, public health nurses have specialized competencies, as described in the *Scope and Standards of Public Health Nursing Practice* (American Nurses Association, 2013). The core public health competencies are divided into the following eight domains:

1. Analytic assessment skills
2. Basic public health sciences skills
3. Cultural competency skills
4. Communication skills
5. Community dimensions of practice skills
6. Financial planning and management skills
7. Leadership and systems thinking skills
8. Policy development and program planning skills

Many of these core public health competencies are provided by nurses who have learned these skills in the workplace while gaining knowledge through years of practice. Rapid changes in public health are providing a challenge to nurses in that neither the time nor the staff is available to provide as much on-the-job training as is needed to learn and upgrade skills and knowledge of staff. Nurses with baccalaureate or master's preparation are needed to provide a strong public health system (see Chapter 1).

CASE STUDY
Sudden Infant Death

Four-year-old David had a near–sudden infant death episode when he was 4 months old. His father was able to revive David with cardiopulmonary resuscitation (CPR) but not before his brain had become anoxic. David was left a blind quadriplegic with little or no ability to communicate, even after having spent many months in a hospital.

When nurse Margaret Moore first started visiting David, he was receiving tube feedings and personal care from his mother. (His father had left the home, saying he could not stand seeing his son in this debilitated state.) David's mother, Brandy Johnson, received emotional support from her mother and sister, who stopped by when they could. David was enrolled three mornings per week in a special education program for children with cerebral palsy and other severe disabilities. Those mornings, Ms. Johnson worked at a minimum-wage job bagging groceries. Some days she made extra money caring for a niece after school in her home. The rest of the time she cared for David; her only outlet was to write mournful poetry when he slept.

Ms. Moore's visits involved checking David's physical status and determining what care and support the two needed. One week she realized that David was getting too big for his car seat because he had grown to 45 pounds, yet regular car seats assumed that a child that size could sit by himself. She had to find a source and some funding for the specially adapted $250 car seat he needed.

Ms. Moore worried about Ms. Johnson's mental health given that she was a young woman alone, with no car, and unable to have the normal experiences of a young woman. The nurse found a community support group for parents of disabled children, located on the bus line, in which parents could share their experiences with one another. She also found a group that met once per month that was interested in poetry writing. Ms. Johnson had trouble getting her calls returned from the program in which she needed to enroll David to get some help caring for her son. Ms. Moore also got no response to her calls to that agency, so she made a visit in person; she was able to get David enrolled quickly.

Created by Deborah C. Conway, Assistant Professor, School of Nursing, University of Virginia.

NATIONAL HEALTH OBJECTIVES

Since 1979 the US Surgeon General has worked with local, state, and federal agencies, the private sector, and the US population to develop health objectives for the nation. These objectives are revisited every 10 years. In 2010 the USDHHS released *Healthy People 2020*. These objectives will guide the work of public health nurses over the next decade.

State health departments play a key role in implementing the *Healthy People* objectives. Examples of state *Healthy People 2020* goals can be located on the *Healthy People* website at http://www.healthypeople.gov/2020/implement/StateSpecificPlans.aspx. State health departments help set local goals using the *Healthy People 2020* objectives as a framework. Knowing that public health departments do not have the resources to accomplish these goals independently, collaboration is essential to quality nursing practice and is encouraged at the local level with existing groups. New partnerships are developed related to specific goals. Communities develop coalitions to address selected objectives, based on community needs, to include all of the local community stakeholders, such as social services, mental health, education, recreation, government, and businesses. Membership varies across communities depending on that community's formal and informal structure. The groups join the coalition for a variety of reasons. For example, businesses see the value of developing a productive workforce that will be of importance to them and the community in the future.

The *Healthy People 2020* objectives are developed to achieve the four major goals of attaining high-quality and longer healthy life, achieving health equity and eliminating health disparities, creating environments that promote good health for all, and promoting quality of life (USDHHS, 2010). Nurses help clients identify unhealthy behaviors and then help them develop strategies to improve their health. Some of the behaviors addressed by nurses are tobacco use, physical activity, and nutritional habits that lead to obesity, all of which affect quality and years of healthy life. Nurses also organize the community to conduct community health assessments to identify where health disparities exist and target interventions to address those disparities. For example, community health assessments may disclose that certain populations are at higher risk for the following:
- Asthma
- Diabetes
- Low immunization rates
- Heavy cigarette smoking
- Exposure to environmental hazards

The following are some *Healthy People 2020* Immunization and Infectious Disease areas of focus:
- Vaccine-preventable infectious diseases
- Emerging antimicrobial resistance
- Human immunodeficiency virus (HIV)
- Acquired immunodeficiency syndrome (AIDS)
- Sexually transmitted diseases (STDs)
- Pneumococcal infections
- Tuberculosis

HEALTHY PEOPLE 2020

The following selected national health objectives relate to the public health infrastructure:
- **PHI-1:** Increase the proportion of federal, tribal, state, and local public health agencies that incorporate core competencies for public health professionals into job descriptions and performance evaluations.
- **PHI-4:** Increase the proportion of 4-year colleges and universities that offer public health or related majors or minors.
- **PHI-13:** Increase the proportion of tribal, state, and local public health agencies that provide or ensure comprehensive epidemiology services to support essential public health services.
- **PHI-14:** Increase the proportion of state and local public health jurisdictions that conduct performance assessment and improvement activities in the public health system using national standards.
- **PHI-15:** Increase the proportion of tribal, state, and local public health agencies that have implemented a health improvement plan and increase the proportion of local health jurisdictions that have implemented a health improvement plan linked with their state plan.

From U.S. Department of Health and Human Services: *Healthy People 2020: national health promotion and disease prevention objectives,* Washington, DC, 2010. USDHHS. Retrieved 6/21/16from http://healthypeople.gov/2020/.

To help clients reduce their risk for acquiring a communicable disease, nurses provide clients with instructions on the use of barrier methods of contraception and information on the hazards of multiple sexual partners and street drug use. Getting a complete sexual history on all clients coming to the health department for services takes special skills but is essential to determine the behaviors that have brought the client to the local health department. Abstinence as a birth control method can be addressed with all populations. Education of young persons before they become sexually active has helped reduce the incidence of some STDs in this population.

FUNCTIONS OF PUBLIC HEALTH NURSES

Nurses in public health have many functions, depending on the needs and resources of an area. **Advocate** is one of the many roles of the nurse. As an advocate, the nurse collects, monitors, and analyzes data and discusses with the client which services are needed and whether the client is an individual, a family, or a group. The nurse and the client then develop the most effective plan and approach to take, and the nurse helps the client implement the plan so the client can become more independent in making decisions and obtaining the services needed.

Case manager is a major role for nurses. Nurses use the nursing process of assessing, planning, implementing, and evaluating outcomes to meet clients' needs. Clear and complex communications are frequently an important component of case management. Other health and social agency participants may not be familiar with the home and community living conditions that are known to the nurse. It is the nurse who has been there and seen the living conditions and who can tell the story for the client or assist the individual or family with the telling of their story. Case managers assist clients in identifying and obtaining the services they need the most at the least cost. For example, a nurse may go into the home to visit a new mother and baby. On assessment, the nurse may find that the mother needs help in finding a new job, child care, and a pediatrician and assistance in finding health insurance. The nurse helps the mother in the following ways:

- Assists with prioritizing the problems
- Helps make a plan for resolving the problems
- Contacts other agencies on behalf of the mother when needed
- Follows up with the mother to see if the problems are being resolved
- Follows up with the agencies, such as social services, to make certain the mother's request to enroll her children in the State Children's Health Insurance Program has been honored

Nurses are a major referral resource. They maintain current information about health and social services available within the community. They know what resources will be acceptable to the client within the social and cultural norms for that group. The nurse educates clients to enable them to use the resources and to learn self-care. Nurses refer to other services in the area, and other services refer to the nurse for care or follow-up. For example, the mother and new baby may be referred to the nurse for postnatal care with postpartum home visit follow-up.

Assessor of literacy is a large part of nursing in public health. Many individuals are limited in their ability to read, write, and communicate clearly. The nurse has to be culturally sensitive and aware of the specific areas of unique problems of clients, such as financial limitations that may in turn limit educational opportunities. Frequently, when persons go to a physician's office, clinic, or hospital, they are clean and neatly dressed. The assumption is made that when they nod at the health care provider, it means that they understand what has been said. This is frequently not the case, but the client is embarrassed to admit that he or she does not understand what has been said. Being illiterate does not mean a person is mentally slow. It is important for the nurse to follow up on the many contacts the individual or family has with medical, social, and legal services to clarify what is understood and to find an answer to the questions that have not been asked by the client or answered by the services.

The nurse is an educator, teaching to the level of the client so that the information received is information that can be used. Patience and repetitions over time are necessary to develop trust and enable the client to use the relationship with the nurse for more information. As educator, the public health nurse identifies community needs (e.g., playground safety, hand hygiene, pedestrian safety, safe-sex practices) and develops and implements educational activities aimed at changing behaviors over time.

Nurses in public health are direct primary caregivers in many situations, both in the clinic and in the community. Where the nurse provides primary care is determined by community assessment and is usually in response to an identified gap to which the private sector is unable to respond, coupled with an assessment of the effect of the gap in services on the health of the population. Examples include the following:

- Prenatal services for uninsured women
- Free or low-cost immunization services for targeted populations
- Directly observed therapy for clients with active TB
- Treatment for STDs

Nurses ensure that direct care services are available in the community for at-risk populations by working with the community to develop programs that will meet the needs of those populations. Currently, no system of outreach service in the medical models of care addresses the multiple needs of high-risk populations. High-risk populations frequently do not understand the medical, social, educational, or judicial system and the professional languages, codes of behavior, or expected outcomes of these services. Clients need a case manager, a health educator, an advocate, and a role model to enable them to benefit from these services and to teach them how to avoid complex and expensive problems in the future. The local nurse in public health fills these roles and many more for this population. These are examples of the difficult clinical issues that nurses face in making ethical and professional decisions.

The nurse's role in public health is unique and essential in many situations. Access to homes gives the nurse information that usually cannot be gathered in the hospital or clinic setting. The nurse learns to ask intimate questions creatively and to seek

EVIDENCE-BASED PRACTICE

Nurse–Family Partnership

The Nurse–Family Partnership home visitation program provides rigorously defined nurse home visits to first-time low-income mothers. It is an evidence-based public health program that has been rigorously evaluated in three randomized, controlled trials. Results demonstrated improvements in birth outcomes, prenatal health, child development, school readiness, and academic achievement, and reductions in child abuse, neglect, and early childhood injuries. A recent study questioned the Nurse–Family Partnership program restriction to only first-time mothers. In this longitudinal, prospective study, researchers Lanier and Jonson-Reid (2014) compared primiparous ($n = 1370$) and multiparous ($n = 1890$) mothers participating a nurse home visiting program, Nurses for Newborns (NFN). Results showed multiparous mothers had higher cumulative risk scores and individual risk factors related to maternal and child health, behavioral health, and violence exposure. A significant trend emerged among more children and greater caregiver stress, maternal depression, and child maltreatment. The researchers found that although the multiparous mothers were at higher risk, they had similar levels of service use as the primiparous mothers. The researchers concluded that programs limited to primiparous mothers were missing a critical opportunity for prevention. Furthermore, programs that serve multiparous mother should incorporate strategies to directly address caregiver stress and postpartum depression.

Nurse Use

The passage of the Patient Protection and Affordable Care Act in 2010 sparked an expansion of evidence-based early childhood home visiting services in the United States. As such, nurses need to explore issues of participant engagement and whom to target with limited resources.

Data from Lanier P, Jonson-Reid M: Comparing primiparous and multiparous mothers in a nurse home visiting prevention program, *BIRTH*, 41(4): 344-352, 2014.

information that will facilitate case management and provide the clinical and social care needed, including other community resources. Careful attention must be paid to privacy and confidentiality in delivering these nursing services. The credibility of the nurse and the agency depends on the professional handling of the public health information by each staff member.

When an emergency or disaster occurs, nurses at the local, state, and federal levels have multiple roles in assessment, planning, implementing, and evaluating needs and resources for the different populations being served. Whether the disaster is local or national, small or large, natural or caused by humans, nurses are skilled professionals essential to the team. As a health care facility, the local public health department has an emergency operations plan, as well as a role in the local, regional, and state disaster plans. In these situations, the nurse is called upon to be the incident commander. Nurses in this role take on functions that include the following:

- Providing education that will prepare communities to cope with disasters
- Establishing mass-dispensing clinics
- Conducting enhanced communicable disease surveillance
- Working with environmental health specialists to ensure safe food and water for disaster victims and emergency workers
- Serving on the local emergency planning committee

Their presence may be required in other regions of the state or country to provide official nursing duties in a time of crisis, such as a hurricane, that requires a lengthy period of recovery. Each governmental jurisdiction has an emergency plan. The public health agency is expected to provide planning and staffing during a disaster. These local emergency preparedness plans may be multigovernmental, which requires coordination among communities.

Essential and unique roles for nurses in public health exist in the area of communicable disease control. Nursing skills are necessary for education, prevention, surveillance, and outbreak investigation. Nurses can do the following:

- Find infected individuals
- Notify contacts
- Refer to other health providers or agencies for care
- Administer treatments
- Educate the individual, family, community, professionals, and populations
- Act as advocate for the clients
- Use state-of-the-art resources to reduce the rate of communicable disease in the community

CHECK YOUR PRACTICE

As a nurse in the local health department, you have been asked to be the incident commander for a recent outbreak of pertussis in the community. What would you do?

The communicable disease role is one of the most important roles for nursing during disasters. During the September 11, 2001 airplane attacks, nurses at the federal, state, and local levels immediately implemented active enhanced surveillance activities. Information about communicable diseases seen at the local level was passed on to the state public health agency and finally to the CDC. At each step, the data were analyzed for evidence of unusual disease trends.

It is important for nurses in public health to practice confidentiality when they have knowledge about an individual, family, communicable disease outbreak, community-level problem, or any special knowledge obtained in the public health work setting.

When October 2001 alerts from the CDC began presenting information about a photo editor in Florida who had been hospitalized with inhalation of anthrax, nurses in public health and hospital infection control practitioners throughout the nation increased activity. Public health response to disasters requires that resources be redirected temporarily from other programs while maintaining programs that will prevent additional outbreaks. Therefore nurses not normally involved in communicable disease activities can be shifted to this function. The exposures resulting from the anthrax-tainted letters presented unprecedented public health challenges. The Washington, DC anthrax exposures resulted in thousands of possible work-related exposures, five cases of inhalation anthrax in the region, and two deaths over a period of months. Public health at the federal, state, and local levels was looked to for coordinated leadership and answers to a situation in which experience was limited and answers were uncertain. Although communicable disease control is a core public health service, the role of public health as incident commander in a widespread public health emergency is a new role. The following were issues to be addressed:

- How to conduct mass treatment in response to a bioterrorism event
- Which jurisdiction is in charge
- How to communicate unclear information to the public
- Who should take antibiotics and for how long and resolving this rapidly across jurisdictional and agency lines

The anthrax exposures are typical of the nature of public health emergencies. They unfold as the communicable disease moves through communities.

Nurses in public health are essential partners in disaster drills. In Virginia, an electrical company has a nuclear plant that requires annual multijurisdictional disaster drills. These disaster planning and practice sessions are an opportunity for local nurses to get to know other agencies' representatives and to let them know what nursing can offer. Because nurses are out in the communities and have assessment skills, they are essential in evaluating how the disaster was handled and in making suggestions about how future events might be managed. To be most effective as disaster responders, nurses have to be a part of the team *before* an emergency. Knowing what type of disaster is likely to occur in a community is essential for planning. Types of disasters vary from place to place, but there is a history of past events and how they were handled, as well as resources and training from regional, state, and federal agencies. Nurses can help educate the public about the individual responsibilities and preparations that can be in place for both the person and the community. Nurses at the local, state, and federal levels work in partnership to accomplish each function (see the Levels of Prevention box on page 502).

QSEN FOCUS ON QUALITY AND SAFETY EDUCATION FOR NURSES

Public Health Nursing at Local, State, and National Levels

Targeted Competency: Teamwork and Collaboration—Function effectively within nursing and interprofessional teams, fostering open communication, mutual respect, and shared decision making to achieve quality patient care. Important aspects of teamwork and collaboration include the following:

- **Knowledge:** Describe scopes of practice and roles of health care team members.
- **Skills:** Integrate the contributions of others who play a role in helping client/family achieve health goals.
- **Attitudes:** Respect the unique attributes that members bring to a team, including variations in professional orientations and accountabilities.

Teamwork and Collaboration Question

Your state has recently been awarded funding from the Centers for Disease Control and Prevention to prevent the spread of viral hepatitis through increased testing, improving access to care, and strengthening surveillance to detect viral hepatitis transmission and disease. You are a staff nurse for the local Public

Health Department and currently serve on the Infectious Disease Prevention (IDP) committee. The IDP committee has been given the responsibility to determine how to best utilize this new funding to effectively meet the objectives of the grant. Consider the following:

- As a staff nurse for the local Public Health Department, what is your role in addressing this initiative within the community? How would your role change if you were a public health nurse working at the state health department?
- In addition to nursing, give examples of other professionals who likely serve on the IDP committee with you. Describe the role of each professional on this committee.
- Identify local and state organizations in your community that you would recommend that the IDP committee collaborate with to develop and implement a response to identified issues.
- Through this grant, your state is addressing several objectives in the *Healthy People 2020* focus area of Immunization and Infectious Diseases. Go to the *Healthy People 2020* website and identify which specific objectives would apply to this initiative.

Prepared by Lisa Turner, PhD, RN, PHCNS-BC, Assistant Professor, Berea College Nursing Program, Berea, Kentucky.

▶ APPLYING CONTENT TO PRACTICE

This chapter focuses on the role of the nurse in public health in local, state, and national health initiatives. The history of public health has changed throughout the decades, and the nurse is currently involved in keeping the community and clients safe from emerging infectious diseases and is more focused on managing disasters. There is an increasing expansion of the functions of public health as well as the roles of the nurse in public health. Not only does the nurse function

as a case manager, referral source, assessor, educator, advocate, and role model to the community and provide direct-care services that may not otherwise be available but now also serves as an incident commander for urgent and emergent situations in the community. Education for the public health nurse is key to assisting the nurse in performing these functions. The competencies needed by the nurse in public health are discussed in each of the previous chapters.

■ PRACTICE APPLICATION

A retirement community in a small town reported to the local health department 24 cases of severe gastrointestinal illness that had occurred among residents and staff of the facility during the past 24 to 36 hours. It was determined that the ill clients became sick within a short, well-defined period and that most recovered within 24 hours without treatment. The communicable disease outbreak team, composed of nurses, public health physicians, and an environmental health specialist, was called to respond to this possible epidemic.

How should they respond to this situation?

A. Call the Centers for Disease Control and Prevention and ask for help with surveillance.
B. Send all the ill persons in the retirement community to the hospital.
C. Evaluate the agent, host, and environment relationships to determine the cause of the problem.
D. Close the dining room and find another source to provide food to the residents.

Answers can be found on the Evolve website.

■ REMEMBER THIS!

- Local public health departments are responsible for implementing and enforcing local, state, and federal public health codes and ordinances while providing essential public health services.
- The goal of the local health department is to safeguard the public's health and improve the community's health status.
- Nursing in community health is the practice of promoting and protecting the health of populations using knowledge from nursing and social and public health sciences.
- Public health is based on the scientific core of epidemiology.
- Marketing of nursing in public health is essential to inform both professionals and the public about the

  opportunities and challenges of populations in public health care.
- A driving force behind nursing changes is the economy and the increase in managed care.
- Nurses need ongoing education and training as public health changes.
- Some of the roles in which nurses function are advocate, case manager, referral source, counselor, primary care provider, educator, outreach worker, and disaster responder.
- Nurses have an important role in helping with local disasters, including planning, staffing, and evaluating events.

ⓔ EVOLVE WEBSITE

http://evolve.elsevier.com/Stanhope/foundations
- Case Study, with Questions and Answers
- NCLEX® Review Questions
- Practice Application Answers

REFERENCES

Agency for Healthcare Research and Quality: *National healthcare quality and disparities report and 5th anniversary update on the national quality strategy*, Rockville, MD, 2015, AHRQ. Retrieved August 2016 from http://www.ahrq.gov/research/findings/nhqrdr/nhqdr15/index.html.

American Nurses Association: *Public health nursing: scope and standards of practice*, Silver Spring, Md, 2013, ANA.

American Public Health Association, Public Health Nursing Section: *The definition and practice of public health nursing: a statement of public health nursing section*, Washington, DC, 2013, APHA.

Centers for Disease Control and Prevention: *Ten public health achievements of first decade of 21st century*, Atlanta, 2011, CDC. Retrieved July 2016 from http://www.cdc.gov/about/history/tengpha.htm/.

Centers for Disease Control and Prevention: *National public health performance standards program (NPHPSP)*, Atlanta, GA, June 2015, CDC. Retrieved July 2016 from http://www.cdc.gov/nphpsp/.

Community Campus Partnerships for Health Board of Directors: *Position Statement of Authentic Partnerships*, 2013. Retrieved from CCPH 2013. Available at https//ccph.memberclickes.net. Accessed May 13, 2015.

Council on Linkages Between Academia and Public Health Practice: *Core competencies for public health professionals*, Washington, DC, 2001, Public Health Foundation.

Council on Linkages Between Academia and Public Health Practice: *Tier 1, tier 2, and tier 3 core competencies for public health professionals*, Washington, DC, 2010, Public Health Foundation. Retrieved September 2012 from http://www.phf.org/resourcestools/documents/core_public_health_competencies_iii.pdf.

Council on Linkages Between Academia and Public Health Practice: *Core competencies for public health professionals*, Washington, DC,

2014, PHF. Retrieved August 2016 from http://www.phf.org/programs/council/Pages/default.aspx/corecompetencies.htm.

Friis RH, Sellers TA: *Epidemiology for public health practice*, Sudbury, MA, ed 5, 2013, Jones and Bartlett.

Institute of Medicine: *The future of public health*, Washington, DC, 1988, National Academies Press.

Institute of Medicine: *Unequal treatment: confronting racial and ethnic disparities in health care*, Washington, DC, 2002, National Academies Press.

Institute of Medicine: *The future of public health in the 21st century*, Washington, DC, 2003, National Academies Press.

Lanier P, Jonson-Reid M: Comparing primiparous and multiparous mothers in a nurse home visiting prevention program, *BIRTH*, 41(4):344–352, 2014.

National Association of County and City Health Officials: *Operational definition of a functional local health department*, 2014. Available at http://www.naccho.org. Accessed August 23, 2014.

Public Health Nursing Section: *Public health interventions: applications for public health nursing practice*, St. Paul, MN, 2001, Minnesota Department of Health.

Rosen G: *History of public health*, Baltimore, MD, 2015, John Hopkins University Press.

Schneider MJ: *Introduction to public health*, ed 5, Burlington, MA, 2017, Jones & Bartlett Learning.

Turnock BJ: *Public health: what it is and how it works*, ed 6, Sudbury, MA, 2015, Jones and Bartlett.

US Department of Health and Human Services: *Healthy People 2010: understanding and improving health*, ed 2, Washington, DC, 2000, US Government Printing Office.

US Department of Health and Human Services: *Healthy People 2020: national health promotion and disease prevention objectives*, 2010. Available at http://www.healthypeople.gov/hp2020/objectives/TopicAreas.aspx. Accessed July 21, 2016.

US Department of Health and Human Services: *The ACA Prevention and Public Health FUND*, 2014. Retrieved from HHS.gov.

World Health Organization [WHO]: *Antimicrobial resistance: global report on surveillance*, Geneva, Switzerland, 2014, WHO Document Production Services. Available at http://www.who.int/drugresistance/documents/surveillancereport/en/. Accessed August 13, 2016.

The Faith Community Nurse

Lisa M. Zerull

OBJECTIVES

After reading this chapter, the student should be able to:

1. Define faith community nursing and wholistic health promotion.
2. Describe the historical roots of nursing and healing ministries as well as professional issues for the future development of faith community nursing.
3. Compare models of faith community nursing with the scope and standards of practice for faith community nursing.
4. Develop awareness of the nurse's role within faith communities for spiritual care, health promotion, and disease prevention.
5. Describe the differences between spirituality and religiosity.
6. Use the nursing process in a faith community to assess, implement, and evaluate programs for healthy congregations using *Healthy People 2020* leading health indicators.

CHAPTER OUTLINE

Definitions in Faith Community Nursing
Historical Perspectives
   Faith Communities
   Faith Nurse Community
   Health Care Delivery
Faith Community Nursing Practice
   Characteristics of the Practice
   Scope and Standards of Faith Community Nursing Practice

Educational Preparation for the Faith Community Nurse
Issues in Faith Community Nursing Practice
   Professional Issues
   Ethical Issues
   Legal Issues
   Financial Issues
National Health Objectives and Faith Communities
Functions of the Faith Community Nurse

KEY TERMS

congregants, 518
congregational model, 511
faith communities, 511
faith community nurse, 510
faith community nurse coordinator, 514
healing, 512

health ministries, 511
holistic/wholistic care, 512
holistic health centers, 513
institutional model, 511
parish nurses, 511
parish nursing, 511
partnerships, 512

pastoral care staff, 512
polity, 517
religiosity 511
spirituality, 511
wellness committee, 512

Parish nursing, now referred to as faith community nursing, has long-established roots in the healing and health professions (Schnepfer, 2016). Historical accounts of nursing document the importance of caring for members of communities. The earliest accounts of concern for others stem from communities of faith. Wholeness in health and being in relationships with the Creator have sustained individuals and groups during times of illness, brokenness, stress, and incurable conditions (Burkhardt and Nagai-Jacobson, 2016; Pappas-Rogich and King, 2014; Royer, 2013). Today these nurses work in close relationships with individuals, families, and faith communities to establish programs and services that significantly affect health, healing, and wholeness (Cherry and Jacob, 2017; Church Health Center, n.d.a; Pappas-Rogich and King, 2014; Royer, 2013; Schnepfer, 2016). Nurses balance knowledge and skill in the role and facilitate the faith community to become a caring place—a place that is a source of health and healing.

Parish or faith community nurses address the universal health problems of individuals, families, and groups of

The authors acknowledge the contribution of Jean Bokinskie to the content of this chapter.

all ages. The members of congregations experience the following:
- Birth
- Death
- Acute and chronic illness
- Growth and development
- Stress
- Dependency concerns
- Challenges of life transitions
- Growth and development
- Decisions regarding healthy lifestyle choices

Faith community nursing or parish nursing is a recognized nursing specialty practice in the community setting, yet it is frequently overlooked when creative strategies are needed for improving the health of individuals and the larger community. According to Balboni et al (2013), only 12% to 14% of nurses reported receiving spiritual care training as part of their nursing education. Nurses often confuse religious practice or religiosity with spirituality and may neglect patients' spiritual needs (O'Brien, 2014). Whereas religiosity relates to "a person's beliefs and behaviors associated with a specific religious tradition or denomination" (O'Brien, 2014), spirituality is "an individual's attitudes and beliefs related to transcendence (God) or to the nonmaterial forces of life and nature" (O'Brien, 2014). Thus additional education in spiritual care to distinguish between the two and to provide an understanding of faith community nursing is needed.

Faith members live in communities that make decisions regarding policies for financing and managing health care and for keeping environments safe and communities healthy for present and future generations. Nurses encourage partnering with other community health resources to arrive at creative responses to health issues and concerns.

Parish, or faith community, nursing is gaining prominence as nurses reclaim their traditions of healing, acknowledge gaps in service delivery, and, along with the rise of nursing centers, affirm the independent functions of nursing (Hickman, 2011). In 1998 the American Nurses Association (ANA) accepted *parish nursing* as the most recognized term for the practice of nurses working with congregations or faith communities. With the Health Ministries Association (HMA), the ANA published the *Scope and Standards of Parish Nursing* (HMA and ANA, 1998). In the 2005 revision of the *ANA Scope and Standards of Practice*, the term *faith community nurse* was adopted to be inclusive of the titles of parish nurse, congregational nurse, health ministry nurse, crescent nurse, or health and wellness nurse (ANA and HMA, 2005). The most recent edition, released in 2012, focuses on faith community nurses but is also aimed at other health care providers, spiritual leaders, families, and members of faith communities (ANA and HMA, 2012).

Although most parish nurses are in Protestant congregations, they may be found in most faith communities, including communities that serve diverse cultures (Solari-Twadell and Hackbarth, 2010). Parish nurses are also serving faith communities in 29 countries around the world, including Australia, Bahamas, Canada, England, Korea, Malaysia, New Zealand, and South Africa (Church Health Center, n.d.b).

DEFINITIONS IN FAITH COMMUNITY NURSING

Faith communities are groups of people who gather in churches, cathedrals, synagogues, or mosques and acknowledge common faith traditions. Parish nursing is the most commonly used term that denotes the professional nursing practice in this context. Parish nurses respond to health and wellness needs of populations of faith communities and are partners with the church in fulfilling the mission of the health ministry. The inclusive term of *faith community nursing*, as adopted by the ANA and the HMA, defines nursing practice with an intentional focus on *spiritual care* as central to promoting "wholistic" health and prevention of illness (ANA and HMA, 2012, p 1).

The faith community includes persons throughout the life span—active and less active members, those confined to homes, or those in nursing homes. Often the faith community's mission also includes individuals and groups in the geographic or common cultural community who are not designated members. The services may be extended to those beyond the congregation. The parish nurse emphasizes the nursing discipline's spiritual dimension while incorporating physical, emotional, and social aspects of nursing with individuals, families, and faith communities.

Health ministries are those activities and programs in faith communities organized around health and healing to promote wholeness in health across the life span (Health Ministries Association, n.d.). The services may be specifically planned or may be more informal. A professional or a layperson may provide them. These services include the following (Gleason, 2015):
- Visiting in the home
- Providing meals for families in crisis or when returning home after hospitalization
- Participating in quilting circles
- Holding regular grief support groups
- Prayers for healing services

Popular parish nurse models include the congregational model, which may be a paid or unpaid model, and the institutional model which may be paid or unpaid (Box 29.1).

The development of a faith community nurse and health ministry program arises from the individual community of faith. The nurse is accountable to the congregation and its governing body. The institutional model includes greater

---

BOX 29.1 Parish Nurse Models

- **Congregation-based model,** in which the nurse is usually autonomous. The development of a parish nurse/health ministry program arises from the individual community of faith. The nurse is accountable to the congregation and its governing body.
- **Institution-based model,** which includes greater collaboration and partnerships. The nurse may be in a contractual relationship with hospitals, medical centers, long-term care establishments, or educational institutions.

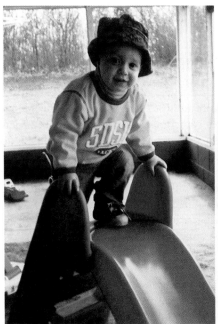
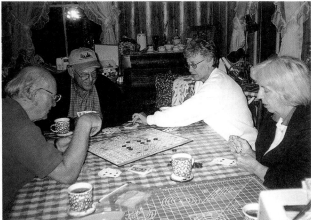

FIG. 29.1 Promoting healthy activities across the life span in church and community activities.

collaboration and partnership; the nurse may be in a contractual relationship with hospitals, medical centers, long-term care establishments, or educational institutions, and may receive a salary. In either model, nurses work closely with professional health care members, faith community pastoral care staff, and lay volunteers who represent various aspects of the life of the congregational community (Pappas-Rogich and King, 2014; Royer, 2013). To promote healing, the nurse builds on strengths to encourage integrating inner spiritual knowledge and healthy lifestyle choices for optimal wellness. The intentional and compassionate presence of a spiritually mature professional nurse in individual or group situations is vital. In this role, providing such holistic care

with congregation populations is important. Holistic/wholistic care is concerned with the relationship of body, mind, and spirit in a constantly changing environment (Mariano, 2016). The nurse and members of the congregation assess, plan, implement, and evaluate programs. The process of providing holistic care is enhanced by an active wellness committee or health cabinet (Royer, 2013).

These committees are most effective when members represent the broad spectrum of the life of the church (Fig. 29.1). The parish nurse uses all the knowledge and skills of this specialty to provide effective services. The outcome is a truly caring congregation that supports healthy, spiritually fulfilling lives. Box 29.2 lists resources for parish nursing.

EVIDENCE-BASED PRACTICE

In this descriptive research project, certified diabetic educators (CDEs) partnered with faith community nurses (FCNs) to mobilize communities to help prevent, identify, and manage diabetes in places where people live, work, and worship. Using an evidence-based chronic care model to enhance positive health lifestyle practices over a 4-week program, CDEs and FCNs used a pre- and posttest evaluation (i.e., biologic measures of body mass index [BMI] and blood pressure with a questionnaire) to identify diabetes self-care activities following interventions of screening, education, and disease management. A convenience sample of 149 participants, primarily white married women over age 65 from low-income urban areas, completed healthy living classes held at 16 different churches in 2008 and 2009. Significant was that 38% of the sample had a diabetes diagnosis, with most participants being overweight (mean BMI 32.5) and prehypertensive (mean BP 136/79). Findings suggest that participants had increased awareness about diet, exercise, and motivation to adopt healthy behaviors based on posttest responses. In this demonstration project, faith community nurses extended the diabetes education, prevention, and management previously limited to two CDEs from a regional health

system. Thus a larger population was reached to promote health through the use of churches as community setting. Additionally, partnering with congregations having faith community nurses is an invaluable and cost-effective strategy for screening and disease management.

Nurse Use
Faith community nurses are encouraged to partner with other care providers to offer screening and education for chronically ill persons in the community, particularly those with limited access to care and follow-up services. This community outreach project to low-income communities in urban New York fostered a positive, trusting client–provider relationship that formed the basis of the clients' motivation to make positive lifestyle changes for better health. Assisting vulnerable individuals to decrease health risks and better manage chronic disease helps empower people to care for themselves. As faith community nurses reach out to their surrounding community, creative strategies and collaboration with other care providers positively influence health attitudes and behaviors, with resultant cost-effective and quality outcomes.

Data from Austin SA, Brennan-Jordan N, Frenn D, et al: Defy diabetes: a unique partnership with faith community/parish nurses to impact diabetes, *J Christ Nurs*, 30: 238-243, 2013.

HISTORICAL PERSPECTIVES

FAITH COMMUNITIES

In the roots of many faith communities are concerns for justice, mercy, and the need for spiritual and physical healing. The appeal for caring, the healing of diseases, and acknowledging periods of illness and wellness are universal. Throughout a major portion of the 20th century, religion played an important role in the lives of many in this country. An important aspect of living one's spirituality and religion is being a part of a community of faith from birth to death, throughout wellness and illness. Participating as individuals or as families, all benefit from the associations with the supportive faith community or congregation (Burkhardt and Nagai-Jacobson, 2016; Pappas-Rogich and King, 2014; Royer, 2013).

To promote healing, the nurse builds on strengths to encourage the connecting and integrating of inner spiritual knowing and healthy lifestyle choices to achieve optimal wellness in the many circumstances faced by individuals and families in life. Intentional and compassionate presence of a spiritually mature professional nurse in individual or group situations is vital. In this role, providing holistic care with congregation populations is important. Holistic care is concerned with the relationship between body, mind, and spirit in a constantly changing environment (Dossey et al, 2013).

Support from members of groups that are meaningful to a person's total well-being aids in recovery and healing (O'Brien, 2014). Asking for help and using strengths from earliest faith traditions, family support, and teachings assist individuals, groups, and communities in interpreting brokenness, disasters, joys, births, deaths, illness, and recovery. Throughout history, health existed at the center of the human interaction with the Creator.

The integration of faith and health within the caring community results in beneficial outcomes. Persons who are assaulted with physical and emotional illness and brokenness and who are able to call on their faith beliefs and religious traditions are able to increase coping skills and realize spiritual growth. These coping skills and spiritual strengths extend beyond the current situation and help with future life challenges and total well-being (O'Brien, 2014).

Some of the major Christian faith communities in the late 19th and early 20th centuries used missionaries to develop multipurpose activities in communities, which included education and health activities along with religious messages. Hospitals were built in the United States and abroad, and underserved populations were targeted. As political and economic forces have changed through the years, so health ministries of the faith communities have altered their approaches. Some groups have identified with community development efforts in helping people empower themselves to meet their needs for food, education, clean environments, social support, and primary health care.

Some groups have also recognized and increased their emphasis on the following:
- Individual responsibility
- The escalating cost of health care
- The need for cost containment
- The increasing numbers of uninsured and underserved
- The ever-increasing dilemma of interpreting the many changes in the health care delivery system
- Issues of domestic violence
- Issues of substance abuse
- Issues with human immunodeficiency virus (HIV)/AIDS

These efforts have been translated into a variety of positions endorsed by the governing bodies of the faith communities.

The holistic health centers of the 1970s emphasized a comprehensive team approach to total health care. The teams in those centers included family and clergy who emphasized personal responsibility for health and encouraged preventive health practices. The formation of parish nursing in the early 1980s built on the strengths of the holistic health centers and focused on the team of nurses and clergy, working with individuals and with their families. Nurses used their abilities to listen to the spoken and unspoken concerns of individuals and made assessments and judgments based on their knowledge of the health sciences and humanities. As with the early history of the development of public health nursing in this country, parish nurses found that health promotion services were needed in underserved and rural areas (Palpant, 2012). Nurses identified the following:
- Gaps in the delivery of service
- Acknowledged strength within persons to increase healing
- The vital role of families in healthy outcomes
- The community support needed for individuals and families

FAITH NURSE COMMUNITY

The beginnings of the parish nurse movement coincided with the following (Hickman, 2011):
- Recognition of more independent functions of the nurse
- Articulation and proliferation of advanced-practice nursing roles

- The growth of nursing centers
- Technological advances
- Diagnosis-related groups (DRGs), which resulted in hospitals discharging clients earlier and clients returning to their homes sicker, with few, if any, caregivers available
- Caregivers faced with multiple tasks of coordinating employment and finances, learning new caregiving tasks, and maintaining former and ongoing family responsibilities
- Increased consumer demand for involvement in health care decisions
- Society's emphasis on individual responsibility for health because of the recognition that many diseases were indeed preventable and health care costs had to be cut
- Recognition that fragmented care and inadequate caregiver training and availability were problems for the disenfranchised, underserved, uninsured, economically well-situated, and better-educated persons
- Challenges faced by suburban and rural families to seek ways to best meet the multiple demands of young children, teens, and aging parents

These numerous interacting and overlapping forces were burdens for the population. Parish nurse services were one way to coordinate care and foster continuity of care. The parish nurse services emphasized health promotion and disease prevention and provided the benefits of holistic care through the supportive faith community.

The mission of the International Parish Nurse Resource Center (IPNRC), now known as the Westberg Institute, is the promotion and development of quality faith community nurse programs through research, education, and consultation (Church Health Center, n.d.c). Information about accessing the Westberg Institute appears in Box 29.2. The Westberg Institute has also endorsed curricula for the parish nurse and faith community nurse coordinator (Church Health Center, n.d.d). Throughout the years, the Westberg Institute has been vigilant in addressing emerging issues such as documentation accountability, certification for faith community nurses, and accreditation concerns (related to the Joint Commission on Accreditation of Healthcare Organizations [The Joint Commission]) for faith community nurses connected with institutional hospital systems.

Nurses functioning as faith community nurses need to have the following:

- Active registered nurse license in the state of practice
- Baccalaureate degree or higher in nursing, with experience in community nursing preferred
- Completion of a foundational education course in faith community nursing
- Specialized knowledge of the spiritual beliefs and practices of the faith community
- Personal spirituality maturity in practice
- Should be organized, flexible, self-starter, and a good communicator

As with other population groups, the faith community nurse attempts to include those persons who are less vocal or visible in the community of faith. If the vision of the congregation extends beyond its immediate membership, those outside of the immediate faith community who would benefit from the services are also potential recipients.

HEALTH CARE DELIVERY

The health care delivery system is challenged to work within parameters of tighter financial constraints while also welcoming advanced technology and addressing new health concerns. Consumer demand for involvement in health care decisions continues to increase, and society emphasizes individual responsibility for health. Simultaneously, consumers have increased interest in their own well-being and have expressed needs for more current health information to be available in a wider variety of formats (Washington et al, 2016; Sarrami-Foroushani et al, 2014). These numerous interacting and overlapping forces are both a challenge and a burden for the population.

In addition to consumer interest and a heightened awareness of responsibility for our own health, health care providers and managed care systems have found it financially advantageous for their participants to be healthy and remain out of the system. Thus with rising costs of care, scarce resources for populations, and the complex system demands on individuals and families to seek health care, the challenge for the consumer now is how to cope with these forces. Consumers and health care providers are still muddling through the complexity and fragmentation of the delivery system as it affects the young, old, and very old; the poor, middle income, and affluent; persons of diverse ethnic origins; and those affected by disparities within society (Washington et al, 2016). Advanced-practice nurses are addressing these consumer needs for primary care by practicing in the faith community setting (Balint and George, 2015).

A primary focus of the nurse in the past few decades has been to coordinate care and to link health care providers, groups, and community resources as the client tries to understand diverse health plans. Negotiating with individuals, agencies, and community partnerships within the complex maze of the broader health care environment demands a knowledgeable and seasoned professional. Nurses are aware of the necessity of collaborative practices and the formation of partnerships to care for groups and individuals throughout the age span. These nurses recognize the need for health promotion and disease prevention at all levels; they regularly assess the need to interpret care plans given to clients by health care providers. They advocate for healthy lifestyle choices in exercise, nutrition, substance use, and stress management. They realize that information and guidance must be available via media and in schools, workplaces, faith communities, and residential neighborhoods. Parish nurses share these and other important nursing functions as they serve populations through faith communities (Cherry and Jacob, 2017; O'Brien, 2014; Pappas-Rogich and King, 2014; Royer, 2013).

FAITH COMMUNITY NURSING PRACTICE
CHARACTERISTICS OF THE PRACTICE

The goal of faith community nursing is to develop and sustain health ministries within faith communities. Health ministries promote wholeness in health and emphasize health promotion and disease prevention, and they do this within the context of linking healing with the person's faith belief and level of spiritual maturity. Parish nurse Ruth Berry, the previous author of this chapter, participated in a 1994 invitational conference that included 26 professionals consisting of nurse educators, practicing parish nurses, and the staff of the IPNRC; their purpose was to discuss and design a document outlining educational guidelines for the rapidly growing new nursing specialty. The final product included the following five characteristics identified as central to the philosophy of parish nursing (Church Health Center, n.d.e):

1. The spiritual dimension is central to the practice of parish nursing. Nursing embodies the physical, psychological, social, and spiritual dimensions of clients into professional practice. Although parish nursing includes all four, it focuses on intentional and compassionate care, which stems from the spiritual dimension of all humankind.

2. The roots of the role balance the knowledge and skills of nursing, using nursing sciences, the humanities, and theology. The nurse combines nursing functions with pastoral care functions. Visits in the office, home, hospital, or nursing home often involve prayer and may include a reference to scripture, symbols, sacraments, and liturgy of the faith community represented by the nurse. The values and beliefs of the faith community are integral to the supportive care given. Nurses also assist with worship services as appropriate within the faith community.

3. The focus of the specialty is the faith community and its ministry. The faith community is the source of health and healing partnerships, which result in creative responses to health and

health-related concerns. Partnerships may be among individuals, groups, and health care professionals within the congregation. They may also be among various congregations or community agencies, institutions, or individuals. Partnerships also evolve as the congregation visualizes its health-related mission beyond the walls, stones, and steeples of its own place of worship.

4. Parish nurse services emphasize the strengths of individuals, families, and communities. Parish nurses endorse this fourth characteristic in their practice. As congregations realize the need for care and care for one another, their individual and corporate relationship with their Creator is often enhanced. This provides additional coping strength for future crisis situations within the family and community.

5. Health, spiritual health, and healing are considered an ongoing, dynamic process. Because spiritual health is central to well-being, influences are evident in the total individual and noted in a healthy congregation. Well-being and illness may occur simultaneously; spiritual healing or well-being can exist in the absence of cure. The philosophy of parish nursing comprises four concepts: spiritual formation, professionalism, shalom as health and wellness, and community, incorporating culture and diversity.

CHECK YOUR PRACTICE

You are working with your home church to provide a primary prevention program for a group of overweight teens. The goal is to reduce their risk of becoming diagnosed as obese. What would you do? What type of program would you implement?

LEVELS OF PREVENTION

Related to Overweight, Obesity, and Physical Activity

Primary Prevention
- Hold classes with youth and parents on healthy eating appropriate for various age levels.
- Promote and encourage age-appropriate activities that include physical exercise in youth group meetings, retreats, summer camps, and nursery programs.
- Encourage a variety of activities and discourage extended inactivity (including television and video games).
- Encourage healthy snacks and meals for youth activities and parenting sessions.
- Write faith community newsletter articles informing parents of the need for adequate exercise and proper nutrition for healthy lifestyles in youth and teen years.
- Encourage parents to be proactive in school parenting councils and in neighborhood recreation leagues to ensure exercise programs and activities for youth.
- Encourage faith community leaders to sponsor a safe indoor and outdoor activity area for neighborhood or at-risk children.

Secondary Prevention
- Provide health assessment and counseling during home visits for health promotion initiated for other family members—such as visits after a hospitalization or a birth.
- Using an attitudinal/behavioral risk survey, identify factors for obesity in the faith community's youth.

- Be available for health counseling for teens before and after youth activities.
- In schools associated with faith communities, assist with height and weight screening to identify youth and teens needing attention and referral.

Tertiary Prevention
- Collaborate closely with faith education teachers, youth ministers, and counselors about sessions that deal with nutrition behavior change, exercise behavior modification, injury prevention guidelines, health problems of overweight young persons, and the advantages of reduced weight, support, stress management, and improved quality of life.
- Follow up and monitor the health care provider's plan of care for young persons who have been identified as overweight; support and encourage them to withstand peer ridicule during behavior changes.
- Facilitate a faith-based activities program for overweight youth that includes age-appropriate exercises, health education, and spiritual development.
- Assist in making choices for behavior change (suggest avoiding calorie-rich or nutritionally lacking foods during school meal and snack times; suggest possible paths for walking and bicycling; identify courts and gyms available for more strenuous exercise).
- Discuss in youth groups and parenting groups the need for loving, caring friends and the support needed for long-term behavior modification programs that are life-long efforts.

The Third Invitational Parish Nurse Educational Colloquium, sponsored by the IPNRC, affirmed assumptions of the practice of parish nursing (IPNRC, 2014). Those gathered affirmed that the term *client* in parish nursing embraces individuals, families, congregations, and communities across the life span. The practice includes the full cultural and geographic community, regardless of ethnicity, lifestyle, sex, sexual orientation, or creed. The nurse in the practice incorporates faith and health and employs the nursing process in providing services to the faith community, as well as to the community served by that faith community. Facilitating collaborative health ministries in the faith communities is an important component of the practice. In addition, the group affirmed that although the curricula stem from a Judeo-Christian theological framework, parish nursing respects diverse traditions of faith communities and encourages adaptation of the programs to these faith traditions.

SCOPE AND STANDARDS OF FAITH COMMUNITY NURSING PRACTICE

Nursing: Scope and Standards of Practice (ANA, 2010) describes what nursing is, what nurses do, and the responsibilities for which they are accountable. This document serves as the template for the specialties within the profession and therefore is the foundation for *Faith Community Nursing: Scope and Standards of Practice* (ANS and HMA, 2012). This revised scope and standards describes the who, what, where, when, why, and how of the practice of faith community nursing. Nurses well versed in the parish nursing practice field compiled this revision of the 1998 *Scope and Standards of Parish Nursing Practice* by a thorough review of the practice, public comments, and dialogue of practicing parish nurses. Specialty areas within professional nursing achieve a major milestone when the standards and scope common to that practice are recognized.

The specialized practice of faith community nursing focuses on intentional *spiritual care* as an integral part of the process of promoting wholistic health and preventing or minimizing illness in the faith community (ANA and HMA, 2012) (see the How To box).

HOW TO Intervene in Maternal and Infant Health

- Visit a family immediately after the birth of a new infant to further assess parenting skills and parent and infant bonding, reinforce a holistic reflection of life transitions, and plan for faith community support as indicated in those areas not addressed by family or other community agencies.
- Augment community prenatal classes or facilitate classes in the faith community stressing growth and development in the prenatal and postnatal period, family transitions, and adequate health monitoring needed by parents, children, and new family members.
- Facilitate an expectant parent support group to reinforce positive health during pregnancy, interpret plans negotiated with the health care provider, promote spiritual reflection of family life transitions, and encourage a connection with the Creator and the beliefs of the faith community; provide emotional, social, and community support to the family.

The *Scope and Standards* delineate examples of the parish nurse's independent functions. These functions are in compliance with and reflect current nursing practice, client health

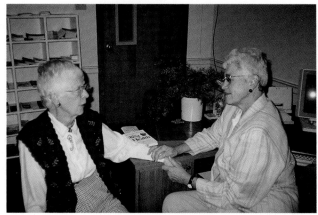

FIG. 29.2 A parish nurse provides support for spiritual and emotional needs as well as physical needs.

promotion needs, professional standards, and the legal scope of professional nursing practice. Nurses function within the nurse practice act of their jurisdiction (state). If dependent functions are practiced, parish nurses must be in compliance with the legal criteria of the jurisdiction's nurse practice act (ANA and HMA, 2012). For example, when influenza vaccine or immunization clinics are offered, appropriate arrangements are made to use nurses from the cooperating agency (health department), or the parish nurse must have a contractual policy agreement with the cooperating agency to provide the immunizations. In addition to a narrative description and glossary of terms, the 1998 document outlines standards of care and standards of professional performance. In keeping with the wise use of persons and materials, standards of professional performance elaborate on the coordination of care and consultation. Faith community nurses are "vital partners in advancing the nation's health initiatives, such as *Healthy People 2020,* to increase the quality of years of healthy life and eliminate health disparities" (ANA and HMA, 2012, p 9) (Fig. 29.2).

EDUCATIONAL PREPARATION FOR THE FAITH COMMUNITY NURSE

Current educational preparation for the parish nurse includes the successful completion of extensive continuing education contact hours or designated coursework in parish nurse preparation at the baccalaureate or graduate level, as well as a thorough grasp of the *Scope and Standards* of the practice (ANA and HMA, 2012). Such preparation is held in colleges, universities, health care institutions, and parish nurse networks across the United States and other countries, as well as online and distance delivery (Church Health Center, n.d.d). Many of these programs are in partnership with the Westberg Institute for ongoing support and revision. These basic programs provide an orientation to the role and functions of the parish nurse as well as worship experiences for the process of ministry (Church Health Center, n.d.d). Parish nurses are then able to adapt this knowledge, combined with an in-depth understanding of the beliefs of their faith tradition, to meet the holistic health needs of their local community of faith. According to

Faith Community Nursing: Scope and Standards of Practice (ANA and HMA, 2012), the preferred minimum preparation for the specialty includes educational preparation at the baccalaureate or higher level with content in community nursing, experience as a registered nurse, knowledge of the health care assets of a community, specialized knowledge of the spiritual practices of a given faith community, and specialized skills and knowledge to implement the *Scope and Standards*. Both the annual Westberg Symposium offered by the IPNRC and the annual meeting of the HMA offer comprehensive sessions and a forum for nurses to network, gain new knowledge, and stay abreast of current resources, trends, and issues in the practice.

Advanced-practice opportunities also enrich a specialty practice. Master's prepared nurses (with a specialization in public health nursing, holistic nursing, or mental health nursing) and nurse practitioners have found niches in parish nursing. Major universities have had creative arrangements for faculty and student clinical options at the undergraduate and graduate levels (Dahlke et al, 2016). A 1500-member congregation in Florida employed a full-time master's prepared nurse certified in holistic nursing by the American Holistic Nurses Association. Faculty practice arrangements at the University of Kentucky (with a 1000-member congregation), collaborations between the Divinity School and nursing programs to form the Health and Nursing Ministries Program at Duke University, University of Colorado faculty arrangements offering opportunities for doctoral and master's level students, and the pioneering Parish Health Nurse program at Georgetown University are notable.

Many parish nurses function in a part-time capacity. Some nurses are responsible for service with several congregations, whereas others engage in parish nursing as part of a full-time commitment in other capacities. Working in several areas adds distinctive perspectives to a parish nurse service. Depending on the practice model, the nurse has a narrowly defined or a wider realm of responsibility. Parish nurse practices may be integrated into a health care facility or into practices that collaborate with related professional practice areas such as health departments or colleges of nursing. Practices in which several parish nurses are supervised by a coordinator have built-in opportunities for sharing, partnering, and mentoring. Parish nurses may also have regional responsibilities that correspond to intermediate governing areas of the faith community. These regions may be clusters of churches or areas such as districts, synods, presbyteries, or jurisdictions.

Parish nurses accept responsibility for ongoing professional education within nursing and pastoral care areas. Preparation and continuing education must continue to include the basics and enrichment courses and updates in the following (Church Health Center, n.d.f):

- Nursing
- Theological/pastoral care field
- Public health
- Medicine
- Sociology
- Cultural diversity
- Human growth and development throughout the life span
- Improving collaboration, negotiation, and coordination skills

- Consultation
- Leadership
- Management
- Research skills

The challenge for the practice is to document trends, maintain and enhance the quality of the preparation and services offered, engage in evidence-based practice, use increased numbers of advanced-practice nurses, network within professional organizations, and become involved in outcomes-oriented research. To remain at the cutting edge of the profession and recognize competency among practitioners, the specialty must pursue professional certification.

ISSUES IN FAITH COMMUNITY NURSING PRACTICE

Every new discipline or care area must be alert to issues of accountability to populations served and to those who entrust the nurse with the responsibility to serve a designated population. This facilitates positive outcomes and avoids conflicts with individual and group rights and state regulations. Considerations include the following:

- Discussions of health promotion plans must include the individual, the family, and the faith community.
- Negotiations with the pastoral staff, congregations, institutions, and the wider community may be involved in job description preparation or program planning.
- Issues such as privacy, confidentiality, group concerns, access, and record management must be discussed with the pastoral staff or the contracting agency at the outset of any parish nurse agreement.

PROFESSIONAL ISSUES

Annual and periodic evaluations are required of parish nurse practices and services needed. These evaluations may be self, peer, congregational, and/or institutional. Personnel committees provide guidance and contribute to the evaluation. They also advocate for parish nurse services and raise awareness with the congregational staff members and programs. Professional appraisal is standard in nursing practice. The appraisals guide professional development and program development and planning.

Because the scope of parish nursing practice is broad and focuses on the independent practice of the discipline, the nurse must consider a wide variety of issues, such as the following:

- Position descriptions
- Professional liability
- Professional education
- Experiential preparation
- Collaborative agreements
- Working with lay volunteers as well as retired professionals

Abiding by the professional nursing code is understood; however, the nurse must also know the polity, expectations, and mission of the particular faith community. The nurse also continually interprets the profession for the faith community.

The nurse is required to be the following:
- Knowledgeable about lines of authority and channels of communication in the congregation and in the collaborative institutions
- Well acquainted with the personnel committees of the congregation
- An advocate for well-being to highlight justice issues in local and national legislation
- A contributor of information to policymakers about the implications for health and well-being for the parish and the local and global communities
- An active participant in political activities that contribute to spiritual growth and healthy functioning

ETHICAL ISSUES

Issues evolve from client, faith community, and professional arenas. The nurse's interventions are guided by professional responsibilities that include the following:
- Code of Ethics for Nurses (ANA, 2015)
- Individual and group rights
- Statements of faith
- Polity of the faith community served

Professional and therapeutic relationships are maintained at all times; consulting and counseling with minors and individual members of the opposite sex are conducted using professional ethical principles. Policies about these issues are established at the outset of the practice with the pastoral team, the wellness committee, the parish nurse, and the local congregation's governing body.

As in other community health situations, the parish nurse, along with the client, does the following:
- Identifies parameters of ethical concerns
- Plans ahead with clients to consider healthy options in making ethical decisions
- Supports clients in their journey to choose alternatives that will strengthen coping skills
- Allows the client to grow stronger in faith and health
- Considers the "virtue ethics, such as caring, forgiveness, and compassion, in their decision making" (ANA and HMA, 2016, p 19)

Communities of faith strive to be caring communities and value the fellowship among their members. However, confidentiality is of utmost importance in parish nursing practice. The parish nurse values client confidentiality while delicately assisting the client and the client's family to "share" concerns with the pastoral staff and fellow congregants. This sharing gains valuable support to promote optimal healing. The nurse is often the staff member who helps the family to the stage of acceptance of a health concern. How much to share and when to share a concern are indeed a private affair and a part of the important journey of healing. A joyous event for one family may be a devastating event or even a depressing reminder of a past event for another family. The celebrations and joys of a healthy new infant one week may raise guilt and ambivalence for congregational members when, within a brief time, another family's long-awaited child dies at birth.

LEGAL ISSUES

As an advocate of client and group rights, the nurse does the following:
- Identifies and reports neglect, abuse, and illegal behaviors to the appropriate legal sources
- Appropriately refers members to pastoral or community resources if the scope of the problem is beyond the realm of the professional nurse
- Refers to another health care professional if conflict between the nurse and client is such that no further progress is possible

The parish nurse who has a positive relationship that values open dialog with the pastoral team will be supported in efforts to select the most appropriate community resources for clients.

The nurse must personally and professionally abide by the parameters of the nurse practice act of the jurisdiction and maintain an active license in that state. The following are additional legal concerns:
- Institutional contractual agreements
- Records management
- Release of information
- Volunteer liability

Resources would include the faith community's legal consultant, the faith community's national position statements, and those of the HMA and IPNRC.

FINANCIAL ISSUES

Innovative arrangements for variations of the basic models mentioned previously call for sustained financial support. The nurse is called on to partner in finding funds and networking with potential supporters. The nurse is accountable for money spent and for fundraising, whether the position is salaried or volunteer. Educational and promotional materials, equipment, travel time, continuing education, and malpractice insurance are selected areas that need to be included in the budget of the parish nurse. If these materials are not budget items, services may be limited, and this needs to be interpreted to the faith community. Money, time, and people are never sufficient to meet the needs of a parish nurse ministry, but it is up to the nurse to use a resource assessment in advance of a project to be able to come to a clear understanding of what is possible given the specific faith community resources (Durbin et al, 2013).

NATIONAL HEALTH OBJECTIVES AND FAITH COMMUNITIES

The *Healthy People 2020* indicators encourage communities to support individuals and families to attain high-quality lives free of preventable diseases across the life span, to reduce health disparities across groups, and to create environments that promote health. Faith communities have long held a position of esteem in communities. One of the oldest and strongest partnerships is that established between communities and religious or faith communities. The Carter Center in Atlanta and the Park Ridge Center for Health, Faith, and Ethics in Chicago collaborated with health care professionals and leaders of faith traditions to identify roles of faith communities to address national health objectives and approaches to improving overall public health.

Because faith communities are rooted in healing traditions and hold issues of justice and mercy as a priority, the *Healthy People 2020* goals to attain high-quality, longer lives free of preventable disease, disability, injury, and premature death; achieve health equity; eliminate disparities and improve the health of all groups; create social and physical environments that promote good health for all; and promote quality of life, healthy development, and healthy behaviors across all life stages can be readily addressed. Because the values of health and faith institutions are closely aligned, evidence of partnering is becoming more prominent and necessary in the current socioeconomic environment. The National Heart, Lung, and Blood Institute and the American Heart Association have long partnered with faith communities and offered resources for programs.

Specific national objectives dealing with nutrition; physical activity; use of tobacco, alcohol, and other drugs; immunization status; environmental health; and injury and violence are within the realm of the health education role of the faith community nurse. Activities include age-appropriate discussions of preventive activities with various groups; classes on the use and misuse of alcohol, tobacco, and other drugs; and discussions regarding responsible sexual behavior in the context of faith values. As an outreach to the surrounding community, the nurse can create an environment within the faith community that promotes health and is a safe setting for activities.

Wellness committees and faith community nurses may regularly review the various health status objectives, make comparisons between national and specific state objectives, and then assess the extent to which the individual faith community member or group is in need of reducing risk. The nurse can do the following:

- Provide regular blood pressure screening and monitoring activities focusing on heart disease and stroke prevention and disability.
- Promote age-appropriate discussion of preventive activities with various groups.
- Describe signs and symptoms of heart attack and stroke in newsletters and post on bulletin boards throughout the facility.
- Coordinate healthy, low-fat meals.
- Encourage youth groups to choose healthy fruits and vegetables as snacks after their activities.
- Coordinate a series of classes for families of adolescents on stress management and sessions on the use and misuse of alcohol, tobacco, and other drugs.
- Encourage or lead a faith-based exercise program for individuals as part of an ongoing faith community activity.

Examples of interventions related to selected portions of *Healthy People 2020* objectives that could be addressed by faith community nurses are listed in the *Healthy People 2020* box.

The faith community's wellness committee also can address other objectives to identify activities in which to engage the entire faith community or surrounding geographic area. Most advantageous for the faith community would be for the faith community nurse, wellness committees, and other interested

HEALTHY PEOPLE 2020

The following objectives relate to nutrition and weight and physical activity and fitness for youth in faith communities:

Nutrition and Weight Status
- **NWS-7:** Increase the proportion of worksites that offer nutrition or weight management classes or counseling.
- **NWS-10:** Reduce the proportion of children and adolescents who are considered obese.
- **NWS-11:** (Developmental) Prevent inappropriate weight gain in youth and adults.
- **NWS-14:** Increase the contribution of fruits to the diets of the population aged 2 years and older.

From U.S. Department of Health and Human Services: *Healthy people 2020: the road ahead*, Rockville, MD, 2010, Office of Disease Prevention and Health Promotion. Retrieved August 2016 from https://www.healthypeople.gov/2020/topics-objectives.

CASE STUDY

Educational Experiences in Parish Nursing

Jeremy Black is the community nursing professor at a school of nursing. Looking for new clinical experiences, Mr. Black was advised to examine parish nursing experiences for his students. He contracted with a Baptist church to bring health services to the church through himself and his students.

With Mr. Black's prompting, volunteers from the church joined together to form the church's Wellness Committee. The goal of the Wellness Committee was to identify the needs of the church members and to provide direction for Mr. Black and his students. Through interviews and surveys, the Wellness Committee and Mr. Black identified "increase knowledge of health promotion activities" as one of the needs the nursing students could address.

Mr. Black decided the nursing students would plan and organize a health fair for the church. Pairs of students were assigned to develop booths. Students were expected to research their topic, develop educational materials, and then teach at the fair. The five booths were blood pressure screening and information, osteoporosis screening and information, body mass index screening and information, self-screening information for certain cancers (e.g., skin, breast), and vision and hearing screenings and information. Mr. Black would provide the necessary equipment for the various screenings.

The health fair was given on a Sunday morning after worship services. Church members walked through and visited booths in which they were interested. Church members commented to the students how nice the booths looked and how glad they were to obtain the information.

persons to engage in partnership activities with community efforts such as health fairs. The teachers, principal, clergy, parent–teacher group, staff, students, wellness council, special education teachers, and recreation leaders are all potential participants. Health fairs are effective strategies for health promotion efforts guided by the *Healthy People 2020* framework (USDHHS, 2010). These and similar activities promote increased health of the entire community, and they include persons of all ages, encourage enthusiasm, offer fellowship and leisure, and reduce duplication of effort.

FUNCTIONS OF THE FAITH COMMUNITY NURSE

Examples of nursing interventions have been cited throughout this chapter. This section summarizes and expands some of the usual functions and describes activities. Nurses carry out their practice in groups or individually. As the faith community nurse plans and provides intentional holistic care, he/she benefits from an awareness of the seven functions of the professional nurse role (Slutz and Wehling, 2013):

1. **Integrator of faith and health:** Assist others to improve spiritual and physical health; assess personal spirituality as well as that of clients. Interventions focus on providing presence, listening, and rituals such as prayer and scripture. *Example:* Use prayer, as appropriate, at the conclusion of each individual encounter or group gathering.

2. **Personal health counselor:** Discuss health problems and recommend interventions as necessary. Therapeutic communication strategies and techniques are utilized to discuss, explore, and guide clients through health concerns. *Example:* Offer blood pressure screenings one Sunday each month, and discuss ways to reduce risk for high blood pressure (e.g., stress reduction, weight management, smoking cessation, healthy eating).

3. **Health educator:** Provide opportunities to learn about health; focus on the teaching role of the nurse; and select resources, utilize strategies, and lead activities to promote health. Use a variety of formats, including seminars, conferences, classes, workshops, individual or group sessions, newsletters, printed materials, bulletin inserts, and bulletin boards, to empower others to be active partners in managing health. *Example:* Create a bulletin board display on whole-person health of body, mind, and spirit, including the connection between faith and health.

4. **Referral agent:** Provide information for referrals to appropriate agencies and services. Maintain an awareness of local agencies, services, and resources and how to make referrals. *Example:* Refer an adult female to a gynecologist for preventative women's care and mammogram.

5. **Health advocate:** Empower congregants to obtain needed health care services. Develop advocacy skills, including expert communication techniques and facilitation and problem-solving skills, and increase knowledge of the health care system, health policy, and access to care in order to assist others. *Example:* Interface with homeless persons accessing congregational resources of food or financial support.

6. **Coordinator of volunteers:** Recruit, train, and supervise volunteers to expand ministry and outreach. Organize a health ministry team to guide and direct faith and health initiatives. Utilize the gifts and talents of congregation and community members. *Example:* Plan an annual health fair with members of the congregational health ministry team, inviting other health care professionals and community agencies to participate and display health resources available in the community.

7. **Developer of support groups:** Establish and facilitate support groups. Increase knowledge of existing support groups to provide referrals as needed. *Example:* Organize a bereavement/grief support group for older adults, including widows and widowers, that may or may not be led by the faith community nurse.

Box 29.3 gives an example of how the parish nurse works with other providers and community resources to meet the health needs of a client. Box 29.4 lists several selected activities of parish nurses.

Several images of the faith community nurse in practice highlight varying settings and professional activities. Central to all interactions is intentional care of the spirit and the healing presence

---

BOX 29.3 Parish Nursing as Healing Ministry: An Adult Daughter's Reflection

What a pleasure to be able to commend [parish nurse's] personal friendship and professional help! Without her support it would have been difficult, if not impossible, for my father to live at home during his last 6 years. But she had, along with his doctor, the sure feeling that it was the right thing for him and that it could be done. When the time came that he needed caregivers around the clock, she skillfully conveyed suggestions in such a way that the caregivers' cultural differences were not a barrier. She helped them grow as caregivers, appreciating their accomplishments, even to having a blackberry-picking "outing" at her home.

My father in his earlier years had been a deacon and had loved visiting shut-ins. It brought him so much happiness that he in turn received his church's caring, healing ministry through his parish nurse. He attended church on Sundays beyond what one would expect of one in his 90s, and almost his last Sunday was the day he celebrated turning 96.

Thank you, [parish nurse], for our "Mission Accomplished"!

With permission, A.F.H.

BOX 29.4 Examples of Parish Nurse Interventions and Activities

- Sharing the joys of a new member in the family; sharing the sorrows of losses
- Anticipating changes in health status or in growth and development
- Being present for questions that seem difficult or unacceptable to ask the health care provider
- Explaining and assisting in considering choices when new living and care arrangements must be made
- Listening to the concerns of a youngster anticipating diagnostic procedures
- Praying with the spouse of a dying parishioner
- Helping individuals and families make decisions regarding advance directives in light of faith beliefs
- Helping teens consider options when overwhelmed with serious life issues
- Providing information, support, and prayer regarding advance directives
- Seeking community resources and opportunities for fitness and nutrition classes
- Working with the wellness committee to ensure that fellowship meals meet the nutritional and spiritual needs of the elderly
- Offering educational opportunities about changes in health care legislation and its influence on the congregation and community
- Accompanying a faith community member to a 12-step meeting
- Participating in worship leadership with the pastoral staff

From Berry R: A parish nurse. In *Office of Resourcing Committees on Preparation for Ministry: a day in the life of . . .: a kaleidoscope of specialized ministries,* Louisville, Ky, 2004, Presbyterian Church (USA), Distribution Management Service.

QSEN FOCUS ON QUALITY AND SAFETY EDUCATION FOR NURSES

The Nurse in the Faith Community

Targeted Competency: Quality Improvement—Use data to monitor the outcomes of care processes, and use improvement methods to design and test changes to continuously improve the quality and safety of health care systems. Important aspects of safety include the following:

- Knowledge: Describe approaches for changing processes of care.
- Skills: Design a small test of change in daily work (using an experiential learning method such as Plan-Do-Study-Act).
- Attitudes: Value measurement and its role in good patient care.

Quality Improvement Question:

You are a parish nurse at a busy urban church. An alarmingly high percentage of your congregation over the age of 65 are diagnosed with type 2 diabetes. The national average of type 2 diabetes in this population is 26%. In your congregation, 30% of your parishioners over the age of 65 have been diagnosed with type 2 diabetes.

You have developed an online educational module for this population about the importance of glycemic control. You've also collaborated with a dietician to offer cooking classes every Sunday afternoon in the church's kitchen. You want to evaluate the effectiveness of these interventions.

Use the program outcomes used by Faith Communities as listed below to evaluate your diabetic program:

Step 1: What is the problem or issue that your diabetes program is designed to address?

Step 2: Identify both short-term and long-term goals for your diabetes program.

Step 3: How would you document the specific program outcomes?

Step 4: Are there best practices that might inform your educational module or your collaborative cooking class with the dietician?

Step 5: How would you evaluate the short-term and long-term goals of your program?

Prepared by Gail Armstrong, PhD(c), DNP, ACNS-BC, CNE, Associate Professor, University of Colorado Denver College of Nursing.

---

of the faith community nurse. Blood pressure screenings offer therapeutic touch as well as assessment for cardiac status, social health, and overall well-being as the parishioner spends time with the nurse (Fig. 29.3). Informal pew-side consultations take place after worship when individuals ask health-related questions or request resource or referral information (Fig. 29.4). Young families require comprehensive support with diverse needs related to age, supportive relationships, childcare support, and parenting. The health educator role requires creative and differing teaching strategies for the nurse based on the ages of individuals or groups being taught. Faith community nurses may organize an annual health fair inviting community partners and service agencies to share resources and promote health ministries to parishioners of all ages. Hospital and institutional care visits provide spiritual and emotional support when unexpected illness and health crisis may challenge coping skills and raise questions about faith and denominational theology. Other interventions, services, or programs provided by the faith community nurse are determined by taking into consideration specific congregation needs and the

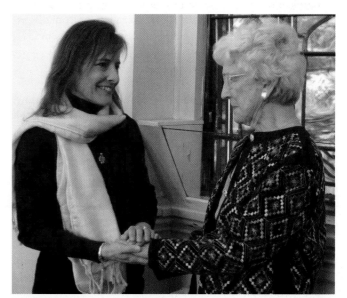

FIG. 29.4 Faith community nurse provides informal pew-side health consultation.

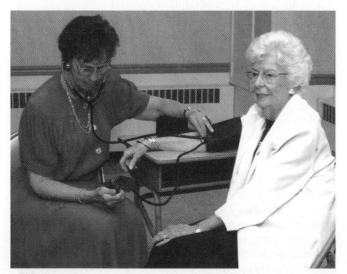

FIG. 29.3 Blood pressure screening in the faith community.

mission, vision, and strategic plan of the congregation matched with the knowledge, skills, and experience as well as time availability of the faith community nurse (part-time versus full-time).

Underlying all of the previously mentioned functions is *pastoral care,* which the nurse fulfills as follows:

- Stresses the spiritual dimension of nursing
- Lends support during times of joy and sorrow
- Guides the person through health and illness throughout life
- Helps identify the spiritual strengths that assist in coping with particular events

The nurse may use hymns, favorite scripture verses, psalms, pictures, church windows, stories, or other images that are important for the individual or group to hold to the connectedness among faith, health, and well-being.

Numerous healthy activities should be encouraged in congregations, and the nurse often works with the congregation to expand its immediate borders to augment services in the community that

promote health and wellness. Congregations are keenly aware that more than half of the members of mainstream churches are part of the growing aging population of our country. Increased numbers of persons who are either uninsured or underinsured are in their communities. Thus services offered may include the following:
- Food pantries
- Daycare for seniors
- Congregate meals
- Preschool and latch-key arrangements
- Tutoring
- Meals on Wheels
- Visits to less-mobile members
- Outreach for vulnerable populations

PRACTICE APPLICATION

The nursing process is a method that can be used to begin program planning and evaluation with faith communities. Such an approach can involve congregational members and parish nurses in a dynamic endeavor to jointly learn about the members' individual health status, as well as that of the faith community and the local and broader geographic community. Parish nurse programs are derived in various ways. Initially, the impetus for parish nursing may stem from an unmet health need within the congregation, from visions of a lay or health professions member concerned about caring within the congregation, or from discussions of a committee dealing with health and wellness issues.

Which of the following activities is most likely to increase the interest and involvement of the congregation's members?
A. Writing a contract for parish nursing services
B. Surveying the faith community's environment
C. Gathering information on leaders and valued activities in the congregation through focus groups of pastoral staff
D. Assessing the needs of the congregational members through a survey
E. Holding a health fair
Answers can be found on the Evolve site.

REMEMBER THIS!

- Faith community nurse services respond to health, healing, and wholeness within the context of the church. Although the emphasis is on health promotion and disease prevention throughout the life span, the spiritual dimension of nursing is central to the practice.
- The nurse partners with the wellness committee and volunteers to plan programs and consider health-related concerns within the faith community.
- To promote a caring faith community, examples of functions of the nurse include personal health counseling, health teaching, facilitating linkages and referrals to congregation and community resources, advocating and encouraging support resources, and providing pastoral care.
- Nurses collaborate to plan, implement, and evaluate health promotion activities considering the faith community's beliefs, rituals, and polity. *Healthy People 2020* guidelines are basic to the partnering for programs.
- Nurses in congregational or institutional models enhance the health ministry programs of the faith communities if carefully chosen partnerships are formed within the congregation, with other congregations, and also with local health and social community agencies.
- Nurses working in the faith community nursing specialty must seek to attain adequate educational and skill preparation and to be accountable to those served and to those who have entrusted the nurse to serve.
- Nurses are encouraged to consider innovative approaches to creating caring communities. These may be in congregations as parish nurses, among several faith communities in a single locale or regionally, or in partnership with other community agencies.
- To be sustained in the role, the nurse needs to heal and nurture herself or himself while supporting individuals, families, and congregation communities in their healing process.

▶▶ APPLYING CONTENT TO PRACTICE

This chapter describes individual, group, and population health in the faith community setting. In Christian traditions, the scriptural story of the Good Shepherd who cares for the whole flock, including the lost or vulnerable until they once again become a part of the flock, is an effective parallel to population focus. The faith community nurse follows this example of care and healing to assess the needs of parishioners and then act as a catalyst to address health indicators of the faith community. The larger faith community is instrumental in providing the structure, place, and resources and may intentionally seek out the vulnerable and marginalized to receive support in healthy environments and become part of the efforts to promote healthy behaviors.

Faith communities often partner with other community or denominational organizations closely aligned with their mission and outreach activities for a common purpose. The organizations may include a health care institution, a childcare or adult daycare center, an immigrant community, a homeless shelter,

a crisis center, a preschool, or local public schools. Depending on desired outcomes, the faith community nurse combines knowledge, skills, and experience in collaboration with others to make a difference for a larger population.

To illustrate, a faith community partners with a hospital, the local agency on aging, and a retirement community to promote older adult health. Key stakeholders gather for discussions on priorities identified from a community needs assessment completed by the hospital. The stakeholders also review suggested prevention and services objectives for older adult health from *Healthy People 2020*. The group considers baseline data and identifies desired outcomes. From discussions, activities and programs are planned, drawing from the collective human and financial resources. In this example, the faith community nurse works with hospital staff to coordinate screenings and health promotion programs held in the congregation setting and at various locations using a mobile health vehicle. Successful disease management programs for diabetes and congestive

ⓔ EVOLVE WEBSITE

http://evolve.elsevier.com/Stanhope/foundations

- Case Study, with Questions and Answers
- NCLEX® Review Questions
- Practice Application Answers

REFERENCES

American Nurses Association: *Nursing: scope and standards of practice,* Silver Spring, MD, 2010, ANA.

American Nurses Association: *Code of ethics for nurses with interpretive statements,* Silver Spring, MD, 2015, ANA.

American Nurses Association and Health Ministries Association: *Faith community nursing: scope and standards of practice,* ed 3, Silver Spring, MD, 2016, ANA.

American Nurses Association and Health Ministries Association: *Faith community nursing: scope and standards of practice,* ed 3, Silver Spring, MD, 2016, ANA.

Austin SA, Brennan-Jordan N, Frenn D, et al: Defy diabetes: a unique partnership with faith community/parish nurses to impact diabetes, *J Christ Nurs* 30:238–243, 2013.

Balboni MJ, Sullivan A, Amobi A, et al: Why is spiritual care infrequent at the end of life? Spiritual care perceptions among patients, nurses and physicians and the role of training. *J Clin Oncol* 31(4):461–467, 2013.

Balint KA, George N: Faith community nursing scope of practice: extending access to healthcare, *J Christian Nursing* 32(1):34–40, 2015.

Berry R: A parish nurse. In *Office of Resourcing Committees on Preparation for Ministry: a day in the life of . . .: a kaleidoscope of specialized ministries,* Louisville, KY, 2004, Presbyterian Church (USA), Distribution Management Service.

Burkhardt MA, Nagai-Jacobson MG: Spirituality and health. In Dossey BM, Keegan L (authors), Barrere CC, Helming MB, Shields DA, Avino K, editors: *Holistic nursing: a handbook for practice,* ed 7, Burlington, MA, 2016, Jones & Bartlett Learning.

Cherry B, Jacob SR: *Contemporary nursing: issues, trends, and management,* ed 7, St. Louis, Missouri, 2017, Elsevier.

Church Health Center: *What is faith community nursing?* n.d.a. Retrieved August 2016 from http://www.churchhealthcenter.org/whatisfaithcommunitynursing.

Church Health Center: *International faith community nursing,* n.d.b. Retrieved August 2016 from http://www.churchhealthcenter.org/internationalfaithcommunitynursing.

Church Health Center: *History and mission,* n.d.c. Retrieved August 2016 from http://www.parishnurses.org/.

Church Health Center: *Courses,* n.d.d. Retrieved August 2016 from http://www.parishnurses.org/.

Church Health Center: *Philosophy of parish nursing,* n.d.e. Retrieved August 2016 from http://www.churchhealthcenter.org/philosophy.

Church Health Center: *Foundations of faith community nursing,* n.d.f. Retrieved August 2016 from http://www.churchhealthcenter.org/forfaithcommunitynurses.

Dahlke S, O'Connor M, Hannesson T, Cheetham K: Understanding clinical nursing education: an exploratory study, *Nurse Education in Practice* 17:145–152, 2016.

Dossey BM, Keegan L: *Holistic Nursing: A Handbook for Practice,* ed 6. Burlington, MA, 2013, Jones & Bartlett.

Durbin NLF, Cassimere M, Howard C, et al: *Faith community nurse coordinator manual: a guide to creating and developing your program,* Memphis, TN, 2013, Church Health Center.

Gleason J: *The pastoral caregiver's casebook, volume 3: ministry in health,* Valley Forge, PA, 2015, Judson Press.

Health Ministries Association: *What is health ministry?* n.d. Retrieved August 2016 from http://hmassoc.org/about-us/what-we-do/.

Health Ministries Association, American Nurses Association: *Scope and standards of parish nursing practice,* Washington, DC, 1998, ANA.

Hickman J: *Fast facts for the faith community nurse: implementing FCN/parish nursing in a nutshell,* New York, 2011, Springer.

International Parish Nurse Resource Center, *Conversation with Maureen Daniels, faith community nurse specialist with the Church Health Center and IPNRC resource,* March 30, 2014.

Mariano C: Holistic nursing: scope and standards of practice. In Dossey BM, Keegan L (authors), Barrere CC, Helming MB, Shields DA, Avino K, editors: *Holistic nursing: a handbook for practice,* ed 7, Burlington, MA, 2016, Jones & Bartlett Learning.

O'Brien ME: *Spirituality in nursing: standing on holy ground,* ed 5, Burlington, MA, 2014, Jones & Bartlett Learning.

Palpant KA: *Health promotion: a collaborative model for faith community nursing, Master's thesis,* 2012, Washington State University. Retrieved 4/20/2013 from https://research.wsulibs.wsu.edu:8443/xmlui/handle/2376/3570.

Pappas-Rogich M, King M: Faith community nursing: supporting Healthy People 2020 initiatives, *J Christian Nursing* 31(4):228–234, 2014.

Royer L: *Empowering the congregational nurse: implementing a faith community nursing practice,* 10-Amazon Inc. Seattle Washington, 2013, CreateSpace Independent Publishing Platform.

Sarrami-Foroushani P, Travaglia J, Debono D, Braithwaite J: Key concepts in consumer and community engagement: a scoping meta-review, *BMC Health Services Research* 14(1):138–157, 2014.

Schnepfer E: Professional issues: a renewed look at faith community nursing, *MEDSURG Nursing* 25(1):62–66, 2016.

Slutz M, Wehling B: Foundation of faith community nursing practice. In *Faith Community Nurse Coordinator Manual: A Guide to Creating and Developing Your Program.* Memphis, 2013, Church Health Center.

Solari-Twadell P, Hackbarth DP: Evidence for a new paradigm of the ministry of parish nursing practice using the nursing intervention classification system, *Nurs Outlook* 58:69–75, 2010.

U.S. Department of Health and Human Services: *Healthy people 2020: the road ahead,* Rockville, MD, 2010, Office of Disease Prevention and Health Promotion. Retrieved August 2016 from https://www.healthypeople.gov/2020/topics-objectives.

Washington K, Oliver D, Gage A, Albright D, Demiris G: A multimethod analysis of shared decision-making in hospice interdisciplinary team meetings including family caregivers, *Palliative Medicine* 30(3):270–278, 2016.

The Nurse in Home Health and Hospice

Karen S. Martin and Kathyrn H. Bowles

OBJECTIVES

After reading this chapter, the student should be able to do the following:

1. Compare different practice models for home- and community-based services.
2. Identify the basic roles and responsibilities of home health, palliative, and hospice nurses.
3. Explain the professional standards and educational requirements for nurses in home health, palliative care, and hospice.
4. Describe the three components of the Omaha System.
5. Explain how nurses in home health, palliative care, and hospice use best practices, evidence-based practice, and quality improvement strategies to improve the care they provide.
6. Cite examples of trends and opportunities in home health, palliative care, and hospice involving technology, informatics, and telehealth.

CHAPTER OUTLINE

History of Home Health and Nursing
Description of Practice Models
  Population-Focused Home Care
  Transitional Care in the Home
  Home-Based Primary Care
  Home Health
  Hospice
  Home Care of the Dying Child
Scope and Standards of Practice
  Direct and Indirect Care
  Nursing Roles in Home Health, Hospice, and Palliative Care
Omaha System
  Description of the Omaha System
Professional Development and Collaboration
  Education and Roles

Certification
Interprofessional Collaboration
Accountability and Quality Management
  Evidence-Based Quality and Performance Improvement
    and Client Safety
  Accreditation
Legal, Ethical, and Financial Aspects of Home Care
  Reimbursement Mechanisms
  Cost-Effectiveness
  Legal and Ethical Issues
Trends and Opportunities
  National Health Objectives
  Family Responsibility, Roles, and Functions
  Technology and Telehealth
  Health Insurance Portability and Accountability Act of 1996

KEY TERMS

accreditation, 534
benchmarking, 534
care coordination, 526
certification, 532
client outcomes, 534
family caregiving, 525

hospice, 526
interprofessional collaboration, 526
Outcomes and Assessment Information
  Set (OASIS), 534
palliative care, 526
prospective payment system, 526

regulations, 531
reimbursement system, 534
skilled care, 530
telehealth, 536
transitional care, 527

This chapter explains the development and current status of nursing in-home care as well as palliative and hospice care. *Home health, palliative, and hospice nursing* refers to care provided by a formal caregiver such as a nurse, speech or physical therapist, or physician within a client's home, as well as the potential for providing services in such settings as work, school,

residential, and acute care facilities. The care offered by formal caregivers is complemented by self-care provided by the client and caregiving by family members and friends. Care provided in the home differs from other areas of health care in that health care providers practice in the client's home environment. The home is where nurses have provided care for more than a century in the United States. Home care enables clients and families to receive health care in their usual home environment, where they may feel more comfortable and where it may be easier to learn how to make health-related lifestyle changes. For clients who are homebound, home care may be a necessity.

Home health care includes disease prevention, health promotion, and episodic illness-related services provided most often to people in their places of residence. Home may be a house, an apartment, a trailer, a boarding and care home, a shelter, a car, or any other place in which someone lives, such as residential facilities for the elderly. This triple-aim model of health care was published in 2008 with the outcome of healthier lifestyles (Berwick et al, 2008).

Home care does not refer only to home health; it is much broader than that. It is an approach to care that is provided in people's homes because theory or research suggests this is the optimum location for certain health and nursing services. Home care includes home health services, in-home hospice services, home visiting by public health nurses, and a variety of home-based health care programs focused on specific populations, such as new mothers, frail elders, and people with certain chronic health problems. Home health nursing is "a specialty area of nursing practice that promotes optimal health and well-being for patients, their families, and caregivers within their homes and communities. Home health nurses use a holistic approach aimed at empowering patients/families/caregivers to achieve their highest levels of physical, functional, spiritual, and psychosocial health. Home health nurses provide nursing services to patients of all ages and cultures and at all stages of health and illness, including end of life" (American Nurses Association [ANA], 2014, p 7).

It is essential to work with the family in the provision of care to an individual client. Family is defined by the individual and includes any caregiver or significant person who assists a client in need of care at home. Family caregiving includes assisting clients to meet their basic needs and providing direct care such as personal hygiene, meal preparation, medication administration, and treatments. Today, caregivers provide care in the home that in the past was provided in a hospital. Caregivers and clients themselves also provide health maintenance care between the visits of the professional provider. Levels of prevention in home care, including health maintenance care, are discussed in the Levels of Prevention box.

Client goals include health promotion, maintenance, and restoration. By maximizing the level of independence and self-care abilities, nurses help their clients function at the highest possible level. In addition, nurses contribute to the prevention of complications in chronically ill persons and help minimize the effects of disability and illness.

In any form of home care, nurses continually assess the client's response to interventions, report their findings to the client's physician or other health care provider as appropriate, and collaborate to modify the treatment plan or interventions as needed. Interventions are modified based on the client's responses. Services are coordinated through an agency obligated to maintain quality care and provide continuity whether that agency is a home health agency, hospice, community nursing program, clinic, or hospital. Thus the range of services provided in home care is extensive.

LEVELS OF PREVENTION
Applied to Home Care

Primary Prevention
- The nurse (1) administers seasonal vaccines, such as flu, or (2) provides case management interventions so clients obtain the vaccines at convenient locations.

Secondary Prevention
- The nurse monitors clients in their homes for early signs of new health problems to initiate prompt treatment. When the nurse works collaboratively with the physician or nurse practitioner, effective interventions can be provided. An example is monitoring clients for medication side effects.

Tertiary Prevention
- The nurse provides instruction about dietary modifications and insulin injections to the newly diagnosed diabetic clients. The purpose of these interventions is to prevent the development of complications from diabetes. Diabetic clients and their families implement the therapeutic plan with the goal of maintaining the highest possible level of health.

Nurses practice autonomously with little structure in the home setting; therefore, competence and creativity are essential (Cherry and Jacob, 2015). The home environment lacks many resources typically found in institutions, so it is essential that nurses have good organizational, critical thinking, communication, and documentation skills; are able to adapt to different settings; and demonstrate interpersonal ability to work with the diverse needs of people in their homes.

When working in a client's home, the nurse is a guest and, to be effective, must earn the trust of the family and establish a partnership with the client and family. Client safety is of utmost concern in home care just as in other health care settings.

HISTORY OF HOME HEALTH AND NURSING

Home care provided by formal caregivers can be traced back to the 19th century (Dieckmann, 2017; Harris, 2012). At that time, ladies' charitable organizations provided care to the sick in their own homes by hiring nurses. By the late 19th and early 20th centuries, Lillian Wald had established the Henry Street Settlement House in New York City and expanded home care to include community health needs. From Wald's Henry Street Settlement House, nurses and social workers visited people in their homes and provided instruction on basic hygiene, assessed health status, educated people about good nutrition, and provided support and immunizations. Although much home care was provided by voluntary organizations such as visiting nurse associations in the early 20th century, it was coordinated with governmental agencies such as health departments (Dieckmann, 2017; Christopher et al, 2016).

Home care began changing from its charitable and public health–oriented beginnings when payers added it to their benefit plans (Dieckmann, 2017; Harris, 2012). Wald persuaded the Metropolitan Life Insurance Company to include home care as a benefit in the early 1900s. Later, home care was included as a benefit for Medicare enrollees following the passage of Medicare legislation in 1965.

Inclusion of home care in the benefit packages of the Metropolitan Life Insurance Company and later in Medicare began to change the nature of the services (Dieckmann, 2017; Harris, 2012). Services focused on clients with specific functional and health problems who could not be cared for elsewhere. Nurses provided more technical care as time progressed. Home health as an industry expanded after the shift to prospective payment for hospital care with the federal Tax Equity and Fiscal Responsibility Act in 1982 (Feder, 2015). This occurred because clients were discharged more quickly from hospitals and needed more high-acuity nursing care in the home. The 1997 federal Balanced Budget Act (Feder, 2015; Huckfeldt et al, 2012) required moving reimbursement for home health services to a prospective payment system, which again meant pressure to care for clients with acute illnesses that were likely to improve. Attention continues to be paid to efficiency and cost-effectiveness of care. This often means that care is targeted toward very specific client populations and is highly organized and closely documented.

Historically, nurses who worked in people's homes were social reformers, living in immigrant communities and providing nursing clinics, health education, and care for the sick. They provided for the nutritional needs of their communities as well as clothing, hygiene, and adequate shelter. They were responsible for developing needed programs and providing necessary services in communities, including prenatal care, postpartum visits to new mothers and babies, hot-lunch school programs, preschool clinics, transportation services, summer camp programs, tuberculosis screening, blood typing, immunization for polio, and "sick room" equipment programs.

This combination of preventive services and illness care shifted after the introduction of Medicare in 1966. The Medicare program emphasized care for more acutely ill people rather than illness prevention and health promotion.

Hospice care, or care of the dying client and his or her significant others, was introduced in the United States in the 1970s by Dr. Florence Wald, dean of the Yale University School of Nursing, with the input of Dr. Cicely Saunders, a British physician who had developed the modern hospice concept in England in the 1960s (ANA and Hospice and Palliative Nurses Association [HPNA], 2014; National Hospice and Palliative Care Organization [NHPCO], 2016). Elisabeth Kübler-Ross's book *On Death and Dying* (1969) highlighted the need to provide more humane and sensitive care at the end of life. The concept of hospice grew out of a commitment to provide compassionate and dignified end-of-life care to people in the comfort of their homes (ANA/HPNA, 2014). Later hospice models included palliative care, which is symptom management, with a focus on care coordination and comprehensive support (NHPCO, 2016), often in specialized inpatient hospice units. Both home-based and inpatient hospice care models share a focus on comfort, pain relief, and mitigation of other distressing symptoms.

DESCRIPTION OF PRACTICE MODELS

Several practice models will be described in this chapter. They are population-focused home care, transitional care in the home, home-based primary care, home health, and hospice

---

QSEN FOCUS ON QUALITY AND SAFETY EDUCATION FOR NURSES

Targeted Competency: Client-Centered Care—Recognize the client or designee as the source of control and full partner in providing compassionate and coordinated care based on respect for client's preferences, values, and needs.

Important aspects of client-centered care include the following:

- **Knowledge:** Demonstrate comprehensive understanding of the concepts of pain and suffering, including physiological models of pain and comfort.
- **Skills:** Elicit expectations of client and family for relief of pain, discomfort, or suffering.
- **Attitudes:** Recognize that client expectations influence outcomes in management of pain or suffering.

Client-Centered Care Question:

Visit a community-based hospice or palliative care unit. Spend time observing the care provided in this setting.

A. How is care provided in this setting different from care you have seen in the acute care setting? In the home-care setting?

B. Notice how nurses and nursing assistants assess pain in this environment.

C. Discuss with the nurses how they address concerns around pain and suffering with clients and families in this environment. How do nurses evaluate clients and families' expectations around pain?

D. Discuss with the nurses differences in care approaches between a community-based hospice or palliative care versus care approaches for home hospice and palliative care. Is there additional education that is required for the client and family because the family often provides some aspects of care for home hospice and palliative care?

Prepared by Gail Armstrong, DNP, ACNS-BC, CNE, Associate Professor, University of Colorado Denver College of Nursing.

(Wepfer, 2011; Sherman and Matzo, 2015). All involve interprofessional collaboration as well as interest in best practices and evidence-based practice. Best practices suggest using the best possible evidence from a variety of sources, including research, experience, and expert practitioners; evidence-based practice suggests increased emphasis on programs of research that demonstrate consistently good outcomes. The models vary regarding the size and extent of participation, focus of the services, target population, research, political involvement, and funding. With each model, nurses have essential roles in the provision of care, documentation of services, program development and management, outcome and effectiveness analysis, and public education.

POPULATION-FOCUSED HOME CARE

Research has demonstrated that home-based approaches to care delivery produce better outcomes for certain populations. Population-focused home care is directed toward the needs of specific groups of people, including those with high-risk health needs such as mental health problems, cardiovascular disease, or diabetes; families with infants or young children; or older adults. These models commonly include structured approaches to regular visits with assessment protocols, focused health education, counseling, and health-related support and coaching for an identified population who share the same health issue. The following discussion describes several approaches to population-focused home care, such as the interprofessional home-care program and

PACE. In one example, Colandrea and Murphy-Gustavson (2012) describe the journey of clients with an identified health issue of heart failure from hospitalization to the home-care program. The interprofessional home-care program provided comprehensive health care and supportive services to clients. The nurses provided counseling, coaching, medication monitoring, referrals, and coordinated care with physicians, psychologists, social workers, dietitians, physical therapists, recreational therapists, and nurse aides. The program was effective in reducing readmission to the hospital for heart failure symptoms.

The Program of All-Inclusive Care for the Elderly (PACE) is a managed care model of integrated health and personal care services (Cortes and Sullivan-Marx, 2016; National PACE Association, 2016). Interprofessional care is provided in adult daycare centers with home-based assessments and supportive services also provided. Because of the model's success, it is now included in Medicare and Medicaid capitation plans.

The population-focused home-care approach uses care-delivery models developed using research evidence to improve health and cost outcomes for high-risk populations (see the Evidence-Based Practice box on page 531, which describes the improving outcomes for high-risk osteoporosis clients).

TRANSITIONAL CARE IN THE HOME

Transitional care programs in the home are designed for populations who have complex or high-risk health problems and are making a transition from one level of care to another (Transitional Care Model, 2014). Examples of high-risk groups for whom transitional care programs have been tested include older adult veterans (Gilmore-Bykovskyi et al, 2014), adults with mental illness (Solomon et al, 2014), adults with heart failure (Feltner et al, 2014), and adults with multiple chronic conditions (Carlos et al, 2016). These programs facilitate a smooth and coordinated health care experience for clients receiving health services across sites of care. An example would be an adult with diabetes who visits an ambulatory care clinic, is hospitalized, and is then discharged home. A transitional care program would involve assessment, planning, teaching, making referrals, and following up on the referrals by nurses at each stage of care to foster independence and self-care. Nursing care might include intensive teaching about self-care and telephone calls to ensure that the client and caregiver understood and were able to implement the instructions (Gilmore-Bykovskyi et al, 2014).

Nurses can facilitate smooth transitions from one level of care to another by working closely with hospital discharge planners (Naylor et al, 2011). Because clients and caregivers may find it difficult to learn while the client is hospitalized, nurses should communicate clearly with discharge planners about the therapeutic plan, medication regimens, what clients have been taught about self-care, and symptoms that should be reported to the physician.

HOME-BASED PRIMARY CARE

Home-based primary care is another form of home-care delivery. The emphasis in these programs is on delivering primary care in the homes of people who have difficulty going to a primary care clinic, community center, or physician's office because of functional or other health problems (Agency for Healthcare Research and Quality, 2014; Stall et al, 2014). One example is the Veterans Affairs Administration Hospital-Based Home Care Program (Edes et al, 2014; US Department of Veteran Affairs [USDVA], 2016). These programs are interprofessional and emphasize self-care; they help clients understand that the care experience is well coordinated across sites of care. Nurses provide health education to clients and caregivers in addition to primary care services such as health assessment, medication management, referrals, case management, and screening for new health problems. Comprehensive home-care services are part of the Veterans Health Administration's goals to create more client-centered care arrangements that promote coordination of the care experience across sites of care (Edes et al, 2014; USDVA, 2016).

House-call programs represent another example of primary care in the home. Nurse practitioners or physicians may provide primary care to clients who would find it difficult to visit a primary-care office because of their health problems, or interprofessional teams that include nurses, physicians, or other health professionals may provide primary care (De Jonge, 2015).

HOME HEALTH

Home health agencies are divided into the following five general categories based on administrative and organizational structures (Fig. 30.1):

- Official
- Private and voluntary
- Combination
- Hospital based
- Proprietary

These categories differ in organization and administration but are similar in terms of the standards they must meet for licensure, certification, and accreditation.

Official or public agencies include those agencies operated by the state, county, city, or other local government units, such as health departments. Nurses employed in these settings may also provide well-child clinics, immunizations, health education programs, and home visits for preventive health care. Official

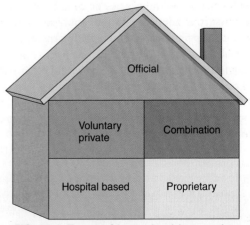

FIG. 30.1 Types of home health agencies.

agencies are funded primarily by tax funds and are nonprofit. Home-care services are reimbursed through Medicare, Medicaid, and private insurance companies.

Voluntary and private agencies are grouped together as nonprofit home health agencies. Voluntary agencies are supported by charities such as United Way; by Medicare, Medicaid, and other third-party payers; and by client payments. Traditionally, visiting nurse associations were the principal type of voluntary home health agency. With the initiation of Medicare in 1966, private nonprofit agencies emerged as alternatives to publicly supported programs.

Boards of directors that represent the communities they serve govern voluntary and private nonprofit agencies. These agencies are nongovernmental organizations and are exempt from federal income tax. Historically, voluntary agencies were responsible for the development of nursing in the home that was based on the client's need for service rather than the ability to pay. In some communities, official and voluntary home health agencies have merged into combination agencies to provide home health care, decrease cost, and prevent duplication of services. The services remain the same, and either the board members come from the two existing agencies or a new board is formed. The nurse may serve in several population-focused nursing roles, as does the nurse in the official type of agency.

In the 1970s, hospital-based agencies emerged in response to the recognized need for continuity of care from the acute care setting and also because of the high cost of institutionalization.

In 1983, implementation of the prospective payment system for acute hospital care by the federal government caused a fundamental change in home care. Costs of care dictated earlier client discharge to control expenses. Home health agencies, including hospital-based agencies, increased in number and developed services to improve quality along with controlling costs (Feder, 2015).

Agencies that are not eligible for income tax exemption are called proprietary (profit-making) agencies. Proprietary agencies can be licensed and certified for Medicare by the state licensing agency. The owner of the agency is responsible for governing. Reimbursement is primarily from third-party payers and individual clients if agencies do not accept Medicare.

The changing environment in home health care has several implications for the nurse providing care in the home. Because clients are discharged from acute care at earlier stages of treatment, a highly skilled level of care at home is needed. For example, many home health agencies provide infusion therapies in the home, such as administration of antibiotics, blood products, chemotherapy, and parenteral nutrition therapies (e.g., see Polinski et al, 2016). To survive in the competitive arena, agencies must continue to provide quality care and be cost-effective without compromising accountability.

CHECK YOUR PRACTICE

You have been participating in clinical practice at a local agency that provides home health, hospice and palliative care services. The staff does not seem to understand the differences in the care provided through each of these services. They have asked you to develop a brief presentation to help staff understand how the services are similar and how they are different. How would you approach this assignment? What would you do?

HOSPICE

Historically, the word *hospice* referred to a place of refuge for travelers. The contemporary meaning refers to palliative care of the very ill and dying, reducing distress from physical, emotional, and spiritual symptoms (Hui et al, 2013). Originating in 19th-century England, the earliest hospices first provided palliative care to terminally ill clients in hospitals and later extended the services into homes. In 1970 the hospice movement in the United States gained momentum in response to awakened public interest generated by Dr. Elisabeth Kübler-Ross's work on death and dying (Kübler-Ross, 1969). Public-sponsored hospices, successful in meeting the special needs of the dying client, attracted the attention of Congress. Medicare reimbursement for hospice services became available in 1982; services not covered by Medicare may be covered by other insurance plans or charitable organizations (Hospice Action Network, 2015; NHPCO, 2015).

Various hospice care models in the United States use institutional services, home care, or both. In addition to prescribed home-care services, core services offered through hospice include volunteers, chaplain support, respite care, financial help with medicines and equipment, and bereavement support for the family after the client's death.

One criterion for hospice is that the disease process or condition has progressed to the extent that further treatment cannot cure. It is the goal of hospice to increase the quality of remaining life. The hospice team is usually medically directed and nurse coordinated. Pain management, symptom control, and emotional support are key interventions.

Hospice provides on-call nursing 24 hours per day to monitor changes in the client's condition and attend to the needs of the client and family. After the death of the client, hospice provides bereavement counseling and services for up to 1 year.

Hospice programs may be integrated with a home health, hospital, or skilled nursing agency, or they may be freestanding (NHPCO, 2015). The philosophy of care requires that the members of the interprofessional team have the knowledge, skill, compassion, and experience to work with the unique needs of this population. The primary goal is to help maintain the client's dignity and comfort (Matzo and Sherman, 2015). Alleviating pain; encouraging the client, family, and friends to communicate with each other about essential sensitive issues related to death and dying; and coordinating care to ensure a comfortable, peaceful death contribute to palliative care. Although providing comfort transcends cultures, nurses should incorporate an understanding of unique cultural values, expectations, and preferences into hospice and palliative care (Paice, 2016).

Health care providers who work with the dying often experience unique stress. Staff stress must be identified and appropriately addressed to help in the delivery of quality care and to maintain the care provider's well-being. Nurses should be aware of signs of physical or emotional fatigue and design their own self-care strategies to prevent these problems (Paice, 2016; Matzo and Sherman, 2015). The hospice nurse needs a firm foundation in home-care skills, knowledge of community resources, the ability to function constructively as a team member, the ability to comfort with death and dying, and the mature ability to meet personal emotional needs as well as the emotional needs of the hospice client and family.

End-of-life care is of great concern to nursing, and many issues are debated by the public (e.g., client choice, available hospice services, reimbursement status, admission criteria, and assisted suicide). The *Code of Ethics for Nurses with Interpretive Statements* (ANA, 2015) and involvement in a formal interdisciplinary ethics committee can assist nurses in resolving these dilemmas (see the How To box).

HOW TO Use a Hospice Approach to Care in Any Setting

The hospice philosophy of care means providing comfort measures to an individual before death. The circumstances of death vary. The individual may be any age, from infancy to the older adult. A nurse may be faced with the death of a single individual or of many people during a limited time. Death may occur in the individual's home, in a hospital setting, or in an uncontrolled setting such as the community. How can nursing care be adapted to any situation? What basic skills of professional caregivers can be applied in any situation or setting? How do caregivers adapt to a hospice home death, inpatient death, or a sudden and unexpected death in which, for example, many people have died as a result of a natural disaster or a terrorist act?

- Be prepared now. Consider your own philosophy of death so that you can assist others without distraction when that time comes.
- Cultures vary in their beliefs about and responses to death. Know the differences in cultural responses so that you can effectively help people in their time of need.
- Death events cannot be totally controlled—even in a hospice environment in which family and friends and the dying individual have been prepared for the death. Expect the unexpected and take cues from the client and the loved ones regarding their needs.
- Shock, disbelief, and crisis reactions occur even with prepared hospice deaths. Ask family and caregivers what they need; provide them with the basics such as food or blankets; provide comfort; if it is not contraindicated, provide the family and friends with personal effects or mementos of the individual; give sensitive, caring support. Sit with them and listen.
- In a disaster, when many people are affected, the philosophy of care is to provide the greatest good to the greatest number of people. In a triage situation, the needs of those with less severe injuries have priority over the needs of those who are closer to death (Mistovich et al, 2013). Responsibilities of caregivers and health professionals will be stretched to the maximum. How do we care for the needs of the dying? How do we attend to the responses of the public to their loved ones? Someone needs to be present to support them. A specified leader to a group of clients must delegate responsibility to a caregiver who can assist the dying and their loved ones.

From Mistovich JJ, Karren KJ, Hafen B: *Prehospital emergency care,* ed 10, New York, 2013, Pearson.

HOME CARE OF THE DYING CHILD

In most situations, the terminally ill child desires to be home with his or her parents in familiar surroundings. That secure place is where families can provide the greatest comfort. The needs of the dying child and family are unique partly because society does not expect death to occur in the young or to have the child die before the parent.

Knowledge of the child's physical, cognitive, psychosocial, and spiritual development will enable the nurse to provide appropriate pain management, assist the child and family to communicate with each other, advocate for their needs in the community, and refer to key players who can offer them assistance, such as volunteers, counselors, or clergy.

Bereavement telephone calls or visits by hospice staff may continue for the family up to 1 year after the death of the child, at anniversaries of the child's death, and on holidays and the child's birthday. The family (including parents, grandparents, and siblings) can participate in community memorial services and support groups that are offered by the hospice program or other bereavement organizations. More research is needed on the most effective nursing interventions for dying children and their families (Ferrell, 2016).

SCOPE AND STANDARDS OF PRACTICE

Nursing is a theory-based and practice-based profession that incorporates art and science. Examples of nursing, family, and systems theories are mentioned and summarized in other chapters of this book. Chapter 10 addresses evidence-based practice; the concept is addressed frequently in this chapter, and two examples are included. Several chapters of this book describe the Quad Council's (2011) eight domains of practice; those domains are linked to information in this chapter in the Linking Content to Practice box. In addition, the Council on Linkages Between Academia and Public Health Practice (2014) provides guidance for future practice.

The nursing process is the theoretical framework used by the ANA, which notes that the nursing process is the essential methodology by which client goals are identified and achieved. The ANA's scope and standards publications, including those for Home Health Nursing and Hospice and Palliative Nursing, are organized according to the nursing process and contain two sections: the Standards of Care and the Standards of Professional Performance (ANA, 2014; ANA and HPNA, 2014). Both include the six steps of the nursing process: assessment, diagnosis, outcomes identification, planning, implementation, and evaluation; the steps are linked to standards and more specific measurement criteria that are stated in behavioral objectives. The standards address quality of care, performance appraisal, education, collegiality, ethics, collaboration, research, and resource use.

Nursing care provided in the home involves both direct and indirect activities.

DIRECT AND INDIRECT CARE

Direct care refers to the actual physical aspects of nursing care—anything requiring physical contact and face-to-face interactions. In home care, direct-care activities include performing a physical assessment on the client, changing a dressing on a wound, giving medication by injection, inserting an indwelling catheter, and providing intravenous therapy. Direct care also involves teaching clients and family caregivers how to perform a certain procedure or task. By serving as a preeminent model, the nurse helps the client and family develop positive health behaviors. When in the home, nurses need to be aware of infection control guidelines for self-protection and to protect the client (see the How To box on infection control).

HOW TO Maintain Infection Control Standards for Home Care

The practice of universal precautions means that all blood and body fluids are treated as potentially infectious. Universal precautions are implemented to prevent exposure and infection of caregivers. It is an important practice because many infections are subclinical.

- Use extreme care to prevent injuries when handling needles, scalpels, and razors. Do not recap, bend, break, or remove the needle from a syringe before disposal. Discard needles and syringes in puncture-resistant containers made of plastic or metal, and dispose of them in a local landfill or as directed by your agency.
- Soiled dressings or other materials contaminated with body fluids should be double bagged in polyethylene garbage bags using two bags, one inside the other as a liner.
- Human immunodeficiency virus (HIV) is easily decontaminated by common disinfectants such as Lysol and is rapidly killed by household bleach. Surfaces can be disinfected with a solution of 1 part bleach to 10 parts water. A new solution must be prepared daily to retain its disinfectant properties. Bathrooms and kitchens can be safely shared with persons infected with HIV, but towels, razors, and toothbrushes should not be shared. Household cleaning can be done in a regular manner unless there are spills of blood or body fluids. If a spill occurs, wear gloves and decontaminate the area by flooding the spill with a disinfectant, then use paper towels to remove visible debris, and reapply the disinfectant.
- Kitchen counters, dishes, and laundry should be cleaned with warm water and detergent after use. Bathrooms may be cleaned with a household disinfectant.
- Hand hygiene is the most important practice in preventing infections. Hand hygiene should be performed before and after providing client care and before and after preparing food, eating, feeding, or using the bathroom.

Nursing care in home health is covered by Medicare and other third-party payers as long as the care being delivered is skilled care. To determine whether a service performed by the nurse is skilled nursing care, several factors are evaluated and must be adequately documented. Examples of skilled nursing services include the following:

- Evaluating a client's health status and condition
- Administering treatments, rehabilitative exercises, and medications; inserting catheters; irrigating colostomies; and providing wound care
- Teaching the client and family to implement the therapeutic plan, such as treatments, therapeutic diets, and taking medications
- Reporting changes in the client's condition to the physician and arranging for medical follow-up as indicated

Indirect care activities are those that a nurse does on behalf of clients to improve or coordinate care. These activities include consulting with other nurses and health care providers in a multidisciplinary approach to care, organizing and participating in client care team conferences, advocating for clients with the health care system and insurers, supervising home health aides, obtaining results of diagnostic tests, and documenting

care. The following example illustrates direct and indirect care activities in a home health agency:

Mr. Jones, 70 years old, was discharged from the hospital yesterday after heart surgery for coronary artery disease. Today he is admitted to home health services for skilled nursing for an assessment of his cardiovascular status. Direct care involves teaching Mr. and Mrs. Jones about medications, exercise, nutrition, and the signs and symptoms of possible postoperative cardiac problems. In addition, the nurse will assess Mr. Jones's cardiovascular status and the healing of his incisions and help him return to an optimal state of functioning. The family's psychosocial adaptation and needs will also be addressed, and Mr. Jones's adjustment to his postsurgical status and his level of self-care will be assessed. The nurse also teaches Mr. Jones how he can prevent an exacerbation of his condition by maintaining medical follow-up and adapting his lifestyle to increase his adherence to the programs established for him. Primary prevention assessment strategies and counseling include environmental issues such as safety in the home and neighborhood, immunizations (e.g., influenza, pneumococcus), and reduction of stress factors. One of the nurse's indirect-care activities might be consulting with the pharmacist about optimal strategies for monitoring and preventing medication side effects. Another would be contacting a social service agency to facilitate Mr. Jones's access to financial assistance for his medications.

NURSING ROLES IN HOME HEALTH, HOSPICE, AND PALLIATIVE CARE

Nurses fulfill roles such as the following:

- Clinician
- Case manager
- Client advocate
- Educator
- Mentor
- Researcher
- Administrator
- Consultant

Nurses in staff positions are clinicians who provide direct nursing care to clients and families. They are also educators because they teach clients and families the "how to" and "why" of self-care.

Nurses function as case managers, coordinating care with and for clients over time and across settings. They function according to client needs, either providing the care to meet those needs or making referrals and coordinating care (Milone-Nuzzo and Hollars, 2017). In some cases, nurses provide disease management services, in which the emphasis is on the use of research evidence, guidelines, and protocols for managing populations with chronic illnesses (Free et al, 2013). Nurse care coordination has been found to improve outcomes for older adults with chronic health problems (Camicia et al, 2013).

Nurses also act as mentors, participating in the ongoing education of their colleagues, both formally, providing in-service education, and informally as team members. Additionally, they may teach classes to community groups regarding health education topics. The researcher role is increasingly important as the efficacy, or quality, and cost-effectiveness of care become mandated by Medicare and other payers. Nurses often provide the data required for clinical or administrative changes to occur within their agencies of employment. There are a variety of opportunities to participate in research. All nurses should use appropriate and current research to improve practice. Staff nurses can participate in research by suggesting clinical problems in need of research and participating in clinical research teams. Research must be a priority in the future if quality and cost-effectiveness are to be maintained. An administrator can be a nurse who has had advanced education with public health experience; requirements are stipulated by both federal and state rules and regulations. Finally, consultants may provide advice and counsel to staff and clients.

The *Code of Ethics for Nurses with Interpretive Statements* (ANA, 2015) is a guide for nurses facing ethical dilemmas. It is the "profession's nonnegotiable ethical standard" (p viii). The home-care nurse acts as a client advocate, maintaining client confidentiality, promoting informed consent, and making and following up on contacts to see that community resources are available to clients. Ethical conflicts and dilemmas are identified and resolved through formal agency mechanisms designed to address such issues. The nurse is responsible for building a trusting relationship with the family, determining whether the home is a safe and appropriate place to provide care for the particular client, and staying abreast of current research and ethical issues related to home care. The nurse acts in the area of professional obligations through political and social reform that affects client-based and population-based care. The client privacy guidelines from the Health Insurance Portability and Accountability Act of 1996 (HIPAA) require ethical conduct by the nurse in the protection of all forms of personal health information (Solve, 2013). This is becoming an even greater concern

EVIDENCE-BASED PRACTICE

Use of a Population-Focused Approach with a High-Risk Population

Outman and colleagues (2012) investigated improving osteoporosis care in high-risk home health clients. Clients with a history of fractures were targeted. The intervention was delivered by home health nurses and included development of a nursing care plan and client teaching materials concerning osteoporosis and antiosteoporosis medications. The intervention was piloted in one field office with 92 home health clients. Results indicated improvement in high-risk clients receiving osteoporosis prescription medications.

Nurse Use

This study shows how home health care nurses can provide effective education for clients at risk and improve treatment management.

From Outman et al: Improving osteoporosis care in high-risk home health patients through a high-intensity intervention, *Contemporary Clinical Trials* 33:206-212, 2012.

as health data are stored and transmitted electronically with electronic health records and electronic billing.

The nurse uses appropriate agency and community resources, including delegating tasks to other caregivers, to provide good benefits at a reasonable cost to the client. The nurse helps the client become an informed consumer to assist in empowerment and self-advocacy. Some health clients have more complicated health needs than in the past, and it is especially important for nurses to work with clients and other home-care professionals to plan clinical interventions carefully to obtain the best possible outcomes.

Home health nurses practice in accordance with *Home Health Nursing: Scope and Standards of Practice* developed by the ANA (2014). Nurses providing hospice care in the home use *Palliative Nursing: Scope and Standards of Practice* (ANA and HPNA, 2014). Periodically, the profession revises the scope of practice and standards of specialty practice to reflect the ongoing changes in the health care system and their effects on nursing care. Other clinical standards of practice from the ANA and specialty professional organizations guide population-focused home care, transitional care in the home, and home-based primary care.

OMAHA SYSTEM

Nurses, other practitioners, managers, and administrators in community settings face urgent practice, documentation, and information management challenges (Martin, 2005; Martin and Kessler, 2017; Topaz et al, 2014). Because of the magnitude and speed of changes in the health care system and developments in information technology, those in community settings face critical needs for the following:

1. Timely, valid, and reliable data that describe clients' demographic characteristics, the severity and acuity of their needs, the type and location of services, and reimbursement methods
2. Timely, valid, and reliable data that quantify the clients receiving care, the services they receive, and the costs and outcomes of that care
3. Verbal and automated methods for nurses to communicate with other nurses and health care practitioners

The ANA (2012) has addressed these challenges; the ANA website summarizes the Omaha System and other recognized terminologies that can describe clinical data, improve and standardize practice, and increase interoperability—the ability to exchange coded data (Thede and Schwirian, 2015).

DESCRIPTION OF THE OMAHA SYSTEM

As early as 1970, the staff and administrators of the Visiting Nurse Association (VNA) of Omaha, Nebraska, began addressing nursing practice, documentation, and information management concerns. At that time, no systematic nomenclature or classification of client problems existed that could be used with a problem-oriented record system, and practitioners were not using computers. These realities provided the incentive for initiating research.

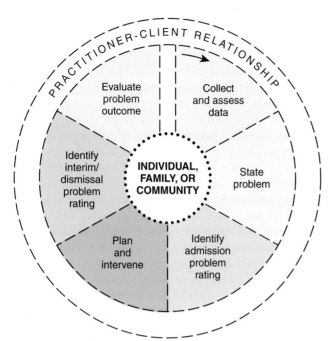

FIG. 30.2 Omaha System model of the problem-solving process. (From Martin KS: *The Omaha System: a key to practice, documentation, and information management,* reprinted, ed 2, Omaha, NE, 2005, Health Connections Press.)

During the next 20 years, the VNA of Omaha staff conducted four extensive, federally funded Omaha System development, reliability, validity, and usability research projects. The result of the research was the Problem Classification Scheme, the Intervention Scheme, and the Problem Rating Scale for Outcomes (Martin, 2005; Martin and Kessler, 2017; The Omaha System, 2016). As shown in Fig. 30.2, the theoretical framework of the Omaha System is based on the dynamic, interactive nature of the nursing or problem-solving process, the practitioner–client relationship, and concepts of diagnostic reasoning, clinical judgment, and quality improvement. The client as an individual, a family, or a community appears at the center of the model; this location shows the many ways the Omaha System can be used and the essential partnership between clients and practitioners.

The Omaha System is the only ANA-recognized terminology developed inductively (initially) by and for practicing nurses in the community. The goals of the Omaha System research were:

1. To develop a structured and comprehensive system that could be both understood and used by members of various disciplines
2. To foster collaborative practice

Therefore the Omaha System was designed to guide practice decisions, sort and document pertinent client data uniformly, and provide a framework for an agency-wide, multidisciplinary clinical information management system capable of meeting the needs of practitioners, managers, and administrators (Martin, 2005; Martin and Kessler, 2017; The Omaha System, 2016). See the tools in Appendix B.4 for the Omaha System Problem Classification Scheme with Case Study Application.

PROFESSIONAL DEVELOPMENT AND COLLABORATION

EDUCATION AND ROLES

Nurses come to home health and hospice from a variety of educational and practice backgrounds. Differences in both experience and educational preparation influence the contributions that nurses make. Home health and hospice nurses should be educated to function at a high level of competency so they can be relied on not only by their professional colleagues but also by the community. A baccalaureate degree in nursing should be the minimum requirement for entry into professional practice in any community health setting.

The nurse with a baccalaureate degree functions in the role of a generalist, providing skilled nursing and coordinating care for a variety of home health clients. The nurse with a master's degree is prepared for the advanced practice role as clinical specialist, nurse practitioner, researcher, administrator, or educator. As home health continues to play a larger role in community nursing practice, the need for specialized nurse clinicians will increase to meet the highly technological and complex care that has been moved from the hospital into the home setting. In managed care, more clinical specialists will be needed to provide case management and to develop programs to meet the needs of the population served by the managed care network. Nurse practitioners can provide primary care to frail older adults and other homebound clients. Educational programs are increasing to prepare nurses for advanced practice roles in home health.

CERTIFICATION

Home health nurses can maintain certification from the American Nurses Credentialing Center (ANCC) if already certified by the organization. The examinations for home health have been retired. The Hospice and Palliative Credentialing Center (HPCC) (2016) will certify hospice and palliative nurses. A baccalaureate degree in nursing is required for the generalist examination and a master's degree for the advanced-practice examinations. Nurses must also demonstrate current practice. In the highly competitive health care environment, certification is expected to become more necessary to ensure the competence and quality of care for the public. In addition there is a Home Health Nursing Association within the HPCC. Nurses can be nominated by their state to receive certification from this organization.

INTERPROFESSIONAL COLLABORATION

The responsibilities and functions of other health professions in home health and hospice are dictated by Medicare regulations, professional organizations, and state licensing boards. Other specialized services can be provided, such as the following:

- Enterostomal therapy
- Podiatry

- Pharmaceutical therapy
- Nutrition counseling
- Intravenous therapy
- Respiratory therapy
- Psychiatric or mental health nursing

Many of these services can be provided on a consulting basis, either in the form of staff education or through direct care. The interprofessional team may be composed of any or all of the following providers:

- Physician
- Physical therapist
- Occupational therapist
- Social worker
- Home health aides
- Speech pathologist

Each client in Medicare-funded home-care programs must be under the current care of a doctor of medicine, podiatry, or osteopathy to certify that the client has a medical problem. The physician must certify a plan of treatment before care is provided to the client.

Successful interprofessional collaboration and functioning depend on numerous factors, including the knowledge, skills, and attitudes of each team member. Factors necessary for successful interprofessional team functioning are shown in Box 30.1. The plan of care should be implemented and reinforced by all involved disciplines. For example, nurses must reinforce the teaching by the physical therapist of the exercise regimen and gait training.

BOX 30.1 Factors for Successful Interprofessional Functioning

Knowledge
1. Understand how the group process can be used to achieve group goals.
2. Understand problem solving.
3. Understand role theory.
4. Understand what other professionals do and how they view their roles.
5. Understand the differences between client levels of acuity across levels of care, including acute care, home care, ambulatory care, and long-term care.

Skill
1. Use principles of group process effectively.
2. Communicate clearly and accurately.
3. Communicate without using the profession's jargon.
4. Express yourself clearly and concisely in writing.

Attitude
1. Feel confident in your role as a professional.
2. Trust and respect other professionals.
3. Share tasks with other professionals.
4. Work effectively toward conflict resolution.
5. Be flexible.
6. Adopt an attitude of inquiry.
7. Be timely.

ACCOUNTABILITY AND QUALITY MANAGEMENT

EVIDENCE-BASED QUALITY AND PERFORMANCE IMPROVEMENT AND CLIENT SAFETY

Quality improvement activities are a crucial part of nursing care delivery. Nurses participate in the following:

- Monitoring care
- Seeing and analyzing opportunities for improving care
- Developing guidelines to improve care
- Collecting data
- Making recommendations
- Implementing activities to enhance quality of care
- Evaluating care and services

Results of these activities are used to make changes in health care delivery. Outcomes to determine quality indexes in Medicare are taken from the OASIS-C database and integrated into Outcome Based Quality Management (OBQI) (Centers for Medicare and Medicaid Services [CMS], 2016a). The OBQI is a quality improvement system for home health care (CMS, 2016b).

Quality management activities include peer review and other forms of performance appraisal. Professional development and lifelong learning are increasing in importance as home care changes rapidly to meet society's health care needs. Both the nurse and the employing agency are encouraged to endorse nursing participation in ongoing professional development, which includes continuing education and competence in home-care nursing. The nurse likewise exhibits collegiality by sharing expertise with others as appropriate and participating in the education and evaluation of students and other colleagues.

Since the beginning of Medicare, home health agencies have monitored the quality of care provided to their clients as a mandatory requirement for certification as a home health agency. All agencies, whether home health, hospice, or a clinic, hospital, or program providing home care, are accountable to their clients, to their reimbursement sources, to themselves as health care providers, and to professional standards.

Clinical data are of great importance in assessing the quality of care. The care and services the client receives and any communication between the physicians and other home health providers must be documented. Increasingly this documentation occurs in electronic health records, often by entering data into a laptop computer while in the home. It is in the clinical record that nurses demonstrate that they are delivering quality care and are also identifying means to improve the quality of care. It is the legal method by which the quality of care can be assessed. This documentation also demonstrates the client's ongoing need for services and shows how the multiple disciplines arrange for continuity and comprehensive care.

As an example, during the initial home visit, the nurse assesses the status of the client and family. This information becomes a permanent part of the clinical record. Subsequent integration of health services must be noted. In addition to clinical notes of all home visits, progress notes must be sent to the client's physician, including the assessment of the client to verify the implementation of the plan of care.

The Outcomes and Assessment Information Set (OASIS) measures outcomes for quality improvement and client satisfaction with care. Funded by the CMS and the Robert Wood Johnson Foundation, OASIS underwent extensive testing and is required for use by Medicare-certified home health agencies (Marrelli, 2012). See **Resource Tool 30A** for one part of this assessment.

The OASIS was revised and renamed in 2016 and is now OASIS-C2 (CMS, 2016c). OASIS data are measured and reported to the CMS on the client's admission to home health care, after an episode of hospitalization, at the time of recertification, and on discharge from care. Data are submitted by each agency to a national databank, and agencies receive both results and comparisons with similar agencies to determine areas needing improvement. See **Resource Tool 30A** for one part of this assessment.

Using the OASIS-C2 data, outcome analysis and improvement strategies can be accomplished through the OBQI framework (CMS, 2016b). The OBQI is a two-stage framework that includes "outcome analysis" and "outcome enhancement" (Fig. 30.3). The first stage, data analysis, enables an agency to compare its performance to a national sample, identify factors that may affect outcomes, and identify final outcomes that show improvement in or stabilization of a client's condition. The second stage, known as *outcome enhancement,* involves the selection of specific client outcomes and then determining strategies to improve care (CMS, 2012). Fig. 30.4 shows the OBQI outcome paradigm. The goal of the OASIS and OBQI is the provision of cost-effective, quality care.

Accrediting organizations also mandate reporting outcomes as a performance standard. Performance improvement programs are based on measurable data, including benchmarking, which means comparing yourself with national standards and guidelines and with other agencies. Clinical guidelines, pathways, and clinical maps are other methods that agencies are using to standardize care and control costs.

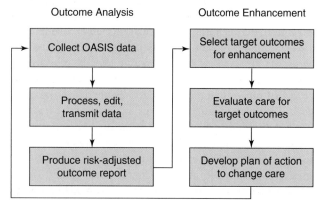

FIG. 30.3 Two-stage OBQI framework. (From Centers for Medicare and Medicaid Services: *Outcome-based quality improvement (OBQI) manual,* Baltimore, Md, 2012, CMS. pp 2.3)

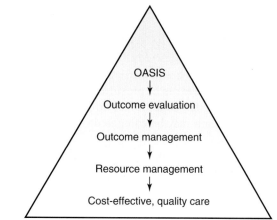

FIG. 30.4 The outcome paradigm. (From Centers for Medicare and Medicaid Services: *Outcome-based quality improvement (OBQI) manual,* Baltimore, MD, 2012, CMS. pp 2.4, 2.10.)

ACCREDITATION

Accreditation is a voluntary process; an agency chooses to participate. The accreditation decision is based on the data in a self-study, the report of a site visit team, and other relevant information. In the future, accreditation may become a requirement for licensure of all home health agencies. Today, home health agencies may be accredited through The Joint Commission (TJC) or the Community Health Accreditation Program (CHAP), initially established by the National League for Nursing and now an independent nonprofit organization. Both organizations look at the organizational structure through which care is delivered, the process of care through home visits, and the outcomes of client care, focusing on improved health status. Performance improvement must be ongoing in the agency.

Ensuring client safety is of primary concern in home health and hospice. Although client safety problems in the home may differ somewhat from those in acute care, they are still serious issues and must be prevented. With the emphasis on self-care by clients and families, safety problems may relate to clients having a good understanding of their health behaviors. Home clients may experience the following:

- Care errors as a result of inaccurate communications around referrals
- Cognitive deficits from health problems
- Socioeconomic problems such as lack of money for food or medications

TJC (2016) has National Patient Safety Goals that apply to all health care organizations, including home care and hospices accredited by TJC.

LEGAL, ETHICAL, AND FINANCIAL ASPECTS OF HOME CARE

REIMBURSEMENT MECHANISMS

The reimbursement system for home health is complicated and standardized. Medicare and Medicaid are the principal funding sources for home health care, with third-party health insurance

TABLE 30.1 Comparison of the Two Major Federally Supported Programs for Home Health Care

Medicare (Title XVIII)	Medicaid (Title XIX)
Federal insurance program administered by the Social Security Administration	Federal and state assistance program administered by the state
Age 65 years and over or disabled	Income-based eligibility
Conditions of participation	Conditions of participation
Homebound status	Not necessarily homebound status
Intermittent service	Intermittent service
Skilled service	Not necessarily skilled service
Restorative program	Custodial and maintenance program
Physician certification	Physician certification
Therapist, medical, or social service	State option: Therapist, medical, or social service
Pays for rental and purchase	Pays for purchase of equipment
Reimbursement by prospective payment	Reimbursement: Maximum allowed at the state level
Based on national rates	Based on a negotiated rate between the federal government and state

providing another major source. Budgeted funds for public health from taxes cover preventive home-care visits to the clients of public health agencies. Other home-care services such as health education, risk reduction, case management, or primary care may be reimbursed from a variety of sources. These include program funds, grants, contracts, and third-party billing.

If a client has both Medicare and Medicaid or a private insurance plan, Medicare is used as the primary payment source provided the services being delivered to the client meet the definition of *skilled*. After Medicare pays, private insurance is used. When the client is no longer eligible for home care under Medicare, the Medicaid benefits can be used. Table 30.1 illustrates the differences between Medicare and Medicaid programs.

COST-EFFECTIVENESS

Because of the increased number of home health agencies and increasing costs, the federal government instituted a prospective payment system on October 1, 2000. This system prevents the abuse or fraudulent use of Medicare funding.

Nurses in many settings are not directly exposed to the financial aspects of health care. In home health, nurses must be "cost-conscious" so that they can explain to clients what Medicare will or will not cover. It is often difficult for older clients to

understand why Medicare will not pay for the nurse to make home visits to take their blood pressure if their condition remains stable. Medicare pays for services only if the client's condition is unstable, the client is homebound, and the client requires skilled, intermittent, and part-time care.

LEGAL AND ETHICAL ISSUES

In any health care system there is the potential for illegal and unethical activity. Much publicity has been given to Medicare fraud and abuse. Examples of such practices include inappropriate use of home health services, inaccurate billing for services, excessive administrative staff, "kickbacks" for referrals, and billing for non-covered medical supplies.

Home health and hospice nurses are confronted with multiple issues in everyday practice. Third-party payers have interpreted the definition of skilled care inconsistently over the years. The nurse must abide by established federal regulations when delivering care to clients, even when the needs are greater than what is reimbursed. The frequency of visits poses another issue. Only intermittent visits are reimbursed. If the frequency increases, then full-time skilled services may be required. Continual reassessment of client and family needs is imperative to avoid inappropriate use and overuse of services. Nurses must be knowledgeable about which medical supplies are covered. This information is readily available, and nurses must work within regulatory guidelines and educate the community as to what should be covered and what is actually covered. Evidence-based nursing practice is essential.

Nurses are at risk for malpractice claims related to the complexity of care needed and actual or alleged negligence from rushed visits or failure to adhere to standards of practice (Neil, 2015). Performance improvement programs, use of evidence-based practice guidelines, and appropriate use of information technology for communication and telehealth are strategies that can help reduce these risks (Neil, 2015).

TRENDS AND OPPORTUNITIES
NATIONAL HEALTH OBJECTIVES

Because nurses are working with clients and families in the home and community, they are in a position to promote the achievement of some of the key *Healthy People 2020* objectives. The nurse can assess the client's status related to key objectives, identify available resources and gaps to meet client needs, and coordinate care with other providers and community agencies.

❤ HEALTHY PEOPLE 2020

The following are examples of national health objectives for the year 2020:
- **AOCBC-11** Reduce hip fractures among older adults.
- **C-1** Reduce the overall cancer death rate.
- **C-13** Increase proportion of cancer survivors beyond 5 years.
- **CKD-9** Reduce kidney failure resulting from diabetes.

- **HD-3** Reduce stroke deaths.
- **HDS-1** (Developmental) Increase overall cardiovascular health in the US population.
- **HDS-5** Reduce the proportion of persons in the population with hypertension.
- **IID-4** Reduce invasive pneumococcal infections.

From US Department of Health and Human Services: *Healthy People 2020: national health promotion and disease prevention objectives*, Washington, DC, 2010, USDHHS. Retrieved August 2016 from https://www.healthypeople.gov/2020/topics-objectives.

The *Healthy People 2020* box highlights the objectives of home health and hospice nurses. Note that many of these objectives relate to lifestyle issues. With appropriate health education, referral to community resources, and follow-up, there is a potential to reduce morbidity and mortality and decrease chronic disabilities. Nurses can make important contributions at one-to-one and population-focused levels.

FAMILY RESPONSIBILITY, ROLES, AND FUNCTIONS

The family plays an important role in the delivery of care in the home. The term *family,* as discussed previously, refers to a caregiver responsible for the client's well-being. Women have traditionally been the caregivers for children and older adults in the United States. Now, however, women are less available to provide this care without assistance because they are often working outside the home. Similarly, other family members may be employed or have multiple obligations, creating new challenges for family caregiving and for nurses designing care delivery strategies in home care.

Home health and hospice programs and reimbursement systems may be set up to provide family services or may reserve those services for families in crisis (Heller et al, 2015). Nurses must find creative ways to include family caregivers as partners in the client's care and must provide the teaching, coaching, and support needed. Nurses should advocate for policy changes when necessary to foster effective evidence-based family care strategies.

Assistance from social support systems helps families cope with the stress of caring for an ill family member. The goal is to maintain the client at home for as long as possible and to provide high-quality care. To do this, resources must be used appropriately and effectively. However, developing a public consensus to resolve these issues has been challenging.

TECHNOLOGY AND TELEHEALTH

The incentives and pressures for cost control and improved health outcomes have increased the development and use of telehealth technology in the home-care setting (Bowles et al, 2012; Radhakrishnan et al, 2016). At the same time, some technologies have been simplified and their reliability increased, facilitating their safe use in the home. Telehealth, parenteral nutrition, chemotherapy, intravenous therapy for hydration and antibiotics, intrathecal pain management, ventilators, apnea monitors, chest tubes, and skeletal traction are examples of current home-care technologies. The home-care nurse must be prepared to evaluate the cost and safety of technology for the home. Clients must be screened and meet specific admission criteria for use of particular technologies.

Telehealth has emerged as a viable and acceptable way to provide health care. Telehealth is defined as sharing health information between the client and clinicians using either synchronous or asynchronous electronic communications via telephone, videophone, or a biometric monitoring unit (Bowles et al, 2012; Radhakrishnan et al, 2016). The technology used

varies to include videoconferencing, the Internet, store-and-forward imaging, streaming media, satellite, wireless communications, and telephone systems. Telehealth equipment and program components include telephone triage and advice and biometric telemonitoring equipment to measure vital signs, cardiac function, and point-of-care diagnostics. The system may or may not include video technology for live interaction (Weinstein et al, 2014). When conducted in the home, it is commonly referred to as *telehomecare.*

Telehealth has been used successfully to improve health outcomes for clients with diabetes (Baron et al, 2016), heart failure (Gorst et al, 2014), chronic obstructive pulmonary disease (Gorst et al, 2014), and chronic wounds (Chanussot-Deprez and Contreras-Ruiz, 2013).

Telemonitoring is increasingly being used with infants, women with high-risk pregnancies, and adults with various health problems. Smart homes are emerging to help the older adult to "age in place." Sensors can monitor activities and detect adverse events such as a fall or lack of movement and trigger a call for help. Medication management devices remind clients to take their medications, dispense medications, and send alerts to providers if devices are not accessed as expected. The next generation of devices is expected to focus on smartphone technology, making telemonitoring even more ubiquitous.

HEALTH INSURANCE PORTABILITY AND ACCOUNTABILITY ACT OF 1996

In 1996 Congress passed the Health Insurance Portability and Accountability Act (HIPAA; Public Law [PL] 104-191), which was initially related specifically to the portability of health insurance. The full scope of the legislation had a far-reaching impact on protecting the privacy and security of personal health information. All health care organizations were required to meet HIPAA federal privacy standards by April 14, 2003. This legislation protects the client's private information through the electronic transfer of health records, allows individuals full access to their personal medical records, provides clear information (informed consent) specifying the medical use of the client's personal health information and records to allow the client to have control over that information, and ensures legal protection, with significant criminal and civic penalties to those individuals or agencies that do not comply with the privacy requirements (US Department of Health and Human Services, n.d.).

More recent federal efforts have stimulated the use of electronic health records (Middleton et al, 2013), and there is a federal mandate to use electronic health records by 2014 (PL 104-191, 2010). This has the potential to make seamless care delivery and client safety more likely, although safeguards need to be included to protect the privacy and confidentiality of personal health information. The Patient Protection and Affordable Care Act provides for home health care services through private insurance plans, Medicare, and long-term care benefits. It also provides for support with activities of daily living.

▶ APPLYING CONTENT TO PRACTICE

The Nurse in Home Health and Hospice

The individuals, families, and communities served by home health, hospice, and palliative care nurses are described throughout this chapter, as are the knowledge, skills, and attitudes of nurses who function well in those settings. The descriptions are evident in the text, clinical examples, boxes, figures, tables, references, and other parts of the chapter. The competencies in this chapter are congruent with the following core competencies of the Quad Council's (2011) Domains of Public Health Nursing: (1) Analytic/Assessment Skills, (2) Policy Development/Program Planning Skills, (3) Communication Skills, (4) Cultural Competency Skills, (5) Community Dimensions of Practice Skills, (6) Basic Public Health Sciences Skills, (7) Financial Planning and Management Skills, and (8) Leadership and Systems Thinking Skills. Students and new graduates cannot be expected to have developed all of these skills when they begin home health or hospice practice. However, as nurses proceed in their career development and gain valuable work experience, they will progress along the novice-to-expert continuum described by the Quad Council (2011).

▌ PRACTICE APPLICATION

The home visit is the hallmark of nursing in home health and hospice. When a nurse enters a client's home, he or she is a guest and must recognize that the services offered can be accepted or rejected. The first visit sets the stage for success or failure. The initial assessment of the client, the support system, and the environment is critical.

What strategies would the nurse consider to develop a trusting relationship during the first visit?

What would be the most important elements to assess in the home environment?

What should the nurse include in the client contract?

How can the nurse assess the preferred learning style?

Answers can be found on the Evolve site.

▌ REMEMBER THIS!

- Home health hospice and palliative care differ from other areas of health care because health care providers practice in the client's environment in a number of types of settings. This unique characteristic affects several components of nursing practice in the home-care setting, including establishing trust, developing care partnerships, selecting interventions, collecting outcomes and data, ensuring client safety, and promoting quality.
- Family members, including any caregiver or significant person who takes the responsibility to assist the client in need of care at home, are an integral part of home health care.
- Home nursing care has its roots in public health nursing, with an emphasis on health promotion, illness prevention, and caring for people in the contexts of their communities.
- Home health, hospice, and palliative care reached a turning point with the arrival of Medicare, which provided regulations for each of these types of health care practice and reimbursement mechanisms.
- Although many think of home health when thinking of home care, there are many other approaches to home care. Five models of practice are described in this chapter: population-focused home care, transitional care in the home, home-based primary care, home health, and hospice and palliative care. Nurses will want to learn about current and new models of care and use those that are most effective for the client situation.
- Home health agencies are divided into the following five general categories on the basis of administrative and organizational structures: official, private and voluntary, combination, hospital based, and proprietary.
- Standards of practice originate from American Nurses Association (ANA) and specialty organizations.
- Demonstration of professional competency is essential for home health and hospice nurses.
- The home health care nurse practices in accordance with *Home Health Nursing: Scope and Standards of Practice* developed by the ANA (2014). Hospice nurses use *Palliative Nursing: Scope and Standards of Practice*, jointly developed by the ANA and the Hospice and Palliative Care Nurses Association (ANA/HPNA, 2014).
- Interprofessional collaboration is a required process in home health and hospice care. It is inherent in the definition of home care.
- In home care, as in other care settings, professionals experience stress associated with changing roles and overlapping responsibilities. In collaborating, home health care providers should carefully analyze one another's roles to determine whether overlapping occurs and adjust the plan of care as needed.
- Since the advent of Medicare, home health, hospice, and palliative care agencies have monitored the quality of care to their clients as a mandatory requirement for certification as a home health agency. All agencies are accountable to clients and families, to their reimbursement sources, to themselves as a health care provider, and to professional standards.
- Nurses in any home setting should work to establish and use quality improvement processes and design care systems to ensure client safety.
- The nurse today faces many challenges. Ethical issues (e.g., reimbursement criteria, access to care), role development (e.g., high-technology nursing, hospice nursing), and opportunities for research (e.g., quality of care, cost-effectiveness, client safety) affect nursing practice in the home.
- Home-care agencies may be accredited through The Joint Commission or the Community Health Accreditation Program.
- The Omaha System was developed and refined through a process of research. Reliability and validity were established for the entire system.

- The Omaha System is unique in that it is the only comprehensive vocabulary developed initially by and for practicing population-focused nurses.
- The Omaha System was designed to follow specific principles. The system consists of a Problem Classification Scheme, an Intervention Scheme, and a Problem Rating Scale for Outcomes.

- The Omaha System offers benefits in three principal areas: practice, documentation, and information management. These areas are of concern to community health educators and students, as well as community health practitioners and administrators.

ⓔ EVOLVE WEBSITE

http://evolve.elsevier.com/Stanhope/foundations
- NCLEX® Review Questions
- Practice Application Answers

REFERENCES

Agency for Healthcare Research and Quality: *Home-based primary care interventions systematic review*, 2014. http://www.effectivehealthcare.ahrq.gov.

American Nurses Association (ANA): *ANA recognized terminologies that support nursing practice*, Silver Spring, MD, 2012, Nursebooks.org. Available at http://www.nursingworld.org/MainMenuCategories/ThePracticeofProfessionalNursing/NursingStandards. Accessed August 17, 2016.

American Nurses Association (ANA): *Home health nursing: scope and standards of practice*, ed 2, Silver Spring, MD, 2014, Nursebooks.org.

American Nurses Association (ANA): *Code of ethics for nurses with interpretive statements*, Silver Spring, MD, 2015, Nursebooks.org.

American Nurses Association and Hospice and Palliative Nurses Association (ANA/HPNA): *Palliative nursing: scope and standards of practice – an essential resource for hospice and palliative nurses*, Silver Spring, MD, 2014, Nursebooks.org.

Baron JS, Hirani S, Newman SP: A randomized, controlled trial of the effects of a mobile telehealth intervention on clinical and patient-reported outcomes in people with poorly controlled diabetes, *J Telemedicine and Telecare* 23(2):197–206, 2016.

Berwick DM, Nolan TW, Whittington J: The triple aim: care, health and cost, *Health Affairs* 27:759–769, 2008.

Bowles KH, O'Connor M, Hanlon A, et al: *Barriers to cost and clinical efficiency with telehomecare and proposed solutions*, eTelemed, 2012. Retrieved August 2016 from http://www.thinkmind.org/index.php?view=article&articleid=etelemed_2012_7_30_40192.

Camicia M, Chamberlain B, Finnie RR, Nalle M, Lindeke LL, Lorenz L, Hain D, Haney KD, Campbell-Heider N, Pecenka-Johnson K, Jones T, Parker-Guyton N, Brydes G, Briggs WT, Cisco MC, Haney C, McMenamin P: The value of nursing care coordination: a white paper of the American Nurses Association, *Nursing Outlook* 61(6):490–501, 2013.

Carlos J, Kasper EW, Williams C, DuBard CA: Incremental benefit of a home visit following discharge for patients with multiple chronic conditions receiving transitional care, *Population Health Management* 19(3):163–170, 2016.

Centers for Medicare and Medicaid Services: *Outcome-based quality improvement (OBQI) manual*, Baltimore MD, 2012, CMS, pp 2–3.

Centers for Medicare and Medicaid Services [CMS]: *Home Health Quality Initiative*, Baltimore MD, 2016a, CMS. Retrieved August 2016 from https://www.cms.gov/Medicare/Quality-Initiatives-Patient-Assessment-Instruments/HomeHealthQualityInits/index.html?redirect=/homehealthqualityinits//.

Centers for Medicare and Medicaid Services [CMS]: *OASIS OBQI*, Baltimore MD, 2016b, CMS. Retrieved August 2016 from https://www.cms.gov/Medicare/Quality-Initiatives-Patient-Assessment-Instruments/HomeHealthQualityInits/HHQIOASISOBQI.html.

Centers for Medicare and Medicaid Services [CMS]: *OASIS User Manuals*, 2016c. Retrieved August 2016 from https://www.cms.gov/Medicare/Quality-Initiatives-Patient-Assessment-Instruments/HomeHealthQualityInits/HHQIOASISUserManual.html.

Chanussot-Deprez C, Contreras-Ruiz J: Telemedicine in wound care: a review, *Advances in Skin and Wound Care* 26(2):78–82, 2013.

Cherry B, Jacob SR: *Contemporary nursing: issues, trends, & management*, ed 7, St. Louis, MO, 2017, Elsevier.

Christopher MA, Hawkey R, Jared MC: Lillian D. Wald: pioneer of public health. In Forrester DA, editor: *Nursing's greatest leaders: a history of activism*, New York, 2016, Springer Publishing Company, LLC.

Colandrea M, Murphy-Gustavson J: Patient care heart failure model: the hospitalization to home plan of care, *Home Healthcare Nurse* 30:337–344, 2012.

Cortes TA, Sullivan-Marx EM: A case exemplar for national policy leadership: expanding Program of All-Inclusive Care for the Elderly (PACE), *J Gerontological Nursing* 42(3):9–14, 2016.

Council on Linkages Between Academia and Public Health Practice: *Core competencies for public health professionals*, Washington, DC, 2014, The Public Health Foundation.

De Jonge KE: *Back to the future: making house calls for better care, reduced costs*, Washington DC, 2015, US Department of Health and Human Services. Retrieved August 2016 from http://www.hhs.gov/blog/2015/08/11/making-house-calls-better-care-reduced-costs.html.

Dieckmann JL: Home health care: a historical perspective and overview. In Harris MD, editor: *Handbook of home health care administration*, Burlington, MA, 2017, Jones & Bartlett Learning.

Edes T, Kinosian B, Vuckovic NH, Nichols LO, Becker MM, Hossain M: Better access, quality, and cost for clinically complex veterans with home-based primary care, *J American Geriatric Society* 62(10):1954–1961, 2014.

Feder J: The missing piece – Medicare, Medicaid, and long-term care. In Cohen AB, Colby DC, Wailoo K, Zelizer JE, editors: *Medicare and Medicaid at 50: Americas entitlement programs in the age of affordable care*, New York, 2015, Oxford University Press.

Feltner C, Jones CD, Cene CW, Zheng Z, Sueta CA, Coker-Schwimmer EJL, Arvantis M, Lohr KN, Middleton JC, Jonas DE: Transitional care interventions to prevent readmissions for persons with heart failure: a systematic review and meta-analysis, *Ann Intern Med* 160(11):774–784, 2014.

Ferrell BR, editor: *Pediatric palliative care*, New York, 2016, HPNA Palliative Nursing Manuals, Oxford University Press.

Free C, Phillips G, Galli L, Watson L, Felix L, Edwards P, Patel V, Haines A: The effectiveness of mobile-health technology-based health behavior change or disease management interventions for health care consumers: a systematic review, *PLOS Medicine* 10(1):e1001362, 2013. https://doi.org/10.1371/journal.pmed.1001362.

Gilmore-Bykovskyi A, Jensen L, Kind AJH: Development and implementation of the Coordinated-Transitional Care (C-TraC) Program, *Fed Pract* 31(2):30–34, 2014.

Gorst SL, Armitage CJ, Brownsell S, Hawley MS: Home telehealth uptake and continued use among heart failure and chronic obstructive pulmonary disease patients: a systematic review, *Annals of Behavioral Medicine* 48(3):323–336, 2014.

Harris M: Home healthcare then and now: a personal experience, *Home Healthcare Nurse* 30:492–496, 2012.

Heller T, Givvons HM, Fisher D: Caregiving and family support interventions: crossing networks of aging and developmental disabilities, *Intellectual and Developmental Disabilities* 53(5):329–345, 2015.

Hospice Action Network: *Hospice compliance/regulatory requirements, with Medicare reimbursement changes 2009-2016*, Alexandria, VA, 2015, Hospice Action Network and National Hospice and Palliative Care Organization. Retrieved August 2016 from http://hospiceactionnetwork.org/linked_documents/get_informed/policy_resources/Regulatory_Timeline.pdf.

Hospice and Palliative Credentialing Center: *Certifications/Candidate Handbooks & Applications*, 2016. Retrieved August 2016 from http://hpcc.advancingexpertcare.org/competence/certifications-handbooks-applications/.

Huckfeldt PJ, Sood N, Escarce JJ, Graowski DC, Newhouse JP: *Effects of Medicare payment reform: evidence from the home health interim and prospective payment systems, National Bureau of Economic Research, NBER working paper no. 17870*, 2012. Retrieved August 2016 from http://www.nber.org/papers/w17870.

Hui D, de la Cruz M, Mori M, et al: Concepts and definitions for "supportive care," "best supportive care," "palliative care," and "hospice care" in the published literature, dictionaries, and textbooks, *Support Care Cancer* 21:659–685, 2013.

Kübler-Ross E: *On death and dying*, New York, 1969, McMillan.

Marrelli TM: *Handbook of home health standards: quality, documentation, and reimbursement*, ed 5, revised reprint, St. Louis, MO, 2012, Mosby.

Martin KS: *The Omaha System: a key to practice, documentation, and information management, reprinted*, ed 2, Omaha, NE, 2005, Health Connections Press.

Martin KS, Kessler PD: The Omaha System: improving the quality of practice and decision support. In Harris MD, editor: *Handbook of home health care administration*, ed 6, Burlington, MA, 2017, Jones and Bartlett Learning.

Matzo M, Sherman DW, editors: *Palliative care nursing: quality care to the end of life*, ed 4, New York, 2015, Springer Publishing Company, LLC.

Middleton B, Bloomrosen M, Dente MA, Hashmat B, Koppel R, Overhage JM, Payne TH, Rosenbloom ST, Weaver C, Zhang J: Enhancing patient safety and quality of care by improving the usability of electronic health record systems: recommendations from AMIA, *J American Medical Informatics Association* 20(e1):e2–e8, 2013.

Milone-Nuzzo P, Hollars ME: Transitioning nurses to home care. In Harris MD, editor: *Handbook of home health care administration*, ed 6, Burlington, MA, 2017, Jones and Bartlett Learning.

Mistovich JJ, Hafen BQ, Karren KJ: *Prehospital emergency care*, ed 10, New York, 2013, Pearson.

National Hospice and Palliative Care Organization (NHPCO): *History of hospice care*, 2016. Retrieved August 2016 from http://www.nhpco.org/history-hospice-care.

NHPCO: *The Medicare Hospice Benefit from the Medicare Payment Advisory Commission. Chapter 12, Report to Congress: Medicare Payment Policy*. March 2015. http://medpac.gov/documents/reports/chapter-12-hospice-services-(march-2015-report).pdf.

National PACE Association: *Understanding the PACE model of care*, Alexandria, VA, 2016, National PACE Association. Retrieved August 2016 from http://www.npaonline.org/start-pace-program/understanding-pace-model-care.

Neil HP: Nursing liability and evidence-based practice, *MedSurg Nursing* 24(5):S10–S210, 2015.

Outman RC, Curtis JR, Locher JL, et al: Improving osteoporosis care in high-risk home health patients through a high-intensity intervention, *Contemp Clin Trials* 33:206–212, 2012.

Paice JA, editor: *Care of the imminently dying*, New York, 2016, HPNA Palliative Nursing Manuals, Oxford University Press.

Patient Protection and Affordable Care Act (PL 104-191): Washington, DC, 2010, Department of Health and Human Services.

Polinski JM, Kowal MK, Gagon M, Brennan TA, Shrank WH: *Home infusion: safe, clinically effective, patient preferred, and cost saving, Healthcare*, 2016. http://dx.doi.org/10.1016/j.hjdsi.2016.04.004i.

Quad Council of Public Health Nursing Organizations: *Core competencies for public health nursing practice*, Washington, DC, 2011, Public Health Foundation.

Radhakrishnan K, Berkley A, Kim M: Barriers and facilitators for sustainability of tele-homecare programs: a systematic review, *Health Services Research* 51(1):48–75, 2016.

Sherman DW, Matzo M, Metheny T: The interprofessional practice of palliative care nursing. In Matzo, M, Sherman, D. *Palliative care in nursing* ed 4, chapter 1, Springer, 2015, New York, pages 3–21.

Solomon P, Hanrahan NP, Hurford M, DeCesaris M, Josey L: Lessons learned from implementing a pilot RCT of transitional care model for individuals with serious mental illness, *Archives of Psychiatric Nursing* 28(4):250–255, 2014.

Solve DJ: HIPAA turns 10: analyzing the past, present, and future impact, *Journal of AHIMA*, 8:22–28, 2013. GWU Legal Studies Research Paper No. 2013-76, GWU Law School Public Law Research Paper No. 2013-75.

Stall N, Nowaczynski M, Sinha SK: Systematic review of outcomes from home-based primary care programs for homebound older adults, *J American Geriatrics Society* 62(12):2243–2251, 2014.

The Joint Commission: *National patient safety goals*, 2016. Retrieved August 2016 from https://www.jointcommission.org/standards_information/npsgs.aspx.

The Omaha System: *Omaha system overview*, 2016. Retrieved August 2016 from http://www.omahasystem.org/overview.html.

Thede LQ, Schwirian PM: Informatics: the standardized nursing terminologies: a national survey of nurses' experience and attitudes – SURVEY II: evaluation of standardized nursing terminologies, *The Online Journal of Issues in Nursing* 21(1), 2015. DOI: 10.3912/OJIN.Vol21No01InfoCol01.

Topaz M, Golfenshtein N, Bowles KH: The Omaha System: a systematic review of the recent literature, *J Am Med Inform Assoc* 21:163–170, 2014.

Transitional Care Model: *About TCM*, Philadelphia, PA, 2014, University of Pennsylvania Nursing Science. Retrieved August 2016 from http://www.transitionalcare.info/about-tcm.

US Department of Health and Human Services: *Health information privacy*, Washington, DC, n.d., USDHHS. Retrieved August 2016 from http://www.hhs.gov/hipaa/index.html.

US Department of Health and Human Services: *Healthy People 2020: national health promotion and disease prevention objectives*, Washington, DC, 2010, US Department of Health and Human Services. Retrieved August 2016 from https://www.healthypeople.gov/2020/topics-objectives.

US Department of Veteran Affairs: *Geriatrics and extended care: home-based primary care*, Washington, DC, 2016, USDVA. Retrieved August 2016 from http://www.va.gov/geriatrics/Guide/LongTermCare/Home_Based_Primary_Care.asp.

Weinstein RS, Lopez AM, Joseph BA, Erps KA, Holcomb M, Barker GP, Krupinski EA: Telemedicine, telehealth, and mobile health applications that work: opportunities and barriers, *The American Journal of Medicine* 127(3):183–187, 2014.

Wepfer VM: Home health nursing: unlocking the door to the heart of wellness, *Home Healthcare Nurse* 29:199–200, 2011.

The Nurse in the Schools

Lisa Pedersen Turner

OBJECTIVES

After reading this chapter, the student should be able to:

1. Discuss professional standards expected of school nurses.
2. Differentiate between the many roles and functions of school nurses.
3. Describe the different variations of school health services and coordinated school health programs.
4. Discuss common health problems of children and adolescents seen in the school setting.
5. Assess the nursing care given in schools in terms of the primary, secondary, and tertiary levels of prevention.
6. Identify future trends in school nursing.

CHAPTER OUTLINE

History of School Nursing
Federal Legislation in the 1970s, 1980s, 1990s, and 2000s
Standards of Practice for School Nurses
Educational Credentials of School Nurses
Roles and Functions of School Nurses
School Nurse Roles
School Health Services
Federal School Health Programs
School Health Policies and Practices Study
School-Based Health Programs

School Nurses and *Healthy People 2020*
Levels of Prevention in Schools
Primary Prevention in Schools
Secondary Prevention in Schools
Tertiary Prevention in Schools
Controversies in School Nursing
Ethics in School Nursing
Future Trends in School Nursing

KEY TERMS

American Academy of Pediatrics (AAP), 543
Americans with Disabilities Act (ADA), 542
case manager, 544
Centers for Disease Control and Prevention (CDC), 545
community outreach, 544
consultant, 544
counselor, 544
crisis teams, 549
direct caregiver, 544
Do-Not-Resuscitate (DNR) orders, 555

emergency plan, 549
health educator, 544
individualized education plans (IEPs), 542
individualized health plans (IHPs), 542
National Association of School Nurses (NASN), 543
PL 93-112 Section 504 of the Rehabilitation Act of 1973, 541
PL 94-142 Education for All Handicapped Children Act, 541
PL 105-17 Individuals with Disabilities Education Act (IDEA), 542

PL 114-95 Every Student Succeeds Act (ESSA), 542
primary prevention, 546
researcher, 545
Safe Kids Campaign, 547
school-based health centers (SBHCs), 546
School Health Policies and Programs Study, 546
school nursing, 541
secondary prevention, 546
tertiary prevention, 546

In the fall of 2015, more than 50.1 million children attended a public school in the United States (35.2 million in prekindergarten through grade 8 and 14.9 million in grades 9 through 12), and an additional 4.9 million students attended a private school (US Department of Education, National Center for Education Statistics [USDE, NCES], 2015). Enrollment in public schools is projected to increase annually over the next 10 years (USDE, NCES, 2016). These children need health care during their school day, and this is the job of the school nurse. There are approximately 61,232 to 73,697 school nurses working in elementary and secondary schools (National Association of School Nurses [NASN], 2016a). The school nurse serves an important role in provided health services and health promotion in the school setting (NASN, 2016b; Schaffer et al, 2016)

It is commonly perceived that school nurses do nothing but put bandages on cuts and soothe children with stomachaches. However, that is not their major role. The NASN defines school nursing as "a specialized practice of professional nursing that advances the well-being, academic success and lifelong achievement of health of students" (NASN, 2016b, p 1) School nurses give comprehensive nursing care to the children and the staff at the school (NASN, 2016b). At the same time, they coordinate the health education program of the school and consult with school officials to help identify and care for other persons in the community (NASN, 2016b). The school nurse gives care to the children not only in the school building itself but also in other settings in which there are children—for example, in juvenile detention centers, in preschools and daycare centers, during field trips, at sporting events, and in the children's homes (Loschiavo, 2015; Selekman, 2012). The school nurse, therefore, must be flexible in providing nursing care, education, and help to those who need it.

This chapter discusses the history of nursing in schools and the functions of school nurses today. In addition, the standards of practice for school nurses are discussed because the nurse takes on a variety of roles. Different types of school health services are reviewed, including government-financed programs. The primary, secondary, and tertiary levels of nursing care that nurses give to children in schools are presented. The most common health problems that the school nurse encounters are also discussed under their appropriate prevention levels. The chapter ends with a discussion of the ethical dilemmas that may arise for school nurses. The future of nursing in schools is predicted for ever-changing communities.

HISTORY OF SCHOOL NURSING

The history of school nursing began with the earliest efforts of nurses to care for people in the community.

- In the late 1800s in England, the Metropolitan Association of Nursing provided medical examinations for children in the schools of London.
- By 1892, nurses in London were responsible for checking the nutrition of the children in the schools (Rosen and Fee, 2015).
- In 1897, nurses in New York City schools began to identify ill children. They then excluded these children from classes so that other children would not be infected (Judd and Sitzman, 2013).
- Many states had laws in the late 1800s mandating that within the schools, nurses teach about the abuse of alcohol and narcotics (Sharma, 2017).

In the early 1900s in the United States, the main health problem in the community was the spread of infectious diseases. On October 1, 1902, in New York City, Lillian Wald's Henry Street Settlement nurses began going into homes and schools to assess children. At first, these public health nurses were in only four schools, caring for about 10,000 children. They made plans to identify children with lice and other infestations and children

with infected wounds, tuberculosis (TB), and other infectious diseases (Judd and Sitzman, 2013; Ruel, 2014).

The need for school nurses was immediately recognized by the health care community.

- By 1910, Teachers College in New York City added a course on school nursing to their curriculum for nurses.
- In 1916 a school superintendent requested that a public health nurse be sent to the schools to care for children of immigrants (Judd and Sitzman, 2013).
- By the 1920s, school nurse teachers were employed by most municipal health departments.
- In the 1940s the nurses were employed mostly by the school districts directly.
- The nurses in the 1940s also provided home nursing and health education for the children and their parents (Judd and Sitzman, 2013).

After World War II and into the 1950s, as a result of the increased use of immunizations and antibiotics, the number of children with communicable disease in schools decreased.

- School nurses then turned their attention to screening children for common health problems and for vision and hearing problems.
- School nurses were less likely to teach health concepts in the children's classrooms and more likely to consult with teachers about health education (Judd and Sitzman, 2013).
- There was an increased emphasis on employee health, and school nurses began screening teachers and other school staff for health problems (Galemore et al, 2016).
- In the 1960s there was an upsurge in the call for higher levels of education for school nurses.
- A position paper delivered at the 1960 American Nurses Association (ANA) convention called for a Bachelor of Science degree in nursing as the minimum educational preparation for school nurses.

Table 31.1 highlights the history of school nursing over the past century.

FEDERAL LEGISLATION IN THE 1970s, 1980s, 1990s, AND 2000s

Community involvement in health in schools was a major thrust in the 1970s and 1980s.

- Counseling and mental health services were added to the responsibilities of school nurses, who began to directly teach children concepts of health.
- Children were no longer just being screened for illnesses (Loschiavo, 2015).
- Because of federal laws that required schools to make accommodations for handicapped children, medically fragile children were attending schools, often for the first time.

One of these laws, Public Law (PL) 93-112 Section 504 of the Rehabilitation Act of 1973, was an important step in helping all children enjoy a normal educational experience (NASN, 2013a). This law was followed by PL 94-142 Education for All Handicapped Children Act, which required that children with disabilities have services provided for them in schools.

TABLE 31.1   Federal Legislation Affecting School Nursing

Law	Effect on School Nurses and Children
1973: PL 93-112, Section 504 of the Rehabilitation Act	Children cannot be excluded from schools because of a handicap. The school must provide the health services that each child needs.
1975: PL 94-142, Education for All Handicapped Children Act	All children should attend school in the least restrictive environment. Requires school district's committee on the handicapped to develop individualized education plans for children.
1992: Americans with Disabilities Act	Persons with disabilities cannot be excluded from activities.
1997: PL 105-17, Individuals with Disabilities Education Act	Educational services must be offered by the schools for all disabled children from birth through age 22 years.
2001: No Child Left Behind Act of 2001	All children must receive standardized education in a healthy environment.
2004: Child Nutrition and WIC Reauthorization Act of 2004	Every local education agency participating in federal school meal programs must establish a school wellness policy.
2010: Healthy, Hunger-Free Kids Act	Authorized $4.5 billion in new funding for federal school meals and child nutrition programs to increase access to healthy food for low-income children
2015: Every Student Succeeds Act (ESSA)	Revision of the No Child Left Behind Act of 2001. Continued focus that all children must receive standardized education in a healthy and safe environment. Provided funds to support Promise Neighborhood activities.

After the passing of the Americans with Disabilities Act (ADA) in 1992, PL 105-17 Individuals with Disabilities Education Act (IDEA) was passed in 1997. Both of these laws required that more children be allowed to attend schools. Schools had to make allowances for children's special needs, which included ensuring that their school experience was in balance with their health care needs by developing individualized education plans (IEPs) and individualized health plans (IHPs). That meant that more children with human immunodeficiency virus (HIV), acquired immunodeficiency syndrome (AIDS), chronic illnesses, or mental health problems were in the classrooms and needed more attention from the school nurse (National Center for Learning Disabilities, 2014). The No Child Left Behind Act (PL 107-110) of 2001 requires a healthy environment in schools, which also affects children who have health problems (USDE, 2015). In 2015 the No Child Left Behind Act was revised, creating the new law PL 114-95 Every Student Succeeds Act (ESSA) (USDE, 2015). The new law, which will take full effect in the 2017–18 school year, continues the focus on healthy and safe schools through its support and partnering with the Promise Neighborhoods program (USDE, 2015). The Promise Neighborhoods program, which began in 2010, seeks to break the cycle of intergenerational poverty in the nation's most distressed communities by creating comprehensive, wrap-around education support services and strong, vibrant school environments (White House, 2015).

Also during the 1990s, the responsibilities of the school nurse were extended to include the development of complete clinics and health care agency centers within or attached to schools (Keeton et al, 2012). These school-based clinics are discussed later in this chapter. By 2002, some school nurses were responsible for several schools, and they gave care under a variety of nursing roles. To address obesity and to promote healthy eating and physical activity through changes in school environments, Congress passed the Child Nutrition and WIC Reauthorization Act of 2004 (PL 108-265, Section 204), which designated that each local education agency (LEA) participating in federal school meal programs,

such as the National School Lunch or Breakfast Program, must establish a local school wellness policy. The Healthy, Hunger-Free Kids Act of 2010 (PL 111-296) authorized funding and set policy for federal school meals and child nutrition programs to increase access to healthy food for low-income children (US Department of Agriculture, 2016). Table 31.2 summarizes the effects of these laws on school nurses and schoolchildren.

TABLE 31.2   High Points in School Nursing History

Decade	Major Events in School Nursing
1890s	English and American nurses are used in schools to examine children for infectious diseases and teach about alcohol abuse.
1900s	Henry Street Settlement in New York City sends nurses into schools and homes to investigate the children's overall health.
1910s	School nursing course added to Teachers College nursing program.
1920s and 1930s	School nurses are employed by community health departments.
1940s	School districts employ school nurses.
1950s	Children are screened in schools for common health problems.
1960s	Educational preparation for school nurses is debated.
1970s	School nurse practitioner programs are begun. Increased emphasis is put on mental health counseling in schools.
1980s	Children with long-term illness or disabilities attend schools.
1990s	School-based and school-linked clinics are started. Total family and community health care is offered.
2000s	School nurses provide comprehensive primary, secondary, and tertiary levels of nursing care. Attention given to federal school meal programs to promote healthy eating and physical activity.

STANDARDS OF PRACTICE FOR SCHOOL NURSES

The professional body for school nurses is the National Association of School Nurses (NASN), headquartered in Washington, DC. This association provides general guidelines and support for all school nurses. Along with the ANA, the NASN revised the scope and standards of professional practice for school nurses in 2011. These standards include assessment, diagnosis, outcomes identification, planning, implementation, and evaluation. In addition, the professional performance standards include quality of practice, education, professional practice evaluation, collegiality, collaboration, ethics, research, resource utilization, leadership, and program management (ANA and NASN, 2011). Box 31.1 summarizes the major concepts addressed in the standards.

In addition to the *Scope and Standards* document, the NASN (2016b) recently released a position statement regarding the role of the school nurse in the 21st century. According to the NASN (2016b), the services provided by the school nurse include the following:

- Leadership: the school nurse leads the development of policies, programs, and procedures for school health series at both an individual and district level and acts as an advocate for the individual student.
- Community/public health: the school nurse provides interventions in each of the levels of prevention, as well as disease surveillance, promoting health equity, and delivering effective cultural competent care to diverse communities.
- Care coordination: the school nurse coordinates student health care between the medical home, family, and school.
- Quality improvement: the school nurse utilizes continuous quality improvement in the nursing process and utilizes research data in his or her practice.

The American Academy of Pediatrics (AAP) developed its own ideas about how nurses function in schools based on its assessment of schoolchildren's health needs (AAP Council on School Health, 2016). In general, the ANA and NASN standards compare very well with those developed by the AAP regarding the provision of health care to students in schools. The AAP Council on School Health (2016) recognizes the important role school nurses play in promoting optimal health and well-being in school-age children in the school setting, noting that the

school nurse often leads the coordinated school health program, and recommends that physicians do the following:

- Advocate for a minimum of one full-time school nurse in every school, with medical oversight from a school physician in every school district.
- Ask school-related questions at each visit, and provide relevant information directly to the school.
- Establish a working relationship with school nurses to improve chronic condition management.
- Include school nurses and important team members in the delivery of health care for children and adolescents.

The goal is for children to obtain complete health care in schools.

EDUCATIONAL CREDENTIALS OF SCHOOL NURSES

The NASN recommends that school nurses be registered nurses licensed through the State Board of Nursing who also have a bachelor's degree in nursing (NASN, 2016c). The NASN (2016c) also supports state school nurse certification, where required, and promotes national certification of school nurses through the National Board for Certification of School Nurses. However, not all nurses have been educated this way. There are no general laws regarding the educational background of school nurses. School nurses in some states are required to be registered nurses, but licensed practical nurses (LPNs) and licensed vocational nurses (LVNs) are also seen in some schools. Although NASN recommends school nurses be baccalaureate prepared, the Association notes that LPNs/LVNs can be a valuable part of the school health team in meeting the increasing number and acuity of student health care needs (NASN, 2015a). Only about half of all US states require some form of additional study for school nurse specialty certification (National Association of State Boards of Education, 2013).

School nurses in some schools may be advanced-practice nurses who specialize in caring for children. They may be nurse practitioners who have specialized in child health nursing (pediatrics), in family nursing, or in the school nurse practitioner role. Clinical nurse specialists who are school nurses also may be found in child health nursing or community or public health nursing. These advanced-practice nurses may be certified by professional organizations such as the ANA or their own professional organizations. Most hold master's degrees in nursing.

School nurses do not start their nursing careers in schools. All have prior experience in nursing—most from working either in hospitals or communities. In addition, most have spent years working with children, so they are aware of their special health needs.

ROLES AND FUNCTIONS OF SCHOOL NURSES

School nurses give care to children as direct caregivers, educators, counselors, consultants, and case managers. As noted earlier, they must coordinate the health care of many students in their schools with the health care that the children receive from their own health care providers and be leaders in the school.

> ### BOX 31.1   Summary of Major Concepts of American Nurses Association and National Association of School Nurses Standards
>
> - Give and evaluate appropriate up-to-date nursing care.
> - Collaborate well with other health providers and school staff.
> - Maintain school health office policies, including privacy and safety of health records.
> - Teach health promotion and maintenance to children, families, and communities.

Modified from American Nurses Association and National Association of School Nurses [ANA and NASN]: *Scope and standards of professional school nursing practice*, ed 2, Silver Spring, MD, 2011, Nursebooks.org.

Having enough adequate school nurse staffing across schools is important. If there are fewer nurses in the schools, the nurses are expected to perform many different functions. It would therefore be possible that they are unable to provide the amount of comprehensive care that the students need (Kerfoot and Douglas, 2013). In *Healthy People 2020 (HP2020)*, objective ECBP-5 states that there should be 1 nurse for every 750 children in each school (US Department of Health and Human Services [USDHHS], 2010). At baseline in 2006, approximately 40% of the nation's schools met that standard, and the target was set to 44.7% of the country's elementary, middle, junior high, and senior high schools having this many nurses by 2020 (USDHHS, 2010). In 2014 this objective was met, with 51.1% of schools meeting this ratio (USDHHS, 2016). Although this is a notable achievement, the NASN states that a one-size-fits-all ratio, such as the 750:1 in *HP2020*, is inadequate to fill the increasingly complex health needs of students and school communities and that all students should have access to a school nurse (NASN, 2015b). Rather, NASN (2015b) purports that determining adequate school nurse staffing ratios is a complex decision making process and should be determined at least annually, using student- and community-specific health data.

SCHOOL NURSE ROLES

Direct Caregiver

The school nurse is expected to give immediate nursing care to the ill or injured child or school staff member. **Direct caregiver** is the traditional role of the school nurse.

Although most school nurses are in public or private schools and give care only during school hours, the nurse in a boarding school gives nursing care to children 24 hours per day and 7 days per week. In boarding schools, the children live at school and go home only for vacations. The nurse also lives at the school and may be on call all the time. The nurse in the boarding school is very important to the children because this nurse is the gatekeeper to their complete health care (Pavletic et al, 2016). The nurse makes all of the health care decisions for the child and has a referral system to contact other health care providers, such as physicians and psychological counselors, if needed.

Health Educator

The school nurse in the **health educator** role may be asked to teach children both individually and in the classroom. The nurse uses different approaches to teach about health, such as instruction concerning proper nutrition or safety information. Many school nurses teach the older elementary girls and boys about the coming changes in their bodies as puberty arrives. Other school nurses may teach the health education classes that are required by the states to be included in the programs (see the How To box on page 546).

Case Manager

The school nurse is expected to function as a **case manager,** helping to coordinate the health care for children with complex health problems. This may include the child who is disabled or chronically ill, who may be seen by a physical therapist, an occupational therapist, a speech therapist, or another health

Increasing Activity Among Schoolchildren

Because of the obesity epidemic in the United States, interventions to increase physical activity and reduce sedentary behaviors have become a priority for public health practitioners. This research study evaluated the feasibility and efficacy of a school nurse–delivered intervention aimed at improving diet and activity and reducing body mass index (BMI) among overweight and obese adolescents. This study used a pair-matched cluster-randomized controlled school-based trial. Six high schools were randomized into either the six-session counseling intervention or the control group. The intervention, "Lookin' Good Feelin' Good," consisted of six one-on-one school nurse–led counseling sessions conducted over 2 months during school hours. Those in the control group had six one-on-one visits with the school nurse over 2 months to be weighed and review informational pamphlets on weight management. Although there was no significant difference in BMI, activity, or caloric intake between the groups at 2 months, those in the intervention group ate breakfast on more days of the week and had a lower intake of sugar than the control group.

Nurse Use

This study indicates that a school nurse–delivered obesity intervention is feasible and may improve select behaviors that may result in obesity.

Data from Pbert L, Druker S, Gapinski MA, et al: A school nurse-delivered intervention for overweight and obese adolescents. *J Sch Health* 83(3): 182-193, 2013.

care provider during the school day. The nurse sets up the schedule for the child's visits so that those appointments do not unnecessarily have a negative effect on the child's academic day.

Consultant

The school nurse is the person who is best able to provide health information to school administrators, teachers, and parent–teacher groups. As a **consultant,** the school nurse can provide professional information about proposed changes in the school environment and their effect on the health of the children. The nurse can also recommend changes in the school's policies or ask community organizations to help make the children's schools healthier places (Loschiavo, 2015; Selekman, 2012).

Counselor

The school nurse may be the person whom children trust to tell important secrets about their health. It is important that as a **counselor,** the school nurse is considered a trustworthy person to whom the children can go if they are in trouble or when they need to talk (Loschiavo, 2015; Selekman, 2012). Nurses in this situation should tell children that if anything they reveal indicates that they are in danger, the parents and school officials must be told. However, privacy and confidentiality, as in all health care, are important. In addition, the school nurse may be the person to help with grief counseling in the schools. (The school crisis team is discussed later in this chapter.)

Community Outreach

When participating in **community outreach,** nurses can be involved in the following (Dyess et al, 2016):

- Community health fairs or festivals in the schools
- Teaching others an influenza immunization program for the school staff

- Promoting a health education fair and a blood pressure screening program
- Initiating a liaison
- Coordinating with local health charities to provide education to the schools

Researcher

Little research has been done on nurses caring for children in the schools. The school nurse is responsible for making sure that the nursing care given is based on solid, evidence-based practice. Outcomes regarding school nurse services need to be studied (NASN, 2016b). Therefore the school nurse, as an educator, is in the right position to do studies as a researcher that advance school nursing practice.

SCHOOL HEALTH SERVICES

School health services vary in their scope. However, there are common parts to the programs.

FEDERAL SCHOOL HEALTH PROGRAMS

The federal government, through the coordination of the Centers for Disease Control and Prevention (CDC),

developed a Coordinated School Health (CSH) program that was widely used in schools since its development in the late 1980s (Centers for Disease Control and Prevention [CDC], 2015a) The CSH program followed a systems-based approach addressing eight components of the school as venues for health promotion and disease prevention (CDC, 2015a). In spring 2013, the CDC and ASCD (formerly known as the Association for Supervision and Curriculum Development) developed the Whole School, Whole Community, Whole Child (WSCC) model, which integrates the eight components of the CSH program with the tenets of a whole-child approach to education (CDC, 2015b; Lewallen et al, 2015) (Fig. 31.1). The new model expanded the components into 10 parts (CDC, 2015b; Lewallen et al, 2015):

1. Health education
2. Nutrition environment and services
3. Employee wellness
4. Social and emotional school climate
5. Physical environment
6. Health services
7. Counseling, psychological, and social services
8. Community involvement
9. Family engagement
10. Physical education and physical activity

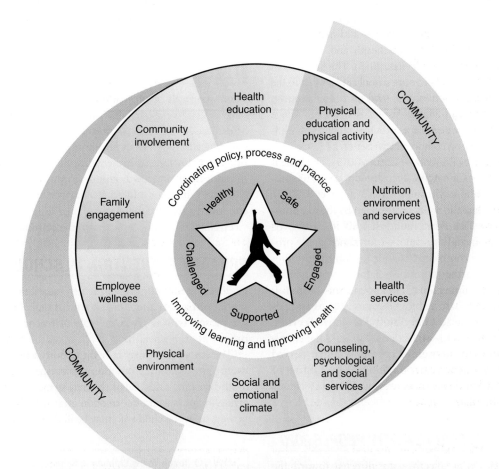

FIG. 31.1 The Whole School, Whole Community, Whole Child (WSCC) model. (From Centers for Disease Control and Prevention: *Whole School, Whole Community, Whole Child (WSCC)*, Atlanta, 2015b, CDC. Retrieved July 2016 from http://www.cdc.gov/healthyschools/wscc/index.htm.)

This expanded model promotes greater alignment, integration, and collaboration between education and health to improve each child's cognitive, physical, social, and emotional development (CDC, 2015b; Lewallen et al, 2015).

SCHOOL HEALTH POLICIES AND PRACTICES STUDY

The national survey that assesses school health policies and practices at the state, district, school, and classroom levels is called the School Health Policies and Programs Study (SHPPS) (CDC, 2015c). This survey assesses the characteristics of the Whole School, Whole Community, Whole Child model (CDC, 2015c). The 2012 survey results are focused at the state and district level, whereas the 2014 survey results are focused at the school and classroom level (CDC, 2015c). Comprehensive results and fact sheets are available at http://www.cdc.gov/healthyyouth/data/shpps/results.htm.

SCHOOL-BASED HEALTH PROGRAMS

Because many schoolchildren may not receive health care services other than screening and first-aid care from the school nurse, the US government began funding school-based health centers (SBHCs) during the 1990s. These are family-centered, community-based clinics run within schools, often in low-income populations (Guide to Community Preventive Services, 2015). These centers provide primary health care services to pre-K–12 students and may offer expanded health services, including mental health and dental care (Guide to Community Preventive Services, 2015). The SBHCs can range in size from small to large. There are school clinics open to the community only during the school year and also health centers that are open 24 hours per day all year. Some SBHCs have a single clinician providing primary care services, whereas others have multidisciplinary teams providing comprehensive services (Clackamas, 2016; Guide to Community Preventive Services, 2015). The Patient Protection and Affordable Care Act of 2010 appropriated $200 million to improve and expand services at SBHCs (Vaughn et al, 2013).

Findings from a systematic review completed by the Community Preventive Service Task Force found that SBHCs improved educational outcomes, including school performance, grade promotion, and high school completion (Guide to Community Preventive Services, 2015). Furthermore, the task force recommended implementing and maintaining SBHCs in low-income communities because they were likely to reduce educational gaps and advance health equity (Guide to Community Preventive Services, 2015). According to the 2013–14 National Census of School-Based Health Centers, there were 2315 SBHCs that served students and communities in 49 of 50 states and the District of Columbia, a 20% increase since the previous 2010–11 census (School-Based Health Alliance, 2015).

SCHOOL NURSES AND *HEALTHY PEOPLE 2020*

Many *Healthy People 2020* objectives are directed toward the health of children. In addition, several refer directly to the care that nurses give to children in schools. The *Healthy People 2020* box lists the objectives that involve school-age children. These

---

♥ **HEALTHY PEOPLE 2020**

The following objectives are related to school health and school nursing:

ECBP-2	Increase the proportion of elementary, middle, and senior high schools that provide comprehensive school health education to prevent health problems in the following areas: unintentional injury; violence; suicide; tobacco use and addiction; alcohol or other drug use; unintended pregnancy, HIV/AIDS, and STD infection; unhealthy dietary patterns; and inadequate physical activity.
ECBP-5	Increase the proportion of the nation's elementary, middle, and senior high schools that have a nurse-to-student ratio of at least 1:750.
IID-10	Maintain vaccination coverage levels for children in kindergarten.
IID-11	Increase routine vaccination coverage levels for adolescents.
IVP-27	Increase the proportion of public and private schools that require students to wear appropriate protective gear when engaged in school-sponsored physical activities.
RD-5	Reduce the number of school days or work days missed among persons with current asthma.

From US Department of Health and Human Services: *Healthy People 2020: topics and objectives,* Washington, DC, 2010, US Government Printing Office. Retrieved July 2016 from https://www.healthypeople.gov/2020/topics-objectives.

---

objectives are concerned with children with disabilities in the schools, the number of children with major health problems, and the ratio of nurses to children in schools. Nurses can accomplish these goals using the three levels of prevention, as discussed next.

LEVELS OF PREVENTION IN SCHOOLS

The three levels of prevention (primary, secondary, and tertiary) have always been a part of health care in schools (Loschiavo, 2015; Selekman, 2012). Primary prevention provides health promotion and education to prevent health problems in children. Secondary prevention includes the screening of children for various illnesses, monitoring their growth and development, and caring for them when they are ill or injured. Tertiary prevention in schools is the continued care of children who need long-term health care services, along with education within the community (Fig. 31.2).

PRIMARY PREVENTION IN SCHOOLS

Children need continued health services in schools. The school nurse sees them on an almost daily basis and is usually the person who is given the role of teaching them about and promoting their health.

The school nurse may have the opportunity to go into the classroom to teach health promotion concepts, such as hand-washing or tooth-brushing skills. He or she may spend time with the teachers, giving them the latest information on healthy lifestyles for children or ways to spot a child who may be ill or in need of counseling.

HOW TO Teach Young Children in School
- Keep the lesson to no more than 20 minutes in length.
- Use a lot of examples, pictures, and stuffed animals in the talk.
- Always remember the developmental stage of the children when teaching them.

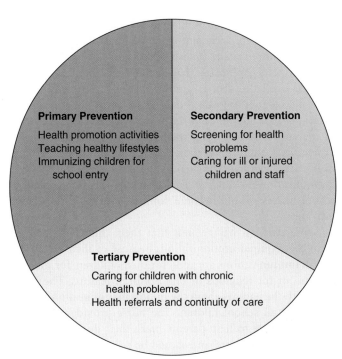

FIG. 31.2 Levels of prevention in schools.

The areas of primary prevention that the school nurse focuses on include preventing childhood injuries, preventing substance abuse behaviors, reducing the risk for the development of chronic diseases, and monitoring the immunization status of children. These primary prevention activities are completed for the population of children in the school. The activities for the population are determined by analysis of the assessments completed on all of the children in the school to determine the most pressing priorities for the population.

School nurses use the nursing process while they care for children in schools. In their primary prevention efforts, they do the following:

- Assess children and families to determine their level of knowledge about health issues.

CASE STUDY

Roles of the School Health Nurse

Samantha Smith is the registered nurse for Green Hills Elementary School and Rising Stars Elementary School. Ms. Smith spends 2.5 days at each school providing health care in the nursing clinics and helping the science teachers incorporate health into their curriculum. This week Ms. Smith is performing vision screenings for kindergarten and grades 1, 3, and 5 at both schools.

At the beginning of the school year, Ms. Smith asked parents to volunteer to help with vision and hearing screenings. Shortly before the day of the vision screening, Ms. Smith met with and trained the five parents who had volunteered to help.

The day before the screening, Ms. Smith spoke to the students in each classroom that would receive screening. She talked to the students about their five senses and how to keep them healthy. Ms. Smith explained the vision screening process so that the students would know what to expect the next day. On the day of the screening, Ms. Smith set up the screening charts and called each grade level separately for screening. Students who failed the screening were rescreened by Ms. Smith and then referred to an ophthalmologist for vision correction.

- Find out whether children are at risk for preventable problems.
- Analyze the assessment findings.
- Make plans to develop teaching plans or health promotion activities.
- Implement these activities.
- Evaluate and revise the plan.

The school nurse focuses on the following areas of primary prevention:

- Preventing childhood injuries
- Preventing substance-abuse behaviors
- Reducing the risk for the development of chronic diseases
- Monitoring the immunization status of children

Prevention of Childhood Injuries

Accidents (unintentional injuries) are the leading cause of death in children and teenagers (Xu et al, 2016). The school nurse educates children, teachers, and parents about preventing injuries. Working with the national Safe Kids Campaign, the school nurse can provide educational programs reminding children to use their seat belts or bicycle helmets to prevent injuries. Other classes can focus on crossing the street, water safety, and fire safety. The school nurse, as the trusted person at school, is able to quickly provide information on injury prevention; most injuries are preventable (Al-Bashtawy et al, 2016).

School nurses also provide information on how to prevent playground injuries. They assess school playgrounds for equipment safety on the basis of the US Consumer Product Safety Commission guidelines (Al-Bashtawy et al, 2016). School nurses also promote bicycle, skateboard, and scooter safety by providing health educational workshops to children and their families. School sports also have the potential to cause injuries to children, and the school nurse is usually involved in deciding with parents and coaches on how to best prevent injuries on the sports field (NASN, 2016d).

These programs can be implemented by the nurse on a community-wide scale. Research has shown that once behaviors of children related to safety are taught, their effects spread quickly throughout the community. This makes the entire community safer (Loschiavo, 2015; Selekman, 2012).

Substance Abuse Prevention Education

Primary prevention interventions by the school nurse include educating children and adolescents about the effects of alcohol and other drugs on their bodies. Preventing use of and promoting "saying no" to drugs have been part of the school health program for many years. Teenagers are taught by the school nurse to stay away from drugs (e.g., marijuana, cocaine, crack, heroin) and alcohol.

There has been an increase in the use of "club drugs" such as lysergic acid diethylamide (LSD), ketamine, gamma-hydroxybutyrate (GHB), Rohypnol, and methylenedioxymethamphetamine (MDMA; Ecstasy). Teaching teenagers about the dangers of all drugs is the responsibility of the school nurse. In addition, the school nurse can teach parents and other members of the community about the latest drug fads, increasing everyone's awareness of these dangerous trends (NASN, 2013b).

Disease Prevention Education

The nurse has the opportunity to teach children healthy life-styles to reduce their risk for disease later in life. For example, children can be taught ways to reduce their risk of becoming obese by teaching and reinforcing healthy nutrition and exercise (Tucker and Lanningham-Foster, 2015). The school nurse can then reinforce the teachers' educational plans or develop the program further for other age groups to teach them how to take care of their heart.

Getting health promotion information to the parents of the children is often a challenge for the school nurse. In Newport, Oregon, the school nurse at one of the elementary schools has a "Nurse's Corner" web page (Lincoln County School District, 2016). On this page, the nurse shares important health information related to school-age children, on subjects such as immunization requirements, flu prevention tips, and school health policies, procedures, and plans. In this way, the school nurse is able to promote the health of not only the schoolchildren but also the community.

Required Vaccinations for Schoolchildren

All states have laws that require that children receive immunizations, or vaccinations, against communicable diseases before they attend school (CDC, 2015d). School nurses must be up to date on the latest laws on immunizations for children in their own state.

For children entering kindergarten, these vaccinations include diphtheria, pertussis, and tetanus (the DPT series); measles, mumps, and rubella (the MMR series); and polio.

The school nurse must keep a complete file of all of the children's vaccination records to meet the state's laws. These files should contain the following:

- Student's name
- Date of birth
- Address
- Telephone number
- Parents' or guardians' names
- Contact information
- Primary health care provider's name, telephone number, and address
- All the vaccinations with the dates the child received booster shots

This makes it easy for the school nurse to find out which children still need immunizations or boosters.

Because children are prevented from attending school if they have not had the required shots, the school nurse must make every effort to find missing data in the immunization record.

- The nurse must contact the parents to get the immunization history for the child.
- Written notes should be sent to each child's home at least 1 year before each new immunization is needed so that the parents have time to get the child to their health care provider for the shots.
- If the parents or guardians do not speak English, these notes should be translated into the family's language.
- If the parents have lost the information that gives the child's immunization history, the nurse should encourage them to contact their physician or nurse practitioner to get it.

Many problems with children not being immunized or having incomplete vaccination records may occur in families who have moved many times or who may not have a regular physician. The parents may have no idea whether the child has even received the shots. Families may not have health care insurance to pay for the immunizations, or they may have insurance that does not pay for preventive care. In these cases, the parents have to pay for the immunizations, which can be expensive. Certain low-income families without health care insurance may qualify for federal programs that provide free immunizations to children. Each state has its own program, so school nurses should become familiar with what their state provides.

Some parents may request that their child be exempted from the required immunizations because of their belief that not all immunizations are good for their children, for medical reasons, or for religious or philosophical reasons. The nurse talks with the parents about the importance of immunizations to protect all schoolchildren. The nurse provides evidence-based literature to help parents make their decision. But the decision is the parents' and should be respected. It is then up to the school administration to determine the admission of the child to the school.

SECONDARY PREVENTION IN SCHOOLS

Because secondary prevention involves caring for children when they need health care, this is the largest responsibility for the school nurse. This includes caring for ill or injured students and school employees. It also involves screening and assessing children and referral to appropriate health agencies or providers. The school nurse uses the nursing process during secondary prevention activities. When an ill or injured child comes to the school's health office, the nurse must immediately assess the child for the degree of illness or injury.

Children seek out the school nurse for a variety of different needs, such as the following:

- Headaches
- Stomachaches
- Diarrhea
- Anxiety over being separated from the parents
- Cuts, bruises, or other injuries

In addition, children may seek reassurance from the school nurse or even appear to hide in the nurse's office. This may be caused by harassment or bullying from other children in the school (NASN, 2014a).

Once the assessment data are gathered, the nurse determines the course of action and follows it through the implementation and evaluation phases. This occurs for direct child health care as well as for screening children for other health problems. If assessment data identify a child as having a health problem, the school nurse continues to follow the nursing process to further care for that child.

Nursing Care for Emergencies in the School

The school nurse cares for children who are injured or become ill in the school. The school nurse should therefore have an emergency plan in place so that a routine can be followed when emergencies occur. This plan should include the following:

- Making an assessment of the emergency and surveying the scene
- Treating the injured or ill children or teachers
- Calling for backup help from the community's emergency medical units if needed

The AAP and the American Health Association (AHA) have recommended that plans be developed in the schools in case of an emergency when a child or staff member needs immediate care. The school nurse should develop this plan so that a staff member in the school, for example, the principal or an athletic coach, can follow it in case the nurse is not in the building at the time of the emergency. The NASN (2014b) recommends the nursing plan for children with special health needs include the following:

- Health care provider orders for 72-hour lockdown or disaster
- A system for retrieving and transporting medications to areas of lockdown or evacuation
- Provision of necessary supplies and food in the classroom or carried with the child or teacher in an evacuation or a 3-day supply in case of a lockdown
- Education of all staff members/substitutes responsible for the child with a special health needs during an emergency
- An alarm system for students with auditory and/or visual needs
- Backup power source for specialized equipment
- Emergency evacuation plan for students with physical, mental, or communication limitations (e.g. visually and/or hearing impaired, students with autism, and English as a second language students).

Furthermore, the AAP Committee on School Health (2008) offers general guidelines for school emergency plans. Such plans should include:

- When to call 9-1-1 for local emergency personnel
- How to make arrangements to transfer a child to the hospital via ambulance in case more care is needed
- If the nurse is not in the school at all times, at least two different staff members identified as responsible for determining whether emergency care is needed. These persons should be educated by the school nurse on proper first-aid techniques so that correct care is given until further help arrives.
- All staff in the schools should be taught standard precautions. These policies should be written into the emergency plan.
- Members of the athletic staff, such as coaches and physical education teachers, should also be up to date on emergency health procedures. If they are not, the school nurse should teach them about the policies and provide a means to review first-aid procedures with them on a regular basis.
- The children in the schools should be taught basic first-aid procedures by the nurse, including standard precautions related to blood exposure. This lesson, depending on the age and grade level of the children, would allow the children to help in a playground accident while the adults are being summoned to the scene.

The Center for Health and Health Care in Schools (2013) recommends that all schools have crisis plans in place to help the children, teachers, parents, and the community cope with the sudden event. Crisis teams are prepared to help everyone respond quickly to the crisis, to ensure the safety of the school, and to follow up on the effects of the crisis on the members of the school (Lerner et al, 2013). The crisis plan includes an administrative policy made either for the entire school district or, if the schools are large, for each individual school. The plan includes the names of the persons on the crisis team: the superintendent of the school district, the school nurse, the guidance counselor, the school psychologist or social worker, teachers, police or school security, clergy from the community, and parents. Plans to obtain and share information can be made quickly (Lerner et al, 2013).

The nurse can help the crisis team make a checklist for everyone to follow that explains what to do in every possible crisis situation. Then, at the end of the crisis, the crisis team will want to take time to counsel all of the people who helped in the crisis, including the teachers, emergency personnel, and parents, as well as the children. That way everyone can talk about the crisis. The crisis plan should be reviewed every year to see what parts of the plan need updating. Drills take place to act out the plan to see how it works and how it can be revised to make it more workable (Lerner et al, 2013).

The nurse may not always be at the school, and the emergency may have to be handled by a teacher, administrator, secretary, custodian, or coach. Therefore all emergency procedures should be written and easily accessible to anyone in the school. Along with the procedures and an emergency manual written or obtained by the school nurse, the following are required:

- An injury or illness log should be maintained by personnel so that the emergency is accurately recorded.
- Procedures should be available for notifying the parents or legal guardians about the emergency, what was done for the child, and where the child was sent if transfer to a hospital or other medical agency was required.

Because nursing care may have to be given to a child or adult in respiratory or cardiac arrest, the nurse must have current certification in cardiopulmonary resuscitation and the use of the automated external defibrillator (AED), which should be available to all school nurses per the AHA (Boudreaux and Broussard, 2012). Other education in the area of emergency nursing would also be helpful to the school nurse, including pediatric advanced life support (PALS) or emergency nursing for pediatrics certification (American Heart Association, 2016).

See Box 31.2 for a list of responsibilities of the school nurse during a disaster.

Emergency Equipment in the School Nurse's Office

The school nurse needs much equipment to deal with emergencies in the school. These needs are based on the guidelines of the AAP (AAP, Committee on School Health, 2008). The health office should have basic items on hand. Necessary equipment includes the following:

- Full oxygen tanks with oxygen masks of different kinds (bag-valve masks, resuscitation masks)
- Splints for sprained or broken limbs
- Cervical spine collars to keep a child's head in proper alignment
- Sterile dressings

Various sizes of these items are needed because children of different ages are in the school. Another recommended item for the nurse's office is an epinephrine autoinjector kit in case a child goes into anaphylactic shock after exposure to an allergen (AAP, Committee on School Health, 2008). This should be locked in a medication cabinet because there is a needle in the kit. The school nurse will need to teach other school personnel how to use the EpiPen autoinjector in an emergency (Murphy, 2014). Of course, gloves should also be available to meet Standard Precautions guidelines. A telephone should be available for calling emergency personnel and parents. Paper and a pen should be next to the phone so that instructions from the emergency personnel can be written. The AED should be located in a central location at the school for easy access in an emergency. It should not be locked in the nurse's office but rather available for school staff to obtain in case the nurse is off site that day.

Giving Medication in School

The school nurse, as part of secondary prevention, may be responsible for giving medications to children during the school day (NASN, 2012a). These may include the following:
- Prescribed medications
- Medications that the parents have asked the school's nurse to give (e.g., cold remedies)
- Vitamins

In all instances, the nurse should develop a series of guidelines to help with the legal administration of medications in the school. Parents should be sure to tell the school nurse if the child is on any medications (NASN, 2012a). The Health Insurance Portability and Accountability Act (HIPAA; PL 104-191) of 1966 requires that all of this information be confidential (Association of State and Territorial Health Officials [ASTHO], 2015; NASN, 2012a).
- The prescribed drug should have the original prescription label on it and be in the original container so that there are no errors.
- A current, signed parental consent form for giving the medication should also be in the student's file (NASN, 2012a).
- A current medication (drug) book should be in the nurse's office so that it can be consulted for information.

The school nurse should also have a means of contacting a pharmacist to ask questions regarding the medication if needed.

QSEN FOCUS ON QUALITY AND SAFETY EDUCATION FOR NURSES

Targeted Competency: Safety—Safety minimizes risk of harm to patients and providers through both system effectiveness and individual performance. Important aspects of safety include the following:
- **Knowledge:** Describe factors that create a culture of safety (such as open communication strategies and organizational error reporting systems).
- **Skills:** Communicate observations or concerns related to hazards and errors to patients, families, and the health care team.
- **Attitudes:** Value own role in preventing errors.

Safety Question:
Imagine you are working as a nurse in an elementary school. Due to budget cuts, you are only at the school 2 days a week. Juan, a student in the third grade, is newly diagnosed with asthma and will have an inhaler at school for emergencies. Your state allows nurses to delegate the administration of inhaler medications to unlicensed personnel. You decide to delegate the administration of Juan's emergency inhaler to his classroom teacher, Mr. Smith. What steps would you take to ensure you safely delegated this medication?

Answer:
First, you would need to establish open communication between Mr. Smith and yourself. After the initial medication training, you can maintain open communication by checking in with Mr. Smith on a regular basis to assess his knowledge and comfort level in administering Juan's inhaler. Second, in the event that Mr. Smith gives Juan a dose from the inhaler, have a system in place to document when and why the medication was given. Periodically review the records to ensure that everything was documented correctly and that the medication was given for appropriate reasons. Last, in the event of a medication error, reflect on what you can do differently to prevent future errors.

Assessing and Screening Children at School

Children should receive screening for vision, hearing, height and weight, oral health, tuberculosis, and scoliosis in the schools. For each of these areas, the school nurse should keep a confidential record of all of the screening results for the children in the school, according to HIPAA rules. In addition, each state has different laws regarding the screenings, and the nurse should be aware of these laws.

Physical examinations to play in a school sport may also be given in the school. The school nurse would arrange for the sports physicals and would help monitor the examinations being done by the school's physician or nurse practitioner.

Screening for tuberculosis in schoolchildren is also done in several states. This can be a problem because the nurse cannot read the Mantoux test, or the tuberculin skin test (TST), until 3 days after it is administered. Often nurses are part time and may not be at the school on the day the child's test needs to be read. Perhaps the best way is to telephone the parents, telling them that the child needs to see the physician or nurse practitioner and that the child will be bringing the information home that day. In this way, the parents can ask the child for the report, and the parents can read the report or, if unable to do so, can provide it to the child's physician or nurse practitioner. With the phone call, the child is aware that the parents expect the report.

Screening Children for Lice

School nurses also must screen children for lice infestation. The prevalence of head lice in US schools is estimated between 6 million to 12 million infestations each year, being found most commonly in children 3 to 11 years of age (CDC, 2013). Infestation is much less common among African Americans than among persons of other races (CDC, 2013). The suggestion that lice are associated with unclean homes in poverty areas is incorrect—getting head lice is not related to the cleanliness of the person or his or her environment (CDC, 2013). Rather, lice are spread through direct contact with the hair of an infested person (head-to-head contact) (CDC, 2013). The school nurse needs to check children for lice because, in many areas, children with lice are excluded from school. Check on the local school district policies. During the "lice check," the nurse must check the children's hair for both lice and nits (NASN, 2016e).

The following are responsibilities of the school nurse (NASN, 2016e):

- Provide accurate health education to the school community about the etiology, transmission, assessment, and treatment of head lice.
- Advocate for school policy that is more caring and less exclusionary (i.e., elimination of "no-nit" school policies).
- Implement intervention strategies that are student-centered.
- Support the current treatment recommendations of the AAP and CDC.
- Participate in research that evaluates the effectiveness of head lice policies and educational programs.

Identification of Child Abuse or Neglect

The school nurse is mandated by state laws to report suspected cases of child abuse or neglect. These laws differ from state to state, and the nurse should be aware of the particular requirements for reporting in each state.

A nurse who identifies a child who may be abused or receives information from a teacher or other staff member that leads to the belief that a child has been abused must contact the appropriate legal authorities and the school's principal. A confidential file should be made about the incident. However, the nurse should let the government authorities, usually the state or county child protection department, look into the suspected case. In all cases, the child should be protected from harm, and those who have no right to know that child abuse or neglect is suspected should not be given any information.

Communicating with Health Care Providers

The school nurse often makes an assessment of a child that requires referral to the child's family physician or other health care provider. The findings from these assessments must be communicated accurately to the child's parent and the provider. The nurse must be able to get the information quickly and accurately to the child's parents. Be aware of the HIPAA privacy rules (ASTHO, 2015).

One way to do this is to write a detailed report about the findings. This information can be given to the child to give to his or her parents. However, the child may lose the report before it gets to them. The information can be mailed to the parents, but this takes more time. Perhaps the best way is to telephone the parents, telling them that the child needs to see the physician or nurse practitioner and that the child will be bringing the information home that day. In this way, the parents can ask the child for the report, and the child is aware that the parents expect it.

Efforts to Prevent Suicide and Other Mental Health Problems

Suicide is the second leading cause of death in adolescents 15 to 19 years of age (Heron, 2016). Recommendations have been made about reducing the incidence of suicide in teenagers. A suicide prevention program contains ideas for the school nurse to use. Suicide prevention must be addressed by school nurses, who can do the following (Ramos et al, 2013):

- Lead educational programs within the schools to emphasize coping strategies and stress management techniques for children and adolescents who have problems and to teach about the risk factors.
- Teach faculty members to look for the risk factors.
- Help organize a peer assistance program to help teenagers cope with school stresses.

If a student threatens suicide at school, the school nurse should intervene by ensuring the safety of the student and by removing him or her from the school situation immediately. While parents are being notified, the nurse should assess the child's suicide risk and refer the child or teenager to crisis intervention or mental health services.

In the unfortunate instance in which a teenager who attended the school has committed suicide, the school nurse is called on to help the school population, both students and teachers, cope with the death. Grief counseling should be set up and coordinated by the school nurse. In addition, further assessments should be made regarding the suicide potential among the deceased teenager's friends because suicide clusters have been seen to occur.

Other mental health problems may affect students. These may include but are not limited to attention deficit/hyperactivity disorders, autism spectrum disorders, anxiety disorders, conduct disorders, depression, bipolar disorder, disordered eating, and substance abuse (NASN, 2013c). Adolescents may have early signs of mental or emotional problems, such as behavior problems in class or severe class or test anxiety. The NASN (2013c) notes that school nurses play a vital role in the assessment, identification, intervention, referral, and follow-up of students in need of mental health services and serve as advocates, facilitators, and counselors of mental health services.

Children who are homeless have special problems. Children who do not have a stable address have probably moved from school to school very frequently. Children whose parents are addicted to drugs or alcohol also can benefit from support from the school nurse. This lack of a stable environment may make it more likely that they may develop mental or emotional problems. The school nurse can be an advocate for these children and their families.

...nce at School

In 2015, in the previous 30 days before the survey, approximately 4.1% of high school students carried a weapon on school property, and 5.6% of high school students missed at least 1 day of school because they felt unsafe (CDC, 2016a). In the year before being surveyed, 6.0% of high school students reported being threatened or injured with a weapon on school property at least once, and 7.8% had been in a physical fight on school property at least once (CDC, 2016a).

In the past several years, school shootings by students have occurred involving other students and teachers. The school nurse may be able to help identify students who will act in this way. Furthermore, the nurse can provide health education classes to help children learn positive ways of dealing with conflict.

Bullying is at the center of attention among child and adolescent advocates. Twenty percent of high school students surveyed reported being bullied while on school property (CDC, 2016a). Since 2007, the incidence of electronic aggression, or "cyberbullying," has risen (Hamm et al, 2015). Physical injury, social and emotional distress, and even death can result from bullying (CDC, 2015e). Students may come to the school nurse complaining of psychosomatic illnesses, such as headaches and stomachaches, due to bullying (NASN, 2014a). Students who are being bullied may feel sad or lose hope and begin considering harming themselves (CDC, 2015e). The school nurse needs to be knowledgeable about bullying and provide leadership to implement bullying prevention strategies, such as increased supervision and antibullying policies (NASN, 2014a). In an effort to reduce the prevalence of bullying, all 50 states now have antibullying laws (stopbullying.gov, 2015).

The school nurse's primary goal is to prevent violence from occurring and prioritize the safety of everyone on the school's campus (NASN, 2013d). Interventions that the nurse can implement to prevent violence include (NASN, 2013d) the following:

- Facilitate student connectedness to the school community.
- Engage parents in school activities that promote connections with their children, and foster communication, problem solving, limit setting, and monitoring of children.
- Support activities and strategies to help establish a climate that promotes and practices respect for others and for the property of others.
- Support policies of zero tolerance for weapons on school property, including school buses.
- Advocate for adult monitoring in the hallways between classes and at the beginning and end of the school day, and the assignment of staff to monitor the playground, cafeteria, and school entrances before and after school.
- Serve as a positive role model, developing mentoring programs for at-risk youth and families.
- Educate students and their parents about gun safety.

If violence occurs, the school nurse should do the following (NASN, 2013d):

- Coordinate emergency response until rescue teams arrive.
- Provide nursing care for injured students.
- Apply crisis intervention strategies that help de-escalate a crisis situation and help resolve the conflict.

- Identify and refer those students who require more in-depth counseling services.
- Participate in crisis intervention teams.

By helping to identify the student who might be considering school violence and by teaching students and teachers about these warning signs in students, the school nurse may be able to help prevent violent actions through education and follow-up of children who need help. The US federal government has many agencies that can be used as resources to help school nurses develop programs in their schools (CDC, 2015e).

TERTIARY PREVENTION IN SCHOOLS

Using the nursing process, the school nurse gives nursing care related to tertiary prevention when working with children who have long-term or chronic illnesses or children with special needs. The nurse participates in developing an IEP for students with long-term health needs. The nurse's responsibilities include the following:

- The nurse must have information about the child's medications to be given during school hours.
- The nurse must know if the child needs any therapy during the school day, such as physical or occupational therapy.
- The nurse must know if the child has a hearing or vision problem.
- The nurse must ask the teacher to seat the child in the best place in the classroom so the child can better see or hear the teacher and other children.

If a child is in a wheelchair or uses crutches, or has a hearing or vision problem, the school building itself may need to be altered so that the child can get around the school and use the restrooms. It is the responsibility of the nurse to tell the school's administrators about any needs such as these.

Children with Allergies

Food and insect sting allergies that result in anaphylaxis are being diagnosed more frequently (NASN, 2014c). Anaphylaxis is a severe allergic reaction that occurs quickly and can be life-threatening. Food allergies affect approximately 4% to 6% of children in the United States (CDC, 2015f). Milk, eggs, fish, shellfish, wheat, soy, peanuts, and tree nuts account for 90% of serious allergic reactions in the United States (CDC, 2015f).

The school nurse must take a leadership role in coordinated care for these students. The school nurse must develop a plan for preventing exposure to a known allergen and responding to an allergy emergency, collaborating with the student, the student's parents, and school personnel to determine the best plan of action (NASN, 2014c). The school nurse must provide annual training to school personnel who are involved with the student (NASN, 2014c). Most states have laws that allow students to carry emergency medication and, if developmentally appropriate, self-administer as needed (NASN, 2014c). Some states allow trained unlicensed assistive personnel to administer the emergency medication if the student is unable to do so and a nurse is not available.

Children with Asthma

Asthma is the leading chronic illness among children and adolescents in the United States, and it is one of the leading causes of absenteeism among children with a chronic illness (CDC, 2015g). Children may be hospitalized with an asthma attack, or they may have just returned home from the hospital. Asthma can also be caused by allergic triggers that affect children in the school. The following are possible culprits:

- Chalk dust from the blackboards
- Molds or mildew in the school
- Dander from pets that live in some classrooms

There also may be concerns about the quality of the air in the school building because many doors are shut. Industrial arts classes and other sources of air pollution are in the school (US Environmental Protection Agency, 2016). The school nurse can keep track of the indoor air quality of the school so that school administrators have data about what can affect the children. Fig. 31.3 contains the questions developed by the US Environmental Protection Agency that the school nurse should answer regarding the air quality of the school.

The nurse uses tertiary prevention when helping children who have asthma. This includes the following (NASN, 2015c):

- Administering or helping children use their inhalers or other asthma rescue medications
- Teaching the teachers, children, and parents about asthma and ways to reduce the factors to which the child may be allergic in the classroom

Many schools have management programs in place to help children with asthma (NASN, 2015c).

Children with Diabetes Mellitus

Diabetes is one of the most common chronic diseases in children and adolescents; nearly 167,000 youth below the age of 20 years have type 1 diabetes (CDC, 2015h). Every year, more than 18,000 children and adolescents are diagnosed with type 1 diabetes (CDC, 2015h). In the last couple of decades, type 2 diabetes mellitus (formerly known as adult-onset diabetes) has been reported among US children and adolescents with increasing frequency (CDC, 2015h). The school nurse must establish a plan of care for children with diabetes. This includes plans to monitor blood glucose and give insulin or other medications during the school day. Special nutritional needs also must be discussed (NASN, 2012b).

Children Who Are Autistic

Because all children are expected to attend some school regardless of their illness, children with autism go to regular schools in most cases. Because a child with autism has severe communication problems, the school nurse helps the child, the teachers, and the parents so that the child's school day is pleasant, as follows (NASN, 2013c):

- The nurse can give the child prescribed medications for mood or prevention of seizures.
- The nurse is responsible for preparing the teachers for the communication problems that the child may have.
- The nurse may recommend the use of sign language, picture boards, or other types of communication devices that are used by the child.
- The nurse can teach the parents about autism.

The nurse can help parents work with others in the health care system so the child can have a positive learning experience at school.

Children Who Have Attention Deficit Hyperactivity Disorder

Children with attention deficit/hyperactivity disorder (ADHD) also attend school. A national survey of parents found that 11% (6.4 million) of children 4 to 17 years of age have been diagnosed with ADHD (CDC, 2016b). The school nurse can help these children learn appropriate behaviors to reduce classroom disruptions (NASN, 2013c).

Children with Special Needs in the Schools

Also attending school are children who need the following:

- Urinary catheterization
- Dressing changes
- Peripheral or central line intravenous catheter maintenance
- Tracheotomy suctioning
- Gastrostomy or other tube feedings
- Intravenous medication

The following are included in the nurse's responsibilities:

- To supervise a health aide who is assigned to the child to care for complex nursing needs
- To provide tertiary care to maintain the child's health
- To maintain the skills needed to assess the child's well-being
- To teach another person in the school how to care for the child in case the nurse is not in the building when the child needs help

It is the responsibility of the school nurse to keep up with the latest health care information through in-service programs (NASN, 2012c).

Children with HIV or AIDS also may attend school. Because of privacy and confidentiality laws, the school nurse may not even know that a child with HIV or AIDS attends the school. In these cases, the nurse may be aware of the child's HIV status either by direct notification from the parents or physician or just by knowing that certain drugs the child is taking during the school day are anti-HIV medications. In all cases, the nurse cannot release that information to anyone.

- As part of regular health education in the school, the school nurse can provide education to the children, school employees, and community about HIV/AIDS prevention and risks.

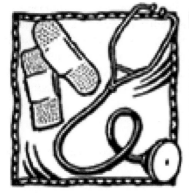

Health Officer/School Nurse Checklist

Name: _____

School: _____

Room or Area: _____ Date Completed: _____

Signature: _____

1. MAINTAINING STUDENT HEALTH

	Yes	No	N/A
1a. Completed health records for each student	☐	☐	☐
1b. Updated health records, as appropriate	☐	☐	☐
1c. Obtained necessary information about student allergies and other health factors	☐	☐	☐
1d. Developed a system to log health complaints (note symptoms, location and time of symptom onset, and exposure to pollutant sources)	☐	☐	☐
1e. Monitored trends in health complaints (especially in timing or location of complaints)	☐	☐	☐
1f. Investigated potential causes of health complaints (for example, school was renovated or refurnished recently; individual recently started working with new or different materials or equipment; new practices or products, such as cleaners or pesticides, were introduced into the school)	☐	☐	☐
1g. Ensured that the school prohibits smoking	☐	☐	☐
1h. Noted any new warm-blooded animals introduced into classrooms	☐	☐	☐
1i. Reviewed and understood indicators of IAQ-related problems	☐	☐	☐

2. HEALTH, IAQ, AND HYGIENE EDUCATION

	Yes	No	N/A
2a. Educated students and staff about the importance of good hygiene	☐	☐	☐
2b. Arranged individual instruction/counseling where necessary	☐	☐	☐
2c. Developed information and education programs for parents and staff	☐	☐	☐
2d. Established an information and counseling program for smokers	☐	☐	☐
2e. Provided literature on smoking and secondhand smoke	☐	☐	☐
2f. Educated school staff, students, and parents on the link between IAQ and health	☐	☐	☐

3. HEALTH OFFICER'S OFFICE

	Yes	No	N/A
3a. Ensured the ventilation system operates properly and supplies adequate quantities of outdoor air (i.e., at least 25 cubic feet per minute of outdoor air per occupant)	☐	☐	☐
3b. Ensured that air filters are clean and properly installed	☐	☐	☐
3c. Ensured that air supply pathways are clear of any obstructions	☐	☐	☐
3d. Determined that air removed from the health office is separated from the ventilation system to avoid affecting other occupied areas of the school	☐	☐	☐

FIG. 31.3 Indoor air quality checklist. (From US Environmental Protection Agency: Indoor air quality tools for schools action kit, Washington, DC, 2015, US EPA. Retrieved July 2016 from https://www.epa.gov/iaq-schools/health-officer-and-school-nurse-checklist-indoor-air-quality-tools-schools.)

- The school nurse also should be part of the school health advisory committee to develop an HIV/AIDS health curriculum that teaches not only about HIV/AIDS prevention but also about the disease itself so that children and families are not afraid to go to school with children who have the disease.
- Continuing education programs can be useful to teach the teachers and parents about the disease.

Children with Do-Not-Resuscitate Orders and the School Nurse

As part of tertiary prevention, the school nurse also maintains the health of children with terminal diseases who go to school. These children have been largely mainstreamed into the regular school population. The Education for All Handicapped Children Act (PL 92-142) stated in 1975 that all children should go to school in the "least restrictive environment" (NASN, 2013a). Therefore children who have Do-Not-Resuscitate (DNR) orders may attend the school, and some may die at school. DNR orders are signed by the parents and the physician according to state law. Under law, the school nurse is bound to obey the DNR order; however, it is not clear how the schools view them. NASN (2014d) recommends that each student with a DNR order have an IHP and an emergency care plan (ECP) developed by the school nurse with input from parents or guardians, the local funeral director, and, when appropriate, the student.

When a child dies in school, the nurse is responsible for helping the children who witnessed the death. The nurse becomes a grief counselor and helps the children and teachers cope with the death. Further education about death and dying given by the school nurse would also help the school community cope with death in the schools.

Homebound Children

Even though the laws regarding persons with disabilities state that all children should go to school, some children cannot do so. Instead, they may be taught in the home or in another institutional setting, such as the hospital. In these situations, the school nurse functions as follows:
- Should be a liaison between the child's teacher, physician, school administrators, and parents regarding the child's needs
- Helps these individuals make up the child's IEP so that it is appropriate for the child and does not remove necessary learning from the plan
- Allows the child to go to school when he or she is able
- Coordinates the child's health care needs and classes

Pregnant Teenagers and Teenage Mothers at School

Many teenage girls who are pregnant attend school. Therefore the school nurse may provide ongoing care to the mother (NASN, 2015d). Although this may appear to be primary prevention, it is tertiary prevention because adolescent pregnancies are considered to be at high risk.

CONTROVERSIES IN SCHOOL NURSING

School nursing has evolved into a complex health care role, and some areas of the field still cause controversy—for example,

birth control education and giving birth control to students in the schools. Because opinions differ relating to sex education and reproductive services in the schools, the school nurse should make an effort to communicate with the community, school board, teachers, parents, and students about what they think about different types of services in the school (NASN, 2012d).

ETHICS IN SCHOOL NURSING

The school nurse may be faced with ethical issues in the schools, such as the following:
- A child may have a DNR order that the parents wish to be used if the child dies at school (see earlier discussion), but following the DNR order may be against the nurse's personal beliefs.
- Perhaps a girl asks the nurse where she can get an abortion and wishes to talk to the school nurse about how she feels, but the nurse is against abortions.
- A teenager asks for emergency contraception, which the nurse does not wish to give.
In these cases the following action should be taken:
- The nurse must give nursing care to the student client and keep personal beliefs out of the discussion.
- If the nurse feels so strongly that he or she cannot work with the situation, another school nurse should be called for help.
- The student should be referred to other health providers who can give the care the student needs.

FUTURE TRENDS IN SCHOOL NURSING

The Patient Protection and Affordable Care Act (ACA) provided exciting opportunities for school nursing, with emphasis on Medicaid enrollment, health promotion, and care coordination. School nurses are in a prime position to advocate for, and assist students and their families to work through, the Medicaid enrollment process to ensure all students have access to care. As more families and students become eligible for Medicaid coverage, and as more private insurance companies recognize the benefit of caring for children at school, more school health services become reimbursable. In addition, there is a recommendation by *Healthy People 2020* that there be 1 nurse for every 750 schoolchildren to ensure all students have access to a school nurse. This is an extremely important issue because of the increasing numbers of children in schools with chronic disease and debilitating illnesses, the increasing numbers of new types of infectious diseases, and the acute-care diseases of childhood.

The ACA emphasized keeping children well by investing in prevention activities to improve health and reduce overall health costs. Since 1900, the school nurse role has focused on keeping students healthy and promoting health. To support community prevention efforts, activities that improve nutrition and increase physical activity, promote healthy lifestyles, and reduce obesity-related conditions and costs are programs in which school nurses are often involved. As the health and education systems evolve, the ability may exist to receive reimbursement for school health services and activities related to community-based prevention, health education, and counseling programs, such as immunizations, integrated behavioral health screening, suicide prevention activities, and substance use programs, to name a few.

The coordinated care models, including accountable care organizations, patient-centered medical homes, health information technology, and electronic health records, offer financial incentives to provide quality care in a cost-effective way. Evidence already exists that school nurses, acting as case managers, improve costs and outcomes in the school setting. The currently existing health care reform provides an opportunity to expand that role. It is hoped that any future changes related to health reform will continue to support and emphasize the work of the school health nurse. Evidence exists that school health nurses have improved the efficiency of care and student health outcomes while also increasing the communication between providers, schools, and families. Future improvement in population health and health care makes the work and expertise of school nurses more important than ever before.

The future of school nursing is strong. The amount of health care being given in the schools is increasing. In the future,

TABLE 31.3 Online Resources for School Nurses	
Organization	**Internet Address**
The American Academy of Child and Adolescent Psychiatry	http://www.aacap.org
American Academy of Pediatrics	http://www.aap.org
National Association of School Nurses	http://www.nasn.org
Center for Health and Health Care in the Schools	http://www.healthinschools.org
Healthy Schools Network	http://www.healthyschools.org

school nursing will use telehealth and telecounseling to teach health education (NASN, 2012e). School nurses will use the Internet to work with children and parents. Online resources are listed in Table 31.3. The school nurse is responsible for keeping up with the latest changes in health care and health practice so that the health of children in the schools can be enhanced by new trends in health care.

▶▶ APPLYING CONTENT TO PRACTICE

This chapter emphasizes the role and functions of the school health nurse and the important contributions nurses have made to population health, past, present, and future. The school nurse engages in all levels of prevention and applies the nursing process as individual children are cared for and as activities are implemented related to population and community health. The federal government has passed several landmark laws mandating that health and health care be addressed within schools. It is recommended that the registered nurse credentials with the baccalaureate degree serve as the basis for employing a school health nurse. Nurse practitioners are also beginning to play a role in school nursing, supporting the work of the registered nurse. Both state and national certification are available and may be required in some states. Within the school the nurse encounters a variety of health issues and will want to be prepared for disaster management as well. A very important and evolving role of the school nurse is participation on interprofessional teams to assure the most comprehensive levels of care and positive health outcomes. If students are healthy, they will be able to learn and become productive members of families, communities, and society as a whole.

▌ PRACTICE APPLICATION

Erin and Sandy, student nurses in their last semester of nursing school, were invited by their former high school to give a talk on nursing as a career at the school's career day. During their presentation, which included a multimedia PowerPoint video section on nursing, a student asked, "Why would I want to be a school nurse? Ours just sits in the office handing out bandages."

How should Erin and Sandy respond?

A. Talk about the many things for which school nurses are responsible.

B. Ask how other high school students in the room feel about this comment.

C. Use the classroom's intercom to ask the school nurse to come to the classroom.

D. Discuss the ways the school nurse prevents injuries from becoming infected.

Answers can be found on the Evolve site.

▌ REMEMBER THIS!

- School nurses provide health care for children and families.
- In the early 1900s, school nurses screened children for infectious diseases.
- By 2002, school nurses provided direct care, health education, counseling, case management, and community outreach.
- The National Association of School Nurses is the professional organization for school nurses.
- School nurses have varying educational levels depending on state laws.

- The US government supports school-based health centers, school-linked programs, and full-service school-based health centers.
- *Healthy People 2020* has objectives to enhance the health of children in the schools.
- Primary prevention provides health promotion and education to prevent childhood injuries and substance abuse.
- The school nurse monitors the children for all of their state-mandated immunizations for school entry.

- Secondary prevention involves screening children for illnesses and providing direct nursing care.
- School nurses develop plans for emergency care in the schools.
- Giving medications to children in the school must be monitored carefully to prevent errors.
- School health nurses are mandated to tell the authorities about suspected cases of child abuse and neglect.

- Tertiary prevention includes caring for children with long-term health needs, including asthma and disabling conditions.
- School nurses carry out catheterizations, suctioning, gastrostomy feedings, and other skills in the schools.
- Some ethical dilemmas in the schools are related to women's health care.
- Some nurses use the Internet to help communicate with children and their families.

ⓔ EVOLVE WEBSITE

http://evolve.elsevier.com/Stanhope/foundations
- Case Study, with Questions and Answers
- NCLEX® Review Questions
- Practice Application Answers

REFERENCES

Al-Bashtawy M, Al-Awamreh K, Gharaibeh H, Al-Kloub M, Batiha A, Alhalaiqa F, Hamadneh S: Epidemiology of nonfatal injuries among schoolchildren, *J of School Nursing (online)* June 2, 2016, doi: 10.1177/1059840516650727.

American Academy of Pediatrics, Committee on School Health: Guidelines for emergency medical care in school, *Pediatrics* 122:887–894, 2008.

American Academy of Pediatrics, Council on School Health: Role of the school nurse in providing school health services, *Pediatrics* 137(6):e20160852, 2016.

American Heart Association: *Pediatric course options*, 2016. Retrieved July 2016 from http://cpr.heart.org/AHAECC/CPRAndECC/Training/HealthcareProfessional/Pediatric/UCM_473190_Pediatric.jsp.

American Nurses Association and National Association of School Nurses [ANA and NASN]: *Scope and standards of professional school nursing practice*, ed 2, Silver Spring, MD, 2011, Nursebooks.org.

Association of State and Territorial Health Officials [ASTHO]: *Public health and schools toolkit: Public health access to student health data: authorities and limitations in sharing information between schools and public health agencies (Issue Brief)*, 2015. Retrieved July 2016 from http://www.astho.org/Programs/Preparedness/Public-Health-Emergency-Law/Public-Health-and-Schools-Toolkit/Public-Health-Access-to-Student-Health-Data/.

Boudreaux S, Broussard L: Sudden cardiac arrest in schools: the role of the school nurse in AED program implementation, *Issues Compr Pediatr Nurs* 35(3-4):143–152, 2012.

Center for Health and HealthCare in Schools: *Emergency preparedness: a quick guide for school staff*, George Washington University, 2013. Retrieved July 2016 from http://www.healthinschools.org/Health-in-Schools/Health-Services/School-Health-Services/School-Health-Issues/Emergency-Preparedness/A-Quick-Guide-for-School-Staff.aspx.

Centers for Disease Control and Prevention [CDC]: *Parasites—Lice—Head Lice*, Atlanta, GA, 2013, CDC. Retrieved July 2016 from http://www.cdc.gov/parasites/lice/head/epi.html.

Centers for Disease Control and Prevention [CDC]: *Expanding the Coordinated School Health Approach*, Atlanta, GA, 2015a, CDC. Retrieved July 2016 from http://www.cdc.gov/healthyschools/wscc/approach.htm.

Centers for Disease Control and Prevention [CDC]: *Whole School, Whole Community, Whole Child (WSCC)*, Atlanta, GA, 2015b,

CDC. Retrieved July 2016 from http://www.cdc.gov/healthyschools/wscc/index.htm.

Centers for Disease Control and Prevention [CDC]: *School Health Policies and Practices Study (SHPPS)*, Atlanta, GA, 2015c, CDC. Retrieved July 2016 from http://www.cdc.gov/healthyyouth/data/shpps/index.htm.

Centers for Disease Control and Prevention: *SchoolVaxView*, Atlanta, GA, 2015d, CDC. Retrieved July 2016 from http://www.cdc.gov/vaccines/imz-managers/coverage/schoolvaxview/index.html.

Centers for Disease Control and Prevention: *Understanding Bullying Factsheet*, Atlanta, GA, 2015e, CDC. Retrieved July 2016 from http://www.cdc.gov/violenceprevention/pdf/bullying_factsheet.pdf.

Centers for Disease Control and Prevention: *Food allergies in schools*, Atlanta, GA, 2015f, CDC. Retrieved July 2016 from http://www.cdc.gov/healthyschools/foodallergies/index.htm.

Centers for Disease Control and Prevention: *Asthma and schools*, Atlanta, GA, 2015g, CDC. Retrieved July 2016 from https://www.cdc.gov/healthyschools/asthma/index.htm.

Centers for Disease Control and Prevention: *Diabetes report card 2014*, Atlanta, GA, 2015h, CDC, USDHHS.

Centers for Disease Control and Prevention: *Youth Risk Behavior Survey: Trends in the behaviors that contribute to violence on school property, National YRBS, 1991-2015*, Atlanta, GA, 2016a, CDC. Retrieved July 2016 from http://www.cdc.gov/healthyyouth/data/yrbs/pdf/trends/2015_us_violenceschool_trend_yrbs.pdf.

Centers for Disease Control and Prevention: *Attention-Deficit/Hyperactivity Disorder (ADHD)—Data & Statistics*, Atlanta, GA, 2016b, CDC. Retrieved July 2016 from http://www.cdc.gov/ncbddd/adhd/data.html.

Clackamas County: *School based health centers*, Oregon City, OR, 2016. Retrieved July 2016 from http://www.clackamas.us/healthcenters/schoolhealth.html.

Dyess SM, Opalinski A, Saiswick K, Fox V: Caring across the continuum: a call to nurse leaders to manifest values through action with community outreach, *Nursing Administration Quarterly* 40(2):137–145, 2016.

Galemore CA, Bowlen B, Combe LG, Ondeck L, Porter J: Whole school, whole community, whole child—calling school nurses to action, *NASN School Nurse* 31(4):216–223, 2016.

Guide to Community Preventive Services: *Promoting health equity through education programs and policies: school-based health centers, Community Preventive Services Task Force*, Atlanta, GA, 2015, CDC.

Hamm MP, Newton AS, Chisholm A, Shulhan J, Milne A, Sundar P, Ennis H, Scott SD, Hartling L: Prevalence and effect of cyberbullying on children and young people: a scoping review of social media studies, *JAMA Pediatr* 169(8):770–777, 2015.

Heron M: Deaths: leading causes for 2013, *National Vital Statistics Reports* 65(2):1–95. Hyattsville, MD, 2016, National Center for Health Statistics.

Judd D, Sitzman K: *A history of American nursing, trends and eras*, ed 2, Sudbury, MA, 2013, Jones and Bartlett.

Keeton V, Soleimanpour S, Brindis CD: School-based health centers in an era of health care reform: building on history, *Curr Probl Pediatr Adolesc Health Care* 42(6):132–158, 2012.

Kerfoot KM, Douglas KS: The impact of research on staffing: An interview with Linda Aiken-Part 1, *Nursing Economic* 31(5): 216–220, 253, 2013.

Lerner MD, Lindell B, Volpe J: *A practical guide for crisis response in our schools*, ed 4, Commack New York, 2013, American Academy of Experts in Traumatic Stress.

Lewallen TC, Hunt H, Potts-Datema W, Zaza S, Giles W: The Whole School, Whole Community, Whole Child Model: a new approach for improving educational attainment and healthy development for students, *J of School Health* 85(11):729–739, 2015.

Lincoln County School District: *Nurse's Corner*, 2016. Retrieved July 2016 from http://www.lincoln.k12.or.us/student_parent/nurses_corner.php.

Loschiavo J: *Fast facts for the school nurse: school nursing in a nutshell*, ed 2, New York, 2015, Springer Publishing Company.

Murphy MK: Emergency anaphylaxis at school, *American Journal of Nursing* 114(9):51–58, 2014.

National Association of School Nurses [NASN]: *Medication administration in the school setting (Position Statement)*, Silver Spring, MD, 2012a, NASN.

National Association of School Nurses [NASN]: *Diabetes management in the school setting (Position Statement)*, Silver Spring, MD, 2012b, NASN.

National Association of School Nurses [NASN]: *Chronic health conditions managed by school nurses (Position Statement)*, Silver Spring, MD, 2012c, NASN.

National Association of School Nurses [NASN]: *School health education about human sexuality (Position Statement)*, Silver Spring, MD, 2012d, NASN.

National Association of School Nurses [NASN]: *The use of telehealth in schools (Position Statement)*, Silver Spring, MD, 2012e, NASN.

National Association of School Nurses [NASN]: *Section 504 and Individuals with Disabilities Education Improvement Act—the role of the school nurse (Position Statement)*, Silver Spring, MD, 2013a, NASN.

National Association of School Nurses [NASN]: *Drug testing in schools (Position Statement)*, Silver Spring, MD, 2013b, NASN.

National Association of School Nurses [NASN]: *Mental health of students (Position Statement)*, Silver Spring, MD, 2013c, NASN.

National Association of School Nurses [NASN]: *School violence, role of the school nurse in prevention (Position Statement)*, Silver Spring, MD, 2013d, NASN.

National Association of School Nurses [NASN]: *Bullying prevention in schools (Position Statement)*, Silver Spring, MD, 2014a, NASN.

National Association of School Nurses [NASN]: *Emergency preparedness and response in the school setting – the role of the school nurse (Position Statement)*, Silver Spring, MD, 2014b, NASN.

National Association of School Nurses [NASN]: *Food allergy management in the school setting, Clinical conversations for the school nurse*, Silver Spring, MD, 2014c, NASN.

National Association of School Nurses [NASN]: *Do not attempt resuscitation (DNAR) – the role of the school nurse (Position Statement)*, Silver Spring, MD, 2014d, NASN.

National Association of School Nurses [NASN]: *Role of the licensed practical nurse/licensed vocational nurse in the school setting (Position Statement)*, Silver Spring, MD, 2015a, NASN.

National Association of School Nurses [NASN]: *School nurse workload: staffing for safe care (Position Statement)*, Silver Spring, MD, 2015b, NASN.

National Association of School Nurses [NASN]: *School nurse—evidence-based clinical guidelines: asthma*, Silver Spring, MD, 2015c, NASN.

National Association of School Nurses [NASN]: *Pregnant and parenting students—the role of the school nurse (Position Statement)*, Silver Spring, MD, 2015d, NASN.

National Association of School Nurses [NASN]: *Frequently asked questions*, 2016a. Retrieved July 2016 from https://www.nasn.org/AboutNASN/FrequentlyAskedQuestions.

National Association of School Nurses [NASN]: *The role of the 21st century school nurse (Position Statement)*, Silver Spring, MD, 2016b, NASN.

National Association of School Nurses [NASN]: *Education, licensure, and certification of school nurses (Position Statement)*, Silver Spring, MD, 2016c, NASN.

National Association of School Nurses [NASN]: *Concussions—the role of the school nurse (Position Statement)*, Silver Spring, MD, 2016d, NASN.

National Association of School Nurses [NASN]: *Head lice management in the school setting (Position Statement)*, Silver Spring, MD, 2016e, NASN.

National Association of State Boards of Education: *State school healthy policy database: requirements for school nurses*, 2013, NASBE. Retrieved July 2016 from http://www.nasbe.org/healthy_schools/hs/bytopics.php?topicid=2130.

National Center for Learning Disabilities: *The state of learning disabilities: facts, trends and emerging issues*, ed 3, New York, 2014, NCLD.

Pavletic AC, Dukes T, Greene JG, Taylor J, Gilpin LB: Health services in boarding school: an oasis of care, counseling, and comfort, *J of School Nursing* (online) May 23, 2016. doi: 10.1177/1059840516649234.

Pbert L, Druker S, Gapinski MA, et al: A school nurse-delivered intervention for overweight and obese adolescents, *J Sch Health* 83(3):182–193, 2013.

Ramos MM, Greenberg C, Sapien R, et al: Behavioral health emergencies managed by school nurses working with adolescents, *J Sch Health* 83(10):712–717, 2013.

Rosen G, Fee E: *A history of public health*, Baltimore, MD, 2015, Johns Hopkins University Press.

Ruel SR: Lillian Wald, *Home Healthcare Nurse* 32(10):597–600, 2014.

Schaffer MA, Anderson LJW, Rising S: Public health interventions for school nursing practice, *J School Nursing* 32(3):195–208, 2016.

School-Based Health Alliance: *2013-14 National Census of School-Based Health Centers*, 2015. Retrieved July 2016 from http://www.sbh4all.org/school-health-care/national-census-of-school-based-health-centers/.

Selekman J, editor: *School nursing: a comprehensive text*, ed 2, Philadelphia, 2012, FA Davis.

Sharma M: *Theoretical foundations of health education and health promotion*, ed 3, Burlington, MA, 2017, Jones and Bartlett Learning.

Stopbullying.gov: *Policies and laws*, 2015, USDHHS. Retrieved July 2016 from http://www.stopbullying.gov/laws/.

Tucker S, Lanningham-Foster LM: Nurse-led school-based child obesity prevention, *J of School Nursing* 31(6):450–466, 2015.

US Department of Agriculture: *School meals: Healthy Hunger-Free Kids Act*, Washington, DC, 2016, USDA. Retrieved July 2016 from http://www.fns.usda.gov/school-meals/healthy-hunger-free-kids-act.

US Department of Education (USDE): *Every Student Succeeds Act (ESSA)*, 2015, USDE. Retrieved July 2016 from http://www.ed.gov/essa?src=rn.

US Department of Education, National Center for Education Statistics [USDE, NCES]: *Fast facts: back to school statistics*, 2015. Retrieved July 2016 from https://nces.ed.gov/fastfacts/display.asp?id=372.

US Department of Education, National Center for Education Statistics [USDE, NCES]: *Fast Facts: Enrollment Trends, Digest of Education Statistics, NCES 2016-006*, Chapter 1, 2016.

US Department of Health and Human Services: *Healthy People 2020: topics and objectives*, Washington, DC, 2010, USDHHS. Retrieved July 2016 from https://www.healthypeople.gov/2020/topics-objectives.

US Department of Health and Human Services: *Chart ECBP-5.1: Total, School Health Policies and Practices Study (SHPPS), Centers for Disease Control and Prevention, National Center for HIV/AIDS, Viral Hepatitis, STD, and TB Prevention (CDC/NCHHSTP)*, 2016. Retrieved July 2016 from https://www.healthypeople.gov/2020/data/Chart/4258?category=1&by=Total&fips=-1.

US Environmental Protection Agency: *Indoor air quality tools for schools action kit*, Washington, DC, 2015, US EPA. Retrieved July 2016 from https://www.epa.gov/iaq-schools/health-officer-and-school-nurse-checklist-indoor-air-quality-tools-schools.

US Environmental Protection Agency: *Asthma facts, EPA-402-F-04-019*, May 2016. Retrieved July 2016 from https://www.epa.gov/sites/production/files/2016-05/documents/asthma_fact_sheet_english_05_2016.pdf.

Vaughn B, Princiotta D, Barry M, Fish H, Schmitz H: *Schools and the Affordable Care Act, National Center of Safe Supportive Learning Environments*, Washington, DC, 2013, US Department of Education.

White House, Office of the Press Secretary: *White House report: the Every Student Succeeds Act*, December 10, 2015. Retrieved July 2016 from https://www.whitehouse.gov/the-press-office/2015/12/10/white-house-report-every-student-succeeds-act.

Xu J, Murphy SL, Kochanek KD, Bastian BA: Deaths: Final Data for 2013, *National Vital Statistics Reports* 64(2):1–95. Hyattsville, MD, 2016, National Center for Health Statistics.

The Nurse in Occupational Health

Bonnie Rogers

OBJECTIVES

After reading this chapter, the student should be able to:

1. Describe the nursing role in occupational health.
2. Describe current trends in the American workforce
3. Use the epidemiological model to explain work–health interactions, and give examples of work-related illness, injuries, and hazards.
4. Complete an occupational health history.
5. Describe the functions of the Occupational Safety and Health Administration and National Institute for Occupational Safety and Health.
6. Describe an effective disaster plan.

CHAPTER OUTLINE

Definition and Scope of Occupational Health Nursing
History and Evolution of Occupational Health Nursing
Roles and Professionalism in Occupational Health Nursing
Workers as a Population Aggregate
    Characteristics of the Workforce
    Characteristics of Work
    Work–Health Interactions
Application of the Epidemiologic Model
    Host
    Agent
    Environment
Organizational and Public Efforts to Promote Worker Health and Safety
    Onsite Occupational Health and Safety Programs
Nursing Care of Working Populations
    Worker Assessment
    Workplace Assessment
Healthy People 2020 Related to Occupational Health
Legislation Related to Occupational Health
Disaster Planning and Management

KEY TERMS

agents, 565
environment, 568
Hazard Communication Standard, 575
host, 564
National Institute for Occupational Safety and Health (NIOSH), 575
occupational health hazards, 571
occupational health history, 570
Occupational Safety and Health Administration (OSHA), 574
work–health interactions, 563
workers' compensation, 561
worksite walk-through, 571

In America, work is viewed as important to our life experiences, with most adults spending about one-third of their time at work (Rogers, 2015). Work—when fulfilling, fairly compensated, healthy, and safe—can help build long and contented lives and strengthen families and communities. Although some workers may never face more than minor adverse health effects from exposures at work, such as occasional eye strain resulting from poor office lighting, every industry grapples with serious hazard. No work is completely risk-free, and all health care professionals should have some basic knowledge about workforce populations, work and related hazards, and methods to control hazards and improve health.

Many substantial changes have occurred in the following:
- The nature of work
- Workplace risks
- The work environment
- Workforce composition and demographics
- Health care delivery mechanisms

An analysis of these trends suggests that work–health interactions will continue to grow in importance, affecting the following:
- How work is done
- How hazards are controlled or minimized
- How health care is managed and integrated into workplace health delivery strategies

As a result, significant developments are occurring in occupational health and safety programs designed to prevent and control work-related illness and injury and to create environments that foster and support health-promoting activities. Occupational health nurses have performed critical roles in planning and delivering worksite health and safety services. In addition, the continuing increase in health care costs and the concern about health care quality have prompted the inclusion of primary care and management of non–work-related health problems in the health services programs. In some settings, family services are also provided. This chapter describes the role of the nurse in relation to the working population.

DEFINITION AND SCOPE OF OCCUPATIONAL HEALTH NURSING

Occupational and environmental health nursing is the specialty practice that provides for and delivers health and safety programs and services to workers, worker populations, and community groups. The practice focuses on promotion and restoration of health, prevention of illness and injury, and protection from work-related and environmental hazards. Occupational and environmental health nurses (OHNs) have a combined knowledge of health and business that they blend with health care expertise to balance the requirement for a safe and healthful work environment with a "healthy" bottom line.

Occupational health nurses work in traditional manufacturing, industry, service, health care facilities, construction sites, and government settings. Their scope of practice is broad and includes the following:
- Worker and workplace assessment and surveillance
- Primary care
- Case management
- Consulting
- Counseling
- Crisis intervention
- Health promotion and risk reduction
- Administration and management
- Research
- Legal–ethical and regulatory monitoring
- Workplace hazard detection
- Community orientation

The knowledge in occupational health and safety is applied to the workforce aggregate.

HISTORY AND EVOLUTION OF OCCUPATIONAL HEALTH NURSING

Ada Mayo Stewart, hired in 1885 by the Vermont Marble Company in Rutland, Vermont, is often considered the first industrial nurse. Riding a bicycle, Miss Stewart visited sick employees in their homes, provided emergency care, taught mothers how to care for their children, and taught healthy living habits (Felton, 1985). In the early days of occupational health nursing, the nurse's work was family centered and holistic. Nursing care for workers in industry began in 1888 and was called *industrial nursing*. A group of coal miners hired Betty Moulder, a graduate of the Blockley Hospital School of Nursing in Philadelphia (later called the Philadelphia General Hospital), to take care of their ailing coworkers and families (American Association of Occupational Health Nurses, 1976).

Employee health services grew rapidly during the early 1900s as companies recognized that the provision of worksite health services led to a more productive workforce. At that time, workplace accidents were seen as an inevitable part of having a job. However, the public did not support this attitude, and a system for workers' compensation arose that remains in place today (McGrath, 1945).

Industrial nursing grew rapidly during the first half of the 20th century. Educational courses and professional societies were established. By World War II there were approximately 4000 industrial nurses (Brown, 1981). The American Association of Industrial Nursing (AAIN), now called the American Association of Occupational Health Nurses, was established as the first national nursing organization in 1942. The aim of the AAIN was to improve industrial nursing education and practice and promote interdisciplinary collaborative efforts (Rogers, 1988).

The passing of several laws in the 1960s and 1970s to protect workers' safety and health led to an increased need for occupational health nurses. In particular, the passing of the landmark Occupational Safety and Health Act in 1970, which created the Occupational Safety and Health Administration (OSHA) and the National Institute for Occupational Safety and Health (NIOSH), discussed later in this chapter, created a large need for nurses at the worksite to meet the demands of the many standards being implemented. The Occupational Safety and Health Act focused primarily on education and research. In 1988 the first occupational health nurse was hired by OSHA to provide technical assistance in standards development, field consultation, and occupational health nursing expertise. In 1993 the Office of Occupational Health Nursing was established within the agency.

ROLES AND PROFESSIONALISM IN OCCUPATIONAL HEALTH NURSING

As American industry has shifted from agrarian (agriculture) to industrial to highly technological processes, the role of the occupational health nurse has continued to change. The focus on work-related health problems now includes the spectrum of human responses to multiple, complex interactions of biopsychosocial factors that occur in community, home, and work environments. The customary role of the occupational health nurse has extended beyond emergency treatment and prevention of illness and injury. The interdisciplinary nature of occupational health nursing has become more critical as occupational health and safety problems require more complex solutions. The occupational health nurse frequently collaborates closely with multiple disciplines, industry management, and representatives of labor.

Occupational health nurses constitute the largest group of occupational health professionals. The most recent national survey of registered nurses indicates that there are approximately 19,000 nurses working in occupational health settings (US Department of Health and Human Service [USDHHS], 2010a; OHN Week, 2016). Their role is unique in that the nurse adapts to an agency's needs as well as to the needs of specific groups of workers.

The professional organization for occupational health nurses is the American Association of Occupational Health Nurses (AAOHN). The AAOHN's mission is comprehensive. The mission is to ensure that occupational and environmental health nurses are seen as the authority on health, safety, productivity, and disability management for worker populations (AAOHN, 2016). It supports the work of the occupational health nurse and advances the specialty. The AAOHN also does the following:

- Promotes the health and safety of workers (see the Evidence-Based Practice box below)
- Defines the scope of practice and sets the standards of occupational health nursing practice
- Develops the *Code of Ethics* with interpretive statements for occupational health nurses
- Promotes and provides continuing education in the specialty
- Advances the profession through supporting research
- Responds to and influences public policy issues related to occupational health and safety

The AAOHN describes 10 job roles for occupational health nurses: clinician, case manager, coordinator, manager, nurse practitioner, corporate director, health promotion specialist, educator, consultant, and researcher (AAOHN, 2012). The majority of occupational health nurses work as solo clinicians, but increasingly, additional roles are being included in the specialty practice. In many companies, the occupational health nurse has assumed expanded responsibilities in job analysis, safety, and benefits management. Many occupational health nurses also work as independent contractors or have their own businesses providing occupational health and safety services to industry, as well as consultation. With the current changes in health care delivery and the movement toward managed care, occupational health nurses will need increased skills in primary care, health promotion, and disease prevention. Occupational health nurses devote much attention to keeping workers and, in some cases, their families healthy and free from illness and worksite injuries. Specializing in the field is often a requirement.

Academic education in occupational health and safety is generally at the graduate level; however, many nurses with an associate degree in nursing (ADN) or a bachelor's degree in nursing (BSN) work in occupational health. Certification in occupational health nursing is provided by the American Board for Occupational Health Nurses. Requirements include experience, continuing education, professional activities, and examination.

WORKERS AS A POPULATION AGGREGATE

The population of the United States was expected to increase from approximately 319 million people in 2014 to an estimated 400 million people by the year 2051 (Colby and Ortman, 2014). In reality, the population grew to approximately 324 million people by 2016 (US Census Bureau, 2016). The US population is becoming older, with the greatest growth among people older than 65 years of age, and a reduction in the number of those younger than 25 years (Ortman et al, 2014). This will be reflected in the workforce, with a decrease in the number of young job seekers. It is estimated that by the year 2024, 47.9% of the workforce will be between the ages of 25 and 54 years, and 38.2% will be older than 55 years (Toossi, 2015). The number of adults ages 65 years and older will more than double between now and the year 2050 (Ortman et al, 2014). By that year, one in five Americans will be an older adult (Ortman et al, 2014).

In 2015 there were more than 148 million workers in the United States (Bureau of Labor Statistics [BLS], 2016). In 2014 workers were employed at over 8 million different worksites (US Department of Labor [USDL], 2014). Neither of these statistics indicates the full number of individuals who have potentially been exposed to work-related health hazards. Although some individuals may currently be unemployed or retired, they continue to bear the health risks for past occupational exposures. The number of affected individuals may be even larger because work-related illnesses are found among spouses, children, and neighbors of exposed workers.

Americans are employed in diverse industries that range in size from one to tens of thousands of employees. Types of industries include the following:

- Traditional manufacturing (e.g., automotive, appliances)
- Service industries (e.g., banking, health care, restaurants)
- Agriculture
- Construction
- Newer high-technology firms, such as computer chip manufacturers

Approximately 50% of business organizations are considered small, employing fewer than 500 people (Caruso, 2015). Although some industries are noted for the high degree of

EVIDENCE-BASED PRACTICE

Promoting the Health and Safety of Workers

Some employers have begun to expand occupational worksite clinics to include more comprehensive primary care and pharmacy services. Shahly et al (2014) did a systematic review of the literature to explore the available evidence regarding worksite primary care clinics, including current rationale, historical trends, prevalence and projected growth, expected health and financial benefits, challenges, and future research directions. The worksite clinic paradigm offers broad office hours, low wait time, long appointment time, personalized and skilled nursing care, and an on-site pharmacy. Reported benefits of the worksite primary-care clinic include reductions in both direct and indirect health care costs, with reductions in workers' compensation, disability, and life insurance claims; employee turnover; absenteeism; and presenteeism. Despite a low amount of peer-reviewed cost–benefit evidence, the broad consensus of available literature over the past 10 years finds that worksite clinics provide convenient and high-quality health care for employees and produce prompt and stably positive return on investment (ROI) for employers. The researchers concluded that a worksite primary-care clinic may offer employees a comprehensive, patient-centered "medical home" that provides accessible, team-based, prevention-focused primary care; reduces socioeconomic health inequalities; and offsets physician shortages in the community. More research is needed regarding standardized methods to quantify and report health outcomes and the ROI of worksite primary-care clinics as well as the impact of these clinics on the national economy and health care crisis.

Nurse Use

Worksite primary-care clinics have the potential to improve several serious problems in the US health care system. Such clinics rely on nurse practitioners and registered nurses in offering primary care services (with physician consultation), education, and preventive services.

Data from Shahly V, Kessler RC, Duncan I: Worksite primary care clinics: a systematic review, *Population Health Management,* 17(5): 306-315, 2014.

hazards associated with their work (e.g., manufacturing, mines, construction, agriculture), no worksite is free of occupational health and safety hazards. The larger the company, the more likely it is to sponsor health and safety programs for employees. Smaller companies are more apt to rely on the external community to meet their needs for health and safety services.

CHARACTERISTICS OF THE WORKFORCE

The US workplace and workforce are rapidly changing (BLS, 2016):
- Jobs in the economy continue to shift from manufacturing to service.
- Longer hours, compressed work weeks, shift work, reduced job security, and part-time and temporary work are realities of the modern workplace.
- New chemicals, materials, processes, and types of equipment are developed and marketed at an ever-increasing pace.
- As the US workforce grows to approximately 163.8 million by the year 2024, it will become older and more racially diverse (Toossi, 2015).
- By the year 2014, minorities represented 21% of the workforce, with 16% represented by Hispanics (BLS, 2015a).
- By the year 2015, women represented approximately 57% of the workforce.

In an era in which it was expected that the demand for workers would outstrip the available supply, businesses were concerned about strategies to increase the health status, employment longevity, and satisfaction of workers. However, the 2008 downturn in the economy changed the picture, with record-high unemployment rates (BLS, 2016). By the year 2024, minorities are projected to constitute 23% of the workforce and women approximately 47% of the workforce (Toossi, 2015). These changes will present new challenges to protecting worker safety and health.

The demographic trends in the US workforce indicate a changing population aggregate that has implications for the prevention services targeted to that group. Major changes in the working population are reflected in the increasing numbers of women, older individuals, and those with chronic illnesses who are part of the workforce. Because of changes in the economy, extension of life span, legislation, and society's acceptance of working women, the proportion of the employed population that these three groups represent will probably continue to grow.

CHARACTERISTICS OF WORK

Over time, there has been a dramatic shift in the types of jobs held by workers. Following the evolution from an agrarian economy to a manufacturing society and then to a highly technological workplace, the greatest proportion of paid employment was in the following occupations:
- Service (e.g., health care, information processing, banking, insurance)
- Professional technical positions (e.g., managers, computer specialists)
- Clerical work (e.g., word processors, secretaries)

Service-producing industries are projected to capture 94.6% of all new jobs added between 2014 and 2024 (BLS, 2015b). Health care occupations and industries are expected to have the fastest job growth and add the most jobs between 2014 and 2024 (BLS, 2015b). Within the industry, health care practitioners and technical occupations and health care support occupations are expected to grow the fastest (BLS, 2015b). This change in the nature of work has been accompanied by many new occupational hazards, such as the following:
- Complex chemicals
- Nanotechnology
- Nonergonomic workstation design (the adaptation of the workplace or work equipment to meet the employee's health and safety needs)
- Job stress
- Burnout
- Exhaustion

In addition, the emergence of the global economy with free trade and multinational corporations has presented new challenges for health and safety programs that are culturally relevant.

WORK–HEALTH INTERACTIONS

The influence of work on health, or work–health interactions, is shown by statistics on illnesses, injuries, and deaths associated with employment. In 2014 nearly 3 million workers reported nonfatal work-related illnesses and injuries, of which over half resulted in lost time from work (BLS, 2015c). Of these, approximately 2% were severe enough to result in temporary or permanent disabilities that prevented the workers from returning to their usual jobs (BLS, 2015c). The ten occupations with the highest incidence rates of nonfatal injuries and illnesses involving days away from work are shown in Fig. 32.1. Occupations involving public safety (patrol officers and firefighters) and highway maintenance were the top three occupations representing days away from work; nursing assistants ranked fifth (BLS, 2015d).

Occupational injuries and illnesses are estimated to cost employers in the United States $225.8 billion in lost wages and lost productivity, administrative expenses, health care, and other costs (Greenwell, 2015). These figures are often described as the "tip of the iceberg" because many work-related health problems go unreported. But even the recorded statistics are significant in describing the amount of human suffering, financial loss, and decreased productivity associated with workplace hazards. The high number of work injuries and illnesses can be drastically reduced. In fact, significant progress has been made in improving worker protection since Congress passed the 1970 Occupational Safety and Health Act. For example, vinyl chloride–induced liver cancers and brown lung disease (byssinosis) from cotton dust exposure have been almost eliminated. Reproductive disorders associated with certain glycol ethers have been recognized and controlled. Fatal work injuries have declined substantially through the years. Notably, since 1970, fatal injury rates in coal miners have been reduced by more than 75% (USDL, 2015a).

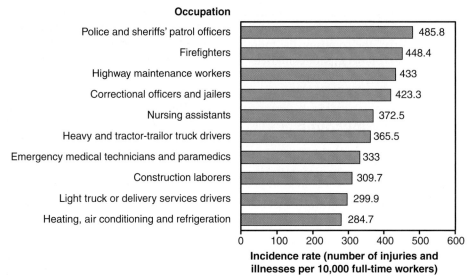

FIG. 32.1 The 10 occupations with the most injuries and illnesses involving days away from work, 2014. (Data from the Bureau of Labor Statistics [BLS]: *Nonfatal occupation injuries and illnesses requiring days away from work, 2014,* BLS News Release USDL 15-2205, 2015d, US Department of Labor.)

The US workplace has been rapidly changing and becoming more diverse. Major changes have been occurring in the following areas:

- In the way work is organized
  - With increased shiftwork
  - With reduced job security
- In part-time and temporary work
- As new chemicals, materials, processes, and equipment (e.g., latex gloves in health care, fermentation processes in biotechnology) continue to be developed and marketed at an ever-accelerating pace

APPLICATION OF THE EPIDEMIOLOGIC MODEL

The epidemiological triad can be used to understand the relationship between work and health (Fig. 32.2).

With a focus on the health and safety of the employed population, the *host* is described as any susceptible human being. Because of the nature of work-related hazards, nurses must assume that all employed individuals and groups are at risk for being exposed to occupational hazards. The agents, factors associated with illness and injury, are occupational exposures that are classified as *biological, chemical, ergonomic, physical,* or *psychosocial* (Box 32.1).

The third element, the environment, includes all external conditions that influence the interaction of the host and agents. These may be workplace conditions such as the following:

- Temperature extremes
- Crowding
- Shiftwork
- Inflexible management styles

The basic principle of epidemiology is that health status interventions for restoring and promoting health are the result of

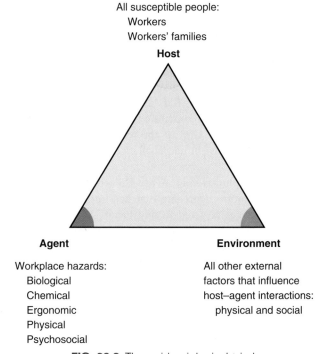

FIG. 32.2 The epidemiological triad.

complex interactions among these three elements. To understand these interactions and to design effective nursing strategies for dealing with them in a proactive manner, nurses must look at how each element influences the others.

HOST

Each worker represents a **host** within the worker population group. Certain host factors are associated with increased risk

- **Biological and infectious hazards.** Infectious and biological agents, such as bacteria, viruses, fungi, or parasites, that may be transmitted via contact with infected patients or contaminated body secretions and fluids to other individuals
- **Chemical hazards.** Various forms of chemicals, including medications, solutions, gases, vapors, aerosols, and particulate matter, that are potentially toxic or irritating to the body system
- **Enviromechanical hazards.** Factors encountered in the work environment that cause or potentiate accidents, injuries, strain, or discomfort (e.g., unsafe or inadequate equipment or lifting devices, slippery floors, workstation deficiencies)
- **Physical hazards.** Agents within the work environment, such as radiation, electricity, extreme temperatures, and noise, that can cause tissue trauma
- **Psychosocial hazards.** Factors and situations encountered or associated with a job or work environment that create or potentiate stress, emotional strain, or interpersonal problems

From Rogers B: *Occupational health nursing: concepts and practice,* St. Louis, MO, 2015, Elsevier.

for adverse response to the hazards of the workplace. These include the following (Rogers, 2015):

- Age
- Gender
- Health status
- Work practices
- Ethnicity
- Lifestyle factors

For example, the population group at greatest risk for experiencing work-related accidents with subsequent injuries is new workers with less than 1 year of experience on the current job (BLS, 2015d). The host factors of age, gender, and work experience combine to increase this group's risk for injury because of characteristics such as risk taking, lack of knowledge, and lack of familiarity with the new job.

Older workers may be at increased risk in the workplace because of diminished sensory abilities, the effects of chronic illnesses, and delayed reaction times.

A third population group that may be very susceptible to workplace exposure is women in their child-bearing years because of the following:

- The hormonal changes during these years
- The increased stress of new roles and additional responsibilities
- Transplacental exposures

These are host factors that may influence this group's response to potential toxins. In addition to these host factors, there may be other, less-understood individual differences in responses to occupational hazard exposures. Even if employers maintain exposure levels below the level recommended by occupational health and safety standards, 15% to 20% of the population may have health reactions to the "safe" low-level exposures (Friis, 2016). This group has been termed *hypersusceptible.* The following are host factors that appear to be associated with this hypersusceptibility:

- Light skin
- Malnutrition

- Compromised immune system
- Glucose 6-phosphate dehydrogenase deficiency
- Serum alpha 1-antitrypsin deficiency
- Chronic obstructive pulmonary disease
- Sickle cell trait
- Hypertension

Individuals who have known hypersusceptibility to chemicals that are respiratory irritants, hemolytic chemicals, organic isocyanates, and carbon disulfide also may be hypersusceptible to other agents in the work environment (Friis, 2016). Although this has prompted some industries to consider preplacement screening for such risk factors, the associations between these individual health markers and hypersusceptible response are unclear.

AGENT

Work-related hazards, or **agents** (see Box 32.1), present potential and actual risks to the health and safety of workers in the millions of business establishments in the United States. Any worksite commonly presents multiple and interacting exposures from all five categories of agents. Table 32.1 lists some of the more common workplace exposures, their known health effects, and the types of jobs associated with these hazards.

Biological Agents

Biological agents are living organisms whose excretions or parts are capable of causing human disease, usually by an infectious process. Biological hazards are common in workplaces such as health care facilities and clinical laboratories in which employees are potentially exposed to a variety of infectious agents, including viruses, fungi, and bacteria. Of particular concern in occupational health are infectious diseases transmitted by humans (e.g., from client to worker or from worker to worker) in a variety of work settings. Blood-borne and airborne pathogens represent a significant class of exposures for the US health care worker. Occupational transmission of blood-borne pathogens (including the hepatitis B and C viruses and the human immunodeficiency virus [HIV]) occurs primarily by means of needlestick injuries but also through exposures to the eyes or mucous membranes (Centers for Disease Control and Prevention [CDC], 2016a).

Transmission of tuberculosis (TB) within health care settings, especially multidrug-resistant TB, has reemerged as a major public health problem. Since 1989, outbreaks of this type of TB have been reported in hospitals, and some workers have developed active drug-resistant TB. In addition, among workers in health care, social service, and corrections facilities who work with populations at increased risk for TB, hundreds have experienced tuberculin skin test conversions. Reliable data are lacking on the extent of possible work-related TB transmission among other groups of workers at risk for exposure.

Many workers in these settings are employed as maintenance workers, security guards, aides, or cleaning people, who tend not to be well protected from inadvertent exposures, which include contaminated bed linen in the laundry, soiled equipment, and trash containing contaminated dressings or specimens

TABLE 32.1 **Selected Job Categories, Exposures, and Associated Work-Related Diseases and Conditions**

Job Categories	Exposures	Work-Related Diseases and Conditions
All workers	Workplace stress	Hypertension, mood disorders, cardiovascular disease
Agricultural workers	Pesticides, infectious agents, gases, sunlight	Pesticide poisoning, "farmer's lung," skin cancer
Anesthetists	Anesthetic gases	Reproductive effects, cancer
Automobile workers	Asbestos, plastics, lead, solvents	Asbestosis, dermatitis
Butchers	Vinyl plastic fumes	Meat wrapper's asthma
Caisson workers	Pressurized work environments	"Caisson disease," "the bends"
Carpenters	Wood dust, wood preservatives, adhesives	Nasopharyngeal cancer, dermatitis
Cement workers	Cement dust, metals	Dermatitis, bronchitis
Ceramic workers	Talc, clays	Pneumoconiosis
Demolition workers	Asbestos, wood dust	Asbestosis
Drug manufacturers	Hormones, nitroglycerin, etc.	Reproductive effects
Dry cleaners	Solvents	Liver disease, dermatitis
Dye workers	Dyestuffs, metals, solvents	Bladder cancer, dermatitis
Embalmers	Formaldehyde, infectious agents	Dermatitis
Felt makers	Mercury, polycyclic hydrocarbons	Mercury poisoning
Foundry workers	Silica, molten metals	Silicosis
Glass workers	Heat, solvents, metal powders	Cataracts
Hospital workers	Infectious agents, cleansers, radiation	Infections, latex allergies, unintentional injuries
Insulators	Asbestos, fibrous glass	Asbestosis, lung cancer, mesothelioma
Jackhammer operators	Vibration	Raynaud's phenomenon
Lathe operators	Metal dusts, cutting oils	Lung disease, cancer
Office computer workers	Repetitive wrist motion on computers and eye strain	Tendonitis, carpal tunnel syndrome, tenosynovitis

(Ito et al, 2016; Occupational Safety and Health Administration [OSHA], 2013; Uppal et al, 2014).

Chemical Agents

More than 300 billion pounds of *chemical agents* are produced annually in the United States. Of the approximately 2 million known chemicals in existence, fewer than 0.1% have been adequately studied for their effects on humans. Of chemicals that have been linked to carcinogens, approximately half test positive as animal carcinogens. Most chemicals have not been studied epidemiologically to determine the effects of exposure on humans (Friis, 2016). As a consequence of general environmental contamination with chemicals from work, home, and community activities, a variety of chemicals are found in the body tissues of the general population (Dong, 2014).

In many workplaces, significant exposure to a daily, low-level dose of chemicals may be below the exposure standards but may still involve a potentially chronic and perhaps cumulative assault on workers' health. Predicting human responses to such exposures is further complicated because several chemicals are often combined to create a new chemical agent. Human effects may be associated with the interaction of these agents rather than with a single chemical. Another concern about occupational exposure to chemicals is effects on reproductive health. Workplace reproductive hazards have become important legal and scientific issues. Toxicity to male and female reproductive systems has been demonstrated from exposure to common agents such as lead, mercury, cadmium, nickel, and zinc, as well as to antineoplastic drugs. Because data for predicting human responses to many chemical agents are inadequate, workers

should be assessed for all potential exposures and cautioned to work preventively with these agents. High-risk or vulnerable workers should be carefully screened and monitored for optimal health protection, such as those workers with latex allergy, which is a widely recognized health hazard (Hawker et al, 2012).

Environmental and Mechanical Agents

Environmental and mechanical agents are agents that can potentially cause injury or illness, that are related to the work process, or that can cause musculoskeletal or other strains that can produce negative health effects when certain tasks are performed repeatedly. Examples are repetitive motions, poor workstation–worker fit, and lifting heavy loads. Carpal tunnel syndrome, tendonitis, and tenosynovitis are the most frequently seen occupational diseases observed in workers who are chronically exposed to repetitive motion. The most frequently reported upper-extremity musculoskeletal disorders affect the hand and wrist region.

In 2014, sprains, strains, and tears were by far the most frequent disabling conditions, accounting for 420,870 days-away-from-work cases and an incidence rate of 38.9 cases per 10,000 full-time workers (BLS, 2015d). Workers who sustained sprains, strains, or tears required a median of 10 days away from work, compared to 9 days for all types of injuries or illnesses. Soreness and bruises accounted for the next more frequently seen injuries (Fig. 32.3) (BLS, 2015d). Overexertion was the most common event or exposure leading to injury, accounting for 33% of total cases, followed by falls, slips, or trips at 27% of cases (BLS, 2015d). The upper extremities (shoulders, arms, wrists, or hand) were the body parts most often affected by disabling work incidents (BLS, 2015d).

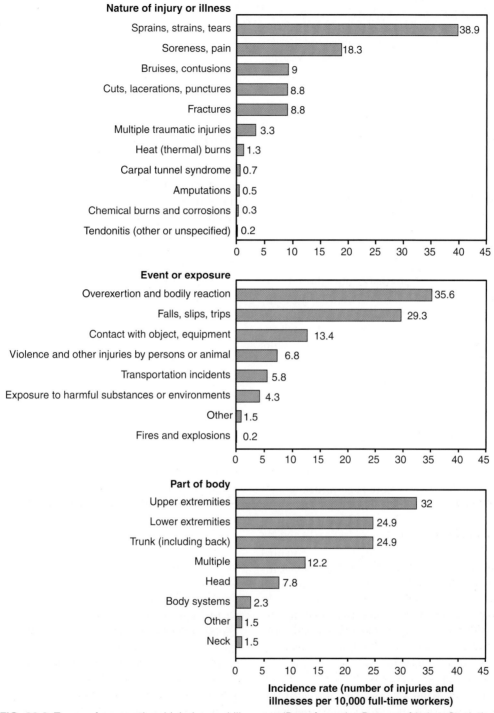

FIG. 32.3 Types of occupational injuries and illnesses (Data from the Bureau of Labor Statistics [BLS]: *Nonfatal occupation injuries and illnesses requiring days away from work, 2014,* BLS News Release USDL 15-2205, 2015d, US Department of Labor.)

Physical Agents

Physical agents are those that produce adverse health effects through the transfer of physical energy. Commonly encountered physical agents in the workplace include the following:

- Temperature extremes
- Vibration
- Noise
- Radiation
- Laser
- Lighting

For example, vibration, which accompanies the use of power tools and vehicles such as trucks, affects internal organs, supportive ligaments, the upper torso, and the shoulder-girdle structure.

Localized effects are seen with handheld power tools; the most common is Raynaud's phenomenon. The control of worker exposure to these agents is usually accomplished through engineering strategies such as eliminating or containing the offending agent. In addition, workers must use preventive actions, such as practicing safe work habits and wearing personal protective equipment when needed. Examples of safe work habits include taking appropriate breaks from environments with temperature extremes and not eating or smoking in radiation-contaminated areas. Personal protective equipment includes the following:

- Hearing protection
- Eye guards
- Protective clothing
- Devices for monitoring exposures to agents such as radiation

This class of agents is considered one of the most easily controlled.

Psychosocial Agents

Psychosocial agents involve conditions that create a threat to the psychological or social well-being of individuals and groups (Rogers, 2015). A psychosocial response to the work environment occurs as an employee acts selectively toward the environment in an attempt to achieve a harmonious relationship. When such a human attempt at adaptation to the environment fails, an adverse psychosocial response may occur. Work-related stress or burnout is fast becoming a significant problem for many individuals (Rogers, 2015). Responses to negative interpersonal relationships, particularly those with authority figures in the workplace, are often the cause of vague health symptoms and increased absenteeism. Epidemiological work in mental health has pointed to environmental variables such as these in the incidence of mental illness and emotional disorder.

The psychosocial environment includes characteristics of the work itself, as well as the interpersonal relationships required in the work setting and shiftwork. An estimated 10% of Americans do some form of shiftwork, which has the potential to lead to a variety of psychological and physical problems, including exhaustion, depression, anxiety, and gastrointestinal disturbance.

Strategies to minimize the adverse effects of shiftwork, such as rotating shifts clockwise, are beneficial. Job characteristics associated with an increased risk for heart disease among clerical and blue-collar workers are low autonomy, poor job satisfaction, and limited control over the pace of work.

Interpersonal relationships among employees and coworkers or bosses and managers are often sources of conflict and stress. Another aspect is *organizational culture*. This refers to the norms and patterns of behavior that are sanctioned within a particular organization. Such norms and patterns set guidelines for the types of work behaviors that will enable employees to succeed within a particular firm. The following are examples (Ehrhart et al, 2014):

- Following organizational norms for working overtime
- Expressing constructive dissatisfaction with management
- Making work a top priority

These factors and the employee's response to them must be assessed if strategies for influencing the health and safety of workers are to be effective.

Nonfatal violence in the health care worker's workplace is a serious problem that seems to be underreported. Much of the study of health care worker violence has been in psychiatric settings; however, reports in other areas, such as the emergency department, have occurred. Risk factors associated with this type of violence must be identified and strategies implemented to reduce the risk (USDL, 2015b).

ENVIRONMENT

Environmental factors influence the occurrence of host–agent interactions and may direct the course and outcome of those interactions. The physical environment involves the geological and atmospheric structure of an area and the source of elements such as water, temperature, and radiation, which may serve as positive or negative stressors. Although aspects of the physical environment (e.g., heat, odor, ventilation) may influence the host–agent interaction, the social and psychological environment can be of equal importance (Merrill, 2016).

New environmental problems continue to arise, such as an increase in industrial wastes and toxins and indoor and outdoor environmental pollution, that present opportunities for significant health threats to the working and general population. The social aspects of the environment encompass the economic and political forces affecting society and its health. This includes factors such as the following:

- Sanitation and hygiene practices
- Housing conditions
- Level and delivery of health care services
- Development and enforcement of health-related codes (e.g., occupational health and safety, pollution)
- Employment conditions
- Population crowding
- Literacy
- Ethnic customs
- Extent of support for health-related research
- Equal access to health care

In addition, addictive behaviors, such as alcohol and substance abuse, and various forms of psychosocial stress may be an outgrowth of negative social environments. Consider an employee who is working with a potentially toxic liquid. Providing education about safe work practices and fitting the employee with protective clothing may not be adequate if the work must occur in a very hot and humid environment. As the worker becomes uncomfortable in the hot clothing, protection may be compromised by the worker rolling up a sleeve, taking off a glove, or wiping his or her face with a contaminated piece of clothing. If the psychosocial norms in the workplace condone such work practices (e.g., "Everyone does it when it's too hot"), the interventions that address only the host and agent will be ineffective.

The epidemiological triad can be used as the basis for planning interventions to restore and promote the health of workers. These efforts are influenced by society and organizational activities related to occupational health and safety (Rogers, 2015).

ORGANIZATIONAL AND PUBLIC EFFORTS TO PROMOTE WORKER HEALTH AND SAFETY

Promotion of worker health and safety is the goal of occupational health and safety programs (Friis, 2016). These programs are offered primarily by the employer at the workplace, but the range of services and the models for delivering them have been changing dramatically over the past few years. In addition to specific services, legislation at the federal and state levels has had a significant effect on efforts to provide a healthy and safe environment for all workers. Recently under the Occupational Safety and Health Act and increased public concern about worker health and safety, companies that do not meet minimal occupational health and safety standards have received citations. Criminal charges have been filed against business owners when preventable work-related deaths occurred. These events have redirected an emphasis on preventive occupational health and safety programming.

Unless a company has OSHA-regulated exposures, business firms are not required to provide occupational health and safety services that meet any specified standards. With few exceptions, there is no legal request for specific services or level of personnel provided by employers to protect worker health and safety. Therefore the range of services offered and the qualifications of the providers of occupational health and safety vary widely across industries. An important stimulus for health and safety programs is avoiding cost that can be attributed to the effectiveness of prevention services, as well as the need to support occupational health and safety and health promotion at the worksite.

ONSITE OCCUPATIONAL HEALTH AND SAFETY PROGRAMS

Optimally, onsite occupational health and safety services are provided by a team of occupational health and safety professionals. The following are core members of this team:
- Occupational health nurse
- Occupational physician
- Industrial hygienist
- Safety professional

The largest group of health care professionals in business settings are occupational health nurses; therefore, the most frequently seen model is that of the one-nurse unit. This nurse collaborates with a community physician or occupational medicine physician who provides consultation and accepts referrals when medical intervention is needed. The collaboration may occur primarily through telephone contact, or the physician may be under contract with the company to spend a certain amount of time on site each week. As companies grow, they are likely to hire the following:
- Additional nurses
- Safety professionals
- Industrial hygienists
- Physicians, part time or on a consultant basis
- Employee assistance counselors
- Physical therapists

> ### BOX 32.2 Scope of Services Provided Through an Occupational Health and Safety Program
> - Health and medical surveillance
> - Workplace monitoring and surveillance
> - Health assessments
> - Preplacement
> - Periodic, mandatory, voluntary assessments and services
> - Transfer of clients or services
> - Retirement and termination
> - Executive
> - Return to work
> - Health promotion
> - Health screening
> - Employee assistance programs
> - Case management
> - Primary health care for workers and dependents
> - Worker safety and health education related to occupational hazards
> - Job task analysis and design
> - Prenatal and postnatal care and support groups
> - Safety audits and accident prevention
> - Workers' compensation management
> - Risk management, loss of control
> - Emergency preparedness
> - Preretirement counseling
> - Integrated health benefits programs

- Health educators
- Physical fitness specialists
- Toxicologists

The services provided by onsite occupational health programs range from those focused only on work-related health and safety problems to a wide scope of services that includes primary care (Box 32.2).

In industries that have exposures regulated by law, certain programs are required, such as respiratory protection or hearing conservation. The ability of a company to offer additional programs depends on the following:
- Employee needs
- Management's attitudes and understanding about health and safety
- Acceptance by the workers
- The economic status of the firm

A significant increase in the number of health promotion and employee assistance programs offered in industry occurred over the past few years. Health promotion programs focus on lifestyle choices that cause risks to health—for example, job stress, obesity, smoking, stress responses, or lack of exercise (O'Donnell, 2014). Employee assistance programs are designed to address personal problems (e.g., marital and family issues, substance abuse, financial difficulties) that affect the employee's productivity. Because such efforts are cost-effective for businesses, they should continue to increase in good economic times.

Similar types of occupational health and safety programs are available on a contractual basis from community-based providers. These may be offered by freestanding industrial clinics, health maintenance organizations, hospitals, emergency clinics, and other health care organizations. In addition, consultants in each discipline work in the private sector (e.g., self-employed, in group practice, in insurance companies) and in the public sector (e.g., in local and state health departments, in departments of labor and industry). These services may be provided onsite, delivered elsewhere in the community, or offered through a mobile van that visits companies. These multiple resources have increased the options for companies that need occupational health and safety services and have also broadened the employment opportunities for health and safety professionals.

NURSING CARE OF WORKING POPULATIONS

The nurse is often the first health care provider seen by an individual with a work-related health problem. Consequently, nurses are in key positions to intervene with working populations at all levels of prevention.

The occupational health nurse practices all levels of prevention (Rogers, 2015). Delivery of primary prevention services to employees is directed toward promoting health and averting a problem. In the occupational health setting, the purpose of health promotion is to maintain or enhance the well-being of individuals or groups of employees and the company in general. This may include programs designed to enhance coping skills or good nutrition and knowledge about potential health hazards both in and outside the workplace.

Health protection (i.e., taking primary prevention measures) is designed to eliminate or reduce the risk for disease to prevent the development of an illness or injury. Walkthroughs by the occupational health nurse and/or other team members to identify workplace hazards are aimed at health protection.

Specific protection programs or interventions often require active participation on the part of the employee. Participation in an immunization program, use of personal protective equipment such as respirators or gloves, and smoking cessation are examples of specific health protection measures.

Secondary prevention occurs after a disease process has already begun. It is aimed at early detection, prompt treatment, and prevention of further limitations. For employees, early detection involves health surveillance and periodic screening to identify an illness at the earliest possible moment in its course and elimination or modification of the hazard-producing situation. Interventions aimed at limiting disability are intended to prevent further harm or deterioration; they include referral for counseling and treatment of an employee with an emotional or mental health problem whose work performance has deteriorated and removal of workers from heavy metal exposure who manifest neurological symptoms.

Tertiary prevention is intended to restore health as fully as possible and assist individuals to achieve their maximum level of functioning. Rehabilitation strategies such as return-to-work programs after a heart attack or limited-duty programs after a cumulative trauma injury are examples of tertiary prevention.

CHECK YOUR PRACTICE

As a student in a public health course, you have been assigned to work with the nurse practitioner in a local industry. The nurse practitioner has noticed an unusual number of respiratory infections among the workers. She has asked you to help her determine the cause of this increasing rate of infections. How could you best help the nurse practitioner? What would you do?

WORKER ASSESSMENT

The initial step of assessment involves the traditional history and physical assessment, emphasizing exposure to occupational hazards and individual characteristics that may predispose the client to the increased health risks of certain jobs. The occupational health history is an indispensable component of the health assessment of individuals (Rogers, 2015) (see Appendix B.3). Because work is a part of life for most people, including an occupational health history in all routine nursing assessments is essential. Many workers in the United States do not have access to health care services in their workplaces. Yet it is not unusual to find health care providers in the community who have little or no knowledge about workplaces or expertise in occupationally related illnesses and injuries. Because of the large number of small businesses that do not have the resources to maintain onsite health care, injured and ill workers are first seen in the public and private health care sector (e.g., in clinics, emergency rooms, physicians' offices, hospitals, health maintenance organizations [HMOs], ambulatory care centers). Nurses are often the first-line assessors of these individuals and perhaps the only contact for education about self-protection from workplace hazards.

Identifying workplace exposures as sources of health problems may influence the client's course of illness and rehabilitation and also prevent similar illnesses among others with potential for exposure (Friis, 2016). Including occupational health data in client assessments begins with recognizing the possible relationship between health and occupational factors. The next step is to integrate into the history-taking procedure some routine assessment questions that will provide the data necessary to confirm or rule out occupationally induced symptoms. Symptoms of hazardous workplace exposures may be indicated by vague complaints involving any body system. These complaints are often similar to common medical problems. The occupational health histories should include the following points:

- A list of current and past jobs the client has held, including specific job titles, or history of exposure

LEVELS OF PREVENTION
Related to Occupational Health

Primary Prevention
Provide education on safety in the workplace to prevent injury.

Secondary Prevention
Screen for hearing loss resulting from noise levels in the plant.

Tertiary Prevention
Work with employees with chronic diabetes to ensure appropriate medication use and blood glucose screening to avoid lost work days.

- Questions about current and past exposures to specific agents and relationships between the symptoms and activities at work
- Other factors that may enhance the client's susceptibility to occupational agents (e.g., life history, such as smoking, underlying illness, previous injury, disability)

Questions about the employee's occupational history can be included in existing assessment tools. The more complete the data collected, the more likely the nurse is to notice the influence of work–health interactions. All employees should be questioned about their employment history. To describe only a current status of "retired" or "housewife" may lead to the omission of needed data. The nurse should be aware that not all workers are well informed about the materials with which they work or about potential hazards. For this reason the nurse must develop basic knowledge about the types of jobs held by clients and the possible hazards associated with them. Because there is an increased likelihood that multiple exposures from other environments such as home and yard may interact with workplace exposures, the nurse should extend the questioning to include this information.

Identifying work-related health problems does not require an extensive knowledge of occupational agents and their effects. A systematic approach for evaluating the potential for workplace exposures is the most effective intervention for detecting and preventing occupational health risks. Fig. 32.4 shows one short assessment tool that can be incorporated into routine history taking. Similar questions can be included in the assessment of workers' spouses and dependents, who may have indirect exposure to occupational hazards.

During these health assessments, the nurse has the opportunity to provide instruction about workplace hazards and preventive measures the worker can use. At the same time, the nurse is obtaining information that will be valuable in optimizing the fit between the worker and the job. Such assessments may be done as follows:

- As preplacement examinations before the client begins a job
- On a periodic basis during employment
- With the onset of a work-related health problem or exposure
- When an employee is being transferred to another job with different requirements and exposures
- At termination
- At retirement

The goal of these assessments is to identify agent and host factors that could place the employee at risk and determine prevention steps that can be taken to eliminate or minimize the exposure and potential health problem. When the health data from such assessments are considered collectively, the nurse may determine some patterns in risk factors associated with the occurrence of work-related injuries and illnesses in a total population of workers. For example, a nurse practitioner in a clinic noted a dramatic increase in the number of dermatitis cases among her clients. When she looked at factors in common among these individuals, she determined that they all worked at a company with solvent exposure commonly associated with dermal irritations. She worked with the union and the company to assess the environment and agent exposure to the employees.

This nursing intervention led to a safer work environment and a decrease in dermatitis in this population group. Such an approach can be used at the company, industry, and community levels. The initial collection of data and the questioning about workplace exposures are vital steps for any intervention.

WORKPLACE ASSESSMENT

The nurse may conduct a similar assessment of the workplace itself. The purpose of this assessment, known as a worksite walk-through or survey, is to learn about the following (Rogers, 2015):
- Work processes and the materials
- Requirements of various jobs
- Presence of actual or potential hazards
- Work practices of employees

Fig. 32.5 shows a brief outline that can be used to guide a worksite assessment.

More complex surveys are performed by industrial hygienists and safety professionals when the purpose of the walk-through is environmental monitoring or a safety audit. However, most occupational health nurses have developed expertise in these areas and include such tasks as part of their functions. For any health care provider who assesses workers, this information makes up an important database. For the onsite health care provider, worksite walk-throughs assist the professional in developing rapport and establishing credibility with the employees.

A worksite survey begins with an understanding of the type of work that occurs in the workplace. All business organizations are classified within the North American Industry Classification System (NAICS) with a numerical code. This code, usually a two-digit to four-digit number, indicates a company's product and therefore the possible types of occupational health hazards that may be associated with the processes and materials used by its employees. NAICS codes are used to collect and report data on businesses. For example, the illness and injury rates of one company are compared with the rates of other companies of similar size with the same NAICS code to determine whether the company is experiencing an excess of illness or injury.

By knowing the NAICS code of a company, a health care professional can access reference books that describe the usual processes, materials, and by-products of that kind of company.

The nurse should review the work processes and work areas by jobs or locations in the workplace. These preliminary data provide clues about what hazards may be present and an understanding of the types of jobs and health requirements that may be involved in a particular industry. A description of the work environment is next and provides an overall picture of the general appearance, physical layout, and safety of the environment. Are safety signs posted and readable where needed? Is clutter or dampness on the floor that could cause slips or falls?

A description of the employee group is vital to understanding the demographics and the work distribution in the company. Knowing about shiftwork and productivity can be helpful in pinpointing potential stressors. Human resources management and corporate commitment to health and safety are necessary to develop a support culture for effective and efficient

I. Present Job

    A. What is your job title? _____

    B. What do you do for a living? _____

    C. How long have you had this job? _____

    D. Describe the specific tasks of this job: _____
        _____

    E. What product or service is produced by the company where you work? _____
        _____

    F. Are you exposed to any of the following on your present job?

Metals	Radiation	Stress
Vapors, gases	Vibration	Others: _____
Dusts	Loud noise	
Solvents	Extreme heat or cold	

    G. Do you feel you have any health problems that may be associated with your work?
        If yes, describe: _____
        _____

    H. How would you describe your satisfaction with your job? _____
        _____

    I. Have any of your coworkers complained of illness or injuries that they associate with their job?
        If yes, describe: _____
        _____

II. All Past Work

    Starting with your first job, please provide the following information:

Job title	Years held	Description of work	Exposures	Injuries/illnesses	Personal protection equipment used

III. Other Exposures

    A. Do you have any hobbies that involve exposure to chemicals, metals, or any of the other agents mentioned
        before? If yes, describe: _____

    B. Are any other members of your household exposed to any of the substances listed above? If yes, describe:
        _____

    C. Do you live near any factories, dump sites, or other sources of pollution? If yes, describe: _____
        _____

FIG. 32.4 Occupational health history form.

Name of company: _____ Date: _____

Address: _____

Telephone: _____

Parent company (if any): _____

Location of corporate offices: _____

SIC code: _____

The Work:

Major products: _____

Major processes and operations, raw materials, by-products: _____

_____

Type of jobs: _____

_____

Potential exposures: _____

_____

Work Environment

General conditions: _____

Safety signs: _____

Physical environment: _____

Worker Population

Employees

Total number: _____ Number in production: _____ Others: _____

% Full-time: _____ % Men: _____ % Women: _____

% First shift: _____ % Second shift: _____ % Third shift: _____

Age distribution: _____

% Unionized: _____ Names of unions: _____

Human Resources Management

Corporate commitment to health

Personnel

Policies/procedures

Input/surveys/committees

Record keeping

Health Data

Work-related illnesses, injuries, deaths per annum: _____

OSHA recordable: _____ Workers' Compensation: _____

Other: _____ Most frequent complaints: _____

Average number of monthly calls to the health unit: _____

Absenteeism rate: _____

Occupation Health and Safety Services

Examinations

Employee assistance

Treatment of illness/injury

Health education

Physical fitness, health promotion activities

Mandatory programs

Safety audits

Environmental monitoring

Health risk appraisal

Screenings

Health promotion

Control Strategies

Engineering

Work practice

Administrative

Personal protective equipment

FIG. 32.5 Worksite assessment guide.

programming. Assessing the status of policies and procedures and assessing opportunities for input into improving service are important to establish the organization's strength in occupational health and safety management. Gathering data about the incidence and prevalence of work-related illnesses and injuries and the cost patterns for these conditions provides useful epidemiological trends. It also targets high-cost areas. It is important to know the types of occupational safety and health services and programs. This will indicate whether required programs are being offered and whether they include strategies for health promotion and disease prevention.

Finally, examining control strategies that are effective in eliminating or reducing exposure is important in determining risk reduction. Engineering controls can reduce worker exposure by modifying the exposure source, such as putting needles in a puncture-proof container (see the How To box).

HOW TO Assess a Worker and the Workplace

Assessing the worker for a work-related problem is a critical practice element. The nurse should do the following:

- *Obtain a complete general and occupational health history with emphasis on workplace exposure assessment, job hazard analysis, and list of previous jobs.*
- *Conduct a health assessment to identify agent and host factors that interact to place workers at risk.*
- *Identify patterns of risk associated with illness and injury.*

Assessing the work environment is necessary to determine workplace exposures that create worker health risk. The nurse should do the following:

- *Understand the work being done.*
- *Understand the work process.*
- *Evaluate the work-related hazards.*
- *Gather data about the incidence and prevalence of work-related illness and injuries and related hazards.*
- *Conduct a walk-through of the work environment.*
- *Examine the prevention and control strategies in place for eliminating exposures.*

CASE STUDY

Occupational Health Nurse in Health Clinic

Brenda Dowell is an occupational health nurse. Ms. Dowell works in the employee health clinic of a teaching hospital. This morning, Cindy True visits Ms. Dowell after accidentally sticking herself with a needle she just used to draw blood from one of her patients.

Ms. True tells Ms. Dowell that she graduated last year from nursing school and has been working on the cancer unit for the past 8 months. Ms. True usually works the night shift, but she was called to fill in for an evening shift nurse who was out sick. Ms. True was not accustomed to the evening shift routine and felt disoriented. One of Ms. True's patients was admitted to the floor 1 hour before her shift started and needed several laboratory tests. The day-shift nurse did not have time to draw blood for the laboratory studies and passed the task on to Ms. True. This was her second time drawing blood for laboratory tests, and she was having difficulty finding the vein. Ms. True was relieved when the blood was finally drawn, but as she was cleaning up her supplies, she felt a sharp tinge of pain in her hand. She looked down and saw the used needle in her finger. The nurse-manager for her unit sent Ms. True to employee health.

Ms. Dowell counsels Ms. True about the risks from needlestick injuries and about the seriousness of Ms. True's exposure and explains the testing for blood-borne pathogens Ms. True will have to undergo.

Work practice controls include good hygiene, waste disposal, and housekeeping. Administrative controls reduce exposure through job rotation, workplace monitoring, and employee training and education. Personal protective control is the last resort and requires the worker to actively engage in strategies for protection, such as the use of gloves, masks, and gowns to prevent exposure to blood and body fluid (Rogers, 2015).

The more information that can be collected before the walk-through, the more efficient will be the process of the survey. After the survey is conducted, the nurse can use the information with the aggregate health data to evaluate the effectiveness of the occupational health and safety program and to plan future programs.

HEALTHY PEOPLE 2020 RELATED TO OCCUPATIONAL HEALTH

Healthy People 2020 identifies the national health objectives aimed at reducing the risk for occupational illnesses and promoting safety. Health education and health protection strategies are proposed to address the needs of large population groups such as the American workforce.

LEGISLATION RELATED TO OCCUPATIONAL HEALTH

The occupational health and safety services provided by an employer are influenced by specific legislation at federal and state levels. Although the relationship between work and health has been known since the 2nd century (Ramazzini, 1713), public policy that effectively controlled occupational hazards was not enacted until the 1960s. The Mine Safety and Health Act of 1968 was the first legislation that specifically required certain prevention programs for workers. This was followed by the Occupational Safety and Health Act of 1970, which established two agencies to carry out its purpose of ensuring "safe and healthful working conditions for working men and women" (PL 91-596, 1970).

Within the context of the Occupational Health and Safety Act, the Occupational Safety and Health Administration (OSHA), a federal agency within the US Department of Labor, was created to develop and enforce workplace safety and health

---

♥ *HEALTHY PEOPLE 2020*

The following are example objectives that focus on occupational health:

OSH-1	Reduce deaths from work-related injuries.
OSH-2	Reduce nonfatal work-related injuries.
OSH-3	Reduce the rate of injury and illness cases.
OSH-4	Reduce pneumoconiosis deaths.
OSH-5	Reduce deaths from work-related homicides.
OSH-6	Reduce work-related assault.
OSH-9	Increase the proportion of employees who have access to worksites that provide programs to prevent or reduce employee stress.

From US Department of Health and Human Services: *Healthy People 2020,* Washington, DC, 2010b, US Government Printing Office.

regulations. OSHA sets the standards that regulate workers' exposure to potentially toxic substances, enforcing these at the federal, regional, and state levels. Specific standards and information about compliance can be obtained from federal, regional, and state OSHA offices (http://www.osha.org).

The National Institute for Occupational Safety and Health (NIOSH) was established by the Occupational Safety and Health Act of 1970 and is part of the Centers for Disease Control and Prevention (CDC). The NIOSH agency identifies, monitors, and educates about the incidence, prevalence, and prevention of work-related illnesses and injuries and examines potential hazards of new work technologies and practices (CDC, 2016b). Although NIOSH and OSHA were both created by the same act of Congress, they have discrete functions (Box 32.3).

Many standards have been established by OSHA and promulgated to protect worker health. One example is the Hazard Communication Standard. This standard is based on the premise that while working to reduce and eliminate potentially toxic agents in the work environment, an important line of defense is to provide the work community with information about hazardous chemicals so as to minimize exposures. The Hazard Communication Standard, which was first established in 1983, requires that all worksites with hazardous substances inventory their toxic agents, label them, and provide information sheets, called *material safety data sheets* (MSDSs), for each agent. In addition, the employer must have in place a hazard communication program that provides workers with education about these agents. This education must include agent identification, toxic effects, and protective measures. Numerous standards have been established by OSHA for specific chemicals and programs. A standard familiar to all health care professionals is the Bloodborne Pathogens Standard.

BOX 32.3 Functions of Federal Agencies Involved in Occupational Health and Safety

Occupational Safety and Health Administration (OSHA)
- Determine and set standards and permissible exposure limits (PELs) for hazardous exposures in the workplace.
- Enforce the occupational health standards (including the right of entry for inspection).
- Educate employers about occupational health and safety.
- Develop and maintain a database of work-related injuries, illnesses, and deaths.
- Monitor compliance with occupational health and safety standards.

National Institute for Occupational Safety and Health (NIOSH)
- Conduct research and review research findings to recommend permissible exposure levels for occupational hazards to OSHA.
- Identify and research occupational health and safety hazards.
- Educate occupational health and safety professionals.
- Distribute research findings relevant to occupational health and safety.

From Centers for Disease Control and Prevention: About NIOSH, Atlanta GA, 2016b, National Institute of for Occupational Safety and Health. Available at https://www.cdc.gov/niosh/about/default.html; United States Department of Labor: About OSHA, Washington DC, 2016, Occupational Safety and Health Administration. Retrieved August 2016 from https://www.osha.gov/about.html.

QSEN FOCUS ON QUALITY AND SAFETY EDUCATION FOR NURSES

Targeted Competency: Evidence-Based Practice—Integrate best current evidence with clinical expertise, client and family preferences, and values for delivery of optimal health care.

Important aspects of evidence-based practice include the following:
- **Knowledge:** Describe reliable sources for locating evidence reports and clinical practice guidelines.
- **Skills:** Locate evidence reports related to clinical practice topics and guidelines.
- **Attitudes:** Value the need for continuous improvement in clinical practice based on new knowledge.

Evidence-Based Practice Question:
Contact the American Association of Occupational Health Nurses and ask what the most pressing trends are in the specialty. Then look at nursing research journals to see if any nursing research is being done to address this trend. If you find nursing research addressing this trend, discuss an article with your classmates about the impact that nurses can have on this issue in occupational health.

Prepared by Gail Armstrong, DNP, ACNS-BC, CNE, Associate Professor, University of Colorado Denver College of Nursing.

Workers' compensation acts are important state laws that govern financial compensation of employees who suffer work-related health problems. These acts vary by state; each state sets rules for the reimbursement of employees with occupational health problems for medical expenses and lost work time associated with the illness or injury. Workers' compensation claims and the experience-based insurance premiums paid by industry have been important motivators for increasing the health and safety of the workplace.

DISASTER PLANNING AND MANAGEMENT

Although disaster planning and management have been functions of occupational health and safety programs, this is an area of new legislation that affects businesses and health professionals. The legislation of the Superfund Amendment and Reauthorization Act (SARA) requires that written disaster plans of industries be shared with key resources in the community, such as fire departments and emergency departments. Concern about disasters—such as the terrorist attacks on the World Trade Center and Pentagon on September 11, 2001, and in Paris, France, in 2015–16; the methyl isocyanate leak in Bhopal, India; the community exposure to chemicals at Times Beach, Missouri; the effects of hurricanes such as Hurricane Matthew that hit the East Coast of the United States in 2016; and the forest fire in Gatlinburg, Tennessee, in 2016, destroying homes and businesses—has mandated more attention to disaster planning.

The goals of a disaster plan are to prevent or minimize injuries and deaths of workers and residents, minimize property damage, provide effective triage, and facilitate necessary business activities. A disaster plan requires the cooperation of different personnel within the company and community. The nurse is often a key person on the disaster-planning team, along with safety professionals, physicians, industrial hygienists, the fire chief, and company management. The potential for disaster (e.g., explosions, fires, leaks) must be identified; this is best achieved by completing an exhaustive chemical and hazard inventory of the workplace. The plant blueprints are critical for correctly identifying substances and work areas that may be hazardous. Worksite surveys are the first step to completing this inventory.

Effective disaster plans are designed by those with knowledge of the work processes and materials, the workers and workplace, and the resources in the community. Specific steps must be detailed for actions to be put in place by specific individuals in the event of a disaster, as follows:

- The written plan must be shared with all who will be involved.
- Employees should be prepared in first aid, cardiopulmonary resuscitation, and fire brigade procedures.
- Plans must be clear, specific, and comprehensive (i.e., covering all shifts and all work areas) and must include activities to be conducted within the worksite and those that require community resources.
- Transportation plans, fire response, and emergency response services should be coordinated with the agencies that would be involved in an actual disaster.
- The disaster plan, emergency and safety equipment, and the first-response team's abilities should be tested at least annually with a drill.
- Practice results should be carefully evaluated, with changes made as needed.
- Hospitals and other emergency services, such as fire departments, should be involved in developing the disaster plan and should receive a copy of the plan and a current hazard inventory.

- The occupational health nurse or another company representative should provide emergency health care providers with updated clinical information on exposures and appropriate treatment.
- It should never be assumed that local services will have current information on substances used in industry.
- Representatives of these agencies should visit the worksite and accompany the nurse on a worksite walk-through so that they are familiar with the operations.

In disaster planning, the nurse often assumes or is assigned to the following:
- Coordinating the planning and implementing efforts
- Working with appropriate key people within the company and in the community to develop a workable, comprehensive plan
- Providing ongoing communication to keep the plan current
- Planning the drills
- Educating the employees, management, and community providers
- Assessing the equipment and services that may be used in a disaster

In the event of a disaster, the nurse should play a key role in coordinating the response. Principles of triage may be used as the response team determines the extent of the disaster and the ability of the company and community to respond. Postdisaster nursing interventions are also critical. Examples include identifying ongoing disaster-related health needs of workers and community residents, collecting epidemiological data, and assessing the cause of recurrence and the necessary steps to prevent it.

▶▶ APPLYING CONTENT TO PRACTICE

This chapter emphasizes the roles and functions of the nurse in occupational health. This dynamic specialty practice is broad and is founded in public health practice, supporting a model of health promotion, risk reduction, protection, and illness prevention. The occupational health nurse must have interprofessional skills and linkages to provide the most effective care and service. The epidemiological model is applied to occupational health and considers the host, agent, and environmental issues that may result in injury or illnesses. The goal is to assess the workplace to prevent injuries or illnesses where possible. In applying the model the nurse uses the nursing process and considers the impact of the workforce characteristics, the characteristics of the work, and work–health interaction in order to work toward a healthy and safe environment. Thus it is important to assess both the worker and the workplace to build this environment. Occupational health nursing has a rich history in the profession, beginning in the 1800s. The roles and functions of the occupational health nurse are many, and the education and certification of the nurse are considered as the nurse seeks a position as an occupational health nurse.

▮ PRACTICE APPLICATION

When an insurance company renovated its claims-processing office area and fitted the workstations with new computers, the company's occupational health nurse noticed an increase in visits to the health unit for complaints of headaches, stiff neck muscles, and visual disturbances consistent with computer usage. To conduct a complete investigation of this problem, the nurse assessed the workers, the new agent (the computers), previously existing potential agents, and the work environment. Interventions focused on designing a program to resolve the health hazard by changing the work process, if possible. In the present example, the first level of intervention was the design of the workstation for better worker use of the computer. Minimizing the possible hazards of the agent involved recommendations for desks, chairs, and lighting designs that would accommodate the individual worker and allow shielding of the monitor. The nursing interventions included strengthening the resistance of the host by prescribing appropriate rest breaks, eye exercises, and relaxation strategies. Recognizing that previous cervical neck injury or impaired vision may increase the risk for adverse effects from computer use, the nurse would include assessment for these factors in employees' preplacement and periodic health examinations.

For the environmental concerns, the nurse educated the manager about the health risks for paced, externally controlled work expectations and recommended alternatives.

This case is an example of which of the following?
A. The application of the occupational health history
B. A worksite assessment or walk-through
C. A work–health interaction

D. The use of the epidemiological triad in exploring occupational health problems
Answers can be found on the Evolve site.

REMEMBER THIS!

- Occupational health nursing is an autonomous practice specialty.
- The scope of occupational health nursing practice is broad, including worker and workplace assessment and surveillance, case management, health promotion, primary care, management and administration, business and finance skills, and research.
- The workforce and workplace are changing dramatically, requiring new knowledge and new occupational health services.
- The type of work has shifted from primarily manufacturing to service and technological jobs.
- Workplace hazards include exposure to biological, chemical, environmental and mechanical, physical, and psychosocial agents.
- The Occupational Safety and Health Act of 1970 states that workers must have a safe and healthful work environment.
- The interdisciplinary occupational health team usually consists of the occupational health nurse, occupational medicine physician, industrial hygienist, and safety specialist.

- Work-related health problems must be investigated and control strategies implemented to reduce exposure.
- Control strategies include engineering, work practice, administration, and personal protective equipment.
- The Occupational Safety and Health Administration enforces workplace safety and health standards.
- The National Institute for Occupational Safety and Health is the research agency that provides grants to investigate the causes of workplace illness and injuries.
- Workers' compensation acts are important laws that govern the financial compensation of employees who suffer work-related health problems.
- The occupational health nurse should play a key role in disaster planning and coordination.
- Academic education in occupational health nursing is generally at the graduate level; however, many nurses with associate degrees in nursing and bachelor's degrees in nursing work in occupational health.

EVOLVE WEBSITE

http://evolve.elsevier.com/Stanhope/foundations
- Case Study, with Questions and Answers
- NCLEX® Review Questions
- Practice Application Answers

REFERENCES

American Association of Occupational Health Nurses [AAOHN]: *The nurse in industry*, New York, 1976, AAOHN.
American Association of Occupational Health Nurses [AAOHN]: *Standards of occupational & environmental health nursing*, 2012, AAOHN. Retrieved August 2016 from http://aaohn.org/page/practice-standards.
American Association of Occupational Health Nurses [AAOHN]: *Fact Sheet*, New York, 2016, AAOHN.
Brown M: *Occupational health nursing*, New York, 1981, MacMillan.
Bureau of Labor Statistics [BLS]: *Labor force statistics by race and ethnicity, 2014, BLS Reports*, Washington, DC, 2015a, Report 1057, US Bureau of Labor Statistics.
Bureau of Labor Statistics [BLS]: *Employment projections: 2014-24, BLS News Release USDL-15-2327*, Washington, DC, 2015b, US Department of Labor.
Bureau of Labor Statistics [BLS]: *Employee-reported workplace injuries and illnesses – 2014, BLS News release USDL-15-2086*, Washington, DC, 2015c, US Department of Labor.
Bureau of Labor Statistics [BLS]: *Nonfatal occupation injuries and illnesses requiring days away from work, 2014, BLS News Release USDL 15-2205*, Washington, DC, 2015d, US Department of Labor.
Bureau of Labor Statistics [BLS]: *Labor force statistics from the current population survey, Table 18b: Employed persons by detailed industry and age*, 2016. Retrieved August 2016 from http://www.bls.gov/cps/cpsaat18b.htm.
Caruso A: *Statistics of US Businesses Employment and Payroll Summary: 2012, Economy-wide Statistics Briefs*, 2015, US Department of Commerce Economics and Statistics Administration, US Census Bureau. Available at http://www.census.gov/content/dam/Census/library/publications/2015/econ/g12-susb.pdf.
Centers for Disease Control and Prevention [CDC]: *Bloodborne infectious diseases: HIV/AIDS, Hepatitis B, Hepatitis C*, Atlanta, GA, 2016a, National Institute of for Occupational Safety and Health.
Centers for Disease Control and Prevention [CDC]: *About NIOSH*, Atlanta, GA, 2016b, National Institute of for Occupational Safety and Health. Available at https://www.cdc.gov/niosh/about/default.html.
Colby SL, Ortman JM: *Projections of the size and composition of the U.S. population: 2014 to 2060, Current Population Reports, P25-1143*, Washington, DC, 2014, US Census Bureau.
Dong MH: *An introduction to environmental toxicology*, ed 3, North Charleston, SC, 2014, CreateSpace Publishing.
Ehrhart MG, Schneider B, Macey WM: *Organizational climate and culture: an introduction to theory, research, and practice*, New York, 2014, Routledge.
Felton J: The genesis of American occupational health nursing, I. *Occup Health Nurs* 33:615–620, 1985.
Friis RH: *Occupational health and safety for the 21st century*, Burlington, MA, 2016, Jones and Bartlett Learning.
Greenwell C: *Worker illness and injury costs U.S. employers $225.8 billion annually, CDC Foundation*, 2015. Retrieved August 2016 from http://www.cdcfoundation.org/pr/2015/worker-illness-and-injury-costs-us-employers-225-billion-annually.
Hawker J, Begg N, Blair I, Reintjes R, et al: *Communicable disease control and health protection handbook*, ed 3, Hoboken, NJ, 2012, Blackwell and Wiley.

Ito Y, Nagao M, Iinuma Y, Matsumura Y, Mishima M: Risk factors for nosocomial tuberculosis transmission among health care workers, *American Journal of Infection Control* 44(5):596–598, 2016.

McGrath B: Fifty years of industrial nursing, *Public Health Nurs* 37:119, 1945.

Merrill RM: *Introduction to epidemiology*, ed 4, Burlington, MA, 2016, Jones & Bartlett Learning.

Occupational Health Nurse (OHN) Week, 2016; Creating a culture of health and safety in the work place, New York, june 21, 2016, AAOHN.

Occupational Safety and Health Administration [OSHA]: *Facts about hospital worker safety*, 2013, US Department of Labor. Available at https://www.osha.gov/dsg/hospitals/documents/1.2_Factbook_508.pdf.

O'Donnell MP: *Health promotion in the workplace*, ed 4, Troy, MI, 2014, Am J of Health Promotion.

Ortman JM, Velkoff VA, Hogan H: *An aging nation: the older population in the United States, Current Population Reports, P25-1140*, Washington, DC, 2014, US Census Bureau.

Ramazzini B: *De Morbis Artifiticum (Diseases of Workers), 1713, Translated by Wright WC*. Chicago 1940, University of Chicago Press, Illinois.

Rogers B: Perspectives on occupational health nursing, *AAOHN J* 36:100–105, 1988.

Rogers B: *Occupational health nursing: concepts and practice*, St. Louis, 2015, Elsevier.

Shahly V, Kessler RC, Duncan I: Worksite primary care clinics: a systematic review, *Population Health Management* 17(5):306–315, 2014.

Toossi M: *Labor force projections to 2024: the labor force is growing, but slowly, Monthly Labor Rev*, Washington, DC, 2015, Bureau of Labor Statistics.

Uppal N, Batt J, Seemangal J, McIntyre SA, Aliyev N, Muller MP: Nosocomial tuberculosis exposures at a tertiary care hospital: a root cause analysis, *American Journal of Infection Control* 42(5):511–515, 2014.

US Census Bureau: *U.S. & world population clocks*, Washington, DC, 2016, USCB. Retrieved August 2016 from http://www.census.gov/popclock/.

US Department of Health and Human Services [USDHHS]: *The registered nurse population: findings from the 2008 national sample survey of registered nurses*, Washington, DC, 2010a, Health Resources and Services Administration. Retrieved August 2016 from http://bhpr.hrsa.gov/healthworkforce/rnsurveys/rnsurveyfinal.pdf.

US Department of Health and Human Services [USDHHS]: *Healthy People 2020*, Washington, DC, 2010b, US Government Printing Office.

US Department of Labor [USDL]: *Commonly used statistics*, 2014, Occupational Safety and Health Administration. Retrieved August 2016 from https://www.osha.gov/oshstats/commonstats.html.

US Department of Labor [USDL]: *Mine safety and health at a glance*, 2015a, Mine Safety and Health Administration. Retrieved August 2016 from http://arlweb.msha.gov/MSHAINFO/FactSheets/MSHAFCT10.asp.

US Department of Labor [USDL]: *Guidelines for preventing workplace violence for healthcare and social service workers*, Washington, DC, 2015b, Occupational Safety and Health Administration, OSHA 3148-04R.

US Department of Labor [USDL]: *About OSHA*, Washington, DC, 2016, Occupational Safety and Health Administration. Retrieved August 2016 from https://www.osha.gov/about.html.

APPENDIXES

APPENDIX A   GUIDELINES FOR PRACTICE

A.1: *The Health Insurance Portability and Accountability Act (HIPAA): What Does It Mean for Public Health Nurses?* (Chapters 1, 2, 3, 7, 8, 28, 30), 580

A.2: Living Will Directive (Chapters 20 and 30), 582

APPENDIX B   ASSESSMENT TOOLS

B.1: Community Assessment Model (Chapters 12 and 22), 583

B.2: Friedman Family Assessment Model (Short Form) (Chapters 18 and 20), 584

B.3: Comprehensive Occupational and Environmental Exposure History (Chapters 6 and 32), 586

B.4: Omaha System Problem Classification Scheme with Case Study Application (Chapter 30), 590

B.5: Cultural Assessment Guide (Chapter 5), 593

APPENDIX C   ESSENTIAL ELEMENTS OF PUBLIC HEALTH NURSING

C.1: Examples of Public Health Nursing Roles and Implementing Public Health Functions (Chapters 1, 10, 12, 28), 594

C.2: American Nurses Association Standards of Practice and Professional Performance for Public Health Nursing (Chapters 1, 2, 4, 17), 601

C.3: Quad Council Public Health Nursing Core Competencies and Skill Levels (Chapters 1, 10, 12, 17, 28), 602

C.4: Minnesota Department of Health Public Health Interventions Wheel (All Chapters), 603

APPENDIX D   HEPATITIS INFORMATION

D.1: Summary Description of Hepatitis A-E (Chapter 27), 606

D.2: Recommendations for Prophylaxis of Hepatitis A (Chapter 27), 608

D.3: Recommended Postexposure Prophylaxis for Percutaneous or Permucosal Exposure to Hepatitis B Virus (Chapter 27), 609

APPENDIX E   GLOSSARY

Guidelines for Practice

A.1 *The Health Insurance Portability and Accountability Act* (HIPAA): What Does It Mean for Public Health Nurses?

Public Health Nursing Practice: Definition—the synthesis of nursing and public health theory applied to promoting and preserving the health of populations. The practice focuses on the community as a whole and on the effect of the community's health status (resources) on the health of individuals, families, and groups. The goal is to prevent disease and disability and promote and protect the health of the community as a whole.

EXPLANATION

- Federal privacy standards were created by the U.S. Department of Health and Human Services (USDHHS) to protect patients' medical records and other health information provided to health plans, doctors, hospitals, and other health care providers.
- These standards took effect on April 14, 2003.
- The *Health Insurance Portability and Accountability Act* sought to reduce the cost of and improve the delivery of health care through the standardization of electronic transactions and the elimination of inefficient paper forms.

PRIVACY RULE

- Protects the confidentiality of individually identifiable health information, whether it is on paper, in computers, or communicated orally.
  - Protected health information (PHI) is the name for this individually identifiable health information.
  - Limits the ways that health plans, pharmacies, hospitals, and other covered entities can use patients' personal medical information.

PATIENT PROTECTIONS

- Patients should be able to see, obtain copies of, and make corrections to their medical records.
- Patients should receive a notice from health care providers regarding how their personal medical information may be used by them and their rights under the privacy regulation. Patients can restrict this use.
- Limits have been set on how health care providers can use individually identifiable health information. Doctors, nurses, and other providers can share information needed to treat a patient. For purposes other than medical care, personal health information generally may not be used.

- Pharmacies, health plans, and other covered entities must obtain an individual's authorization before disclosing patient information for marketing purposes.

PUBLIC HEALTH SERVICES AND PROTECTED HEALTH INFORMATION

Overview: Although protection of health information is important, PHI is used for the public good by health officials to identify, monitor, and respond to disease, death, and disability among populations. Examples of ways PHI is used include public health surveillance, program evaluation, terrorism preparedness, outbreak investigations, direct health services, and public health research. Public health authorities have taken precautions in the past to protect the privacy of individuals and will continue to do so under HIPAA. The privacy rule, however, still permits PHI to be shared for important public health purposes.

PERMITTED PROTECTED HEALTH INFORMATION DISCLOSURES TO A PUBLIC HEALTH AUTHORITY WITHOUT AUTHORIZATION

- Reporting of disease, injury, and vital events
- Conducting public health surveillance, investigations, and interventions
- Reporting child abuse or neglect to a public health or other government authority legally authorized to receive such reports
- Reporting to a person subject to the jurisdiction of the U.S. Food and Drug Administration (FDA) concerning the quality, safety, or effectiveness of an FDA-related product or activity for which that person has responsibility
- To a person who may have been exposed to a communicable disease or may be at risk for contracting or spreading a disease or condition, when legally authorized to notify the person as necessary to conduct a public health intervention or investigation
- To an individual's employer, under certain circumstances and conditions, as needed for the employer to meet the

requirements of the Occupational Safety and Health Administration, Mine Safety and Health Administration, or similar state law

HEALTH INSURANCE PORTABILITY AND ACCOUNTABILITY ACT AND NURSING RESEARCH

Definitions

Covered entity: A health plan, a health care clearinghouse, or a health care provider who transmits any health information in electronic form.

Individually Identifiable Health Information (IIHI): Information about an individual regarding his or her physical or mental health, the provision of health care, or the payment for the provision of health care and that identifies the individual.

- It is the covered entity's obligation not to disclose the information improperly when a researcher seeks data that includes PHI.

A covered entity can disclose IIHI for research purposes under any of the following conditions:

1. The IIHI pertains only to deceased persons.
2. The IIHI can be examined for reviews preparatory to research if it is not removed from the covered entity.
3. Information that has been deidentified can be disclosed; this information is no longer considered IIHI and thus is not covered by HIPAA.
4. Data must be disclosed as part of a limited data set if the researcher has a data use agreement with the covered entity.
5. The researcher has a valid authorization from the research subject to disclose IIHI.
6. An institutional review board or privacy board has waived the authorization requirement.

Creating Data

Researchers may also be creating IIHI. If the researcher is part of a covered entity, any PHI obtained by any means is covered by HIPAA, and the researcher and his or her institution are bound by HIPAA regulations. Most universities with nursing schools will be hybrid entities (i.e., some parts of the university are a covered entity and some are not). Researchers should check their institution's policies.

Disclosing Data

Nurse researchers should be aware that sharing data with colleagues and students may constitute disclosures of IIHI and they should conform to HIPAA regulations. In this case, the researcher is the holder of the IIHI and can disclose it only under appropriate conditions:

1. Patients agree to specific disclosures in the initial authorization.
2. Former patients sign an additional authorization.
3. An institutional review board or privacy board waives the need for authorization.
4. The holder allows the colleague to review the data to prepare a research protocol if the colleague takes no information away.
5. A holder enters the data in a limited data set and signs a data use agreement with the recipient.
6. A holder deidentifies the data and shares it freely.

From Begley EB, Ware JM, Hexem SA, Papposelli K, Thomson K, Penn MS, Aquino GA: Personally identifiable information in state laws: Use, release, and collaboration at health departments, *American Journal of Public Health,* Published online ahead of print June 22, 2017: e1–e5. doi:10.2105/AJPH.2017.303862; Bernstein AB, Sweeney MH: *Public health surveillance data: legal, policy, ethical, regulatory, and practical issues, Morbidity and Mortality Weekly Report,* 61(03): 30-34, 2012. Retrieved July 2017, from https://www.cdc.gov/mmwr/preview/mmwrhtml/su6103a7.htm?s_cid%3Dsu6103a7_x; Centers for Disease Control and Prevention: *HIPAA privacy rule and public health, MMWR* 52(S-1): 1-12, 2003. Retrieved July 2017, from http://www.cdc.gov/mmwr/preview/mmwrhtml/su5201a1.htm; Goldstein ND, Sarwate AD: Privacy, security, and the public health researcher in the era of electronic health record research, *Online J of Public Health Informatics,* 8(3): e207, 2016; Institute of Medicine (2009): *Beyond the HIPAA privacy rule: enhancing privacy, improving health through research,* Washington, DC: National Academies Press; Jacobson PD, Wasserman J, Botoseneaunu A, Silverstein A, Wu HW: The roles of law in public health preparedness: Opportunities and challenges, *J Health Politics Policy Law* 37(2): 297-328, 2012; Olsen DP: HIPAA privacy regulations and nursing research, *Nurs Res* 52: 344-348, 2003; U.S. Department of Health and Human Services: Health information privacy: public health. Washington, DC, 2003, USDHHS. Retrieved July 2017 from http://www.hhs.gov/ocr/privacy/hipaa/understanding/special/publichealth/index.html.

A.2 Living Will Directive

Living Will Directive

My wishes regarding life-prolonging treatment and artificially provided nutrition and hydration to be provided to me if I no longer have decisional capacity, have a terminal condition, or become permanently unconscious have been indicated by checking and initialing the appropriate lines below. By checking and initialing the appropriate lines, I specifically:

Designate _____ as my health care surrogate(s) to make health care decisions for me in accordance with this directive when I no longer have decisional capacity. If _____ refuses or is not able to act for me, I designate _____ as my health care surrogate(s).

Any prior designation is revoked.

If I do not designate a surrogate, the following are my directions to my attending physician. If I have designated a surrogate, my surrogate shall comply with my wishes as indicated below:

_____ Direct that treatment be withheld or withdrawn, and that I be permitted to die naturally with only the administration of medication or the performance of any medical treatment deemed necessary to alleviate pain.

_____ DO NOT authorize that life-prolonging treatment be withheld or withdrawn.

_____ Authorize the withholding or withdrawal of artificially provided food, water, or other artificially provided nourishment or fluids.

_____ DO NOT authorize the withholding or withdrawal of artificially provided food, water, or other artificially provided nourishment or fluids.

_____ Authorize my surrogate, designated above, to withhold or withdraw artificially provided nourishment or fluids, or other treatment if the surrogate determines that withholding or withdrawing is in my best interest; but I do not mandate that withholding or withdrawing.

In the absence of my ability to give directions regarding the use of life-prolonging treatment and artificially provided nutrition and hydration, it is my intention that this directive shall be honored by my attending physician, my family, and any surrogate designated pursuant to this directive as the final expression of my legal right to refuse medical or surgical treatment, and I accept the consequences of the refusal.

If I have been diagnosed as pregnant and that diagnosis is known to my attending physician, this directive shall have no force or effect during the course of my pregnancy.

I understand the full import of this directive and I am emotionally and mentally competent to make this directive.

Signed this _____ day of _____, 20____.

Signature and address of the grantor.

_____

In our joint presence, the grantor, who is of sound mind and eighteen (18) years of age, or older, voluntarily dated and signed this writing or directed it to be dated and signed for the grantor.

_____

Signature and address of witness.

_____Signature and address of witness.

OR

_____

_____ County

Before me, the undersigned authority, came the grantor who is of sound mind and eighteen (18) years of age, or older, and acknowledged that he voluntarily dated and signed this writing or directed it to be signed and dated as above.

Done this _____ day of _____, 20____.

_____

Signature of Notary Public or other.

_____

Date commission expires.

Execution of this document restricts withholding and withdrawing of some medical procedures. Consult State Revised Statutes or your attorney.

B.1 Community Assessment Model

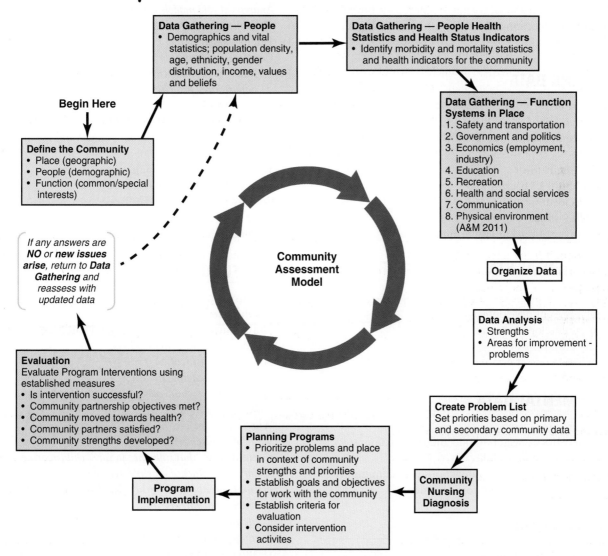

Using the figure above, the first step of the community assessment is to define the community. To do this, geographic boundaries, the population within the boundaries, the purpose of the assessment, and a data collection plan will be identified. Census blocks or tracts and geopolitical boundaries such as city or county lines will allow for collection of consistent data about the region under study. Included in "place" is the type of terrain or environment, the climate, the history of the area, and its size. The population is the next identifier. How does your assessment define those within the community? Are they members of a specific group or the population in general? What data are available for the assessment and where will you seek your sources? In essence, the identification of the community's members comprise the "client" within these boundaries.

What is the local history? Who were the original settlers and how has the community developed over time? Is it an area of growth or decline? Are original families still living in the area or has the early population been replaced? History can reveal a lot about customs and mores that could influence the health of the community.

From Stanhope M, Lancaster L: *Public health nursing: Population-centered health care in the community,* ed 9, St. Louis, 2016, Elsevier.

.2 Friedman Family Assessment Model (Short Form)

Before using the following guidelines in completing family assessments, two words of caution are in order. First, not all areas included below will be germane for each of the families visited. The guidelines are comprehensive and allow depth when probing is necessary. The student should not feel that every subarea needs to be covered when the broad area of inquiry poses no problems to the family or concern to the health worker. Second, by virtue of the interdependence of the family system, one will find unavoidable redundancy. For the sake of efficiency, the assessor should try not to repeat data, but to refer the reader back to sections where this information has already been described.

IDENTIFYING DATA

1. Family name
2. Address and phone
3. Family composition (see Family Composition Form on p. 613)
4. Type of family form
5. Cultural (ethnic) background
6. Religious identification
7. Social class status
8. Family's recreational or leisure-time activities

DEVELOPMENTAL STAGE AND HISTORY OF FAMILY

9. Family's present developmental stage
10. Extent of developmental tasks fulfillment
11. Nuclear family history
12. History of family of origin of both parents

ENVIRONMENTAL DATA

13. Characteristics of home
14. Characteristics of neighborhood and larger community
15. Family's geographic mobility
16. Family's associations and transactions with community
17. Family's social support network (ecomap)

FAMILY STRUCTURE

18. Communication patterns
    Extent of functional and dysfunctional communication (types of recurring patterns)
    Extent of emotional (affective) messages and how expressed
    Characteristics of communication within family subsystems
    Extent of congruent and incongruent messages
    Types of dysfunctional communication processes seen in family
    Areas of open and closed communication
    Familial and external variables affecting communication

19. Power structure
    Power outcomes
    Decision-making process
    Power bases
    Variables affecting family power
    Overall family system and subsystem power

20. Role structure
    Formal role structure
    Informal role structure
    Analysis of role models (optional)
    Variables affecting role structure

21. Family values
    Compare the family to American or family's reference group values and/or identify important family values and their importance (priority) in family
    Congruence between the family's values and the family's reference group or wider community
    Congruence between the family's values and family member's values
    Variables influencing family values
    Values consciously or unconsciously held
    Presence of value conflicts in family
    Effect of the above values and value conflicts on health status of family

FAMILY FUNCTIONS

22. Affective function
    Family's need-response patterns
    Mutual nurturance, closeness, and identification
    Separateness and connectedness

23. Socialization function
    Family child-rearing practices
    Adaptability of child-rearing practices for family form and family's situation
    Who is (are) socializing agent(s) for child(ren)?
    Value of children in family
    Cultural beliefs that influence family's child-rearing patterns
    Social class influence on child-rearing patterns
    Estimation about whether family is at risk for child-rearing problems and, if so, indication of high-risk factors
    Adequacy of home environment for children's needs to play

24. Health care function
    Family's health beliefs, values, and behavior
    Family's definitions of health-illness and their level of knowledge
    Family's perceived health status and illness susceptibility
    Family's dietary practices
    Adequacy of family diet (recommended 24-hour food history record)
    Function of mealtimes and attitudes toward food and mealtimes

Shopping (and its planning) practices
Person(s) responsible for planning, shopping, and preparation of meals
Sleep and rest habits
Physical activity and recreation practices (not covered earlier)
Family's drug habits
Family's role in self-care practices
Medically based preventive measures (physicals, eye and hearing tests, and immunizations)
Dental health practices
Family health history (both general and specific diseases—environmentally and genetically related)
Health care services received
Feelings and perceptions regarding health services

Emergency health services
Source of payments for health and other services
Logistics of receiving care

FAMILY STRESS AND COPING

25. Short- and long-term familial stressors and strengths
26. Extent of family's ability to respond, based on objective appraisal of stress-producing situations
27. Coping strategies utilized (present/past)
    Differences in family members' ways of coping
    Family's inner coping strategies
    Family's external coping strategies
28. Dysfunctional adaptive strategies utilized (present/past; extent of usage)

Family Composition Form

Name (Last, First)	Gender	Relationship	Date and Place of Birth	Occupation	Education
1. (Father)					
2. (Mother)					
3. (Oldest child)					
4.					
5.					
6.					
7.					
8.					

From Friedman MM, Bowden VR, Jones EG: *Family nursing: research, theory, and practice,* ed 5, 2003. Electronically reproduced by permission of Pearson Education, Inc., Upper Saddle River, New Jersey.

B.3 Comprehensive Occupational and Environmental Exposure History

Taking an Exposure History

Exposure History Form

Part 1. Exposure Survey   **Name:** _____ **Date:** _____

Please circle the appropriate answer.   **Birth date:** _____ **Sex (circle one):** Male   Female

1. Are you currently exposed to any of the following?

   metals   no   yes

   dust or fibers   no   yes

   chemicals   no   yes

   fumes   no   yes

   radiation   no   yes

   biologic agents   no   yes

   loud noise, vibration, extreme heat or cold   no   yes

2. Have you been exposed to any of the above in the past?   no   yes

3. Do any household members have contact with metals,
   dust, fibers, chemicals, fumes, radiation, or biologic agents?   no   yes

If you answered *yes* to any of the items above, describe your exposure in detail—how you were exposed, to what you were exposed. If you need more space, please use a separate sheet of paper.

4. Do you know the names of the metals, dusts, fibers, chemicals, fumes, or radiation that you are/were exposed to?   no   yes   → If *yes*, list them below.

5. Do you get the material on your skin or clothing?   no   yes

6. Are your work clothes laundered at home?   no   yes

7. Do you shower at work?   no   yes

8. Can you smell the chemical or material you are working with?   no   yes

9. Do you use protective equipment such as gloves, masks, respirator, or hearing protectors?   no   yes   → If *yes*, list the protective equipment used.

10. Have you been advised to use protective equipment?   no   yes

11. Have you been instructed in the use of protective equipment?   no   yes

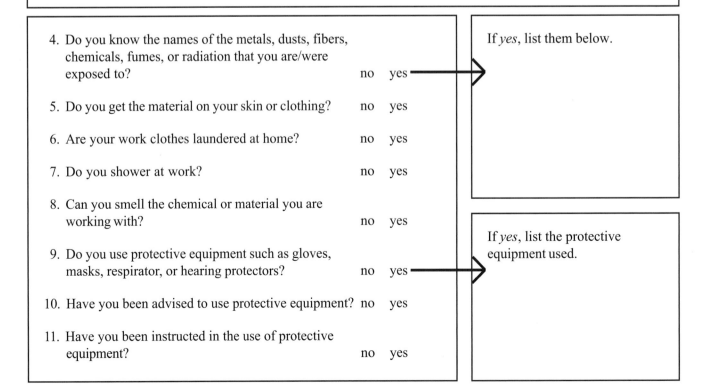

12. Do you wash your hands with solvents? no   yes

13. Do you smoke at the workplace? no   yes   At home? no   yes

14. Are you exposed to secondhand tobacco smoke at the workplace? no   yes   At home? no   yes

15. Do you eat at the workplace? no   yes

16. Do you know of any co-workers experiencing similar or unusual symptoms? no   yes

17. Are family members experiencing similar or unusual symptoms? no   yes

18. Has there been a change in the health or behavior of family pets? no   yes

19. Do your symptoms seem to be aggravated by a specific activity? no   yes

20. Do your symptoms get either worse or better at work? no   yes
                                             at home? no   yes
                                       on weekends? no   yes
                                       on vacation? no   yes

21. Has anything about your job changed in recent months (such as duties, procedures, overtime)? no   yes

22. Do you use any traditional or alternative medicines? no   yes

23. Have you or your child ever eaten non-food items such as paint, plaster, dirt and/or clay? no   yes

---

If you answered *yes* to any of the questions, please explain.

Part 2. Work History

A. Occupational Profile

Name: _____

Birth date: _____ **Sex:** Male   Female

The following questions refer to your current or most recent job:

Job title: _____   Describe this job: _____

Type of industry: _____   _____

Name of employer: _____   _____

Date job began: _____   _____

Are you still working in this job? yes   no   _____

If *no*, when did this job end? _____   _____

Fill in the table below listing all jobs you have worked, including short-term, seasonal, part-time employment, and military service. Begin with your most recent job. Use additional paper if necessary.

Dates of Employment	Job Title and Description of Work	Exposures*	Protective Equipment

*List the chemicals, dusts, fibers, fumes, radiation, biologic agents (i.e., molds or viruses) and physical agents (i.e., extreme heat, cold, vibration, or noise) that you were exposed to at this job.

Have you ever worked at a job or hobby in which you came in contact with any of the following by breathing, touching, or ingesting (swallowing)? If *yes*, please check the circle beside the name.

O Acids	O Chloroprene	O Methylene chloride	O Styrene
O Alcohols (industrial)	O Chromates	O Nickel	O Talc
O Alkalies	O Coal dust	O PBBs	O Toluene
O Ammonia	O Dichlorobenzene	O PCBs	O TDI or MDI
O Arsenic	O Ethylene dibromide	O Perchloroethylene	O Trichloroethylene
O Asbestos	O Ethylene dichloride	O Pesticides	O Trinitrotoluene
O Benzene	O Fiberglass	O Phenol	O Vinyl chloride
O Beryllium	O Halothane	O Phosgene	O Welding fumes
O Cadmium	O Isocyanates	O Radiation	O X-rays
O Carbon tetrachloride	O Ketones	O Rock dust	O Other (specify)
O Chlorinated naphthalenes	O Lead	O Silica powder	
O Chloroform	O Mercury	O Solvents	

B. Occupational Exposure Inventory   *Please circle the appropriate answer.*

1. Have you ever been off work for more than 1 day because of an illness related to work?   no   yes

2. Have you ever been advised to change jobs or work assignments because of any health problems or injuries?   no   yes

3. Has your work routine changed recently?   no   yes

4. Is there poor ventilation in your workplace?   no   yes

Part 3. Environmental History   *Please circle the appropriate answer.*

1. Do you live next to or near an industrial plant, commercial business, dump site, or nonresidential property?   no   yes

2. Which of the following do you have in your home?
   Please circle those that apply.
   Air conditioner   Air purifier   Central heating (gas or oil?)   Gas stove   Electric stove
   Fireplace   Wood stove   Humidifier

3. Have you recently acquired new furniture or carpet, refinished furniture, or remodeled your home?   no   yes

4. Have you weatherized your home recently?   no   yes

5. Are pesticides or herbicides (bug or weed killers; flea and tick sprays, collars, powders, or shampoos) used in your home or garden, or on pets?   no   yes

6. Do you (or any household member) have a hobby or craft?   no   yes

7. Do you work on your car?   no   yes

8. Have you ever changed your residence because of a health problem?   no   yes

9. Does your drinking water come from a private well, city water supply, or grocery store?

10. Approximately what year was your home built?_____

11. Does your food come from somewhere other than a grocery store?   no   yes

If you answered *yes* to any of the questions, please explain.

From the U.S. Department of Health and Human Services Agency for Toxic Substances and Disease Registry: *ATSDR Case Studies in Environmental Medicine Taking an Exposure History*, Course WB 2579, 2015. Retrieved July 2017 from https://www.atsdr.cdc.gov/csem/csem.asp?csem=33&po=9.

B.4 Omaha System Problem Classification Scheme with Case Study Application

DOMAINS AND PROBLEMS OF THE OMAHA SYSTEM PROBLEM CLASSIFICATION SCHEME

Environmental Domain

Material resources and physical surroundings both inside and outside the living area, neighborhood, and broader community:
- Income
- Sanitation
- Residence
- Neighborhood/workplace safety

Psychosocial Domain

Patterns of behavior, emotion, communication, relationships, and development:
- Communication with community resources
- Social contact
- Role change
- Interpersonal relationship
- Spirituality
- Grief
- Mental health
- Sexuality
- Caretaking/parenting
- Neglect
- Abuse
- Growth and development

Physiological Domain

Functions and processes that maintain life:
- Hearing
- Vision
- Speech and language
- Oral health
- Cognition
- Pain
- Consciousness
- Skin
- Neuro-musculo-skeletal function
- Respiration
- Circulation
- Digestion-hydration
- Bowel function
- Urinary function

- Reproductive function
- Pregnancy
- Postpartum
- Communicable/infectious condition

Health-Related Behaviors Domain

Patterns of activity that maintain or promote wellness, promote recovery, and decrease the risk of disease:
- Nutrition
- Sleep and rest patterns
- Physical activity
- Personal care
- Substance use
- Family planning
- Health care supervision
- Medication regimen

CATEGORIES OF THE OMAHA SYSTEM INTERVENTION SCHEME

Teaching, Guidance, and Counseling

Activities designed to provide information and materials, encourage action and responsibility for self-care and coping, and assist the individual, family, or community to make decisions and solve problems.

Treatments and Procedures

Technical activities such as wound care, specimen collection, resistive exercises, and medication prescriptions that are designed to prevent, decrease, or alleviate signs and symptoms for the individual, family, or community.

Case Management

Activities such as coordination, advocacy, and referral that facilitate service delivery; promote assertiveness; guide the individual, family, or community toward the use of appropriate community resources; and improve communication among health and human service providers.

Surveillance

Activities such as detection, measurement, critical analysis, and monitoring intended to identify the individual, family, or community's status in relation to a given condition or phenomenon.

TARGETS OF THE OMAHA SYSTEM INTERVENTION SCHEME

- anatomy/physiology
- anger management
- behavior modification
- bladder care
- bonding/attachment
- bowel care
- cardiac care
- caretaking/parenting skills
- cast care
- communication
- community outreach worker services
- continuity of care
- coping skills
- day care/respite
- dietary management
- discipline
- dressing change/wound care
- durable medical equipment
- education
- employment
- end-of-life care
- environment
- exercises
- family planning care
- feeding procedures
- finances
- gait training
- genetics
- growth/development care
- home
- homemaking/housekeeping
- infection precautions
- interaction
- interpreter/translator services
- laboratory findings
- legal system
- medical/dental care
- medication action/side effects
- medication administration
- medication coordination/ordering
- medication prescription
- medication set-up
- mobility/transfers
- nursing care
- nutritionist care
- occupational therapy care
- ostomy care
- other community resources
- paraprofessional/aide care
- personal hygiene
- physical therapy care
- positioning
- recreational therapy care
- relaxation/breathing techniques
- respiratory care
- respiratory therapy care
- rest/sleep
- safety
- screening procedures
- sickness/injury care
- signs/symptoms—mental/emotional
- signs/symptoms—physical
- skin care
- social work/counseling care
- specimen collection
- speech and language pathology care
- spiritual care
- stimulation/nurturance
- stress management
- substance use cessation
- supplies
- support group
- support system
- transportation
- wellness
- other

CASE STUDY MARTHA P.: OLDER WOMAN LIVING IN A DETERIORATING HOME

Joan B. Castleman, RN, MS, Clinical Associate Professor
College of Nursing, University of Florida
Gainesville, Florida

Information Obtained During the First Visit/Encounter

Martha P. was a 93-year-old woman who lived by herself in a deteriorating house. She had kyphosis and arthritis that contributed to her unsteady gait. Martha rarely used her cane in her house, but steadied herself by holding on to furniture.

When a student nurse arrived, Martha was shivering under a thin blanket. Boxes filled with old papers were stacked along the walls. The student nurse asked Martha if she had wood for the stove that heated the house. She replied that she ran out of wood yesterday. "I don't know what I'm going to do, but I'm not leaving this house." She reported that people from a church had brought the last load of wood. The student asked permission to contact Concerned Neighbors, a volunteer organization that could provide firewood. Martha was pleased. The student expressed concern that the boxes of paper, especially those near the stove, were a fire hazard. "Those boxes have been there for years, and I use them to light the stove." When the student asked if she could help Martha move the four boxes near the stove to the other wall, she grudgingly agreed.

The student nurse noted that Martha was wearing a "Lifeline necklace," a fall alert system, and asked about her history of falls. Martha described how she moved around her home and fell in the bathroom last week when she was trying to take a sponge bath. She pushed the button, and "two nice gentlemen from the fire department came to pick me up." The student and Martha walked around her house. They talked about where she fell in the past, how fortunate she was not to have injuries, and ways to decrease her risk of falling in the future. Martha was willing to have a personal care assistant visit weekly to help her with a bath and shampoo as long there was no charge. Before leaving, the student took Martha's vital signs and blood pressure and noted that they were within normal limits. The student called Concerned Neighbors and arranged for firewood to be delivered that day; the student also telephoned a local health assistance organization to schedule a home health aide to provide personal care for the next week. Although Martha sounded grumpy, she asked the student to return.

Omaha System Problem Rating Scale for Outcomes

Concept	1	2	3	4	5
Knowledge: Ability of the client to remember and interpret information	No knowledge	Minimal knowledge	Basic knowledge	Adequate knowledge	Superior knowledge
Behavior: Observable responses, actions, or activities of the client fitting the occasion or purpose	Not appropriate behavior	Rarely appropriate behavior	Inconsistently appropriate behavior	Usually appropriate behavior	Consistently appropriate behavior
Status: Condition of the client in relation to the objective and subjective defining characteristics	Extreme signs/symptoms	Severe signs/symptoms	Moderate signs/symptoms	Minimal signs/symptoms	No signs/symptoms

APPLICATION OF THE OMAHA SYSTEM

Domain: Environmental

Problem: Residence (High Priority)
Problem Classification Scheme
Modifiers: Individual and actual
Signs/symptoms of actual:
Inadequate heating/cooling
Cluttered living space
Unsafe storage of dangerous objects/substances
Intervention Scheme
Category: Teaching, guidance, and counseling
Targets and client-specific information:
Safety (moved boxes away from stove; Martha unwilling to dispose of papers)
Category: Case management
Targets and client-specific information:
Other community resource (referred to Concerned Neighbors; arranged delivery of firewood)
Category: Surveillance
Targets and client-specific information:
Housing (needed wood)
Problem Rating Scale for Outcomes
Knowledge: 2—minimal knowledge (not aware/unwilling to recognize fire hazards)
Behavior: 2—rarely appropriate behavior (unable/unwilling to make changes)
Status: 2—severe signs/symptoms (residence was livable but needed changes)

Domain: Physiological

Problem: Neuromusculoskeletal Function (High Priority)
Problem Classification Scheme
Modifiers: Individual and actual
Signs/symptoms of actual:
Limited range of motion
Decreased balance
Gait/ambulation disturbance
Intervention Scheme
Category: Teaching, guidance, and counseling
Targets and client-specific information:
Mobility/transfers (ways to decrease risk of falling, absence of injuries, continue wearing " Lifeline necklace")
Category: Surveillance
Targets and client-specific information:

Mobility/transfers (how, when falls occurred)
Signs/symptoms—physical (falls/injuries; vital signs, blood pressure)
Problem Rating Scale for Outcomes
Knowledge: 2—minimal knowledge (knew few options to decrease falls)
Behavior: 2—rarely appropriate behavior (had not used cane in the house; did wear and use the "Lifeline necklace")
Status: 3—moderate signs/symptoms (activities restricted, fell last week)

Domain: Health-Related Behaviors

Problem: Personal Care (High Priority)
Problem Classification Scheme
Modifiers: Individual and actual
Signs/symptoms of actual:
Difficulty with bathing
Difficulty shampooing/combing hair
Intervention Scheme
Category: Teaching, guidance, and counseling
Targets and client-specific information:
Personal hygiene (needed help with bathing, shampoo)
Category: Case management
Targets and client-specific information:
Paraprofessional/aide care (referred to health assistance organization for home health aide)
Problem Rating Scale for Outcomes
Knowledge: 3—basic knowledge (knew she needed to bathe, but was not aware of assistance)
Behavior: 3—inconsistently appropriate behavior (tried to take a sponge bath)
Status: 3—moderate signs/symptoms (cannot bathe safely without help)

This case illustrates use of the Omaha System with a client in the home. Talk with your classmates and other colleagues about how this form of documenting care would help guide your practice as a home care nurse, ensuring the highest quality possible and client safety.

From Martin KS: *The Omaha System: a key to practice, documentation, and information management,* reprinted, ed 2, Omaha, Neb, 2005, Health Connections Press.

B.5 Cultural Assessment Guide

There must be an awareness of your own ethnocultural heritage, both as a person and as a nurse. In addition, an awareness and sensitivity must be developed to the health beliefs and practices of a client's heritage. This awareness and sensitivity can be developed through careful assessment of a client's heritage and cultural beliefs. The factors that must be explored during a multicultural nursing assessment are as follows:

CULTURAL IDENTITY, ANCESTRY, AND HERITAGE

- Place of birth of patient and his or her parents/ancestors
- Reason for immigration

Ethnohistory

- Length of time in the United States
- Age of immigration
- Degree of acculturation

Social Organization

- Living arrangements
- Family composition, definition, and degree of contact with family members
- Position in the family hierarchy and decision making
- Social support
- Family roles, expectations of each other, gender-appropriate roles
- Extent of family participation in the care desired

Socioeconomic Status

- Occupation before and after immigration
- Educational attainment
- Type of residence
- Medical insurance
- Primary care provider, other care providers and specialists used

BIOCULTURAL ECOLOGY AND HEALTH RISKS

- Purpose of visit/consultation/hospitalization
- Perceived cause of the problem
- Terms used to describe problem, feelings

- Preponderance of the problem within the family and community
- Folk treatment
- Effect of the problem on self and family
- Expectations of care to be provided
- Presence of health risks

LANGUAGE AND COMMUNICATION

- Languages spoken and written
- Preferred language when speaking and reading
- Need and preference for an interpreter (gender, age, etc.)
- Literacy level and English proficiency

RELIGION AND SPIRITUALITY

- Religion, spiritual leader, contact for religious/spiritual leader
- Religious/spiritual needs
- Religious rituals observed
- Dietary practices observed

CARING BELIEFS AND PRACTICES

- Measures to promote health
- Caring practices when sick
- Practices relevant to activities of daily living
- Folk and professional healers sought
- Healing modalities used for problem
- Expectations about care to be given
- Hygiene, dietary, and mobility concerns
- Age and gender considerations
- Beliefs and practices with regard to life transitions

EXPERIENCE WITH PROFESSIONAL HEALTH CARE

- Evaluations of previous experiences
- Attributes of valued caregivers

From Potter PA, Perry AG, Stockert P, Hall A: *Essentials for Nursing Practice*, ed 8, St. Louis, Missouri, 2015, Mosby.

Essential Elements of Public Health Nursing

C.1 Examples of Public Health Nursing Roles and Implementing Public Health Functions

This document is intended to clearly present the role of public health nurses in one state. Nurses are members of multidisciplinary public health teams in a changing health care environment. The following matrices present the role of public health nursing in one state. The following definitions were used to develop these matrices.

Essential Elements of public health and nursing are considered the three pillars or building blocks for the public health infrastructure. These are assessment, assurance, and policy development. There are 10 essential services to be provided to support the public health infrastructure:

1. **Monitor** health status to identify community health problems.
2. **Diagnose and investigate** health problems and health hazards in the community.
3. **Inform, educate, and empower** people about health issues.
4. **Mobilize** community partnerships to identify and solve health problems.
5. **Develop policies and plans** that support individual and community health efforts.
6. **Enforce** laws and regulations that protect health and ensure safety.
7. **Link** people to needed personal health services and assure the provision of health care when otherwise unavailable.
8. **Assure** a competent public health and personal healthcare workforce.
9. **Evaluate** effectiveness, accessibility, and quality of personal and population-based health services.
10. **Research** for new insights and innovative solutions to health problems.

Public Health Function is defined as a broad public health activity needed to ensure a strong, flexible, accountable public health infrastructure. It may require a multidisciplinary team to carry out.

Public Health Nurse Role is the activity the public health nurse is responsible for, either alone or as a member of a team, to accomplish the stated public health functions (essential elements). This can be the public health nurse at the local level or at the state level. The nurse participates in these functions depending upon the level of education of the nurse. The nurse also adheres to the scope and standards of public health nursing practice (ANA, 2013)—see discussion in C.2.

State Role is what public health nurses need from the state level to do their jobs (e.g., policy, aggregate data, training). This refers to any Central Office program or staff, not just nurses.

A process can be implemented that would involve all public health nurses in a state. Although the timeline to completion may be lengthened when nurses at local and state levels are participating, it will ensure that the final document represents a consensus developed through creative open dialog.

From American Public Health Association: Ten Essential Public Health Services, Washington, DC, 2017, Retrieved July 2017 from https://www.apha.org/about-apha/centers-and-programs/quality-improvement-initiatives/national-public-health-performance-standards-program/10-essential-public-health-services, and CDC, National Public Health Performance Standards Program, Atlanta, Ga, 2015, Retrieved July 2017 from https://www.cdc.gov/nphpsp/ .

This is how one state might have defined and described the application of the standards to PHN practice.

Standard 1: Conduct Community Assessment: Systematically collect, and make available health-related data for the purpose of identifying and responding to community- and state-level public health concerns for conducting epidemiological and other population-based studies.

Public Health Function	PHN Roles	State Roles
Develop frameworks, methodologies, and tools for standardizing data collection and analysis and reporting across all jurisdictions and providers.	• Provide, review, and comment on proposed methodologies and tools for data collection. • Field test tools and methods.	• Collaborate with professional organizations and academic and governmental institutions to develop and test tools and methods. • Provide educational opportunities in areas of and use of tools. • Work with local level agencies to standardize definitions, data collected, etc., across jurisdictions and among all stakeholders (schools, community-based organizations, and private providers). • Provide aggregated data to the local level in a timely and accurate manner. • Provide census tract–level aggregated data to the local level.

Standard 2: Population Diagnosis and Priorities: The public health nurse analyzes the assessment data to determine the population diagnoses and priorities.

Public Health Function	PHN Roles	State Roles
Collect and analyze data.	• Collaborate with the community to identify population-based needs and gaps in service. • Analyze data and needs, knowledge, attitudes, and practices of specific populations. • Identify patterns of diseases; illness and injury and develop or stimulate development of programs to respond to identified trends.	• Provide national and state comparisons to be used with local data to obtain trends and assist localities in documenting need, progress, etc., to attain standard outcomes.

Standard 3: Outcomes Identification: The public health nurse identifies expected outcomes for a plan that is based on population diagnoses and priorities.

Public Health Function	PHN Roles	State Roles
Promote competency in public health issues throughout the health delivery system.	• Provide educational and technical assistance in areas such as case management and appropriate treatment and control of communicable diseases to the community.	• Develop appropriate regulatory, educational, and technical assistance programs. • Provide technical assistance and training to local health departments for local forecasting and interpretation of data.
Collect data.	• Participate in data collection with a target population. • Ensure that the data collection system supports the objectives of programs serving the community by participating in the design and operation of data collection systems. • Collect data via surveys, polls, interviews, and focus groups that will enable assessment of the community's perception of health status and understanding of how the system works and how to obtain needed service.	• Work with localities (health districts, private providers, other state and local agencies) to develop standard data elements and definitions across jurisdictions and among all stakeholders, especially for consistency in coding of population-based data. • Identify data collection and analytic issues related to monitoring the impact of health system changes such as costs and benefits of record linkage, strategies for ensuring confidentiality, and strategies for analyzing trends in health within a broader social and economic context. • Advocate for uniform data collection from all managed care plans so that outcomes and health trends can be analyzed and tracked and sentinel events reported.

Continued

Standard 3: Outcomes Identification:—cont'd

Public Health Function	PHN Roles	State Roles
Analyze data to ensure the accurate diagnosis of health status, identification of threats to health, and assessment of health service needs.	• Participate in a systematic approach to convert data into information that will identify gaps in service at the local and state level and will lead to action. • Monitor health status indicators to identify emerging problems and facilitate community-wide responses to identified problems. • Facilitate data analysis as part of a local collaborative effort.	• Develop a systematic, integrated statewide approach to converting data into information that directs action. • Ensure that resources to analyze data, such as hardware and software, are available at the local level. • Work with localities (health districts, private providers, other state and local agencies) to address issues related to variable access to technology, confidentiality issues. • Educate and train currently employed public health nurses in areas of epidemiology and population-based services.
Monitor health status indicators for the entire population and for specific population groups and/or geographic areas.	• Identify target populations that may be at risk for public health problems such as communicable diseases and unidentified and untreated chronic diseases. • Conduct surveys or observe targeted populations such as preschools, child care centers, and high-risk census tracks to identify health status. • Monitor health care utilization of vulnerable populations at the local and regional level.	• Develop methodology for identification, measurement, and analysis of key indicators of health care utilization of vulnerable populations.
Monitor and assess availability, cost-effectiveness, and outcomes of personal and population-based health services.	• Identify gaps in services (e.g., a neighborhood with deteriorating immunization rates may indicate a lack of available primary care services). • Ensure that all receive the same quality of care, including comprehensive preventive services. • Monitor the impact of health system reforms on vulnerable populations. • Evaluate the effectiveness and outcomes of care. • Plan interventions based on the health of the overall population, not just for those in the health care system. • Identify interventions that are effective and replicable.	• Develop analyses that demonstrate the cost effectiveness of investment in public health services. • Develop protocols and technical assistance for ensuring accountability of Medicaid-managed care plans and other government-funded plans for service delivery and overall health status of their covered populations. • Identify standard theoretical, methodological, and measurement issues that are specific to population subgroups for monitoring the impact of health system changes on vulnerable populations.
• Disseminate information.	• Disseminate information to the public on community health status, including how to access and use the services appropriately. • Disseminate information to other health care providers regarding gaps in services or deteriorating health status indicators.	• Ensure a mechanism for public accountability of performance and outcomes through public dissemination of information and, in particular, ensure that underservice, a risk inherent in capitated plans, is measurable through available data. • Ensure that information is provided to communities, local health departments, managed care plans, and other appropriate state agencies.

Standard 4: Planning: The public health nurse develops a plan that reflects best practices by identifying strategies, action plans, and alternatives to attain expected outcomes.

Public Health Function	PHN Roles	State Roles
Develop programs that prevent, contain, and control the transmission of diseases and danger of injuries (including violence).	• Provide community-wide preventive measures in the form of health education and mobilization of community resources. • Ensure isolation/containment measures when necessary. • Ensure adequate preventive immunizations. • Implement programs that control the transmission of diseases and danger of injuries during disasters.	• Work with local jurisdictions to develop tools such as videos, PSAs, and/or posters that local jurisdictions can use. • Work with local jurisdictions to develop disaster plans for the control of the transmission of diseases and danger of injuries during disasters. • Facilitate state-level partnerships that promote health, healthy lifestyles, and wellness (individual and family).

Standard 4: Planning:—cont'd

Public Health Function	PHN Roles	State Roles
Develop regulatory guidelines for the prevention of targeted diseases.	• Implement regulatory measures. • Implement OSHA Guidelines for Bloodborne Pathogens and the Prevention of the Transmission of TB in Health Care Settings. • Serve as a clearinghouse or source of information.	• In partnership with localities, develop regulatory guidelines.
Develop methods/tools for the collection and analysis of health-related data (occurrence of mortality and morbidity relating to both communicable and chronic diseases, injury registries, sentinel event establishment, environmental quality, etc.).	• Provide reporting guidelines and consultation regarding disease prevention, diagnosis, treatment, and follow-up of cases/contacts to physicians and institutions (emergency department, university and secondary school student health, prisons, industries, etc.). • Conduct/participate in community needs assessments to determine customer/provider knowledge deficits and perceptions of need. • Provide education to individuals, providers, targeted populations, etc., in response to knowledge deficits, disease outbreaks, toxic waste emissions, etc. • Provide individual follow-up/case management of communicable diseases that are transmitted by air, water, food, and fomites (TB, hepatitis A, salmonella, and staphylococcus, etc.).	• Develop standard methodology and tools for the collection and analysis of health-related data. • Provide training in the area of data collection and analysis. • Evaluate activities and outcomes of interactions. • Work in partnership with localities to develop programs based on data analysis needs.
Develop programs that promote a safe environment in the home.	• Provide childhood lead poisoning screenings and follow-up. • Teach clients to inspect homes for safety violations and toxic substances and to practice safe behaviors; assist families to access/use available resources/safety devices. • Assess/teach regarding safe food selection, preparation, and storage. • Train/supervise volunteers/auxiliary personnel in the performance of the above tasks. • Teach families that all men, women, and children have a right to a safe environment free of physical and mental abuse.	• Provide consultation and technical assistance to state and local organizations regarding laws and regulations that protect health and ensure safety. • In partnership with localities, develop and evaluate educational programs.
Develop programs that promote a safe environment in the workplace.	• Provide consultation in the implementation of OSHA regulations relating to occupational exposure to diseases. • Provide educational programs related to healthy lifestyles (smoking cessation, back protection, etc.). • Ensure provision of screenings for individuals to determine baselines and the occurrence of infectious diseases and preventable deterioration of health and function: hearing, back soundness, lung capacity, RMS indicators, PPDs, etc. • Assist in policy/practice development to address the prevention of the above. • Provide immunizations.	• Monitor and assist localities to implement prevention activities. • Assist localities in developing and evaluating educational programs. • Monitor outcomes of screening activities and evaluate interventions.
Develop programs that promote a safe environment in the school setting.	• Provide consultations on the implementation of OSHA regulations relating to occupational exposure to diseases. • Provide educational programs related to healthy lifestyles (smoking cessation, etc.). • Ensure provision of screenings for students to determine baselines and the occurrence of infectious disease and preventable deterioration of health and function. • Assist in policy/practice development to address prevention of the above. • Provide immunizations.	• Develop guidelines that ensure accountability in meeting standards set forth. • Ensure that policy is developed to protect children in the school environment. • Monitor the immunization status of children and provide immunizations during outbreaks and evaluate activities.

Continued

Standard 4: Planning: —cont'd

Public Health Function	PHN Roles	State Roles
Develop programs that promote a safe environment in the community.	• Identify population clusters exhibiting an unhealthy environment; provide consultation/group education regarding preventive measures. • Participate in the development of local disaster plans to ensure provision of safe water, food, air, and facilities. • Respond in time of natural disasters such as floods, tornadoes, and hurricanes. • Participate in developing plans for shelter management during disasters, especially "Special Needs" shelters that may require nursing staff.	• In times of disaster, facilitate the availability of resources across jurisdictions. • Have a statewide plan. • Ensure that localities have developed plans to protect the public in time of national and/or other disasters. • Coordinate efforts statewide. • Assist localities in responding. • Evaluate efforts.
Develop and issue standards that guide regulations and program development, and mandate policy. Develop protocols to ensure accountability of all health care providers, public and private. Provide in-service to all providers of health care services.	• Survey worksites, schools, institutions, etc., for compliance to regulations that protect health and ensure safety. • Provide technical assistance, i.e., interpretation, implementation, and evaluation processes. • Share and implement knowledge gained in in-services.	• Develop a systematic evaluation tool for the collection of data to measure trends. • Assist localities in developing standards to mandate accountability. • Provide consultation/technical assistance to localities.

Standard 5 encompasses the elements of implementation, coordination, health education and health promotion, consultation, and regulatory activities. Each element is described and the table that follows integrates and applies these five elements.

Standard 5: Implementation: The public health nurse implements the identified plan by partnering with others.

Standard 5A: Coordination: The public health nurse coordinates programs, services, and other activities to implement the identified plan.

Standard 5B: Health Education and Health Promotion: The public health nurse employs multiple strategies to promote health, prevent disease, and ensure a safe environment for populations.

Standard 5C: Consultation: The public health nurse provides consultation to various community groups and officials to facilitate the implementation of programs and services.

Standard 5D: Regulatory Activities: The public health nurse identifies, interprets, and implements public health laws, regulations, and policies.

Public Health Function	PHN Roles	State Roles
Promote informed decision making of residents about things that influence their health on a daily basis.	• Exert influence through contact with individuals and community groups. • Accept and issue challenges concerning healthy lifestyles to all contacts. • Reinforce and reward positive informed decisions made for healthy lifestyles.	• Develop and monitor standards to determine changes in behavior.
Promote effective use of media to encourage both personal and community responsibility for informed decision making.	• Be a resource for the community. • Gather data and address findings as appropriate. • Work with community groups to promote accurate information for healthy lifestyles through the media. • Utilize current information and other agencies' resources to maximize information accessible to the public.	• Assist localities to provide current information to community organizations and other state organizations. • Serve as a resource for localities and work with media.
Develop a public awareness/marketing campaign to demonstrate the importance of public health to overall health improvement and its proper place in the health delivery system. Develop public information and education systems/programs through partnerships.	• Provide education to special groups, e.g., local politicians, school boards, PTAs, churches, civic groups, and news media, regarding the benefits of preventive health. • Provide educational sessions/programs to the public regarding the components of healthy lifestyles. • Access grants/other funding sources to promote healthy lifestyle decisions (e.g., cervical and breast cancer prevention; bike helmets, hypertension). • Provide/promote teaching for individuals and families at every opportunity (home, clinic, community settings).	• Develop training activities to assist localities in marketing. • Assist localities in developing and evaluating educational programs. • Assist localities in funding. • Hold regional/state training sessions. • Evaluate outcomes and plan ongoing educational systems/programs.

Standard 5:—cont'd

Public Health Function	PHN Roles	State Roles
Ensure accessibility to health services that will improve morbidity, decrease mortality, and improve health status outcomes.	• Provide family-centered case management services for high-risk and hard-to-reach populations that focus on linking families with needed services. • Improve access to care by forming partnerships with appropriate community individuals and entities. • Increase the influence of cultural diversity on system design and on access to care, as well as on individual services rendered. • Ensure that translation services are available for the non-English-speaking populations. • Participate in ongoing community assessment to identify areas of concern and needs for rules. • Provide outreach services that focus on preventing epidemics and the spread of disease, such as tuberculosis and sexually transmitted diseases.	• Provide funds in cooperation with the locality. • Ensure policy development that includes case management and is culturally sensitive. • Provide adequate ongoing continuing education for the staff (especially in areas common to all localities). • Participate in state-level contract development to ensure that contracts with health plans require and include incentives for health plans to offer and deliver preventive health services in the minimum benefits package. • Educate financing officials about the roles of public health both in performing core public health services and in ensuring access to personal health services.
Provide direct services for specific diseases that threaten the health of the community and develop programs that prevent, contain, and control the transmission of infectious diseases.	• Plan, develop, implement, and evaluate: Sexually transmitted disease services Communicable disease services HIV/AIDS services Tuberculosis control services • Develop and implement guidelines for the prevention of the above targeted diseases.	• Establish standards/criteria for personal health care. • Work with local health departments to assist in developing infrastructure and management techniques to facilitate record-keeping and appropriate financial monitoring and tracking systems, which enable local health departments to enter into contractual arrangements for preventive health and primary care services.
Provide health services, including preventive health services, to high-risk and vulnerable populations (e.g., the uninsured working poor), and in geographic areas in which primary health care services are not readily accessible or available in a privatized setting. Provide leadership to stimulate the development of networks or partnerships that will ensure the availability of comprehensive primary health care services to all, regardless of the ability to pay. Initiate collaboration with other community organizations to ensure the leadership role in resolving a public health issue.	• Provide coordination, follow-up, referral, and case management as indicated. • Integrate supportive services, such as counseling, social work, and nutrition, into primary care services. • Assess the existing community medical capacity for referral and follow-up. • Advocate for improved health. • Disseminate health information. • Build coalitions. • Make recommendations for policy implementation or revision. • Facilitate resources that manage environmental risk and maintain and improve community health. • Provide information for a community group working on impacting policy at the local, state, or federal level. • Use results of community health assessments to stimulate the community to develop a plan to respond to identified gaps in service.	• Continue to work at the state and local level to build primary and preventive health services capacity, particularly in traditionally underserved areas, to ensure availability to providers and primary care sites essential to primary care access. • Facilitate the establishment and enhancement of statewide high-quality, needed health services. • Administer quality improvement programs. • Use information-gathering techniques of assessment to assist policy/legislature activities to develop needed health services and functions that require statewide action or standards. • Recommend programs to carry out policies.

The above was adapted and excerpted from the work of Diane B. Downing and the Virginia Public Health Nurses, 2013 by Marcia Stanhope.

Standard 6: Evaluation: The public health nurse evaluates the health status of the population.

Public Health Function	PHN Roles	State Roles
Ensure ongoing prevention research relating to biomedical and behavioral aspects of health promotion and prevention of disease and injury. Implement pilot or demonstration projects.	• Develop outcome measures. • Identify research priorities for target communities and develop and conduct scientific and operations research for health promotion and disease/injury prevention. • Develop and implement linkages with academic centers, ensuring that clients and populations who participate in research projects benefit as a result of the research.	• Provide training in the area of measuring program effectiveness. • Support evaluations and research that demonstrate the benefits of public health, as well as the consequences of failure to support public health interventions.

C.2 American Nurses Association Standards of Practice and Professional Performance for Public Health Nursing

THE STANDARDS OF PRACTICE FOR PUBLIC HEALTH NURSING

Standard 1: Assessment: The public health nurse collects comprehensive data pertinent to the health status of populations.

Standard 2: Population Diagnosis and Priorities: The public health nurse analyzes the assessment data to determine the population diagnoses and priorities.

Standard 3: Outcomes Identification: The public health nurse identifies expected outcomes for a plan specific to the population or situation.

Standard 4: Planning: The public health nurse develops a plan that prescribes strategies and alternatives to attain expected outcomes.

Standard 5: Implementation: The public health nurse implements the identified plan.

Standard 5A: Coordination of Care: The public health nurse coordinates care delivery.

Standard 5B: Health Teaching and Health Promotion: The public health nurse employs multiple strategies to promote health and a safe environment.

Standard 5C: Consultation: The public health nurse provides consultation to influence the identified plan, enhance the abilities of others, and effect change.

Standard 5D: Prescriptive Authority: *Not applicable*

Standard 5E: Regulatory Activities: The public health nurse participates in applications of public health laws, regulations, and policies.

Standard 6: Evaluation: The public health nurse evaluates the progress toward attainment of outcomes.

STANDARDS OF PROFESSIONAL PERFORMANCE FOR PUBLIC HEALTH NURSING

Standard 7: Ethics: The public health nurse practices ethically.

Standard 8: Education: The public health nurse attains knowledge and competence that reflect current nursing practice.

Standard 9: Evidence-Based Practice and Research: The public health nurse integrates evidence and research findings into practice.

Standard 10: Quality of Practice: The public health nurse contributes to quality nursing practice.

Standard 11: Communication: The public health nurse communicates effectively in a variety of formats in all areas of practice.

Standard 12: Leadership: The public health nurse demonstrates leadership in the professional practice setting and the profession.

Standard 13: Collaboration: The public health nurse collaborates with the population, and others in the conduct of nursing practice.

Standard 14: Professional Practice Evaluation: The public health nurse evaluates her or his own nursing practice in relation to professional practice standards and guidelines, relevant statutes, rules, and regulations.

Standard 15: Resource Utilization: The public health nurse utilizes appropriate resources to plan and provide nursing and public health services that are safe, effective, and financially responsible.

Standard 16: Environmental Health: The public health nurse practices in an environmentally safe, fair, and just manner.

Standard 17: Advocacy: The public health nurse advocates for the protection of the health, safety, and rights of the population.

C.3 Quad Council Public Health Nursing Core Competencies and Skill Levels

The Quad Council of Public Health Nursing Organizations is an alliance of the four national nursing organizations that address public health nursing issues: the Association of Community Health Nurse Educators (ACHNE), the American Nurses Association's Congress on Nursing Practice and Economics (ANA), the American Public Health Association—Public Health Nursing Section (APHA), and the Association of State and Territorial Directors of Nursing (ASTDN). In 2000, prompted in part by work on educating the public health workforce being done under the leadership of the Centers for Disease Control and Prevention (CDC), the Quad Council began the development of a set of national public health nursing competencies. In 2011 the "Core Competencies for Public Health Nursing" was updated to reflect the changes seen in the revised "Core Competencies for Public Health Professionals."

The approach utilized by the Quad Council was to start with the Council on Linkages between Academia and Public Health Practice (COL) "Core Competencies for Public Health Professionals" and to determine their application to three levels of public health nursing practice: the basic or generalist level (Tier 1), the specialist or mid-level (Tier 2), and the executive and/or multi-systems level (Tier 3). These tiers were defined on a continuum, meaning that PHN practice within each tier assumes the mastery of the competencies of the previous tier. In developing the competencies. The Quad Council members concurred that the generalist level would reflect preparation at the baccalaureate level.

The core competencies are further described within eight skill domains. These domains are: (1) Analytic and Assessment Skills, (2) Policy Development/Program Planning Skills, (3) Communication Skills, (4) Cultural Competence Skills, (5) Community Dimensions of Practice, (6) Public Health Science Skills, (7) Financial Planning and Management Skills, and (8) Leadership and Systems Thinking Skills. The "Quad Council PHN Competencies" document is designed for use with other documents. It complements the "Definition of Public Health Nursing" adopted by the APHA's Public Health Nursing Section in 1996 and the *Scope and Standards of Public Health Nursing* (Quad Council, 2000, and the competencies were used in the development of the ANA Scope and Standards, revised, 2013). Differentiating PHN competencies at the generalist, specialist, and executive levels will help clarify the PHN specialty for both the discipline of nursing and the profession of public health. In addition, the ability to identify PHN competencies should facilitate collaboration among public health nurses and other public health professionals in education, practice, and research to improve the public's health.

The Quad Council determined that although the Council on Linkages competencies were developed with the understanding that public health practice is population focused and public health nursing is also population focused, one of the unique contributions of public health nurses is the ability to apply these principles at the individual and family level *within the context of population-focused practice.*

These competencies can be found on the ASTDN website: http://www.achne.org/files/Quad%20Council/QuadCouncil-CompetenciesforPublicHealthNurses.pdf.

C.4 Minnesota Department of Health Public Health Interventions Wheel

Public Health Interventions

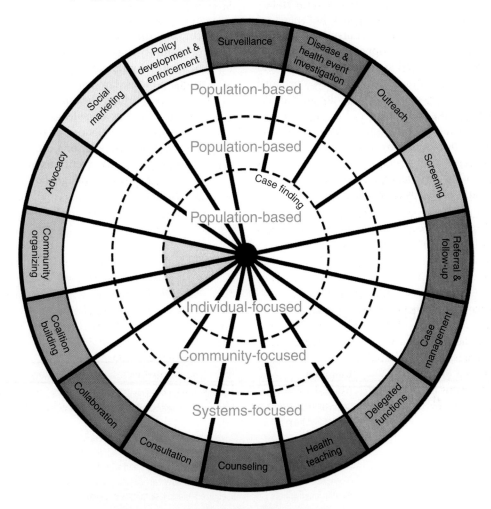

March 2001

**Minnesota Department of Health
Division of Community Health Services
Public Health Nursing Section**

Minnesota Department of Health Public Health Intervention Wheel. (From Section of Public Health Nursing, Minnesota Department of Health: *Public health interventions*, 2001. Retrieved July 2017 from http://www.health.state.mn.us/divs/opi/cd/phn/docs/0301wheel_manual.pdf)

DEFINITION OF POPULATION-BASED PRACTICE

Population-Based Practice

1. **Focuses on entire populations**

   A **population** is a collection of individuals who have one or more personal or environmental characteristics in common.[1]

A **population-of-interest** is a population essentially healthy but who could improve factors that promote or protect health.

A **population-at-risk** is a population with a common identified risk factor or risk exposure that poses a threat to health.

Population-based practice always begins with identifying everyone who is in the population-of-interest or the population-at-risk. It is not limited to only those who seek service or who are poor or otherwise vulnerable.

[1]Williams, CA, Highriter ME: Community health nursing: population focus and evaluation, Public Health Rev 7(3-4):197-221, 1978.

2. **Is grounded in an assessment of the population's health status**

   Population-based practice reflects the priorities of the community. Community priorities are determined through an assessment of the population's health status and a prioritization process.

3. **Considers the broad determinants of health**

   Population-based practice focuses on the entire range of factors that determine health rather than just personal health risks or disease. Health determinants include income and social status, social support networks, education, employment and working conditions, biology and genetic endowment, physical environment, personal health practices and coping skills, and health services.

4. **Emphasizes all levels of prevention**

   Prevention is anticipatory action taken to prevent the occurrence of an event or to minimize its effect after it has occurred.[2] Not every event is preventable, but every event does have a preventable component. Primary prevention promotes health or keeps problems from occurring; secondary prevention detects and treats problems early; tertiary prevention keeps existing problems from getting worse. Whenever possible, population-based practice emphasize primary prevention.

5. **Intervenes with communities, systems, individuals, and families**

   Population-based practice intervenes with communities, with the systems involving the health of communities, and/or with the individuals and families that comprise communities. Community-focused practice changes community norms, attitudes, awareness, practices, and behaviors. Systems-focused practice changes organizations, policies, laws, and power structures of the systems that affect health. Individual/family-focused practice changes knowledge, attitudes, beliefs, values, practices, and behaviors of individuals (identified as belonging to a population), alone or as part of a family, class, or group. Interventions at each level of practice contribute to the overall goal of improving population health status.

---

[2]Turnock, BJ: Public health: what it is and how it works, ed. 5, Burlington, MA, 2012, Jones & Bartlett Learning.

PUBLIC HEALTH INTERVENTIONS WITH DEFINITIONS

Public Health Intervention	Definition
Surveillance	Describes and monitors health events through ongoing and systematic collection, analysis, and interpretation of health data for the purpose of planning, implementing, and evaluating public health interventions. (Modified from *MMWR*, 1988.)
Disease and other health event investigation	Systematically gathers and analyzes data regarding threats to the health of populations, ascertains the source of the threat, identifies cases and others at risk, and determines control measures.
Outreach	Locates populations-of-interest or populations-at-risk and provides information about the nature of the concern, what can be done about it, and how services can be obtained.
Screening	Identifies individuals with unrecognized health risk factors or asymptomatic disease conditions in populations.
Case finding	Locates individuals and families with identified risk factors and connects them with resources.
Referral and follow-up	Assists individuals, families, groups, organizations, and/or communities to identify and access necessary resources in order to prevent or resolve problems or concerns.
Case management	Optimizes self-care capabilities of individuals and families and the capacity of systems and communities to coordinate and provide services.
Delegated functions	Directs care tasks that a registered professional nurse carries out under the authority of a health care practitioner as allowed by law. Delegated functions also include any direct care tasks that a registered professional nurse entrusts to other appropriate personnel to perform.
Health teaching	Communicates facts, ideas, and skills that change knowledge, attitudes, values, beliefs, behaviors, and practices of individuals, families, systems, and/or communities.
Counseling	Establishes an interpersonal relationship with a community, a system, family, or individual intended to increase or enhance their capacity for self-care and coping. Counseling engages the community, a system, family, or individual at an emotional level.
Consultation	Seeks information and generates optional solutions to perceived problems or issues through interactive problem solving with a community, system, family, or individual. The community, system, family, or individual selects and acts on the option best meeting the circumstances.

Public Health Intervention	Definition
Collaboration	Commits two or more persons or organizations to achieve a common goal through enhancing the capacity of one or more of the members to promote and protect health. (Modified from Henneman EA, Lee J, Cohen J: Collaboration: a concept analysis, *J Advan Nurs* 21:103-109, 1995.)
Coalition building	Promotes and develops alliances among organizations or constituencies for a common purpose. It builds linkages, solves problems, and/or enhances local leadership to address health concerns.
Community organizing	Helps community groups to identify common problems or goals, mobilize resources, and develop and implement strategies for reaching the goals they collectively have set. (Modified from Minkler M, editor: *Community organizing and community building for health*, New Brunswick, NJ, 1997, Rutgers University Press.)
Advocacy	Pleads someone's cause or acts on someone's behalf, with a focus on developing the community, system, individual, or family's capacity to plead their own cause or act on their own behalf.
Social marketing	Utilizes commercial marketing principles and technologies for programs designed to influence the knowledge, attitudes, values, beliefs, behaviors, and practices of the population-of-interest.
Policy development	Places health issues on decision makers' agendas, acquires a plan of resolution, and determines needed resources. Policy development results in laws, rules and regulations, ordinances, and policies.
Policy enforcement	Compels others to comply with the laws, rules, regulations, ordinances, and policies created in conjunction with policy development.

THREE LEVELS OF PUBLIC HEALTH PRACTICE

Public health interventions are population-based if they consider all levels of practice. This concept is represented by the three inner rings of the model. The inner rings of the model are labeled community-focused, systems-focused, and individual/family-focused.

A population-based approach considers intervening at all possible levels of practice. Interventions may be directed at the entire population within a community, the systems that affect the health of those populations, and/or the individuals and families within those populations known to be at risk.

Levels	Definition
Population-based **community-focused** practice	Changes community norms, community attitudes, community awareness, community practices, and community behaviors. They are directed toward entire populations within the community or occasionally toward target groups within those populations. Community-focused practice is measured in terms of what proportion of the population actually changes.
Population-based **systems-focused** practice	Changes organizations, policies, laws, and power structures. The focus is not directly on individuals and communities but on the systems that affect health. Changing systems is often a more effective and long-lasting way to affect population health than requiring change from every individual in a community.
Population-based **individual-focused** practice	Changes knowledge, attitudes, beliefs, practices, and behaviors of individuals. This practice level is directed at individuals, alone or as part of a family, class, or group. Individuals receive services because they are identified as belonging to a population-at-risk.

(From Section of Public Health Nursing, Minnesota Department of Health: Public Health Interventions, 2001, available at http://www.health.state.mn.us/divs/opi/cd/phn/docs/0301wheel_manual.pdf.)

Hepatitis Information

D.1 Summary Description of Hepatitis A-E

Type	Definition	Risk	Symptoms	Precautions	Prevention of Spread
A	Liver disease caused by picornavirus; commonly called "infectious hepatitis"	Live in house with infected person Have sexual contact with someone who has hepatitis A infection Are men who have sexual encounters with other men Use recreational drugs, whether injected or not Travel to or live in countries with a high prevalence of hepatitis A virus Have clotting-factor disorders, such as hemophilia Are household members or caregivers of a person infected with hepatitis A virus	Loss of appetite Nausea Vomiting Fever Fatigue Stomach pain Joint pain Gray-colored stools Dark urine Jaundice	Stricter handwashing by foodhandler Improved sanitary conditions Improved personal hygiene	Hepatitis A vaccine
B	A major cause of acute and chronic liver disease that can lead to cirrhosis and hepatocellular cancer; "serum hepatitis"	Exposure to human blood Live with a person who has hepatitis B Inject drugs or share needles, syringes, or other injection equipment Have a sex partner infected with hepatitis B virus Have multiple sex partners Are men who have sexual encounters with other men Is infant born to infected mother Are on hemodialysis	Jaundice Loss of appetite Nausea Vomiting Fatigue Gray-colored stools Dark urine Abdominal pain Joint pain	Vaccinate: • Babies at birth • Anyone having sex with an infected person • People with multiple sex partners • Anyone with a sexually transmitted disease • Men who have sexual encounters with other men • People who inject drugs • People who live with someone with hepatitis B infection • People with chronic liver disease, end-stage renal disease, or HIV infection • Health care and public safety workers exposed to blood • Travelers to certain countries	Hepatitis B vaccine
C	Virus causing chronic liver disease, found in blood, caused by non-A and non-B hepatitis virus May develop cirrhosis and liver failure	Drug injection Exposure to human blood Hemodialysis patients Receipt of blood transfusion Multiple sex partners Live with person with hepatitis C infection	Same as hepatitis B infection	Do not take blood, organs, tissue, or sperm from person with hepatitis C infection Do not share personal items that may have come into contact with an infected person's blood, such as toothbrushes, razors, nail clippers, or other items possibly contaminated with blood (including needles) Do not get tattoos or body piercings from an unlicensed facility or in an informal setting Cover open sores or other skin breaks	Practice safe sex Have only one sex partner Routine screening of blood/other donors No vaccine currently available

Type	Definition	Risk	Symptoms	Precautions	Prevention of Spread
D	An incomplete virus requiring hepatitis B virus to be present to cause infection. This results in a more severe acute liver disease, leading to chronic liver disease with cirrhosis	Injection drug users Hemophilia clients Developmentally disabled persons who are hospitalized	Same as hepatitis B	Avoid sexual contact with injection drug users Do not use needle used by others Proper sterilization technique in institutions	Individual screening for hepatitis B virus Blood screening for hepatitis B and hepatitis D viruses Early vaccination for hepatitis B virus No vaccine currently available for hepatitis D infection
E	Enterically transmitted non-A and non-B hepatitis virus. Usually acute and does not usually cause chronic disease	Ingestion of fecally contaminated water Pregnant women International travelers Persons in Asia, Middle Eastern, African, and Central American countries	Same as hepatitis B	Avoid contaminated waters	No vaccine available at this time

Data from Centers for Disease Control and Prevention (CDC) (2015): *Hepatitis A: general information*, Publication NO. 21-1072. Retrieved July 2017 from https://www.cdc.gov/hepatitis/hav/pdfs/hepageneralfactsheet.pdf; CDC (2016): *Hepatitis B: general information.* Retrieved July 2017 from https://www.cdc.gov/hepatitis/hbv/pdfs/hepbgeneralfactsheet.pdf; CDC (2015): *Hepatitis C: general information.* Retrieved July 2017 from https://www.cdc.gov/hepatitis/hcv/pdfs/hepcgeneralfactsheet.pdf; CDC (2015): *Viral Hepatitis: Hepatitis D.* Retrieved July 2017 from https://www.cdc.gov/hepatitis/hdv/index.htm; CDC (2009): *Viral Hepatitis: Hepatitis E.*Retrieved July 2017 from https://www.cdc.gov/hepatitis/hev/index.htm.

D.2 Recommendations for Prophylaxis of Hepatitis A

General information: Both vaccines for hepatitis A and hepatitis B are highly effective with nearly 100% of all adults who receive the vaccine. For prevention of hepatitis A two doses of vaccine given 5 months apart are recommended for complete protection. Persons who have been exposed to hepatitis A virus (HAP) recently and who have not been vaccinated should be given a single dose of single-antigen hepatitis A vaccine or immune globulin (IG) as soon as possible and within 2 weeks of the exposure. *Note:* The guidelines vary by age and health status, so consult the Centers for Disease Control and Prevention website under Hepatitis A for specific information. Read the following section for who requires protection with either IG or hepatitis A vaccine after exposure.

1. *Close personal contacts:* This includes close personal contacts of persons who have been confirmed by a blood test to have hepatitis A infection and persons in the household, including babysitters or caretakers, as well as those with whom the person has sexual contacts or shares illicit drugs.

2. *Daycare centers.* Daycare facilities with children in diapers can be important settings for hepatitis A virus (HAV) transmission. IG or hepatitis A vaccine should be administered to all staff and attendees of daycare centers or homes if (1) one or more hepatitis A cases are recognized among children or employees or (2) cases are recognized in two or more households of center attendees. When an outbreak (hepatitis cases in three or more families) occurs, IG or hepatitis A vaccine should also be considered for members of households whose diapered children attend. In centers not enrolling children in diapers, IG need be given only to classroom contacts of an index case.

3. *Schools.* Contact at elementary and secondary schools is usually not an important means of transmitting hepatitis A virus. Routine administration of IG or hepatitis A vaccine is not indicated for pupils and teachers in contact with a patient. However, when epidemiological study clearly shows the existence of a school- or classroom-centered outbreak, IG or hepatitis A vaccine may be given to those who have close personal contact with patients.

4. *Institutions for custodial care.* Living conditions in some institutions, such as prisons and facilities for the developmentally disabled, favor transmission of HAV. When outbreaks occur, giving IG or hepatitis A vaccine to residents and staff who have close contact with patients with hepatitis A infection may reduce the spread of the disease. Depending on the epidemiological circumstances, prophylaxis can be limited or can involve the entire institution.

5. *Hospitals.* Routine hepatitis A postexposure prophylaxis is not routinely indicated when a single case occurs. Rather, sound hygienic practices should be emphasized. Staff education should point out the risk for exposure to hepatitis A virus and emphasize precautions regarding direct contact with potentially infective materials. Outbreaks of hepatitis A infection among hospital staff occur occasionally, usually in association with an unsuspected index patient who is fecally incontinent. Large outbreaks have occurred among staff and family contacts of infected infants in neonatal intensive care units. In outbreaks, prophylaxis of persons exposed to feces of infected patients may be indicated.

6. *Offices and factories.* Routine hepatitis A postexposure prophylaxis is not indicated under the usual office or factory conditions for persons exposed to a fellow worker with hepatitis A infection. Experience shows that casual contact in the work setting does not result in virus transmission.

7. *Common-source exposure.* IG or hepatitis A vaccine might be effective in preventing foodborne or waterborne hepatitis A if exposure is recognized in time. However, postexposure prophylaxis is not recommended for persons exposed to a common source of hepatitis infection after cases have begun to occur in those exposed, because the 2-week period during which prophylaxis is effective will have been exceeded.

If a food handler is diagnosed as having hepatitis A infection, common-source transmission is possible but uncommon. Prophylaxis should be administered to other foodhandlers but is usually not recommended for patrons. However, IG or hepatitis A vaccine administration of patrons may be considered if (1) the infected person is directly involved in handling, without gloves, foods that will not be cooked before they are eaten; (2) the hygienic practices of the foodhandler are deficient; and (3) patrons can be identified and treated within 2 weeks of exposure. Situations in which repeated exposures may have occurred, such as in institutional cafeterias, may warrant stronger consideration of IG or hepatitis A vaccine use.

D.3 Recommended Postexposure Prophylaxis for Percutaneous or Permucosal Exposure to Hepatitis B Virus

Vaccination and Antibody Response Status of Exposed Person	HBsAg-Positive Source	HBsAg- Negative Source	Source not Tested or Status Unknown
Unvaccinated	HBIG × 1; initiate hepatitis B vaccine series	Initiate hepatitis B vaccine series	Initiate hepatitis B vaccine series
Previously vaccinated	No treatment	No treatment	No treatment
Known responder*	HBIG × 2 or HBIG × 1 and initiate revaccination	No treatment	If known high-risk source, treat as if source were HBsAg positive
Known nonresponder			
Antibody response unknown	Test exposed person for anti-HBs 1. If adequate,* no treatment 2. If inadequate,* HBIG × 1 and vaccine booster	No treatment	Test exposed person for anti-HBs 1. If adequate,* no treatment 2. If inadequate,* initiate revaccination

Centers for Disease Control and Prevention: Recommendations for Identification and Public Health Management of Persons with Chronic Hepatitis B Virus Infection
Source: MMWR, September 19, 2008; 57(RR—8):1-20
(Not an ACIP statement, but an important new recommendation from CDC).
*Responder is defined as a person with adequate levels of serum antibody to hepatitis B surface antigen (e.g., anti-HBs >10 mIU/ml); inadequate response to vaccination defined as serum anti-HBs <10 mIU/ml.
HBsAg, Hepatitis B surface antigen; *HBIG,* hepatitis B immune globulin; dose 0.06 ml/kg intramuscularly; *anti-HBs,* antibody to hepatitis B surface.

Glossary

abortion   Termination of a pregnancy by spontaneous or induced expulsion of a human fetus during the first 12 weeks of gestation.

accountability   Being legally, morally, ethically, and socially answerable to someone for something you have done.

accreditation   Credentialing process used to recognize health care agencies or educational programs for provision of quality services and programs.

acquired immunity   Resistance acquired by a host as a result of previous natural exposure to an infectious agent; it may be induced by passive or active immunization.

acquired immunodeficiency syndrome (AIDS)   AIDS is caused by the human immunodeficiency virus (HIV); it affects only humans, and HIV weakens the immune system by destroying important cells (CD4) that fight disease and infection.

active immunization   Administration of all or part of a microorganism to stimulate an active response by the host's immunological system, resulting in complete protection against a specific disease.

addiction treatment   Focuses on the addiction process by helping clients view addiction as a chronic disease and assisting them in making lifestyle changes to halt the progression of the disease.

adoption   Action of taking a child by choice into a relationship; to take voluntarily as one's own child.

advance directives   Written or oral statements by which a competent person makes known his or her treatment preferences or designates a surrogate decision maker.

advanced practice nurses   Nurses with advanced education beyond the baccalaureate degree who are prepared to manage and deliver health care services to individuals, families, groups, communities, and populations; includes clinical nurse specialists, nurse practitioners, nurse midwives, nurse anesthetists, and others.

advanced practice nursing (APN)   Nurses who hold graduate preparation in a nursing specialty area.

advocacy   Set of actions undertaken on behalf of another while supporting the other's right to self-determination; activities for the purpose of protecting the rights of others while supporting the client's responsibility for self-determination; involves informing, supporting, and affirming a client's self-determination in health care decisions.

advocate   One who works to protect the rights of the client while supporting the client's responsibility for self-determination. Nurses may function as advocates for vulnerable populations by working for the passage and implementation of policies that will result in improved public health services for these populations. An example would be a nurse who serves on a local coalition for uninsured people and works toward development of a plan for sharing the provision of free or low-cost health care by local health care organizations and providers.

affective domain   Domain of learning that includes changes in attitudes and the development of values.

affirming   Ratifying, asserting, or giving strength to the declarations of self or others.

Affordable Care Act   Law enacted March 23, 2010 that put in place comprehensive health insurance reforms.

Agency for Healthcare Research and Quality (AHRQ)   Division of the U.S. Department of Health and Human Services, formerly known as the Agency for Healthcare Policy and Research (AHCPR), whose mission is to support research designed to improve the outcomes and quality of health care, reduce its costs, address patient safety and medical errors, and broaden access to services.

agent   Causative factor, such as a biological or chemical agent, invading a susceptible host through an environment favorable to produce disease.

aggregate   Population or defined group.

alcohol   Oldest and most widely used psychoactive drug in the world; also known as ethyl alcohol or ethanol.

Alcoholics Anonymous (AA)   Lay, self-help group that practices a 12-step approach to recovery for persons with alcoholism.

alcoholism   Addiction to alcohol.

American Academy of Pediatrics (AAP)   Professional organization for pediatricians that sets policy statements for child health.

American Association of Colleges of Nursing (AACN)   National organization founded in 1969 whose members are baccalaureate and higher degree nursing education programs. The Association serves as the national voice for these programs.

American Nurses Association (ANA)   National association for registered nurses in the United States, founded in 1896 as the Nurses' Associated Alumnae of the United States and Canada.

American Public Health Association (APHA)   National organization founded in 1872 to facilitate interdisciplinary efforts and promote public health.

American Red Cross   National organization founded in 1881 through the efforts of Clara Barton that today seeks to reduce human suffering through health, safety, and disaster-relief programs in affiliation with the International Committee of the Red Cross.

Americans with Disabilities Act **(ADA)**   Act passed in 1990 that mandated that individuals with mental and physical disabilities be brought into the mainstream of American life.

analytic epidemiology   Form of epidemiology that investigates causes and associations between factors or events and health.

andragogy   Art and science of teaching adults and individuals with some knowledge about a health-related topic.

anorexia nervosa   Intense fear of becoming obese, with disturbance in body image, resulting in strict dieting and excessive weight loss.

anthrax   Acute disease caused by the spore-forming bacterium, *Bacillus anthracis*.

assault   Violent physical or verbal attack.

assertiveness   Ability to state one's own needs.

assessment   Systematic data collection about a population. This includes monitoring the population's health status and providing information about the health of the community.

assessor   Health professional who uses data in a systematic way to help identify needs, questions to be addressed, abilities, and available resources.

assurance   Public health role of making sure that essential community-oriented health services are available.

attack rate   Type of incidence rate defined as the proportion of persons who are exposed to an agent and who develop the disease, usually for a limited time in a specific population.

audit process   Six-step process used to recognize health care agencies or educational programs for provision of quality services and programs.

autonomy   Freedom of action as chosen by an individual.

behavioral risk   Personal health habits and behaviors (e.g., diet patterns) that contribute to individual and family health status.

benchmarking   Comparing national standards and guidelines with other agencies.

beneficence   Ethical principle that is complementary to nonmaleficence and requires that we "do good" and prevent or avoid doing harm. We are limited by time, place, and talents in the amount of good we can do. We have general obligations to perform those actions that maintain or enhance the dignity of other persons whenever those actions do not place an undue burden on health care providers. Health care professionals have special obligations of beneficence to clients.

bias In determining causality, a systematic error because of the way the study is designed, how it was carried out, or some unplanned events that occurred and affected the study.

bioethics Branch of ethics that applies the knowledge and processes of ethics to the examination of ethical problems in health care.

biological risk Potential health danger for a person who may be prone to certain illnesses because of inherited genetics or family lifestyle patterns.

biological terrorism Intentional release of viruses, bacteria, or other agents for the purpose of harming or killing.

biological variations Physical, biological, and physiological differences that exist and distinguish one racial group from another.

block grants Predetermined amount of money based on previous spending and availability of funds that is given to a state by the federal government for designated purposes such as state health care programs.

blood alcohol concentration (BAC) Also called blood alcohol level (BAL); the amount of alcohol in the blood, commonly expressed as grams of alcohol per 100 milliliters of blood. Most state legal limits of intoxication while driving are 0.08% or 0.1%.

board of nursing Group created in each state by legislation known as a state nurse practice act. The board is made up of nurses and consumers who operationalize, implement, and enforce the statutory law by writing explicit statements (called rules) regarding nursing and nursing practice.

Breckinridge, Mary Pioneering nurse who established the Frontier Nursing Service to deliver community health services to families in rural Kentucky.

brief interventions Interventions that are sometimes made by health care professionals who are not treatment experts and that have been found to be effective in helping alcohol, tobacco, and other drug abusers and persons with addictions reduce their consumption or follow through with treatment referrals. They can have six parts: feedback, responsibility, advice, menu of options, empathy, and self-efficacy.

bulimia Persistent concern with body shape and weight. Recurrent episodes of binge eating followed by extreme methods to prevent weight gain such as purging, fasting, or vigorous exercise.

C

capitation Payment system whereby one fee is charged the client to pay for all services received or needed.

care coordination Linking clients with services.

care management Program or process that established systems and monitors the health status of individuals, families, and groups. The program or process develops planning and intervention activities, as well as targeted evaluation outcomes for the client and program.

caregiver burden Physical, psychological, emotional, social, and financial problems that can be experienced by those who provide care for impaired others.

CareMaps Tool developed by Zander showing cause and effect and identifying expected client or family and staff behaviors against a timeline.

case fatality rate Proportion of persons diagnosed with a specific disorder who die within a specified time.

case management Interchangeable term with care management. A client service including the following activities: screening, assessment, care planning, arranging for, and coordinating service delivery, monitoring, reassessment, evaluation, and discharge. Case management is a process that enhances continuity and appropriateness of care. It is most often used with clients whose health problems are actually or potentially chronic and complex. Includes the activities implemented with individual clients in the system.

case manager Nurse who works to enhance continuity and provide appropriate care for clients whose health problems are actually or potentially chronic and complex. School nurse who performs general activities concerning health problems of the children. Builds on the basic functions of the traditional role and adapts new competencies for managing the transition from one part of the system to another or to home.

case registers Systematic registration of acute, chronic, and contagious diseases.

case-control study Epidemiologic study design in which subjects with a specified disease or condition (cases) and a comparable group without the condition (controls) are enrolled and assessed for the presence or history of an exposure or characteristic.

categorical programs and funding Federal, state, or local funds used to conduct a specific program such as tuberculosis screening, HIV/AIDS home care, or prenatal care. The money cannot be used for any other program or purpose.

causal inference Using epidemiological, clinical, statistical, and other scientific evidence to judge if a causal association exists between two or more factors or events. Guidelines for evaluation of evidence are often used in making causal inference. Different levels of evidence may be required for different settings, for example, clinical decisions versus policy determinations.

Centers for Disease Control and Prevention (CDC) Branch of the U.S. Public Health Service whose primary responsibility is to propose, coordinate, and evaluate changes in the surveillance of disease in the United States.

certification Mechanism, usually by means of a written examination, that provides an indication of professional competence in a specialized area of practice.

change agent Nursing role that facilitates change in client or agency behavior to more readily achieve goals. This role stresses gathering and analyzing facts and implementing programs.

change partner Nursing role that facilitates change in client or agency behavior to more readily achieve goals. This role includes the activities of serving as an enabler-catalyst, teaching problem-solving skills, and acting as an activist advocate.

charter Mechanism by which a state governmental agency grants corporate status to institutions with or without rights to award degrees.

chemical, biological, radiological, nuclear, and explosive (CBRNE) Describes the full spectrum of munitions used to create a human-made disaster.

chemical terrorism Intentional release of hazardous chemicals into the environment for the purpose of harming or killing.

child abuse Active forms of maltreatment of children.

child maltreatment Any act or series of acts of commission or omission by an adult that results in harm, potential for harm, or threat of harm to a child.

child neglect Physical or emotional neglect. Physical neglect refers to the failure to provide adequate food, clothing, shelter, hygiene, or necessary medical care; emotional neglect refers to the omission of basic nurturing, acceptance, and caring essential for healthy personal development.

chlamydia Sexually transmitted disease caused by the organism *Chlamydia trachomatis,* which can damage a woman's reproductive organs. Infections may be asymptomatic and if untreated result in severe morbidity.

chronic illness Illness in which a cure is not expected and nursing activities address function, wellness, and psychosocial issues.

client outcomes Changes in client health status as a result of care or program implementation.

code of ethics Moral standards that specify a profession's values, goals, and obligations.

codependency Condition characterized by preoccupation and extreme dependency (emotionally, socially, and sometimes physically) on a person. Eventually this dependence on another person becomes a pathological condition that affects the person in all of his or her relationships.

cognitive domain Domain of learning that includes memory, recognition, understanding, and application and is divided into a hierarchical classification of behaviors.

cohesion Attraction between individual members and between each member and the group.

cohort study Epidemiological study design in which subjects without an outcome of interest are classified according to past or present (or future) exposures or characteristics and followed over time to observe and compare the rates of some health outcome in the various exposure groups.

collaboration Mutual sharing and working together to achieve common goals in such a way that all persons or groups are recognized and growth is enhanced.

Collaborative Model for School Health a school health services delivery model developed by CDC which includes 8 categories of services, interprofessional and community partnerships.

common source outbreak Outbreak in which a group is exposed to a common noxious influence such as the release of noxious gases.

common vehicle Transportation of the infectious agent from an infected host to a susceptible host via water, food, milk, blood, serum, or plasma.

communicable diseases Diseases of human or animal origin caused by an infectious agent and resulting from transmission of that agent from an infected person, animal, or inanimate source to a susceptible host. Not all communicable diseases are communicated from host to host. For example, tetanus is transmitted from an inanimate source to a person but then cannot be passed from the infected person to another person.

communicable period Time or times when an infectious agent may be transferred from an infected source directly or indirectly to a new host.

communitarianism Maintains that abstract, universal principles are not an adequate basis for moral decision making. History, tradition, and concrete moral communities should be the basis of moral thinking and action.

community People and the relationships that emerge among them as they develop and use in common some agencies and institutions and a physical environment.

community assessment Process of critically thinking about the community and getting to know and understand the community as a client. Assessments help identify community needs, clarify problems, and identify strengths and resources.

community health Meeting collective needs by identifying problems and managing interactions within the community and larger society. The goal of community-oriented practice.

community health nursing A term often interchanged with public health nursing or nursing practice in the community, with the primary focus on the health care of a community and the effect of the community health status on individuals, families, and groups. The goal is to preserve, protect, promote, or maintain health.

community health problems Actual or potential difficulties within a target population with identifiable causes and consequences in the environment.

community health strengths Resources available to meet a community health need.

community index Summary of the health features of a community that enables us to determine health care delivery needs.

community outreach Role of a nurse who gives care outside one defined setting.

community participation Involvement of members of the community in decision making and planning for meeting their needs.

community partnership Collaborative decision-making process participated in by community members and professionals.

community-based Occurs outside an institution. Services are provided to individuals and families in a community.

community-based nursing Provision of acute care and care for chronic health problems to individuals and families in the community.

community-oriented nursing Nursing that has as its primary focus the health care of either the community or a population of individuals, families, and groups.

community-oriented practice Clinical approach in which the nurse and community join in partnership and work together for healthful change. Broader in scope than community-based practice. A form of care in which the nurse provides health care after doing a community diagnosis to determine what conditions need to be altered so that individuals, families, and groups in the community can stay healthy.

compliance Processes for ensuring that permitting requirements are met.

comprehensive services Health services focusing on more than one health problem or concern.

concurrent audit Method of evaluating the quality of ongoing care through appraisal of the nursing process.

confidentiality Information kept private, such as between the health care provider and client.

conflict Opposite of harmony; a state of interference that people want to guard against; antagonistic points of view.

conflict management Process of assisting clients in resolving issues between competing needs and resources.

confounding Bias that results from the relationship between both the outcome and study factor (exposure or characteristic) and some third factor not accounted for in analysis.

congregants People who gather as part of a faith community of the congregation of a church.

congregational model Parish nurse arrangement in an individual community of faith in which the nurse is accountable to the congregation and its governing body.

consequentialism Approach whereby the right action is the one that produces the greatest amount of good or the least amount of evil in a given situation.

constituency Group or body that patronizes, supports, or offers representation.

constitutional law Branch of law dealing with the organization and function of a government.

consultant Someone who provides professional advice, services, or information.

consumer confidence report (CCR) Report that began in 1996 when Congress amended the *Safe Drinking Water Act* to add a provision that required all community water systems to deliver a brief annual water quality report to their customers. The CCR includes information on the water source, the levels of any detected contaminants, and compliance with drinking water rules, plus some educational material. The

rationale for these reports is that consumers have a right to know what is in their drinking water. The reports help consumers make informed choices that affect their health.

consumer price index (CPI) Basic indicator of inflation—a measurement of inflation by comparison of prices overall and of categories of consumed goods and services purchased by urban wage earners and their families over a certain period.

continuous quality improvement (CQI) Approach to managing quality that emphasizes continual improvement in real time, empowering employees to manage quality themselves, including client and family perceptions of quality and making changes in organizational systems to enable workers to provide high-quality services.

contracting Making an agreement between two or more parties involving a shift in responsibility and control toward a shared effort by client and professional as opposed to an effort by the professional alone.

cooperation Working together or associating with others for a common benefit; a common effort.

coordinating Conscious activity of assembling and directing the work efforts of a group of health providers so that they can function harmoniously in the attainment of the objective of client care.

counselor Role of a nurse when mental health support is provided.

covered lives Persons enrolled in a health care plan who are eligible for services under that plan.

credentialing Mechanism to produce performance of acceptable quality by individuals or by programs of education and service.

crisis poverty Situation of hardship and struggle; it may be transient or episodic and can result from lack of employment, lack of education, domestic violence, or similar issues. These issues can lead to persistent poverty.

crisis teams School staff designated to deal with crises at school.

critical paths Planning technique that focuses on activities, best use of time and resources, and estimated time to complete activities. The technique can be used for planning programs or individual client care as it is related to a specific diagnosis.

cross-sectional study Epidemiological study in which health outcomes and exposures or characteristics of interest are simultaneously ascertained and examined for an association in a population or sample, providing a picture of existing levels of all factors.

cross-tolerance Condition in which tolerance to one drug results in a decreased response to another drug in the same general category.

cultural accommodation Negotiation with clients to include aspects of their folk practices with the traditional health care system to implement essential treatment plans.

cultural attitudes Beliefs and perspectives that a society values.

cultural awareness Appreciation of and sensitivity to a client's values, beliefs, practices, lifestyle, and problem-solving strategies.

cultural blindness When differences between cultures are ignored and persons act as though these differences do not exist.

cultural brokering Advocating, mediating, negotiating, and intervening between the client's culture and the biomedical health care culture on behalf of clients.

cultural competence Interplay of factors that motivates persons to develop knowledge, skill, and ability to care for others.

cultural conflict Perceived threat that may arise from a misunderstanding of expectations between clients and nurses when neither is aware of their cultural differences.

cultural desire Nurse's intrinsic motivation to provide culturally competent care.

cultural encounter Interaction with a client related to all aspects of his or her life.

cultural imposition Process of imposing one's values on others.

cultural knowledge Information necessary to provide nurses with an understanding of the organizational elements of cultures and to provide effective nursing care.

cultural nursing assessment Systematic way to identify the beliefs, values, meanings, and behaviors of people while considering their history, life experiences, and the social and physical environments in which they live.

cultural preservation Use by clients of those aspects of their culture that promote healthy behaviors.

cultural repatterning Working with clients to make changes in health practices when the clients' cultural behaviors are harmful or decrease their well-being.

cultural shock Feeling of helplessness, discomfort, and disorientation experienced by an individual attempting to understand or effectively adapt to another cultural group that differs in practices, values, and beliefs. It results from the anxiety caused by losing familiar sights, sounds, and behaviors.

cultural skill Effective integration of cultural knowledge and awareness to meet the needs of clients.

culture Learned ways of behaving that are communicated by one group to another to provide tested solutions to vital problems.

cumulative risks Additive effects of multiple risk factors.

customer Consumer of products or services.

D

data collection Process of acquiring existing information or developing new information.

data gathering Process of obtaining existing, readily available data.

data generation Development of data, frequently qualitative rather than numerical, by the data collector.

database Collection of gathered and generated data.

Declaration of Alma-Ata Resolution supporting primary health care for all people by 2000.

deinstitutionalization Effort to move long-term psychiatric patients out of the hospital and back into their own community.

delayed stress reactions Occur after a disaster and can include exhaustion and an inability to adjust to postdisaster routines.

demand management Program that provides to consumers, at the point at which they are deciding how to enter the health care system, information and support to access care.

democratic leadership Type of leadership characterized by being cooperative in nature in which all members can be involved in decision making and planning.

denial Primary symptom of addiction. The person may lie about use, play down use, and blame; may also use anger or humor to avoid acknowledging the problem to self and to others.

deontology Ethical theory that bases moral obligation on duty and claims that actions are obligatory irrespective of the good or bad consequences that they produce. Because humans are rational, they have absolute value. Therefore, persons should always be treated as ends in themselves and never only as means.

depressants Drugs that reduce the activity of the central nervous system.

descriptive epidemiology Form of epidemiology that describes a disease according to dimensions of person, place, and time.

determinants Factors that influence the risk of or distribution of health outcomes.

determinants of health Range of personal, social, economic, and environmental factors that influence health status (*Healthy People 2020*).

detoxification Process of allowing time for the body to metabolize or excrete accumulations of a drug. It is often called *social detoxification* if the withdrawal symptoms are not life-threatening and do not require medication, or medical detoxification if the symptoms require medical management.

devolution Process of shifting, planning, delivering, and financing responsibility for programs from the federal to the state level.

diagnosis-related groups (DRGs) Patient classification scheme that defines 468 illness categories and the corresponding health care services that are reimbursable under Medicare.

direct caregiver Role of a nurse giving health care to the ill or injured.

directly observed therapy (DOT) System of providing medications for persons with tuberculosis infection in which the client is monitored to ensure that the medication is taken and to maximize adherence to the treatment.

disadvantaged People who lack adequate resources that other people may take for granted.

disaster Human-caused or natural event that causes destruction and devastation that cannot be alleviated without assistance.

disaster medical assistance teams (DMATs) Teams of specially-trained civilian physicians, nurses, and other health care personnel who are sent to a disaster.

disaster responders People who work as members of a team in a disaster to feed back information to relief workers to facilitate rapid rescue and recovery.

disease Indication of a physiological dysfunction or a pathological reaction to an infection.

disease management Proactive treatment approach, focused on a specific diagnosis, that seeks to manage a chronic health condition and minimize acute episodes in a population.

disease prevention Activities that have as their goal the protection of people from becoming ill because of actual or potential health threats.

disease surveillance Ongoing systematic collection, analysis, interpretation, and dissemination of specific health data for use in public health.

disenfranchisement Sense of social isolation; a feeling of isolation from mainstream society.

distribution Pattern of a health outcome in a population; the frequencies of the outcome according to various personal characteristics, geographic regions, and time.

distributive justice Requires that there be a fair distribution of the benefits and burdens in society based on the needs and contributions of its members. This principle requires that consistent with the dignity and worth of its members and within the limits imposed by its resources, a society must determine a minimal level of goods and services to be available to its members.

district nursing System in public health nursing in which a nurse was assigned to a geographic district in a town to provide a variety of health services for its residents.

district nursing association Founded in Liverpool, England, by philanthropist William Rathbone to provide nursing care for poor and suffering people similar to the care that his terminally ill wife had received.

do-not-resuscitate (DNR) orders Physician's orders to not medically intervene when death is about to occur.

drug addiction Pattern of abuse characterized by an overwhelming preoccupation with the use (compulsive use) of a drug and securing its supply and a high tendency for relapse if the drug is removed.

drug dependence Physiological change in the central nervous system as a result of chronic drug use.

durable power of attorney Legal way for a client to designate someone else to make health care decisions when he or she is unable to do so.

dysfunctional families Family units that inhibit clear communication within family relationships and do not provide psychological support for individual members.

E

ecological model Multidimensional model of determinants of health and disease that spans many levels from individual genetic and physiologic characteristics to broader contextual influences (e.g., neighborhood characteristics and social context). This model encompasses a broader spectrum of systems and etiological factors than the web of causality model and includes a life span perspective.

economic risk Possible danger to a family's health determined by the relationship between family financial resources and the demands on those resources.

economics Social science concerned with the problems of using or administering scarce resources in the most efficient way to attain maximum fulfillment of society's unlimited wants.

education Establishment and arrangement of events to facilitate learning.

educator Nurse who provides information to clients or staff for the purpose of facilitating learning.

effectiveness Measure of an organization's performance as compared with its philosophy, goals, and objectives.

efficiency Process of meeting goals in a way that minimizes costs and maximizes benefits.

elder abuse Form of family violence against older members. It may include neglect and failure to provide adequate food, clothing, shelter, and physical and safety needs; it can also include roughness in care and actual violent behavior toward the elderly.

electronic medical record (EMR) Client safety–oriented system in which patient information is digital, privacy protected, and interchangeable.

elimination Focuses on removing a disease from a large geographic area such as a country or region of the world.

emergency plan Procedures to effectively give care in a crisis situation.

emergency support functions (ESFs) Fifteen functions used in a federally declared disaster. Each function is headed by a primary agency.

emerging infectious diseases Diseases in which the incidence has increased in the past two decades or has the potential to increase in the near future.

emotional abuse Extreme debasement of a person's feelings so that he or she feels inept, uncared for, and worthless.

emotional neglect The omission of the basic nurturing, acceptance, and caring essential for healthy personal development.

empowerment Helping people acquire the skills and information necessary for informed decision making and ensuring that they have the authority to make decisions that affect them.

enabling Act of shielding or preventing the addict from experiencing the consequences of the addiction. Also applies to shielding individuals from the consequences of their actions more generally.

endemic Disease or an event that is found to be present (occurring) in a population in which there is a persistent (usual) presence with low to moderate disease or event cases; the constant presence of an infectious disease within a specific geographic area.

enforcement Occurs when formal actions are taken to control environmental damage. Examples include fines or penalties, suspension of specific operations, or closure of the facility.

environment All of the factors internal and external to the client that constitute the context in which the client lives and that influence and are influenced by the host and agent–host interactions; the sum of all external conditions affecting the life, development, and survival of an organism; for public health, refers to all factors that constitute the context in which persons or

animals live and that influence and are influenced by the host and agent–host interactions.

environmental control Ability of individuals to control nature and to influence factors in the environment that affect them.

environmental epidemiology Study of the effect on human health of physical, chemical, and biological factors in the external environment.

environmental justice Equal protection from environmental hazards for individuals, groups, or communities regardless of race, ethnicity, or economic status. This applies to the development, implementation, and enforcement of environmental laws, regulations, and policies and implies that no population of people should be forced to shoulder a disproportionate share of negative environmental effects of pollution or environmental hazard because of a lack of political or economic strength levels.

environmental risk social and economic issues that affect family health.

environmental standards Norms that impose limits on the amount of pollutants or emissions produced. The Environmental Protection Agency establishes minimum standards, but states are allowed to be stricter.

epidemic Rate of disease clearly in excess of the usual or expected frequency in that population; occurrence of a disease within an area that is clearly in excess of expected levels (endemic) for a given period; the occurrence of an infectious agent or disease within a specific geographic area in greater numbers than would normally be expected.

epidemiologic triangle Infectious agent, host, and environment.

epidemiology Science that explains the strength of association between exposures and health effects in human populations; the study of the distribution and factors that determine health-related states or events in a population and the use of this information to control health problems.

eradication Irreversible termination of all transmission of infection by extermination of the infectious agents worldwide.

established groups Existing group of persons linked by membership and group purpose.

ethic of care Belief in the morality of responsibility in relationships that emphasize connection and caring.

ethical decision making Making decisions within an orderly framework that considers context, ethical approaches, client values, and professional obligations.

ethical dilemmas Puzzling moral problems in which a person, group, or community can envision morally justified reasons for both taking and not taking a certain course of action.

ethical issues Moral challenges facing the nursing profession.

ethics Branch of philosophy that includes both a body of knowledge about the moral life and a process of reflection for determining what persons ought to do or be, regarding this life.

ethnicity Shared feeling of peoplehood among a group of individuals.

ethnocentrism Belief that one's own group or culture is superior to others.

evaluation Systematic and logical way to examine a program and make decisions about how to improve the program; provision of information through formal means such as criteria, measurement, and statistics, from asking rational judgments about outcomes of care.

evaluation of processes a type of evaluation which monitors the progress of a program by assessing the degree to which objectives are met or activities are being conducted. It occurs on an ongoing basis while a program exists.

evaluation of program effectiveness Examination of the level of client and provider satisfaction with a program.

event Occurrence of a phenomenon of health that can be discretely characterized; it can be environmental, occupational, or biological, naturally occurring, or person induced.

evidence-based medicine Being "aware of the evidence on which one's practice is based, the soundness of the evidence, and the strength of inference the evidence permits" (Guyatt and Rennie, 2002, p xiv).

evidence-based nursing "An integration of the best evidence available, nursing expertise, and the values and preferences of the individuals, families, and communities who are served" (Honor Society of Nursing, Sigma Theta Tau, *Position Statement*, 2005).

evidence-based practice Includes the best available evidence from a variety of sources, including research studies, evidence from nursing experience and expertise, and evidence from community leaders.

evidence-based public health Public health endeavor "for making decisions on the basis on the best available evidence, using data and information systems, applying program planning frameworks, engaging the community in decision making, conducting evaluation and disseminating what has been learned" (Brownson et al, 2009, p 175).

F

faith communities Distinct groups of people acknowledging specific faith traditions and gathering in churches, cathedrals, synagogues, or mosques.

family Two or more individuals who depend on one another for emotional, physical, and/or financial support. Members of a family are self-defined.

family caregiving Assisting the client to meet his or her basic needs and providing direct care such as personal hygiene, meal preparation, medication administration, and treatments.

family crisis Situation in which the demands of the situation exceed the resources and coping capacity of the family.

family demographics Study of the structure of families and households and the family-related events, such as marriage and divorce, that alter the structure through the number, timing, and sequence of the events.

family functions Behaviors or activities performed to maintain the integrity of the family unit and to meet the family's needs, individual members' needs, and society's expectations.

family health   Condition including the promotion and maintenance of physical, mental, spiritual, and social health for the family unit and for individual family members; dynamic, changing, relative state of well-being that includes the biological, psychological, sociological, cultural, and spiritual factors of the family system.

family nursing   Specialty area that has a strong theory base and consists of nurses and families working together to ensure the success of the family and its members in adapting to responses to health and illness.

family nursing assessment   Comprehensive family data collection process used to identify the major problems facing the family.

family nursing diagnosis   Central issue of concern with the family; this directs the interventions.

family nursing theory   Theory whose function is to characterize, explain, or predict phenomena (events) evident within family nursing.

family structure   Characteristics of the individual members (i.e., gender, age, number) who constitute the family unit.

farm residency   Residency outside the area zoned as "city limits"; usually infers involvement in agriculture.

Federal Income Poverty Guidelines   Definition of poverty drafted by the Social Security Administration in 1964. The federal government defines poverty in terms of income, family size, the age of the head of household, and the number of children younger than 18 years. The guidelines change annually to be consistent with the consumer price index.

federal poverty guideline   Income level for a certain family size that the federal government uses to define poverty.

federal public health agencies   Federal-level government agencies that develop regulations to implement policies formulated by Congress and provide a significant amount of funding to state and territorial health agencies for public health activities.

fee-for-service   List of health care services with monetary or unit values attached that specifies the amounts third parties must pay for specific services.

feminist ethics   Knowledge and critique of classical ethical theories developed by men and women; entails knowledge about the social, cultural, political, economic, environmental, and professional contexts that insidiously and overtly oppress women as individuals, or within a family, group, community, or society.

feminists   Women and men who hold a worldview advocating economic, social, and political status for women that is equivalent to that of men.

fetal alcohol syndrome (FAS)   Condition that may occur when a woman has consumed alcohol regularly during pregnancy (about six drinks per day). Infants tend to be of low birthweight and intellectually disabled and may have behavioral, facial, limb, genital, cardiac, or neurological impairments.

five I's   Five conditions believed to adversely affect the aging experience: intellectual impairment, immobility, instability, incontinence, and iatrogenic drug reactions.

forensic nursing   Nursing care individuals and communities receive in response to injury in situations where health and law intersect.

formal group   Those with a defined membership and a specific purpose.

formative evaluation   Ongoing evaluation instituted for the purpose of assessing the degree to which objectives are met or activities are being conducted.

Frontier Nursing Service (FNS)   Provides community health services to rural families in eastern Kentucky. Beginning in 1925, Mary Breckinridge developed outpost centers throughout the mountain areas in Kentucky to provide midwifery and nursing, medical, and dental care. A hospital was opened in 1928 in Hyden, Kentucky.

functional families   Family units that provide autonomy and are responsive to the particular interests and needs of individual family members.

G

genital herpes   Caused by the herpes simplex virus 2 (HSV-2) and is considered a chronic disease that is transmitted through direct exposure and infects the genitalia and surrounding skin. Infection is characterized by painful lesions that present as vesicles and progress to ulcerations on the male and female genitals, buttocks, or upper thighs.

genital warts   Most common sexually transmitted disease in the United States; is characterized by papular-type growths that are caused by the genital human papillomavirus.

genomics   Study of the genes in the human genome and their interactions with other genes and the physical environment and their influence of cultural and psychosocial factors.

goals   End or terminal point toward which intervention efforts are directed.

gonorrhea   Sexually transmitted disease caused by a bacterium, *Neisseria gonorrhoeae*, that infects the mucous membranes of the genitourinary tract, rectum, and pharynx. It is transmitted through genital–genital contact, oral–genital contact, and anal–genital contact.

grading the strength of evidence   Determining the quality, quantity, and consistency of all evidence and research studies to make recommendations for practice.

gross domestic product (GDP)   Statistical measure used to compare health care spending among countries.

group   Collection of interacting individuals who have a common purpose or purposes.

group culture   Composite of the group norms that come to dictate perceptions and behaviors.

group purpose   Reason two or more people come together; it may be subtle or obvious and is easily stated by members.

group structure   Particular arrangement of group parts that constitute the whole.

gynecological age   Number of years from menarche.

H

hallucinogens   Also known as psychedelics; drugs that stimulate the nervous system and produce varied changes in perception and mood.

harm reduction   Also called harm minimization; a public health approach to substance abuse problems. This approach acknowledges, without judgment, that licit and illicit drug use is a reality, and the focus of interventions is to minimize these drugs' harmful effects rather than to simply ignore or condemn them; also to facilitate responsible use of substances.

Hazard Communication Standard   "Right-to-know" standard that requires all manufacturing firms to inventory toxic agents, label them, develop information sheets, and educate employees about these agents.

healing   Strengthening the inner spiritual connectedness and choosing healthy lifestyles.

health   State of complete physical, mental, and social well-being; not merely the absence of disease or infirmity (World Health Organization, 1986a, p 1).

Health Belief Model   Popular individual level health promotion model that has six components used to assess what motivates a person to do something.

health care–acquired infections (HAIs)   Infections acquired during hospitalization or developed within a health care setting; they may involve clients, health care workers, visitors, or anyone who has contact with a health care setting.

health care rationing   Method to reduce health care costs by controlling the use of health care services and technologies.

health disparities   "A particular type of health difference that is closely linked with social, economic and/or environmental disadvantage" (*Healthy People 2020*).

health economics   Branch of economics concerned with the problems of producing and distributing the health care resources of the nation in a way that provides maximum benefit to the most people.

health educator   Role of a nurse in providing instruction on health topics.

health literacy   Extent to which people have the ability to obtain, process, and understand basic health information and services to make informed decisions about their health.

health ministries   Activities and programs in faith communities directed at improving the health and well-being of individuals, families, and communities across the life span.

health policy   Public policy that affects health and health services. Delineates options from which individuals and organizations make their health-related choices. Made within a political context.

Health Professional Shortage Areas (HPSAs)   Geographic areas that have insufficient numbers of health professionals according to criteria established by the federal government. It often consists of rural areas in which a physician, nurse practitioner, or nurse in community health provides services to residents who live in several counties.

health program planning Five-step process of formulating a plan, conceptualizing, detailing, evaluating, and implementing.

health promotion Activities that have as their goal the development of human attitudes and behaviors that maintain or enhance well-being.

health risk appraisal Process of identifying and analyzing an individual's prognostic characteristics of health and comparing them with those of a standard age group, thereby making it possible to predict a person's likelihood of prematurely developing the health problems that have high morbidity and mortality in this country.

health risk reduction Application of selected interventions to control or reduce risk factors and minimize the incidence of associated disease and premature mortality. Risk reduction is reflected in greater congruity between appraised and achievable ages.

health risks Factors that determine or influence whether disease or other unhealthy results occur.

health status indicators Quantitative or qualitative measures used to describe the level of well-being or illness present in a defined population or to describe related attributes or risk factors.

hepatitis A virus (HAV) Liver disease caused by the hepatitis A virus (HAV) and primarily transmitted by the fecal–oral route, by either person-to-person contact or through consuming contaminated food or water. The clinical course of hepatitis A ranges from mild to severe and often requires prolonged convalescence. The onset is usually characterized by acute fever, nausea, lack of appetite, malaise, and abdominal discomfort, followed after several days by jaundice.

hepatitis B virus (HBV) Severe liver disease infection caused by hepatitis B virus (HBV) and transmitted through percutaneous (skin puncture) or mucosal contact with infectious blood or body fluids. Infection results in a clinical picture that ranges from a self-limited acute infection to a chronic infection that can develop into cirrhosis, liver failure, liver cancer, and death.

hepatitis C virus (HCV) Liver disease caused by the hepatitis C virus (HCV) that is transmitted through exposure to the blood of an infected person. Hepatitis C virus infection may present with such mild symptoms that it goes unrecognized, and in most affected persons it becomes a silent, chronic infection.

herd immunity Immunity of a group or community.

HIV antibody test Laboratory procedure that detects antibodies to human immunodeficiency virus (HIV). Enzyme-linked immunosorbent assay (ELISA) is the test commonly used in screening blood for the antibody to HIV; the Western blot is used as a confirmatory test.

holistic care Understanding the body, mind, and spirit relationship of persons in an environment that is always changing.

holistic health centers Comprehensive health teams that include family and clergy and encourage personal responsibility for health and preventive health practices.

holoendemic Highly prevalent problem found in a population commonly acquired early in life. The prevalence of this problem decreases as age increases.

home visits Provision of community health nursing care where the individual resides.

homeless persons Federal government defines a homeless person as one who lacks a fixed, regular, and adequate address or has a primary nighttime residence in a supervised publicly or privately operated shelter for temporary accommodations.

homicide Killing of one human being by another.

horizontal transmission Person-to-person spread of infection through one or more of the following routes: direct or indirect contact, common vehicle, airborne, or vector-borne.

hormone replacement therapy (HRT) Hormone combination of estrogen and progesterone used for postmenopausal women who have not had a hysterectomy.

hospice Palliative system of health care for terminally ill people; it takes place in the home with family involvement under the direction and supervision of health professionals, especially the visiting nurse. Hospice care takes place in the hospital when severe complications of terminal illness occur or when the family becomes exhausted or does not fulfill commitments.

host Human or animal that provides adequate living conditions for any given infectious agent; living human or animal organism in which an infectious agent can exist under natural conditions; the combined human potential of the people living in a community.

human capital Combined human potential of the people living in a community; measure of macroeconomic theory that involves improving human qualities, such as health, and is a focus for developing and spending money on goods and services because health is valued, it increases productivity, enhances the income-earning ability of people, and improves the economy.

human immunodeficiency virus (HIV) Virus that causes acquired immunodeficiency syndrome (AIDS) and HIV infection.

human papillomavirus (HPV) More than 100 types of HPV exist, and more than 40 can infect the genital area. Most HPV infections do not have symptoms and they go unrecognized; however, oncogenic or high-risk HPV caused by types 16 and 18 are the cause of cervical cancers. HPV also causes genital warts.

human-made disasters Destruction or devastation caused by humans.

hyperendemic Disease or event that is found to have a persistently (usually) high number of cases.

I

immigrants People who come into a new country to settle there.

immunization Process of protecting an individual from a disease through introduction of a live, killed, or partial component of the invading organism into the individual's system.

implementation Carrying out a plan that is based on careful assessment of need.

incest Sexual abuse among family members, typically a parent and a child.

incidence In epidemiology, the number of new cases of infection or disease that occur in a defined population in a specified period of time.

incidence proportion Proportion of the population at risk who experience the event over some period of time.

incidence rate Frequency or rate of new cases of an outcome in a population; it provides an estimate of the risk of disease in that population over the period of observation.

incubation period Time interval beginning with invasion by an infectious agent and continuing until the organism multiplies to sufficient numbers to produce a host reaction and clinical symptoms.

individualized education plans (IEPs) Plans to decide educational accommodations for disabled children.

individualized health plans (IHPs) Plans to decide the health needs of disabled children in school.

indoor air quality Measure of the breathable air inside a habitable structure or conveyance. A measure of the chemical, physical, or biological contaminants in indoor air.

infection State produced by the invasion of a host by an infectious agent. Such infection may or may not produce clinical signs.

infectiousness Measure of the potential ability of an infected host to transmit the infection to other hosts.

inflation Sustained upward trend in the prices of goods and services.

informal group Common form of group in which the members may have multiple ties to one another and the purposes are unwritten yet understood by the members.

informant interviews Directed conversation with selected members of a community about community members or groups and events; a direct method of assessment.

informing Communication process in which the nurse interprets facts and shares knowledge with clients.

inhalants Substances, often common household chemicals, that are inhaled by drug users. Inhalants fall into four categories: volatile organic solvents, aerosols, volatile nitrites, and gases; they are inhaled from bottles, aerosol cans, or soaked cloth.

in-home phase Actual visit of the nurse to the home; it gives the nurse the opportunity to assess the family's neighborhood and community resources, as well as the home and family interactions.

initiation phase First contact between the nurse and the family. It provides the foundation for an effective therapeutic relationship.

injection drug use Includes intravenous and subcutaneous drug injection; the latter is usually over the abdominal area. Injection drug use often includes both sharing and reusing of needles.

injection drug users (IDUs) Persons who inject drugs by intravenous or subcutaneous methods.

The sharing of paraphernalia to prepare or inject the drug can result in transmission of blood-borne pathogens, such as human immunodeficiency virus.

institutional model Parish nurse arrangement in a larger partnership under contract with hospitals, medical centers, long-term care facilities, or educational institutions.

instructive district nursing Early term for visiting nursing. Begun in Boston, it emphasized health education and care to families.

integrative review Form of a systematic review that does not have the summary statistics found in the meta-analysis because of the limitations of the studies that are reviewed and can be done by one individual.

intensity Use of technologies, supplies, and health care services by or for the client.

interdependent Involvement among different groups or organizations within the community that are mutually reliant on each other.

intermittent or continuous source Cases may be exposed periodically or uninterrupted over a period of days or weeks.

interprofessional collaboration Working agreement in which each home health care provider carefully analyzes his or her role in determining the best plan for the client's care.

intervention activities Means or strategies by which objectives are achieved and change is effected.

intimate partner violence (IPV) See spouse abuse.

J

judicial law Law based on court or jury decisions.

justice Ethical principle that claims that equals should be treated equally and those who are unequal should be treated differently according to their differences.

L

leadership Influencing others to achieve a goal.

learning Process of gaining knowledge and skills that lead to behavioral changes.

legislation Bills introduced by Congress for the purpose of establishing laws that direct policy.

legislative staff Individual or groups of individuals who perform duties such as research and writing, which helps the legislator move policy ideas through the legislative processes and into law.

levels of prevention Three-level model of interventions based on the stages of disease, designed to halt or reverse the process of pathological change as early as possible, thereby preventing damage.

liability Obligation an individual has incurred or might incur through any act or failure to act, or responsibility for conduct falling below a certain standard that is the cause of client injury.

licensure Legal sanction to practice a profession after attaining the minimum degree of competence to ensure protection of public health and safety.

life care plan Customized, medically based document that provides assessment of all present and future needs (i.e., medical, financial, psychological, vocational, spiritual, physical, and social), including services, equipment, supplies, and living arrangements for a client (Llewellyn and Leonard, 2009).

life-event risks Age-related risks to a person's health that often occur during transitions from one developmental stage to another.

linguistically appropriate health care Communicating health-related assessment and information in the recipient's primary language when possible and always in a language the recipient can understand.

living will Document that allows a client to express wishes regarding the use of medical treatments in the event of a terminal illness.

local public health agencies Agencies responsible for implementing and enforcing local, state, and federal public health codes and ordinances and providing essential public health programs to a community.

long-term care Care designed to help a person with basic activities of daily living that is given to individuals over a sustained period of time.

long-term evaluation Geared toward following and assessing the behavior of an individual, family, community, or population over time.

low birth weight Birthweight of less than 5½ pounds.

M

mainstream smoke Smoke inhaled and exhaled by the smoker after it is drawn through the cigarette.

maintenance functions Behaviors that provide physical and psychological support and therefore hold the group together.

maintenance norms Norms that create group pressures to ensure affirming actions for members and are helpful in maintaining comfort.

malpractice lawsuits Approach to quality assurance imposed on the health care system by the legal system.

managed care Health care financing mechanism designed to control costs by influencing the ways, type, and amount of care that clients receive. Method of organizing multiple health care services together along a continuum of care—for example, from physician's office, to hospital, to home health, to nursing home. The client pays for services through an insurance plan. Integrated system for providing health care services in which consumers must abide by certain rules designed to achieve cost savings.

MDMA (Ecstasy) Semisynthetic drug classified as a mood elevator that produces feelings of empathy, openness, and well-being.

means testing Method used to assess whether a client's income level qualifies him or her for Medicare and/or Medicaid.

mediator Role in which the nurse acts to assist parties to understand each other's concerns and to determine their conclusions concerning the issues. The mediator has no authority to decide on behalf of another.

Medicaid Jointly sponsored state and federal program that pays for medical services for the aged, poor, blind, disabled, and families with dependent children.

medical technology Set of techniques, drugs, equipment, and procedures used by health care professions in the delivery of medical care to individuals.

Medicare Federally funded health insurance program for the elderly and disabled and persons with end-stage renal disease.

menopause Permanent cessation of menstruation resulting from loss of ovarian follicular activity.

mental health Ability to engage in productive activities and positive relationships and to adapt to change and cope with adversity.

mental illness Refers to all diagnosable mental disorders; it can affect persons of all ages, races, cultures, socioeconomic levels, and educational levels and persons of both genders.

meta-analysis Specific method of statistical synthesis used in some systematic reviews, in which the "results from several studies are quantitatively combined and summarized" (Rychetnik et al, 2003, p 542).

methyl mercury Organic form of mercury. Methyl mercury may be formed when inorganic mercury enters lakes and combines with bacteria. It can then build up in the tissues of fish. Larger and older fish tend to have the highest levels of methyl mercury. Methyl mercury is highly toxic to humans and causes multiple adverse effects. It is a potent neurotoxicant.

Metropolitan Life Insurance Company Life insurance company that paid for or directly provided home nursing services for its beneficiaries and their families from 1909 to 1952.

migrant farmworker Person whose primary employment is in agriculture on a seasonal basis, who has been employed in that work within the past 2 years, and who has a temporary abode.

Migrant Health Act Legislation passed in the United States in 1962 that provides support for clinics serving agricultural workers. Grants were given to community-based and state organizations in the United States and its territories to enable them to provide culturally sensitive, comprehensive medical services to migrant and seasonal farmworkers and their families. In 2002, 670,000 people received services from the funds from the *Migrant Health Act*.

migrant health centers Federally funded primary care centers to serve migrant populations.

mitigation Actions or measures to prevent a disaster from occurring or to reduce the severity of its effects.

mixed outbreak Outbreak with a common source followed by secondary exposures related to person-to-person contact, as in the spreading of influenza.

monitoring Periodic or continuous surveillance or testing to determine the level of compliance with statutory requirements and/or pollutant levels in various media or in humans, plants, and animals.

moral distress Uncomfortable state of self when one is unable to act ethically.

morality Shared and generational societal norms about what constitutes right or wrong conduct.

N

narrative review Review done on published papers that support the reviewer's particular point of view or opinion and used to provide a general discussion of the topic reviewed.

National Assessment of Adult Literacy (NAAL) Largest literacy assessment study done in the United States.

National Association of School Nurses (NASN) Professional organization for school nurses that sets standards and guidelines for them.

National Health Security Strategy (NHSS) Connected public health and medical preparedness, response and recovery strategies.

National Health Service Corps (NHSC) Commissioned corps of health personnel who provide care in designated underserved areas.

National Institute for Occupational Safety and Health (NIOSH) Branch of the U.S. Public Health service that is responsible for investigating workplace illnesses, accidents, and hazards.

National Institute of Nursing Research (NINR) One of the National Institutes of Health charged with promoting the growth and quality of research in nursing.

National League for Nursing (NLN) National nursing organization that began in 1893 as the American Society of Superintendents of Training Schools of Nursing and later the National League for Nursing Education. The NLN initially established nurse training standards and promoted collegial relations among nurses.

National Notifiable Disease Surveillance System (NNDSS) Voluntary system monitored by the Centers for Disease Control and Prevention that includes 52 infectious diseases or conditions with case definitions that are considered important to the public's health.

National Organization for Public Health Nursing (NOPHN) Organized in 1912 to improve the education and standards of public health nursing and to help the public understand the importance of this type of nurse.

National Response Framework (NRF) Successor to the national response plan. NRF presents the guiding principles to enable all response partners to prepare for and provide a unified national response to diseases and emergencies.

natural disasters Destruction or devastation caused by natural events.

natural history of disease Course or progression of a disease process from onset to resolution.

natural immunity Species-determined innate resistance to an infectious agent.

needs assessment Systematic appraisal of type, depth, and scope of problems as perceived by clients, health providers, or both.

negative predictive value Proportion of persons with a negative test who are disease free.

neglect Failure to act as an ordinary, prudent person; conduct contrary to that of a reasonable person under a specific circumstance; the failure of a caregiver to provide services that are necessary for the physical and mental health of an individual.

negotiating Working with others in a formal way to achieve agreement on areas of conflict, using principles of communication, conflict resolution, and assertiveness.

neighborhood nurse Also known as block nurse; the nurse responds to a defined community or "locality."

neighborhood poverty Refers to spatially defined areas of high poverty, characterized by dilapidated housing and high levels of unemployment.

Nightingale, Florence English nurse who is credited with establishing nursing as a profession.

nonfarm residency Residence within an area zoned as "city limits."

nongonococcal urethritis (NGU) Inflammation of the urethra from microorganisms other than *Neisseria gonorrhoeae; Chlamydia trachomatis* has been implicated as the cause of 50% of cases. In men the symptoms of NGU are dysuria and urethral discharge.

nonmaleficence Principle, according to Hippocrates, that requires that we do no harm. It may be impossible to avoid harm entirely, but this principle requires that health care professionals act according to the standards of due care and try to cause the least amount of harm possible.

nonpoint source Diffuse pollution source (i.e., without a single point of origin or not introduced into a receiving stream from a specific outlet). The pollutants may be carried off the land by storm water. Examples of nonpoint sources are traffic, fertilizer or pesticide run-off, and animal wastes.

nonverbal communication Use of body language or gestures to convey information that cannot or may not be indicated verbally.

norms Standards that guide, regulate, and control.

nurse practice act State law that governs the practice of nursing.

O

obesity In children, when the body mass index is at or above the 95th percentile for children of the same age and sex when plotted on the Centers for Disease Control and Prevention growth charts.

objectives Precise behavioral statement of the achievement that will accomplish partial or total realization of a goal; includes the date by which the achievement is expected to be completed.

occupational health hazards Dangerous processes, conditions, or materials within a work environment that can result in harm to an employee.

occupational health history Questions added to a health assessment that provide data necessary to rule out or confirm job-induced symptoms or illnesses.

Occupational Safety and Health Administration (OSHA) Federal agency charged with improving worker health and safety by establishing standards and regulations and by educating workers.

Office of Homeland Security Office of the executive branch designed to protect citizens from terrorist threats or attacks, including bioterrorism.

official health agencies Agencies operated by state or local governments to provide a wide range of public health services, including community and public health nursing services.

outbreak Change (increase) in a disease and/or an event from expected levels to levels that are clearly in excess of expected levels.

outbreak detection Identifying a rise in the frequency of a disease above the usual occurrence of the disease.

outcome Change in client health status as a result of care or program implementation.

Outcomes and Assessment Information Set (OASIS) Instrument to collect client data for doing outcome assessments in home health.

outreach workers Health workers who make a special, focused effort to find people with specific health problems for the purpose of increasing their access to health services.

overweight In children, when the body mass index is at or above the 85th percentile and lower than the 95th percentile.

P

palliative care Alleviating symptoms of, meeting the special needs of, and providing comfort for the dying clients and their families by the nurse.

pandemic Worldwide outbreak of an epidemic disease; refers to the epidemic spread of the problem over several countries or continents (e.g., the SARS outbreak).

parish nurse coordinator Parish nurse who has completed a certificate program designed to develop the nurse as a coordinator of a parish nursing service.

parish nurses Nurses who respond to health and wellness needs within the faith context of populations of faith communities and are partners with the church in fulfilling the mission of the health ministry.

parish nursing Community-based and population-focused professional nursing practice with faith communities to promote whole person health to its parishioners, usually focused on primary prevention.

participant observation Conscious and systematic sharing in the life activities and occasionally in the interests and activities of a group of persons; observational methods of assessment; a direct method of data collection.

partner notification Identifying and locating contacts of persons who have been diagnosed with a transmissible disease to notify them of their exposure and to encourage them to seek medical treatment.

partnerships Relationships between individuals, groups, or organizations in which the parties are working together to achieve a joint goal; it is often used synonymously with coalitions and alliances, although partnerships usually have focused goals, such as jointly providing a specific program. Partnerships generally involve shared power.

passive immunization Immunization by a transfer of a specific antibody from an immunized person to one who is not immunized.

pastoral care staff Faith community leaders, including clergy, nurses, and educational and youth ministry staff.

paternity Fatherhood.

Patient Self-Determination Act Law that requires providers who receive Medicare and Medicaid payments to give their clients written information regarding their legal options for treatment choices if they become incapacitated.

patriarchal leadership Paternal style in which one person has the final authority to make decisions about the direction and movement of the group.

pedagogy Art and science of teaching children and individuals with little knowledge about a health-related topic.

pelvic inflammatory disease (PID) Infection of the female reproductive organs, specifically the fallopian tubes and endometrium, resulting in infertility or ectopic pregnancy. Acute symptoms and signs include lower abdominal pain, increased vaginal discharge, urinary frequency, vomiting, and fever. PID most often results from untreated sexually transmitted diseases and other infections of the female reproductive system.

permitting First step in the process of controlling pollution. A process by which the government places limits on the amount of pollution emitted into the air or water.

persistent bioaccumulative toxins (PBTs) Highly toxic, long-lasting substances that can build up in the food chain to levels that are harmful to human health and cause environmental harm. These contaminants can be transported long distances and move readily from land to air and water.

persistent organic pollutants (POPs) Toxic substances composed of organic (carbon-based) chemical compounds and mixtures. They include industrial chemicals such as polychlorinated biphenyl (PCB) and pesticides such as dichlorodiphenyltrichloroethane (DDT). They are primarily products and by-products from industrial processes, chemical manufacturing, and resulting wastes. These pollutants are persistent in the environment and have the ability to travel through the air and water to regions far from their original source. POPs are highly toxic; at very low concentrations they can injure wildlife and human health.

persistent poverty Refers to individuals and families who remain poor for long periods.

pesticide exposure Health risk to farmworkers who work in fields that have been treated with pesticides. Residue from pesticides also enters farmworkers' homes and their food. Risks include mild psychological and behavioral deficits and acute severe poisoning that can result in death.

physical abuse One or more episodes of physical aggression, often resulting in serious physical damage to the internal organs, bones, central nervous system, or sense organs.

physical neglect Failure to provide adequate food, proper clothing, shelter, hygiene, or necessary medical care.

PL 93-112 Section 504 of the *Rehabilitation Act* of 1973 Federal law requiring services for persons with handicaps.

PL 94-142 *Education for All Handicapped Children Act* Federal law requiring education for all children with handicaps.

PL 105-17 *Individuals with Disabilities Education Act* (IDEA) Federal law requiring that educational services must be provided for disabled children from birth through age 22 years.

planning process Systematic approach to selecting and carrying out a series of actions to achieve a goal.

point epidemic Concentration in space and time of a disease event, such that a graph of the frequency of cases over time shows a sharp point, usually suggestive of a common exposure.

point source Stationary location or fixed facility from which pollutants are discharged; any single identifiable source of pollution (e.g., a pipe, ditch, ship, ore pit, factory smokestack).

point-source outbreak A pattern of occurrence in which all persons exposed become ill at the same time, during one incubation period.

police power States' power to act to protect the health, safety, and welfare of their citizens.

policy Settled course of action to be followed by a government or institution to obtain a desired end.

policy development Providing leadership in developing policies that support the health of the population.

politics Art of influencing others to accept a specific course of action.

polity Policy, governances, expectations, and mission of a specific faith community.

polysubstance use or abuse Use of drugs from different categories together or at different times to regulate how the person feels.

population Collection of people who share one or more personal or environmental characteristics. The population can be a collection of individuals, families, or groups that share common health issues.

population-centered practice Nurse and community seek healthful change together through an ongoing series of health-promoting changes.

population-focused Emphasizes populations who live in a community.

population-focused practice Core of public health, a practice that emphasizes health protection, health promotion, and disease prevention of a population.

positive predictive value Proportion of persons with a positive screening or diagnostic test who do have the disease (the proportion of "true positives" among all who test positive).

post-visit phase After a home visit is concluded, the nurse documents the visit and the services provided.

poverty Refers to having insufficient financial resources to meet basic living expenses. These expenses include cost of food, shelter, clothing, transportation, and medical care.

Precaution Adoption Process Model (PAPM) Health promotion model that has seven stages a person goes through in making changes in behavior, ranging from being unaware of the issue to maintaining the new behavior.

prejudice Emotional manifestation of deeply held beliefs about other groups; it involves negative attitudes.

preparedness Advance preparation to cope with a disaster.

prevalence proportion Measure of existing disease in a population at a given time.

prevention Strengthening a person, family, or community's resources to ensure that a disruption does not occur.

pre-visit phase Contact between the nurse and the family before an actual home visit is made.

primary care Providing of integrated, accessible health care services by clinicians who are accountable for addressing a large majority of personal health care needs, developing a sustained partnership with patients, and practicing in the context of family and community.

primary caregivers Health care professionals who are primarily responsible for providing for the health care needs of clients.

primary health care (PHC) Combination of primary care and public health care made universally accessible to individuals and families in a community, with their full participation, and provided at a cost that the community and country can afford (World Health Organization, 1978).

primary health care services Both primary care and public health services that are designed to meet the basic needs of people in communities at an affordable cost.

primary prevention Type of intervention that seeks to promote health and prevent disease from the beginning; involves health promotion and education.

principlism Approach to problem solving in bioethics that uses the principles of respect for autonomy, beneficence, nonmaleficence, and justice as the basis for organization and analysis.

problem analysis Process of identifying problem correlates and interrelationships and substantiating them with relevant data.

problem prioritizing Evaluating problems and establishing priorities according to predetermined criteria.

problem solving Process of seeking to find solutions to situations that involve difficulty or uncertainty.

problem-purpose-expansion method Way to broaden limited thinking that involves restating the problem and expanding the problem statement so that different solutions can be generated.

process Ongoing activities and behavior of health care providers engaged in conducting client care.

process evaluation That aspect of the evaluation that examines the dynamic component of the educational program and is used throughout the implementation of the program.

Professional Review Organization (PRO) Organizations established by law to monitor the delivery of health care to clients of Medicare, Medicaid, and Maternal and Child Health programs and to monitor the implementation of prospective reimbursement.

program Health care service designed to meet identified health care needs of clients.

program evaluation Collection of methods, skills, and activities necessary to determine whether a service is needed, likely to be used, conducted as planned, and actually helps people.

promoter Advocacy role in which the nurse partners with the client and promotes the client's rights to make his or her own decision.

propagated outbreak Outbreak that does not have a common source and spreads gradually from person to person over more than one incubation period.

proportion Type of ratio in which the denominator includes the numerator.

proportionate mortality ratio Proportion of all deaths resulting from a specific cause.

prospective payment system (PPS) Diagnosis-related group payment mechanism for reimbursing hospitals for inpatient health care services through Medicare. Mechanism whereby Medicare will pay home health agencies a set amount of money to care for a client who meets the criteria of 1 of 80 home health resource groups (the diagnosis is based on severity, functional status, and number of services needed).

prostate cancer Second most common cancer among men in the United States; sometimes hard to diagnose because of a lack of symptoms.

psychoactive drugs Drugs that affect mood, perception, and thought.

public health Organized community efforts designed to prevent disease and promote health. It links disciplines, builds on the science of epidemiology, and focuses on the community; organized efforts designed to fulfill society's interest in ensuring conditions in which people can be healthy. It can be what members of society do collectively to ensure conditions that support health.

public health core functions These include assessment, policy development, and assurance.

public health economics Focuses on the producing, distributing, and consuming of goods and services as related to public health.

public health nurses deliver services within the framework of ever-constricting resources coupled with emerging and complex public health issues. This requires the efficient, equitable, and evidence-based use of resources.

public health nursing Specialty of nursing that is defined as, "The practice of promoting and protecting the health of populations using knowledge from nursing, social, and public health sciences" (APHA Public Health Nursing Section, 1996, p 1).

public health programs Programs designed with the goal of improving a population's health status.

Q

quality Continuously striving for excellence while adhering to set specifications or guidelines.

quality assurance Monitoring the activities of client care to determine the degree of excellence attained in the implementation of the activities.

R

race Biological designation whereby group members share distinguishing features (e.g., skin color, bone structure, genetic traits such as blood groupings).

racism Form of prejudice that refers to the belief that persons who are born into particular groups are inferior in intelligence, morals, beauty, and self-worth.

randomized controlled trial (RCT) Generally ranks as the highest level of evidence followed by other RCTs, nonrandomized clinical trials, prospective cohort studies, case-control studies, case reports, and expert opinion (Russell-Babin, 2009).

rape Sexual intercourse forced on an unwilling person, which may include threat of bodily injury or loss of life.

rapid needs assessment Form of assessment used in a disaster that immediately takes into account the scope of the problem and the needs of those affected, as well as determining what resources are needed to intervene.

rate Measure of the frequency of a health event in a defined population during a specified period.

Rathbone, William British philanthropist who founded the first district nursing association in Liverpool. With Florence Nightingale, he advocated for district nursing throughout England.

reality norms Group members' perceptions of reality, on which daily behavior is based; influence decision-making and action-taking processes.

recognition Process by which one agency accepts the credentialing status of and the credentials conferred by another agency.

recovery Last stage in a disaster; when agencies join to restore the economic and civic life of the community.

referral resource Agency or source in the community with whom nurses communicate and to which clients are sent for assistance.

regulations Specific statements of law that relate to and clarify individual pieces of legislation.

reimbursement system Process by which home health care agencies receive payment, either by the client or three major funding sources: Medicare, Medicaid, and third-party funding.

reliability Precision, stability, agreement, or replicability of a measuring instrument when repeatedly used; an indication of consistency from time to time or from person to person.

research utilization "The process of transforming research knowledge into practice" (Stetler, 2001, p 272) and "the use of research to guide clinical practice" (Estabrooks, Winther, and Derksen, 2004, p 293).

researcher Role of a nurse to investigate phenomena related to health.

resilience Ability to withstand many forms of stress and deal with several problems simultaneously without developing health problems.

resistance Ability of the host to withstand infection.

respect for autonomy Based on human dignity and respect for individuals and allows them to choose those actions and goals that fulfill their life plans unless those choices result in harm to another.

response Organized actions to deal with a disaster.

retrospective audit Method of evaluating the quality of care through appraisal of the nursing process after the client's discharge from the health care system.

retrospective reimbursement Method of payment to an agency based on units of service delivered.

return on investment Improved health outcomes as a result of the resources provided for a program or intervention. Resources include money, providers, time, equipment.

right to know Right of citizens to have direct access to information about issues of environmental concern, such as information on the quality of drinking water, the use of food additives, and chemical use in the workplace and community.

risk Probability of some event or outcome occurring within a specified period of time.

risk assessment Qualitative and quantitative evaluation of the risk posed to human health or the environment by the actual or potential presence or use of specific pollutants.

risk communication Exchange of information about health or environmental risks among, for example, risk assessors and managers, the general public, news media, and interest groups.

risk management Designed to reduce the liability on the part of an agency or individual by assisting employees to act in accordance with set guidelines and procedures.

risk sharing a process in which the third party payers and the provider share the risk of the costs of managing disease.

role model Person who is an example of professional or personal behavior for others.

role structure Arrangement of group member positions according to the expected functions of members.

root cause analysis Technique for identifying prevention of error strategies and developing a culture of safety.

rural Communities having fewer than 20,000 residents or fewer than 99 persons per square mile.

rural–urban continuum Residences ranging from living on a remote farm, to a village or small town, to a larger town or city, to a large metropolitan area with a "core inner city."

S

Safe Kids Campaign Federal program to provide education to children about safety.

safety net providers Those community providers that offer services to the uninsured and underinsured.

School Health Policies and Programs Study 2006 (SHPPS 2006) Federal study of school health programs funded by the Centers for Disease Control and Prevention.

school-based health centers (SBHCs) Federal program providing health care, dental care, and mental health care to children and families in schools.

school-linked program School health program run by a community health agency.

screening Application of a test to people who are as yet asymptomatic for the purpose of classifying them with respect to their likelihood of developing a particular disease.

secondary analysis Analysis using previously gathered data.

secondary health care services Services designed to detect and treat disease in the early acute stage.

secondary prevention Intervention that seeks to detect disease by screening and providing health care early in its progression (early pathogenesis) before clinical signs and symptoms become apparent in order to make an early diagnosis and begin treatment.

secondhand smoke A combination of sidestream smoke and mainstream smoke. It is also known as environmental tobacco smoke, or ETS. Smoke that comes off a cigarette from the outside rather than being drawn through the cigarette.

secular trends Long-term patterns of morbidity or mortality (i.e., over years or decades).

selected membership group Group in which members share a common concern or interest.

sensitivity Extent to which a test identifies those individuals who have the condition being examined.

sentinel Surveillance system that monitors key health events when information is not otherwise available or in vulnerable populations to calculate or estimate disease morbidity.

sentinel method Uses outcome measures to evaluate the quality of care; based on epidemiologic principles.

set Expectation, including unconscious expectation, as a variable determining a person's reaction to a drug.

setting Environment—physical, social, and cultural—as a variable determining a person's reaction to a drug.

setting for practice Community.

settlement houses Neighborhood centers providing social and health services.

severe acute respiratory syndrome (SARS) Previously unknown disease of undetermined etiology and no definitive treatment that was reported in early 2003 in places such as China and Hong Kong.

sexual abuse Coerced sexual acts ranging from fondling to rape or sexual degradation; it can happen to children or adults and be perpetrated by anyone inside or outside the family.

sexual assault nurse examiner Nurses trained in sexual assault examination who perform the physical examination in the emergency department to gather evidence (e.g., hair samples, skin fragments beneath the victim's fingernails, evidence from pelvic examinations using colposcopy) for criminal prosecution of sexual assault.

sexual debut First intercourse.

sexual victimization Suffering from a destructive or injurious sexual action.

sexually transmitted diseases (STDs) Communicable diseases such as gonorrhea, chlamydia, and HIV infection that can be transmitted by sexual activity. The Centers for Disease Control and Prevention uses the term *sexually transmitted diseases,* other sources may refer to this collection of diseases as *sexually transmitted infections.*

Shattuck Report First attempt to describe a model approach to the organization of public health.

short-term evaluation Focuses on identifying behavioral effects of health education programs and determining whether changes are caused by the educational program.

sidestream smoke A combination of sidestream smoke and mainstream smoke. It is also known as environmental tobacco smoke, or ETS. Smoke that comes off a cigarette from the outside rather than being drawn through the cigarette.

skilled care Care provided to a client that requires the knowledge and skill of a registered nurse.

smallpox Acute contagious febrile disease caused by a pox virus and characterized by skin eruption with pustules, sloughing, and scar formation.

social determinants of health Reflect social factors and the physical conditions in the environment in which people are born, live, learn, play, work, and age *(Healthy People 2020).*

social justice Based on the principles of equality in which the worth of every member is respected and valued.

social organization Way in which a cultural group structures itself around the family to carry out role functions.

social risks Risky social situations that can contribute to the stressors experienced by families. If adequate resources and coping processes are not available, breakdowns in health can occur.

***Social Security Act* of 1935** Enacted to protect the welfare and health of Americans, the Act included funds for education and employment of public health nurses.

space Physical distance between individuals during an interaction.

Special Supplemental Nutrition Program for Women, Infants and Children (WIC) Special supplemental food program administered by the Department of Agriculture through the state health departments; it provides nutritious foods that add to the diets of pregnant and nursing women, infants, and children younger than 5 years. Eligibility is based on income and nutritional risk as determined by a health professional.

specificity Extent to which a test identifies those individuals who do not have the disease or condition being examined.

sporadic Problems with an irregular pattern with occasional cases found at irregular intervals.

spouse abuse Physical, emotional, or sexual mistreatment of a partner or former partner.

Standard Precautions Procedures to prevent exposure to blood-borne diseases.

state public health agency Each of the U.S. states and territories has a single identified official state public health agency, managed by a state health commissioner.

stereotyping Basis for ascribing certain beliefs and behaviors about a group to an individual without giving adequate attention to individual differences.

***Stewart B. McKinney Homeless Assistance Act* of 1994** PL 100-77 passed in 1987 officially involved the federal government in meeting the needs of homeless persons. It was intended to respond to the range of emergency needs facing homeless Americans, such as food, shelter, and health care.

stimulants Drugs that increase the activity of the central nervous system, causing wakefulness.

strategic planning Process by which client needs, specific provider strengths, and agency and community resources are successfully matched to offer a service to the community.

structure Component in quality improvement that measures the setting and instruments used to provide care.

subpopulations Subsets of the population who share similar characteristics. For example, people older than 65 years who live in a residential home would be a subpopulation of a larger population of older persons in the community.

substance abuse Use of any substance that threatens a person's health or impairs his or her social or economic functioning.

suburbs Areas adjacent to a highly populated city.

sudden infant death syndrome Sudden death of an infant under 1 year of age, which remains unexplained after a thorough case investigation, including performance of a complete autopsy, examination of the death scene, and review of the clinical history.

suicide Act or an instance of taking one's own life voluntarily and intentionally.

summative evaluation Method used to assess program outcomes or as a follow-up of the results of program activities.

***Superfund Amendment and Reauthorization Act* (SARA)** law passed to assist in clean up of nation's uncontrolled hazardous waste.

supporting Upholding the client in making decisions about care or about entering the health care system.

surveillance Systematic and ongoing observation and collection of data concerning disease occurrence to describe phenomena and detect changes in frequency or distribution.

surveys Method of assessment in which data from a sample of persons are reported to the data collector.

syndronic surveillance systems Systems developed to monitor illness syndromes or events, such as increased numbers of medication purchases, trips to physicians or emergency departments, or orders for cultures or radiographs, as well as rising levels of school or work absenteeism, which may indicate that an epidemic is developing hours or days before disease clusters are recognized or specific diagnoses are made and reported to public health agencies.

syphilis Infectious sexually transmitted disease caused by a bacterium, *Treponema pallidum;* it is characterized by the appearance of a single or many sores called chancres that may involve any tissue. If untreated, the disease can progress from primary to secondary to late or latent stages. Relapses are frequent, and after the initial chancre and secondary symptoms, syphilis may exist without symptoms for years. Late stage syphilis can be serious and cause death.

systematic review Summary of the research evidence that relates to a specific question and to the effects of an intervention.

T

target of practice Population group for whom healthful change is sought.

task function Behaviors that focus or direct movement toward the main work of the group.

task norm Group's commitment to return to the central goals of the group when it has strayed from its purpose.

telehealth Organized health care delivery approach to do triage and provide advice, counseling, and referral for a client with a health problem using phones or computers with cameras. The client is usually in the home, and the nurse is at an office, health care facility, or phone bank location. Health information sent from one site to another by electronic communication.

Temporary Assistance to Needy Families (TANF) Formerly called Aid to Families with Dependent Children (AFDC), a federal and state program to provide financial assistance to needy children deprived of parental support because of death, disability, absence from the home, or in some states, unemployment. This program mandates that women heads-of-household find employment to retain their benefits.

termination phase When the purpose of a home visit has been accomplished, the nurse reviews with the family what has occurred and what has been accomplished. This provides a basis for planning further home visits.

tertiary health care services Services designed to limit the progression of disease or disability.

tertiary prevention Continued long-term health care. Intervention that begins once the disease is obvious; the aim is to interrupt the course of the disease, reduce the amount of disability that might occur, and begin rehabilitation.

testicular cancer Commonly identified solid malignant mass (tumor) found in the testicles of men.

third-party payers Reimbursement made to health care providers by an agency other than the client for the care of the client (e.g., insurance companies, governments, employers).

time Refers to past, present, and future times, as well as to the duration of, and period between, events. Some cultures assign greater or lesser value to events that occurred in the past, occur in the present, or will occur in the future.

timelines Landmarks of an episode of health or illness care from initial encounter to the transfer of accountability to the client or another health care agency.

tolerance In pharmacology, the need for increasing doses of a drug over time to maintain the same effect.

total quality management (TQM) Approach to managing the quality of care through appraisal of the nursing process after the client's discharge from the health care system.

toxicology Basic science that studies the health effects associated with chemical exposures.

tracer method Way to evaluate the quality of care that measures both process and outcome.

transitions Movement from one developmental or health stage or condition to another; may be a time of potential risk for families.

Transtheoretical Model (TTM) Health promotion model that looks at the stages of change a person goes through when changing behavior. The stages move from precontemplation to termination of the change process.

triage Process of separating casualties and allocating treatment based on the victim's potential for survival.

tuberculosis (TB) Infectious disease caused by a bacterium, *Mycobacterium tuberculosis*. It is transmitted by airborne droplets, resulting in pulmonary symptoms and wasting. Infection can be latent and asymptomatic, later progressing to active infection.

U

U.S. Department of Health and Human Services (USDHHS) Regulatory agency of the executive branch of government charged with overseeing the health and welfare needs of U.S. citizens. The federal agency most heavily involved in health and welfare.

unintentional injuries Any injuries sustained by accident such as falls, fires, drowning, suffocation, poisoning, sports or recreation, or motor vehicle accidents.

Universal Precautions Strategy to prevent exposure to pathogens transmitted through blood and other body fluids by requiring blood and body fluids from *all clients* to be handled as if they were infected with such pathogens.

urban Geographic areas described as nonrural and having a higher population density, more than 99 persons per square mile; cities with a population of at least 20,000, but fewer than 50,000.

use management Continual process of evaluating the appropriateness, necessity, and efficiency of health service over a period of time.

utilitarianism Ethical theory based on the weighing of morally significant outcomes or consequences regarding the overall maximizing of good and minimizing of harm for the greatest number of people.

utilization review Review that is directed toward ensuring that care is actually needed and cost is appropriate for the level of care provided.

V

vaccines Preparation of killed microorganisms, living attenuated organisms, or living fully virulent organisms that is administered to produce or artificially increase immunity to a particular disease.

validity Accuracy of a test or measurement; how closely it measures what it claims to measure. In a screening test, validity is assessed in terms of the probability of correctly classifying an individual with regard to the disease or outcome of interest, usually in terms of sensitivity and specificity.

value Ideas of life, customs, and ways of behaving that members of a society regard as desirable.

vectors Nonhuman organisms, often insects, that either mechanically or biologically play a role in the transmission of an infectious agent from source to host.

veracity Truth telling.

verbal communication Use of language in the form of words within a grammatical structure to express ideas and feelings and to describe objects.

vertical transmission Passing the infection from parent to offspring via sperm, placenta, milk, or contact in the vaginal canal at birth.

violence Nonaccidental acts, interpersonal or intrapersonal, that result in physical or psychological injury to one or more of the people involved.

virtue ethics Asks "What kind of person should I be?" and purports that people should be allowed to flourish as human beings.

virtues Acquired traits of character that dispose humans to act in accord with their natural good.

visiting nurse associations Agencies staffed by nurses who provide care for patients and families, most often in the home.

vulnerability Results from the interaction of internal and external factors that cause a person to be susceptible to poor health.

vulnerable populations Those with increased risk for developing poor health outcomes.

W

Wald, Lillian First public health nurse in the United States and an influential social reformer. She founded the Henry Street Settlement (later the Visiting Nurse Service of New York).

web of causality Complex interrelations of factors interacting with each other to influence the risk for or distribution of health outcomes.

wellness committee Health cabinet supporting healthy, spiritually fulfilling lives; it is made up of a nurse and members of the congregation.

wife abuse See spouse abuse.

windshield survey Community assessment, the motorized equivalent of a physical assessment for an individual; windshield refers to looking through the car windshield as the nurse in community health drives through the community collecting data.

withdrawal Physical and psychological symptoms that occur when a drug upon which a person is dependent is removed.

Workers' Compensation Compensation given to an employee for an injury that occurred while the employee was working.

work-health interactions Influence of work on health shown by statistics on illnesses, injuries, and deaths associated with employment.

worksite walk-through Assessment of the workplace conducted by the nurse.

World Health Organization (WHO) Arm of the United Nations that provides worldwide services to promote health.

wrap-around services Social and economic services provided, either directly or through referrals, in addition to available comprehensive health services. In this way, social and economic services that will help ensure the effectiveness of health services are "wrapped around" health services.

A

Abortion, 402
Abuse, 440–448
  child. *see* Child abuse.
  elders. *see* Elder abuse.
  emotional, 443, 447
  financial, in older adults, 447
  power and control aspect of, 441, 441b
  during pregnancy, 446
  as a process, 445–447
  psychological, in older adults, 447
  sexual, 400–401, 444–445
  substance. *see* Substance abuse.
  types of family, 441–447
Abusive parenting, 404
Access to health care, 38, 41b, 504
  among special groups
    adults of color, 350
    migrant farmworkers, 374
  for prisoners, 117
  in rural *versus* urban areas, 375–376
Accidents, 336–339, 337t
  motor vehicle, 336
  prevention of, 338–339, 338b
  sports-related, 336, 338f
Accommodating behaviors, 232b
Accreditation
  approaches to quality improvement, 280–281
  of home health and hospice, 534
Acquired immunity, 458
Acquired immunodeficiency syndrome (AIDS)
  caring for clients with, 481–482
  in children, 340, 482
  in homeless population, 397–398
  incidence as indicator of community health status, 207, 207b
  as last stage on the long continuum of HIV infection, 479
  in migrant farmworkers, 384
  rates in urban *versus* rural communities, 377
Action, in continuous quality improvement program, 287f, 288–289
Active immunization, 458
Active surveillance system, 260
ACTS (assess, collaborate, train and survey), 189
Addiction. *see also* Alcohol, tobacco, and other drug (ATOD) problems; Substance abuse.
  genetic factors in, 422–423
  recovery from, 428
Addiction treatment, 428–429
Adequacy, aspects of program evaluation, 273, 274b
Administration on Aging (AOA), 343
Adolescents
  homeless, 399
  injuries and accidents in, 337–338
  with mental illness, 406–407
  nutritional needs during pregnancy, 403, 403t
  poverty in women, 395
  trends in sexual behavior and pregnancy, 399–404
Adoption, options for teens, 402

Adult Children of Alcoholics (ACOA) groups, 429
Adult day health, 352
Adults
  with mental illness, 406–407
  with serious mental illness, 407–408, 408b
  suicides rates in, 407
Advance directives, types of, 343
Advanced practice nurses (APNs)
  reimbursement of, 120–121
  title protection of, 121
  trends in, 36
Advocacy/advocates
  in constituency, 229–230
  in cultural brokering, 78
  cultural competence and, 74
  definition of, 61
  for environmental health, 100–101
  ethics and, 61
  for health care reform, 61–62
  impact of, 231
  nursing, 121–122
  process of, 229–230
    affirming, 230
    informing, 230, 232b
    nursing, 229t
    supporting, 230
    systematic problem solving, 230–231, 231b
  in public health code of ethics, 60
  skills needed by case managers, 226f, 229–231
  for social justice, 365
  for vulnerable population, 365, 368
Affective domain of learning, 184
Affirming role in advocacy, 230
Affordable Care Act, 29, 503
  health care system and, 38, 45t
African Americans
  demographic trends of, 35
  of different cultures, 69
  health care needs and risks of rural, 381t
  history in public health nursing, 19, 23, 23f
  mental health needs of, 409
Agencies, influencing health, 110–114
Agency for Healthcare Research and Quality (AHRQ), 112–113, 175b
  defining quality, 279
  on grading evidence in EBP, 176
Agent-host-environment interaction, 155–156, 155b, 155f
Agents
  classification of, 261b
  in epidemiologic triangle, 88, 155, 155b, 155f
  in occupational health epidemiological triad, 564f, 565–568, 565b, 566t
    biological, 564f, 565–566, 565b
    chemical, 564f, 565b, 566
    environmental and mechanical, 564f, 565b, 566, 567f
    physical, 564f, 565b, 567–568
    psychosocial, 564f, 565b, 568
Age-related risk, 315–316, 315t, 316b
Age-specific rate, 154, 154t

Aggregate
  in case management, 222–223
  definition of, 205
  in public health nursing, 7
Aging
  considerations in health education, 190–191
  within family, 296
  mental health issues with, 408
Aikenhead, Sister Mary Augustine, 17
Air pollution, 92–93, 92f
  point and nonpoint sources, 92
Air quality, indoor, 92–93
Al-Anon, 429
Alateen, 429
Alcohol, Smoking, and Substance Involvement Screening Test (ASSIST), 425
Alcohol, tobacco, and other drug (ATOD)
  problems, 415–432, 430b
  in adolescents, 322b
  assessment of, 425, 425b
  case study of, 429b
  codependency and family involvement in, 427–428
  definitions of, 417
  high-risk groups in, 426–427
    adolescents, 426
    injection drug users, 427
    older adults, 426–427
    pregnancy, 427
    use of illicit drugs, 427
  illicit drug use, 421–422
    amphetamines and methamphetamines, 421–422
    cocaine, 421
    marijuana, 422
    opioids, 421
    street drugs, 422
  nurse's role in, 429–430
  predisposing and contributing factors to, 422–423
  prevention of
    primary prevention, 423–425, 423b, 425b
    secondary prevention, 425–428
    tertiary prevention, 428–429
  psychoactive drugs, 417–420
    alcohol, 417–418
    caffeine, 420, 420t
    tobacco, 418–419, 418f, 419f
  scope of, 416–417
Alcohol abuse
  chronic, 418
  detoxification for, 428
  high risk groups
    adolescents, 426
    older adults, 408
  in homeless population, 397
  in older adults, 426–427
  during pregnancy, 348
  in rural populations, 377
Alcoholics anonymous (AA), 429
Alcoholism
  definition of, 417
  genetics and, 417–418

Al-Gasseer, Naeema, 110
Allergies, school nursing and, 552–553
Alternative healers, cultural variations in, 70t
Alzheimer's disease, 405
American Academy of Pediatrics (AAP), 543, 543b
American Association of Colleges of Nursing (AACN), 26
American Association of Occupational Health Nurses (AAOHN)
  history of, 561
  mission of, 561–562
American Community Survey, 159
American Nurses Association (ANA), 25–26, 504
  on parish or faith community, 511
  on policy process, 117–118
  on quality assurance, 278
American Public Health Association (APHA), 21, 117–118
  on community health nursing, 206
  defining public health nursing by, 7
American Red Cross (ACR), history of, 20
Americans with Disabilities Act, 343, 406, 542
Amphetamines, 421–422
Analytic epidemiology, 148, 163–165, 163t
Andragogy, definition of, 190–191
Anorexia nervosa, 347
Anthrax, 464, 501
  outbreak of, 107
Antigenicity, 458, 458b
Anxiety disorders, 405
  in adults, 407
  in children and adolescents, 339
  in migrant populations, 384
Asian Americans
  immigration statistics of, 66
  mental health needs of, 409
Assault, 437
Assertiveness, in conflict management, 231–232
Assessment Protocol for Excellence in Public Health (APEXPH), 210, 270, 270b
Assessments
  in case management nursing process, 225t
  of causality, 167
  of children at school, 550
  in cultural nursing, 80–81
  ethical principles of, 57–58
  in family nursing, 302b
  of health problems in community, 160b
  of individual health problems, 161b
  of needs in educational process, 185, 185b
  as public health core function, 5
  questions in public health nursing, 8, 8b
  tools, Friedman Family Assessment Model, 305–306
  of vulnerable populations, 367–368, 367b
Assessor, of literacy role of public health nurses, 506
Assisted living, 352
Association of State and Territorial Health Officials (ASTHO), 210
Assurance. see also Access to health care.
  ethical principles of, 58–59
  as public health core function, 5, 9
Asthma, 340, 341
  children with, 553, 553b, 554f
Attack rate, as basic concept in epidemiology, 153

Attention deficit disorder with or without hyperactivity disorders (ADD/ADHD)
  in children and adolescents, 339
  school nursing caring for, 553
Attitude scales, 272
Audit process, for quality of care, 283b, 284
Autism spectrum disorder, in children and adolescents, 339
Autonomy, 233
  in public health code of ethics, 60
  respect as ethical principle, 54, 54b
Avoiding behaviors, 232b

B

"Baby boomers," 35, 212b
Balanced Budget Act of 1997, 120–121, 363–364, 526
Bath salts, 422
Behavioral Risk Factor Surveillance System (BRFSS), 159
Behavioral risks, 313, 321–322, 322b, 322f
  assessment of, 322–323
Behaviors
  alterations in children and adolescents, 339
  family health and, 315b, 321
Benchmarking, 534
Beneficence
  ethical principle of, 54, 54b
  principle for case managers, 233
Berry, Ruth, 514–515
Betts, Virginia Trotter, 110
Bias, 166–167
Bioecological systems theory, 300–301, 301f
Bioethics
  definition of, 50
  history of, 50–51
Biological agents, in occupational health epidemiological triad, 564f, 565–566, 565b
Biological risk, 313, 315–316, 315t, 316b
  assessment of, 316–318
Biological terrorism, 256
Biological variations, cultural differences in, 70t, 72
BioSense, 246
Bioterrorism
  agents of, 463–465
    anthrax, 464
    smallpox, 464–465
  and disaster management, 236–237, 241b
  epidemiological clues of, 262b
  response networks and, 260b
  surveillance for agents of, 460
BioWatch, 245
Bipolar disorder, in children and adolescents, 339, 405
Birth control, 400
Blinding, 177
Block grants, 107
Blood alcohol concentration (BAC), 418
Blood-borne pathogens, hepatitis B, 488
Bloodborne Pathogens Standard, 575
Board of nursing, 115
Breast cancer, as women's health concern, 348
Breckinridge, Mary, 22–23, 22b, 22f
Brief interventions, FRAMES acronym for drug and alcohol abuse, 429–430, 430b
Bronfenbrenner, Urie, on bioecological systems theory, 300, 301f

Bubonic plague, 255
Bulimia, 347
Bull's-eye lesion, 470
Bullying, 552

C

Caffeine, 417, 420, 420t
Campbell Collaboration, 174, 175b
Cancer
  in adults, 346–347
  in children, 340
Capitation, 143
Carbon monoxide, 93
Cardiovascular disease, in adults, 345
Care coordination, in hospice care, 526
Care ethics, 56, 57b
Care management
  definitions of, 223–224
  strategies of, 223b
Caregiver burden, 343
Caregiving, of family, 525
CareMaps, 227
Case fatality rate, 154–155, 154t
Case law, 115
Case management, 221–235
  case manager roles, 226b
    advocacy, 226f, 229–231, 229t
    collaboration, 232
    conflict management, 231–232, 232b
    with vulnerable populations, 370–371, 371f
  case study of, 232b
  community models of, 228–229
  concepts of, 222–228
  coordinating activities within, 223
  definitions of, 223–224, 223b
  ethical issues in, 232–234, 234b
  examples of conditions, 228b
  knowledge domains for, 226b
  legal issues in, 232
  model of, 226f
  and the nursing process, 224, 225f, 225t
  in rural settings, 223
  six "rights" of, 226
  working with vulnerable populations, 366, 370b
Case management and community health primary health care (COPHC), addressing rural health disparities, 387
Case management plans, 227
Case manager, 505–506
  advocacy skills needed by, 226f, 229–231, 229t
  essential skills for, 229–231
  knowledge and skill requirements for, 225–226
  risk for, 233b
  roles of, 226b
    collaboration, 232
    conflict management, 231–232, 232b
  school nurses as, 544
  tools of, 226–228
Case registers, 270–271
Case-control studies, epidemiologic, 163t, 164–165
Categorical programs and funding, 114
Causal inference, 167, 167b
Cause-specific rate, 154–155, 154t
Center for Reviews and Dissemination (CRD), 174, 175b

Centers for Disease Control and Prevention (CDC), 111, 175b
  on biological agent information, 245–246
  on evaluation process, 271, 271f
  guidelines for planning health fairs, 187, 187b, 188f
  on HIV/AIDS, 479
  list of national notifiable infectious diseases, 460–461
  Public Health Information Network, 246
  resources for nurses in rural and migrant populations, 388b
  on "ten great public health achievements," 457
  Youth Risk Behavior Surveillance System instrument, 313
Centers for Medicare and Medicaid Services (CMS), 3–4, 107, 113
Cerebral palsy, 340
Certification
  in approaches to quality improvement, 281
  of home health nurses, 532
Change, stages of, 430b
Change agents, 216
Change partners, 216
Charter, 281
Chemical, biological, radiological, nuclear, and explosive (CBRNE) threats, 239
Chemical agents, in occupational health epidemiological triad, 564f, 565b, 566
Chemical Safety Information, Site Security, and Fuels Regulatory Act, 99–100b
Chemical terrorism, 256
Chemoprophylaxis, prevention strategies for adults, 349b
Chickenpox, versus smallpox, 464, 464b
Child abuse, 441–443, 441b, 443b
  indicators of, 443
  risk factors for, 442b
  school nurse identifying, 551
  sexual, 444
Child maltreatment, 339
Child neglect, defining, 444
Child sexual abuse, 444
Childhood dental caries, case study on, 38b
Childhood injuries, prevention of, 547
Children
  changing demographics of, 334
  disasters effect on, 247, 247b, 247f
  environmental health assessment in, 95–97, 95t
  handwashing for, 340, 340b
  lead-based paint and, 85, 85f
  major public health issues of, 334–341
    acute illnesses as, 340
    alterations of behavior as, 339
    chronic health conditions as, 340–341
    maltreatment as, 339
    mental health problems as, 339
    obesity as, 334–336
  mental illness in, 406–407
  of migrant workers, 384–385
  poverty and health effects on, 395, 395b
  rural versus urban health rates of, 378
  sexual abuse, 444
  with special needs, 553–555
  target areas for prevention in, 341–343
    environmental health hazards as, 85f, 342–343
    immunizations as, 342
    nutrition as, 342
    smoking as, 341–342

Children's Health Insurance Program (CHIP), 66–67
Children's Health Insurance Program Reauthorization Act of 2009 (CHIPRA), 363
Chlamydia, 483–484t, 485–486
Cholera, early epidemiology work on, 149, 149t
Chronic disease
  in adults, 345–347
  in children, 340–341
  common types of
    cancer as, 346–347
    cardiovascular disease as, 345
    diabetes as, 346
    hypertension as, 345, 345b
    mental illness as, 346
    stroke as, 346
  Healthy People 2020 selected objectives relevant to, 345b
  in older adults, 344
Chronosystems, 301, 301f
Cigarettes, electronic, 419–420, 420b
Cities Readiness Initiative, 246
Citizenship, 58
Civil immunity, 117
Civil Works Administration (CWA), 23
Clarification, in client value illumination, 231
Clean Air Act, 92, 99–100b
Clean Water Act (CWA), 99–100b
Client-centered care, competency definition of, 11b
Client outcomes, accountability and quality management, 534
Client populations, specifying the size and distribution of, 268
Clients
  needs assessment, 266, 266b
  specifying the size and distribution of, 268
  use of term in parish nursing, 516–515
Climate change, 89–90, 90b, 90f
Clinical record, 290
Clinical trials, 165–166
Clostridium botulinum, 469t
Clostridium perfringens, 469t
Coal miners, health care needs and risks of rural, 381t
Cocaine, 421
Cochrane Database of Systematic Reviews, 175b
Cochrane Library, 174
Cochrane Public Health Group, 174, 175b
Code of Ethics for nurses, 59–60
Code of Ethics for Nursing (ANA)
  on advocacy role in nursing, 229
  on compassion and respect, 229
  ethical issues in case managers, 232–233
Code of Ethics for Public Health, 60–61, 60b
Code of regulations, 121
Codeine, 421
Codependency, issues with addiction, 427–428
Cognitive domain of learning, 184
Cohesion, definition of, 196
Cohort studies, epidemiologic, 163, 163t, 164f
Collaboration
  behaviors, 232b
  in public health nursing, 508b
  teamwork and
    in case management, 232
    competency definition of, 11b
Common law, 115
Common source outbreak, 261

Common vehicle, 459
Communicable diseases, 456
  deaths caused by, 457
  disease development of, 459
  diseases of travelers, 474–475
  emerging, 461–462, 461t
  and epidemiologic triangle, 458, 458f
  foodborne. see Foodborne diseases.
  Healthy People 2020 objectives related to, 457, 458b
  historical and current perspectives of, 456–458
  history of, 17, 24
  list of reportable, 460–461
  modes of transmission of, 459
  multisystem approach to control, 463
  nurse's role in providing preventive care for, 491–495, 491b
  parasitic, 472–474, 473t
  prevention and control of, 462–463
  spectrum of, 459–460
  transmission of, 458–460
  vaccine-preventable, 465–468
  vector-borne, 470–472
  waterborne, 468–470, 468b
Communicable period, 459
Communication
  in cultural diversity, 70–71
  effective, 120
  risk, in environmental health, 98
  skills, core competencies for educators, 200b
Communities
  as client and partner, 206–207
  community-based nursing and, 11–12, 12b
  comprehensive services in, 364–365
  conceptual definition of, 205
  Healthy People 2020 and, 209, 210b
  how disasters affect, 246–248
  identifying problem in, 214–215
  partnerships, 209–210
  as setting for practice, 1, 10, 205
  system categories within, 205b
  as target of practice, 205
  types of, 204, 204b
  WHO definition of, 204
  wrap-around services in, 364
Community assessment
  case study and examples of, 212b
  checklist of, 218b
  concepts of, 205t
  confidentiality during, 214
  consensus set of health status indicators, 207, 207b
  core competencies, 204
  data collection and interpretation in, 211–212
  evaluation and, 203–220
  of health access parity and program planning, 267b
  issues, 214
  steps in, 211
  of vulnerable populations, 367–368, 367b
  websites' usefulness in, 214b
Community care model (CCM), for adults, 352
Community care settings, 352–353
  adult day health as, 352
  assisted living as, 352
  home health and hospice as, 352
  long-term care and rehabilitation as, 352–353
  senior centers as, 352, 352f

Community competence, 208
Community Emergency Response Team (CERT), 39–42, 241–242
Community facilities, violence and, 436
Community forum, 268t
Community groups
　formal or informal, 196
　nurses choosing, 195–196, 198–199, 198f
Community health, 501
　assessment of, 211–214, 211b
　concept of, 207–209
　nursing application to. *see* Community-focused nursing process.
　personal safety in, 217–218
　planning for, 215–216
　process, 208–209, 208t
　status, 207, 207b
　strategies and resources to improve, 210–211
　structure, 207–208
Community Health Accreditation Program (CHAP), 534
Community health agency records, for documentation, 290
Community Health Assessment and Group Evaluation (CHANGE) Tool, 210
Community health nursing, 15–32, 26b, 29b, 30b
　cultural influences in, 65–83, 73b
　definition of, 1–2
　for vulnerable populations, 364–371, 365b
Community health planning, program management, 266
Community health problems, identifying during assessment process, 212
Community health strengths, identifying during assessment process, 212
Community indexes, 270–271
Community mental health centers (CMHCs), 406
Community outreach, school nurses' role in, 544–545
Community partnerships, 209–210
Community reconnaissance, 214, 214b
Community resources, for families, 329–330
Community trials, 166
Community-based nursing (CBN), 11–12
　versus community-oriented nursing, 1–2, 2–3t
　definition of, 1, 12b
Community-based settings, 1
Community-Campus Partnerships for Health (CCPH), 498–499, 499b
Community-focused nursing process
　assessment process. *see* Community assessment.
　establishing goals and objectives in, 215–216
　evaluation of, 217f
　identifying intervention activities in, 216
　implementation in, 216
　outcomes of, 217
　overview of, 211–217
　problem analysis in, 215
　problem prioritizing in, 215
Community-oriented nursing, 10–11
　case study of, 10b
　challenges for the future in, 12, 12b
　versus community-based nursing, 1–2, 2–3t
　definition of, 1–2, 12b
　evidence-based practice (EBP) methods for, 178–179
　versus public health nursing, 6, 7b
Community-oriented practice, 207

Compassionate Investigational New Drug Program, 422
Competencies
　cultural, 73–77, 74b
　definition of, 74
　for faith community nurses, 517
　in public health code of ethics, 60
　QSEN definition of nurses, 11b
Competing behaviors, 232b
Compliance, to environmental standards, 100
Comprehensive Environmental Response, Compensation, and Liability Act (CERCLA or Superfund), 99–100b
Comprehensive services, for vulnerable populations, 364–365
Compromising behaviors, 232b
Concurrent audits, 284
Condoms, 400, 492
Conduct disorders, in children and adolescents, 339
Confidentiality. *see also* Health Insurance Portability and Accountability Act.
　in case management, 231–232, 233b
　during community assessment process, 214
　in public health code of ethics, 60
Conflict management
　case manager role in, 231–232, 232b
　in groups, 199
Confounding factor, 166–167
Congenital predisposition, 368
Congenital syphilis, 485
Congregants, 518
Congregational-based parish nursing model, 511–512, 511b
Congress, 106
Consequentialism, 53
Constituency, advocacy in, 229–230
Constitutional law, 115
Consultant, school nurses as, 544
Consumer confidence report (CCR), 94
Consumer price index (CPI), 393–394
Continuous quality improvement (CQI), quality assurance and, 277, 280b, 282–286
Continuous source outbreak, 261
Contraceptive, 347, 400
Contracting
　advantages and disadvantages of, 328
　contingency, 327
　definition of, 327
　for family health risks, 327–328
　noncontingency, 327
　phases and activities in, 327t
　process of, 327
　purposes of, 327
Co-occurring disorders, substance abuse and mental illness, 407
Cooperation, in conflict management, 231–232
Coordinating activities, within case management, 223
Core-based statistical area (CBSA), 375
Correctional health, legal issues in, 117
Cost *versus* quality, 177
Cost-effectiveness, of home health and hospice, 535
Costs. *see also* Financing.
　factors influencing health care, 136–137
　　chronic illness and, 137
　　demographics, 136
　　technology and intensity, 136–137, 137t
　　trends in health care spending, 135–136, 135f, 135t

Counselor, school nurses as, 544
Credentials, educational, of school nurses, 543
Crimean War, 17, 149
Criminal offenders, sexually transmitted infections (STIs) in, 156b
Crisis
　disasters. *see* Disaster management.
　family, 314
　teams in schools, 549
Crisis poverty, homelessness and, 397
Critical paths, in case management, 222–223, 223b
Cross-sectional studies, epidemiologic, 163t, 165
Crude mortality (death) rate, 154, 154t
Cryptosporidium, 462t
Cultural accommodation, 77–78, 77b
Cultural attitudes, definition of, 393
Cultural awareness, 75, 75b
Cultural blindness, 79
Cultural brokering, 78
Cultural competence, 73–77, 74b
　Campinha-Bacote on
　　cultural awareness, 75, 75b
　　cultural desire, 77
　　cultural encounter, 76, 77f
　　cultural knowledge, 75–76, 76b
　　cultural skill, 76, 76f
　development of, 74–77, 77b
　framework of stages of competence, 75t
　inhibitors to developing, 78–80
　nursing interventions of, 77–78
　　cultural accommodation, 77–78, 77b
　　cultural brokering, 78
　　cultural preservation, 77
　　cultural repatterning, 78
　standards of, 74
Cultural conflict, 79–80
Cultural considerations, in health education, 190–191
Cultural desire, Campinha-Bacote on, 77
Cultural diversity, mental illness and, 70–73, 70t, 71b, 409
Cultural encounter, Campinha-Bacote on, 76, 77f
Cultural imposition, 79
Cultural knowledge, Campinha-Bacote on, 75–76
Cultural nursing assessment, 80–81, 80b
Cultural preservation, 77
Cultural relativism, 79
Cultural repatterning, 78
Cultural shock, definition of, 80
Cultural skill, Campinha-Bacote on, 76, 76f
Cultural value, 68–69
Culturally Appropriate Resources and Education Clinic (C.A.R.E.), 68
Culturally competent organizations, building, 81
Culture, 68–69
　communication and
　　directness, 69f
　　indirect approach, 69f
　definition of, 68
　linguistically appropriate health care, 365
　organizational elements of, 69
　sexual violence and, 438–439
Cumulative incidence rate, 152
Cumulative Index to Nursing and Allied Health (CINAHL), 174
Cumulative risks, 358

D

DARE Project, 424
"DARN-CAT" mnemonic, 188–189
Data, international and national sources of, 109t
Data collection
    in community assessment, 211–212
        methods of, 212–214
    for other purposes, 159
    routinely collected data, 159
Data gathering, during community assessment, 212
Data generation, during community assessment, 212
Database, of community assessment, 214–215
Date rape, 438
Deadbeat dad, 395
Deadbeat parent, 395
Death
    Kübler-Ross's book on, 526
    leading causes of, in 2013, 149
Death certificates, 159
Death rates, as indicator of community health status, 207, 207b
Decision making
    ethical, 51–59, 53f
    for older adults, 344
Declaration of Alma-Ata, 33
Deinstitutionalization, of mentally ill patients, 406
Delano, Jane, 21
Delayed stress reactions, international relief workers, 250
Delinquency, in children and adolescents, 339
Delirium, in adults, 344–345
Demand management, in case management, 222–223
Dementia, in adults, 344–345
Democratic leadership, 198
Demographics
    of American children, 334
    family, 295
    health care system trends and, 35–36
    workers as population aggregate and, 571–574
Denial, symptom of addiction, 425
Dental disease, in migrant farmworkers, 384
Dental health, prevention strategies for, 349b
Deontology, ethical theory of, 53–56, 54b
Department of Agriculture, 113
Department of Commerce, 109t
Department of Defense, 113
Department of Homeland Security (DHS), 41–42, 238
Department of Justice, 113
Department of Labor, 109t, 113
Depressants, 417
Depression
    in adults, 344–345
    in children and adolescents, 339, 405
    in migrant populations, 384
    in older adults, 408
    in rural populations, 378
Depression-era, public health during, 23
Descriptive epidemiology, 148, 160–162, 162b
Determinants of health
    in family health, 315b
    of health event, 148, 163
Detoxification, for alcohol, tobacco, and other drug (ATOD) problems, 428
Developmental theories, family life cycle theory, 299–300, 300b, 300t

Devolution, from federal to state, 107
Diabetes
    case study on learning domains, 185b
    in migrant farmworkers, 384
    in rural populations, 377
Diabetes mellitus
    in adults, 344–345, 346
    childhood obesity and, 335, 335b
    in children, 340
    school nursing and, 553
Diagnosis-related groups (DRGs), 133
Diagnostic and Statistical Manual of Mental Disorders, 5th edition, 339
Diarrheal diseases, suffered by travelers, 474–475
Diet
    recommendations for child obesity prevention, 335–336, 335b, 336t
    reducing family health risks, 321
Dietary practices, assessment of, 72b
Digital rectal examination (DRE), 349
Dioxin, 101
Diphtheria, 21
Direct care, in home health and hospice, 529–530
Direct caregiver, school nurses as, 544
Directly observed therapy (DOT), 490, 494
Disadvantaged population, definition of, 358–359
Disaster management, 252b, 236–254. see also Disasters.
    cycle of, 239–251, 239f
    disaster medical assistance teams (DMATs), 241–242
    evidence-based practice of, 249b
    future of, 251–252
    international relief efforts in, 250
    mass casualty exercises, 243–244, 244b
    plans in occupational health, 575–576
    response to bioterrorism, 245–246
    role of nurse in, 239–249
    shelter management, 249–250
    stress reactions
        in community, 248
        in individuals, 246–248, 246b
Disaster medical assistance teams (DMATs), 241–242
Disaster responders, 507
Disaster workers, psychological stress of, 250
Disasters. see also Disaster management.
    definition of, 236–239, 237f
    HSPD 21: Public Health and Medical Preparedness, and National Health Security Strategy (NHSS), 238
    human-made, 236, 237–238
    natural, 236–237
    populations at greatest risk for disruption after, 247b
    stress response to, 405
    types of, 237b
Discrimination, against migrant farmworkers, 384
Disease management
    in case management, 222–223
    philosophy of, 227
Disease prevention, 33–34
    definition of, 34b
    Healthy People 2020 goals of, 44
Disease surveillance, 255–258
    definitions and importance of, 255–256
    national notifiable diseases, 258–259, 258–259b

Diseases
    chronic. see Chronic disease.
    definition of, 456
    investigations of, 261–262
    natural history of, 156
    prevention education in school, 548
Disenfranchisement
    advocacy, as ethical principle of public health nursing, 60
    as aspect of vulnerability, 359
Disparities
    cultural competence and, 73–74
    definition of, 34b
    environmental health, 101
Dissenters, 230
Distribution, of health event patterns, 148, 163
Distributive justice
    case study of, 59b
    ethical principle of, 54, 54b, 55b
District nursing, history of, 17, 17t
District nursing association, founded by William Rathbone, 18
Diversity. see also Culture.
    in public health code of ethics, 60
DNA testing, 318
Documentation
    of migrant farmworkers, 384
    to reduce risks case manager, 233b
Domestic violence. see Intimate partner violence.
Donabedian's model, 285
Do-not-resuscitate (DNR) orders, 343, 555
Down syndrome, 340
Drug abuse, in older adults, 408
Drug addiction, definition of, 417
Drug dependence, definition of, 417
Drug testing, 426
Duke University Center for Spirituality, Theology, and Health, 513b
Durable power of attorney, 343
Dysfunctional families, 297

E

Earthquakes, 236–237, 405
Eating disorders
    in children and adolescents, 339
    as women's health concern, 347
Ebola-Marburg viruses, 462t
Ecologic fallacy, 165
Ecological model, Institute of Medicine's population health, 155–156
Ecological studies, 163t, 165
Ecomap, 320–321, 320f
Economic risks
    affecting family health risks, 319
    affecting mental health in rural versus urban areas, 378
Economics, 125–127
    definition of, 126–127
    factors influencing health care costs, 136–137
        chronic illness and, 137
        demographics, 136
        technology and intensity, 136–137, 137t
    future of nursing practice and, 143–144, 144b
    health care payment systems and, 142–143
        for health care organizations, 142–143
        for health care practitioners, 143

Economics (*Continued*)
  primary prevention and, 130
  public health and, 126–127
  trends in health care spending and, 135–136, 135f, 135t
Ecstasy, 422
Education
  definition of, 184
  of faith community nurse, 516–517
  home visit to address family health risks, 323
  needs, of pregnant teenagers, 404
  for parish nursing, 519b
  requirements for occupational health nurses, 562, 575b
Educational credentials, of school nurses, 543
Educator, nurse as, 506
Effectiveness
  aspects of program evaluation, 274, 274b
  claims by American Nurses Association, 143
Efficiency
  aspects of program evaluation, 273–274, 274b
  claims by American Nurses Association, 143
Egalitarian theory, 55b
Ehrlichiosis, 456
Elder abuse, definition of, 344, 447
Electronic cigarettes, 419–420, 420b
Electronic medical record
  definitions of, 34b
  technological trends in, 37
Electronic nicotine delivery systems, 419–420
Elimination
  of disease, 462–463
  problems, in children and adolescents, 339
Emergencies
  equipment, in school nurse's office, 549–550
  in school, nursing care for, 548–549, 550b
Emergency plan, by school nurses, 548–549
Emergency Planning and Community Right to Know Act (EPCRA), 99–100b
Emergency Support Functions (ESFs), 244
Emerging infectious diseases, factors of, 461–462, 461t, 462t
Emotional abuse
  in children, 443
  in older adults, 447
Emotional neglect, defining child, 444
Employee assistance programs (EAPs), 426
Employers, private support and, 141
Employment, statistics in U.S., 562
Empowerment
  cultural brokering and, 78
  cultural competence and, 74
  through advocacy, 230
Enabling, defining addict, 427–428
Endemic, definition of, 261, 460
End-of-life care, in nursing, 529
Enforcement, of environmental standards, 99
Environment, 84–85
  defining epidemiologic triangle, 88, 155, 155b, 155f
  factor, in transmission of communicable diseases, 459
  living, of vulnerable populations, 368
  in occupational health epidemiological triad, 564f, 568
Environmental agents, in occupational health epidemiological triad, 564f, 565b, 566, 567f
Environmental control, 72

Environmental epidemiology, 88
Environmental health, 84–104, 86b
  advocacy of, 100–101
  assessment of, 90–97, 91b
    air, 92–93, 92f
    children, 95–97, 95t
    food, 94
    land, 94
    right to know, 94
    risk, 94–95
    water, 93–94
  historical context of, 86
  problems in rural areas, 379–380
  referral resources for, 101
  resources, 93b
  roles for nurses in, 86b, 102
  threats in health care industry, 101
Environmental health hazards, as prevention target area for children, 342–343
Environmental health sciences, 87–89
  epidemiology as, 88, 88f
  multidisciplinary approaches to, 88–89, 89b
  toxicology as, 87–88, 87b
Environmental justice, 101
Environmental Protection Agency (EPA)
  National Environmental Policy Act (NEPA), 99–100b
  on six common air pollutants, 84–85
Environmental risks, 313, 319–320
  assessment of, 320–321, 320f
  reducing, 97–100
    ethics, 98
    government environmental protection, 99–100, 99–100b
    risk communication, 98
Environmental standards, 100
Epidemics, 152
  definition of, 261, 460
Epidemiologic triangle, 155–156, 155b, 155f
  causal factors from, 261–262
  of communicable diseases, 458, 458f
  in environmental health, 88
Epidemiological data, 159, 272
Epidemiological studies, determining if problems exist, 153b
Epidemiological triad, in occupational health, 564, 564f
Epidemiology, 150b
  analytic, 148, 163–165
  basic concepts in, 151–157
    attack rate, 153
    epidemiologic triangle, 155b
    incidence and prevalence compared, 153
    levels of preventive interventions, 156–157
    measures in morbidity and mortality, 151–155
    measures of incidence, 152
    mortality rates, 153–155, 154t
    prevalence proportion, 152–153
    rates, proportions, and risk, 151–152
  basic methods in, 159–160
    comparison groups, 160
    data sources, 159
    rate adjustment, 159–160
  case studies of, 150–151b, 157b
  causality, 166–167
    assessment for, 167
    bias, 166–167
    statistical associations, 166

Epidemiology (*Continued*)
  definitions of, 148
  descriptive, 148, 160–162, 162b
  distribution and determinants in, 148, 163
  in environmental health science, 88, 88f
  experimental studies in, 165–166
  history of, 149–150, 149t
  of human immunodeficiency virus, 480–481, 481f
  nurses use of, 150–151
  nursing applications of, 167
  origin of term, 148
  screening in, 157–159
  studies in, 163t
Eradication, of disease, 462–463
Erectile dysfunction, as men's health concern, 350
Escherichia coli infections, 456, 462t, 469–470
"Essential Nursing Competencies and Curricula Guidelines for Genetics and Genomics," 150
Established groups, 199
Ethical decision making, 51–59, 53f
  ethical principles and theories in, 53–57
  rationale for steps of, 52t
Ethical dilemmas, definition of, 51–52
Ethical issues
  definition of, 51–52
  in faith community nursing, 518
Ethics
  care ethics and, 56, 57b
  case studies on, 55b, 59b, 60b
  consequentialism, 53
  definition of, 50
  deontology, 53–56, 54b
  in environmental health, 98
  feminist, 56–57, 57b
  history of, 50–51
  issues in older adults, 344
  principles of, 54, 54b
  principlism and, 54, 56b
  in public and community health nursing practice, 49–64, 56b, 59b, 62b
  public health nursing core functions and, 57–59
  related to adult health, 343–344
  utilitarianism, 53–56, 54b
  virtue ethics and, 56, 56b
Ethnicity, 70
  considerations in health education, 190–191
Ethnocentrism, definition of, 79
Evaluations
  in case management nursing process, 225t
  in community-focused nursing process, 217f
  in continuous quality improvement program, 287f, 288–289
  definition of, 266
  of educational process, 194–195
  formative, 266b
  of health and behavioral changes, 195
  levels of, 266b
  process
    in program management, 271, 271f
    specifying objectives, 271–272
  summative, 266b
Evaluative studies, of quality improvement, 285–286
Event
  defining magnitude of, 261
  outbreak patterns, 256
  risks of unhealthy, 313

Evidence
  approaches to finding, 174–176
    integrative review, 174
    meta-analysis, 174
    narrative review, 174
  grading and evaluating strength and quality of, 176
  types of, 172–173
Evidence-based medicine, 171
  history and paradigm shift of, 172
Evidence-based nursing, definition of, 171
Evidence-Based Nursing Journal, 175b
Evidence-based practice (EBP), 7b, 179b, 170–181, 171b. *see also* Evidence-based practice (EBP) boxes.
  barriers to, 173
  case study of, 179b
  current perspectives of, 177–179
  definition of, 171
  eight steps in process, 173b
  evaluating evidence, 176–177
  history of, 171–172
  implementation of, 173, 177
  individual differences in, 178
  methods for community-oriented nursing practice, 178–179
  as norm in nursing today, 1
  to public health nursing, 179, 180t
  resources for implementing, 175b
  steps in, 173–174
Evidence-based practice (EBP) boxes
  on behavior change counseling (BCC), 194b
  on case management, 224b
  on community partnership for mammogram screening, 210b
  on government health care functions, 108b
  on health access parity and program planning, 267b
  on homelessness and gender, 399b
  on infectious disease prevention, 465b
  on Massachusetts health care system, 35b
  on obesity, 341b
  on promoting health and safety of workers, 562b
  on Temporary Assistance for Needy Families (TANF), 11b
  on undocumented immigration, 382b
  on vaccination to prevent transmission of human papillomavirus (HPV), 492b
Evidence-Based Practice for Public Health Project, 175b
Evidence-based protocols, 176b
Evidence-based public health, definition of, 171
Exercise
  for osteoporosis, 348
  recommendations for child obesity prevention, 335–336, 335b
  reducing family health risks, 321
Exosystems, 301, 301f
Experimental studies, epidemiologic, 165–166

F

Faith communities
  definition of, 511
  historical perspectives in, 513
  national health objectives of, 518–519, 519b
Faith community nurse, 510–523, 521b, 522–523b
  educational preparation for, 516–517
  functions of, 520–522, 520b, 521f

Faith community nurse coordinator, 514
Faith community nursing
  characteristics of, 514–515, 515b
  definition of, 511–512
  evidence-based practice in, 512b
  historical perspectives of, 513–514
  issues in, 517–518
    ethical issues, 518
    financial issues, 518
    legal issues, 518
    professional issues, 517–518
  levels of prevention in, 515b
  philosophy of, 514–515
  scope and standards of, 516
Faith nurse community, 513–514
Families. *see also* Family health risks; Family nursing.
  in alcohol, tobacco, and other drug (ATOD) problems, 427–428
  characteristics of healthy, 297b
  definition of, 295, 525
  dysfunctional, 297
  ecomap in, 320–321, 320f
  functional, 297
  health history of, 311–312, 318b
  nursing theory, 299, 299f
    bioecological systems theory, 300–301, 301f
    developmental and life cycle theory, 299–300, 300b, 300t
    systems theory, 299
  obesity prevention recommendations for, 335b
  Patient Protection and Affordable Care Act, 306
  practice focusing on, 10–12
  responsibility, roles, and functions, in home health and hospice, 536
  social and family policy challenges, 306–307
  strategies for prevention related to, 328b
Family and Medical Leave Act, 343
Family caregiving, by home health nurses, 351, 525
Family crisis, 314
Family demographics, 295
Family functions, 295, 295b
Family health, 297, 312–313
  definitions related to, 315b
  legal issues with, 117
  Neuman Systems Model in, 312–313
  six categories of risk factors. *see* Family health risks.
Family health policy, 311
Family health risks, 310–332
  appraisal of, 314–323
  behavioral (lifestyle) risk, 321–322, 322b, 322f
    assessment of, 322–323
  biological and age-related risk, 315–316, 315t, 316b
    assessment of, 316–318
  community resources in, 329–330
  concepts in, 312–314
  early approaches to, 311–312
  ecomap, 320–321, 320f
  economic risk, 319
  environmental risk, 319–320
    assessment of, 320–321, 320f
  genetics and, 318–319
  nursing interventions and, 314–323
  reduction of, 323–329
    contracting with families for, 327–328
    empowering families for, 328–329
    home visits for, 323–327
  social risks and, 319

Family homicide, 437
Family life-cycle stages, 315, 315t
Family nursing, 307b. *see also* Families; Family health risks.
  approaches to, 297–299, 298f, 299f
  in community, 294–295
  definition of, 294
  home visiting safety tips, 302, 302b
  theoretical frameworks for, 299–301
    bioecological systems theory, 300–301, 301f
    developmental and life cycle theory, 299–300, 300b, 300t
    systems theory, 299–300
  working with families, 301–305
    assessment, 302b
    case presentation, 303
    case study on, 303–304b, 305b
    data collection, 301
    designing family interventions, 303–304, 303b
    evaluation of plan, 304–305, 305b
    interviewing the family and defining problem, 302–303, 302b
    making an appointment, 302, 302b
Family nursing assessment, 305–306, 305b
Family nursing theory, 299, 299f
  bioecological systems theory, 300–301, 301f
  developmental and life cycle theory, 299–300, 300b, 300t
  systems theory, 299
Family organization, cultural variations in, 70t
Family stress theory, 316
Family structure, 295–296, 296b, 296f
  in adolescent sexual behavior and pregnancy, 401
Family violence, 440–448
  development of abusive patterns in, 440–441
  firearm accidents and, 448
  nursing interventions for, 448–451, 448b
  types of, 441–447
    child abuse as, 441–443, 441b, 442b, 443b, 444b
    child neglect as, 444
    intimate partner violence, 445–447, 446b, 447b
    sexual abuse as, 444–445
Farm residency
  children's health and, 379
  health care needs and risks of rural, 381t
  as part of rural definition, 375
  pesticide exposure and, 379, 379b
Federal Emergency Relief Administration (FERA), 23
Federal government, role in US health care of, 106
Federal health agencies, US Department of Health and Human Services. *see* US Department of Health and Human Services.
Federal income poverty guidelines, 393–394, 394t
Federal Insecticide, Fungicide, and Rodenticide Act (FIFRA), 99–100b
Federal legislation
  examples of, 343
  in school nursing, 541–542, 542t
Federal public health agencies, 499
  roles of, 499–500
Federal system, health care system and, 39–42, 40f, 42t
Fee-for-service, 143

Feminist ethics, 56–57, 57b
Feminists, 56–57
Fetal alcohol syndrome (FAS), 427
Financial issues
    abuse in older adults, 447
    in faith community nursing, 518
Financial records, 290
Financing
    of health care, 138–142
        other public support, 140
        private support, 140–142
        public health, 140
        public support, 138–140, 138t
    payment systems, 142–143
        for health care organizations, 142–143
        for health care practitioners, 143
Flakka, 422
Fliedner, Pastor Theodor, 17
Focus groups, 268t
Follower role, in groups, 197b
Food, environmental health assessment of, 94
Food consumption patterns, assessment of, 72b
Food Quality Protection Act (FQPA), 95–96, 96b,
    99–100b
Food stamps, 393–394
Foodborne diseases, 468–470, 468b
    affecting travelers, 474
    salmonellosis as, 469
    World Health Organization (WHO) on,
        468
Foreign-born persons, four categories of, 66–67
Forensic nursing, 439
Formal groups, 196
Formative evaluation, 266b
Frankel, Dr. Lee, 21
Fraud, in case management, 233b
Freedom of Information Act, 94
Friedman Family Assessment Model, 305–306
Frontier areas, health care shortage in, 379
Frontier Nursing Service (FNS), 22–23, 22b
Functional families, 297

G

Gardner, Mary, 20
Gatekeeper role, in groups, 197b
Genetic predisposition, 368
Genetics
    alcohol use disorders and, 417–418
    epidemiology and, 150, 150b
    family health risks and, 318–319, 318b
Genital herpes, 483–484t, 486
Genital warts, 483–484t, 486
Genogram, 316, 317f
Genomics, 318
Geographic information systems (GIS), for
    environmental health studies, 88
Geographic variations, in descriptive
    epidemiology, 161
German measles, 466
Gestational diabetes
    incidence of, 348
    as women's health concern, 348
Global warming, 89
Globalization, definition of, 34b
Goals, establishing in community-focused nursing
    process, 215–216
Gold standard, 158
Gonorrhea, 482–485, 483–484t

Government, 105–124, 122b
    branches of, 106
    community resources for families, 329–330
    definition of, 106
    family policy challenges and, 306
    federal health agencies and, 110–113
    health care functions of, 108–109
        direct services, 108
        financing, 108
        information, 108, 109t
        policy setting, 108
        public protection, 108–109
    impact on nursing, 114
    role of, in US health care, 106–109
Government environmental protection, 99–100,
    99–100b
Grading the strength of evidence, 176
Great Recession, 38
Green-card holders, 66–67
Greenhouse effect, 89
Gross domestic product (GDP), 135
Group culture, 197
Group purposes, 196
Groups
    case example of, 199b
    cohesion in, 196
    conflict, 199–200
    definitions and concepts of, 196–198
    evaluation of, 200
    formal and informal, 196
    leadership
        behaviors associated with, 197–198
        core competencies for educators, 200b
    maintenance norms in, 197
    nurses choosing community, 198–199, 198f
    practice focusing on, 10–12
    role structures of, 197, 197b
    task function of, 196
    tools in health education, 195–200
Gun violence, 339
Guyatt, Gordon, 172
Gynecological age, 403

H

H1N1 and H3N2 viruses, 462t, 467
Haiti earthquake of 2010, 251–252
Halfway houses, 428–429
Handwashing, importance of, 340, 340b
Hantavirus, 462t
Harm reduction model, for ATOD problems, 416,
    423
Hawes, Bessie M., 23
Hazard Communication Standard, 94, 575
Hazards. see also Environmental health hazards;
    Occupational health hazards.
    assessment by occupational health nurses, 571
    Bloodborne Pathogens Standard, 575
    categories of work-related, 564, 565b
    Hazard Communication Standard, 575
    workplace, 560
Healing, in faith community nurse, 511–512,
    520–521, 520b
Health, 33
    culture, diversity, and social determinants of,
        73–77, 359–361, 360f
    definition of, 34b
    life span, effects across the, 394–396
Health Belief Model (HBM), 193

Health care
    costs, factors influencing, 136–137
    factors affecting resource allocation in,
        127–129
        access to health services, 128–129
        Healthy People 2020, 129, 129b
        poor, 128
        rationing, 129
        uninsured, 127–128
Health care delivery, in faith community nursing,
    514
Health Care Financing Administration
    (HCFA), 107
Health care policy, family health and, 311
Health care practices, legal issues affecting, 117
    correctional health, 117
    home care and hospice, 117
    occupational health, 117
    school and family health, 117
Health care providers, school nursing and, 551
Health care rationing, 127
Health care systems, 33–48, 45b
    access to, 38, 41b
    barriers to integration of, 43–44, 43b
    cost and, 38
    federal system and, 39–42, 40f, 42t
    forces influencing changes in, 43
    local system and, 42–43
    organization of, 39–43
    primary health care on, 44
    public health system in, 39
    quality of, 37b, 38–39
    social and economic trends of, 36
    state system and, 42
    technological trends in, 36–37
    workforce trends in, 36
Health Care Without Harm campaign, 101
Health care-acquired infections (HAIs), 475
Health departments, state and local, 113–114
Health disparities
    definition of, 358
    Healthy People 2020 goals regarding, 358,
        359b
Health economics, definition of, 126–127
Health education
    barriers to learning in, 189
    case study on domains of learning, 185b
    core communication competencies of, 200b
    cultural, age, and ethnic considerations of,
        190–191
    developing effective programs, 189, 190f
    educational process, 185–195
        designing clear educational programs, 190b
        evaluation of, 194–195
        goals and objectives of, 186
        identity needs of, 185–186
        motivational interviewing of, 188–189,
            188b
        needs assessment of, 185, 185b
        select strategies and methods of, 186–187,
            186f
        TEACH mnemonic, 186b
        use of technology in, 194
    educator-related barriers of, 191–192
    guidelines for planning health fairs in, 187,
        187b, 188f
    instructive district nursing in, 18, 18f
    learner-related barriers of, 192–194

Health education (*Continued*)
  objectives for *Healthy People 2020,* 183, 183b
  skills of effective educator of, 187–188
  use of plain language in, 189b
  for vulnerable populations, 366
Health educators
  role of public health nurses, 504
  school nurses as, 544
Health fairs, guidelines for planning, 187, 187b, 188f
Health impact pyramid, 5, 5f
Health insurance. *see also* Patient Protection and Affordable Care Act.
  evolution of, 140–141, 140b
  uninsured. *see* Uninsured population.
Health Insurance Portability and Accountability Act (HIPAA), 107, 142
  on home health and hospice, 536–537
  on teen pregnancy, 306
Health literacy, 192
Health maintenance organizations (HMOs), 141–142, 142b
Health ministries
  in characteristics, of faith community nursing practice, 514–517
  definition of, 511
Health Ministries Association (HMA)
  defining faith community nursing, 511
  resources for parish nursing, 513b
Health perception, cultural variations in, 70t
Health policy
  definition of, 106, 117
  outcomes of, methods of influencing of, 119–120
  related to adult health, 343–344
Health problems
  in community
    assessment of, 160b
    existence, 153b
  in individual, assessment of, 161b
Health Professional Shortage Areas (HPSAs), 377
Health program planning
  defining the problem and assessing client need, 266
  needs assessment, 266
Health promotion, 33–34
  definition of, 34b
  Healthy People 2020 on, 44–45, 44b
Health Resources and Services Administration (HRSA), 111
Health risk appraisal, 313
Health risk reduction, 313–314, 314f
Health risks, across the life span, 313, 333–356, 353b
  adolescents, 337–338
  in adults, 344–350
    cancer as, 346–347
    cardiovascular disease as, 345
    chronic disease as, 345–347
    diabetes as, 346
    health status indicators and, 345
    hypertension as, 345, 345b
    mental illness as, 346
    stroke as, 346
    weight control and, 347
  among special groups of adults, 350–351
    color, 350
    incarcerated, 350

Health risks, across the life span (*Continued*)
    lesbian and gay, 350
    with physical and mental disabilities, 350–351
  children
    acute illnesses as, 340
    alterations of behavior and mental health problems as, 339
    children and, 334
    chronic health conditions as, 340–341
    injuries and accidents as, 336–339, 338b
    maltreatment as, 339
    obesity as, 334–336, 334t, 335b, 336t, 337b
  infants, 337
  preschoolers, 337
  school-age children, 337
  toddlers and, 337
Health screening, prevention strategies for adults and, 349b
Health Services Pyramid, 5, 5f
Health status, in vulnerable populations, 362
Health status indicators, 345
  for community assessment, 207, 207b
Healthy, Hunger-Free Kids Act of 2010 (PL 111-296), 542
Healthy People 2000, versus Healthy People 2010 and *Healthy People 2020,* 109b
Healthy People 2010, versus Healthy People 2000 and *Healthy People 2020,* 109b
Healthy People 2020, 503–504, 505b
  on behavioral (lifestyle) health risk assessment, 322
  cancer and, 347
  on case management, 224, 224b
  on childhood obesity prevention, 336
  on community consortium and partners, 209, 210b
  economic influences, 129, 129b
  epidemiology to analyze goals of, 148, 148b
  ethics and, 59b
  on evidence-based practice care decisions, 179, 179b
  example of measurable national health objective, 272b
  on faith communities, 518–519, 519b
  on families and family nursing, 307, 307b
  on family health risk, 312, 312b
  gun violence and, 339
  on health access parity and program planning, 267b
  on health disparities, 358, 359b
  on health education, 183, 183b, 184b
  on health promotion and disease prevention, 186
  on health risk, categorizing, 313
  versus Healthy People 2000 and *Healthy People 2010,* 109
    comparison of, 109b
  history of, 28b
  human immunodeficiency virus infection and, 478–479, 479b
  major health issues and chronic disease of adults and, objectives for, 345b
  national health objectives of, 505, 505b
  objectives, 238–239
  overview and goals of, 9b
  on poor and homeless people, adolescent reproductive health, and mental illness, 398b
  on promoting health/preventing disease, 44, 44b

Healthy People 2020 (*Continued*)
  quality health care and, 290, 290b
  on rural health, 388–389, 388b
  school nurses and, 544, 546, 546b
  secondhand smoke and, 419
  substance abuse and, 416, 426b
  on vulnerable populations, 358, 359b
  women's reproductive health and, 347
Heart disease, in adults, 344–345
Helping Patients Who Drink Too Much: A Clinician's Guide, 425
Hemophilia, children and, 340
Henry Street Settlement, 6, 31
Hepatitis, 487–489
  case study on, 488b
  profiles, 487t
Hepatitis A virus (HAV), 487, 487t, 488b
Hepatitis B virus (HBV), 487–488, 487t
Hepatitis C virus (HCV), 487t, 489
Herd immunity, 127, 459
Heroin, 421
Herpes simplex virus 2, 483–484t, 486
High blood pressure (HBP), in adults, 345
Highly active antiretroviral therapy (HAART), 473, 479, 481
Hippocrates, 149
Hispanics, mental health needs of, 409
Historical cohort studies, 164
Historical perspectives, of faith community nursing, 513–514
History
  of American Red Cross (ACR), 20
  of community health nursing, 15–32
  of evidence-based practice, 171–172
  of infectious diseases, 456–458
  milestone, in public health, 17, 17t, 25t, 27–28t
HIV antibody test, 481
Holistic health centers, historical perspectives of, 513
Holistic/wholistic care
  in faith and community nursing practice, 516, 516f
  in parish nursing model, 511–512
Holoendemic, definition of, 261
Home care, 525
  legal issues with, 117
Home health, 352
Home health agencies, 527, 527f, 528b
Home health and hospice, 524–539, 537b
  definition of, 524–525
  direct and indirect care, 529–530
  of dying child, 529
  Healthy People 2020 in, 535, 535b
  history of, 525–526
  infection control standards for, 530b
  legal and ethical issues in, 535
  levels of prevention in, 525b
  nursing roles in, 530–531, 531b, 532
  population-focused, 526–527
  quality and safety education for nurses in, 526b
  reimbursement mechanisms, 534–535
  transitional care in, 527
  universal precautions in, 530b
Home health and nursing
  accountability and quality management of, 533–534
  history of, 525–526
  interprofessional collaboration in, 532–533, 533b

Home health care, 525
  history of, 26, 31
Home visits, for family health risks, 323–327
  advantages and disadvantages of, 323
  process of, 323–327, 323t
    in-home phase in, 325–326, 325b, 326f
    initiation phase in, 323–324
    postvisit phase in, 326–327
    previsit phase in, 324–325
    termination phase in, 326
  purpose of, 323
Home-based primary care, 527
Homebound, school nursing and, 555
Homeland Security Act of 2002, 238
Homeless person, 397
  adolescents, 399
  effect of, on health, 397–398
  older adults, 399
  pregnant woman, 398
  with serious mental illness, 407–408
Homelessness, 392–414
  at-risk populations and, 398–399
  case example for, 396b
  concept of, 396–399, 396b
  levels of prevention related to, 409
  as vulnerable population, 361, 361f
Homicide, 436–437
Honor Society of Nursing, Sigma Theta Tau
    International, 171, 175b
Horizontal transmission, 459
Hormone replacement therapy, for menopause, 348
Hospice, 352
  accountability and quality management of,
    533–534
  definition of, 528
  of dying child, 529
  Healthy People 2020 in, 535, 535b
  interprofessional collaboration in, 532–533,
    533b
  legal and ethical issues in, 117, 535
  models, 526
  philosophy of care, 528, 529b
  reimbursement mechanisms, 534–535
Hospice nurse, 528–529
Hospital Compare, 39
Hospital-based agencies, as home health agencies,
    528
Host factor, transmission of communicable
    diseases, 458–459
Hosts
  in epidemiological triangle, 88, 155, 155b, 155f
  in occupational health epidemiological triad,
    564–565, 564f
House of Representatives, 106
House-call programs, 527
"How to" boxes
  apply case management strategies, 411b
  assess socioeconomic problems resulting from
    substance abuse, 425b
  assess workers and workplace, 574, 574b
  on building professional, community, and
    client partnerships, 388b
  conduct a sentinel evaluation, 286b
  determine the relative safety of a drug for
    personal or client use, 424b
  determine usefulness of websites, 214b
  develop program plans, 267–268b
  develop protocol, 176b

"How to" boxes (*Continued*)
  do program evaluation, 274b
  evaluate the concept of homelessness, 396b
  gather disaster information, 249b
  help families complete a family health history,
    318b
  identify community systems, 205b
  identify key informants, 213b
  intervene with vulnerable populations, 369b,
    370b
  making an appointment with the family, 302b
  obtain a quick community assessment, 214b
  plan for the assessment process, 302b
  prepare for the home visit and initiation phase,
    324b
  prevent infectious diseases in home, 463b
  promote interactions between the teen mother
    and her baby, 396b
  Red Cross, 240b
  set up community-based activities aimed at
    substance abuse prevention, 423b
  tuberculin skin test, 490b
HSPD 21: Public Health and Medical Preparedness,
    and *National Health Security Strategy*
    (NHSS), 238
Human abuse, 433–454
Human capital, 130, 359
Human Genome Project, 150
Human immunodeficiency virus (HIV), 462t,
    479–482
  among criminal offenders, 156b
  epidemiology and surveillance of, 480–481, 481f
  Healthy People 2020 and, 478–479, 479b
  incubation period of, 479
  in migrant farmworkers, 384
  natural history of, 479–480
  symptoms, transmission, and emergence of, 462t
  test counseling, 493–494
  testing for, 481
  transmission of, 480, 480b
  in vulnerable populations, 358, 366
Human papillomavirus infection
  genital warts and, 483–484t, 486–487
  symptoms, transmission, and emergence of,
    462t
Human rights, in cultural competence, 74
Human-made disasters, 236, 405
Hurricane Katrina, 246
Hydrophobia, 472
Hygiene. *see also* Handwashing.
  history of public health, 16, 18f
Hyperendemic, definition of, 261
Hypertension, adults and, 345, 345b
Hypothermia, in homeless persons, 399

I

"I PREPARE" mnemonic, 91, 91b
Iatrogenic drug reactions, in adults, 344–345
Illegal aliens, 66, 67
Illegal drugs, as bad drugs, 416
Illicit drugs
  amphetamines and methamphetamines as,
    421–422
  cocaine as, 421
  marijuana as, 422
  opioids as, 421
  street drugs as, 422
  use of, 421–422, 427

Illnesses
  focus, 1, 2–3t
  occupational injuries and, types of, 566, 567f
Immigrants. *see also* Migrant health.
  health issues in, 66–68
  unauthorized, 67
Immobility, in adults, 344–345
Immunity, natural, host factors and, 458
Immunization
  childhood schedule, 465
  on *Healthy People 2020,* 505
  measles, 465–466
  police powers requiring, 106
  policies for, case study on, 114b
  prevention strategies for adults and, 349b
  as prevention target area for children, 342
  as primary prevention, 156
  for program management, 267, 269f
Impact, aspects of program evaluation, 274, 274b
Implementation
  in case management nursing process, 225t
  in community-focused nursing process, 216
Impotence, 350
Incarcerated adults, 350
Incest, 444
Incidence proportion, 152
Incidence rate, 152
Incident commander, 507
Incineration, of waste products, 97
Incontinence, in adults, 344–345
Incubation period
  definition of, 459
  of human immunodeficiency virus infection,
    479
Indicators approach, 268t
Indirect care, in home health and hospice,
    529–530
Individualized education plans (IEPs), 542
Individualized health plans (IHPs), 542
Individuals
  practice focusing on, 10–12
  private support and, 141
Indoor air quality, 92–93
Industrial hygienists, 97, 97b
Industrial nursing, 20, 561
Industrial revolution, 16
Industrialization, in public health, 16
Infant care, teaching teens on, 404
Infant mortality ratio, definition and example of,
    154t, 155
Infants
  developmental considerations in, injuries and
    accidents and, 337
  health care in rural areas for, 377–378
  sudden infant death syndrome and, 340
Infectious agents
  transmission of communicable diseases, 458
  types of, 261b
Infectious disease
  deaths caused by, 457
  disease development of, 459
  diseases of travelers, 474–475
  emerging, 461–462, 461t
  epidemiology work on, 150
  foodborne. *see* Foodborne diseases.
  Healthy People 2020 objectives related to, 457,
    458b
  history of, 27

Infectious disease (*Continued*)
  list of reportable diseases in, 460–461
  modes of transmission of, 459
  parasitic, 472–474, 473t
  prevention and control of, 455–477, 475b
  spectrum of, 459–460
  vaccine-preventable, 465–468
  vector-borne, 470–472
  waterborne, 468–470, 468b
Infectivity, 458, 458b
  definition of, 261b
Inflation, rate of, 126
Influenza, 467–468, 467b
  pandemic of 1918, 21
  symptoms, transmission, and emergence of, 462t
  vaccines for, 467–468
Influenza A H5N1 virus, 462t
Informal groups, 196
Informant interviews, during community assessment, 212
Informatics, competency definition of, 11b
Informing role in advocacy, 230, 230b, 231b, 232b
In-home phase, in home visits, 323t, 325–326, 325b
Initiation phase, in home visits, 323–324, 323t
Injection drug users, as high-risk group, for alcohol, smoking, and other drug (ATOD) problems, 427
Injuries, 336–339, 337t
  childhood, prevention of, 547
  occupational, illnesses and, types of, 566, 567f
  prevention of, 338–339, 338b
  sports and, 336
  unintentional, 336
Insecticides
  dangers of, 85
  exposure to, 85
Instability, in adults, 344–345
Institute of Medicine (IOM)
  on environmental health, 86
  goals for evidence-based practice (EBP), 170
  on priorities for public health, 501
  quality of health care and, 38–39
Institutional model, parish nursing model, 511–512, 511b
Instructive district nursing, 18
Insurance, in family, access of, 319–320
Integrative review, 174
Integrator of faith and health, in faith communities, 520
Integrity, definition of, 57–58
Intensity, 130–131
  technology and, 136–137, 137t
Interdependent, community and, 205
Interfaith Health Program of the Carter Center, 513b, 518–519
Intermittent source outbreak, 261
International Classification of Diseases (ICD), secular trends and, 161
International organizations, 110
International Parish Nurse Resource Center (IPNRC), 514
International relief efforts, 250
International relief workers, delayed stress reactions, 250
Interpretation, in continuous quality improvement program, 287f, 288–289

Interpreter, selecting and using, guidelines for, 68b
Interprofessional collaboration, in home health and nursing, 526, 532–533, 533b
Interracial families, 69
Interstate Nurse Licensure Compact, 116
Intervention activities, in community-focused nursing process, 216
Intervention Wheel, 179
Interventions
  description in evidence-based practice studies, 177
  typology for classifying by level scientific evidence, 176t
Interview, informant, during community assessment, 212
Interviewing, motivational, 188–189, 188b
Intestinal parasitic infections, 473
Intimate partner violence, 445–447, 446b, 447b
  process of response to, 445
  sexual abuse in, 446
  signs of, 445
  during teen pregnancy, 402–403
Invasiveness, 458, 458b
Iron deficiency, during pregnancy, 403–404

J

Judicial law, 115
"Just say no" approach, 424, 427
Justice, principle for case managers, 233

K

Key informant, 268t
Knowledge, in public health nursing, 508b
Knowledge, skills, and attitudes (KSAs)
  in case management, 227b
  in evidence-based practice (EBP) example, 178b
  informatics to improve, 168b
Krokodil, as street drug, 422
Kübler-Ross, Elisabeth, 526, 528

L

Land, environmental health assessment of, 94
Landfilling, of waste products, 97
Language barriers
  in immigrants, 67
  for migrant health care, 384
Latent syphilis, 485
Law(s), 122b, 105–124. *see also* Legislation.
  bills and, 118f, 119
  common, 115
  constitutional, 115
  definition of, 106, 114
  federal legislation, examples of, 343
  health care and, 114–115
  judicial, 115
  legislation and, 115
  regulation and, 115, 119f
  specific to nursing practice, 115–116
    professional negligence in, 116, 116b
    scope of practice in, 115–116
Lawful permanent residents, 66–67
Lead exposure, reduction of, 97, 98b
Lead-based paint poisoning
  in children, 85, 85f
  multidisciplinary approach to, 88–89
Leadership
  democratic, 198
  patriarchal, 198

Learning
  affective domain in, 184
  barriers, 192–194
  case study on domains of, 185b
  cognitive, affective and psychomotor domains in, 184
  cultural, age and ethnic considerations in, 190–191
  definition of, 184
  example format of, 187b
  nature of, 184–185
  psychomotor domain in, 184–185
Legal immigrants, 66–67
Legal issues
  affecting health care practices, 117
    correctional health in, 117
    home care and hospice in, 117
    occupational health in, 117
    school and family health in, 117
  in faith community nursing, 518
  liability issues in case management, 232–234, 233b
  older adults and, 344
Legionella pneumophila, 462t
Legislation, 115
  federal, examples of, 343
  Occupational Safety and Health Act, 574
  for older adults, 344
  related to adult health, 343–344
  Sheppard-Towner Act, 108, 109b
  state nurse practice act and, 115
  tips for action, 120b
Legislative action, 119–121
Legislative staff, 119
Legislators, 119
  visits with, tips for, 120b
  writing to, tips for, 120b
Length of follow-up, 177
Lesbian, gay, bisexual, and transgendered (LGBT) families, as vulnerable population, 328–329
"Let's Move!" campaign, 335–336
Level of scientific evidence, typology for classifying interventions by, 176t
Levels of prevention
  for cardiovascular disease, 167b
  in epidemiology, 156
  for infectious diseases, 463b
  for mental illness, 409–410, 410b
  for obesity, 297b
  for pesticide exposure, 380b
  program planning and evaluation, 273b
  in public health, 11b
  for quality management, 289b
  related to case management, 231b, 232b
  in strategies for prevention related to families, 328b
  using evidence-based practice, 177b
  using health education, 187b
  for vulnerable populations, 366–367, 367b
Liability, issues in case management, 232, 233b
Liberal democratic theory, 55b
Libertarian theory, 55b
Liberty Mutual Insurance Company, case management principles and conditions, 228, 228b
Lice, screening children for, 551
Licensure
  in approaches to quality improvement, 280
  requirements for, 115–116

Life care plans, in case management, 228, 228b
Life cycle theory, developmental and, for families, 299–300, 300b, 300t
Life expectancy, 345
Life span, health risks across, 333–356, 353b
    adolescents, 337–338
    in adults, 344–350
        cancer as, 346–347
        cardiovascular disease as, 345
        chronic disease as, 345–347
        diabetes as, 346
        health status indicators and, 345
        hypertension as, 345, 345b
        mental illness as, 346
        stroke as, 346
        weight control and, 347
    among special groups of adults, 350–351
        adults of color, 350
        incarcerated adults, 350
        lesbian and gay, 350
        with physical and mental disabilities, 350–351
    children, 334
        acute illnesses, 340
        alterations of behavior and mental health problems as, 339
        chronic health conditions as, 340–341
        injuries and accidents as, 336–339, 337t, 338b
        maltreatment as, 339
        obesity as, 334–336, 334t, 335b, 336t, 337b
    effects of poverty and health across, 394–396
    infants, 337
    mental illness across, 404–405
    preschoolers, 337
    school-age children, 337
    toddlers, 337
Life-cycle stages, family health risk and, 315, 315t
Lifestyle
    family health risks in, 321–322, 322b, 322f
        assessment of, 322–323
    in migrant population, 382–383
    and prevention of obesity in children, 335–336, 335b
Linguistically appropriate health care, 365
Literacy levels, low, 192
Living will, 343
Local health departments, 113–114
Local public health agencies, 499–500
    functions, 500b
Local system, health care systems and, 42–43
Longitudinal study. *see* Prospective cohort study.
Long-term care, 352–353
Long-term evaluation, of behavioral and health education, 195
Low-birth-weight, with teen pregnancy, 402
Lyme disease, 456, 459f, 470–471, 471b
Lysergic acid diethylamide (LSD), as street drug, 422, 547

M

Macrosystems, 301, 301f
"Mad cow disease," 456
Mainstream smoke, 419
Maintenance functions, in groups, 196
Maintenance norms, 197
Maintenance specialist role, in group, 197b
Malaria, 474
    history of, 16
Malpractice, defined, 116

Malpractice lawsuit, 283–284
Managed care, 39, 141
    for mental health, 405–406
Managed care arrangements, private support and, 141–142, 142b
Managed care organizations (MCOs), 277
Marijuana, 422
Marine Hospital service, 16–17
Marital rape, 438
Master's prepared nurses, 517
Material safety data sheet (MSDS), 94, 575
Mature minors doctrine, 338
McIver, Pearl, 24
Means testing, 136
Measles, 207, 207b, 465–466
    outbreak of, Centers for Disease Control and Prevention and, 111
Mechanical agents, in occupational health epidemiological triad, 564f, 565b, 566, 567f
Media, violence and, 435
Mediator, nurse advocates as, 229
Medicaid, 37, 106–107, 128, 139–140, 139f
    Centers for Medicare and Medicaid Services (CMS) and, 3–4, 107, 113
    in community resources, 329–330
    for families with limited resources, 319–320
    history of, 363
    non-qualification for, 394
Medical Reserve Corps (MRC), 241–242
Medical savings accounts, private support and, 142
Medical technology, 130–131
Medicare, 106–107, 136, 138–139, 139f
    Balanced Budget Act and, 526
    Centers for Medicare and Medicaid Services (CMS) and, 3–4, 107, 113
    comparison with, 535t
    Outcomes and Assessment Information Set (OASIS), 534, 534f
    prescription drug benefit policy and, 121
Medication, in school, school nursing and, 550
Medline, 174
Men
    alcohol and, 418
    health concerns of, 348–350
        cancers as, 349–350
        erectile dysfunction as, 350
    young, paternity and, 401, 401f
Menopause, as women's health concern, 348
Mental health, 404–405
    community mental health centers (CMHCs), 406
    levels of prevention related to, 410b
    in rural *versus* urban populations, 378–379
    sources of information and help for, 409b
    and stress due to terror and disasters, 404–405
Mental illness, 392–414
    across life span, 404–405
    in adolescents, 339
    in adults, 346
    at-risk populations for, 406–409
        adults, 407
        adults with serious mental illness, 407–408
        children and adolescents, 406–407
        cultural diversity, 409
        older adults, 408–409
    in children, 339
    definition and statistics in U.S., 404–409
    deinstitutionalization, 406

Mental illness (*Continued*)
    impact of, 405
    levels of prevention related to, 409
    prevalence rate for, 346
    school nursing and, 551
    sources of information and help for, 409b
Meperidine, 421
Mercury-containing products, reducing use of, 101
Mesosystems, 301, 301f
Meta-analysis, 174
Methadone, 421
    maintenance programs for, 428
Methamphetamines, 421–422
Methylmercury, 101
Metropolitan, micropolitan *versus,* 375
Metropolitan Life Insurance Company, 21, 526
Mexican population, cultural considerations to, 385
Mexican-born immigrants, 66
Micropolitan, metropolitan *versus,* 375
Microsystems, 301, 301f
Migrant and seasonal farmworkers (MSFWs), 382
    resources for nurses in, 388b
Migrant farmworkers
    characteristics of, 380–382
    children of, 384–385
    definition of, 382
    health care needs and risks of rural, 381t
    housing for, 383–384
    lifestyle of, 382–383
Migrant health, 374–391
    characteristics of, 376
    cultural considerations in, 385–386
    issues in, 383–384
    pesticide exposure in, 379, 379b
Migrant Health Act, 383–384
Migrant health centers, 383–384
Minnesota Department of Public Health, 179
Minnesota Model of Public Health, 257
Minority populations
    mental health needs of, 409
    migrant farmworkers as, 380–385
Mitigation, disaster management of, 239, 239b
Mixed outbreak, 261
Mobile health clinics, 380
Mobilizing for Action through Planning and Partnership (MAPP), 209, 260–261, 270, 270b
Monitoring, environmental standards, 100
Moral distress, definition of, 49–50
Morality
    ethics and, 50
    moral character and, 50–51
Morbidity, as basic concept in epidemiology, 151–155
Morbidity and Mortality Weekly Report (MMWR), 111
Morbidity data, for surveillance, 257
Morphine, 421
Mortality, as basic concept in epidemiology, 151–155
Mortality data, for surveillance, 257
Mortality rates, as basic concept in epidemiology, 153–155, 154t
Motivational interviewing, 188–189, 188b
Motor vehicle accidents, 336
    adolescents and, 337–338
    infants and, 337
    in rural populations, 377
Moulder, Betty, 561

Multifactorial etiology, of diseases, 149
Mushrooms, as street drug, 422
My Health Companion (MHC), 377

N

Narrative review, 174
Nation, health of, 312
National Advisory Council for Nursing Education
    and Practice (NACNEP), 111
National Assessment of Adult Literacy (NAAL), 192
National Association of School Nurses (NASN),
    school nurses and, 543, 543b
National Center for Chronic Disease Prevention
    and Health Promotion, 210
National Center for Farmworker Health, Inc.
    (NCFH), 388b
National Center for Health Statistics, 159
National Environmental Education Act, 99–100b
National Environmental Policy Act (NEPA),
    99–100b
National Environmental Public Health Tracking
    Network, 89–90
National Guideline Clearinghouse, 175b
National Health and Nutrition Examination
    Survey (NHANES), 159
National Health Interview Survey (NHIS), 159
National Health Security Strategy (NHSS), of
    HSPD 21: Public Health and Medical
    Preparedness, 238
National Healthcare Quality and Disparities
    Report, 503–504
National Hospital Discharge Survey (NHDS), 159
National Incident Management System (NIMS),
    245, 245b
National Institute for Occupational Safety and
    Health (NIOSH), 561, 575, 575b
National Institute of Nursing Research (NINR),
    26–27, 108, 112
National Institutes of Health (NIH), 106–107, 112
National League for Nursing (NLN), 25–26
National Notifiable Disease Surveillance System,
    111
National notifiable diseases, 258–259, 258–259b
National Organization for Public Health Nursing
    (NOPHN), 20
National Preparedness Goal, 238
National Preparedness Guidelines (NPG), 238
National Prevention, Health Promotion, and
    Public Health Council, 3
National Prevention and Health Promotion
    Strategy, 3
National Response Framework, 238, 244–245
National Rural Health Association (NRHA),
    resources for nurses in rural and migrant
    populations, 388b
Native Alaskans
    health care needs and risks of rural, 381t
    mental health needs of, 409
Native Americans
    health care needs and risks of rural, 381t
    mental health needs of, 409
Natural disasters, 237
Natural history of disease, 156
Natural immunity, 458
Needs assessment
    definition of, 266, 266b
    develop a program plan, 267–268b
    in educational process, 185, 185b

Negative predictive value, 159
Neglect
    in childhood linked to adult health and mental
        health, 406
    in children, 444
    in older adults, 344, 447
    school nursing and, 551
Negligence, professional, 116, 116b
Negligent referrals, in case management, 233b
Negotiating, in conflict management, 231–232
Neighborhood poverty, 394
Neonatal mortality rate, 154t
Neuman Systems Model, in family health,
    312–313
Neural tube defects, preconceptual counseling
    and, 347–348
NHSS. *see* The National Health Security Strategy.
Nicotine, 418
    electric delivery systems for, 419–420
Nicotine gum, 429
Nicotine inhalers, 429
Nicotine nasal spray, 429
Nicotine patches, 429
Nicotine replacement therapy, 429
Nightingale, Florence, 50–51
    early epidemiology work by, 149
    on environmental health, 86
    role in history of nursing, 17
    work in community of Crimea, 203–204
Noncitizens, in United States, 66
Nonconcurrent cohort, 163t
Noncontingency contract, 327
Noncustodial parents, 395
Non-English-speaking refugees, challenges and
    barriers in, 68
Nonfarm residency, 375
Nongonococcal urethritis (NGU), 483–484t, 485
Nonimmigrants, 67
Nonmaleficence
    ethical principle of, 54, 54b
    principle for case managers, 233
Nonpoint sources, of air pollution, 92
Nontraditional healing practices, 67
Nonverbal communication, cultural variations in,
    70–71, 70t
Norms, 197
North American Industry Classification System
    (NAICS), 571
Nurse
    examining their beliefs regarding vulnerable
        groups, 393b
    levels of prevention for mental illness, 409–410,
        410b
    political activities and, 120
    quality and safety education for, 57b, 410b
    role of
        in policy process, 117–122
        to poor, homeless, mentally ill people,
            410–412, 412b
Nurse practice act, 115
Nurse-client relationship, in rural and migrant
    health care, 385
Nurse-family partnership, 506b
Nursing. *see also* "How to" boxes.
    Code of Ethics for, 59–60
    defining advocacy role of, 229
    evidence-based practice (EBP). *see* Evidence-
        based practice (EBP) boxes.

Nursing (*Continued*)
    examining their beliefs regarding vulnerable
        groups, 393
    shifting paradigms to evidence-based practice
        (EBP), 172
Nursing: Scope and Standards of Practice (ANA,
    2010), 516
Nursing advocacy, 121–122
Nursing approaches, to family health risk
    reduction, 323–329
    contracting with families in, 327–328, 327t
    empowering families in, 328–329
    home visits in, 323–327, 323t, 324b, 325–326b,
        325b, 326f
Nursing homes, 353
Nursing interventions, family health risks and,
    314–323
Nursing practice, 498–509
Nursing process
    advocacy and, 229t
    case management and, 224, 225f
    community-focused. *see also* Community
        assessment.
        assessment process. *see* Community
            assessment.
    evaluation of, 217, 217f
    goals and objectives in, establishing,
        215–216
    implementation in, 216
    intervention activities in, identifying, 216
    outcomes of, 217
    overview of, 211–217
    problem analysis in, 215
    problem prioritizing in, 215
Nursing services, reimbursement for, 143
Nutrition, 72–73, 72b, 72t
    needs during teen pregnancy, 403–404, 403t
    and prevention of obesity in children, 335–336,
        335b
    as prevention target area for children, 342
Nutritional practices, 72–73
Nutting, Mary Adelaide, 20–21

O

Obesity
    in adults, 344–345, 347
        interventions for, 347
    in children, 334–336, 334t
        prevention of, recommendations for, 335b,
            336t, 337b
    faith community nursing and, 515b
    in family health risks, 321
    in rural populations, 377
Objectives
    establishing, in community-focused nursing
        process, 215–216
    levels of program, 272
    in program planning process, 271
    specifying, 271–272
OBQI outcome paradigm, 534, 534f
Observational studies, epidemiologic, 165
Obsessive-compulsive disorder, 405
Obstructers, 230
Occupational and environmental health nursing,
    definition and scope of, 561
Occupational health
    Healthy People 2020 related to, 574, 574t
    in legal issues, 117

Occupational health (*Continued*)
    legislation related to, 574–575, 574b, 575b
    problems in rural areas, 379–380
Occupational health hazards
    assessment by occupational health nurses, 571
    Bloodborne Pathogens Standard and, 575
    Hazard Communication Standard and, 575
    workplace, 571
    work-related, categories of, 564, 565b
Occupational health history, assessment of, 570, 572f
Occupational health nurse, 560–578, 576b
    case study, 574b
    disaster planning and management and, 575–576
    epidemiologic model application of, 564–568, 564f, 565b
    history and evolution of, 561
    onsite programs for, 569–570, 569b
    promotion of worker health and safety, organizational and public efforts for, 569–570
    roles and professionalism in, 561–562
    ten job roles for, 562
    worker assessment by, 570–571, 572f, 574b
    workers as population aggregate, 562–564
    working populations, nursing care of, 570–574, 570b
    workplace assessment by, 571–574, 573f, 574b
Occupational health nursing, 20
    definition and scope of, 561
    history and evolution of, 561
Occupational Safety and Health Act, 99–100b, 561, 563, 569, 574, 575
Occupational Safety and Health Administration (OSHA), 110, 561, 574–575, 575b
Office of Homeland Security, 114
Official health agencies, 24
Older adults
    abuse of, 447–448, 447b
    disaster stress responses in, 247, 247b
    as high-risk group, for alcohol, smoking, and other drug (ATOD) problems, 426–427
    homeless, 399
    mental illness in, 408–409
    poverty and health care in, 395
    Program of All-Inclusive Care for the Elderly (PACE), 527
    in rural environments, 387
    substance abuse in, 408
Older Americans Act, 343
Omaha System, 531–532, 532f
Opioids, 421
Opium, 421
Opportunistic infections, of parasitic diseases, 473–474
Oral rehydrating therapy (ORT), 157
Organizational cultures, 568
Organizations, influencing health, 110–114
Osteoporosis
    prevention for, 348
    as women's health concern, 348
Outbreak, 261
Outbreak detection, 261
Outbreak investigation, 261–262
    conduct, 262b
    defining magnitude of event in, 261
    objectives of, 261–262
    patterns of occurrence in, 261
    when to investigate, 262

Outcome
    in case management nursing process, 225t
    community health, 207
    in continuous quality improvement program, 287f, 288, 288b
    in evidence-based practice studies, 177
    in quality assurance measure, 285, 286t
    statements in program management, 272
Outcomes and Assessment Information Set (OASIS), 534, 534f
Outreach workers, 500
Over-the-counter (OTC) drugs, as good drugs, 416
Overweight. *see also* Obesity.
    adults as, 347
    children as, 334, 334t
    faith community nursing and, 515b
Oxycodone, 421

P

Pacific Islander Americans, mental health needs of, 409
Palliative care, definition of, 526
Pan American Health Organization, 110
Pandemic, definition of, 261, 460
Pandemic and All-Hazards Preparedness Reauthorization Act (PAHPRA), 238
Panic disorder, 405
Papanicolaou (Pap) smears, 157, 158
Parasites, causing malaria, 474
Parasitic diseases, 472–474
    opportunistic infections of, 473–474
Parish nurses
    definition of, 511
    education of, 516–517
    functions of, 520–522
    interventions and activities, examples of, 520b
Parish nursing
    case study of, 519b
    definition of, 510
    in faith community nursing, 511, 511b
    historical perspectives of, 513
    philosophy of, 514–515
    resources for, 513b
Participant observation, 212
Partner notification, 494
Partner pressure, teen pregnancy and, 400
Partnerships
    communities, 209–210
    definition of, 209
    nurse-family, 506b
    in parish nursing model, 511–512
    principles of, 499b
Passive immunization, 458
Passive participation, 209
Passive surveillance system, 260
Pastoral care staff, 511–512
Paternity, 401, 401f
Pathogenicity, 458, 458b
    definition of, 261b
Patient oriented evidence that matters (POEM), 177
Patient Protection and Affordable Care Act, 31, 34, 106–107, 503–504, 555
    health reform for American families, 306
Patient Safety Act of 1997, 120–121
Patient Self-Determination Act of 1990, 343
Patriarchal leadership, 198

Paying health care organizations, 142–143
Peacemaker role, in groups, 197b
Pedagogy, definition of, 190–191
Peer pressure, teen pregnancy and, 400
Pelvic inflammatory disease (PID), 482, 483–484t
Penicillin, history of, 24
Permitting process, in controlling pollution, 99–100
Persistent bioaccumulative toxins (PBTs), 101
Persistent organic pollutants (POPs), 101
Persistent poverty, 394
    homelessness and, 397
Person, in descriptive epidemiology, 160–161
Personal health counselor, in faith communities, 520
Personal Responsibility and Work Opportunity Reconciliation Act, 343–344
Personal safety, in community practice, 217–218
Perspectives on the program, 268
Pertussis, 466–467
Pesticides
    children and, 85
    exposure, risks to rural health, 379, 379b
    on food, 95–96, 96f
Philosophy of care, of hospice, 528, 529b
Phobias, 405
Physical activity
    faith community nursing and, 515b
    for hypertension, 345
    recommendations for child obesity prevention, 335–336, 335b
    for reducing family health risks, 321
Physical agents, in occupational health epidemiological triad, 564f, 565b, 567–568
Physical dependence, defined, 417
Physical environment, family health and, 315b
Physical examinations, school nursing and, 550
Physical neglect, 444
"PICOT" format, for evidence-based practice (EBP), 173–174
PL 93-112 Section 504 of the Rehabilitation Act of 1973, 541
PL 94-142 Education for All Handicapped Children Act, 541
PL 105-17 Individuals with Disabilities Education Act (IDEA), 542
PL 114-95 Every Student Succeeds Act (ESSA), 542
Place, in descriptive epidemiology, 161
Planned Approach to Community Health (PATCH), 210, 270, 270b
Planning, in case management nursing process, 225t
Planning process, 266
    definition of community health program, 266–270
Playground safety, guidelines for, 338–339, 338b
Pneumocystis jiroveci, 462t
Point epidemic, 161–162
Point source outbreak, 261
Point sources, of air pollution, 92
Police power, 106
Policy
    definition of, 106
    development of, as public health core function, 5, 8
        process of, 9b
        process of, nurse's role in, 117–122

Policy activism, 105–124, 122b
Policy development, ethical principles of, 58
Policy issue, in nurses, for draft legislation and
    provide testimony, 321
Polio, 465
Politics
    definition of, 106
    nursing advocacy and, 121–122
Polity, in faith community nursing, 517
Pollution Prevention Act (PPA), 99–100b
Polysubstance use or abuse, 424
Polyvinyl chloride (PVC) plastics, 101
Population
    defining in field of epidemiology, 151b
    defining in public health nursing, 7
    demographic trends and, 35
    of interest in evidence-based studies, 176
    violence and, 436
Population health, 3
Population-centered nursing practice, definition
    of, 206
Population-focused home care, 526–527
Population-focused nursing practice, 5–9, 8b
    defined, 8
Population-focused services, 10
Positive predictive value, 159
Postneonatal mortality rate, 154t
Posttraumatic stress disorder (PTSD), 405
    in veterans, 363
Postvisit phase, in home visits, 323t, 326–327
Poverty, 392–414
    definition of, 393–396
    factors contributing to U.S., 394
    in family health risks, 319
    federal poverty guideline for, 361
    homelessness and, concept of, 396–399
    as indicator, of community health status, 207,
        207b
    levels of prevention, 409
    life span, effects across the, 394–396
    neighborhood and persistent, 394
    violence and, 436
    vulnerability causing, 361
Precaution Adoption Process Model (PAPM),
    193–194
Precautionary Principle, 85, 85b
Precedent, 115
Preconceptual counseling, 347–348
Predictive value negative, 159
Predictive value positive, 159
Preferred provider organizations (PPOs),
    141–142, 142b
Pregnancy
    abuse during, 446
    case study regarding migrant health care,
        386b
    drug use during, 427
    homelessness and, 398
    teenagers, school nursing and, 555
    trends in, 399–404
Pregnancy Risk Assessment Monitoring System
    (PRAMS), 159
Prejudice, 79, 79b
Preschoolers, developmental considerations for,
    injuries and accidents and, 337
Prescription drug benefit policy, 121
Presidential Policy Directive 8: National
    Preparedness (PPD-8), 238

Prevention
    of alcohol, tobacco, and other drug (ATOD)
        problems
        primary, 423–425, 425b
            drug education in, 423–425, 424b
            levels of, 424b
        secondary, 425–428
            drug testing in, 426
        tertiary, 428–429
            addiction treatment in, 428–429
            detoxification in, 428
            smoking cessation programs in, 429
            support groups in, 429
    of diabetes, 346
    of infectious diseases, 463
    levels of, 61b, 502b
        for cardiovascular disease in women, 346b
        using health education, 187b
    levels using evidence-based practice (EBP),
        177b
    nurse and, 409–410
    of osteoporosis, 348
    of sexually transmitted diseases, 347
    stage of disaster management, 239, 239b
    strategies for adults, 349b
    target areas for children, 341–343
        environmental health hazards as, 342–343
        immunizations as, 342
        nutrition as, 342
        smoking as, 341–342
    Task Force on Community Preventative
        Services, 175b
    using health education, 187b
    in vulnerable populations, 366–367, 367b,
        368–369
Prevention-effectiveness analyses (PEAs), 130
Prevention-oriented practice, 1–14
Preventive interventions, levels of, 156–157
Previsit phase, in home visits, 323t, 324–325
Primary care
    definition of, 34b, 39
    home-based, 527
Primary caregivers, in public health nurses,
    506
Primary health care (PHC), 33
    definition of, 34b
Primary infection, from human
    immunodeficiency virus, 479
Primary prevention
    case study of, 157b
    of communicable diseases, 491–493, 491b
    defining in epidemiology, 156
    of infectious diseases, 463, 463b
    of obesity, 297b
    program planning and evaluation, 273b
    in public health, 11b
    related to case management, 231b, 232b
    using evidence-based practice, 177b
    using health education, 187b
    for vulnerable populations, 366, 367b
Primary syphilis, 485
Primary-care system, 39
    public health and, 43–45
Principlism, 54, 56b
Problem analysis, in community-focused nursing
    process, 215
Problem prioritizing, in community-focused
    nursing process, 215

Problem solving
    advocacy and, 230–231, 231b
    problem-purpose-expansion method, 231, 231b
Problem-purpose-expansion method, 231, 231b
Process
    in continuous quality improvement program,
        287–288, 287f
    in quality assurance measure, 285, 286t
Process evaluation, of educational programs,
    194–195
Professional issues, in faith community nursing,
    517–518
Professional negligence, 116, 116b
Professional review organizations, on approaches
    to quality improvement, 285
Program, defining community health, 266
Program evaluation, 270–274, 274b
    aspects of, 273–274
    benefits of, 270–271
    case study of, 271b
    process of, 271, 271f
    sources of, 272–273
Program management, 265–275
    evaluation process, 271, 271f
    formulation of objectives, 271–272
    immunization case example, 267, 269f
    name the problem, 269
    needs assessment tool, 268, 268t
    nursing process *versus*, 265
    program planning, benefits of, 266
Program of All-Inclusive Care for the Elderly
    (PACE), 527
Program planning
    benefits of, 266
    case study, 271b
    definition of problem and need, 266–269
    developing of, 267–268b
    evaluate problem solutions, 270
    models for public health, 270
    objectives and activities for alternatives, 269
    solution, choosing the, 270
Program records, 272
Progress, aspects of program evaluation, 273,
    274b
Project BioShield, 246
Project DARE, 424
Promoter, nurse advocates as, 229
Propagated outbreak, 261
Proportionate mortality ratio, 154t, 155
Proportions, as basic concept in epidemiology,
    151–152
Propoxyphene, 421
Proprietary agencies, as home health agencies, 528
Prospective cohort study, epidemiologic, 163–164,
    163t
Prospective payment system, in home health and
    nursing, 526
Prospective reimbursement, 142
Prostate cancer, as men's health concern, 349
Prostate-specific antigen (PSA) test, 349
Provider service records, 290
Psychoactive drugs, 417–420
    alcohol as, 417–418
    caffeine as, 420, 420t
    tobacco as, 418–419, 418f, 419f
Psychological abuse, in older adults, 447
Psychological dependence, defined, 417
Psychomotor domain, of learning, 184–185

Psychosocial agents, in occupational health epidemiological triad, 564f, 565b, 568
Public health, 3–4, 98, 498–509
  from the 1970s to the present, 26–30
  Code of Ethics for, 60–61, 60b
  during Colonial and New Republic period, 16–17
  core function of, 4. *see also* Public health nursing core functions.
  definition of, 3, 34b
  during depression-era, 23
  early, 16
  essential services of, participation as public health nurse in, 6b
  evidence-based practice (EBP) nursing in, 179, 180t
  history and trends of, 500–501
  Intervention Wheel and, 179
  levels of prevention in, 11b
  milestone, in history, 17, 17t, 25t, 27–28t
  mission of, 4
  nurses in, 502b
  prevention measures in, 3
  primary goal of, 7
  primary-care system and, 43–45
  scopes, standards, and roles of nursing in, 501–502
  in United States, 4f
Public health economics, 126–127
Public health nurses, 206, 501
  education requirements for, 504, 504b
  functions of, 505–508, 507b, 508b
  knowledge requirements for, 504, 504b
Public health nursing (PHN), 508b
  assessor of literacy in, 506
  changing roles in, 5–6
  Code of Ethics, 50–51
  versus community-oriented nursing, 6, 7b
  community-oriented nursing and, 1–2
  definition of, 2–3, 7, 12b
  goals of, 7
  history of, 6
  issues and trends in, 503–504
  process of, 7b
  specialty of, distinguishing of, 7b
Public health nursing core functions
  assessment as, 57–58
  assurance as, 58–59
  ethics and, 57–59
  policy development as, 58
Public Health Nursing Section (PHNS), 21
Public health professionals, core competencies for, 204, 204b
Public health programs, 498
Public Health Security and Bioterrorism Preparedness and Response Act, 107
Public health service (PHS), 16–17, 24f
  creation of, 106–107
Public health surveillance, 256
Public health system, 39, 42b
Public Health Threats and Emergencies Act (US Law, 2000), 107
Public policies, affecting vulnerable populations, 363–364
PubMed, 175b

Q

Quad Council of Public Health Nursing Organizations, in disease surveillance, 257

Quality, 276. *see also* Quality and Safety Education for Nurses (QSEN) boxes.
  Agency for Healthcare Research and Quality on, 279
  definitions of, 276, 279
  five groups and, 279
  Institute of Medicine on, 38–39, 279
  and nursing practice, 278–279
  staff review committees on, 284
Quality and Safety Education for Nurses (QSEN) boxes, 113b
  on client-centered care and education, 185b
  competencies in, 11b
  on cultural influences, in nursing, in community health, 80b
  as evidence-based practice example, 178b
  on informatics for targeted competency, 168b
  on migrant health care, 386b
  on quality care for vulnerable populations, 365b
  on quality improvement, 289b
  on teamwork and collaboration, 227, 227b
Quality assurance, 276
  case study on, 289b
  continuous quality improvement and, 277, 280b
  total quality management and, 277, 279–280
Quality improvement
  approaches to, 280–289
    accreditation in, 280–281
    certification in, 281
    credentialing in, 280
    customer and, 282, 282b
    Donabedian's model on, 285
    evaluative studies in, 285–286
    evidence-based practice on, 283b
    licensure in, 280
    professional review organizations in, 285
    risk management in, 285
    sentinel method in, 286, 286b
    staff review committees in, 284
    total quality management in, 282–286
    tracer method in, 285–286
    utilization review on, 284–285
  competency definition of, 11b
Quality improvement organization, 278

R

Rabies, 472
Race, 69, 69f
Racism, 79, 79b
Randomization, 177
Randomized controlled trial (RCT), definition of, 172
Rape, 437–439
  on college campuses, 438
  date, 438
  marital, 438
  prevention of, 438
  victims of, mental health services for, 439
Rapid needs assessment, 248
Rates
  adjustment of, 159–160
  as basic concept in epidemiology, 151–152
Rathbone, William, 18
Ratio, risk and, 152
Rationing health care, 129
Reality norms, 197

Reciprocity, 280
Recognition, 281
Records, for documentation, 289–290
Recovery, stage of disaster management, 250–251
Recycle, 97
Red Cross Rural Nursing Service, 374–375
Referral agent, in faith communities, 520
Referral resources, 506
  for environmental health, 101
Refugees
  definition of, 67
  non-English-speaking, challenges and barriers in, 68
Regulations, 115
  Code of regulations, 121
  nursing roles and, 530–531
  process of, 121
  writing of, 119f, 121
Regulatory action, 121
Rehabilitation, 352–353
Reimbursement system, for home health, 534–535
Relative risk, 164
Relevance, aspects of program evaluation, 273, 274b
Reliability, in screening, 158, 158b
Religion, organized, violence and, 435–436
Religiosity, 511
Replacement, 35
Reproductive health, women and, 347–348
Research
  federal government and, 108
  medical, domination of men in, 343
Research utilization, definition of, 171
Researcher, school nurses as, 545
Resilience
  family health and, 297
  of vulnerable populations, 358, 362
Resistance, of host factor, 458
Resource Conservation and Recovery Act (RCRA), 99–100b
Resources, for implementing evidence-based practice (EBP), 175b
Respect
  for autonomy, 54, 54b
  in public health code of ethics, 60
Respondeat superior, doctrine of, 116
Retrospective audit, 284
Retrospective cohort studies, epidemiologic, 163t, 164
Retrospective reimbursement, 142
Return on investment, 130
Reuse, 97
Risk assessment, in environmental health, 94–95
Risk communication, in environmental health, 98
Risk exposure, issues in case management, 233b
Risk factors, as indicator, of community health status, 207, 207b
Risk management, 97
  on approaches to quality improvement, 285
Risk sharing, between payers and providers, 227
Risks
  as basic concept in epidemiology, 151–152, 358
  cumulative, 358
  environmental health, 98
  relative, 164
Rockefeller Sanitary Commission, 21
Rocky Mountain Spotted Fever (RMSF), 471
Rogers, Lina, 20

Role model, in nurse, 506
Role structures, in groups, 197
Routinely collected data, 159
Rubella, 466
Rules of transformation, 316
Rural health, 374–391
    barriers to, 380b
    characteristics of rural life, 376b
    definition of, 375
    delivery issues and barriers to, 380
    Healthy People 2020 objectives regarding, 388–389, 388b
    needs and risks of select aggregates to, 381t
    nursing care in, 387, 387b, 388b
    pesticide exposure to, 379
    technology use in, 388–389
Rural populations
    characteristics and cultural considerations for, 376, 376b
    health status of, 376–379
    urban populations *versus,* 375–376
Rural-urban continuum, 375, 375f

S

Sackett, David, 172
Safe Drinking Water Act (SDWA, 99–100b
Safe Kids Campaign, 547
Safer sex, 492–493
Safety. *see also* Quality and Safety Education for Nurses (QSEN) boxes.
    competency definition of, 11b
    and managing quality, 276–293
    personal, in community practice, 217–218
    quality improvement and, 39
Safety net providers, 128–129
Salmon, Marla, 110
Salmonella infections, 457, 503
Salmonellosis, 469
Salvia, as street drug, 422
Same-sex couples, 329
Sample selection, to determine quality of evidence, 177
Sample size, to determine quality of evidence, 177
Sanitation
    early epidemiology work on, 149
    history of public health, 17
Scarlet fever, 21
Schizophrenia, 405–406
School, health practices in, legal issues with, 117
School Health Policies and Programs Study (SHPPS), 546
School maladaptation, in children and adolescents, 339
School nurses, 540–559, 556b
    educational credentials of, 543
    Healthy People 2020 and, 546, 546b
    online resources for, 556t
    quality and safety education for, 550b
    roles and functions of, 543–545, 544b, 547b
    standards of practice for, 543, 543b
School nursing, 20
    controversies in, 555
    definition of, 541
    ethics in, 555
    federal legislation in, 541–542, 542t
    federal school health programs and, 545–546, 545f
    future trends in, 555–556

School nursing (*Continued*)
    history of, 20, 541–542, 542t
    levels of prevention, 546–555, 547f
        primary prevention, 546–548, 546b
        secondary prevention, 548–552
        tertiary prevention, 552–555
    school health policies and practices study and, 546
    school-based health programs and, 546
School violence, 435
School-age children, developmental considerations for, injuries and accidents and, 337
School-based health centers (SBHCs), 546
School-based health programs, 546
Schooling, during teen pregnancy, 404
Scope and Standards of Parish Nursing Practice, 516
Scope and Standards of Public Health Nursing Practice
    ANAs, 30
    domain of core public health competencies, 504
Scope of practice, 115–116
Screening, 157–159
    characteristics of successful, 158b
    of children at school, 550
        for lice, 551
    reliability, 158, 158b
    sensitivity and specificity of, 158–159
    validity, 158–159, 158b
Secondary analysis, of community data, 213
Secondary healthcare services, Health Services Pyramid and, 5
Secondary prevention
    of child abuse, 297b
    defining in epidemiology, 157
    of infectious diseases, 463, 463b
    interventions at, 157
    program planning and evaluation, 273b
    in public health, 11b
    related to case management, 231b, 232b
    for sexually transmitted disease, 491b, 493–494, 494b
    using evidence-based practice, 177b
    using health education, 187b
    for vulnerable populations, 366, 367b
Secondary syphilis, 485
Secondhand smoke, 419, 419f
Secular changes, 161–162
Secular trends, 161
Sedentary lifestyle, high obesity risks and children and, 335, 335b
Selected membership group, 199
Self-care practices, cultural variations in, 70t
Self-determination, nurse advocates role in promoting, 231
Self-esteem, problem behaviors in children and, 339
Senate, 106
Senior centers, 352, 352f
Sensitivity, in screening, 158–159
Sentinel method, on quality improvement, 286, 286b
Sentinel surveillance system, 260
Series testing, 159
Serious mental illness
    adults with, 407–408, 408b
    caregiving issues with, 408–409
    homeless person with, 407–408

Service, as nursing value, 58
Set, drug user, 422
Setting, drug use and, 422
Setting for practice, community as, 1, 10, 205
Settlement houses, 18–19
Severe acute respiratory syndrome (SARS), 457, 462t, 501
Sexual abuse, 444–445
    history and teen pregnancy, 400–401
Sexual activity, teen pregnancy and, 400
Sexual assault, rates in rural and migrant health areas, 378
Sexual assault nurse examiner (SANE), 439
Sexual behavior, pregnancy and trends in, 399–404
Sexual debut, 400
Sexual victimization, 400–401
Sexual violence, 437–439
    cultural differences related to, 438–439
    emotional harm from, 438
    physical injuries from, 438
Sexually transmitted diseases (STDs), 480b, 482–487, 483–484t
    chlamydia, 483–484t, 485–486
    genital herpes, 483–484t, 486
    genital warts, 483–484t, 486
    gonorrhea, 482–485
    herpes simplex virus 2, 483–484t
    in homeless adolescent, 399
    human papilloma virus (HPV), 483–484t
    nongonococcal urethritis (NGU), 483–484t, 485
    nurse's role in providing preventive care for, 491–495, 491b
    partner notification, 494
    pelvic inflammatory disease (PID) in, 482
    prevention of, 347
    syphilis, 483–484t, 485, 485f
Sexually transmitted infections (STIs), evidence-based practice on, 156b
Shattuck Report, 17
Shelters
    in disaster situations, 249
    for homelessness, 396
Sheppard-Towner Act, 21–22, 108, 109b
Short-term evaluation, of behavioral and health education, 195
Side-stream smoke, 419
Skilled care, 530
Skills, in public health nursing, 508b
Sleep disorders, in children and adolescents, 339
Sleet (Scales), Jessie, 19
Smallpox, 464–465
    vaccinations for, 114
Smoking
    cessation programs for, 429
    evidence-based practice on laws regarding, 108b
    harm reduction model and, 416
    limiting, for osteoporosis, 348
    as prevention target area for children, 341–342
Snow, John, early epidemiology work on cholera by, 149, 149t
SNS. *see* Strategic National Stockpile.
Snuff, 419
Social change process, nurse's role and, 216
Social determinants, of health, 359–361, 360f
Social environment, family health and, 315b
Social isolation, family violence and, 441

Social justice, 365
  in cultural competence, 74
Social mandate, for health care, 222
Social organization, in cultural diversity, 71
Social risks, to family health, 319
Social Security Act, 24, 106–107, 363
Social Security Administration, disability defined
  by, 351
Socioeconomic status, 128
Sodium, excessive amount of, in family health
  risks, 321
Sources of error, in screening, 158
Sovereign immunity, 116
Space, in cultural diversity, 71
Special interest groups and, 122
Special needs, children with, school nursing and,
  553–555
Special Supplemental Nutrition Program for
  Women, Infants, and Children (WIC), 319–320
Special surveillance system, 260
Specificity
  in causal inference, 167b
  in screening, 158–159
Spice, as street drug, 422
Spina bifida, 340
Spiritual care, by faith community nurses, 516,
  516b, 516f
Spirituality, 511
Sporadic problems, 261
Spouse abuse, 445
Staff review committees, 284
Standard population, 160
Standard precautions, in preventive care for
  communicable disease, 494–495
Standards of Practice for Case Management,
  232–233
Staphylococcus aureus, 469t
State Children's Health Insurance Program
  (SCHIP), 37, 107, 329–330, 363
State health departments, 113–114
State notifiable diseases, 259–260
State nurse practice act, 115
State public health agency, 499
State system, health care system and, 42
Statistical associations, of causality, 166
Statute law, 115
Stereotyping, 78–79
Stewart, Ada Mayo, 20, 561
Stewart B. McKinney Homeless Assistance Act of
  1994, 396
Stimulants, 417
  detoxification for, 428
Strain, family caregiving and, 351
Strategic National Stockpile (SNS), 246
Strategic planning, definition of program, 266
Street drugs, 422
Streptococcus pneumoniae, 503
Streptococcus pyogenes, 456
Stress
  in childhood linked to adult health, 362
  family caregiving and, 351
  family stress theory in, 316
  management of, in family health risks, 321
  in migrant farmworkers, 382
  in migrant populations, 384
  related to terror and disasters, 405
  in rural *versus* urban populations, 378
  violence and, 434

Stroke, in adults, 344–345, 346
Structure
  in continuous quality improvement program,
    286–287, 287f
  in quality assurance measures, 285
Subpopulations, defined, 7
Substance abuse, 416
  case-control study of, adolescent suicides and,
    164, 164t
  in children and adolescents, 339
  defined, 417
  factors that contribute to, 416
  in family health risks, 322
  Healthy People 2020 and, 416, 426b
  and mental illness in adults, 407
  in older adults, 408
  teen pregnancy and, 400
  vulnerable populations and, 358, 363
Substance-abuse prevention education, school
  nursing and, 547
Suburbs, 376
Sudden infant death syndrome, 340
Suicide, 439–440
  adolescents and, 338
    case-control study of, substance abuse and,
      164, 164t
  and mental illness in adolescents and young
    adults, 406
  prevention of, 440
  school nursing and, 551
Summative evaluation, 266b
Sun protection, for skin cancer prevention,
  346–347
Superfund Amendments and Reauthorization Act
  (SARA), 99–100b
  on disaster plans in occupational health,
    575
Supplemental Nutrition Program for Women,
  Infants, and Children (WIC), 393–394
Support groups, for alcohol, tobacco, and other
  drug (ATOD) problems, 429
Supporters, 230
Supporting role in advocacy, 230
Surgeon General, 109
Surveillance, 255–264
  active system, 260
  collaboration among partners, 256–257
  of communicable diseases, 460–461, 460b
  data sources for, 257–258
  epidemiology and, of human immunodefi-
    ciency virus, 480–481, 481f
  features of, 256b
  interventions and protection via, 262, 262b
  for national notifiable diseases, 258–259,
    258–259b
  nurse competencies and, 257
  objective of, 258b
  passive system, 260
  purposes of, 256, 256b
  sentinel system, 260
  for state notifiable diseases, 259–260
  syndromic system, 260, 260b
  systems, types of, 260
Surveillance data, 159
Survey of existing agencies, 268t
Surveys, 268t
  to gather community data, 213–214
  windshield, 211, 213t

Sustainability, aspects of program evaluation, 274,
  274b
Syndromic surveillance system, 260, 260b
Syphilis, 207, 207b, 483–484t, 485, 485f
Syria, civil war in, 251–252
Systematic review, 174

T

Target of practice, community as, 205
Task Force on Community Preventative Services,
  175b, 177b
Task functions, in groups, 196
Task norm, 197
Task specialist role, in groups, 197b
TEACH mnemonic, 186b
Teach-back, definition of, 189
Teamwork
  and collaboration, in case management, 227b
  competency definition of, 11b
  in public health nursing, 508b
Technological trends, in health care system,
  36–37
Technology
  in environmental health, 87–88
  in home health and hospice, 536
  and intensity, 136–137, 137t
  use in rural health, 388–389, 389b
Teen pregnancy, 392–414
  early identification of, 402
  levels of prevention related to, 409
  prevention of, 306
  special issues in caring for, 402–404
    gynecological age, 403
    infant care, 404, 404b
    low birth weight, 402
    nutrition, 403–404, 403t
    schooling and educational needs, 404
    violence, 402–403
  and trends in sexual behavior, 399–404
Teenage mothers, school nursing and, 555
Telehealth/telemedicine, 226–227, 330, 388–389,
  536
Telehomecare, 330
  in home health and hospice, 536
Telemedicine, 330
Telemonitoring, in home health and hospice,
  536
Temporary Assistance for Needy Families (TANF)
  program, 7b, 319–320, 329–330, 343–344,
  364, 393–394
Termination phase, in home visits, 323t, 326
Terrorist attacks
  biological or chemical, 245
  stress responses following, 405
  on World Trade Center and Pentagon, 575
Tertiary healthcare services, Health Services
  Pyramid and, 5
Tertiary prevention
  of child abuse, 297b
  of infectious diseases, 463, 463b
  interventions at, 157
  program planning and evaluation, 273b
  in public health, 11b
  related to case management, 231b, 232b
  for sexually transmitted disease, 491b, 494–495
  using evidence-based practice, 177b
  using health education, 187b
  for vulnerable populations, 366, 367b

Testicular cancer, as men's health concern, 349–350

The Joint Commission (TJC), on disease management organizations, 227

The National Health Security Strategy (NHSS), 243–244

Third-party payers, 130

Three R's for Reducing Environmental Pollution, 97

Tick-borne diseases, 456, 471f

Time
  component of descriptive epidemiology, 161–162
  cultural perception variations regarding, 70t

Time perception, and cultural diversity, 71–72

Timelines of treatment, 233b

Tobacco
  electronic nicotine delivery systems and, 419–420, 420b
  as psychoactive drug, 418–419, 418f, 419f

Toddlers, developmental considerations for, injuries and accidents and, 337

Tolerance, to alcohol, 418

Tornadoes, 236–237

Total quality management (TQM), 282–286
  quality assurance and, 277, 279–280
  traditional management model and, 281t

Touch, cultural variations in, 70t

Toxic Substances Control Act (TSCA), 99–100b

Toxicity, 458, 458b

Toxicology, as environmental health science, 87–88, 87b

TOXNET, 87–88

Tracer method, 285–286

Tracking Network, 89–90

Traditional quality assurance, approaches to quality improvement, 281t, 283–285

Transitional care, in home, 527

Transitions, 315

Transmission, of human immunodeficiency virus, 480, 480b

Transtheoretical Model (TTM), 193–194

Trauma, in homeless population, 397–398

Travelers, diseases of, 474–475

Triage
  in occupational health disasters, 575–576
  process during disasters, 239

Tsunamis, 236

Tuberculosis, 489–491
  case study of, 462b, 491b
  history of, 16, 17t
  incidence as indicator, of community health status, 207, 207b
  in rural and migrant populations, 384
  screening for, school nursing and, 550
  skin test, 490, 490b, 490f

24-hour skilled care at home, 353

Typhoid, 21

U

Ultraviolet rays, reduce exposure to, 97

Unauthorized immigrants, 67

Underage drinking, 426

Unemployment, violence and, 434

Unhealthy event, 313

Uninsured persons, access to health care and, 38

Uninsured population, vulnerability of, 361

Unintentional injuries, 336

United Nations, as source of data, 109t

United States, health care in, 34

Urban populations
  characteristics and cultural considerations for, 376
  rural populations versus, 375–376
  suburbs and, 376

Urine testing, for drugs, 426

U.S. Preventive Services Task Force (USPSTF), 157, 175b

US census, 159

US Constitution, 108–109, 114

US Department of Health and Human Services (USDHHS), 39–42, 40f, 42t, 110–113, 499
  Agency for Healthcare Research and Quality (AHRQ) and, 112–113
  and governmental role in health care, 106
  Health Resources and Services Administration (HRSA) and, 111
  National Institutes of Health (NIH) and, 106–107, 112
  rural and migrant health resources, 388b
  as source of data, 109t

US health care, governmental role in, 106–109
  trends and shifts in, 106–108

US health system, context of, 130–135, 131f
  21st century, challenges for, 133–135, 134b
  first phase and, 131
  fourth phase, 133
  second phase and, 131–132
  third phase and, 132

US Public Health Service, 3

Use management, in case management, 222–223, 223b

Utilitarianism, 53–56, 54b

Utilization review, 284–285

V

Vaccines
  childhood schedule, 465
  importance for prevention, 465
  measles, 465–466
  for school children, 548

Validity, in screening, 158–159, 158b

Values
  clarification of client, 231
  cultural, 68–69
  cultural imposition and, 79
  ethical decision making and, 52

Vancomycin-resistant Staphylococcus aureus (VRSA), 456–457

Vaping, 420

Vector-borne disease, 470–472

Vectors, of transmission, 459

Veracity, principle for case managers, 233

Verbal communication, cultural variations in, 70–71, 70t

Vertical transmission, 459

Veterans
  health care of, 362–363
  homelessness among, 397

Vibrio parahaemolyticus, 469t

Violence, 433–454
  definition of, 434
  family, 440–448
    development of abusive patterns in, 440–441
    types of, 441–447
  against individuals or oneself, 436–440
    assault as, 437
    homicide as, 436–437
    rape as, 437–439
    sexual violence as, 437–439
    suicide as, 439–440
  nursing interventions for, 448–451, 448b
  prevention of, 450b, 451
  reducing, objective for, 434b
  risk factors of, identification of, 448, 449f, 450b
  school nursing and, 552
  social and community factors influencing, 434–436
    community facilities in, 436
    education in, 435
    media in, 435
    organized religion in, 435–436
    population in, 436
    work in, 434–435, 435b
  during teen pregnancy, 402–403
  victims of, community resources for, 451, 451b

Viral hepatitis, 487, 487t

Virtue ethics, 56, 56b

Virtues, 56

Virulence, 458, 458b
  definition of, 261b

Visiting nurse associations, history of, 18, 25f

Visiting Nurse Quarterly, 20

Visiting nurses, 18, 18f, 206

Vital records, 159

Voluntary agencies, 528

Vulnerability, 357–373
  definition of, 358–359
  factors contributing to, 359–363
  outcomes of, 363

Vulnerable groups, attitudes, beliefs, and media communication about, 393

Vulnerable populations, 357–373, 366b
  assessment issues of, 367–368, 367b
  case management for, 366, 370b
  case study of, 368b
  community health nursing for, 364–371, 365b, 370f
  definition of, 358
  groups of, 358b
  lesbian, gay, bisexual, and transgendered families as, 328–329
  levels of prevention for, 366–367, 367b
  planning and implementing care for, 368–371, 369b, 370b
  public policies affecting, 363–364
  social determinants of health in, 359–361, 360f
  teenage parent families at risk in, 329b
  uninsured population, 361

W

Wald, Lillian, 6, 18–19, 19b, 19f
  case management and, 224
  in home health and nursing, 525
  roles and achievements as first public health nurse, 203–204

Walking, for hypertension, 345
Wars, 405
Water, environmental health assessment of, 93–94
Water discharge, of waste products, 97
Waterborne diseases, 468–470, 468b
    affecting travelers, 474
    outbreaks and pathogens, 470
Web of causality, 155–156
Websites, usefulness of, in community assessment, 214b
Weight control, in adults, 347
Weight gain, during teen pregnancy, 403
Welfare reform, 343–344
Wellness committee
    in national health objectives and faith communities, 519
    in parish nursing model, 511–512, 512f
West Nile virus (WNV), 461, 462t
Westberg Institute for Faith Community Nursing, 513b, 514
Whelan, Linda Tarr, 110
Whole School, Whole Community, Whole Child (WSCC) model, school nursing and, 545, 545f
Whooping cough, 466
Wife abuse, 445
Williams, Carolyn, 110
Windshield surveys, 91, 211, 213t

Withdrawal, defined, 417
Women
    alcohol and, 418
    of childbearing age, negative effect of poverty in, 395
    health care in rural areas, 377–378, 378b
    health concerns of, 347–348
        breast cancer as, 348
        eating disorders as, 347
        gestational diabetes as, 348
        menopause as, 348
        osteoporosis as, 348
        reproductive health as, 347–348
    My Health Companion on, 377
Women, Infants, and Children (WIC), 329–330
    Special Supplemental Nutrition Program for, 319–320
Work
    characteristics of, 563
    violence and, 434–435, 435b
Worker's compensation
    history of, 561
    occupational health scope of services and, 569b, 575
Workforce
    characteristics of, 563
    health, 36
Work-health interactions, 563–564, 564f

Workplace
    reducing environmental health risks in, 97
    worksite walk-through or survey and, 571, 573f
Works Progress Administration (WPA), 23
Worksite walk-through, 571, 573f
World Health Assembly (WHA), 110
World Health Organization (WHO), 110
    on foodborne illnesses, 468
    on mental health, 405
    on primary health care, 44
    as source of data, 109t
    World Health Report and, 110
World Health Report, 110
World Trade Center and Pentagon, terrorist attacks on, 107, 501, 575
Worldviews on Evidence-Based Nursing, 175b
Wrap-around services, 364

Y

Young men, paternity and, 401, 401f
Youth Risk Behavior Surveillance System (YRBSS), 159, 313, 399

Z

Zika virus, 471–472
    outbreak of, 111, 112f
Zoonoses, 472